# ANTIVIRAL AGENTS
# AND
# VIRAL DISEASES OF MAN

*Third Edition*

# ANTIVIRAL AGENTS
## AND
# VIRAL DISEASES OF MAN

*Third Edition*

Editors

**George J. Galasso, Ph.D.**
*Associate Director for Extramural Affairs*
*Office of the Director*
*National Institutes of Health*
*Bethesda, Maryland*

**Richard J. Whitley, M.D.**
*Professor of Pediatrics, Microbiology and Medicine*
*Department of Pediatrics*
*University of Alabama at Birmingham*
*Birmingham, Alabama*

**Thomas C. Merigan, M.D.**
*Becker Professor of Medicine and Head*
*Division of Infectious Diseases*
*Stanford University School of Medicine*
*Stanford, California*

**Raven Press New York**

**Raven Press, 1185 Avenue of the Americas, New York, New York 10036**



Made in the United States of America

**Library of Congress Cataloging-in-Publication Data**

Antiviral agents and viral diseases of man.—3rd ed. / editors, George J. Galasso, Richard J. Whitley, Thomas C. Merigan.
p. cm.
Includes bibliographical references.
ISBN 0-88167-588-1
1. Virus diseases—Chemotherapy. 2. Antiviral agents.
I. Galasso, George J. II. Whitley, Richard J. III. Merigan, Thomas C., 1934– .
[DNLM: 1. Antiviral Agents. 2. Virus Diseases. WC 500 A633]
RC114.5.A55 1990
616.9′25061—dc20
DNLM/DLC
for Library of Congress 89-10800
CIP

The material contained in this volume was submitted as previously unpublished material, except in the instances in which some of the illustrative material was derived.

Great care has been taken to maintain the accuracy of the information contained in the volume. However, neither Raven Press nor the editors can be held responsible for errors or for any consequences arising from the use of the information contained herein.

Some of the names of products referred to in this book may be registered trademarks or proprietary names, although specific reference to this fact may not be made. However, the use of a name without designation is not to be construed as a representation by the publisher or editors that it is in the public domain. In addition, the mention of specific companies or of their products or proprietary names does not imply endorsement or recommendation on the part of the publisher or editors.

Materials appearing in this book prepared by individuals as part of their official duties as U.S. Government employees are not covered by the above-mentioned copyright.

# Preface to the Third Edition

This Third Edition has undergone extensive revision from the previous editions. It was precipitated by the gratifying advances made in the field of antiviral research—advances that have resulted from new approaches in the areas of drug development and Acquired Immune Deficiency Syndrome (AIDS).

The First Edition (1979) lauded the initiation of a new field in the control of viral infectious diseases. It cited the beneficial effects of idoxuridine ointment for the topical treatment of herpetic keratitis, and of adenine arabinoside against herpetic keratitis and herpes encephalitis. It lamented the lack of acceptance for amantadine and hoped for the potential of interferon. With this beginning, we presented a text intended for the widest audience of scientists interested in antivirals: the clinician, the laboratory scientist, and the student. The First Edition anticipated the entering of a new era in the development and application of antivirals. It intended to herald substantial new progress and to stimulate some to pursue studies in this relatively new field.

The Second Edition (1984) acknowledged significant progress which included the new drug acyclovir, but regretted that antiviral agents still remained a novelty to the practice of medicine. The Second Edition was basically an update of the First Edition, hoping to provide the necessary information, as well as identify fertile fields, for further research.

In the intervening years, new crystallographic techniques have provided the opportunity to investigate the anatomy of the outer structure of the virus. Whereas the earlier editions aspired to targeted development of antivirals in addition to the serendipitous screening techniques, the new techniques for targeted development are now rapidly being refined. The devastating expedience of AIDS provided the impetus and the funds to pursue these techniques with a greatly expanded effort. This Third Edition (1990) witnesses the availability of new drugs such as azidothymidine against AIDS, ribavirin for respiratory syncytial infections, dihydroxy propoxymethyl guanine (DHPG) for ocular cyclomegalovirus infection, and a clinical use for interferon. It is anticipated that before this edition is published, rimantadine for influenza will also be licensed.

We are therefore confident that at long last antivirals are no longer a novelty in the clinical armamentarium. This volume has thus been revised to stress the clinical aspects and use of antiviral agents. Although it is still intended for the student and laboratory investigator, this edition should be of increased benefit to the clinician interested in the proper usage of the available and promising agents.

*George J. Galasso*
*Richard J. Whitley*
*Thomas C. Merigan*

# Preface to the Second Edition

Since the first edition of this book, much progress has been made with antiviral agents and in antiviral therapy; witness the fact that acyclovir did not appear in the first edition index. Yet antiviral agents remain novel in clinical medicine. Their proper application is complex due to the interweaving of virus replication with host processes. Other relevant progress, in addition to the several new agents currently under study, include the impact of the new biotechnology that has made a considerable contribution to viral diagnosis and new insights in immunology that have led to a better understanding of pathogenesis of disease. It is our hope that the second edition of this book will acquaint the reader with the contemporary agents and current concepts of the diseases they manage, indications for therapy, parameters responsive to therapy, and in general, the state of the art of antiviral agent development and application. It is also our expectation that this book will serve as a guidepost for future directions of development, identifying both fertile fields and dead-end areas.

The prediction in the preface of the First Edition has proven correct: we do have new antiviral agents available to the clinician. Progress will continue to be steady. Time will divulge what the ultimate limitations are for the control of viral disease. The standards and effective strategies are identified so that antiviral therapy can continue to advance on a sound, rational basis.

We expect that there will be greater efforts in the development of targeted antiviral agents and that many of the planned clinical studies will result in clinically effective drugs. As in all clinical matters, drug usage will ultimately depend on the discretion of the individual physician and the patient's responses. New, unanticipated applications and side effects of drugs will continue to appear as biologically active therapeutic agents are made available and are accepted by those who care for patients. Hence, this book is presented as a contemporary picture of a continually changing perspective.

This Second Edition will be useful to the student, laboratory scientist, and clinician. The student will glean an overview of virology, the diseases caused by viruses, and the role of antivirals. The laboratory scientist is presented the necessary background for further effective and efficient development of new agents. A reasonable strategy for the development of new agents is presented. Finally, the physician providing primary care should benefit by having access to this contemporary knowledge of viral diseases and their management as seen today.

*George J. Galasso*
*Thomas C. Merigan*
*Robert A Buchanan*

# Preface to the First Edition

There is no question that antivirals are important for modifying infections in man. Viral infections are among the greatest causes of human morbidity and resulting economic loss; this, together with the rapid advances being made in other areas of clinical management, accentuates the increasing need for measures to control viral infections. In many instances, the immunologic manipulation of patients that is required for optimal treatment of certain diseases renders the patients extremely susceptible to infections that are not often seen in otherwise healthy populations.

In the past, antivirals usually have been discovered by fortuitous means. Screening programs, in many instances seeking other products such as anticancer agents, have yielded compounds with some potential; these have then been developed by means of tissue culture and animal model systems to determine the feasibility of applying them clinically as antiviral drugs. The development of antivirals has been slow because their effectiveness is closely related to cellular metabolism. Simply put, viral replication is intracellular, and it involves the use of cellular functions for viral synthesis. Until we fully understand viral replication and can clearly uncouple it from normal cellular metabolic processes, tailored antivirals cannot be developed.

Of equal importance to the field is a thorough understanding of the pathogenesis of disease. Recent developments in diagnostic techniques not only have permitted more accurate diagnosis but also have vastly improved our understanding of the natural history of viral diseases. It is only through such understanding that the feasibility of antivirals can be determined.

A third consideration in antiviral development is the basic issue of whether or not they will work. Some experience in this area has been gained with idoxuridine. This compound, in ointment form, has been licensed for a number of years for topical treatment of herpetic keratitis; however, systemic administration has been both ineffective and toxic. Very little experience has been accumulated with other compounds. However, the past 2 years have seen considerable advances in chemoprophylaxis and chemotherapy. Although amantadine has been licensed for prophylaxis against Asian influenza (H2N2) since the late sixties, it was not until 1976 that it became licensed for use against all influenza A strains. Vidarabine ointment has recently been licensed for topical treatment of herpetic keratitis, including cases refractory to idoxuridine. This compound has also been licensed for systemic use against herpes encephalitis.

Interferon was shown in late 1976 to hold some promise in treatment of chronic active hepatitis as well as herpes zoster. Suddenly progress is accelerating, and good news is being heard after a long wait. Several other studies are under way to evaluate the clinical roles of vidarabine and vidarabine monophosphate, interferon and ribavirin, and other antivirals against a spectrum of viral diseases. On the immunologic front, smallpox has fallen by the wayside and become a disease of historical interest only.

It is through advances in all these areas that control of viral disease can be extended beyond the level achieved with vaccines. This book was developed with these problems in mind. Significant progress has been made in all these areas, and the time seems appropriate for a text reviewing the progress and the potential of antiviral research.

Another consideration important in the planning of this text was identification of the audience to whom it is directed. It should be of value to the widest audience of scientists interested in antivirals; it is not intended solely for clinicians or laboratory scientists. It is not a compendium of diseases and information about how they should be treated, nor is it a list of antivirals and their modes of action. Rather, it attempts a synthesis of these areas, discussing the clinical, diagnostic, epidemiologic, pharmacologic, and molecular biologic aspects of the interrelationships of viruses, antivirals, and disease, with particular emphasis on antivirals that are currently available and disorders in which antivirals may be of value if they can be developed. The book is intended for those who will most need it in the coming years: the medical student/resident who is interested in infectious diseases, the clinician who will inform him of the current state of the art, the microbiologist who will apprise him of new developments in the field, and the research scientist who, it is hoped, will be encouraged to undertake further work in the field.

In order to reach such a wide and diverse audience, all aspects of antiviral work must be covered. In order to understand how an antiviral is to be of value in the clinic, one must understand viral replication. Therefore, we begin with the basics of virology, the biology of viral infections, and the pharmacology of antiviral action. If antivirals are to be of value, it is important that rapid and accurate diagnosis be made; we must understand the diagnostic tools available so that we can do more than say that the patient has a fever and the flu. We then proceed to the pathogenesis of various diseases and the roles of antivirals in their control. This is done by means of arbitrary divisions, on the basis of organ systems whenever possible. There are many instances of overlap, but this is not considered to be undesirable. In many instances it is done for completeness and emphasis, as well as for strength when different disciplines must contribute.

The practical aspects of using antivirals must be addressed if the goal is clinical application. Some exciting new developments are also described, even though their practical applications are still being developed. This is particularly pertinent in the case of exogenous interferon. It is our assumption that if an antiviral is found to be efficacious and of clinical importance, the mechanisms for making it economically feasible will be found.

The reader will notice that the chapters in this book vary somewhat in terms of length, organization, and style. These variations arise from the differing natures of the topics being discussed. We have elected to maintain these differences, since the state of the art varies widely from one area to another.

We anticipate that we are entering a new era in the development and application of antivirals. It is hoped that this book will be useful in coordinating many factors and much new knowledge at this pivotal point. We believe that the next several years will see great progress in antiviral developments and applications. If this book enlightens some and, more important, stimulates a few to pursue studies in this field, its intended goal will be accomplished.

*George J. Galasso*
*Thomas C. Merigan*
*Robert A. Buchanan*

# Contents

# Contributors

**Charles A. Alford, Jr., M.D.** *Professor of Pediatrics, Department of Pediatrics, The University of Alabama at Birmingham, UAB Station, 752 CHT, Birmingham, Alabama 35294*

**Ann M. Arvin, M.D.** *Associate Professor, Department of Pediatrics, Stanford University School of Medicine, Stanford, California 94305-5119*

**Robert B. Couch, M.D.** *Professor, Departments of Microbiology, Immunology, and Medicine, Baylor College of Medicine, One Baylor Place, Houston, Texas 77030*

**Adrian M. Di Bisceglie, M.D.** *Guest Scientist, Liver Diseases Section, National Institute of Diabetes and Digestive and Kidney Diseases, National Institutes of Health, Bethesda, Maryland 20892*

**Raphael Dolin, M.D.** *Professor of Medicine, Infectious Diseases Unit, University of Rochester School of Medicine and Dentistry, Rochester, New York 14642*

**Judith Falloon, M.D.** *Critical Care Medicine Department, National Institutes of Health, Bethesda, Maryland 20892*

**George J. Galasso, Ph.D.** *Associate Director for Extramural Affairs, Office of the Director, National Institutes of Health, Bethesda, Maryland 20892*

**Diane E. Griffin, M.D., Ph.D.** *Professor, Departments of Medicine and Neurology, Johns Hopkins University School of Medicine, Baltimore, Maryland 21205*

**Jay H. Hoofnagle, M.D.** *Director, Division of Digestive Diseases and Nutrition, National Institute of Diabetes and Digestive and Kidney Diseases, National Institutes of Health, Bethesda, Maryland 20892*

**John W. Huggins, Ph.D.** *Department of Antiviral Studies, Virology Division, United States Army Medical Research Institute of Infectious Diseases, Fort Detrick, Maryland 21701-5011*

**Earl R. Kern, Ph.D.** *Departments of Pediatrics, Comparative Medicine, and Microbiology, School of Medicine, The University of Alabama at Birmingham, Birmingham, Alabama 35294*

**Oscar L. Laskin, M.D.** *Director, Clinical Pharmacology, Merck, Sharp & Dohme Research Laboratories, Rahway, New Jersey 07065,* and *Adjunct Associate Professor of Medicine and Clinical Pharmacology, Cornell University Medical College, New York, New York 10021*

**Henry Masur, M.D.** *Critical Care Medicine Department, Warren G. Magnuson Clinical Center, National Institutes of Health, Bethesda, Maryland 20892*

**Thomas C. Merigan, M.D.** *Head, Division of Infectious Diseases, Stanford University School of Medicine, Stanford, California 94305*

**Gregory J. Mertz, M.D.** *Associate Professor, Division of Infectious Diseases, Department of Medicine, University of New Mexico School of Medicine, 2211 Lomas NE, Albuquerque, New Mexico 87131*

**Mostafa A. Nokta, M.D., Ph.D.** *Assistant Professor, Infectious Diseases Unit, Department of Medicine, The University of Texas Medical Branch, Route H-82, Galveston, Texas 77550-2774*

**Deborah Pavan-Langston, M.D.** *Department of Ophthalmology, Harvard Medical School,* and *Massachusetts Eye and Ear Infirmary, 243 Charles Street, Boston, Massachusetts 02114*

**Richard B. Pollard, M.D.** *Professor of Medicine, Department of Internal Medicine and Microbiology, The University of Texas Medical Branch, Route H-82, Galveston, Texas 77550-2774*

**Gerald V. Quinnan, Jr., M.D.** *Center for Biologics Evaluation and Research, Food and Drug Administration, 8800 Rockville Pike, Bethesda, Maryland 20892*

**Richard C. Reichman, M.D.** *Associate Professor, Departments of Medicine, Microbiology, and Immunology, University of Rochester Medical Center, 601 Elmwood Avenue, Rochester, New York 14642*

**Douglas D. Richman, M.D.** *Professor, Departments of Pathology and Medicine, 3350 LaJolla Village Drive, University of California at San Diego,* and *Veterans Administration Medical Center, San Diego, California 92161*

**Iain S. Sim, Ph.D.** *Department of Oncology and Virology, Hoffmann-La Roche Inc., 340 Kingsland Street, Nutley, New Jersey 07110-1199*

**Stephen E. Straus, M.D.** *Head, Medical Virology Section, Laboratory of Clinical Investigation, National Institute of Allergy and Infectious Diseases, National Institutes of Health, Bethesda, Maryland 20892*

**John Treanor, M.D.** *Assistant Professor of Medicine, Infectious Diseases Unit, University of Rochester School of Medicine and Dentistry, 601 Elmwood Avenue, Rochester, New York 14642*

**Richard J. Whitley, M.D.** *Professor of Pediatrics, Microbiology and Medicine, Departments of Pediatrics and Microbiology, University of Alabama at Birmingham Medical Center, Children's Hospital Tower, Suite 653, 1600 Seventh Avenue South, Birmingham, Alabama 35294*

**Robert H. Yolken, M.D.** *Professor of Pediatrics, Eudowood Division of Infectious Diseases, Johns Hopkins University School of Medicine, CMSC 1101, 600 North Wolfe Street, Baltimore, Maryland 21205*

*Antiviral Agents and Viral Diseases of Man, 3rd Edition,* edited by G. J. Galasso, R. J. Whitley, and T. C. Merigan, Raven Press, Ltd., New York © 1990.

# 1

# Virus Replication: Target Functions and Events for Virus-Specific Inhibitors

Iain S. Sim

*Department of Oncology and Virology, Hoffmann-La Roche Inc., Nutley, New Jersey 07110*



The synthesis of 5-iodo-2′-deoxyuridine and the subsequent successful development of this compound as a treatment for herpes keratitis was a landmark in the discovery of antiviral agents. At the time, this achievement may have led many to believe that the conquest of viral diseases was almost within grasp. This was not the case. In spite of intensive efforts in chemical synthesis and compound screening, the rewards have been few. This is in marked contrast to the field of antibacterial therapy, where the past few years have seen the introduction of a large number of improved antibiotics with potent broad-spectrum antibacterial properties, good therapeutic ratios, and very favorable pharmacokinetic properties. Third-generation cephalosporins and quinolones, among others, provide the clinician with a wide array of agents for the treatment of troublesome bacterial infections. In contrast, the number of antiviral agents available are still few in number, are restricted in their spectrum of activity and, in some cases, have a narrow ratio of efficacy to toxicity.

The reasons for the lack of success in the development of safe and effective antiviral agents are numerous. The intracellular localization of the virus and its utilization of host cell functions for replication make the discovery of virus-specific inhibitors particularly challenging. In contrast, bacteria can grow and divide, by and large, independent of the host and, consequently, offer many (organism-specific) targets for inhibitors. The routine screening of synthetic compounds and microbial and plant extracts against virus-infected cells in culture has yielded many entities that have proven to lack specificity for the virus target and, consequently, to be unacceptably toxic to the host. Random screening has led to the discovery of a few clinically useful, nontoxic compounds. Subsequent mechanism of action studies have shown these compounds to act via a virus-specific function.

It is now clear that whereas virus replication is dependent on many functions of the host cell, successful replication requires virus-coded and, hence, virus-specific proteins. The number and function of these proteins vary from one virus type to another but, in many cases, are sufficiently different from their cellular counterparts to warrant consideration as potential targets for selective inhibitors.

Recombinant DNA technology has unlocked a powerful array of techniques and reagents that are being used to define in detail virus-specific events in the replicative cycle. The discovery of antiviral agents need no longer be dependent on blind screening of compounds; selected viral targets can be identified, defined, examined in isolation, and incorporated into tests that will more rapidly lead to the identification of those drugs whose action is selective for the virus and reject compounds that are inhibitors of vital host cell functions. Although the role of the molecular biologist in the discovery of antiviral agents will be of great importance in the future, the contribution of other disciplines will be essential as well. It seems likely that the discovery of safe and effective antiviral agents will be the product of multidisciplinary teams that include molecular biologists, biochemists, and protein and physical chemists as well as the virologists and medicinal chemists traditionally associated with such efforts.

The impact of molecular biology on antiviral drug discovery can be seen most clearly in the field of retrovirology, particularly in the quest for antiviral drugs for the treatment of human immunodeficiency virus (HIV) infection. Azidothymidine (AZT) is the only antiviral agent presently approved for treatment of Acquired Immune Deficiency Syndrome (AIDS) and severe AIDS-related complex (ARC). Although its discovery probably owes more to the judicious selection of compounds for screening in whole cell/virus assays than to the application of the target-oriented, rational approach to drug discovery, the description of the replicative cycle of HIV, the characterization of the physical and biological properties of the virus-coded proteins, and the development of a detailed understanding of the mechanisms of viral pathogenesis all promise to offer a basis for the selection of antiviral compounds that will be more effective and possess a greater therapeutic margin than the current agents.

This chapter illustrates the broad potential for the discovery of selective antiviral agents by briefly considering some of the virus-specific functions that may be targeted. The molecular biology of each virus of clinical importance will neither be described separately nor in detail (there are many excellent texts to which the reader may turn for such information). Rather, general principles will be illustrated, drawn from areas of study where our knowledge of a particular viral target function is well defined. The potential of certain viral proteins to serve as targets for inhibitors has been revealed by mechanism-of-action studies on compounds discovered by the more traditional screening approaches; examples of such compounds will be given to illustrate the validity of the belief that the development of selective antiviral agents is an achievable goal if carefully designed target assays are used for compound screening in conjunction with rational drug design and synthesis.

The viral replication cycle and processes that will be considered as potential molecular targets for selective antiviral agents are shown in Fig. 1. These events will be broken down and examined as follows: (a) virus attachment to cell membranes and entry into the cell; (b) virus uncoating; (c) synthesis of viral messenger RNA (mRNA); (d) viral protein synthesis and maturation; (e) replication of genomic DNA and RNA; and (f) assembly and release of infectious particles.

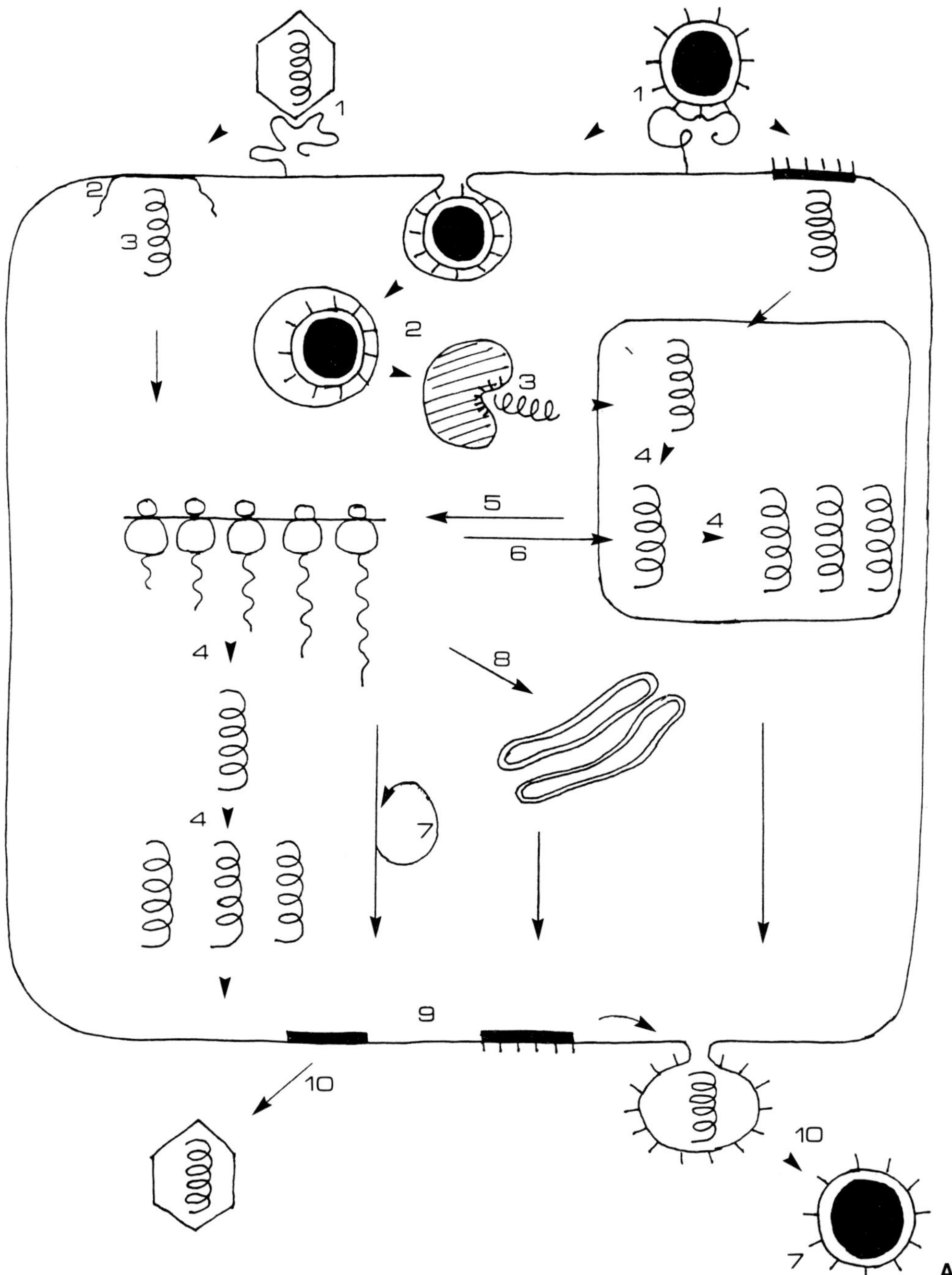


**FIG. 1.A:** Replication of RNA viruses. Many virus-specific events may be targeted by selective inhibitors, including virus attachment to the cellular receptor (*1*); entry of the virion into the cell by direct penetration or fusion (*2*); uncoating of the virion (*3*); transcription of viral RNA by virus-coded RNA polymerase (*4*); translation of mRNA (*5*); modulation of RNA transcription by viral transactivating proteins (*6*); proteolytic cleavage of capsid proteins by virus-specified proteases (*7*); protein modification (*8*); and virus particle assembly and release (*9,10*).

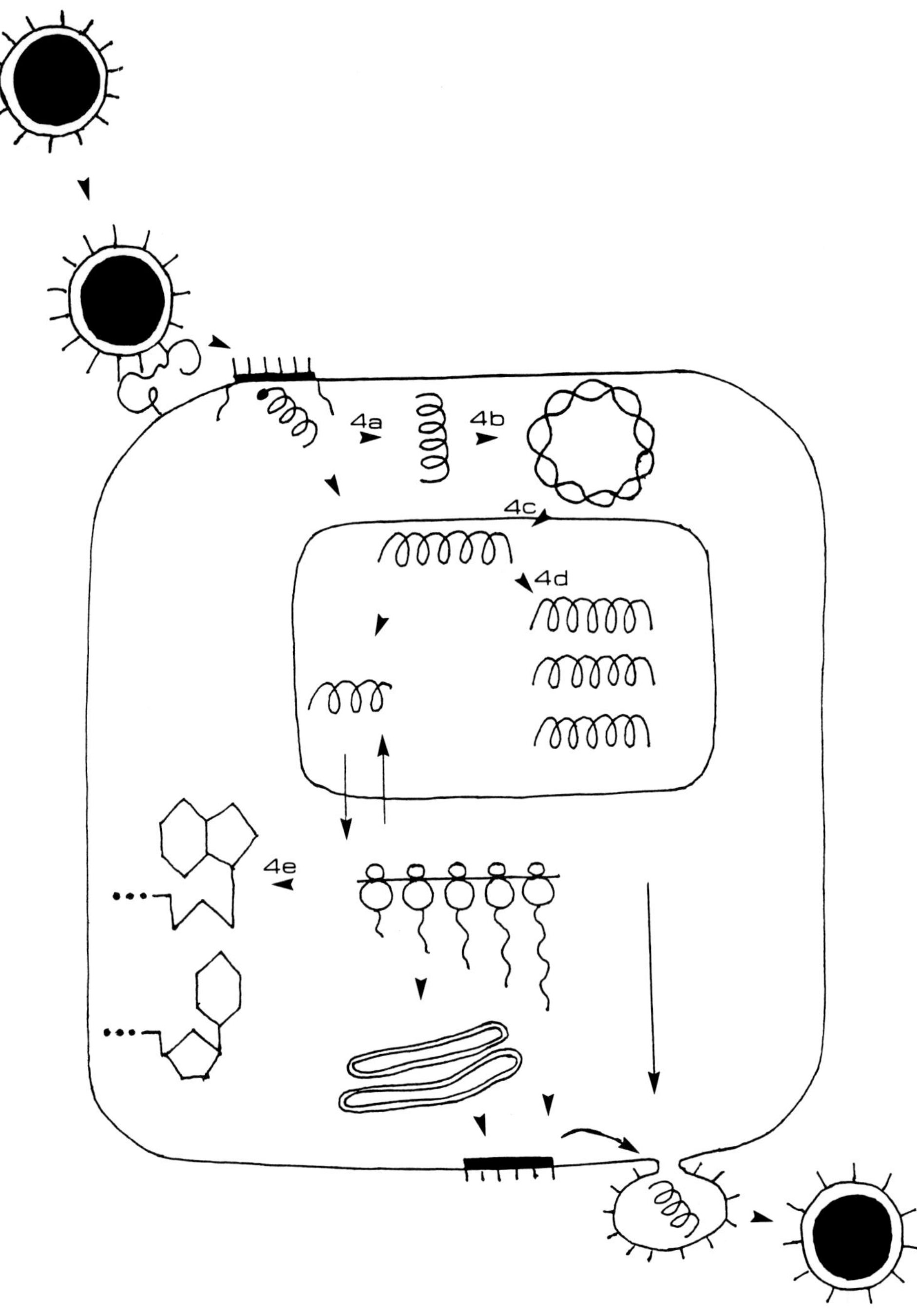


**B**

**FIG. 1.B:** Replication of DNA viruses, including retroviruses. In addition to the inhibition of events common to the replication of both DNA and RNA viruses, the synthesis of viral DNA may be selectively targeted by antiviral agents. Inhibitors of DNA synthesis may act at any of several points, including retroviral reverse transcriptase (*4a*), RNaseH (*4b*), and endonuclease (*4c*); virus-coded DNA polymerase (*4d*); and virus-specific enzymes responsible for the metabolism of DNA synthesis precursors (*4e*).

## INITIATION OF INFECTION

To infect a cell and successfully initiate replication of its genome, a virus must first attach to the exterior of a cell, penetrate through the cell membrane, and disassemble (uncoat), releasing the nucleic acid and associated proteins in a form that can interact with cellular components involved in transcription and translation. It seems logical that these early events should be a focus for antiviral intervention since prevention of cellular uptake of virus is likely to be the most beneficial strategy; in this way, cells will be spared from the potentially destructive effects of virus invasion. The early events in virus infection can be divided into three phases: attachment, penetration, and uncoating (for reviews, see refs. 1 and 2). The many virus types can be differentiated in terms of size, symmetry, the presence or absence of lipid envelope, etc., and distinguished at the molecular level by the sequences of the structural capsid and envelope proteins. Although there may be differences in the details of how each virus initiates infection of the host cell, the underlying principles may be similar for many viruses. A few examples will be given to illustrate how the discovery of antiviral agents, acting at the initial stage of infection, may be accomplished.

### Attachment

Many viruses are strongly restricted as to the host(s) and tissue(s) that they can infect. This tropism is not fortuitous but is the result, at least in part, of the requirement for a specific receptor to be present on the surface of the host cell in order that viral attachment may occur and the process of infection be initiated. The presence of an attachment protein on the exterior of the virion that can bind with high affinity to the cellular receptor serves to enhance the chances of contact between virus and cell, which might otherwise be diminished by charge effects, particle motion, and dilution. The presence or absence of attachment sites on cells of different origin was first recognized as a reason that poliovirus only infects cells of primate origin (3). Since that time evidence for the existence of specific viral receptors on susceptible cells has been gathered with a large variety of viruses, although the identity of only a few such receptors has been determined to date.

It seems reasonable to suggest that viruses have exploited normal components of the cell membrane as attachment sites. This is supported by the recent discovery of the CD4 complex as the receptor for HIV (for a review, see ref. 4) and by earlier studies that revealed an association of the Epstein-Barr virus (EBV) receptor with the type 2 complement receptor (CR2), which binds C3d. In the latter instance, initial studies revealed that both receptors are coordinately expressed on a number of cell lines and freshly isolated lymphocyte fractions (5–7); EBV and C3 receptors co-cap with each other but not with a variety of other cell surface structures (8); membranes stripped of either receptor will not bind the opposite ligand (9); and cells treated with C3 or anti-C3 antibody will not bind EBV (5,10). More recently, CR2, one of the two C3 receptors on B cells, has been shown to be responsible for the binding of EBV to human B lymphocytes (11,12), and early studies that implicated the major viral glycoprotein, gp350, in binding of EBV to the cell receptor (13) have been substantiated by the demonstration of *in vitro* binding of isolated gp350 to CR2 (14,15). This interaction of viral attachment protein to cellular receptor may be mediated by a region of gp350 that is homologous in sequence to a fragment of C3. With the identification of the components responsible for attachment of EBV to the host cell, it is now possible to develop approaches to block the interaction and prevent virus infection. This is reinforced by the observation that certain monoclonal antibodies to gp350 (16) or to CR2 (17) block binding of EBV to B lymphocytes and prevent infection.

Early clinical observations identified the important role of T-helper cells in AIDS (18), and the tropism of HIV for CD4+ cells was revealed by studies of virus infection of cells in culture (19). The use of monoclonal antibodies has confirmed the role of the CD4 antigen as the receptor for virus attachment of T-helper cells (20,21); other cell types that can be infected with HIV, such as monocyte/macrophages (22,23), glial cells (24) and colorectal cells (25), have also been shown to express the CD4 antigen or to contain RNA homologous to CD4 mRNA. This information has been utilized by others to demonstrate that a soluble form of the CD4 antigen inhibits HIV infection by binding to the virus attachment protein (gp120) and that it may be useful as a therapeutic agent (26–29).

The use of soluble receptor of high molecular weight as a therapeutic agent may not always be practical because of the limited bioavailability and potential antigenicity of such molecules. It may be possible, however, to discover lower molecular weight antagonists using rational drug design based on an understanding of the important domains of the native receptor. For example, the receptor site for the attachment of HIV has now been located more precisely to the first and second immunoglobulin domains of CD4, and certain amino acids have been identified as being particularly important in binding of gp120 (30–36). This has provided the basis for the synthesis of defined, lower molecular weight polypeptides that block the interaction between the CD4 receptor and the HIV attachment protein (37,38). Random screening has revealed the antiviral activity of sulfated polysaccharides such as dextran sulfate and heparin, which inhibit the binding of HIV to its cellular receptor (39,40), although such screening does not distinguish between compounds that bind to the virus attachment protein and those that mask the cell receptor. Since the cellular protein that serves as the receptor for viral attachment fulfills other important physiological roles, as is clearly evident in the case of CD4, receptor blockade by compounds such as dextran sulfate and heparin may result in other, undesirable pharmacological effects.

The identification of the domains of the viral proteins responsible for attachment of the virion to the cellular receptor is not a simple task. Antibodies that neutralize virus infectivity may not necessarily bind to epitopes that participate directly in receptor binding. Antibody binding may prevent virus attachment through steric hinderance or, alternatively, result in a conformational change of the virion protein such that events in the infection process subsequent to viral attachment to the cell are blocked. As examples, it is now evident that antibodies that neutralize influenza virus infectivity do not recognize the receptor binding domain of the viral hemagglutinin (HA), and neutralizing antirhinovirus antibodies are excluded from the canyon of the viral capsid into which the cellular receptor is thought to penetrate. The data on the structure of the influenza HA (for a review, see ref. 41) and the rhinovirus capsid will be briefly reviewed here to illustrate general principles. Efforts to map binding domains of the HIV gp120 (42–44) are also likely to provide the basis for design of antiviral agents that are selectively targeted to the viral attachment protein.

Three-dimensional x-ray structure studies of the influenza virus HA (45) suggested the presence of a receptor-binding pocket at the end of the molecule, distal to the point of insertion in the viral envelope. Analysis of mutants of influenza virus that had "drifted" with respect to susceptibility to antibody neutralization revealed that amino acids located within the proposed binding pocket did not change, whereas others at the periphery of the pocket had undergone substitution. On the other hand, mutant HAs that differed from wild-type in their receptor binding exhibited an amino acid substitution in the proposed receptor-binding pocket (46). Most recently, x-ray crystallography has been used to describe the structure of the HA complexed to sialic acids (47); the nature of the sialic acids responsible for virus binding also has been more precisely defined (48). These data should provide the basis for the design of antiviral antagonists that bind in the pocket of the HA and block virus attachment to the receptor.

Although human rhinoviruses occur as many different serotypes, competition binding studies have shown that many isolates share the same receptor and that the virus isolates can be assigned to either of two mutually exclusive receptor-binding groups (49,50). The three dimensional structure of the rhinovirus capsid has been determined separately (51). These studies revealed the presence of a groove, or canyon, in the surface of the capsid, and it is proposed that this region, inaccessible to immunoglobulin, may serve as the site for interaction with the cellular receptor. This has been supported by further studies with mutant viruses in which substitutions of defined amino acids in the capsid protein that makes up the canyon resulted in altered receptor binding and virus infectivity (52). The apparent conservation of the capsid domain responsible for receptor binding makes this viral structure an attractive target for antiviral agents. The design of these agents may be facilitated by knowledge of the overall structure of the binding site and, specifically, of the residues required for direct interaction with the cellular receptor.

### Penetration and Fusion

Penetration of the cell following viral attachment may be brought about by any of a number of mechanisms. The enveloped viruses seem, for the most part, to rely on a process of fusion between the viral envelope and the cell membrane. The site at which fusion occurs seems to depend on the particular virus type and may be either at the cell surface or at the membrane of an intracellular vesicle or endosome. Nonenveloped viruses may be taken up by direct penetration (translocation) (1). A third mechanism for virus uptake may, in certain rare circumstances, be the result of specific antibody binding and the uptake of virus/antibody complexes into cells, primarily of the monocyte/macrophage lineage, through Fc receptors.

If, as has been proposed above, virus attachment occurs as the consequence of binding of virus to a cellular receptor that is required at the cell membrane to perform other functions necessary to the cell, then it seems reasonable to argue that the subsequent uptake of virus into the cell might emulate the responses that follow the binding of the normal ligand to the cellular receptor. A large number of physiologically important ligands, e.g., $\beta_2$-macroglobulin, epidermal growth factor, insulin, and low-density lipoprotein, are taken up into cells by a process known as "receptor-mediated endocytosis" or "adsorptive endocytosis." Briefly, receptor-attached proteins coalesce in regions of the cell surface known as "coated pits" and are subsequently internalized in clathrin-coated vesicles named "receptosomes." The receptosome containing its protein cargo is translocated to the perinuclear region of the cell where the Golgi and Golgi endoplasmic reticulum lysosome (GERL) complexes further process the protein. The compartment is acidified by proton pumps that reside within the membrane, and the ultimate degradation of the internalized protein probably involves fusion of the receptosome with newly forming lysosomes in the GERL system. This route of cell entry is followed by a number of viruses such as Semliki Forest virus (SFV) (53–55), influenza virus (56–59), and vesicular stomatitis virus (VSV) (60). In contrast, in the case of HIV and the paramyxoviruses, the fusion of the viral envelope appears to occur at the cell membrane in the absence of receptor-mediated endocytosis (61–65).

Although interference with receptor-mediated endocytosis might seem an unrewarding strategy for the development of virus-specific agents, there is some evidence to suggest that the process of fusion necessary to liberate the nucleocapsid from the virion into the cytoplasm may be an event to target. Membrane fusion is mediated by a hydrophobic region of the fusion (F) protein of the paramyxoviruses and of the HA of influenza virus. In each case, the protein is synthesized as an inactive precursor that is cleaved upon insertion into the membrane of the infected cell (66,67), with the amino terminus of the newly generated polypeptide ($F_1$ and $HA_2$, respectively) being rich in hydrophobic amino acids. Under appropriate conditions of pH (neutral or alkaline in the case of the paramyxoviruses, acid in the case of influenza virus), the fusion domain undergoes a conformational change that exposes the hydrophobic region, permitting fusion of the envelope to the cell membrane (68–70). There is strong conservation of the primary amino acid sequence of the *N* terminus of $HA_2$ among isolates of influenza virus, and considerable homology between the fusion domain of the influenza virus protein and that of the paramyxoviruses (71–73, and refs. therein). Protein sequence analysis has revealed a repeating triplet of hydrophobic amino acids at the *N* terminus of the HIV glycoprotein gp41 (74), and sequence similarities to the paramyxovirus fusion proteins (75) suggest that this domain may also mediate fusion of the viral envelope. This hypothesis is supported by the observation that a mutation affecting this region of the HIV gp41 interferes with fusion (42). The likely role of the hydrophobic sequence of the Sendai fusion protein led Richardson et al. (76) to synthesize oligopeptides of homologous sequences such as Z-Phe-Phe-Gly and Z-Gly-Leu-Phe-Gly (where Z is a carbobenzoxy protecting group, and Phe, Gly, and Leu are phenylalanine, glycine, and leucine, respectively). They successfully demonstrated that these peptides inhibited the replication of a number of paramyxoviruses, as well as influenza virus, in cell culture (76), and bound to cell membranes and inhibited cell fusion (77). Many similar peptides had been synthesized previously, and certain entities were shown to have activity against measles virus (78). However, the efficacy of these oligopeptides in animal models of virus infection has not been tested, and it remains to be determined whether this approach will yield compounds that have pharmacokinetic and safety properties desirable in antiviral agents.

In concluding this discussion on viral penetration and fusion, it is appropriate to review the action of amantadine (1-adamantanamine) and its derivative rimantadine ($\alpha$-methyl-1-adamantanemethylamine), which are effective clinical agents in the prevention and treatment of influenza virus A infections. Both agents are generally well tolerated in patients (see Chapter 10 for a detailed discussion of their safety and efficacy) and exhibit a high degree of selectivity in their antiviral action, such that even the replication of influenza virus B is not inhibited by either compound. Other lysosomotropic amines such as ammonium chloride, methylamine, and chloroquine have been shown to exert similar effects, inhibiting the early phase of infection by SFV and VSV as well as influenza virus (79). Addition of amine to cells at the same time as virus resulted in the inhibition of infection. However, if amine was added as early as 10 min after the virus, the extent of inhibition was substantially reduced, consistent with the passage of virus particles through the amine-sensitive lysosomal uncoating phase. These observations have led to the conclusion that the action of the lysomotropic amines, including rimantadine and amantadine, is to act as buffering ions, inhibiting the decline in pH in the secondary lysosomes and consequently preventing pH-dependent membrane fusion. As lipophilic amines, amantadine and rimantadine can diffuse into cells in uncharged form; they then accumulate in lysosomes where protonation leads to their conversion to nondiffusible charged forms that remain entrapped within the lysosomal vesicle. The result is a rapid (<2 min after addition to cells) rise in intralysosomal pH to 6.0–6.5 (80). Ammonium chloride and chloroquine are well-known inhibitors of receptor-mediated endocytosis; they also disrupt coated vesicles within the cell (81,82).

Although the mechanism of antiviral action proposed above seems plausible, others have proposed more recently that the buffering effect of amantadine and rimantadine is artifactual, occurring only at drug concentrations in excess of those required for antiinfluenza virus activity *in vivo* (83,84). Without a doubt, amantadine-resistant viruses can be generated in which there are mutations in the gene coding for the HA that result in altered dependence on pH for fusion (85). However, such mutants are obtained following treatment with high concentrations of amantadine. *In vitro* studies with amantadine at concentrations that more closely mimic drug levels achieved *in vivo* have yielded resistant viruses that consistently exhibit substitutions in amino acids in the transmembrane region of the $M_2$ protein (84). That this latter type of mutant virus is more relevant to the mechanism of action of amantadine is supported by the observations of others who demonstrated that rimantadine-resistant influenza viruses isolated from infected children treated with rimantadine also exhibited the same amino acid substitution in the $M_2$ protein (86). The role of the $M_2$ protein in the influenza virus particle and its influence on fusion of the envelope and uncoating are not known. It is encouraging to note, however, that amantadine and rimantadine apparently exert their antiviral effect through interaction with at least one virus-coded protein. If the mechanism of action of these compounds can be more fully understood, it is conceivable that other compounds can be found that exert an antiviral effect on other enveloped viruses, acting on the proteins of those viruses that are functionally equivalent to the influenza virus $M_2$ protein.

### Uncoating

In order to initiate cellular infection, viruses need not only penetrate cells but also need to disassemble the genome from its protein capsid, a process known as "uncoating." The end result is the appearance of the naked viral genome in a form and, ultimately, at the correct geographical location within the cell suitable for transcription. As we have seen, uncoating of enveloped viruses that enter the cell by receptor-mediated endocytosis is now thought to occur primarily in lysosomes or prelysosomal GERL-associated receptosomes, whereas other enveloped viruses uncoat as they fuse with and penetrate through the cell membrane. The mechanism of uncoating of the nonenveloped viruses is poorly understood. In the case of adenovirus, for example, the penton capsomere is shed as the virus penetrates the cell membrane, whereas other capsid proteins remain associated with the genome in the cytoplasm and are only shed when the DNA enters the nucleus (87). Studies with another class of nonenveloped virus, the picornaviridae, have indicated that the initial phases of uncoating occur while the virus is still bound to its receptor. As the virus becomes progressively more tightly bound, the particles lose one of the capsid proteins, VP4. The VP4-deficient "A" particles have a lower density, are sensitive to digestion by proteases and can be eluted in a noninfectious form from cell membranes. Subsequent dissociation of other capsid proteins leads to release of RNA and empty capsids (B particles).

A number of compounds have been described whose action appears to be at the level of viral uncoating. Among the earliest examples of agents acting by this mechanism is rhodanine (2-thio-4-oxothiazolidine), which was shown to block the uncoating of echovirus 12 by stabilizing the nucleocapsid and preventing VP4 release (88). Interestingly, penetration was not inhibited, nonmodified virions being present as an abortive infection in the cytoplasm. Subsequently, a number of classes of compound have been reported to inhibit the uncoating and replication of both enteroviruses and rhinoviruses (e.g., see refs. 89–91). Of particular interest is arildone, a lipophilic aryloxy alkyl diketone, that selectively inhibits the replication of poliovirus 2 (92) as well as rhinovirus and herpes simplex virus (HSV) types 1 and 2 (93,94). Experiments aimed at elucidating the mode of action of arildone revealed that neither adsorption of virus to cells nor penetration was inhibited; arildone did bind to the icosahedral viral capsid—stabilizing the particle and preventing intracellular uncoating (92,95). Careful structure/activity optimization has yielded more active derivatives, particularly WIN 51711 (96), which is inhibitory to several rhinovirus and enterovirus serotypes, by inhibiting virus uncoating (97,98).

The determination of the three-dimensional structure of human rhinovirus type 14 by x-ray diffraction studies (51) and the deduction of the amino acid sequences of the virus proteins (99,100) have facilitated a more detailed analysis of the mechanism of action of WIN 51711. It is hypothesized that the site of binding of the virus to the cellular receptor is within a canyon encircling each of the vertices of the capsid. The amino acids that make up the receptor-binding region are highly conserved, whereas viral mutants that are capable of escaping from neutralization by monoclonal antibodies arise as a result of amino acid substitutions at epitopes on the exposed surface of the viral particle (101,102). Crystallographic studies of inhibitor bound to the virus have revealed the location of WIN 51711 to be within a hydrophobic pocket at the base of the canyon. The broad spectrum of action of the compound may be explained by its binding within a structurally conserved domain; its mechanism of action may be related to (a) a restriction of changes in particle conformation usually required for uncoating and/or (b) the blocking of the putative channel in the floor of the canyon through which ions flow during uncoating (103). The activity of several analogs of WIN 51711 can be related to their relative ability to enter the virion pocket, whereas amino acid substitutions in drug-resistant mutant viruses are predicted to sterically hinder inhibitor binding (103,104).

Studies of the type described above may be generally applied to the search for specific antiviral agents. Using the techniques developed with the picorna viruses, it may be possible to design antiviral agents that bind to conserved domains of the capsid proteins of other viruses of interest. Although further refinement of compound structure may be necessary in order to obtain inhibitors that have the properties required of clinically useful agents (e.g., bioavailability, tissue penetration), there is good reason to be optimistic that compounds with broad-spectrum antiviral activity can be obtained for the treatment, for example, of rhinovirus infections, where the development of effective vaccines seems beyond reach. The structural similarity of the icosahedral capsid proteins of several animal and plant viruses has led Rossmann (105) to propose that the eight-stranded antiparallel β-barrel protein structure present in these viruses may also occur in the HIV p24 structural protein. Moreover, the general absence of this structural feature from host cell proteins makes it an attractive target for the design of selective antiviral agents. Clearly, appropriate studies to identify inhibitors of HIV with a mechanism of action similar to that of WIN 51711 are warranted.

## REPLICATION

In this section, some of the many events in the cycle of virus replication that lead to the production of new viral genomes and structural proteins will be considered. The assembly of these components into infectious daughter virions will be considered in the following section. It would be beyond the scope of this review to describe in detail the many strategies that have been adopted by viruses to ensure the replication of their genetic material and the production of proteins that are necessary to form the structure of the new virions. In brief, viruses have evolved a number of mechanisms for encoding their genetic material, using both DNA and RNA, which may be either double- or single-stranded. The genome may be segmented, even diploid in the case of the retroviruses, where an intermediate DNA copy is made, and, when present as RNA, may be of plus or minus sense. From this diversity of strategies, a range of solutions to the problem of ordering viral transcription and translation, as well as genome replication, within the infected cell has arisen. The sequence of events and their precise timing vary from one class of virus to another. However, for the purposes of defining circumstances that might be points for chemotherapeutic intervention, transcription, translation, and genome replication will be considered separately. Clearly, such an approach is an oversimplification, when, in reality, there are complex interrelationships among these events.

### Transcription

#### *Virus-Specific Transcriptases*

Some viruses, such as the herpesviruses and adenovirus (large, double-stranded DNA genome) and the human retroviruses (which transcribe RNA from a DNA proviral genome that is integrated into the host cell chromosome) utilize host cell RNA polymerase in the synthesis of mRNA. Inhibition of this vital cell enzyme would seem to be an unrewarding strategy for the discovery of selective antiviral agents. The poxviruses contain a virus-specific RNA polymerase within the virion core, and certain RNA viruses code for their own unique RNA polymerase, which may be synthesized in the infected cell early in the replicative cycle (e.g., picornaviruses, togaviruses, and coronaviruses) or may be a structural component of the infecting virion (e.g., ortho- and paramyxoviruses, rhabdoviruses).

Studies on poliovirus, encephalomyocarditis virus, and foot and mouth disease virus provide ample evidence for the presence of a virus-specific RNA-dependent, RNA polymerase in picornavirus-infected cells. Briefly, upon infection, the virion RNA (vRNA) is first translated to supply the proteins necessary for further transcription of the genome. RNA synthesis occurs via the replication intermediate, a structure consisting of full-length template with some six to eight nascent daughter strands, and is primed by a viral protein/uridylic acid complex, VPg-pUpU. Transcription requires the viral polymerase ($3C^{pol}$) and a host cell factor. The identity of the host factor and its relevance *in vivo* remain uncertain; based on an *in vitro* analysis, some authors have suggested that it may be a terminal uridylyltransferase (106,107). The minus sense transcripts function as templates for the synthesis of additional positive strands. The latter may be transcribed, or may serve either as mRNA or as genomic RNA for packaging. The fate of the positive-strand RNAs may be determined by the presence of the 5′-terminal VPg. It is well established that mRNA recovered from polysomes does not bear a viral protein cap (108,109); a cellular enzyme capable of cleaving VPg from RNA has been observed (110). Also detected in picornavirus-infected cells is a double-stranded replicative form, whose role in the overall model of transcription remains uncertain (111).

A number of compounds have been described with antiviral activity in cell culture and/or *in vivo* against picornaviruses, some of which appear to inhibit RNA synthesis, e.g., guanidine (112–114), 4′,5-dihydroxy-3,3′,7-trimethoxyflavone (115), and 3-methylquercetin (116). However, there is little evidence that they are specific inhibitors of the virus RNA polymerase, and progress in this area has generally been disappointing. Nonetheless, the important role of this enzyme in viral replication makes it an attractive target for specific antiviral agents. As the mechanism of poliovirus RNA transcription is better understood, it will be possible to construct more informative systems for *in vitro* compound assessment. More important, perhaps, since poliovirus infection is readily prevented by immunization, it will become easier to develop equivalent assays for other picornaviruses, such as the rhinoviruses, where the absence of effective vaccines makes the need for chemotherapy more pressing. It seems likely that such advances in molecular biology will make the search for selective inhibitors of the viral polymerases more productive.

Influenza virus encloses a complex of three proteins (PB1, PB2 and PA) within the virus particle that together with the nucleocapsid form the RNA polymerase complex responsible for the production of polyadenylated mRNA early in the replication cycle (117; for reviews, see refs. 118 and 119). The virus has evolved a remarkable strategy for the synthesis of capped mRNA in which host cell mRNA is used as a primer, the 5′ cap together with approximately 10–15 nucleotides being transferred to the virus product (120,121). PB2 recognizes the 5′-terminal cap structure of RNAs, whereas PB1 is the transcription/initiation protein that adds GMP residues to the 3′ ends of the primer fragment (122–125). Priming can also be demonstrated *in vitro* by employing disrupted, purified virus together with exogenous mRNA (126,127), which suggests that one of the viral proteins in the transcriptase complex also functions as an endonuclease. This activity had not been assigned to any of the polymerase proteins, and the role of PA is unclear. RNA synthesis occurs exclusively within the nucleus (128), and further analysis has suggested that the nonstructural protein NS1, which is synthesized in abundance early in the replication cycle (128), also localizes within the nucleus (129–131). It is tempting to speculate that this protein may also play a role in the regulation of influenza virus transcription.

These observations suggest that a mechanism-based approach to the development of influenza virus inhibitors is possible. Several groups have demonstrated the inhibition of the transcriptase *in vitro* by cap-like structures, 2′-deoxy-dinucleotides, oligonucleotides of defined sequence, and homo- and heteropolynucleotides; in some instances, virus replication in cell culture and in infected animals was also inhibited (132–136). Although none of these early attempts to develop effective antiviral agents has resulted in useful products, largely because the compounds penetrate cells poorly or are not bioavailable *in vivo*, there is good reason to be optimistic that the transcriptase complex can be the target for selective inhibition. A number of other chemical approaches to the inhibition of the influenza polymerase have been described, although they do not discriminate between the transcriptase and replicase activities of the polymerase complex. Pyrophosphate analogs and substituted methylene diphosphonates have been reported as inhibitors (137–139), and ribavirin, which has broad-spectrum antiviral activity *in vitro* (for a review, see ref. 140) and is effective against experimental influenza virus infections *in vivo* (for a review, see ref. 141), has been shown to be an inhibitor of the influenza polymerase when present as ribavirin triphosphate (142,143). However, ribavirin has other antimetabolic effects that may account for its antiinfluenza virus activity (144–146), and the phosphonates and thiophosphates do not appear promising candidates for clinical use. Nonetheless, the inhibitory activity exhibited by these compounds against influenza virus illustrates the potential of the approach to selective antiviral activity.

With regard to the *Paramyxoviridae*, infection by measles and mumps viruses has been controlled to a substantial extent by vaccination. In contrast, respiratory syncytial virus and the parainfluenza viruses, for which there are no adequate vaccines or chemotherapeutic agents, are a continuing cause of significant morbidity. These viruses are dissimilar to the influenza viruses inasmuch as the negative sense genome is not segmented. The genes [which are similarly ordered in measles virus, parainfluenza virus 3, and respiratory syncytial virus (147–153)] are transcribed from nonoverlapping cistrons that contain discrete start and stop sequences at each end. The large (L) protein, which is thought to contain the polymerase active site (154), and the nucleoprotein (NP) and phosphoprotein (P), which appear to play ancillary roles in transcription, are found within the transcriptase complex. The functioning of this complex is not well understood but may be analogous to that of VSV, which appears to have a similar replication strategy. Capping and methylating activities have not been assigned to any of the virion proteins. A number of compounds have been examined for antiviral activity against respiratory syncytial virus (e.g., see refs. 155–157 and refs. therein), but there is no compelling evidence that these nucleoside analogs are selectively targeted to the viral transcriptase. On the contrary, it is possible that these agents, which are inhibitory to several virus types, are acting at the level of host cell functions. It is likely that we shall have to develop a better understanding of the structure and function of the transcriptase complex, and establish appropriate *in vitro* assays before systematic attempts to discover compounds that are specific inhibitors of the transcriptase can be initiated.

### *Viral Transactivators of Transcription*

One of the most rapidly evolving fields of molecular virology is the elucidation of the role of certain viral proteins in the transactivation of transcription. Several viruses, including the human retroviruses and herpesviruses (which shall be discussed here), papillomavirus, and adenovirus, code for transactivators of transcription. These proteins can be considered as molecular targets for chemotherapeutic agents, although their potential remains untested; to date, no inhibitors that are active by such a mechanism have been described.

#### *Human Retroviruses*

The human retroviruses—human T-lymphotropic virus types I and II (HTLV-I and HTLV-II) and HIV—each code for a protein (termed tax in the case of HTLV-I and HTLV-II and tat in HIV) that stimulates gene expression directed by the respective viral long terminal repeat (LTR) (158–160). In addition, hepatitis B virus (HBV), which replicates by reverse transcription via an RNA intermediate, also codes for a transactivating protein (161,162). For the purposes of discussing strategies for therapeutic intervention, only the HIV-1 protein, tat, will be considered, although there are undoubtedly differences among the retroviral transactivating proteins. (For a detailed discussion of the control of gene expression in the human retroviruses, see ref. 163.) Importantly, it has been shown that tat is required for HIV replication: viral genomes in which the *tat* gene has been deleted are unable to produce new virus (164,165). However, the mechanism(s) by which gene expression is activated by tat remains unclear. Early observations suggested that transactivation could be explained by posttranscriptional events

(166,167), whereas others suggested that the mechanism was bimodal, involving both transcriptional and translational control (168), or occurred exclusively at the level of transcription (169).

HIV tat acts on a sequence called the "transactivating responsive element" (TAR) (170), which has been mapped to a region encompassing the start site for transcription (167,168). There are inverted repeat sequences within the TAR region that may form a stable RNA stem-loop structure (171,172). The tat may specifically relieve a block in transcriptional elongation caused by such a structure (173,174), although specific binding of tat to this region has not been reported and transactivation does not require *de novo* protein synthesis (175). Only the first 58 of the 84 amino acids that comprise full-length tat are required for activity (176), and mutagenesis experiments have revealed certain functional domains within the protein (177,178). Structural analysis of purified tat suggests the protein exists as a dimer, with metal ions acting as bridges in cooperation with cysteine-rich zinc fingers (179).

These studies have demonstrated the potential of tat as a molecular target for a chemotherapeutic agent. Tat appears to be an indispensible function for virus replication, and, therefore, it is suggested that a tat antagonist will exert an antiviral effect. Although the activity of tat has not been demonstrated *in vitro,* enough is known of the probable mechanism of action to permit the design of appropriate screens that will detect specific inhibitors. Finally, further analysis of the structure of the protein and identification of other factors (possibly cellular in origin) with which it interacts may provide the stimulus for the design of potential inhibitory compounds.

Finally, it is pertinent to note that the level of HIV transcription may be enhanced by the action of factors other than tat. These factors, which bind to enhancer regions 5′ of, and distinct from, the TAR region, may be viral in origin, [e.g., HSV immediate early gene products ICP0 and ICP4 (180,181), an EBV immediate early gene product (182), the adenovirus E1A 13S protein (183), the HBV X protein (184)] or cellular in origin (185–187). Although the activation of HIV transcription by these factors has important implications for understanding viral reactivation and pathogenesis, it is not clear at this time that these heterologous viral transactivating factors act by a common mechanism(s) that would define a suitable approach for the discovery of selective antiviral agents. Furthermore, inhibiting cellular transactivating factors that operate on the viral LTR would probably adversely affect normal cellular processes since they, most likely, are similarly regulated.

### *Herpesviruses*

The concept of temporal regulation of gene expression by viruses with early functions (those genes that are transcribed before replication of the genome) and late functions (transcribed after genome replication has started) is well established. Early genes can be described as "immediate early" if transcription occurs in the absence of a requirement for *de novo* protein synthesis or "delayed early" if virus protein synthesis is prerequisite for their expression. This temporal control of virus gene expression is achieved by positive and negative regulation of gene expression by viral proteins acting on upstream promoter-regulatory sequences and adjacent noncoding sequences. To date, it has not been possible to define compounds that exert an antiviral effect through specific perturbation of these regulatory mechanisms. Therefore, only general principles will be illustrated. This can be done with a detailed description of events in HSV infection, which has been well studied, although transcriptional activation has also been reported for human cytomegalovirus (HuCMV), EBV, and Varicella Zoster virus (VZV) (188–191).

There are three classes of virus polypeptide in HSV-infected cells—α, β and γ—that are synthesized sequentially and in a coordinated manner (192). These classes correlate with immediate early, early, and late gene expression. The α and β proteins are mainly nonstructural polypeptides; the γ class contains the major structural polypeptides. The synthesis of the α polypeptides does not require prior protein synthesis in the infected cell, whereas the synthesis of β polypeptides is dependent on prior α polypeptide synthesis and γ polypeptides require prior β polypeptide synthesis (192). This regulation of virus polypeptide synthesis appears to be the result of control at the level of mRNA transcription, which itself is ordered and regulated (193,194). The expression of the immediate early genes (α polypeptides) is transactivated by a virion polypeptide (VP16) (195,196) and requires the regulatory sequence TAATGARAT in the target gene for its action. However, VP16 does not bind directly to DNA but appears to act cooperatively with the cellular transcription factor OTF-1 (197–199). The expression of the delayed early and late genes (β and γ polypeptides) is regulated in a complex manner by the products of at least two (ICP0 and ICP4) of the five immediate early genes. These proteins can act independently or in a cooperative manner; they may also be autoregulatory (200–203). Transactivation of transcription *in vitro* using a partially purified α protein has been reported (204,205), and the protein has been partially characterized with respect to its physicochemical characteristics (206) and functional domains (207).

Clearly, further studies are needed to define more precisely the mechanism of action of these proteins, as well as to determine the role of host cell proteins. In the case of VP16, for example, studies with mutant forms of the protein suggest that the domain responsible for binding to cellular factors is separate from that directly responsible for transactivating the immediate early genes (208) and that the expression of mutant forms of VP16 can block the lytic infection cycle of HSV. Thus, there seems to be good reason to believe that these events will prove useful targets for chemotherapeutics as previously proposed (209).

### *Early and Late Gene Expression: Other Regulatory Mechanisms*

Before leaving the subject of early and late gene expression, there are two other examples, in the human retroviruses and in influenza virus, that are worthy of mention. In the one instance, analysis of gene expression among the human retroviruses points to viral control of levels of spliced versus unspliced mRNAs. As a consequence, certain nonstructural proteins are translated from extensively spliced messages in high abundance early after reactivation, whereas the larger, structural proteins are translated from unspliced or singly spliced messages at later times. In the second example, it is recognized that certain influenza virus proteins are expressed in relatively high abundance early in the cycle, whereas other proteins predominate later. The means by which this level of control is achieved is not known, but appears to be at the level of RNA transcription. In the case of the human retroviruses, the identification of a virus-coded protein that is required for infectivity leads one to the postulate that selective inhibitors of its function may be discovered; in the case of influenza virus replication, the available data strongly argue that additional research may reveal the underlying control process and suggest a mechanism-based approach to antiviral drug discovery. Our knowledge in each of these areas will be reviewed briefly here; we do not know whether drug discovery in either or both of these areas has a high likelihood of success.

Each of the human retroviruses express a gene—*rex* in the case of HTLV-I and HTLV-II, and *rev* (previously *art* or *trs*) in the case of HIV—whose phenotype is to control the relative abundance of proteins expressed from spliced versus unspliced messages. The data that have been obtained with HIV will be described to illustrate the point, although without doubt there will be differences in detail among the human retroviruses.

Early studies showed that the expression of HIV capsid and envelope genes was negatively regulated and that an additional gene was necessary to overcome the repression (166,210). Moreover, mutagenesis experiments have indicated that this gene appears to be essential for virus replication (211,212); they provide a strong argument for the selection of rev as a molecular target for an antiviral agent. Although rev is functional in relieving the negative repression of gene expression when supplied in *trans,* its action appears to be different from that of the tat protein. First, the rev-responsive sequences appear to be located within the coding region of the envelope gene (213) rather than close to the start site of transcription. Second, the action of rev appears to differentiate between proteins translated from multiply spliced mRNAs and those coded by unspliced or singly spliced mRNAs. The exact mechanism of action of rev remains uncertain. Some workers have reported that substantial levels of gag and env mRNAs are synthesized in the absence of rev and propose that its action, therefore, is at a posttranscriptional level (210,214); others propose that rev functions to increase the levels of unspliced or singly spliced mRNAs (166) at the expense of levels of the highly spliced mRNAs that code for full-length tat and for rev itself (215). The role of host protein(s), if any, in the action of rev is not defined, and, in the absence of a good understanding of the action of rev, the rational design of inhibitors is not possible. On the other hand, the design of cell-based assays that can be used in random screens to identify inhibitors is now possible, and, in this context, it is pertinent to note that nuclear extracts from HIV-infected cells have been shown to inhibit the splicing of a synthetic premessenger RNA that incorporates sequences from the HIV *env* gene *in vitro* (216). This result is consistent with the observations of others who have shown that rev is localized predominantly in the nucleus (217). However, although it is by no means certain that the inhibitory activity observed *in vitro* can be attributed to the action of rev, studies such as these do further the search for *in vitro* assays of rev action, such systems being important components of any program that is designed to discover specific inhibitors of rev as well as define its mechanism of action more precisely.

The genome of influenza virus comprises eight RNA segments that separately code for 10 proteins (genes 7 and 8 each yield a second, spliced message). In addition, the genome is single-stranded and of negative sense. Messenger RNAs are transcribed from vRNAs, which are synthesized *de novo* from complementary templates; these, in turn, are copied from the input virus genome. It is well established that during virus infection, the pattern of viral protein synthesis changes during the replication cycle. Thus, the NP and the nonstructural protein NS1 are synthesized in high abundance early in the replication cycle, whereas other proteins, most notably the matrix (M1) protein, are present in greater amounts at later times. The high abundance of the "early" proteins correlates with the levels of their corresponding mRNAs, whereas the disproportionately high levels of these early messages appears to match the relative abundance of the corresponding vRNAs, at least at early times (128) and possibly throughout the replication cycle (218). Since there are approximately equal proportions of template RNAs of each species present (128,218,219), the control of early and late protein synthesis rests primarily at the level of transcription of vRNAs. Although it is unclear how transcription from template RNA is controlled, it remains possible that viral proteins play a key role in this regulation. If this is indeed so, then a mechanism-based approach to the design of antiinfluenza virus agents that are targeted to a virus-specific event might be suggested.

### *Capping of Virus mRNAs*

Virtually all eukaryotic mRNAs contain a 5′ cap of the general structure $m^7G(5')ppp(5')N_1pN_2p$ where the nucleosides $N_1$ and $N_2$ may be purines or pyrimidines, and methylated or nonmethylated. Most viral mRNA is similarly capped (for a review, see ref. 220), although $N_1$ is generally a purine. There is one particularly notable exception in the picornaviruses, where the message terminates in the sequence *pUpUpA* (108,109,221). We can define three strategies for capping. First, as we have already seen, influenza virus scavenges for capped host cell messengers to serve as primers for the synthesis of its own mRNA. The cap-binding domain on the viral transcriptase and the viral-coded endonuclease are potential molecular targets for the selective inhibitors. Second, a number of viruses have capping enzymes [RNA guanylyltransferase and RNA (guanine-7)-methyltransferase] within the virion as well as an RNA polymerase, e.g., vaccinia (222) and reovirus (223), which may also be amenable to specific inhibition. The third arrangement is the use of host cell capping enzymes, as is presumed to be the case for several viruses, e.g., herpes.

Although the virus-coded capping enzymes represent legitimate targets for selective inhibition, the design of inhibitors of the various cellular methyl transferases would seem to be an unrewarding approach in view of the potential for toxicity. *S*-Adenosylmethionine is the source of methyl groups used by many methyltransferases for the alkylation of a variety of substrates including guanine and adenine bases in the mRNA cap. *S*-Adenosylhomocysteine (SAH) hydrolase represents a critical point in this metabolic pathway since its inhibition results in increased SAH levels, which in turn blockade methyltransferase reactions. Considerable effort has been directed to the discovery of SAH hydrolase inhibitors with antiviral activity (for a review, see ref. 224), but such an approach would seem unlikely to yield compounds that are sufficiently selective for the virus-infected cell to warrant their clinical use, except perhaps in the most severe viral infections.

## Virus Protein Synthesis and Maturation

A number of strategies for the inhibition of virus mRNA synthesis have been proposed in this review. To proceed a step further and define conditions for the selective inhibition of translation of virus messengers has proved more difficult. For example, general protein synthesis inhibitors in general are as likely to exhibit toxicity to the host as to exert an antiviral effect. However, one approach that may be of value in specifically inhibiting virus protein synthesis is the use of antisense oligonucleotides. If, however, we look beyond the initial event of protein synthesis to the process of protein maturation, then further opportunities for targeting specific antiviral compounds become apparent. Each of these approaches is considered below.

### *Inhibitors of mRNA Translation: Antisense RNA*

An approach to specific inhibition of virus replication that has undergone a substantial revival in interest over the past few years is the design of antisense inhibitors for the control of mRNA expression. Briefly, it is hypothesized that oligodeoxyribonucleotides (ODN) of a sequence complementary to a viral RNA can be used to inhibit virus replication. This strategy is based on the observations of Zamecnik and Stephenson (225), who demonstrated that a tridecamer, complementary to 13 nucleotides of the 3′ and 5′ reiterated sequences of Rous sarcoma virus RNA, was capable of inhibiting virus production in cell culture. The oligonucleotide exhibited sequence-specific inhibition of mRNA translation *in vitro* (226). As we shall see, however, it still remains to be shown that antisense ODN are effective in virus-infected cells as a result of hybridization to the complementary mRNA and, consequently, inhibition of translation. Therefore, it can only be assumed at this time that this molecular approach is relevant to inhibition of viral protein synthesis. (For a more general review of the antisense approach, see ref. 227.)

Despite the lack of definitive proof of the hypothesized mechanism of action of such antisense DNAs, considerable success has been achieved in the application of this approach to inhibition of virus replication in cell culture. Several groups have reported the inhibition of HIV (228–233), HSV (234), influenza virus (235), and VSV (236,237) replication in cell culture. Because of the perceived susceptibility of unmodified 2′-deoxy-ODN to nuclease attack and because of cell permeability concerns, several chemical types of antisense ODN have now been developed, e.g., ODN methylphosphonates, phosphorothioates, and phosphoramidates. This notwithstanding, 2′-deoxy-ODN have been shown to be antiviral in cell culture in unmodified form (228,230), or when covalently linked to polylysine (237) or to an intercalating agent (235).

Antisense RNAs have been shown to inhibit viral protein synthesis in infected, treated cells as well as *in vitro* translation systems (234,236,237), although inhibitory effects were not necessarily restricted to the viral protein whose mRNA was the putative target for the antisense RNA. This latter observation may be explained by the coordinated regulation of the synthesis of viral proteins. On the other hand, studies with the phosphorothioates suggest that the effect may not, in every instance, be one of antisense inhibition since the greatest antiviral (HIV) effect was obtained with homopolymeric deoxycytidine (231). The compound effectively inhibited *de novo* DNA synthesis in acute HIV infections, but failed to inhibit viral p24 antigen production in chronically infected cells. These results are reminiscent of earlier reports of the *in vitro* inhibition of the reverse transcriptase of murine retroviruses and of the influenza virus transcriptase by polynucleotides.

Problems of delivery of an antisense molecule to the virus-infected cell in the host have yet to be overcome. A parenteral route of administration seems to be the most likely to be successful, but the stability of such molecules *in vivo* and the extent to which they will be distributed within the body remain uncertain. However, before leaving this subject, it is appropriate to consider briefly one case where a natural antisense mechanism may be involved in the regulation of virus replication. Several groups of workers have reported the presence of a new class of viral transcripts in the cells of mice, rabbits, and humans that are latently infected with HSV-1 (238–242). The gene for at least one of these transcripts overlaps the 3′ end of the gene for the immediate early protein ICP0, and its transcript is complementary to ICP0 mRNA. Several alternative roles for the anti-ICP0 transcript in maintaining the latent infected state have been suggested (240); most intriguing is the possibility that the transcript functions as a natural antisense RNA, down-regulating the expression of the immediate early mRNA. Maintenance of the latent state may then be seen in terms of continued suppression of viral immediate early gene expression by an antisense agent, with reactivation occurring when the levels of the positive sense, immediate early gene product exceed those of the antisense. Prophylactic administration of a similar synthetic antisense agent of the ODN type may thus help to maintain the balance in favor of restricted gene expression and continued latency.

### *Inhibition of Virus Protein Maturation*

During the replication cycle of a number of viruses, protein maturation by posttranslational modification is essential if new infectious virions are to be produced. Such modifications may involve cleavage of a larger molecular weight precursor protein to yield the mature polypeptide. Alternatively, or in addition, proteins may be acylated, glycosylated, sulfated, or phosphorylated. Failure to complete such protein maturation may result in an incomplete replicative cycle or the production of defective virions that are incapable of initiating further infection. Our knowledge of these events is still limited, but some potential targets for chemotherapy are beginning to emerge.

#### *Posttranslational Cleavage*

The synthesis of viral proteins as large molecular weight precursors and the cleavage of these proteins to mature functional forms have been observed in the replication of many viruses. For the purposes of defining specific targets for antiviral chemotherapy, we can distinguish two different maturation processes, though to do so risks oversimplification.

In the first case, certain viral polypeptides that are destined for incorporation into the envelope of the mature virion are synthesized in a precursor form and are cleaved by membrane-associated proteases of cellular origin. Such maturation is essential for viral infectivity, as has been clearly demonstrated in the case of influenza virus (67,243,244) and the paramyxoviruses (66,245,246). It seems likely that the cleavage of the HIV envelope precursor glycoprotein gp160 to yield gp120 and gp41 is similarly mediated. In each case, the newly-created amino terminus (of $HA_2$ in the case of influenza virus, $F_1$ of the paramyxoviruses, and gp41 of HIV) is characterized by a cluster of hydrophobic amino acids that are involved in fusion of the virus envelope to the cell membrane in the early stages of virus infection. The trypsin-like protease (247) and arginine carboxypeptidase (248,249), which are responsible for cleavage of the influenza virus hemagglutinin, and the proteases responsible for the cleavage of the fusion proteins of the paramyxoviruses (66,245) are host cell enzymes. Therefore, although general protease inhibitors have been shown to inhibit the production of infectious influenza virus (250,251) and respiratory syncytial virus (252,253), it seems unlikely that, in this instance, truly virus-specific inhibitors can be developed.

By contrast, in several viral systems, e.g., picornaviruses, retroviruses, and togaviruses, the cytoplasmic or virion-associated processing of precursor polypeptides is brought about by virally encoded proteases that, theoretically at least, offer the prospect of unique targets for selective antiviral agents. We shall briefly consider two examples of posttranslational processing, those in poliovirus and HIV infection. (For a more detailed review of viral proteases and the events in protein maturation, see ref. 254.) Although there are marked differences in the detail of events, both in timing within the replicative cycle and in complexity, some fundamental principles for antiviral drug design can be established.

The polycistronic poliovirus RNA is translated from a single initiation site into a precursor polypeptide that is hydrolyzed in a series of steps to yield the nonstructural proteins and the mature virus polypeptides (255). Protein processing occurs within the cell in three phases: cotranslational cleavage that releases the capsid precursor from the nascent polypeptide, secondary cleavage that processes both structural and nonstructural precursor proteins, and maturation cleavage of the capsid. At each level, distinct viral proteases are involved in the catalytic event, and the scissile bond is clearly defined. Primary cleavage in poliovirus is mediated by the viral protease 2A, the putative active site of which contains cysteine and histidine residues, suggesting it to be a cysteine proteinase (256). This is supported by the observation that the enzyme can be inhibited *in vitro* by compounds characterized as inhibitors of cysteine proteases (257). The enzyme, which cuts at a tyrosine-glycine (Tyr-Gly) bond, appears to function intramolecularly, although it is also active if supplied in trans (256,258). Since the sequence Tyr-Gly occurs at several other sites within the viral polyprotein that are not subject to cleavage, it must be assumed that the substrate specificity of protease 2A is dependent on structural determinants, which may be primary or secondary in nature, that extend on either side of the scissile bond. Sequence analysis suggests a requirement for threonine (Thr) at P2 (259) in poliovirus, whereas in the rhinoviruses, for example, the inferred P2-P1-P1′ sequences are Thr-Ala-Gly, Ser-Tyr-Gly, and Asn-Val-Gly (where Ser, Asn, and Val represent serine, asparagine, and valine, respectively) (260,261).

Most recently, the isolation and purification of the 2A protease has been described, together with an *in vitro* assay for the characterization of its action (257). Thus, the elements necessary to explore in greater detail the substrate specificity of the enzyme and to begin to design potential inhibitors are available. It seems reasonable to expect that potent inhibitors of the picornaviral 2A protease will be described in the near future, although careful refinement of structures may be necessary to yield compounds that selectively inhibit the viral enzyme, with minimal activity against cellular counterparts.

Secondary cleavage of picornavirus proteins is affected by a second viral protease, 3C. The enzyme, which is highly conserved in sequence and predicted secondary structure among the picornaviruses (262,263), is possibly a cysteine protease, as is protease 2A. However, in the case of the 3C enzyme, cleavage occurs exclusively at a Gln-Gly bond (where Gln represents glutamine) (264,265). The cleavage site must be further defined, however, since not all Gln-Gly bonds in the viral protein are subject to proteolytic attack. In other picornaviruses, either of the two amino acids flanking the scissile bond may be replaced, e.g., Gln for glutamic acid in rhinovirus, and Gly for alanine (Ala) or Ser in rhinovirus and the cardioviruses. As was argued for the viral enzyme 2A, in the case of protease 3C there is sufficient information to warrant attempts to design inhibitors that are selective for the picornaviral proteases with useful antiviral activity.

The retroviral genome comprises, in order from 5′ to 3′, the genes *gag, pol,* and *env* that code for, respectively, the structural proteins of the capsid; the enzymes reverse transcriptase, ribonuclease H (RNaseH), and integrase that are necessary for transcription of the genome and integration of the proviral DNA into the host cell chromosome; and the glycoproteins of the viral envelope. There may be other genes, e.g., the oncogenes of the transforming retroviruses and the regulatory genes of HIV, but they are of less importance in this context. Located either at the carboxy terminus of the *gag* gene, as is the case in the avian retroviruses, or at the amino terminus of the *pol* gene in the mammalian retroviruses (for a review, see ref. 266) including HIV (267), are sequences that code for a protease. The importance of the protease for viral infectivity has been demonstrated in many systems but may be exemplified by a description of the events in HIV replication.

The HIV gag protein is synthesized as a 56kDa polyprotein and the *pol* products as a gag-pol fusion protein, which results from an infrequent translational frameshift (268).

By this mechanism, the structural gag protein is produced in high abundance relative to the catalytic pol proteins. The immature gag and gag-pol proteins assemble at the membrane of the infected cell and are packaged into budding virions. In contrast to the intracellular processing of the virion proteins observed in the picornaviruses, the HIV protease becomes functional within the virion as it is released from the surface of the infected cell. Active enzyme can be obtained as a 10–11-kDa polypeptide, but the larger gag-pol fusion protein also retains catalytic activity, presumably so that autocatalysis may first occur (269,270,271). The viral protease cleaves gag and gag-pol substrates at specific sites to yield the smaller molecular weight structural proteins p17, p24, p9, and p7, as well as the catalytic proteins required for reverse transcription and integration of the genome. In the absence of a functional protease, virus particles are produced, but they are not infectious (272). Thus, it is possible that specific inhibitors of this viral protease may be effective antiviral agents.

Several pieces of evidence point to the retroviral protease being of the aspartyl type, including comparisons of amino acid sequence with that of known aspartyl proteases (273–275), site-specific mutagenesis of putative active site aspartyl residues (271,272,276), and inhibition by aspartyl protease inhibitors (277,278). Short synthetic peptides may be used as substrates for the isolated enzyme, cleavage occurring at sites corresponding to the authentic cut sites in the viral gag and pol proteins (279–281), whereas modified peptides serve as inhibitors (279). Inhibitors may be designed using structural models of the viral enzyme or, more pragmatically, by the synthesis of derivatives of known inhibitors such as pepstatin, and of analogs of the amino acid sequence(s) surrounding the polyprotein cleavage sites. In this regard, the cleavage sites for the HIV protease have been determined to center on several classes of amino acid clusters, including Phe-Pro, (or Tyr-Pro) Met-Met, and X-Phe-Leu (where Pro and Met are proline and methionine, respectively, and X is a variable hydrophobic amino acid) (282,283). Of these, Phe-Pro may be favored as the starting point for drug design since it appears not to be a cleavage site preferred by human aspartyl proteases. Nonetheless, since there are several such enzymes in the host, including renin, pepsin, and capthepsin D, refinement of inhibitor structure for selective inhibition of the viral enzyme will be necessary if this approach is to yield safe antiviral agents.

### *Glycosylation*

The viral envelope found in several RNA and DNA viruses consists of a combination of membrane components of the infected cell and virus-specific glycoproteins. Most viral glycoproteins contain oligosaccharide side chains that are attached by *N*-glycosidic linkages to asparagine residues within a sequence Asn-X-Thr or Asn-X-Ser (X being a variable amino acid) within the polypeptide chain. Glycosylation is initiated in the rough endoplasmic reticulum where preformed oligosaccharides are coupled to the nascent polypeptide chain. Trimming of the newly added oligosaccharide by glucosidase I and II and mannosidase may then occur, followed by further addition of sugars by glycosyltransferases (for a review, see ref. 284). The sugar moieties that remain in the mature form may depend on the structure of the polypeptide per se and the nature of the host cell.

Several compounds have been described as inhibitors of protein glycosylation, with consequent antiviral effects against a number of viruses (285). The mechanism of action varies from compound to compound and reportedly includes inhibition of the synthesis of the precursor dolichol-linked oligosaccharide (e.g., tunicamycin), inhibition of glucosidase I (e.g., castanospermine, 1-deoxynorijimycin), and of mannosidase (e.g., 1-deoxymannorijimycin, swainsonine). The consequences of the failure to produce mature glycoprotein seem to vary from one virus/host cell system to another. Broadly speaking, the effects of inhibiting protein glycosylation have been reported to be either an increased susceptibility of the nonglycosylated protein to proteolytic cleavage, as was observed in influenza virus-infected cells (286); inefficient intracellular transport of the protein to the cell surface, seen to be the case for the VSV G protein (287); or inhibition of virus assembly and infectivity, as with SFV (288) and HSV (289,290).

More recently, it has been reported that treatment of HIV-infected cells with castanospermine results in a reduction of virus infectivity and inhibition of viral gp120-dependent cell fusion (291). In addition, accumulation of aberrant forms of both gp120 and precursor gp160 were observed, and there was a change in the relative amounts of gp160 vs gp120 in the treated, infected cell, suggesting a failure of protein maturation. Treatment of HIV-infected cells with 1-deoxynorijimycin, but not with 1-deoxymannorijimycin, also results in the inhibition of syncytium formation between virus-infected and CD4-bearing cells and reduces the output of infectious virus (292). Exposure to 1-deoxynorijimycin resulted in the formation of aberrant forms of both gp120 and gp160 that exhibited an increased molecular weight relative to the normal forms in untreated cells, although the ratio of the two species remained unchanged by the treatment. However, it is clear from the studies reviewed above that relatively high concentrations of the inhibitors castanospermine and 1-deoxynorijimycin were required in order to achieve a biological effect. Chemical modification of these lead compounds could result in more powerful inhibitors, as has already been demonstrated for 1-deoxynorijimycin (293,294).

Since the mode of action of these compounds is ostensibly the inhibition of a cellular function rather than the direct interaction with a virus gene product, there is an obvious concern that such inhibitors will adversely affect the glycosylation of proteins of uninfected cells with consequent toxicity to the treated host. In this context, it is of interest to note that 1-deoxynorijimycin has been used clinically without adverse effects, either as a single dose or in short-term repeated doses, as an experimental therapeutic for type II diabetes (295–297), whereas the adverse metabolic effects of castanospermine could be reversed in rats by the coadministration of glucose (298). On the other hand, although some studies have suggested that glycosylation inhibitors could exert an antiviral effect in cell culture in the absence of toxicity to the host cell (291,292,299), others have shown that glucosidase inhibitors affect expression of constitutive cellular glycoproteins at the cell surface (300). Nonetheless, the possibility remains that a selective inhibition of glycoprotein synthesis in the virus-infected cell may be achieved. Such a circumstance may arise if, for example, the function of the virus glycoprotein is exquisitely sensitive to changes in the oligosaccharide structure or if there is a virus-directed component that modulates glycosylation in the infected cell. In this regard, the sialyl and galactosyl transferases in the HSV-infected cell were shown to have altered kinetic properties compared with the corresponding activities in the uninfected cell (301), suggesting that there may be virus control of glycosylation through modification of host cell glycosyl transferases.

In conclusion, these results leave us with some uncertainty as to whether the inhibition of events during viral protein glycosylation is a worthwhile strategy for the discovery of antiviral agents. It is possible that new molecules will be identified in time that are selective inhibitors of viral glycoprotein synthesis and, consequently, are efficacious antivirals. However, considerable attention will have to be devoted to monitoring for toxic effects both *in vitro* and *in vivo*.

## DNA Synthesis

By far the most fruitful area of research for the discovery of antiviral agents has been in the field of DNA synthesis inhibitors. The majority of compounds that are approved for clinical use fall within this class, principally for the treatment of infections caused by HSV. It is no coincidence that when HIV was recognized as the etiologic agent of AIDS, nucleosides were the most prevalent type of compound reported to have antiviral activity. AZT was the first of these agents to demonstrate clinical efficacy in AIDS and severe ARC (302,303), and several additional analogs are presently in clinical trial (304).

The successful discovery of the anti-herpetics and anti-HIV agents underscores the suitability of the viral DNA polymerases, including reverse transcriptases, as molecular targets. That is not to say that the approach is without difficulties or that the discovery of nucleosides that are inhibitors of these viral enzymes is trivial. On the contrary, it has proven to be an exceedingly challenging task to obtain compounds that are potent inhibitors of the target viral enzyme without significantly affecting the function of the corresponding cellular DNA polymerases or other enzymes necessary for the supply of DNA synthesis intermediates, and it is likely that many more unsuccessful compounds have been synthesized and tested than the reports in the literature would lead us to believe.

In this discussion of molecular targets, it is not necessary to give an account of the many nucleosides that have been evaluated as antiviral agents. Such a task would be the subject for an entire chapter in itself, and drug discovery in this area, particularly inhibitors of HIV reverse transcriptase, is moving at such a rapid pace that any review would quickly be outdated. Rather, the principles and the problems can be illustrated by focusing upon a few examples drawn from the herpesviruses and HIV. It should be noted, however, that modest clinical success has also been achieved in the treatment of HBV infection with nucleoside antivirals (see Chapter 12), and it is reasonable to assume that these agents act at the level of the viral DNA polymerase. It has been established that replication of the HBV genome occurs through an RNA intermediate (305,306), but systematic studies and characterization of the isolated polymerase have not been possible until recently (307). Further progress in this area can be reasonably expected in the not-too-distant future. In time, it may also be possible to apply the principles of targeted drug discovery to the selection of inhibitors of adenovirus DNA synthesis. This virus codes for its own DNA polymerase, although there are also proteins of cellular origin in the replication complex. On the other hand, the inhibition of DNA synthesis may not be an appropriate target in all DNA virus infections. For example, it seems likely, by analogy to the polyomaviruses and to SV40, that papillomavirus DNA replication is dependent on the host cell DNA polymerase α. If this is the case, then the use of DNA synthesis inhibitors as antiviral agents for the papovaviruses would seem to be inappropriate. An exception to this may be the treatment of certain superficial papillomavirus-induced warts where the potential toxicity to the host may be limited by topical administration of the agent directly on to the lesion.

### *Herpesviruses*

Many pyrimidine and purine nucleosides and nucleoside analogs have been evaluated for anti-herpes virus activity (for reviews, see refs. 308–311). Among those compounds that have shown considerable promise are the 5-substituted-2′-deoxyuridines, the fluorarabinonucleosides, and the acyclic purine nucleosides, of which acyclovir (ACV) has proven to be particularly useful. An aspect to their action that many of these compounds have in common is their selective phosphorylation by viral thymidine kinase. Although not a target for inhibition per se, the enzyme functions as a specific gate, permitting the entry of antiviral nucleosides into the metabolic pathway of precursors leading to DNA synthesis in the virus-infected cell.

The critical importance of thymidine kinase in the action of selective anti-herpetics has been discussed previously (209) and can be simply illustrated by a comparison of the action of acyclovir (9-[2-hydroxyethoxymethyl]guanine) (ACV) with its congener DHPG (9-[(1,3-dihydroxy-2-propoxy)methyl] guanine). ACV, which is inhibitory to the replication of HSV, is dependent on phosphorylation by viral thymidine kinase for its action because it is a poor substrate for the cellular enzyme (312–314). As the triphosphate, ACV has a greater affinity for the herpesvirus DNA polymerase compared to the cellular enzyme (313,315), prevents chain elongation once incorporated into the nascent viral DNA (316), and causes the virus DNA polymerase to remain bound to the template (315). ACV is also inhibitory to EBV (317,318) and to VZV (319), each of which codes for a thymidine kinase (320,321), but not to HuCMV, for which no viral thymidine kinase has been reported. In contrast, the spectrum of activity of DHPG encompasses HuCMV as well as HSV and EBV (322–324), but the compound appears to be significantly more toxic than ACV *in vivo*.

The difference in spectrum of antiviral activity of these compounds and the greater toxicity of DHPG are related in large measure to the degree to which the compounds are selectively anabolized by virus-coded enzymes. In the HSV-infected cell, ACV and DHPG share a common mechanism of action: both are phosphorylated by the viral thymidine kinase to the respective monophosphate derivatives and, subsequently, to the di- and triphosphates by cellular kinases (314,324,325). On the other hand, further analysis has suggested that DHPG may also be phosphorylated by a host cell deoxyguanosine kinase (326). The elevated levels of this cellular kinase in HuCMV-infected cells may contribute to the antiviral potency of DHPG, but the possibility remains that significant quantities of the compound may also be phosphorylated in uninfected cells. When this is coupled with the observation that the differences in affinity of DHPG-triphosphate for the viral DNA polymerases compared to cellular DNA polymerase α is much less than for ACV-triphosphate (327–329), then DHPG-induced inhibition of cellular DNA synthesis and consequent toxicity are readily explained.

In summary, the thymidine kinases of the herpesviruses represent an important vehicle for ensuring the selective entry of antimetabolites into the metabolic pathways of the virus-infected cell. In the case of HuCMV, where no such virus-coded enzyme appears to exist, there is a need to develop inhibitors that can be anabolized by cellular enzymes, but which must, as the active drug form, show high selectivity for the viral DNA polymerase, the ultimate target enzyme. It remains to be determined whether this goal can be met, but studies of mutant virus enzymes and a greater appreciation of the structure of the enzyme active site (330,331) may facilitate drug design. Also desirable is the development of new therapeutic agents that have enhanced antiviral potency and improved pharmacokinetics while retaining high selectivity for the viral thymidine kinase and DNA polymerase. In this context, it is interesting to refer to several recently described acyclic nucleosides that have antiherpetic activities (332–337). One analog, 2HM-HBG, is particularly interesting in view of its greater inhibitory activity against VZV than ACV

(338). The enhanced antiviral activity of 2HM-HBG is attributed, as least in part, to its greater affinity for the virus thymidine kinase compared to ACV and more rapid phosphorylation; at the same time, selectivity for the viral thymidine kinase, compared to the cellular mitochondrial counterpart, is retained.

The emergence of drug-resistant strains of virus under the appropriate selective conditions is usually considered to be good evidence that a compound acts on a virus-specific function. In view of the requirement for both a viral thymidine kinase and DNA polymerase for the action of ACV, it should be no surprise to learn that ACV-resistant mutant viruses have been isolated, both in the laboratory under selective conditions and in clinical practice from treated patients. Although such a discovery may be gratifying for the theoretician, the emergence of drug resistance during treatment of infected patients is of considerable concern to the clinician. The nature of the mutations that lead to ACV resistance have been reviewed previously (339), and the clinical impact of such viruses will be discussed elsewhere in this volume. It need only be noted here that some, but not all, ACV-resistant viruses are cross-resistant to other nucleoside antiviral agents. Consequently, there remains a strong need to identify other molecular targets for inhibition of herpesvirus replication and to develop other therapeutics that have dissimilar mechanisms of action.

The HSV thymidine kinase is a multifunctional complex with additional deoxycytidine kinase (340), thymidylate kinase (341), and nucleoside phosphotransferase (342) activities. It has been proposed that thymidine kinase may itself be a target for direct inhibition, although the antiviral activity of a compound effective by such a mechanism may only be observed *in vivo* since the enzyme is not absolutely required for virus growth in cell culture (209). The multifunctional nature of HSV thymidine kinase suggests that there is considerable scope for the design of inhibitors. There have been at least two reports using somewhat different chemical approaches of thymidine kinase inhibitors (343,344). These results suggest that it may be possible to obtain selective antiviral agents active by this mechanism. The herpesvirus genome has a large coding capacity with nearly 80 virus-specified proteins being present in the infected cell. There is biochemical and, in some cases, genetic evidence that several of these proteins (in addition to thymidine kinase and DNA polymerase) are involved in the pathways to DNA replication. One such protein, the virus-coded ribonucleotide reductase, will be considered here in more detail, but other enzymes such as the viral alkaline DNase (345–347), dUTPase, uracil-DNA glycosylase (348), and DNA topoisomerase (349–351) may also be candidates for more detailed study.

There is ample evidence that HSV, EBV, and VZV each code for a unique ribonucleotide reductase that is present in the infected cell (352–359). The enzyme is composed of two nonidentical subunits, as is the mammalian cellular counterpart (360,361), and there are certain other structural and mechanistic homologies between the two enzymes. However, there are also clear differences between the viral and cellular ribonucleotide reductases in their respective biochemical properties (359,362), and genetic evidence indicates that the viral enzyme is necessary for replication (355,357,363,364).

Taken together, these observations suggest that the herpesvirus ribonucleotide reductase represents an appropriate molecular target for antiviral agents. Several distinct chemical approaches to inhibition of the viral enzyme have been described (for a review, see ref. 365), of which, two contrasting strategies will be discussed here. In the first case, a number of peptides have been reported that presumably inhibit the association of the two subunits (366,367). Such peptides, homologous in sequence to the carboxy terminus of the H2 subunit of the HSV ribonucleotide reductase, inhibit enzyme activity *in vitro,* although antiviral activity has not been reported. The peptides described to date are unlikely to be useful pharmacological agents because of their weak inhibitory activity and poor bioavailability. However, careful optimization of sequence may yield more potent molecules (368), and the use of peptide mimetics may result in compounds that are antiviral *in vitro* and *in vivo*. Compounds of the second type to be considered, the thiosemicarbazones, are most likely active site inhibitors. Compounds of this class, typified by 2-acetylpyridine thiosemicarbazone, are antiviral *in vitro* (369–371) and *in vivo* (372). Although 2-acetylpyridine thiosemicarbazone shows minimal selectivity for HSV-1 ribonucleotide reductase compared to the human cell equivalent (371), structural optimization of this lead compound may result in the identification of compounds that are both potent and specific inhibitors of the virus enzyme.

### *Retroviruses*

The discovery of the first nucleosides with antiherpetic activity was, by and large, serendipitous, and the synthesis of additional analogs and the refinement of structure/activity relationships empiric. The path to the discovery of antiviral agents targeted to the DNA polymerase activity of the HIV reverse transcriptase has, so far, been similar. AZT and 2′,3′-dideoxycytidine (ddC), both of which are effective inhibitors of HIV in cell culture, were discovered by compound screening (373,374); the use of these compounds in the clinic for the treatment of HIV infection is discussed in Chapter 15. As their respective 5′-triphosphates, AZT and ddC inhibit the viral reverse transcriptase *in vitro* (375–377), but both compounds have exhibited marked, though different, toxicities in clinical use (304,378). The mechanistic basis for these toxicities is not known at this time and may relate to inhibition of cellular DNA synthesis by direct action on the host polymerases, or through effects on intermediary metabolism in one or more different pathways. In this context, it is interesting to note that ddCTP is a powerful inhibitor of DNA polymerase $\gamma$ (379).

Earlier studies using retroviruses of murine and avian origin identified compounds of a number of chemical classes, other than dideoxynucleosides, as inhibitors of reverse transcriptase, e.g., the rifamycins (380), polynucleotides (for a review, see ref. 381), modified pyrimidines (382), and quinone antibiotics (383), although selectivity of action could not be or was not always demonstrated. Some of these compounds may be important leads for the discovery of HIV reverse transcriptase inhibitors, as may be the case for rifabutin, a semisynthetic rifamycin derivative that inhibits HIV reverse transcriptase *in vitro* and is antiviral in cell culture (384). However, considerable effort will undoubtedly continue to be devoted to the optimization of the action of the dideoxynucleosides. It is valid to ask, therefore, whether or not the processes of rational drug design can be used with greater effect to obtain highly selective inhibitors of HIV reverse transcriptase. In this context, the discovery of AZT probably owes much to good fortune (although this does not diminish in any way the significance of this most important achievement), and the search for analogs at present still depends more on empiricism than rational design. However, there is good reason to be optimistic that the tools necessary for a program of rational inhibitor design are obtainable. Several groups have reported the molecular cloning and expression of the gene for reverse transcriptase in prokaryotic hosts (385–389). This, in turn, has made it possible to begin structure/function studies using mutant proteins (390,391) as well as physicochemical analysis of wild-type enzyme (392). The combination of such functional analyses with additional studies of the biochemistry of the

DNA polymerase activity and of enzyme/inhibitor interactions (393–396) are likely to provide the basis for the discovery of more effective and specific inhibitors of reverse transcriptase.

In concluding this brief discussion, mention should also be made of the retrovirus-coded RNaseH and integrase activities whose function is essential for the synthesis and integration of double-stranded proviral DNA into the host genome. In HIV, the RNaseH function has been found to reside in a 15-kDa protein fragment that comprises the carboxy terminus of the 66-kDa reverse transcriptase polypeptide. Reverse transcriptase is found as a 66/51-kDa heterodimer in the virus particle, the result of cleavage of the 15-kDa peptide from one polypeptide during maturation (387,397–399). RNaseH activity is attributable principally to the heterodimer, which also contains DNA polymerase activity, although nonprocessive cleavage of RNA has also been detected in the isolated 15-kDa peptide (399). Effective inhibitors of this RNaseH activity have not been described to date, but it is reasonable to expect that such compounds will be revealed by additional studies. By analogy with other retroviruses, the HIV *pol* gene would be expected to code for an endonuclease, or integrase, activity in addition to protease (see above) and reverse transcriptase/RNaseH. Endonuclease is predicted to occur at the 3′ end of *pol*, and, consistent with this, 31- and 34-kDa proteins have been identified in extracts of virus-infected cells and expressed from cloned fragments of the HIV *pol* gene (400,401). By analogy with other retroviruses, the site of cleavage of circularized HIV DNA by endonuclease would be expected to be sequence specific and to map to the region corresponding to the junction between the long terminal repeats (402,403). Two strategies for the discovery of specific inhibitors of viral endonuclease are readily apparent. In the first case, inhibitors may be designed based on the sequence of bases surrounding the cleavage site; alternatively, inhibitors may be sought using isolated recombinant enzyme in a random screen that measures inhibition of the cleavage of a DNA substrate of an appropriate sequence. In either case, it can be expected that inhibitors of the viral endonuclease should be identified.

## RNA Synthesis

In this section, the opportunities for the inhibition of genomic RNA synthesis will be considered. The RNA viruses invariably code for a unique RNA polymerase. In the negative-strand RNA viruses, this enzyme is a structural protein found in the virion; the enzyme is a nonstructural protein that is synthesized as an early translation product of the positive-strand RNA viruses. The inhibition of viral RNA polymerases has been discussed already in the context of mRNA transcription (see above); compounds that act at this level would also affect genomic RNA synthesis. This section will, therefore, focus on the regulation of RNA synthesis. During the replication cycle, there is a switch from the synthesis of mRNA to genomic RNA. This regulation of the class of RNA synthesized is observed in both the positive- and negative-strand RNA viruses, and it seems plausible that this change is virus-controlled. If this is indeed the case, then there may be opportunities for intervention with a virus-specific inhibitor.

Many human pathogens are to be found among the positive-strand RNA viruses that include the picornaviruses, the togaviruses, and the coronaviruses. Although the overall strategy for replication may be similar among these viruses, there are also many differences in detail, many of which are still not well understood. In general terms, the incoming vRNA first acts as mRNA to direct the synthesis of viral proteins, including an RNA-dependent RNA polymerase. This virus-coded enzyme copies the genomic RNA to give template RNA of negative sense. This template is transcribed in turn to give positive sense RNA, which may function either as genomes for assembly into new virions or serve as additional messages. In the replication of the coronaviruses and togaviruses, the new messages may be less than full length as a result of initiation of transcription at an internal site in the negative strand. The precise nature of the controls that determine whether transcription is initiated at internal sites or at the 3′ end of the template remains to be determined. A role for virus-specific factors would suggest the opportunity for intervention with selective inhibitors.

An even more intriguing picture of events is emerging from studies of the picornavirus-infected cell, where all RNA synthesized *de novo* is full length and where there must, therefore, be discrimination between mRNA and positive-strand template/genomic RNA. It would seem that the positive sense RNA is partitioned between replication complexes, where it functions as a template for the synthesis of additional minus sense RNA, and the free form, in which it serves as mRNA. As viral protein synthesis increases, the amount of positive sense RNA committed to function as mRNA decreases, as does the production of negative strands in the replication complex, and positive-strand RNA is packaged into virions. It is of interest to us to know how these processes are regulated, inasmuch as a greater appreciation of the role of unique virus proteins in the regulation of RNA synthesis may suggest strategies for the discovery of selective RNA synthesis inhibitors. Part of the answer may lie in the observation that vRNA and RNA that is sequestered in the replication complexes are capped with the virus protein VPg, whereas mRNA is free of this structure (see above). If removal of this cap structure is mediated by a host enzyme, then one could speculate that modulation of this activity during the replication cycle could account for the relative abundance of mRNA. On the other hand, viral factors may also play an important role in directing RNA synthesis and determining the fate of positive strands. Additional studies of these unique processes may be very rewarding in helping to define molecular targets for inhibition.

There is also regulation of RNA synthesis in the negative-strand viruses. The case of influenza virus will be discussed here since it is the best understood, although our knowledge is still far from complete. Three classes of RNA are also recognized in the influenza virus-infected cell: full length, negative sense vRNA; full length, positive sense RNA that is complementary to vRNA (cRNA); and capped, prematurely terminated, polyadenylated mRNA (also of positive sense). Both cRNA and mRNA are transcribed from vRNA, but the relationships among these species is complex; the relative abundance of the various species of RNA and their fate appear to be highly regulated (128). The change from the synthesis of mRNA to cRNA requires virus protein synthesis (219), and it is interesting to note that the relative abundance of the virus proteins changes during the replication cycle such that, for example, the NP and nonstructural protein NS1 predominate early, whereas the M protein appears later. The manner in which the relative proportions of the various viral mRNAs, and hence the proportions of the corresponding proteins, is regulated has been discussed above. It would not be surprising if the balance between mRNA and cRNA synthesis and the fate of vRNA were also coordinately regulated by these same proteins.

Some recent observations have begun to shed light on the mechanism whereby a switch occurs from the synthesis of one class of RNA to another. First, studies of influenza virus RNA transcription in isolated nuclear extracts have suggested that the viral NP protein in particular may be important in overcoming the termination signal that must be suppressed for the synthesis of full-length cRNA (404). Second, it has been known for some time that the

5′ and 3′ ends of influenza virus RNAs are complementary in sequence and highly conserved. The complementarity of terminal sequences is found also in other negative-strand viruses, such as the arenaviruses and bunyaviruses, from which it may be inferred that this feature is of some importance. It has now been shown that vRNA isolated from influenza virions may adopt a circular conformation, the 5′ and 3′ termini of the genome forming a panhandle that is stabilized by the presence of virus protein (405). These panhandle stuctures are also found in the infected cell in high abundance at times when vRNA is transcribed to mRNA, but, less frequently, late in the infection when virus assembly occurs. One possible role of the panhandle may be to serve as a signal for termination of transcription at the polyadenylation site for mRNA (405); the destabilization of the structure may be necessary for the switch from mRNA synthesis to full-length cRNA synthesis to occur. Two alternative approaches to virus-specific inhibition are then possible: (a) increase the strength of the RNA-protein interaction so that the switch to cRNA synthesis is prevented, or (b) destabilize the panhandles and abort transcription prematurely.

## VIRUS ASSEMBLY

The events that immediately lead to the assembly and release of mature virus particles are probably the least well understood of all aspects of virus replication. Not surprisingly, there are few reports of compounds that selectively inhibit the events of assembly; some studies have suggested that amantadine may act at a late phase in the replication of the avian influenza viruses as well as at the early fusion/uncoating stage of the human influenza viruses (84), and the bichlorinated pyrimidines may inhibit the assembly of picornaviruses, vaccinia virus, and HSV (406).

For the purposes of this review, we can broadly divide the processes of assembly into two parts: (a) assembly of virus capsids and packaging of the viral genome; and (b) trafficking and membrane localization of envelope glycoproteins, and virus budding and release. Each of these will be considered in turn. Maturation of the retrovirus particle after release from the infected cell by a virion protease has been discussed earlier.

### Capsid Assembly and Genome Packaging

It is now generally accepted that the morphogenesis of virus particles is, for the most part, a self-regulated process. The assembly of viral capsids from basic subunits has been most easily followed among viruses that have icosahedral symmetry, e.g., the picornaviruses. A detailed description of the assembly of the several types of viral capsid is beyond the scope of this review. Although there are differences in detail for each virus structural type, the events seem to follow the same general pathway. The virus capsid is assembled from multiple subunits that are composed of repeating copies of a few proteins. Assembly of these units to form complete, albeit noninfectious, capsids can occur in the absence of genomic nucleic acid. It is not clear, however, whether the empty particle represents an intermediate in the pathway to full infectious capsid assembly, or is an artifact or by-product. Nor is it entirely clear how, and at what stage in the assembly process, the virus genome is packaged within the capsid. The role of host-derived "morphopoietic" factors has been implied by some studies but has not been substantiated.

We now have some insight into the mechanism whereby capsid proteins are transported to the site of assembly. Several studies have shown that the *N*-terminus of the picornavirus capsid precursor protein is covalently bound to myristic acid (407, and refs. therein). A similar situation is seen in the case of the gag polyprotein of the mammalian retroviruses. In the latter instance, myristylation appears to be essential for the transport of gag protein to the cell membrane and for the assembly of capsids (408). A similar function has been proposed for the myristylation of the picornavirus capsid protein, compatible with the observation that assembly of capsids occurs in close proximity to smooth membranes of the host cell.

Genomes are probably transported to the site of capsid assembly as part of a nucleoprotein complex, but the details of packaging process are poorly understood. One problem that is particularly intriguing relates to the viruses with segmented genomes. In influenza virus, for example, the infectious virion must contain at least one copy of each of the eight RNA species that make up the entire genome. It is not clear if this is achieved by the careful selection of only one copy of each RNA for encapsidation or if many RNAs are incorporated into the virion, such that the majority of particles will have at least one of each species present. A recent study has suggested that conformation of the RNA, which can adopt a panhandle structure, may itself serve as a signal for packaging (405). The mechanism whereby segments are sorted, however, remains unresolved.

Inhibitors of myristylation (either of the enzymes required for the addition of the myristic acid or of the factors that participate in the transport of myristylated viral proteins to their target membranes) may seem, at least superficially, to be a promising approach for the development of antiviral agents. However, the enzymes involved in myristylation, although not well understood, are likely to be cellular in origin. This inference is based in part on the observation that several membrane proteins of cellular origin are also myristylated. Furthermore, there is strong conservation of amino acid sequence of these viral and cellular proteins immediately downstream of the myristylation site (407, 409–411). It seems prudent to reserve judgment on the suitability of the processes of myristylation and the transport of such labeled proteins as targets for antiviral agents until a greater appreciation of these events is gained. Similarly, if the events of capsid assembly are to be targets for antiviral agents, then a more detailed understanding of the protein/protein and protein/nucleic acid interactions that drive the process will be required. Recombinant DNA techniques will probably provide new ways to examine the processes of assembly, whereas three-dimensional structural studies may yield the insights into contact and association domains of the proteins that will permit the design of antagonists.

### Glycoprotein Transport and Budding

The assembly of enveloped viruses occurs at cellular membranes in precise locations that are characteristic and distinctive for each particular class of virus. For example, the herpesviruses mature by budding at the inner nuclear membrane, whereas members of the coronavirus group assemble at the rough endoplasmic reticulum. Yet other viruses assemble at the plasma membrane where there is also order, such that within polarized cells, i.e., cells with distinct apical and basolateral domains, virus assembly occurs only at one of these surfaces. In this latter instance, retroviruses and rhabdoviruses, for example, mature from the basolateral domains, whereas the ortho- and paramyxoviruses mature at the apical surface (412,413).

It seems likely that the site of virus assembly and budding is coincident with and determined by the localization of the viral envelope glycoprotein (413,414). The mechanism by which the viral glycoproteins are targeted to specific membranes or domains is poorly understood but most probably is an extension of normal cellular processes (for a review, see ref. 415). Studies on the localization of the influenza virus HA suggest that the information required to specify the particular membrane domain to which the protein should be translocated is contained within the protein itself. Thus, in a mixed infection of polarized cells with influenza virus and VZV, which separately localize in the apical and basolateral domains, respectively, the polarities of glycoprotein transport and virus assembly was maintained, at least at early times postinfection (416). Others have used recombinant DNA techniques to study glycoprotein expression within the cell in the absence of other (homologous) virus proteins. Roth et al. (417) demonstrated that the characteristic apical expression of the influenza virus HA when expressed from an SV40 vector was maintained in the absence of other viral proteins. Further information on the signal sequences within the proteins that determine protein sorting may come from studies on the expression of mutant virus glycoproteins in which amino acid insertions or deletions are engineered (418–420). An alternative approach has been the expression of chimeric proteins that derive domains from more than one virus that differ in their membrane localization pattern (421,422).

The nature of the recognition sequence(s) is still not yet resolved, but what is emerging is the use of transport signals that are essentially cellular in nature. At present, therefore, there seem to be few, if any, opportunities for selective intervention. However, as in so many other areas of viral replication, virus-specific components may become apparent and strategies for the design of specific inhibitors may be revealed when the processes are better understood.

During the assembly of the enveloped viruses, the capsid proteins accumulate at the cell membrane immediately adjacent to the site of glycoprotein insertion. Recognition of the cytoplasmic tails of the membrane-bound viral glycoproteins by the capsid proteins, specifically by the matrix protein, may facilitate the association. The developing virus particle buds through the membrane, emerging on the other side generally as a mature virion. The mechanics of budding are poorly understood and are often dismissed as the reverse of the endocytotic process whereby the virus particle initially enters the cell. In the case of endocytosis, it was argued that inhibition of an event that was essentially cellular in origin would not be an attractive target for the development of antiviral agents. A similar argument may be put forward for "reverse endocytosis." It is clear, however, that much additional work is required to understand the events of virus budding before they can be considered or dismissed as points of intervention in the replicative cycle. It has been proposed that interferon may inhibit the budding of retroviruses from the infected cell. Additional studies of this effect may be particularly informative.

In influenza virus infection, there is one additional virus-specific function, the neuraminidase, that remains to be considered. Several roles have been proposed for this protein, which cleaves carbohydrate chains at the terminal sialic acid residue, including release of the newly budded virus particle from the infected cell. Much is known of the structure of the enzyme from x-ray and site-directed mutagenesis studies (423–426), and a competitive inhibitor of the enzyme with anti-influenza virus activity is known (427). Together these observations represent an important foundation on which to build a program of drug design and synthesis.

## CONCLUSIONS

This brief description of the molecular biology and biochemistry of virus replication has highlighted the existence of a wide variety of potential molecular targets for new selective antiviral agents. The view that virus-specific inhibitors are not achievable can now be seen to be unduly pessimistic and ill-founded. On the other hand, our attempts to date to bring safe and effective antiviral agents into clinical use must be viewed as merely scratching at the surface. For several of the potential targets that have been proposed, there remains a considerable void in our knowledge, and much work remains to be done before these opportunities can be fully exploited. Many of the advances in general pharmacology have been facilitated by the availability of active inhibitors and antagonists, and it seems likely that progress in the elucidation of the underlying molecular principles of virus replication will proceed hand-in-hand with the discovery of selective antiviral agents.

Although the emergence of HIV as a human pathogen is a tragedy in so many respects, the need to discover effective antiviral agents to combat AIDS has served as a stimulus for molecular virology and antiviral research that promises to have a therapeutic impact extending far beyond retrovirology or even virology in general. No attempt has been made here to consider the relative merits of the various molecular targets as the focus for novel chemotherapeutics, and the exploitation of several particular ones may be a goal beyond reach for some time to come. However, many novel approaches to antiviral therapy will undoubtedly be explored in the treatment of AIDS, and the most successful may be extended to other virus diseases. Although approaches of the past that have proved fruitful, such as nucleoside inhibitors of DNA and RNA polymerases, will continue to be the focus of attention, it is reasonable to expect that a number of the alternative targets discussed here will be the basis of effective novel second-generation antiviral agents.

## ACKNOWLEDGMENT

I gratefully acknowledge Dr. Michael Sherman for his thorough review of the manuscript and his many thoughtful suggestions for improvement. I thank my colleagues Dr. Karl Frank and Dr. Mary Graves for their helpful comments, Gerri Carter for secretarial support, and Nelson Gonzalez for his assistance in compiling the bibliography.

## REFERENCES

1. Dimmock NJ. Initial stages in infection with animal viruses. *J Gen Virol* 1982;59:1–22.
2. Mims CA. Virus receptors and cell tropisms. *J Infect* 1986;12:199–203.
3. McLaren LC, Holland JJ, Syverton JT. The mammalian cell-virus relationship. I attachment of poliovirus to cultivated cells of primate and non-primate origin. *J Exp Med* 1959;109:475–85.
4. Sattentau QJ, Weiss RA. The CD4 antigen: physiological ligand and HIV receptor. *Cell* 1988;52:631–3.
5. Jondal M, Klein G, Oldstone MBA, Bokish V, Yefenof E. Surface markers on human B and T lymphocytes. VIII. Association between complement and Epstein-Barr virus receptors on human lymphoid cells. *Scand J Immunol* 1976;5:401–10.
6. Klein G, Yefenof E, Falk K, Westman A. Relationship between Epstein-Barr virus (EBV)-production and the loss of the EBV receptor/complement receptor complex in a series of sublines derived from the same original Burkitt's lymphoma. *Int J Cancer* 1978;21:552–60.
7. Jøhnsson V, Wells A, Klein G. Receptors for the complement C3d component and the Epstein-Barr virus are quantitatively coexpressed on a series of B-cell lines and their derived somatic cell hybrids. *Cell Immunol* 1982;72:263–76.
8. Yefenof E, Klein G, Jondal M, Oldstone MBA. Surface markers on Human B- and T-lymphocytes. IX. Two-color immunofluorescence studies on the association between EBV receptors and complement receptors on the surface of lymphoid cell lines. *Int J Cancer* 1976;17:693–700.
9. Yefenof E, Klein G. Membrane receptor stripping confirms the association between EBV receptors and complement receptors on the surface of human B lymphoma lines. *Int J Cancer* 1977;20:347–52.
10. Yefenof E, Klein G, Kvarnung K. Relationships between complement activation, complement binding, and EBV absorption by human hematopoietic cell lines. *Cell Immunol* 1977;31:225–33.
11. Fingeroth JD, Weiss JJ, Tedder TF, Strominger JL, Bird PA, Fearon DT. Epstein-Barr virus receptor of human B lymphocytes is the C3d receptor CR2. *Proc Natl Acad Sci USA* 1984;81:4510–6.
12. Frade R, Barel M, Ehlin-Henriksson B, Klein G. gp-140, the C3d receptor of human B lymphocytes, is also the Epstein-Barr virus receptor. *Proc Natl Acad Sci USA* 1985;82:1490–3.

13. Wells A, Koide N, Klein G. Two large virion envelope glycoproteins mediate Epstein-Barr virus binding to receptor-positive cells. *J Virol* 1982;41:286–97.
14. Nemerow GR, Mold C, Schwend VK, Tollefson V, Cooper NR. Identification of gp350 as the viral glycoprotein mediating attachment of Epstein-Barr virus (EBV) to the EBV/C3d receptor of B cells: sequence homology of gp350 and C3 complement fragment C3d. *J Virol* 1987;61:1416–20.
15. Tanner J, Weiss JJ, Fearon D, Whang Y, Kieff E. Epstein-Barr virus gp350/220 binding to the B lymphocyte C3d receptor mediates adsorption, capping, and endocytosis. *Cell* 1987;50:203–13.
16. Thorley-Lawson DA, Geillinger K. Monoclonal antibodies against the major glycoprotein (gp350/220) of Epstein-Barr virus neutralize infectivity. *Proc Natl Acad Sci USA* 1980;77:5307–11.
17. Nemerow GR, Wolfert R, McNaughton ME, Cooper NR. Identification and characterization of the Epstein-Barr virus receptor on human B lymphocytes and its relationship to the C3d complement receptor (CR2). *J Virol* 1985;55:347–51.
18. Gottlieb MS, Schroff R, Schanker HM, et al. Pneumocystis carinii pneumonia and mucosal candidiasis in previously healthy homosexual men. Evidence of a new acquired cellular immunodeficiency. *New Engl J Med* 1981;305:1425–31.
19. Klatzmann D, Barre-Sinoussi F, Nugeyre MT, et al. Selective tropism of lymphadenopathy associated virus (LAV) for helper-inducer T lymphocytes. *Science* 1984;225:59–63.
20. Dalgleish AG, Beverley PCL, Clapham PR, Crawford DH, Greaves MF, Weiss RA. The CD4 (T4) antigen is an essential component of the receptor for the AIDS retrovirus. *Nature* 1984;312:763–7.
21. Klatzmann D, Champagne E, Chemeret S, et al. T-lymphocyte T4 molecule behaves as the receptor for human retrovirus LAV. *Nature* 1984;312:767–8.
22. Levy JA, Shimabukuro J, McHugh T, Casavant C, Stites D, Oshiro L. AIDS-associated retroviruses (ARV) can productively infect other cells besides human T helper cells. *Virology* 1985;147:441–8.
23. Nicholson JKA, Cross GD, Callaway CS, McDougal JS. *In vitro* infection of human monocytes with human T lymphotropic virus type III/lymphadenopathy-associated virus (HTLV-III/LAV). *J Immunol* 1986;137:323–9.
24. Cheng-Meyer C, Rutka JT, Rosenblum ML, McHugh T, Stites DP, Levy JA. Human immunodeficiency virus can productively infect cultured human glial cells.*Proc Natl Acad Sci USA* 1987;84:3526–30.
25. Adachi A, Koenig S, Gendelman HE, et al. Productive, persistent infection of human colorectal cell lines with human immunodeficiency virus. *J Virol* 1987;61:209–13.
26. Smith DH, Bryn RA, Marsters SA, Gregory T, Groopman JE, Capon DJ. Blocking of HIV-1 infectivity by a soluble, secreted form of the CD4 antigen. *Science* 1987;238:1704–7.
27. Deen KC, McDougal JS, Inacker R, et al. A soluble form of CD4 (T4) protein inhibits AIDS virus infection. *Nature* 1988;331:82–4.
28. Fisher RA, Bertonis JM, Meier W, et al. HIV infection is blocked *in vitro* by recombinant soluble CD4. *Nature* 1988;331:76–8.
29. Hussey RE, Richardson NE, Kowalski M, et al. A soluble CD4 protein selectively inhibits HIV replication and syncytium formation. *Nature* 1988;331:78–81.
30. Berger EA, Fuerst TR, Moss B. A soluble recombinant polypeptide comprising the amino-terminal half of the extracellular region of the CD4 molecule contains an active binding site for human immunodeficiency virus. *Proc Natl Acad Sci USA* 1988;85:2357–61.
31. Clayton LK, Hussey RE, Steinbrich R, Ramachandran H, Husain Y, Reinherz EL. Substitution of murine for human CD4 residues identifies amino acids critical for HIV-gp120 binding. *Nature* 1988;335:363–6.
32. Landau NR, Warton M, Littman DR. The envelope glycoprotein of the human immunodeficiency virus binds to the immunoglobulin-like domain of CD4. *Nature* 1988;334:159–62.
33. Mizukami T, Fuerst TR, Berger EA, Moss B. Binding region for human immunodeficiency virus (HIV) and epitopes for HIV-blocking monoclonal antibodies of the CD4 molecule defined by site-directed mutagenesis. *Proc Natl Acad Sci USA* 1988;85:9273–7.
34. Peterson A, Seed B. Genetic analysis of monoclonal antibody and HIV binding sites on the human lymphocyte antigen CD4. *Cell* 1988;54:65–72.
35. Richardson NE, Brown NR, Hussy RE, Vaid A, et al. Binding site for human immunodeficiency virus coat protein gp120 is located in the $NH_2$-terminal region of T4 (CD4) and requires the intact variable-region-like domain. *Proc Natl Acad Sci USA* 1988;85:6102–6.
36. Traunecker A, Luke W, Karjalainen K. Soluble CD4 molecules neutralize human immunodeficiency virus type 1. *Nature* 1988;331:84–6.
37. Jameson BA, Rao PE, Kong LI, et al. Location and chemical synthesis of a binding site for HIV-1 on the CD4 protein. *Science* 1988;240:1335–9.
38. Lifson JD, Hwang KM, Nara PL, et al. Synthetic CD4 peptide derivatives that inhibit HIV infection and cytopathicity. *Science* 1988;241:712–6.
39. Baba M, Pauwels R, Balzarini J, Arnout J, Desmyter J, De Clercq E. Mechanism of inhibitory effect of dextran sulfate and heparin on replication of human immunodeficiency virus *in vitro*. *Proc Natl Acad Sci USA* 1988;85:6132–6.
40. Mitsuya H, Looney DJ, Kuno S, Ueno R, Wong-Staal F, Broder S. Dextran sulfate suppression of viruses in the HIV family: inhi-

bition of virion binding of CD4[+] cells. *Science* 1988;240:646–9.
41. Wiley DC, Skehel JJ. The structure and function of the hemagglutinin membrane glycoprotein of influenza virus. *Ann Rev Biochem* 1987;56:365–94.
42. Kowalski M, Potz J, Basiripour L, et al. Functional regions of the envelope glycoprotein of human immunodeficiency virus type 1. *Science* 1987;237:1351–5.
43. Lasky LA, Nakamura G, Smith DH, et al. Delineation of a region of the human immunodeficiency virus type 1 gp120 glycoprotein critical for interaction with the CD4 receptor. *Cell* 1987;50:975–85.
44. Nygren A, Bergman T, Matthews T, Jörnvall H, Wigzell H. 95- and 25-kDa fragments of the human immunodeficiency virus envelope glycoprotein gp120 bind to the CD4 receptor. *Proc Natl Acad Sci USA* 1988;85:6543–6.
45. Wilson IA, Skehel JJ, Wiley DC. Structure of the haemagglutinin membrane glycoprotein of influenza virus at 3 Å resolution. *Nature* 1981;289:366–73.
46. Rogers GN, Paulson JC, Daniels RS, Skehel JJ, Wilson IA, Wiley DC. Single amino acid substitutions in influenza haemagglutinin change receptor binding specificity. *Nature* 1983;304:76–8.
47. Weis W, Brown JH, Cusack S, Paulson JC, Skehel JJ, Wiley DC. Structure of the influenza virus haemagglutinin complexed with its receptor, sialic acid. *Nature* 1988;333:426–31.
48. Suzuki Y, Nagao Y, Kato H, et al. Human influenza A virus hemagglutinin distinguishes sialyloligosaccharides in membrane-associated gangliosides as its receptor which mediates the adsorption and fusion processes of virus infection. *J Biol Chem* 1986;261:17057–61.
49. Abraham G, Colonno RJ. Many rhinovirus serotypes share the same cellular receptor. *J Virol* 1984;51:340–5.
50. Colonno RJ, Callahan PL, Long WJ. Isolation of a monoclonal antibody that blocks attachment of the major group of human rhinoviruses. *J Virol* 1986;57:7–12.
51. Rossmann MG, Arnold E, Erickson JW, et al. Structure of a human common cold virus and functional relationship to other picornaviruses. *Nature* 1985;317:145–53.
52. Colonno RJ, Condra JH, Mizutani S, Callahan PL, Davies M-E, Murcko MA. Evidence for the direct involvement of the rhinovirus canyon in receptor binding. *Proc Natl Acad Sci USA* 1988;85:5449–53.
53. Helenius A, Kartenbeck J, Simons K, Fries E. On the entry of Semliki Forest virus into BHK-21 cells. *J Cell Biol* 1980;84:404–20.
54. White J, Helenius A. pH-dependent fusion between the Semliki Forest virus membranes and liposomes. *Proc Natl Acad Sci USA* 1980;77:3273–7.
55. Marsh M, Bolzau E, Helenius A. Penetration of Semliki Forest virus from acidic prelysosomal vacuoles. *Cell* 1983;32:931–40.
56. Maeda T, Ohnishi S-I. Activation of influenza virus by acidic media causes hemolysis and fusion of erythrocytes. *FEBS Lett* 1980;122:283–7.
57. Matlin KS, Reggio H, Helenius A, Simons K. The infective entry of influenza virus into MDCK-cells. *J Cell Biol* 1981;91:601–13.
58. White J, Matlin K, Helenius A. Cell fusion by Semliki Forest, influenza, and vesicular stomatitis viruses. *J Cell Biol* 1981;89:674–9.
59. Yoshimura A, Ohnishi S-I. Uncoating of influenza virus in endosomes. *J Virol* 1984;51:497–504.
60. Matlin KS, Reggio H, Simons K, Helenius A. The pathway of vesicular stomatitis entry leading to infection. *J Mol Biol* 1982;156:609–31.
61. Stein BS, Gowda SD, Lifson JD, Penhallow RC, Bensch KG, Engleman EG. pH-independent HIV entry into CD4-positive T cells via virus envelope fusion to the plasma membrane. *Cell* 1987;49:659–68.
62. Maddon PJ, McDougal JS, Clapham PR, et al. HIV infection does not require endocytosis of its receptor, CD4. *Cell* 1988;54:865–74.
63. Bratt MA, Gallaher WR. Preliminary analysis of the requirements for fusion from within and fusion from without by Newcastle disease virus. *Proc Natl Acad Sci USA* 1969;64:536–43.
64. Howe C, Morgan C. Interactions between Sendai virus and human erythrocytes. *J Virol* 1969;3:70–81.
65. Fernie BF, Gerin JL. Immunochemical identification of viral and non-viral proteins of the respiratory syncytial virus virion. *Infect Immun* 1982;37:243–9.
66. Scheid A, Choppin PW. Identification of biological activities of paramyxovirus glycoproteins. Activation of cell fusion, hemolysis, and infectivity by proteolytic cleavage of an inactive precursor protein of Sendai virus. *Virology* 1974;57:475–90.
67. Lazarowitz SG, Choppin PW. Enhancement of the infectivity of influenza A and B viruses by proteolytic cleavage of the hemagglutinin polypeptide. *Virology* 1975;68:440–54.
68. Hsu M-C, Sheid A, Choppin PW. Activation of the Sendai virus fusion protein (F) involves a conformational change with exposure of a new hydrophobic region. *J Biol Chem* 1981;256:3557–63.
69. Hsu M-C, Scheid A, Choppin PW. Enhancement of membrane-fusing activity of Sendai virus by exposure of the virus to basic pH is correlated with a conformational change in the fusion protein. *Proc Natl Acad Sci USA* 1982;79:5862–6.
70. Skehel JJ, Bayley PM, Brown EB, et al. Changes in the conformation of influenza virus hemagglutinin at the pH optimum of virus-mediated membrane fusion. *Proc Natl Acad Sci* 1982;79:968–72.
71. Gething MJ, White JM, Waterfield MD. Purification of the fusion protein of Sendai virus: analysis of the $NH_2$-terminal sequence gener-

ated during precursor activation. *Proc Natl Acad Sci USA* 1978;75:2737–40.
72. Collins PL, Huang YT, Wertz GW. Nucleotide sequence of the gene encoding the fusion (F) glycoprotein of human respiratory syncytial virus. *Proc Natl Acad Sci USA* 1984;81:7683–7.
73. Wiley DC. Viral Membranes. In: Fields BN, Knipe DM, Chanock RM, Melnick JL, Roizman B, Shope RE, eds. *Virology*. New York: Raven Press, 1985:45–67.
74. Gallaher WR. Detection of a fusion peptide sequence in the transmembrane protein of human immunodeficiency virus. *Cell* 1987;50:327–8.
75. Gonzalez-Scarano F, Waxham MN, Ross AM, Hoxie JA. Sequence similarities between human immunodeficiency virus gp41 and paramyxovirus fusion proteins. *AIDS Res Hum Retroviruses* 1988;3:245–52.
76. Richardson, CD, Scheid A, Choppin PW. Specific inhibition of paramyxovirus and myxovirus replication by oligopeptides with amino acid sequences similar to those at the *N*-terminal of the $F_1$ or $HA_2$ viral polypeptides. *Virology* 1980;105:205–22.
77. Richardson CD, Choppin PW. Oligopeptides that specifically inhibit membrane fusion by paramyxoviruses: studies on the site of action. *Virology* 1983;131:518–32.
78. Miller FA, Dixon GJ, Arnett G, et al. Antiviral activity of carbobenzoxy di- and tripeptides on measles virus. *Appl Microbiol* 1968;16: 1489–96.
79. Miller DK, Lenard J. Antihistaminics, local anesthetics, and other amines as antiviral agents. *Proc Natl Acad Sci USA* 1981;78:3605–9.
80. Ohkuma S, Poole B. Fluorescence probe measurement of the intralysosomal pH in living cells and the perturbation of pH by various agents. *Proc Natl Acad Sci USA* 1978;75: 3327–31.
81. Maxfield FR, Willingham MC, Davis PJA, Pastan I. Amines inhibit the clustering of $\alpha_2$-macroglobulin and EGF on the fibroblast cell surface. *Nature* 1979;277:661–3.
82. Rothman JE, Fine RE. Coated vesicles transport newly synthesized membrane glycoproteins from endoplasmic reticulum to plasma membrane in two successive stages. *Proc Natl Acad Sci USA* 1980; 77:780–4.
83. Hay AJ, Wolstenholme AJ, Skehel JJ, Smith MH. The molecular basis of the specific anti-influenza action of amantadine. *EMBO J* 1985;4:3021–4.
84. Hay AJ, Zambon MC, Wolstenholme AJ, Skehel JJ, Smith MH. Molecular basis of resistance of influenza A viruses to amantadine. *J Antimicrob Chemother* 1986;18(suppl B):19–29.
85. Daniels RS, Downie JC, Hay AJ, et al. Fusion mutants of the influenza virus hemagglutinin glycoprotein. *Cell* 1985;40:431–9.
86. Belshe RB, Smith MH, Hall CB, Betts R, Hay AJ. Genetic basis of resistance to rimantadine emerging during treatment of influenza virus infection. *J Virol* 1988;62:1508–12.
87. Phillipson L, Lonberg-Holm K, Pettesson U. Virus-receptor interaction in an adenovirus system. *J Virol* 1968;2:1064–75.
88. Rosenwirth B, Eggers HJ. Early processes of echovirus 12-infection: elution, penetration, and uncoating under the influence of rhodanine. *Virology* 1979;97:241–55.
89. Bauer DJ, Selway JWT, Batchelor JF, Tisdale M, Caldwell IC, Young DAB, 4′,6-dichloroflavan (BW683C), a new anti-rhinovirus compound. *Nature* 1981;292:369–70.
90. Ishitsuka H, Ninomiya YT, Ohsawa C, Fujiu M, Suhara Y. Direct and specific inactivation of rhinovirus by chalcone Ro 09-0410. *Antimicrob Agents Chemother* 1982;22:617–21.
91. Andries K, Dewindt B, De Brabander M, Stokbroekx R, Janssen PAJ. In vitro activity of R-61837, a new antirhinovirus compound. *Arch Virol* 1988;101:155–67.
92. McSharry JJ, Caliguiri LA, Eggers HJ. Inhibition of uncoating of poliovirus by arildone, a new antiviral drug. *Virology* 1979;97:307–15.
93. Diana GD, Salvador UJ, Zaley ES, et al. Antiviral activity of some β-diketones. 2. Aryloxy alkyl diketones. *In vitro* activity against both RNA and DNA viruses. *J Med Chem* 1977;20:757–61.
94. Kim KS, Sapienza VJ, Carp RI. Antiviral activity of arildone on deoxyribonucleic acid and ribonucleic acid viruses. *Antimicrob Agents Chemother* 1980;18:276–80.
95. Caliguiri LA, McSharry JJ, Lawrence GW. Effect of arildone on modifications of poliovirus *in vitro*. *Virology* 1980;105:86–93.
96. Diana GD, McKinlay MA, Otto MJ, Akullian V, Oglesby C. [[(4,5-Dihydro-2-oxazolyl) phenoxy]alkyl]isoxazoles. Inhibitors of picornavirus uncoating. *J Med Chem* 1985;28: 1906–10.
97. Otto MJ, Fox MP, Fancher MJ, Kuhrt MF, Diana GD, McKinlay MA. *In vitro* activity of WIN 51711, a new broad-spectrum antipicornavirus drug. *Antimicrob Agents Chemother* 1985;27:883–6.
98. Fox MP, Otto MJ, McKinlay MA. Prevention of rhinovirus and poliovirus uncoating by WIN 51711, a new antiviral drug. *Antimicrob Agents Chemother* 1986;30:110–6.
99. Stanway G, Hughes PJ, Mountford RC, Minor PD, Almond JW. The complete nucleotide sequence of a common cold virus: human rhinovirus 14. *Nucleic Acids Res* 1984;12:7859–75.
100. Callahan PL, Mizutani S, Colonno RJ. Molecular cloning and complete sequence determination of RNA genome of human rhinovirus type 14. *Proc Natl Acad Sci USA* 1985;82: 732–6.
101. Sherry B, Rueckert R. Evidence for at least two dominant neutralization antigens on human rhinovirus 14. *J Virol* 1985;53:137–43.
102. Sherry B, Mosser AG, Colonno RJ, Rueckert RR. Use of monoclonal antibodies to identify four neutralization immunogens on a common cold picornavirus, human rhinovirus 14. *J Virol* 1986;57:246–57.
103. Smith TJ, Kremer MJ, Luo M, et al. The site

of attachment in human rhinovirus 14 for antiviral agents that inhibit uncoating. *Science* 1986;233:1286–93.

104. Badger J, Minor I, Kremer MJ, et al. Structural analysis of a series of antiviral agents complexed with human rhinovirus 14. *Proc Natl Acad Sci USA* 1988;85:3304–8.
105. Rossmann MG. Antiviral agents targeted to interact with viral capsid proteins and a possible application to human immunodeficiency virus. *Proc Natl Acad Sci USA* 1988;85:4625–7.
106. Andrews NC, Levin D, Baltimore D. Poliovirus replicase stimulation by terminal uridylyltransferase. *J Biol Chem* 1985;260:7628–35.
107. Andrews NC, Baltimore D. Purification of a terminal uridylyltransferase that acts as host factor in the *in vitro* poliovirus replicase reaction. *Proc Natl Acad Sci USA* 1986;83:221–5.
108. Fernandez-Munoz R, Darnell JE. Structural difference between the 5′ termini of viral and cellular mRNA in poliovirus-infected cells: possible basis for the inhibition of host protein synthesis. *J Virol* 1976;18:719–26.
109. Hewelt MJ, Rose JK, Baltimore D. 5′-Terminal structure of poliovirus polyribosomal RNA is pUp. *Proc Natl Acad Sci USA* 1976;73:327–30.
110. Ambros V, Baltimore D. Purification and properties of a HeLa cell enzyme able to remove the 5′-terminal protein from poliovirus RNA. *J Biol Chem* 1980;255:6739–44.
111. Takeda N, Kuhn RJ, Yang C-F, Takegami T, Wimmer E. Initiation of poliovirus plus-strand RNA synthesis in a membrane complex of infected HeLa cells. *J Virol* 1986;60:43–53.
112. Tamm I, Eggers HJ. Specific inhibition of replication of animal viruses. *Science* 1963;142:24–33.
113. Caliguiri LA, Tamm I. Action of guanidine on the replication of poliovirus RNA. *Virology* 1968;35:408–17.
114. Tershak DR. Inhibition of poliovirus polymerase by guanidine *in vitro*. *J Virol* 1982;41: 313–8.
115. Ishitsuka H, Ohsawa C, Ohiwa T, Umeda I, Suhara Y. Antipicornavirus flavone Ro 09-0179. *Antimicrob Agents Chemother* 1982;22:611–6.
116. Castrillo JL, Carrasco L. Action of 3-methylquercetin on poliovirus RNA replication. *J Virol* 1987;61:3319–21.
117. Braam J, Ulmanen I, Krug RM. Molecular model of a eucaryotic transcription complex: functions and movements of influenza P proteins during capped RNA-primed transcription. *Cell* 1983;34:609–18.
118. Lamb RA, Choppin PW. The gene structure and replication of influenza virus. *Ann Rev Biochem* 1983;52:467–506.
119. McCauley JW, Mahy BWJ. Structure and function of the influenza virus genome. *Biochem J* 1983;211:281–94.
120. Krug RM, Broni BA, Bouloy M. Are the 5′ ends of influenza viral mRNAs synthesised *in vivo* donated by host mRNAs? *Cell* 1979;18:329–34.
121. Caton AJ, Robertson JS. Structure of the host-derived sequences present at the 5′ ends of influenza virus mRNA. *Nucleic Acids Res* 1980;8:2591–603.
122. Ulmanen I, Broni BA, Krug RM. Role of two of the influenza virus core P proteins in recognizing cap 1 structures ($m^7$GpppNm) on RNAs and in initiating viral RNA transcription. *Proc Natl Acad Sci USA* 1981;78:7355–9.
123. Ulmanen I, Broni BA, Krug RM. Influenza virus temperature-sensitive cap ($m^7$GpppNm)-dependent endonuclease. *J Virol* 1983;45:27–35.
124. Blaas D, Patzelt E, Kuechler E. Cap-recognizing protein of influenza virus. *Virology* 1982;116:339–48.
125. Horisberger MA. Identification of a catalytic activity of the large basic P polypeptide of influenza virus. *Virology* 1982;120:279–86.
126. Bouloy M, Plotch SJ, Krug RM. Globin mRNAs are primers for the transcription of influenza viral RNA *in vitro*. *Biochemistry* 1978;75:4886–90.
127. Plotch SJ, Bouloy M, Krug RM. Transfer of 5′-terminal cap of globin mRNA to influenza viral complementary RNA during transcription *in vitro*. *Proc Natl Acad Sci USA* 1979;76: 1618–22.
128. Shapiro GI, Gurney Jr. T, Krug RM. Influenza virus gene expression: control mechanisms at early and late times of infection and nuclear-cytoplasmic transport of virus-specific RNAs. *J Virol* 1987;61:764–73.
129. Briedis DJ, Conti G, Munn EA, Mahy BWJ. Migration of influenza virus-specific polypeptides from cytoplasm to nucleus of infected cells. *Virology* 1981;111:154–64.
130. Young JF. Desselberger U, Palese P, Ferguson B, Shatzman AR, Rosenberg M. Efficient expression of influenza virus NS1 nonstructural proteins in *Escherichia coli*. *Proc Natl Acad Sci USA* 1983;80:6105–9.
131. Smith GL, Levin JZ, Palese P, Moss B. Synthesis and cellular location of the ten influenza polypeptides individually expressed by recombinant vaccinia viruses. *Virology* 1987;160: 336–45.
132. Krug RM, Broni BA, LaFiandra AJ, Morgan MA, Shatkin AJ. Priming and inhibitory activities of RNAs for the influenza viral transcriptase do not require base pairing with the virion template RNA. *Proc Natl Acad Sci USA* 1980;77:5874–8.
133. Smith JC, Raper RH, Bell LD, Stebbing N, McGeoch D. Inhibition of influenza virion transcriptases by polynucleotides. *Virology* 1980;103:245–9.
134. Potter CW, Teh CZ, Harvey L, Jennings R. The antiviral activity of amantadine and poly ($C,S^4U$) on influenza virus infection of infant rats. *J Antimicrob Chemother* 1981;7:575–84.
135. Round EM, Stebbing N. Antiviral effects of single-stranded polynucleotide inhibitors of the influenza virion-associated transcriptase against influenza virus infection of hamsters and ferrets. *Antiviral Res* 1981;1:237–48.

136. Stridh S, Öberg B, Chattopadhyaya J, Josephson S. Functional analysis of influenza RNA polymerase activity by the use of caps, oligonucleotides and polynucleotides. *Antiviral Res* 1981;1:97–105.
137. Stridh S, Helgstrand E, Lannero B, Misiorny A, Stening G, Öberg B. The effect of pyrophosphate analogues on influenza virus RNA polymerase and influenza virus multiplication. *Arch Virol* 1979;61:245–50.
138. Cload PA, Hutchinson DW. The inhibition of the RNA polymerase activity of influenza virus A by pyrophosphate analogues. *Nucleic Acids Res* 1983;11:5621–8.
139. Hutchinson DW, Naylor M, Cullis PM. Thioanalogues of inorganic pyrophosphate inhibit the replication of influenza virus A *in vitro*. *Antiviral Res* 1985;5:67–73.
140. Sidwell RW. Ribavirin: *in vitro* antiviral activity. In: Smith RA, Kirkpatrick W, eds. *Ribavirin. A broad spectrum antiviral agent*. New York: Academic Press, 1980:23–42.
141. Allen LB, Review of *in vivo* efficacy of ribavirin. In: Smith RA, Kirkpatrick W, eds. *Ribavirin. A broad spectrum antiviral agent*. New York: Academic Press, 1980:43–58.
142. Eriksson B, Helgstrand E, Johansson NG, et al. Inhibition of influenza virus ribonucleic acid polymerase by ribavirin triphosphate. *Antimicrob Agents Chemother* 1977;11:946–51.
143. Wray SK, Gilbert BE, Knight V. Effect of ribavirin triphosphate on primer generation and elongation during influenza virus transcription *in vitro*. *Antiviral Res* 1985;5:39–48.
144. Streeter DG, Witkowski JT, Khare GP, et al. Mechanism of action of 1-β-D-ribofuranosyl-1,2,4-triazole-3-carboxamide (Virazole), a new broad-spectrum antiviral agent. *Proc Natl Acad Sci USA* 1973;70:1174–8.
145. Smith RA. Mechanisms of action of ribavirin. In: Smith RA, Kirkpatrick W, eds. *Ribavirin. A broad spectrum antiviral agent*. New York: Academic Press, 1980:99–118.
146. Wray SK, Gilbert BE, Noall MW, Knight V. Mode of action of ribavirin: effect of nucleotide pool alterations on influenza virus ribonucleoprotein synthesis. *Antiviral Res* 1985;5:29–37.
147. Dickens LE, Collins PL, Wertz GW. Transcriptional mapping of human respiratory syncytial virus. *J Virol* 1984;52:364–9.
148. Richardson CD, Berkovich A, Rozenblatt S, Bellini WJ. Use of antibodies directed against synthetic peptides for identifying cDNA clones, establishing reading frames, and deducing the gene order of measles virus. *J Virol* 1985;54:186–93.
149. Sanchez A, Banerjee AK. Cloning and gene assignment of mRNAs of human parainfluenza virus 3. *Virology* 1985;147:177–86.
150. Collins PL, Dickens LE, Buckler-White A, et al. Nucleotide sequences for the gene junctions of human respiratory syncytial virus reveal distinctive features of intergenic structure and gene order. *Proc Natl Acad Sci USA* 1986;83:4594–8.
151. Dowling PC, Blumberg BM, Menonna J, et al. Transcriptional map of the measles virus genome. *J Gen Virol* 1986;67:1987–92.
152. Rima BK, Baczko K, Clarke DK, et al. Characterization of clones for the sixth (L) gene and a transcriptional map for morbilliviruses. *J Gen Virol* 1986;67:1971–8.
153. Spriggs MK, Collins PL. Human parainfluenza virus type 3: messenger RNAs, polypeptide coding assignments, intergenic sequences, and genetic map. *J Virol* 1986;59:646–54.
154. Blumberg BM, Crowley JC, Silverman JI, Menonna J, Cook SD, Dowling PC. Measles virus L protein evidences elements of ancestral RNA polymerase. *Virology* 1988;164:487–97.
155. De Clercq E, Montgomery JA. Broad-spectrum antiviral activity of the carbocyclic analog of 3-deazadenosine. *Antiviral Res* 1983;3:17–24.
156. De Clercq E, Bergstrom DE, Holy A, Montgomery JA. Broad-spectrum antiviral activity of adenosine analogues. *Antiviral Res* 1984;4:119–33.
157. Kawana F, Shigeta S, Hosoya M, Suzuki H, De Clercq E. Inhibitory effects of antiviral compounds on respiratory syncytial virus replication *in vitro*. *Antimicrob Agents Chemother* 1987;31:1225–30.
158. Chen ISY, Slamon DJ, Rosenblatt JD, Shah NP, Quan SG, Wachsman W. The x gene is essential for HTLV replication. *Science* 1985;229:54–8.
159. Felber BK, Paskalis H, Kleinman-Ewing C, Wong-Staal F, Pavlakis GM. The pX protein of HTLV-I is a transcriptional activator of its long terminal repeats. *Science* 1985;229:675–9.
160. Sodroski J, Rosen C, Wong-Staal F, et al. *Trans*-acting transcriptional regulation of human T-cell leukemia virus type III long terminal repeat. *Science* 1985;227:171–3.
161. Miller RH, Robinson WS. Common evolutionary origin of hepatitis B virus and retroviruses. *Proc Natl Acad Sci USA* 1986;83:2531–5.
162. Spandau DF, Lee C-H, *Trans*-activation of viral enhancers by the hepatitis B virus X protein. *J Virol* 1988;62:427–34.
163. Franza BR, Cullen BR, Wong-Staal F. *The control of human retrovirus gene expression*. New York: Cold Spring Harbor Laboratory, 1988.
164. Dayton AI, Sodroski JG, Rosen CA, Goh WC, Haseltine WA. The *trans*-activator gene of the human T cell lymphotropic virus Type III is required for replication. *Cell* 1986;44:941–7.
165. Fisher AG, Feinberg MG, Josephs SF, et al. The *trans*-activator gene of HTLV-III is essential for virus replication. *Nature* 1986;320: 367–71.
166. Feinberg MB, Jarrett RF, Aldovini A, Gallo RC, Wong-Staal F. HTLV-III expression and production involve complex regulation at the levels of splicing and translation of viral RNA. *Cell* 1986;46:807–17.
167. Rosen CA, Sodroski JG, Goh WC, Dayton AI, Lippke J, Haseltine WA. Post-transcriptional regulation accounts for the *trans*-activation of

the human T-lymphotropic virus type III. *Nature* 1986;319:555–9.
168. Cullen BR. *Trans*-activation of human immunodeficiency virus occurs via a bimodal mechanism. *Cell* 1986;46:973–82.
169. Peterlin BM, Luciw PA, Barr PJ, Walker MD. Elevated levels of mRNA can account for the trans-activation of human immunodeficiency virus. *Proc Natl Acad Sci USA* 1986;83: 9734–8.
170. Rosen CA, Sodroski JG, Haseltine WA. The location of *cis*-acting regulatory sequences in the human T cell lymphotropic virus type III (HTLV-III/LAV) long terminal repeat. *Cell* 1985;41:813–23.
171. Okamoto T, Wong-Staal F. Demonstration of virus-specific transcriptional activator(s) in cells infected with HTLV-III by an *in vitro* cell-free system. *Cell* 1986;47:29–35.
172. Muesing MA, Smith DH, Capon DJ. Regulation of mRNA accumulation by a human immunodeficiency virus *trans*-activator protein. *Cell* 1987;48:691–701.
173. Kao S-Y, Calman AF, Luciw PA, Peterlin BM. Anti-termination of transcription within the long terminal repeat of HIV-1 by *tat* gene product. *Nature* 1987;330:489–93.
174. Feng S, Holland EC. HIV-1 *tat trans*-activation requires the loop sequence within *tar*. *Nature* 1988;334:165–7.
175. Jeang K-T, Shank PR, Kumar A. Transcriptional activation of homologous viral long terminal repeats by the human immunodeficiency virus type 1 or the human T-cell leukemia virus type 1 tat proteins occurs in the absence of *de novo* protein synthesis. *Proc Natl Acad Sci USA* 1988;85:8291–5.
176. Seigel LJ, Ratner L, Josephs SF, et al. Trans-activation induced by human T-lymphotropic virus type III (HTLV III) maps to a viral sequence encoding 58 amino acids and lacks tissue specificity. *Virology* 1986;148:226–31.
177. Garcia JA, Harrich D, Pearson L, Mitsuyasu R, Gaynor RB. Functional domains required for tat-induced transcriptional activation of the HIV-1 long terminal repeat. *EMBO J* 1988;7:3143–7.
178. Sadaie MR, Rappaport J, Benter T, Josephs SF, Willis R, Wong-Staal F. Missense mutations in an infectious human immunodeficiency viral genome: functional mapping of *tat* and identification of the *rev* splice acceptor. *Proc Natl Acad Sci USA* 1988;85:9224–8.
179. Frankel AD, Bredt DS, Pabo CO. Tat protein from human immunodeficiency virus forms a metal-linked dimer. *Science* 1988;240:70–3.
180. Mosca JD, Bednarik DP, Raj NBK, et al. Herpes simplex virus type-1 can reactivate transcription of latent human immunodeficiency virus. *Nature* 1987;325:67–70.
181. Mosca JD, Bednarik DP, Raj NBK, et al. Activation of human immunodeficiency virus by herpesvirus infection: identification of a region within the long terminal repeat that responds to a trans-acting factor encoded by herpes simplex virus 1. *Proc Natl Acad Sci USA* 1987;84;7408–12.
182. Kenney S, Kamine J, Markovitz D, Fenrick R, Pagano J. An Epstein-Barr virus immediate-early gene product trans-activates gene expression from the human immunodeficiency virus long terminal repeat. *Proc Natl Acad Sci USA* 1988;85:1652–6.
183. Rice AP, Mathews MB. Trans-activation of the human immunodeficiency virus long terminal repeat sequences, expressed in an adenovirus vector, by the adenovirus E1A 13S protein. *Proc Natl Acad Sci USA* 1988;85:4200–4.
184. Seto E, Yen TSB, Peterlin BM, Ou J-H. Trans-activation of the human immunodeficiency virus long terminal repeat by the hepatitis B virus X protein. *Proc Natl Acad Sci USA* 1988;85:8286–90.
185. Franza Jr. BR, Josephs SF, Gilman MZ, Ryan W, Clarkson B. Characterization of cellular proteins recognizing the HIV enhancer using a microscale DNA-affinity precipitation assay. *Nature* 1987;330:391–5.
186. Nabel G, Baltimore D. An inducible transcription factor activates expression of human immunodeficiency virus in T cells. *Nature* 1987;326:711–3.
187. Tong-Starksen SE, Luciw PA, Peterlin BM. Human immunodeficiency virus long terminal repeat responds to T-cell activation signals. *Proc Natl Acad Sci USA* 1987;84:6845–9.
188. Everett RD, Dunlop M. *Trans* activation of plasmid-borne promoters by adenovirus and several herpes group viruses. *Nucleic Acids Res* 1984;12:5969–78.
189. Spaete RR, Mocarski ES. Regulation of cytomegalovirus gene expression: $\alpha$ and $\beta$ promoters are *trans* activated by viral functions in permissive human fibroblasts. *J Virol* 1985;56:135–43.
190. Stinski MF, Roehr TJ. Activation of the major immediate early gene of human cytomegalovirus by *cis*-acting elements in the promoter-regulatory sequence and by virus-specific *trans*-acting components. *J Virol* 1985;55:431–41.
191. Lieberman PM, O'Hare P, Hayward GS, Hayward SD. Promiscuous *trans* activation of gene expression by an Epstein-Barr virus-encoded early nuclear protein. *J Virol* 1986;60:140–8.
192. Honess RW, Roizman B. Regulation of herpesvirus macromolecular synthesis I. Cascade regulation of the synthesis of three groups of viral proteins. *J Virol* 1974;14:8–19.
193. Clements JB, Watson BR, Wilkie NM. Temporal regulation of herpes simplex virus type 1 transcription: location of transcripts on the viral genome. *Cell* 1977;12:275–85.
194. Jones PC, Roizman B. Regulation of herpesvirus macromolecular synthesis VIII. The transcription program consists of three phases during which both extent of transcription and accumulation of RNA in the cytoplasm are regulated. *J Virol* 1979;31:299–314.
195. Batterson W, Roizman B. Characterization of

the herpes simplex virion-associated factor responsible for the induction of α gènes. *J Virol* 1983;46:371–7.
196. Campbell MEM, Palfreyman JW, Preston CM. Identification of herpes simplex virus DNA sequences which encode a *trans*-acting polypeptide responsible for stimulation of immediate early transcription. *J Mol Biol* 1984;180:1–19.
197. McKnight JLC, Kristie TM, Roizman B. Binding of the virion protein mediating gène induction in herpes simplex virus 1-infected cells to its cis site requires cellular proteins. *Proc Natl Acad Sci USA* 1987;84:7061–5.
198. Gerster T, Roeder RG. A herpesvirus transactivating protein interacts with transcription factor OTF-1 and other cellular proteins. *Proc Natl Acad Sci USA* 1988;85:6347–51.
199. Preston CM, Frame MC, Campbell MEM. A complex formed between cell components and an HSV structural polypeptide binds to a viral immediate early gene regulatory DNA sequence. *Cell* 1988;52:425–34.
200. Watson RJ, Clements JB. Characterization of transcription-deficient temperature-sensitive mutants of herpes simplex virus type 1. *Virology* 1978;91:364–79.
201. Preston CM. Control of herpes simplex virus type 1 mRNA synthesis in cells infected with wild-type virus or the temperature-sensitive mutant *tsK*. *J Virol* 1979;29:275–84.
202. O'Hare P, Hayward GS. Evidence for a direct role for both the 175,000- and 110,000-molecular-weight immediate-early proteins of herpes simplex virus in the transactivation of delayed-early promoters. *J Virol* 1985;53:751–60.
203. O'Hare P, Hayward GS. Three *trans*-acting regulatory proteins of herpes simplex virus modulate immediate-early gene expression in a pathway involving positive and negative feedback regulation. *J Virol* 1985;56:723–33.
204. Beard P, Faber S, Wilcox KW, Pizer LI. Herpes simplex virus immediate early infected-cell polypeptide 4 binds to DNA and promotes transcription. *Proc Natl Acad Sci USA* 1986;83:4016–20.
205. Pizer LI, Tedder DG, Betz JL, Wilcox KW, Beard P. Regulation of transcription *in vitro* from herpes simplex virus genes. *J Virol* 1986;60:950–9.
206. Metzler DW, Wilcox KW. Isolation of herpes simplex virus regulatory protein ICP4 as a homodimeric complex. *J Virol* 1985;55:329–37.
207. Paterson T, Everett RD. Mutational dissection of the HSV-1 immediate-early protein Vmw175 involved in transcriptional transactivation and repression. *Virology* 1988;166:186–96.
208. Friedman AD, Triezenberg SJ, McKnight SL. Expression of a truncated viral *trans*-activator selectively impedes lytic infection by its cognate virus. *Nature* 1988;335:452–4.
209. Sim IS, McCullagh KG. Potential targets for selective inhibition. In: Harden MR, ed. *Approaches to antiviral agents*. Basingstoke: MacMillan Press Ltd. 1985:15–56.
210. Sodroski J, Goh WC, Rosen C, Dayton A, Terwilliger E, Haseltine W. A second post-transcriptional *trans*-activator gene required for HTLV-III replication. *Nature* 1986;321:412–7.
211. Sadaie MR, Benter T, Wong-Staal F. Site-directed mutagenesis of two trans-regulatory genes (*tat*-III, *trs*) of HIV-1. *Science* 1988;239:910–3.
212. Terwilliger E, Burghoff R, Sia R, Sodroski J, Haseltine W, Rosen C. The *art* gene product of human immunodeficiency virus is required for replication. *J Virol* 1988;62:655–8.
213. Rosen CA, Terwilliger E, Dayton A, Sodroski JG, Haseltine WA. Intragenic cis-acting *art* gene-responsive sequences of the human immunodeficiency virus. *Proc Natl Acad Sci USA* 1988;85:2071–5.
214. Knight DM, Flomerfelt FA, Ghrayeb J. Expression of the *art*/*trs* protein of HIV and study of its role in viral envelope synthesis. *Science* 1987;236:837–40.
215. Malim MH, Hauber J, Fenrick R, Cullen BR. Immunodeficiency virus *rev trans*-activator modulates the expression of the viral regulatory genes. *Nature* 1988;335:181–3.
216. Gutman D, Goldenberg CJ. Virus-specific splicing inhibitor in extracts from cells infected with HIV-1. *Science* 1988;241:1492–5.
217. Cullen BR, Hauber J, Campbell K, Sodroski JG, Haseltine WA, Rosen CA. Subcellular localization of the human immunodeficiency virus *trans*-acting *art* gene product. *J Virol* 1988;62:2498–501.
218. Smith GL, Hay AJ. Replication of the influenza virus genome. *Virology* 1982;118:96–108.
219. Hay AJ, Lomniczi B, Bellamy AR, Skehel JJ. Transcription of the influenza virus genome. *Virology* 1977;83:337–55.
220. Banerjee AK. 5′-Terminal cap structure in eukaryotic messenger ribonucleic acid. *Microbiol Rev* 1980;44:175–205.
221. Nomoto A, Lee YF, Wimmer E. The 5′ end of poliovirus mRNA is not capped with $m^7G(5')ppp(5')Np$. *Proc Natl Acad Sci USA* 1976;73:375–80.
222. Ensinger MJ, Martin SA, Paoletti E, Moss B. Modification of the 5′-terminus of mRNA by soluble guanylyl and methyl transferases from vaccinia virus. *Proc Natl Acad Sci USA* 1975;72:2525–9.
223. Shatkin AJ. Methylated messenger RNA synthesis in vitro by purified reovirus. *Proc Natl Acad Sci USA* 1974;71:3204–7.
224. Keller BT, Borchardt RT. Inhibition of 5-adenosylmethionine-dependent transmethylation as an approach to the development of antiviral agents. In: De Clercq E, Walker RT, eds. *Antiviral drug development. A multidisciplinary approach,* New York: Plenum Press, 1988: 123–38.
225. Zamecnik P, Stephenson M. Inhibition of Rous sarcoma virus replication and cell transformation by a specific oligodeoxynucleotide. *Proc Natl Acad Sci USA* 1978;75:280–4.
226. Stephenson M, Zamecnik P. Inhibition of Rous

sarcoma viral RNA translation by a specific oligodeoxynucleotide. *Proc Natl Acad Sci USA* 1978;75:285–8.
227. Stein CA, Cohen JS. Oligodeoxynucleotides as inhibitors of gene expression: a review. *Cancer Res* 1988;48:2659–68.
228. Zamecnik PC, Goodchild J, Taguchi Y, Sarin PS. Inhibition of replication and expression of human T-cell lymphotropic virus type III in cultured cells by exogenous synthetic oligonucleotides complementary to viral RNA. *Proc Natl Acad Sci USA* 1986;83:4143–6.
229. Agrawal S, Goodchild J, Civeira MP, Thornton AH, Sarin PS, Zamecnik PC. Oligodeoxynucleoside phosphoramidates and phosphorothioates as inhibitors of human immunodeficiency virus. *Proc Natl Acad Sci USA* 1988;85:7079–83.
230. Goodchild J, Agrawal S, Civeira MP, Sarin PS, Sun D, Zamecnik PC. Inhibition of human immunodeficiency virus replication by antisense oligodeoxynucleotides. *Proc Natl Acad Sci USA* 1988;85:5507–11.
231. Matsukura M, Shinozuka K, Zon G, et al. Phosphorothioate analogs of oligodeoxynucleotides: inhibitors of replication and cytopathic effects of human immunodeficiency virus. *Proc Natl Acad Sci USA* 1987;84:7706–10.
232. Sarin PS, Agrawal S, Civeira MP, Goodchild J, Ikeuchi T, Zamecnik PC. Inhibition of acquired immunodeficiency syndrome virus by oligodeoxynucleoside methylphosphonates. *Proc Natl Acad Sci USA* 1988;85:7448–51.
233. Zaia JA, Rossi JJ, Murakawa GJ, et al. Inhibition of human immunodeficiency virus by using an oligonucleoside methylphosphonate targeted to the *tat*-3 gene. *J Virol* 1988;62:3914–7.
234. Smith CC, Aurelian L, Reddy MP, Miller PS, Ts'o POP. Antiviral effect of an oligo(nucleoside methylphosphonate) complementary to the splice junction of herpes simplex virus type 1 immediate early pre-mRNAs 4 and 5. *Proc Natl Acad Sci USA* 1986;83: 2787–91.
235. Zerial A, Thuong NT, Hélène C. Selective inhibition of the cytopathic effect of type A influenza viruses by oligodeoxynucleotides covalently linked to an intercalating agent. *Nucleic Acids Res* 1987;15:9909–19.
236. Agris CH, Blake KR, Miller PS, Reddy MP, Ts'o POP. Inhibition of vesicular stomatitis virus protein synthesis and infection by sequence-specific oligodeoxyribonucleoside methylphosphonates. *Biochemistry* 1986;25: 6268–75.
237. Lemaitre M, Bayard B, Lebleu B. Specific antiviral activity of a poly(L-lysine)-conjugated oligodeoxyribonucleotide sequence complementary to vesicular stomatitis virus N protein mRNA initiation site. *Proc Natl Acad Sci USA* 1987;84:648–52.
238. Rock DL, Nesburn AB, Ghiasi H, et al. Detection of latency-related viral RNAs in trigeminal ganglia of rabbits latently infected with herpes simplex virus type 1. *J Virol* 1987;61:3820–6.
239. Spivack JG, Fraser NW. Detection of herpes simplex virus type 1 transcripts during latent infection in mice. *J Virol* 1987;61:3841–7.
240. Stevens JG, Wagner EK, Devi-Rao GB, Cook ML, Feldman LT. RNA complementary to a herpesvirus α gene mRNA is prominent in latently infected neurons. *Science* 1987; 235:1056–9.
241. Steiner I, Spivack JG, O'Boyle II DR, Lavi E, Fraser NW. Latent herpes simplex virus type 1 transcription in human trigeminal ganglia. *J Virol* 1988;62:3493–6.
242. Wechsler SL, Nesburn AB, Watson R, Slanina S, Ghiasi H. Fine mapping of the major latency-related RNA of herpes simplex virus type 1 in humans. *J Gen Virol* 1988;69:3101–6.
243. Lazarowitz SG, Compans RW, Choppin PW. Influenza virus structural and nonstructural proteins in infected cells and their plasma membranes. *Virology* 1971;46:830–43.
244. Klenk H-D, Rott R, Orlich M, Blödorn J. Activation of influenza A viruses by trypsin treatment. *Virology* 1975;68:426–39.
245. Scheid A, Choppin PW. Protease activation mutants of Sendai virus. Activation of biological properties by specific proteases. *Virology* 1976;69:265–77.
246. Scheid A, Choppin PW. Two disulfide-linked polypeptide chains constitute the active F protein of paramyxoviruses. *Virology* 1977;80: 54–66.
247. Lazarowitz SG, Compans RW, Choppin PW. Proteolytic cleavage of the hemagglutinin polypeptide of influenza virus. Function of the uncleaved polypeptide HA. *Virology* 1973; 52:199–212.
248. Garten W, Bosch FX, Linder D, Rott R, Klenk H-D. Proteolytic activation of the influenza virus hemagglutinin: the structure of the cleavage site and the enzymes involved in cleavage. *Virology* 1981;115:361–74.
249. Garten W, Klenk H-D. Characterization of the carboxypeptidase involved in the proteolytic cleavage of the influenza haemagglutinin. *J Gen Virol* 1983;64:2127–37.
250. Zhirnov OP, Ovcharenko AV, Bukrinskaya AG. Proteolytic activation of influenza WSN virus in cultured cells is performed by homologous plasma enzymes. *J Gen Virol* 1982;63:469–74.
251. Zhirnov OP, Ovcharenko AV, Bukrinskaya AG. Protective effect of protease inhibitors in influenza virus infected animals. *Arch Virol* 1982;73:263–72.
252. Dubovi EJ, Geratz JD, Tidwell RR. Inhibition of respiratory syncytial virus by bis(5-amidino-2-benzimidazolyl)methane. *Virology* 1980; 103:502–4.
253. Dubovi EJ, Geratz JD, Shaver SR, Tidwell RR. Inhibition of respiratory syncytial virus-host cell interactions by mono- and diamidines. *Antimicrob Agents Chemother* 1981;19:649–56.
254. Kräusslich H-G, Wimmer E. Viral proteinases. *Ann Rev Biochem* 1988;57:701–54.
255. Jacobson MF, Baltimore D. Polypeptide cleav-

ages in the formation of poliovirus proteins. *Proc Natl Acad Sci USA* 1968;61:77–84.
256. Toyoda H, Nicklin MJH, Murray MG, et al. A second virus-encoded proteinase involved in proteolytic processing of poliovirus polyprotein. *Cell* 1986;45:761–70.
257. König H, Rosenwirth B. Purification and partial characterization of poliovirus protease 2A by means of a functional assay. *J Virol* 1988;62:1243–50.
258. Nicklin MJH, Kräusslich HG, Toyoda H, Dunn JJ, Wimmer E. Poliovirus polypeptide precursors: expression *in vitro* and processing by exogenous 3C and 2A proteinases. *Proc Natl Acad Sci USA* 1987;84:4002–6.
259. Nicklin MJH, Toyoda H, Murray MG, Wimmer E. Proteolytic processing in the replication of polio and related viruses. *Biotechnology* 1986;4:33–42.
260. Duechler M, Skern T, Sommergruber W, et al. Evolutionary relationships within the human rhinovirus genus: comparison of serotypes 89, 2, and 14. *Proc Natl Acad Sci USA* 1987;84:2605–9.
261. Kowalski H, Maurer-Fogy I, Zorn M, Mischak H, Kuechler E, Blaas D. Cleavage site between VP1 and P2A of human rhinovirus is different in serotypes 2 and 14. *J Gen Virol* 1987;68:3197–200.
262. Argos P, Kamer G, Nicklin MJH, Wimmer E. Similarity in gene organization and homology between proteins of animal picornaviruses and a plant comovirus suggest common ancestry of these virus families. *Nucleic Acids Res* 1984;12:7251–67.
263. Werner G, Rosenwirth B, Bauer E, Seifert J-M, Werner F-J, Besemer J. Molecular cloning and sequence determination of the genomic regions encoding protease and genome-linked protein of three picornaviruses. *J Virol* 1986; 57:1084–93.
264. Kitamura N, Semler BL, Rothberg PG, et al. Primary structure, gene organization and polypeptide expression of poliovirus RNA. *Nature* 1981;291:547–53.
265. Semler BL, Anderson CW, Kitamura N, Rothberg PG, Wishart WL, Wimmer E. Poliovirus replication proteins: RNA sequence encoding P3-1b and the sites of proteolytic processing. *Proc Natl Acad Sci USA* 1981;78:3464–8.
266. Dickson C, Eisenman R, Fan H, Hunter E, Teich N. In: Weiss RA, Teich NM, Varmus HE, Coffin JM, eds. *Molecular biology of tumor viruses*. Cold Spring Harbor, New York: Cold Spring Harbor Laboratory, 1982:513.
267. Kramer RA, Schaber MD, Skalka AM, Ganguly K, Wong-Staal F, Reddy P. HTLV-III gag protein is processed in yeast cells by the virus pol-protease. *Science* 1986;231:1580–4.
268. Jacks T, Power MD, Masiarz FR, Luciw PA, Barr PJ, Varmus HE. Characterization of ribosomal frameshifting in HIV-1 *gag-pol* expression. *Nature* 1988;331:280–3.
269. Debouck C, Gorniak JG, Strickler JE, Meek TD, Metcalf BW, Rosenberg M. Human immunodeficiency virus protease expressed in *Escherichia coli* exhibits autoprocessing and specific maturation of the gag precursor. *Proc Natl Acad Sci USA* 1987;84:8903–6.
270. Graves MC, Lim JJ, Heimer EP, Kramer RA. An 11-kDa form of human immunodeficiency virus protease expressed in *Escherichia coli* is sufficient for enzymatic activity. *Proc Natl Acad Sci USA* 1988;85:2449–53.
271. Mous J, Heimer EP, Le Grice SFJ. Processing protease and reverse transcriptase from human immunodeficiency virus type 1 polyprotein in *Escherichia coli*. *J Virol* 1988;62:1433–6.
272. Kohl NE, Emini EA, Schleif WA, et al. Active human immunodeficiency virus protease is required for viral infectivity. *Proc Natl Acad Sci USA* 1988;85:4686–90.
273. Toh H, Ono M, Saigo K, Miyata T. Retroviral protease-like sequence in the yeast transposon Tyl. *Nature* 1985;315:691–2.
274. Pearl LH, Taylor WR. A structural model for the retroviral proteases. *Nature* 1987;329: 351–4.
275. Katoh I, Yasunaga T, Ikawa Y, Yosinaka Y. Inhibition of retroviral protease activity by an aspartyl proteinase inhibitor. *Nature* 1987; 329:654–6.
276. Le Grice SFJ, Mills J, Mous J. Active site mutagenesis of the AIDS virus protease and its alleviation by *trans* complementation. *EMBO J* 1988;7:2547–53.
277. Nutt RF, Brady SF, Darke PL, et al. Chemical synthesis and enzymatic activity of a 99-residue peptide with a sequence proposed for the human immunodeficiency virus protease. *Proc Natl Acad Sci USA* 1988;85:7129–33.
278. Seelmeier S, Schmidt H, Turk V, von der Helm K. Human immunodeficiency virus has an aspartic-type protease that can be inhibited by pepstatin A. *Proc Natl Acad Sci USA* 1988;85:6612–6.
279. Billich S, Knoop M-T, Hansen J, et al. Synthetic peptides as substrates and inhibitors of human immune deficiency virus-1 protease. *J Biol Chem* 1988;263:17905–8.
280. Darke PL, Nutt RF, Brady SF, et al. HIV-1 protease specificity of peptide cleavage is sufficient for processing of gag and pol polyproteins. *Biochem Biophys Res Commun* 1988;156:297–303.
281. Schneider J, Kent SBH. Enzymatic activity of a synthetic 99 residue protein corresponding to the putative HIV-1 protease. *Cell* 1988;54: 363–8.
282. Henderson LE, Copeland TD, Sowder RC, Schultz AM, Oroszlan S. Analysis of proteins and peptides purified from sucrose gradient banded HTLV-III. *UCLA Symp Mol Cell Biol* 1988;71:135–47.
283. Henderson LE, Benveniste RE, Sowder R, Copeland TD, Schultz AM, Oroszlan S. Molecular characterization of gag proteins from simian immunodeficiency virus ($SIV_{Mne}$). *J Virol* 1988;62:2587–95.
284. Fuhrmann U, Bause E, Ploegh H. Inhibitors of

oligosaccharide processing. *Biochem Biophys Acta* 1985;825:95–110.
285. Klenk H-D, Schwarz RT. Viral glycoprotein metabolism as a target for antiviral substances. *Antiviral Res* 1982;2:177–90.
286. Schwarz RT, Klenk H-D. Inhibition of glycosylation of the influenza virus hemagglutinin. *J Virol* 1974;14:1023–34.
287. Leavitt R, Schlessinger S, Kornfeld S. Impaired intracellular migration and altered solubility of nonglycosylated glycoproteins of vesicular stomatitis virus and Sindbis virus. *J Biol Chem* 1977;252:9018–23.
288. Schwarz RT, Rohrschneider JM, Schmidt MFG. Suppression of glycoprotein formation of Semliki Forest, influenza, and avian sarcoma virus by tunicamycin. *J Virol* 1976; 19:782–91.
289. Spivack JG, Prusoff WH, Tritton TR. A study of the antiviral mechanism of action of 2-deoxy-D-glucose: normally glycosylated proteins are not strictly required for herpes simplex virus attachment but increase viral penetration and infectivity. *Virology* 1982; 123:123–38.
290. Svennerholm B, Olofsson S, Lunden R, Vahlne A, Lycke E. Adsorption and penetration of enveloped herpes simplex virus particles modified by tunicamycin or 2-deoxy-D-glucose. *J Gen Virol* 1982;63:343–9.
291. Walker BD, Kowalski M, Goh WC, et al. Inhibition of human immunodeficiency virus syncytium formation and virus replication by castanospermine. *Proc Natl Acad Sci USA* 1987;84:8120–4.
292. Gruters RA, Neefjes JJ, Tersmette M, et al. Interference with HIV-induced syncytium formation and viral infectivity by inhibitors of trimming glucosidase. *Nature* 1987;330:74–7.
293. Hettkamp H, Legler G, Bause E. Purification by affinity chromatography of glucosidase I, an endoplasmic reticulum hydrolase involved in the processing of asparagine-linked oligosaccharides. *Eur J Biochem* 1984;142:85–90.
294. Karpas A, Fleet GWJ, Dwek RA, et al. Aminosugar derivatives as potential anti-human immunodeficiency virus agents. *Proc Natl Acad Sci USA* 1988;85:9229–33.
295. Joubert PH, Venter CP, Joubert HF, Hillebrand I. The effect of a 1-deoxynorijimycin derivative on post-prandial blood glucose and insulin levels in healthy black and white volunteers. *Eur J Clin Pharmacol* 1985;28:705–8.
296. Joubert PH, Bam WJ, Manyane N. Effect of an α-glucosidase inhibitor (BAY m 1099) on post-prandial blood glucose and insulin in type II diabetics. *Eur J Clin Pharmacol* 1986;30:253–5.
297. Schnack C, Roggla G, Luger A, Schernthaner G. Effects of the α-glucosidase inhibitor 1-deoxynorijimycin (BAY m 1099) on postprandial blood glucose, serum insulin and C-peptide levels in type II diabetic patients. *Eur J Clin Pharmacol* 1986;30:417–9.
298. Saul R, Ghidoni JJ, Molyneux RJ, Elbein AD. Castanospermine inhibits α-glucosidase activities and alters glycogen distribution in animals. *Proc Natl Acad Sci USA* 1985;82:93–7.
299. Spivack JG, Prusoff WH, Tritton TR. Dissociation of the inhibitory effects of 2-deoxy-D-glucose on vero cell growth and the replication of herpes simplex virus. *Antimicrob Agents Chemother* 1982;22:284–8.
300. Nichols EJ, Manger R, Hakomori S, Herscovics A, Rohrschneider LR. Transformation by the v-fms oncogene product: role of glycosylational processing and cell surface expression. *Mol Cell Biol* 1985;5:3467–75.
301. Olofsson S, Khanna B, Lycke E. Altered kinetic properties of sialyl and galactosyl transferases associated with herpes simplex virus infection of GMK and BHK cells. *J Gen Virol* 1980;47:1–9.
302. Fischl MA, Richman DD, Grieco MH, et al. The efficacy of azidothymidine (AZT) in the treatment of patients with AIDS and AIDS-related complex *New Engl J Med* 1987;317: 185–91.
303. Yarchoan R, Berg J, Brouwers P, et al. Response of human-immunodeficiency-virus-associated neurological disease to 3′-azido-3′-deoxythymidine. *Lancet* 1987;i:132–5.
304. Yarchoan R, Perno CF, Thomas RV, et al. Phase 1 studies of 2′,3′-dideoxycytidine in severe human immunodeficiency virus infection as a single agent and alternating with zidovudine (AZT). *Lancet* 1988;i:76–81.
305. Summers J, Mason WS. Replication of the genome of a hepatitis B-like virus by reverse transcription of an RNA intermediate. *Cell* 1982;29:403–15.
306. Miller RH, Marion PL, Robinson WS. Hepatitis B viral DNA-RNA hybrid molecules in particles from infected liver are converted to viral DNA molecules during an endogenous DNA polymerase reaction. *Virology* 1984;139:64–72.
307. Bevand MR, Laub O. Two proteins with reverse transcriptase activities associated with hepatitis B virus-like particles. *J Virol* 1988; 62:626–8.
308. De Clercq E. Synthetic pyrimidine nucleoside analogous. In: Harden MR, ed. *Approaches to antiviral agents*. Basingstoke: MacMillan Press Ltd., 1985:57–99.
309. Holy A. Synthetic purine nucleoside analogues. In: Harden MR, ed. *Approaches to antiviral agents*. Basingstoke: MacMillan Press Ltd., 1985:101–34.
310. De Clercq E. Molecular targets for selective antiviral chemotherapy. In: De Clercq E, Walker RT, eds. *Antiviral drug development, a multidisciplinary approach*. New York: Plenum Press, 1988:97–122.
311. Robins RK, Revankar GR. Design of nucleoside analogs as potential antiviral agents. In: De Clercq E, Walker RT, eds. *Antiviral drug development, a multidisciplinary approach*. New York: Plenum Press, 1988:11–36.
312. Schaeffer HJ, Beauchamp L, de Miranda P,

Elion GB, Bauer DJ, Collins P. 9-(2-Hydroxyethoxymethyl)guanine activity against viruses of the herpes group. *Nature* 1978;272:583–5.
313. Elion GB, Furman PA, Fyfe JA, de Miranda P, Beauchamp L, Schaeffer HJ. Selectivity of action of an antiherpetic agent, 9-(2-hydroxyethoxymethyl)guanine. *Proc Natl Acad Sci USA* 1977;74:5716–20.
314. Fyfe JA, Keller PM, Furman PA, Miller RL, Elion GB. Thymidine kinase from herpes simplex virus phosphorylates the new antiviral compound, 9-(2-hydroxyethoxymethyl) guanine. *J Biol Chem* 1978;253:8721–7.
315. Derse D, Cheng Y-C, Furman PA, St. Clair MH, Elion GB. Inhibition of purified human and herpes simplex virus-induced DNA polymerases by 9-(2-hydroxyethoxymethyl)guanine triphosphate. *J Biol Chem* 1981;256:11447–51.
316. Furman PA, St. Clair MH, Fyfe JA, Rideout JL, Keller PM, Elion GB. Inhibition of herpes simplex virus-induced DNA polymerase activity and viral DNA replication by 9-(2-hydroxyethoxymethyl)guanine and its triphosphate. *J Virol* 1979;32:72–7.
317. Colby BM, Shaw JE, Elion GB, Pagano JS. Effect of acyclovir [9-(2-hydroxyethoxymethyl)guanine] on Epstein-Barr virus DNA replication. *J Virol* 1980;34:560–8.
318. Datta AK, Colby BM, Shaw JE, Pagano JS. Acyclovir inhibition of Epstein-Barr virus replication. *Proc Natl Acad Sci USA* 1980;77:5163–6.
319. Biron KK, Elion GB. *In vitro* susceptibility of varicella-zoster virus to acyclovir. *Antimicrob Agents Chemother* 1980;18:443–7.
320. Littler E, Zeuthen J, McBride AA, et al. Identification of an Epstein-Barr virus-coded thymidine kinase. *EMBO J* 1986;5:1959–66.
321. Fyfe JA. Differential phosphorylation of (E)-5-(2-bromovinyl)-2′-deoxyuridine monophosphate by thymidylate kinases from herpes simplex viruses types 1 and 2 and varicella zoster virus. *Mol Pharmacol* 1982;21:432–7.
322. Ashton WT, Karkas JD, Field AK, Tolman RL. Activation by thymidine kinase and potent antiherpetic activity of 2′-nor-2′-deoxyguanosine (2′NDG). *Biochem Biophys Res Commun* 1982;108:1716–21.
323. Smith KO, Galloway KS, Kennell WL, Ogilvie KK, Radatus BK. A new nucleoside analog, 9-[[2-hydroxy-1-(hydroxymethyl)ethoxy]methy]-guanine, highly active *in vitro* against herpes simplex virus types 1 and 2. *Antimicrob Agents Chemother* 1982;22:55–61.
324. Cheng Y-C, Huang E-S, Lin J-C, et al. Unique spectrum of activity of 9-[(1,3-dihydroxy-2-propoxy)methyl]-guanine against herpesviruses *in vitro* and its mode of action against herpes simplex virus type 1. *Proc Natl Acad Sci USA* 1983;80:2767–70.
325. Smee DF, Boehme R, Chernow M, Binko BP, Matthews TR. Intracellular metabolism and enzymatic phosphorylation of 9-(1,3-dihydroxy-2-propoxymethyl)guanine and acyclovir in herpes simplex virus-infected and uninfected cells. *Biochem Pharmacol* 1985;34:1049–56.
326. Smee DF. Interaction of 9-(1,3-dihydroxy-2-propoxymethyl)guanine with cytosol and mitochondrial deoxyguanosine kinases: possible role in anti-cytomegalovirus activity. *Mol Cell Biochem* 1985;69:75–81.
327. Frank KB, Chiou J-F, Cheng Y-C. Interaction of herpes simplex virus-induced DNA polymerase with 9-(1,3-dihydroxy-2-propoxymethyl)-guanine triphosphate. *J Biol Chem* 1984;259:1566–69.
328. St. Clair MH, Miller WH, Miller RL, Lambe CU, Furman PA. Inhibition of cellular α DNA polymerase and herpes simplex virus-induced DNA polymerases by the triphosphate of BW759U. *Antimicrob Agents Chemother* 1984;25:191–4.
329. Mar E-C, Chiou J-F, Cheng Y-C, Huang E-S. Inhibition of cellular DNA polymerase α and human cytomegalovirus-induced DNA polymerase by the triphosphates of 9-(2-hydroxyethoxymethyl)guanine and 9-(1,3-dihydroxy-2-propoxymethyl)guanine. *J Virol* 1985;53:776–80.
330. Gibbs JS, Chiou HC, Bastow, KF, Cheng Y-C, Coen DM. Identification of amino acids in herpes simplex virus DNA polymerase involved in substrate and drug recognition. *Proc Natl Acad Sci USA* 1988;85:6672–6.
331. Reid R, Mar E-C, Huang E-S, Topal MD. Insertion and extension of acyclic, dideoxy, and ara nucleotides by herpesviridae, human α and human β polymerases. *J Biol Chem* 1988;263:3898–904.
332. Larsson A, Alenius S, Johansson N-G, Öberg B. Antiherpetic activity and mechanism of action of 9-(4-hydroxybutyl)guanine. *Antiviral Res* 1983;3:77–86.
333. Larsson A, Öberg B, Alenius S, et al. 9-(3,4-Dihydroxybutyl)guanine, a new inhibitor of herpesvirus multiplication. *Antimicrob Agents Chemother* 1983;23:664–70.
334. Tippie MA, Martin JC, Smee DF, Matthews TR, Verheyden JPH. Anti-herpes simplex virus activity of 9-[4-hydroxy-3-(hydroxymethyl)-1-butyl]guanine. *Nucleosides Nucleotides* 1984;3:525–35.
335. Larsson A, Stenberg K, Ericson A-C, et al. Mode of action, toxicity, pharmacokinetics, and efficacy of some new antiherpesvirus guanosine analogs related to buciclovir. *Antimicrob Agents Chemother* 1986;30:598–605.
336. Boyd MR, Bacon TH, Sutton D, Cole M. Antiherpesvirus activity of 9-(4-hydroxy-3-hydroxymethylbut-l-yl)guanine (BRL 39123) in cell culture. *Antimicrob Agents Chemother* 1987;31:1238–42.
337. Boryski J, Golankiewicz B, De Clercq E. Synthesis and antiviral activity of novel N-substituted derivatives of acyclovir. *J Med Chem* 1988;31:1351–5.
338. Abele G, Eriksson B, Harmenberg J, Wahren B. Inhibition of varicella-zoster virus-induced

DNA polymerase by a new guanosine analog, 9-[4-hydroxy-2-(hydroxymethyl)butyl]guanine triphosphate. *Antimicrob Agents Chemother* 1988;32:1137–42.
339. Larder BA, Darby G. Virus drug-resistance: mechanisms and consequences. *Antiviral Res* 1984;4:1–42.
340. Jamieson AT, Gentry GA, Subak-Sharpe JH. Induction of both thymidine and deoxycytidine kinase activity by herpes viruses. *J Gen Virol* 1974;24:465–80.
341. Chen MS, Prusoff WH. Association of thymidylate kinase activity with pyrimidine deoxyribonucleoside kinase induced by herpes simplex virus. *J Biol Chem* 1978;253:1325–7.
342. Jamieson AT, Hay J, Subak-Sharpe JH. Herpesvirus proteins: induction nucleoside phosphotransferase activity after herpes simplex virus infection. *J Virol* 1976;17:1056–9.
343. Nutter LM, Grill SP, Dutschman GE, Sharma RA, Bobek M, Cheng Y-C. Demonstration of viral thymidine kinase inhibitor and its effect on deoxynucleotide metabolism in cells infected with herpes simplex virus. *Antimicrob Agents Chemother* 1987;31:368–74.
344. Sim IS, Picton C, Cosstick R, Jones AS, Walker RT, Jaxa Chamiec A. Inhibition of the herpes simplex virus thymidine kinase by 5′-substituted thymidine analogues. Comparison of the types 1 and 2 enzymes. *Nucleosides Nucleotides* 1988;7:129–135.
345. Hoffmann PJ, Cheng Y-C. The deoxyribonuclease induced after infection of KB cells by herpes simplex virus type 1 and type 2. 1. Purification and characterization of the enzyme. *J Biol Chem* 1978;253:3557–62.
346. Clough W. Deoxyribonuclease activity found in Epstein-Barr virus producing lymphoblastoid cells. *Biochemistry* 1979;18:4517–21.
347. Ripalti A, Landini MP. Human cytomegalovirus-associated DNase and the specific immune response in different clinical conditions. *Biochem Pharmacol* 1988;37:1873–4.
348. Caradonna SJ, Cheng Y-C. Induction of uracil-DNA glycosylase and dUTP nucleotidohydrolase activity in herpes simplex virus-infected human cells. *J Biol Chem* 1981;256:9834–7.
349. Biswal N, Feldan, P, Levy CC. A DNA topoisomerase activity copurifies with the DNA polymerase induced by herpes simplex virus. *Biochem Biophys Acta* 1983;740:379–89.
350. Leary K, Francke B. The interaction of a topoisomerase-like enzyme from herpes simplex virus type 1-infected cells with non-viral circular DNA. *J Gen Virol* 1984;65:1341–50.
351. Muller MT, Bolles CS, Parris DS. Association of type 1 DNA topoisomerase with herpes simplex virus. *J Gen Virol* 1985;66:1565–74.
352. Henry BE, Glaser R, Hewetson J, O'Callaghan DJ. Expression of altered ribonucleotide reductase activity associated with the replication of the Epstein-Barr virus. *Virology* 1978;89: 262–71.
353. Huszar D, Bacchetti S. Partial purification and characterization of the ribonucleotide reductase induced by herpes simplex virus infection of mammalian cells. *J Virol* 1981;37:580–8.
354. Langelier Y, Buttin G. Characterization of ribonucleotide reductase induction in BHK-21/C13 syrian hamster cell line upon infection by herpes simplex virus (HSV). *J Gen Virol* 1981;57:21–31.
355. Dutia BM. Ribonucleotide reductase induced by herpes simplex virus has a virus-specified constituent. *J Gen Virol* 1983;64:513–21.
356. Gibson T, Stockwell P, Ginsburg M, Barrell B. Homology between two EBV early genes and HSV ribonucleotide reductase and 38K genes. *Nucleic Acids Res* 1984;12:5087–99.
357. Preston VG, Palfreyman JW, Dutia BM. Identification of a herpes simplex virus type 1 polypeptide which is a component of the virus-induced ribonucleotide reductase. *J Gen Virol* 1984;65:1457–66.
358. Davison AJ, Scott JE. The complete DNA sequence of Varicella-Zoster virus. *J Gen Virol* 1986;67:1759–816.
359. Spector T, Stonehuerner JG, Biron KK, Averett DR. Ribonucleotide reductase induced by varicella zoster virus. Characterization, and potentiation of acyclovir by its inhibition. *Biochem Pharmacol* 1987;36:4341–6.
360. Cohen EA, Charron J, Perret J, Langelier Y. Herpes simplex virus ribonucleotide reductase induced in infected BHK-21/C13 cells: biochemical evidence for the existence of two non-identical subunits, H1 and H2. *J Gen Virol* 1985;66:733–45.
361. Frame MC, Marsden HS, Dutia BM. The ribonucleotide reductase induced by herpes simplex virus type 1 involves minimally a complex of two polypeptides (136K and 38K). *J Gen Virol* 1985;66:1581–7.
362. Averett DR, Lubbers C, Elion GB, Spector T. Ribonucleotide reductase induced by herpes simplex type 1 virus. Characterization of a distinct enzyme. *J Biol Chem* 1983;258:9831–8.
363. Goldstein DJ, Weller SK. Herpes simplex type 1-induced ribonucleotide reductase activity is dispensable for virus growth and DNA synthesis: isolation and characterization of an ICP6 *lacZ* insertion mutant. *J Virol* 1988;62:196–205.
364. Goldstein DJ, Weller SK. Factor(s) present in herpes simplex virus type 1-infected cells can compensate for the loss of the large subunit of the viral ribonucleotide reductase: characterization of an ICP6 mutant. *Virology* 1988;166:41–51.
365. Spector T. Inhibition of ribonucleotide reductases encoded by herpes simplex viruses. *Pharmacol Ther* 1985;31:295–302.
366. Cohen EA, Gaudreau P, Brazeau P, Langelier Y. Specific inhibition of herpesvirus ribonucleotide reductase by a nonapeptide derived from the carboxy terminus of subunit 2. *Nature* 1986;321:441–3.
367. Dutia BM, Frame MC, Subak-Sharpe JH, Clark WN, Marsden HS. Specific inhibition of herpesvirus ribonucleotide reductase by synthetic peptides. *Nature* 1986;321:439–41.

368. Gaudreau P, Michaud J, Cohen EA, Langelier Y, Brazeau P. Structure-activity studies on synthetic peptides inhibiting herpes simplex virus ribonucleotide reductase. *J Biol Chem* 1987;262:12413–6.
369. Shipman Jr. C, Smith SH, Drach JC, Klayman DL. Antiviral activity of 2-acetylpyridine thiosemicarbazones against herpes simplex virus. *Antimicrob Agents Chemother* 1981;19:682–5.
370. Spector T, Averett DR, Nelson DJ, et al. Potentiation of antiherpetic activity of acyclovir by ribonucleotide reductase inhibition. *Proc Natl Acad Sci USA* 1985;82:4254–7.
371. Turk SR, Shipman Jr C, Drach JC. Selective inhibition of herpes simplex virus ribonucleoside diphosphate reductase by derivatives of 2-acetylpyridine thiosemicarbazone. *Biochem Pharmacol* 1986;35;1539–45.
372. Shipman Jr. C, Smith SH, Drach JC, Klayman DL. Thiosemicarbazones of 2-acetylpyridine, 2-acetylquinoline, 1-acetylisoquinoline, and related compounds as inhibitors of herpes simplex virus in vitro and in a cutaneous herpes guinea pig model. *Antiviral Res* 1986;6:197–222.
373. Mitsuya H, Weinhold KJ, Furman PA, et al. 3′-Azido-3′-deoxythymidine (BW A509U): an antiviral agent that inhibits the infectivity and cytopathic effect of human T-lymphotropic virus type III/lymphadenopathy-associated virus *in vitro*. *Proc Natl Acad Sci USA* 1985;82:7096–100.
374. Mitsuya H, Broder S. Inhibition of the *in vitro* infectivity and cytopathic effect of human T-lymphotropic virus type III/lymphadenopathy-associated virus (HTLV-III/LAV) by 2′,3′-dideoxy-nucleosides. *Proc Natl Acad Sci USA* 1986;83:1911–5.
375. Furman PA, Fyfe JA, St. Clair MH, et al. Phosphorylation of 3′-azido-3′-deoxythymidine and selective interaction of the 5′-triphosphate with human immunodeficiency virus reverse transcriptase. *Proc Natl Acad Sci USA* 1986;83:8333–7.
376. Chen MS, Oshana SC. Inhibition of HIV reverse transcriptase by 2′,3′-dideoxynucleoside triphosphates. *Biochem Pharmacol* 1987; 36:4361–2.
377. Mitsuya H, Jarrett RF, Matsukura M, et al. Long-term inhibition of human T-lymphotropic virus type III/lymphadenopathy-associated virus (human immunodeficiency virus) DNA synthesis and RNA expression in T cells protected by 2′,3′-dideoxynucleosides *in vitro*. *Proc Natl Acad Sci USA* 1987;84:2033–7.
378. Richman DD, Fischl MA, Greico MH, et al. The toxicity of azidothymidine (AZT) in the treatment of patients with AIDS and AIDS-related complex. *New Engl J Med* 1987;317: 192–7.
379. Starnes MC, Cheng Y-C. Cellular metabolism of 2′,3′- dideoxycytidine, a compound active against human immunodeficiency virus *in vitro*. *J Biol Chem* 1987;262:988–91.
380. Wu RS, Wolpert-DeFilippes MK, Quinn FR. Quantitative structure-activity correlations of rifamycins as inhibitors of viral RNA-directed DNA polymerase and mammalian α and β DNA polymerases. *J Med Chem* 1980;23: 256–61.
381. Pitha PM, Pitha J. Polynucleotide analogs as inhibitors of DNA and RNA polymerases. *Pharmacol Ther* 1978;2:247–60.
382. Wright GE, Brown NC. Inhibition of RNA-directed DNA polymerase from avian myeloblastosis virus by a 5-benzyl-6-aminouracil. *Biochem Biophys Res Commun* 1985;126: 109–16.
383. Oogose K, Hafuri Y, Takemori E, Nakata E, Inouye Y, Nakamura S. Mechanism of inhibition of reverse transcriptase by quinone antibiotics. *J Antibiot* (Tokyo) 1987;40:1778–81.
384. Anand R, Moore JL, Curran JW, Srinivasan A. Interaction between rifabutin and human immunodeficiency virus type 1: inhibition of replication, cytopathic effect, and reverse transcriptase *in vitro*. *Antimicrob Agents Chemother* 1988:32:684–8.
385. Tanese N, Sodroski J, Haseltine WA, Goff SP. Expression of reverse transcriptase activity of human T-lymphotropic virus type III (HTLV-III/LAV) in *Escherichia coli*. *J Virol* 1986; 59:743–5.
386. Farmerie WG, Loeb DD, Casavant NC, Hutchison III CA, Edgell MH, Swanstrom R. Expression and processing of the AIDS virus reverse transcriptase in *Escherichia coli*. *Science* 1987;236:305–8.
387. Hansen J, Schulze T, Moelling K. RNase H activity associated with bacterially expressed reverse transcriptase of human T-cell lymphotropic virus III/lymphadenopathy-associated virus. *J Biol Chem* 1987;262:12393–6.
388. Larder B, Purifoy D, Powell K, Darby G. AIDS virus reverse transcriptase defined by high level expression in *Escherichia coli*. *EMBO J* 1987;6:3133–7.
389. Le Grice SFJ, Beuck V, Mous J. Expression of biologically active human T-cell lymphotropic virus type III reverse transcriptase in *Bacillus subtilis*. *Gene* 1987;55:95–103.
390. Larder BA, Purifoy DJM, Powell KL, Darby G. Site-specific mutagenesis of AIDS virus reverse transcriptase. *Nature* 1987;327:716–7.
391. Hizi A, McGill C, Hughes SH. Expression of soluble, enzymatically active, human immunodeficiency virus reverse transcriptase in *Escherichia coli* and analysis of mutants. *Proc Natl Acad Sci USA* 1988;85:1218–22.
392. Lowe DM, Aitken A, Bradley C, et al. HIV-1 reverse transcriptase: crystallization and analysis of domain structure by limited proteolysis. *Biochemistry* 1988;27:8884–9.
393. Camerman A, Mastropaolo D, Camerman N. Azidothymidine: crystal structure and possible functional role of the azido group. *Proc Natl Acad Sci USA* 1987;84:8239–42.
394. Cheng Y-C, Dutschman GE, Bastow KF, Sarngadharan MG, Ting RYC. Human immunodeficiency virus reverse transcriptase. General

properties and its interactions with nucleoside triphosphate analogs. *J Biol Chem* 1987;262:2187–9.
395. St. Clair MH, Richards CA, Spector T, et al. 3′-Azido-3′-deoxythymidine triphosphate as an inhibitor and substrate of purified human immunodeficiency virus reverse transcriptase. *Antimicrob Agents Chemother* 1987;31:1972–7.
396. Majumdar C, Abbotts J, Broder S, Wilson SH. Studies on the mechanism of human immunodeficiency virus reverse transcriptase. Steady-state kinetics, processivity, and polynucleotide inhibition. *J Biol Chem* 1988;263:15657–65.
397. Veronese FDM, Copeland TD, DeVico AL, et al. Characterization of highly immunogenic p66/p51 as the reverse transcriptase of HTLV-III/LAV. *Science* 1986;231:1289–91.
398. Johnson MS, McClure MA, Feng D-F, Gray J, Doolittle RF. Computer analysis of retroviral *pol* genes: assignment of enzymatic functions to specific sequences and homologies with nonviral enzymes. *Proc Natl Acad Sci USA* 1986;83:7648–52.
399. Hansen J, Schulze T, Mellert W, Moelling K. Identification and characterization of HIV-specific RNase H by monoclonal antibody. *EMBO J* 1988;7:239–43.
400. Lightfoote MM, Coligan JE, Folks TM, Fauci AS, Martin MA, Venkatesan S. Structural characterization of reverse transcriptase and endonuclease polypeptides of the acquired immunodeficiency syndrome retrovirus. *J Virol* 1986;60:771–5.
401. Steimer KS, Higgins KW, Powers MA, et al. Recombinant polypeptide from the endonuclease region of the acquired immune deficiency syndrome retrovirus polymerase (*pol*) gene detects serum antibodies in most infected individuals. *J Virol* 1986;58:9–16.
402. Skalka AM, Duyk G, Longiaru M, DeHaseth P, Terry R, Leis J. Integrative recombination—a role for the retroviral reverse transcriptase. *Cold Spring Harbor Symp Quant Biol* 1984;49:651–9.
403. Grandgenett DP, Vora AC. Site-specific nicking at the avian retrovirus LTR circle junction by the viral pp32 DNA endonuclease. *Nucleic Acids Res* 1985;13:6205–21.
404. Beaton AR, Krug RM. Transcription antitermination during influenza viral template RNA synthesis requires the nucleocapsid protein and the absence of a 5′ capped end. *Proc Natl Acad Sci USA* 1986;83:6282–6.
405. Hsu M-T, Parvin JD, Gupta S, Krystal M, Palese P. Genomic RNAs of influenza viruses are held in a circular conformation in virions and in infected cells by a terminal panhandle. *Proc Natl Acad Sci USA* 1987;84:8140–4.
406. La Colla P, Marcialis MA, Flore O, Sau M, Garzia A, Loddo B. Specific inhibition of virus multiplication by bichlorinated pyrimidines. *Ann NY Acad Sci* 1977;284:294–304.
407. Chow M, Newman JFE, Filman D, Hogle JM, Rowlands DJ, Brown F. Myristylation of picornavirus capsid protein VP4 and its structural significance. *Nature* 1987;327:482–6.
408. Rein A, McClure MR, Rice NR, Luftig RB, Schultz AM. Myristylation site in $Pr65^{gag}$ is essential for virus particle formation by Moloney murine leukemia virus. *Proc Natl Acad Sci USA* 1986;83:7246–50.
409. Aitken A, Cohen P, Santikarn S, et al. Identification of the $NH_2$-terminal blocking group of calcineurin B as myristic acid. *FEBS Lett* 1982;150:314–8.
410. Carr SA, Biemann K, Shoji S, Parmelee DC, Titani K. *n*-Tetradecanoyl is the $NH_2$-terminal blocking group of the catalytic subunit of cyclic AMP-dependent protein kinase from bovine cardiac muscle. *Proc Natl Acad Sci USA* 1982;79:6128–31.
411. Ozols J, Carr SA, Strittmatter P. Identification of the $NH_2$-terminal blocking group of NADH-cytochrome $b_5$ reductase as myristic acid and the complete amino acid sequence of the membrane-binding domain. *J Biol Chem* 1984; 259:13349–54.
412. Rodriguez-Boulan E, Sabatini DD. Asymmetric budding of viruses in epithelial monolayers: a model system for study of epithelial polarity. *Proc Natl Acad Sci USA* 1987;75:5071–5.
413. Roth MG, Srinivas RV, Compans RW. Basolateral maturation of retroviruses in polarized epithelial cells. *J Virol* 1983;45:1065–73.
414. Rodriguez-Boulan E, Pendergast M. Polarized distribution of viral envelope proteins in the plasma membrane of infected epithelial cells. *Cell* 1980;20:45–54.
415. Garoff H. Using recombinant DNA techniques to study protein targeting in the eucaryotic cell. *Ann Rev Cell Biol* 1985;1:403–45.
416. Roth MG, Compans RW. Delayed appearance of pseudotypes between vesicular stomatitis virus and influenza virus during mixed infection of MDCK cells. *J Virol* 1981;40:848–60.
417. Roth MG, Compans RW, Giusti L, et al. Influenza virus hemagglutinin expression is polarized in cells infected with recombinant SV40 viruses carrying cloned hemagglutinin DNA. *Cell* 1983;33:435–43.
418. Doyle C, Roth MG, Sambrook J, Gething M-J. Mutations in the cytoplasmic domain of the influenza virus hemagglutinin affect different stages of intracellular transport. *J Cell Biol* 1985;100:704–14.
419. Doyle C, Sambrook J, Gething M-J. Analysis of progressive deletions of the transmembrane and cytoplasmic domains of influenza hemagglutinin. *J Cell Biol* 1986;103:1193–204.
420. Roth MG, Gundersen D, Patil N, Rodriguez-Boulan E. The large external domain is sufficient for the correct sorting of secreted or chimeric influenza virus hemagglutinins in polarized monkey kidney cells. *J Cell Biol* 1987;104:769–82.
421. McQueen NL, Nayak DP, Jones LV, Compans RW. Chimeric influenza virus hemagglutinin containing either the $NH_2$ terminus or the COOH terminus of G protein of vesicular stomatitis virus is defective in transport to the cell surface. *Proc Natl Acad Sci USA* 1984;81: 395–9.

422. Puddington L, Woodgett C, Rose JK. Replacement of the cytoplasmic domain alters sorting of a viral glycoprotein in polarized cells *Proc Natl Acad Sci USA* 1987;84:2756–60.
423. Colman PM, Varghese JN, Laver WG. Structure of the catalytic and antigenic sites in influenza virus neuraminidase. *Nature* 1983;303:41–4.
424. Varghese JN, Laver WG, Colman PM. Structure of the influenza virus glycoprotein antigen neuraminidase at 2.9 Å resolution. *Nature* 1983;303:35–40.
425. Lentz MR, Air GM. Loss of enzyme activity in a site-directed mutant of influenza neuraminidase compared to expressed wild-type protein. *Virology* 1986;148:74–83.
426. Lentz MR, Webster RG, Air GM. Site-directed mutation of the active site of influenza neuraminidase and implications for the catalytic mechanism. *Biochemistry* 1987;26:5351–8.
427. Palesse P, Schulman JL. Inhibition of influenza and parainfluenza virus replication in tissue culture by 2-deoxy-2,3-dehydro-*N*-trifluoroacetylneuraminic acid (FANA). *Virology* 1974;59:490–8.

*Antiviral Agents and Viral Diseases of Man, 3rd Edition*, edited by G. J. Galasso, R. J. Whitley, and T. C. Merigan, Raven Press, Ltd., New York © 1990.

# 2

# Pathogenesis of Viral Infections

Mostafa A. Nokta, *Richard C. Reichman, and Richard B. Pollard

*Division of Infectious Diseases, Department of Medicine, The University of Texas Medical Branch, Galveston, Texas 77550; and *Infectious Diseases Unit, University of Rochester, Rochester, New York 14642*



Viral infections of humans occur frequently and individuals undergo multiple infectious events, some simultaneously. In many cases, the infections are asymptomatic; however, they can lead to illnesses with a wide range of severity. Several factors affect the outcome of a particular infection. Among those are factors relating to the degree of virulence of the virus, the amount of virus or inoculum, and the route of transmission. The dose of virus and the route of entry are important determinants of the outcome of infection, as exemplified by rabies virus. Under the usual conditions prevailing in nature, rabies transmission to humans occur after skin puncture in bites. However, if the virus concentration is extremely high, as occurs in certain bat-infested caves or in certain laboratory situations, airborne transmission can occur (1–3). Direct inoculation of certain viruses, e.g., herpes simplex virus (HSV), intracerebrally into experimental animals can also cause fatal infections, whereas peripheral inoculation of higher doses do not (4). The condition of the host, age (4–9), immune status, genetic makeup (9–11), and life-style can be important in determining the outcome of the infection. Newborns are more susceptible to severe and disseminated HSV infections than are adults. On the other hand there are other viruses such as influenza, polio, Epstein-Barr (EBV), cytomegalovirus (CMV), and mumps, in which the severity of infection may increase with age. Life-style may also affect pathogenesis, as exemplified by groups with special risk behaviors, such as drug abusers and male homosexuals. These groups are more vulnerable to viral infections such as hepatitis B virus (HBV). CMV, HSV, EBV, and human immunodeficiency virus (HIV) the causative agent of acquired immunodeficiency syndrome (AIDS). The interactions of multiple infectious agents in a single individual may affect the pathogenesis, resulting in an accelerated course of infection (12,13). Other determinants that influence virus pathogenesis are nutritional status, exercise, and, possibly, emotional stress (14–16). Malnourished children are more susceptible to severe measles infections than are well-fed children (17). Exercise has been associated with severe polio infections among vigorous athletes.

The availability of vectors and common vehicles for transmission of viruses in the environment adds to the ease in which infections are spread. Viruses can be transmitted through water, food, air, and insects, not only from patients with clinical illness but also from unrecognized healthy carriers. The advancement of medical technology itself has not been without hazards in that novel methods of transmission have been introduced that did not exist before. Transmission of CMV and HIV from infected organs to transplant recipients (18–23) have been reported. Two corneal transplant recipients are known to have died of rabies, diagnosed by autopsy. Both happened to receive their grafts from the same donor, who died earlier of an unidentified illness (24). Creutzfeldt-Jakob disease following human dura mater grafting (25), as well as hepatitis B and HIV infection (developing into AIDS in some cases) following artificial insemination have also been described (26,27).

In the past 40 years, much progress has occurred in understanding the ecology and control of virally induced diseases, especially after the introduction of tissue culture techniques and methods of virus isolation, purification, and characterization (28,29). The major approach for prevention and control of viral infections has been by stimulation of the host's specific immune responses against particular viruses by vaccines. Killed virus vaccines have helped control polio, influenza, rabies viruses, and HBV, whereas live virus vaccines have been successfully employed against polio, smallpox, yellow fever, measles, mumps, and rubella. Killed virus antigens may trigger a protective response that can be transient or relatively prolonged. Live attenuated viruses, in contrast, establish true infections that are contained by host immune defense mechanisms. A summary of currently available vaccines is shown in Table 1. The limited infections induced with live virus vaccines provide a large antigenic load that results in durable protection.

Despite the success of vaccination, many

**TABLE 1.** *Immunoprophylaxis of virus infections*

| Virus | Vaccine | | Passive antibody | |
|---|---|---|---|---|
| | Attenuated | Inactivated | Normal globulin | Hyperimmune globulin |
| Polio | + | + | − | Not available |
| Influenza | Experimental | + | − | − |
| Mumps | + | Immunosuppressed or pregnant | − | + |
| Measles | + | Not recommened | + | − |
| RSV | Not recommended | − | − | − |
| Rabies | − | + | − | + |
| Yellow fever | + | − | − | − |
| Rubella | + | Experimental | − | Experimental |
| Smallpox (+ vaccinia)[a] | + | − | − | + |
| Adenovirus 4.7 | Experimental | + | − | − |
| HSV | Experimental | Experimental | − | − |
| VZV | Experimental | − | − | + |
| CMV | Experimental | − | − | Experimental |
| Hepatitis A | Experimental | − | + | − |
| Hepatitis B | − | + | − | + |

[a]Not recommended for routine use

viral diseases are not responsive to this approach. Among those, members of the picornaviruses (other than polio) have large antigenic variation, which makes vaccine development impossible at present because of the lack of common epitopes that produce cross-strain immunity. With others, e.g., members of the herpes virus group (HSV, CMV, EBV), the problems of latency, reactivation, teratogenesis, and oncogenicity create potential problems of live virus vaccines. In spite of great advancements in the isolation, purification, and cloning of viral antigens, the successful introduction of efficient and safe vaccines for many infections does not appear to be possible in the immediate future.

Another approach for the control of viral infections is the use of antiviral drugs. This is especially important in diseases with a high incidence of morbidity and mortality. In contrast to the major advancements in antibacterial chemotherapy, antiviral drug development is in an early phase, and many severe viral illnesses have no specific therapy available. In Chapter 1, potential target sites for antiviral therapy are discussed. In this chapter, much of the current information on the pathogenesis of viral infections and virus/host relationships will be described; understanding of these processes and interactions could help design and introduce effective antivirals and new therapeutic modalities.

## SPREAD

The infection itself, the spread of virus in the body, and the severity of the infection are influenced by the availability of receptors, the nature of the receptors, and the target organ. Viruses can bind to cells specifically through productive receptors (30), leading to infection. Nonspecific binding can also occur, especially among enveloped viruses. Any component of the cell surface, such as lipids, carbohydrates, or proteins, can serve as a receptor. Viruses can also bind to inanimate surfaces such as glass, nitrocellulose, and carbon, and this binding is potentiated by cations and inhibited by antisera. This type of nonspecific binding does not relate to the *in vivo* virus/host relationship.

Viruses can bind to cells, and, yet, a productive infection may not ensue. The virus may not be internalized, or is internalized and its replication is blocked at a later step. Specific binding is genetically determined by both the virus as well as the host, and certain virions have molecules that are complementary to their receptors on host cells.

Several good examples have been described that demonstrate viral tropism toward a particular receptor. Structural similarities between the mammalian β-adrenergic and reovirus type 3 receptors have been reported (31). The β-adrenergic receptors are immunoprecipitable by antireovirus antibodies, and exhibit identical molecular masses and isoelectric points with reovirus receptor obtained from murine thymoma cells. The reovirus receptor also binds the β-antagonist iodohydroxybenzylpindolol, and this binding can be blocked by the β-agonist isoproterenol.

The syndrome of AIDS is characterized by gradual depletion of CD4 positive cells (32). The HIV has been shown to have specific tropism to cells expressing CD4 molecules on their surface, and these molecules appear to be the receptor for HIV. Monoclonal antibodies against CD4 antigen have been shown to block infection of the cell, whereas other monoclonals against other activated T-4 cell markers failed to do so (33,34). The prevention of infection was documented by showing inhibition of reverse transcriptase activity.

Rabies virus, a pathogen of the central nervous system (CNS), apparently adapted itself to overcome natural blood and brain barriers by using the acetylcholine receptor at the neuromuscular junction as its receptor (35). The virus then spreads in a retrograde fashion, slowly to the brain.

EBV has also been reported to share the same receptor with the third component of complement (36,37). EBV is the causative agent of heterophile positive infectious mononucleosis and is highly associated with African Burkitt lymphoma, another lymphoproliferative disorder, as well as nasopharyngeal carcinoma.

The first step in the complex process of viral pathogenesis after entering the host is attachment and adsorption of the virus to the host cells. Viruses can infect and replicate at the site of entry to the body, then shed virus from that site. The infection may be localized, with systemic spread through the body never occurring, as it does with rhinoviruses, the causative agents of the common cold. In this case, the virus remains localized to the upper respiratory tract and causes disease at the site of implantation which, in this case, serve as the target organ. Rhinoviruses appear to be largely limited to the nasal mucosa because of their preference for replicating at temperatures (33–34°C) lower than those present in the lower respiratory tract. Other viruses that fall into the category of agents that replicate only at the site of entry include influenza viruses, affecting the respiratory tract, some of the alimentary tract infections (picorna viruses and rotaviruses), and skin infections (warts and molluscum contagiosum).

Viruses can spread locally by extracellular or intracellular spread. The extracellular spread occurs when the virus is shed into the extracellular fluid and subsequently infects adjacent cells. Intracellular spread occurs when infected cells fuse with neighboring cells, allowing the virus to escape host defenses. Most viruses spread extracellularly, but some spread both extracellularly and intracellularly, as with herpes viruses, paramyxoviruses, and poxviruses. Local spread can be facilitated by local lymphatics and by the presence of migratory cells such as lymphocytes and macrophages.

In disseminated virus infections, following replication at the site of implantation, the virus is shed into the local lymphatics and blood capillaries, causing a transient primary viremia (Table 2). The virus then reaches its target organ where it infects the tissues and causes local disease. At that point, the virus can also be shed into the circulation, causing a secondary viremia and further spread of the virus to other organs. Prime examples of viral infections with viremic spread are measles, smallpox, and poliomyelitis. Viremic dissemination may result from the spread of virus within circulating leukocytes and erythrocytes, or in a cell-free form in plasma. Some viruses have highly specific leukocyte carriers. EBV associates only with B-lymphocytes (38,39), whereas CMV prefers monocytes and granulocytes (40–42). Colorado tick fever virus prefers erythrocytes (43), whereas HBV and many enteroviruses circulate free in plasma. Viruses have also been isolated from blood platelets, although the significance of this relationship remains unproven.

The other major route of systemic spread is by nerves. This type of spread occurs with rabies virus, HSV, varicella zoster vi-

**TABLE 2.** *Modes of virus dissemination*

| Mode | Virus |
|---|---|
| Viremia | |
| Plasma | Togaviruses |
| | Picornaviruses (polio, Coxsackie) |
| | HBV |
| Leukocyte | CMV |
| | EBV |
| | VZV |
| | Measles |
| | HTLV |
| | HIV |
| | Dengue |
| | Adenovirus |
| | Rubella |
| Erythrocyte | Colorado tick fever |
| Nerve | Rabies |
| | HSV |
| | VZV |
| Direct spread | Influenza |
| | Parainfluenza |
| | RSV |

rus, and occasionally with poliomyelitis (5,44). With rabies, the virus replicates at the site of implantation, then spreads locally to gain access to the peripheral nerves, after which it spreads centripetally to the CNS, the site of disease. After reaching the CNS, the virus spreads centrifugally by peripheral nerves to the site of shedding, the salivary glands. Neuronal travel is also critical to the development of HSV and varicella-zoster virus latency and subsequent recurrences. In experimental animals, footpad inoculation of HSV is followed by axonal spread to sciatic spinal ganglia, spinal cord, and brain (45,46). Latent virus is maintained within spinal ganglia, and during reactivation, viral nucleic acid synthesis can first be observed in these areas. In humans, explant culture techniques also clearly indicate that latent HSV is maintained within trigeminal and sacral ganglia (8). How herpes simplex, on rare occasions, also spreads into the brain to cause a characteristic temporal-lobe encephalitis has not been clearly defined, although a direct route via olfactory nerves has been postulated (5).

## HOST RESISTANCE

### Natural Barriers

Viral infections, to become established, have first to overcome the existing natural barriers. The first obstacle is the intact skin, which is covered by a layer of dead keratinized cells that does not support viral replication. In order to produce infection through skin, viruses have to enter through breached areas or be inoculated by needle sticks or insect bites. Some specialized tissues lined with mucous membranes have ciliated epithelium that create a barrier against virus attachment and penetration. Other mucous linings also have nonspecific viral inhibitors (lipids, polysaccharides, proteins, lipoproteins, and glycoproteins) that provide further protection against viral attachment. Other primary barriers along certain mucous membranes include gastric acidity and gastrointestinal enzymes or bile that can disrupt lipoprotein envelopes. The endothelial cells that separate the blood from other tissues creates barriers to virus spread, e.g. the blood-brain barrier. Normally, these barriers are impermeable to viruses, unless the virus penetrates by replicating directly in endothelial cells.

### Immune Responses

#### *Nonspecific Immune Response*

##### *Macrophages*

Once initial implantation and infection occur, the next barrier a virus must overcome is the macrophage or other phagocytic cell. Many experimental studies indicate that the course of subsequent infection depends on the results of the initial virus-macrophage encounter (9,47,48). Adult mouse macrophages are able to ingest and destroy intraperitoneally inoculated HSV. This has been referred to as "intrinsic resistance" of macrophages (48,49). The mouse macrophages also produce interferons and possibly other soluble factors that limit local virus replication (4). Among those are tumor necrosis factor (TNF) and lymphotoxin. Recently, both lymphokines have been shown to exert antiviral activity (50). The TNF-induced antiviral activity has been demonstrated against encephalomyocarditis virus (EMC), HSV, and HIV (51). This activity was shown to be enhanced in the presence of interferon-$\gamma$. Peritoneal macrophages from infant mice are less able to take on the characteristics of activated cells and less able to contain and destroy ingested virus. As a result, herpesviruses replicate in neonatal macrophages, disseminate, and may cause fatal infections, whereas in adults, infection is localized to the peritoneum and is rapidly contained. Transfer of macrophages from adult to neonatal mice confers protection against HSV (4). In humans, a similar pattern of macrophage maturation may be important in age-dependent resistance to HSV and other agents (8). Macrophages serve as ubiquitous cells that phagocytize and destroy many viruses. Later, infected macrophages may also serve in the host response as effector cells. This will be discussed in a subsequent section.

### *Interferons*

Interferon was first described in 1957. At that time, it was characterized as a biological substance, produced by virus-infected cells, which inhibited viral replication (52). Although the existence of interferon was initially questioned, the observations of Isaacs and Lindenmann (52) were subsequently confirmed, and in the early 1970s sufficient quantities of crude interferon-α preparations were available to conduct clinical trials (53–55). In recent years, new technologies have led to the production of large quantities of purified interferons utilizing cell culture and recombinant DNA techniques. These developments have produced new insights into the biochemistry, molecular biology, and clinical application of these molecules.

*Classification and Biological Characteristics.* Interferons are generally designated as either "natural" or "recombinant DNA-derived." Natural interferons are produced by stimulation of certain types of cells, whereas recombinant DNA-derived preparations are produced by expression of interferon that which have been inserted into foreign cell systems, most commonly *Escherichia coli*. Interferons characteristically have the following properties (56): (a) they are specific for the phylogenetic family in which they are produced, (b) they inhibit replication of almost all known viruses, (c) they inhibit replication of some viruses more effectively than others, (d) they require ongoing cellular RNA and protein synthesis for action, (e) they repress genetic functions of infected cells, (f) they are prevented from acting by specific antibodies, (g) they induce a specific set of effector molecules, and (h) cellular activation by interferon preparations decays over hours or days after their removal.

There are three major classes of interferons, including (a) interferon-α (IFN-α), (b) interferon-β (IFN-β), and (c) interferon-γ (IFN-γ) (57,58). Many subtypes of the α class have been described, although only two subtypes of β (1 and 2) and one γ species have been identified. Interferon-α and -β genes cluster on chromosome 9. These two classes of interferons also share a cell surface receptor whose gene is located on chromosome 21 and have marked amino acid homologies. In contrast, the γ gene is located on chromosome 12; interferon-γ cell receptor is on chromosome 6, and this interferon shows no homology with the α and β classes (59,60). Assignment of interferons to the three major classes is based on their antigenic and molecular relatedness, as well as on the cell types that produce them and by the agents that induce their production. Alpha interferons are produced by B lymphocytes, null lymphocytes, and macrophages/dendritic cells after exposure to foreign eukaryotic, tumor, or virus-infected cells. Beta interferons are produced by epithelial cells and fibroblasts following exposure to viral and other foreign nucleic acids. Interferon-γ is produced by T lymphocytes and macrophages after exposure to foreign antigens to which the host has been previously exposed or by exposure to T cell mitogens (61).

*Alpha Interferons.* Alpha interferons constitute a family of structurally related molecules (62–64). Genetic sequences for at least 23 different IFN-α subtypes are encoded in human DNA, and at least 14 are expressed (65–70). Molecular weights range from 16,000 to 27,000 (71–75). Alpha interferons contain 165–166 amino acids and are rich in leucine and glutamic acid/glutamine residues. Amino acid sequences of interferon-α share approximately 70% homology (76,77), with notable conservation of cysteines at positions 1, 29, 98/99, and 138/139. These residues appear to be involved in the formation of disulfide bonds (78). Some species of interferon-α are glycosylated, although most are not (79).

Recombinant DNA-derived alpha interferons have been purified from *E. coli* extracts using a variety of procedures, including crystallization (80) and ion exchange and monoclonal antibody affinity chromatography (81,82). The most extensively studied and clinically evaluated alpha interferons are α-2a and α-2b. Each of these interferons consist of 165 amino acids, and they are identical with the exception of residue 23 (77,83).

*Beta Interferons.* Natural human interferon-β derived from diploid fibroblasts was the first interferon to be purified (84). Both of the two interferon-β subtypes that are encoded in the DNA of humans are expressed *in vivo* (85). These molecules are glycosylated and consist of 166 amino acids with a molecular weight of approximately 19,000. Recombinant DNA-derived interferon-β has a molecular weight and amino acid composition that is similar to natural interferon-β with the exception that the DNA-derived product has a cysteine at position 17 (86). Beta interferons share considerable amino acid homology with alpha interferons.

*Gamma Interferons.* Both natural and recombinant DNA-derived gamma interferons have been purified (87–90). Only one gene for interferon-γ has been identified in human DNA. In general, interferon-γ consists of 146 amino acids, but posttranslational processing may alter this number. Molecular weights ranging from 15,500 to 25,000 have been observed and appear to be due to differences in extent of glycosylation (88,91).

*Biological Properties.* Interferons exhibit a large number of biological properties that can be categorized in general as (a) antiviral, (b) antiproliferative, and (c) immunomodulatory. In addition, characteristic toxicities are observed when significant quantities of exogenous interferons are administered to animals or humans (see Chapter 7). Prior to the availability of highly purified interferon preparations, it was believed that many of these interferon-associated effects were caused by impurities in the crude preparations that were utilized in early *in vitro* and *in vivo* systems. However, most of these effects have subsequently been reproduced with highly purified preparations of both natural and recombinant DNA-derived interferons.

Different interferon preparations within a major class often have different biological properties. For example, although all fractions of one purified natural interferon-α preparation were found to contain both antiviral and antiproliferative activity (92), ratios of antiviral to antiproliferative activity varied from one fraction to another (92,93). Similar observations were made when purified recombinant interferons became available (94). These results suggest that antiviral and antiproliferative effects of interferons are mediated through different mechanisms. In addition to these and other observations of differential antiproliferative and antiviral effects (95–97), varying activities of different interferon preparations have also been demonstrated in assays of cytotoxicity and natural killer cell activity (98–100) and in induction of expression of some tumor cell antigens (101–104).

Another major effect of interferons is their modulation of antigens of the major histocompatibility complex (MHC) on cell surfaces. All interferons induce an increase in surface expression of class I MHC antigens, whereas class II antigens are stimulated predominantly by interferon-γ (105,106). Expression of receptors for the crystallizable fragment of immunoglobulin (Fc) may also be stimulated by interferon (107), and alterations in such surface antigens may represent an important mechanism by which interferon exerts its biological effects.

Interferon combinations may produce both synergistic and antagonistic antiviral and antiproliferative effects (108). In addition, different interferons may potentiate the activities of other cytokines on both proliferative and antiviral assays (109).

*Quantitation.* Assays of interferons present in cell culture supernatants or body fluids have generally been performed employing methods to quantitate biological activity. More recently, because of the availability of highly purified interferon preparations, interferons have been quantitated using immunologic techniques (110,111). Although more rapid and easier to perform than biological assays, immunologic techniques may detect interferons that have little biological activity. Measurement of biologically active interferons may be particularly important in determination of the presence of neutralizing antiinterferon antibodies (112,113).

The interferon bioassay consists of the following steps: (a) exposure of virus susceptible cells to serial dilutions of an interferon preparation for a prescribed period of time at a physiological temperature, (b) washing the cells to remove unbound interferon, (c) challenge of the cells with an appropriate dose of infectious virus, and (d) measurement of the amount of viral growth in interferon-treated cultures compared to simultaneously sham-challenged cultures (56). A variety of methods of bioassay are available including inhibition of virus-specific cytopathic effects in tissue culture, reduction of the number and size of foci of viral destruction (such as plaques), reduction in the yield of infectious virus, reduction in the yield of virus-associated enzymes, decreases in the ability of surviving cells to take up a vital dye, or inhibition of RNA synthesis (114). International Reference Preparations are utilized to standardize these bioassays. Recently, criteria have been established to standardize biological assays of neutralizing antibodies to interferon preparations (115).

*Mechanisms of Action.* Precise molecular mechanisms for the antiviral, antiproliferative, and immunomodulatory effects of interferon are not completely understood, and this is an area of active ongoing research. The mechanisms by which interferons exert their antiviral effects have been studied most thoroughly. The majority of these studies have focused on alpha and beta interferons.

For interferons to exert their antiviral effects, they must first bind to specific cell receptors. Cells that do not possess receptors are unresponsive to interferon (116–118). In addition, antisera directed against interferon receptors can be used to inhibit antiviral activity (119,120). Although binding of interferon to its receptors is necessary for cellular activation, it is not sufficient. Following interferon binding to cell receptors, a variety of polypeptides are produced (61). Production of these polypeptides is associated with inhibition of viral replication. Although virus attachment, penetration, and uncoating, are unaffected by interferon, synthesis of early virus-specific products of both DNA and RNA viruses is inhibited. Studies of both RNA and DNA viruses indicate that inhibition of translation and virion assembly appear to be the principal modes of the antiviral effects of interferons. Several enzyme systems that are induced by interferon have been shown to interfere with viral protein synthesis. These include (a) 2′, 5′, oligoadenylate synthetase, which catalyzes the synthesis of oligonucleotides, which activate endoribonucleases that produce cleavage of both viral and cellular RNA; (b) a protein kinase that phosphorylates elongation initiation factor (EIF) 2-α, which in turn appears to inhibit the binding of methionyl tRNA to ribosomes (this inhibition discriminates cellular from viral mRNA); (c) 2′, 5′ phosphodiesterase system that catalyzes tRNA degradation, thus further inhibiting protein synthesis; and (d) indoleamine 2, 3 dioxygenase, an enzyme that is known to degrade intracellular tryptophan. The first two of these systems appear to depend on activation by double-stranded RNA, which is not normally thought to be present in cells that are not infected by viruses.

Viral-induced interferon is usually produced at the same time the viral progeny is released, thus protecting neighboring cells against viral infection. The interferon response is the earliest appearing host defense, takes place within a few hours of infection, and is followed by the antibody response within the next few days.

Interferons may play a critical early role in the limitation of virus infection, either by inducing antiviral cellular proteins or by modulating host responses such as natural killer (NK) cytotoxicity.

There is evidence from both experimental animals and humans that when passively administered prophylactically or very early after infection, interferons can beneficially alter the course of infection (121, 122). Moreover, administering antiinterferon sera to animals during the course of certain infections can worsen the outcome (11,123). Experiments on the inherent resistance of certain inbred mouse strains also indicate critical differences in the sensitivity of host cells to the antiviral effects of interferon (124). Studies in rhesus monkeys suggest that passive interferon production may protect the animals against vaccinia challenge even when the virus is resistant to interferon *in vitro,* presumably by modifying host responses (125).

Interferons have potent and diverse immunomodulatory effects, which include activation of macrophages, augmentation of NK cytotoxicity, antibody-dependent cellular cytotoxicity, or T-cell cytotoxicity, and alterations of cell motility (121,126–128). Under certain circumstances, interferons can also inhibit primary and secondary antibody responses, diminish delayed hypersensitivity and proliferative responses of lymphocytes, depress leukocyte migration inhibition, and inhibit monocyte maturation.

These multiple influences are not necessarily contradictory but suggest the importance of defining laboratory conditions for individual experiments and the need for caution in interpreting interferon effects in a given model. Several factors influence whether immunoenhancement or suppression follows interferon administration, including timing of interferon exposure relative to antigen presentation, the dose of interferon, the type of interferon (129), and the genetic makeup of the host.

The interactions of interferons and NK cells have received considerable attention. Recent studies indicate that viruses such as HSV-1 and influenza can themselves induce NK cells to produce interferon, which, in turn, can augment NK cytotoxicity (130). Interferon may recruit pre-NK cells from inactive populations, as well as enhance the activity of already functional NK cells (131). Once again, however, caution is necessary in extrapolating the meaning of *in vitro* assays to protection *in vivo.* The clinical administration of interferons has not led to predictable augmentation of NK cell cytotoxicity in peripheral blood leukocytes of recipients (132).

The interferons are important in regulation of the immune response. Thus, they may be found in the sera from virally infected individuals. They have also been described in sera from patients with dysfunctions of immune regulation. Interferons have been noted in sera from patients with systemic lupus erythematosis, rheumatoid arthritis, Sjorgen's syndrome, vasculitis, Behçet's syndrome, and AIDS.

The interferons can modify the outcome of viral infections. They can reduce the severity of infection, thus assisting the specific host defenses in eliminating the organisms. They also have been noted to have some deleterious effects. For example, it has been shown that the interferon produced in response to lymphocytic choriomeningitis (LCM) virus in neonatal mice was responsible for the development of glomerulonephritis in those mice (133,134). Another example is the accentuation of arena virus infection in monkeys by interferon inducers (135). Other experiments have also suggested a possible role for interferon in the pathogenesis of acute bronchiolitis in infants, which is associated with respiratory syncytial virus. It is thought that the pathogenesis of the infection is not solely due to the viral agent, but that other immunologic mechanisms such as immunoglobulin E (IgE) and cell-mediated immune responses may also contribute. Interferon-γ can be detected in sera from 49% of infants with bronchiolitis (136,137), and this in turn may augment immunologic and inflammatory reactions in this condition. It is noteworthy to mention that interferon can also modify and enhance IgE-mediated histamine release.

### *NK Cells*

Another early host defense mechanism that may influence viral pathogenesis is mediated by NK cells. Natural cytotoxicity is mediated by many types of cells that express surface receptors for the Fc portion of IgG, which can be stained with monoclonal antibodies directed at specific surface markers. The cytotoxicity is inherent in that it does not require the prior exposure of the host to the particular virus.

NK cells have been described in a variety of species including humans (6,131,138,139) and may be important in limiting the early spread of viruses. Athymic nude mice, deficient in T-lymphocyte function, can still resist many viral infections, and this resistance can be overcome by antisera directed against NK cells. Interferon may augment NK cell activity both *in vitro* and *in vivo,* by increasing the pool of active cells that will kill infected target cells and by other mechanisms (131,140). NK cytotoxicity may or may not be virus-specific and appears to be mediated by bone-marrow-derived cells that, in humans, appear in blood as large granular lymphocytes (LGL) (141). This cell population constitutes 5–15% of human peripheral blood lymphocytes (PBLs). Certain observations suggest that these cells may be of T-lymphocyte lineage; e.g., they have low affinity receptors for erythrocytes, and they can respond to interleukin 2 (141). However, certain cell surface markers are also shared with monocyte macrophages (138), making their actual origins uncertain.

The overall importance of NK cytotoxicity in recovery from viral infections remains unclear. Cells infected by a variety of viruses are more sensitive to NK lysis than their uninfected counterparts (142). In mice, genetic resistance to certain viruses correlates well with NK activity (6). In certain other viral infections of mice, NK activity does not appear to play an important role in recovery (143). In humans, NK cells may also play a role in early antiviral defense mechanisms. Preliminary studies indicate that certain individuals with a propensity for infection, such as infants and patients with Chediak-Higashi syndrome, have defects in NK cytotoxic mechanisms (144). Activated NK cells have been noted in humans during acute viral infection including EBV, measles, mumps, and CMV. Moreover, recovery from certain infections, such as CMV in transplant recipients, may involve generation of NK cytotoxic responses (145).

All three types of interferon can enhance NK cell activity similarly. In the presence of virus, interferon production has been attributed solely to LGL without participation of any other cells. The interferon affects NK activity by increasing the number of LGL able to bind to the target cells, increasing the proportion of the cytotoxic cells within the LGL population attaching to target cells, by accelerating the kinetics of cell lysis, and by increasing the recycling ability of NK cells.

### *Complement*

The complement system is capable of mediating a number of biological activities. Its components consist of 20 different plasma proteins. Once triggered, they go into a cascade of an orderly and sequentially regulated series of interactions. There are two activation pathways, a classical unit and an alternative one. The classical pathway is triggered by IgM or IgG antibodies in complex with specific antigens, including viruses. But this pathway can also be activated in the absence of antibodies by a number of physically diverse chemicals, as well as viruses (146). The alternative pathway also is activated by viruses (147). Although this activation does not require antibodies, the presence of antibodies enhances the complement response. A number of viruses can directly activate the complement system in the absence of antibodies (148). Retroviruses, EBV, and Newcastle disease virus directly and efficiently trigger the classical pathway (149–151). Sindbis virus can activate either pathway (152).

Consequent to complement activation, the complement proteins are deposited on the viral surface or envelope. These proteins mask structures required for virus adsorption into susceptible cells, thus reducing virus infectivity. Neutralization in this manner, with complement components C3 and C4, has been observed with a number of viruses including influenza, HSV, EBV, infectious bronchitis, and vaccinia (148,153,154). Complement can also inactivate enveloped viruses by direct viral lysis. Although this occurs *in vitro,* virus lysis *in vivo* has not been demonstrated. Immune-mediated complement lysis will be discussed in another section.

### Specific Immune Responses

#### Humoral Immunity

Viral antigens induce a similar sequence of antibody responses, as do other antigens. Five classes of antibodies are immunologically and physicochemically recognized: IgG, IgM, IgA, IgE, and IgD. Only IgG, IgM, and IgA are involved in virus neutralization. Early after infection, IgM humoral antibody titers start to rise and often reach maximum titers within the first 4 weeks after initial exposure, then decrease to low or undetectable levels.

The fact that IgA is found in excessive amounts on the mucous membrane as compared to serum suggests local production by plasma cells underlying the epithelium. Thus, it may be reasonable to administer vaccines locally for viruses that may multiply at such localized areas, e.g., intranasal spray of influenza vaccine and the oral administration of the polio vaccine. Only IgG antibodies can transverse the placenta, thus conferring a short-term passive immunity for the newborn. IgA can assist in passive immunity since it can be secreted in the mother's milk. The presence of IgM antiviral antibody often indicates a recent or ongoing infection. Reactivated infections may or may not be associated with IgM antibody increases. Rises in IgG antibodies often parallel those of IgM antibodies, but persist for much longer periods, often for years. The most marked antibody responses are often seen following systemic infections with viremia. In virus infections that occur on mucous membranes, secretory IgA antibodies are also produced. These may prevent subsequent reinfection with the same virus, but diminish with time, e.g., influenza and polio.

Antibodies are made to a variety of virus-associated antigens, both internal and surface in location. Antibodies to surface glycoproteins appear particularly important determinants of virus immunity, as determined by passive transfer experiments in animals. The roles of specific antigens and specific antibodies in pathogenesis have recently become easier to dissect with the development of hybridoma monoclonal antibody technology (28,29).

Most antibody responses against virus antigens are thymus dependent, whereas some are thymus independent (155–157). Thus, hosts with T-cell deficiencies may make adequate antibodies to certain viral antigens and not to others. Patients with humoral antibody deficiencies, such as hypogammaglobulinemia, are unusually susceptible to certain viruses in which antibodies are particularly important in recovery, such as hepatitis and enteroviruses. Chronic enterovirus meningitis has been a problem in these individuals (158), whereas infections contained primarily by T-cell mechanisms, such as those caused by herpesviruses, pose little problem. A corollary of this is that virus infections involving cell lysis and spread through the extracellular environment are more likely to be affected by circulating antibody than are virus infections where the organisms are strongly cell-associated, e.g., HIV.

A distinction must also be made between recovery from infection and prevention of subsequent infection. Circulating antibody is often a relatively late response in the course of acute infection and may not have an important role in the recovery process against many viruses. However, relatively little antibody can often prevent infection from occurring or progressing. This is the rationale for prophylactic γ globulin use in the prevention or amelioration of a variety of infections including hepatitis, varicella, and rabies. Even in infections where humoral immunity probably has little role in recovery, such as varicella, prophylactic varicella-zoster immune globulin can be useful in high-risk patients (159,160).

How do antibodies protect? They may cover critical viral sites of attachment, may alter viral charge, or cause virus aggregation (Table 3). In addition, even after virus adsorption, subsequent penetration or uncoating can sometimes be inhibited (161). The complement system augments antibody in the humoral arm of the immune response. Antibody and complement together play an important role in neutralizing free virus, and both together are frequently more effective than either alone. Complement and antibody may also act together in several of the above mentioned mechanisms to inhibit virus, including coating the virus, preventing attachment to virus receptors, or facilitating aggregation of the virus particles (155,161,162). Opsonization of the particles by phagocytic cells bearing C3b receptors may also be facilitated by antibody and complement. In addition, complement, in the presence of antibody, may lyse certain viruses with lipid envelopes or lyse virus-infected cells. Virus-infected cells can activate the alternate complement pathway (163), and antibody to the virus can enhance the deposition of C3b on the cell surface (161,162), increasing lytic sites on cell membranes.

Most observations on antibody/complement interactions in viral infections have been made *in vitro*. However, there is also evidence that these mechanisms may be operative *in vivo*. Decomplementation of mice by cobra venom factor increases the severity of influenza and Sindbis virus encephalitis, and delays the clearance of rabies vi-

**TABLE 3.** *Role of antibody in host defenses against viruses*

| Factors | Mechanism of antiviral activity |
|---|---|
| Virus + antibody | Block attachment<br>Decrease penetration<br>Decrease uncoating on initiation of replication<br>Increase clearance |
| Virus + antibody − C | Damage to virus coat<br>Lysis of virus-infected cell<br>Enhance block in attachment and penetration<br>Enhance clearance |
| Virus-cell + antibody + lymphocyte | Cell cytotoxicity |
| Virus-cell + antibody + monocyte macrophage | Cell cytotoxicity |

rus (164–166). As yet, however, there is little compelling evidence that humans with various complement deficiencies have an increased susceptibility to virus infections.

### *T-Cell Mediated Immunity*

The most convincing evidence suggesting the importance of the thymus-dependent (T-cell) immune compartment in resistance to virus infection comes from experiments of nature. Children or adults with T-cell deficiencies have an extraordinary susceptibility to certain viruses, particularly those of the herpes group, vaccinia, and measles (167–170). Patients with iatrogenic T-cell deficiencies, such as transplant recipients, have similar enhanced susceptibilities, as do animals that are thymus-deficient or have suppressed T-cell function (167,171, 172). In contrast, neither animals nor humans with depressed T-cell function appear unusually susceptible to enteroviruses, influenza, hepatitis, or certain togaviruses.

Not only does ablation of T-cell function in experimental animals enhance susceptibility to certain viruses, restoration of immunity through adoptive transfer of T cells is possible. A number of studies have shown that in herpes or pox virus infections, transfer of sensitized T lymphocytes is far more effective in transferring resistance than transfer of antibody (173,174).

As early as 3–4 days following murine infections with Sindbis virus, ectromelia, or CMV, sensitized T cells are detectable within lymph nodes. The sensitized lymphocytes may act in a variety of ways (Table 4). On contact with antigen, T lymphocytes may produce a variety of lymphokines, including interferon-γ and various macrophage-activating factors. Interferon-γ may itself inhibit virus replication or augment various cytotoxic responses. Chemotactic lymphokines attract activated macrophages, which then also help in viral clearance. The importance of these factors in recovery is suggested by the observation that interferon's appearance in varicella zoster vesicular (VZV) fluid is the best correlate of recovery (175).

**TABLE 4.** *Role of T-lymphocytes in antiviral responses*

| |
|---|
| Lysis of virus-infected cells |
| Immunoregulatory function in antibody production |
| Production of interferon-γ |
| Production of lymphokines for chemotaxis and activation of macrophages |

Perhaps the most important role for T lymphocytes in viral infections is as cytotoxic effector cells. The protective effects of primed cytotoxic T-lymphocytes (CTL) have been well established by protective transfer experiments in mice (174). Humans also generate CTL *in vivo* and following induction of secondary responses *in vitro*. Both mouse and human CTL responses are closely linked to and restricted by the major histocompatibility loci, making cytotoxicity assays in humans difficult to perform. Nevertheless, human CTL responses have been reported in measles, influenza, CMV, EBV, and mumps virus infections, among others (176–182). In bone marrow and kidney transplant recipients infected with CMV, the appearance of CMV-specific CTLs has been correlated with a good outcome; patients unable to mount specific CTL responses fare poorly (144).

### *Antibody-Dependent Cellular Cytotoxicity*

Antibody-dependent cellular cytotoxicity (ADCC) combines both humoral and cellular mechanisms, though the immunologic specificity is conferred by specific antibodies (181). It is mediated by leukocytes that have receptors for the Fc portion of IgG, but do not themselves bear surface immunoglobulin. The cells may be comprised of several subpopulations, which are functionally described as K cells, despite the absence of a definable surface marker. Lysis of target cells occurs once effector K cells attach to the Fc portion of IgG bound to cell-surface antigens. Only small amounts of antibody are required in humans for ADCC, and the phenomenon is not histocompatibility leukocyte antigen (HLA) restricted. It may be particularly important in the control of viruses that mature at cell membranes or insert antigens onto cell surfaces. Interferon may also augment ADCC, and distinctions between ADCC and NK cytotoxicity often are difficult.

It is possible that NK cells play an early role in the attack against virus-infected cells. The CTLs are important in terminating acute infections, and ADCC is important in preventing significant reinfection.

#### *Macrophages as Effectors*

In addition to serving as initial barriers limiting early infection, mononuclear phagocytes in both blood and tissue may have other functions in antiviral responsiveness. They may process viral antigens to allow more effective immune responses and may themselves serve as effector cells. Macrophages are critical components of inflammatory responses. They respond to chemotactic stimuli generated at foci of infection and may become activated by interferons or other products of virus/lymphocyte interactions. They may, themselves, produce interferon or other biologically active antiviral substances such as lysosomal hydrolases and arginase (130,183,184) or may act as cytotoxic cells in ADCC. This form of macrophage resistance has been referred to as "extrinsic resistance," i.e., the ability to inhibit virus replication in other cells that are normally permissive, and contrasts with intrinsic resistance, mentioned earlier, wherein the macrophage itself is nonpermissive for virus replication (48,49). Different macrophage subtypes may be involved in intrinsic and extrinsic resistance (185). Both have been clearly shown to be important features of antiviral resistance in experimental animals, although studies of human macrophage have only recently been performed.

### Virus-Induced Lymphocyte Dysfunction

The methods by which viruses induce hyporesponsiveness have been studied in many systems (Table 5). CMV infection has been associated with alterations in the general immune response. During acute CMV mononucleosis, lymphocyte proliferation and interferon responses to certain mitogens and antigens are depressed (186,187). The ability to generate T-cell cytotoxic responses against allogeneic cells is also diminished (41). In convalescence, these responses return to normal. Other responses, e.g., granulocyte phagocytosis and chemotaxis, NK cytotoxicity, and antibody production, remain intact (188,189). Thus, the major CMV-induced defects appear to involve T-lymphocyte function, which may account for the increased susceptibility of certain CMV-infected populations to neoplasms and superinfections with fungi and protozoa (168,190–192). Attempts to further define the mechanisms involved in CMV-induced T-cell dysfunction have shown that infected monocytes may act as suppressor cells (40) and that significant alterations in T-lymphocyte subset populations occur (41,193,194). The number of T8+ ("suppressor-cytotoxic") cells is markedly increased in number, whereas the T4+ ("helper-inducer") cells are diminished. The degree of these alterations reflect the severity of infection and is mir-

**TABLE 5.** *Possible mechanisms of virus-induced hyporesponsiveness*

| |
|---|
| Induction of suppressor macrophages |
| Selective proliferation of suppressor lymphocytes |
| Selective destruction or inactivation of helper or effector lymphocytes |
| Induction of soluble suppressor factors from lymphocytes or macrophages |
| Induction of blocking or enhancing antibodies |

rored by the decrease in lymphocyte proliferative responses.

Infections with HIV are also associated with lymphocyte dysfunction. This virus is associated with AIDS (195,196) and has a special tropism for T lymphocytes that express CD4 molecules (32). The infection of the T4 cells with HIV apparently leads to cell death, with eventual selective depletion of the T helper inducer T-cell subpopulation (32) and inversion of the T4/T8 cell ratios (32,197). As a result, a progressive state of immune suppression develops in these patients.

A number of immune parameters have been described to be impaired in HIV-infected patients and have been attributed directly or indirectly to the lack of sufficient and/or functional T4 cells (198). There have been reports that T cells from AIDS patients do not respond normally to IL-2 (199) and had decreased IL-2 receptor (IL-2R) expression (200), defective IL-2 production (201–203), and impairment of interferon-γ production (204,205).

In other infections, the mechanisms of hyporesponsiveness may vary (206). For example, measles is associated with T-lymphocyte hyporesponsiveness, but no T-cell subset abnormalities (207). Infections with EBV are associated with circulating soluble suppressor factors (208), whereas such factors have not been observed in patients with CMV infections. Infection with LCM may interfere with T-cell maturation (209). Finally, lymphocytes may be made that are directed against uninfected target cells. This has been shown for murine retrovirus models, where infection of T lymphocytes can cause those cells to become cytolytic for autologous uninfected fibroblasts (210). Whether similar virus-infected autoaggressive T-lymphocyte responses occur in humans is unknown (211).

### Genetic Resistance

Susceptibility to virus infection can be influenced by the genetic makeup of the host. The genetic resistance to particular virus-induced diseases has been extensively studied in mice. To date, genes conferring specific virus resistance against particular diseases have been identified in three DNA virus and five RNA virus families (212–218). Resistance of mice to influenza A viruses, for example, is controlled by the *Mx* gene, which is an autosomal dominant allele. This gene has been identified in A2G mice. Virus titers were always 100-fold less in A2G tissue than in other mice lacking this gene. Immunosuppression of A2G mice does not enhance their ability to replicate virus or alter their resistance to diseases induced by influenza virus (214).

Another example is the resistance of Princeton Rockefeller Institute (PRI) mice to flavivirus-induced encephalitis. They carry an autosomal dominant allele that allows the virus to replicate in mouse tissue but with a titer of 10,000-fold less than normal; the spread of the infection is slower than normal and self-limited (212).

Other examples have also been described for murine leukemia viruses, measles, rabies, CMV, HSV, and polyoma (212–218).

The majority of these genes map distant from *H-2* loci and do not act through the host's immune defenses. They code for products that interact with a unique event characteristic for a particular virus. This interaction could occur at any step from virus adsorption through virus assembly and progeny release. Similar genes in humans probably exist, although they are difficult to identify.

## CONSEQUENCES OF VIRAL INFECTIONS

The sequence of events that follow a virus infection are variable, and several virus/host interactions can occur. These interactions can affect the host and/or the virus. For the host, as shown in Table 6, the infection may result into a subclinical, acute, or persistent infection, as well as oncogenic transformation and immune-mediated viral

**TABLE 6.** *Potential outcomes of infection for virus and host*

| |
|---|
| Host exposed but resistant; no infection |
| Acute infection with (a) virus elimination or (b) host death |
| Persistent latent infection with intermittent reactivation either (a) spontaneously or (b) during immunosuppression |
| Chronic persistent carrier state, either (a) asymptomatic or (b) with late-onset disease |
| Oncogenesis |
| Virus triggers later immunological disease |

diseases. For the virus, the infection may lead to immune selection and antigenic variation.

## Host

### *Subclinical and Acute Infections*

Once infection is established within cells, complex interactions between the viral parasite and the host will determine the outcome. As in any battle between invader and invaded, there may be three results: one or the other is destroyed, or there is some accommodation between the two. In the simplest form of infection, either the virus kills the patient or the host eliminates the virus (Table 4). Smallpox is an example of this interaction as, although the survivor may be left with scars of infection, no persistent or latent virus remains. It is largely because of this simple virus/host relationship that smallpox eradication programs have been so successful (183). Had there been reservoirs of latent human or latent animal variola virus infection, the results would have been far different.

In acute self-limited viral infections, as in smallpox, influenza, polio, and measles, the virus enters the body and spreads to the target organs, where it multiplies. After an incubation period that ranges from 2 days to months (hepatitis B), during which viral multiplication reaches a certain level, signs and symptoms of disease appear. During the incubation period, host defense mechanisms, specific and nonspecific, become mobilized to rid the host of the infection. The infection is usually eliminated 2–3 weeks following the onset of symptoms. The host is usually infectious, and virus can be isolated from various sites towards the end of the incubation period and for a few days after the onset of disease. Subclinical infections undergo a similar pattern of pathogenic events and contagiousness but without overt manifestations of clinical disease. Some viruses, such as measles and smallpox, always exclusively cause acute disease.

### *Persistent Infections*

In another form of virus/host interaction, virus persistence is established. In one form of persistence, the virus becomes latent with evidence of or lacking evidence of demonstrable intermittent reactivation. Persistent latent infections are infections with intermittent acute episodes of disease between which the virus is usually not demonstrable.

The prototype viruses for this type of relationship are the herpes group, although similar patterns may exist for adenoviruses and other agents. For each herpesvirus, one or more cell types may harbor latent virus genetic information. HSV and VZV appear to reside in neural ganglion cells (45,46,219), whereas EBV persists in B lymphocytes and possibly nasopharyngeal epithelium (38,39). CMV latent sites are not as well defined, but epithelial, lymphoid, fibroblastic, and reticuloendothelial cells of multiple organs are possible reservoirs.

How an individual virus establishes a latent infection within a cell remains unclear. Viral DNA can integrate within host DNA or exist in an extrachromosomal plasmid form. Viral expression may relate to many factors, both exogenous and endogenous. In certain models of herpesvirus' latency and activation, latent states correlate with heavily methylated viral DNA and reactivation is accompanied by demethylation of viral DNA (220). Whatever the molecular mechanisms underlying persistence, the sine qua non for its maintenance is inadequate expression of virus-associated antigens to allow host recognition and elimination. Viral antigen recognition may be prevented because the antigens are not produced, as in true latent infection, or because blocking factors, such as antibodies, inhibit an effective response. Antibodies, together with complement components, may redistribute viral antigens on cell membranes and promote shedding of these antigens, leaving the cell free of antigenic targets for immune destruction (221,222).

Occasionally, latent virus infections become activated only when there is a significant alteration in host immune responsiveness. Activation of herpes viruses, particularly CMV and HSV, is exceedingly common during T-lymphocyte depression, often with devastating consequences to the host (168). This is exemplified in immunocompromised patients after organ transplant, those with malignancies, and in AIDS (223–229).

Sometimes viral expression occurs after years of latency without any definable immunosuppression. Measles virus infection or vaccination with measles vaccine of young children may be followed by an inapparent CNS latency and then, later, reexpression, culminating in the development of subacute sclerosing *Pan* encephalitis (SSPE) (230). SSPE is a rare disease of childhood and adolescence. The mechanism of its pathogenesis remains unclear, although there is some evidence that it might be due to acute infection in early childhood in conjunction with the presence of passively transferred maternal antimeasles antibody. The antibodies are thought to protect infected cells against complement-mediated cell lysis and immune-lymphocyte–mediated cell killing, leading to virus persistence (230–235). Another example is herpes zoster following infection with VZV, which usually occurs during childhood, causing chicken pox. After the child recovers from the disease, the virus remains hidden and is not eliminated from the body. Reactivation of VZV leads to development of herpes zoster in adulthood. High levels of specific neutralizing antibody to the virus can be found in the patient's serum. Whether transient virus-specific immunosuppression occurs under these circumstances is unclear (236–238).

In a different form of persistent infection, chronic virus carrier states may become established. Chronic infections are those infections where the virus is always demonstrable and often shed; it follows an acute or subclinical infection, after which the host fails to eliminate the virus.

LCM virus infections of mice and HBV infections of humans are the best-studied examples. If certain strains of mice are infected with noncytopathogenic LCM virus while immunologically immature or immunosuppressed, chronic viremic carrier states may ensue (239). Although no effective immune response is induced, antibodies may be produced against certain virus-associated antigens (240). Infectious virus-antibody complexes circulate and may deposit in periarteriolar regions. Viremia occasionally persists for months, years, or even the life of the host. Often the host remains asymptomatic despite carrying, and often excreting, high titers of infectious virus. Sometimes disease ensues after long periods of viral presence, as a result of loss of this endosymbiotic relationship, due to a deposition of immune complexes, or by still other undefined mechanisms.

HBV chronic carrier states in humans are extremely common. Up to 15% of the population in certain countries are HBV carriers, often as a result of neonatal infection. As with the LCM carrier state in mice, most HBV carriers are asymptomatic; however, periarteritis syndromes may follow years of HBV carriage, by mechanisms that remain uncertain (241).

CMV is also secreted in urine of asymptomatic children, some of whom are in the convalescent phase, but most have no history of CMV illness. This is due to subclinical infection. Between 9.4% and 29% of children younger than 5 years old are CMV shedders, and 9.5–15% of children 5–15 years old are also culture-positive in the general population (242–249).

Vertical transmission of infectious virus can occur from carrier mothers to newborn offspring, and infections can be perpetuated from generation to generation, e.g., HBV. Sometimes, latent viruses can also be vertically transmitted, as in the case of retrovirus proviral DNA in several species. Such proviral DNA may or may not become activated in later life. Activation is occasionally associated with development of neoplasms or other diseases, and the activated viruses may, in turn, be oncogenic for other hosts of the same or differing species (250,251).

Another form of persistent infections are those with a long incubation period that is followed by a slowly progressive disease which is usually lethal. These are examples of slow infections. HIV (the causative agent of AIDS), visna virus of sheep, and feline immunodeficiency virus belong to this group. All of them cause a slow progressive fatal disease in their hosts. HIV after infection remains latent in an integrated provirus form in some cells and in other cells maintains a low level of expression. The time frame from infection to the onset of the disease is variable (up to at least 8 years). During this period, a gradual depletion of T cells take place. These cells carry the CD4 molecule, which is the high-affinity receptor for HIV. The rate of this depletion determines the length of the incubation period and the severity of disease (32,198).

One of the most interesting and least understood host/parasite interactions occurs with the so-called slow viruses associated with progressive subacute spongiform encephalopathies. In humans, such agents have been implicated in kuru and Creutzfeldt-Jakob disease, whereas in other species, similar agents cause scrapie and transmissible mink encephalopathy (5,252). The nature of the infectious agents involved remains obscure, and names such as "prions" or "virions" have been coined to define them (253,254). They are exquisitely small transmissible agents and are resistant to procedures that usually inactivate viruses. Of great interest, they appear nonimmunogenic and, thus, establish a unique virus/host relationship. Usually they cause disease only after years of apparently asymptomatic incubation, during which they may replicate to high titers within the nervous system. They have a long incubation period, which may be as long as 30 years. After the onset of the disease, death ensues within 3–9 months. Kuru is confined to an area in New Guinea where the inhabitants had the ritual cannibalistic tradition of eating the brain of the dead. The incidence of the disease has been declining in the past 20 years due to a change in their cannibalistic habits. Creutzfeldt-Jakob disease, on the other hand, is a sporadic rare disease with a familial pattern of inheritance in at least 10% of cases and has a worldwide distribution. Approaches to therapy of these unusual agents will depend on better understanding of how they replicate in the host. Immunological approaches appear unlikely to be useful at the present time.

Another form of slow virus infections are those caused by papovaviruses. Papovaviruses may remain latent for years following childhood infection. Once T-lymphocyte hyporesponsiveness develops, either as a result of exogenous therapy, as in transplant recipients, or because of endogenous factors—e.g., during cancer or AIDS—these viruses reactivate and may cause disease. Progressive multifocal leukoencephalopathy (PML), a usually fatal neurological disorder resulting from activated JC papovavirus infection, occurs virtually exclusively under these conditions of immunodeficiency (255,256) and has been reported frequently in patients with HIV infections. These varied examples illustrate the fundamental point that virus/host interactions are multiple and complex. Our ability to develop therapeutic or prophylactic approaches to individual infections depends on an understanding of how the particular virus affects the host response and is affected by it. Of particular importance is better definition of the mechanisms involved in viral latency. Until it is possible to eradicate established latent infections, the development of universally effective antiviral therapies will not be possible.

### *Oncogenesis*

Several members of DNA and RNA virus families have oncogenic capabilities. This has been shown both in animals and humans, *in vitro* and *in vivo*. Tumor viruses can transform cells *in vitro* and induce tumors experimentally, and some are natural causes of cancers in animals. The strongest associations of human malignancies and viruses are those between human T-cell leukemia/lymphoma virus type I (HTLV-I) and adult T-cell leukemia lymphoma (257–259) and between EBV and African Burkitt's lymphoma (38,39,260) and nasopharyngeal carcinoma (261,262). Also, a strong association exists between chronic HBV infection and liver carcinoma (263,264) and between papilloma virus infection and cervical carcinoma, penile cancer, and benign genital warts (265). Other potential virus-cancer links, but hard to prove, are those between HSV-2 and cervical carcinoma (266,267) and between CMV and cancer of the prostate, cervix, colon, and Kaposi's sarcoma (167,268–272).

The mechanisms involved in viral oncogenesis are under intense investigation. Both viral and cellular oncogenes have been identified, although the former may actually be cellular oncogenes derived by virus passage in cells. Oncogenesis may involve translocation of oncogenes to loci within infected cells where they are not inhibited by normal cellular repressor mechanisms (188,258). The most extensively studied mechanisms of oncogene activation by chromosomal translocation are those associated with Burkitt's lymphoma (273–275). In that instance, a reciprocal translocation between chromosomes 8 and 14 is present in approximately 75% of the cases. In the remainder of the cases, the translocation is between chromosome 8 and either 2 or 22. The proto-oncogene homologue of the retroviral v-*myc* oncogene, c-*myc,* is mapped to the terminal portion of 8. The genes coding for the immunoglobulin heavy and light chains map to chromosomes 2, 14, and 22, which are involved in these translocations. These translocations are transcriptionally active, and immunoglobulin genes are brought into juxtaposition with the c-*myc* gene, resulting in deregulation of the oncogene. Viral genes can also influence the expression of cellular oncogenes by integrating at sites close to these oncogenes. This would activate and amplify their expression by releasing them from normal regulatory control. Oncogene products from nonhuman retroviruses may have enzymatic activity that might alter signal transduction of second messenger system (276,277). Some encode for nuclear proteins that bind to double-stranded DNA and are thus suspected of influencing transcription. Another class that includes v-*sis* is closely related to the platelet-derived growth factor (PDGF) (278,279), and others, like v-*erb* and v-*fms,* have nucleotide sequence similarities with epidermal growth factor (EGF) and mouse macrophage colony stimulating factor (CSF-1) receptors, respectively (280,281). Amplification of these oncogenes may lead to transformation and uncontrolled cellular proliferation. Viruses might also serve as mutagen promoters of oncogenesis, which might explain their association with certain tumors in the absence of detectable residual viral genomes; in this type of relationship, they act as "hit and run" oncogenes (267). It is thought that HSV-2 may be associated with cancer of the cervix by such a mechanism.

### *Immune-Mediated Pathogenic Mechanisms*

Although in most circumstances immune responses limit virus replication and promote recovery, occasionally they may actually contribute to worsening disease. This may come about by at least two mechanisms: (a) deposition of immune complexes or (b) production of aberrant antibodies, effector lymphocytes, or interferons (Table 7). The latter may result in autoimmune reactivity, with resultant damage to normal tissue. Deposition of complexes between viral antigens and antibodies, resulting in tissue damage, has been described in a variety of situations, particularly in murine models of LCM, as discussed earlier, and in retrovirus leukemia (241,282,283). Over extended periods, such complexes may localize in kidneys, choroid plexus, and blood vessels, initiating a sequence that activates complement, increases capillary permeability, releases platelet-activating factors and vasoactive amines, and results in further organ damage. Immune complexes may occur in certain human infections as well, including HBV, HIV, EBV mononucleosis, and CMV infections (242,284–286). Rarely are these complexes associated with detectable tissue damage in humans, and the relevance of their detection during viral infections is unclear. More recently, AIDS-related glomerulopathy has been described with overt clinical manifestations characteristic of nephrotic syndrome with focal segmental sclerosis (FSS). This is thought in many instances to be due to mesangial deposition of immune complexes (287).

**TABLE 7.** *Possible mechanisms of virus-induced autoimmunity*

| |
|---|
| Afferent limb of immune response |
|   Release of sequestered antigens |
|   Cell membrane alterations |
|     Direct enzymatic attack |
|     Interference with cell membrane biosynthesis |
|     Derepression of developmental antigens |
|     Loss of tolerance-inducing antigens |
|   Cross-reactivity between virus and host antigens |
| Efferent limb of immune response |
|   Alteration of T-B or T-T cell interactions |
|     Termination or bypass of T-cell tolerance |
|     Inhibition of suppressor T cells |
|   Direct proliferative stimulation of autoaggressive cells |
|   Nonspecific adjuvant effect |

A link between EBV infection and rheumatoid arthritis has long been suspected but not proven (288,289), due to the elevation of antibodies to EBV in the sera and synovial fluids of those patients. Susceptibility to rheumatoid arthritis is linked to the expression of a particular nucleotide sequence of class II histocompatibility antigens HLA DR4 and HLA DR1 (290,291). This same nucleotide sequence is part of the gp 110 nucleocapsid glycoprotein that is detected in EBV-infected cells that have been induced by viral replication..This presents evidence for the possibility of altered immune recognition during EBV infection that might trigger some episodes of rheumatoid arthritis (292).

Although there is no hard evidence for autoimmune phenomenon in the pathology of AIDS, there are reports that associate it concurrently with Reiter's syndrome and psoriasis (293,294). Others have mistakenly diagnosed cases of systemic lupus erythematosis as AIDS due to the common features they share (295,296).

Heightened T-cell immunity may also contribute to disease (297). In murine models, the use of antilymphocyte serum often potentiates viral infection if administered before virus, whereas when administered late in infection, it may delay death (171). These studies suggest that T cells protect early in the course of infection, but late in the course of infection they may contribute to pathogenesis. Lymphocytic choriomeningitis of mice is the prototype virus-induced immunologic disease (240). A functional T-cell immune response is required for acute disease. Newborns or immunologically suppressed animals do not develop fatal meningoencephalitis following intracerebral injection of virus, whereas immunologically competent mice do. Adoptive transfer of competent T lymphocytes can restore the disease potential in chronically infected animals (298,299). It is possible that interferon produced by sensitized lymphocytes contributes to LCM pathogenesis (299). A number of unusual aberrant host responses are triggered by viruses, causing clinical syndrome.

Direct infection of human lymphoid cells or macrophages by viruses may have profound effects on immune function, ranging from hyporesponsiveness, to autoimmunity, to neoplasia. Many viruses readily infect lymphoid cells, including HSV (140,300–303), HIV, EBV (38,39), measles (304), rubella (305), dengue (306), adenovirus (307), mumps (308), HTLV (259,260), and the recently described human herpes virus 6. Others, such as CMV, HSV, HIV, dengue, and influenza, infect monocyte-macrophages (4,40,309,310). Many of these virus infections are accompanied by altered host immune functions including antibody production, lymphocyte proliferation, and cellular cytotoxicity. Lymphocyte function has been found to be altered in humans during a variety of virus infections, including measles, HIV, HBV, influenza, and CMV and EBV (187,311,312). Viral alteration of immune function may reflect the effects of viruses on specialized subpopulations of lymphoid cells. Different viruses have tropisms for various lymphocyte subsets. For example, EBV specifically infects and transforms B lymphocytes, whereas HIV infection has specificity for the T4+ (helper) lymphocyte subpopulation.

Perturbations of lymphocyte function can, on the other hand, sometimes activate latent viruses resident within these cells. Chronic antigenic stimulation, as occurs during graft versus host reactions or host versus graft reactions, can induce the release of murine retroviruses (251,313,314) and, possibly, CMV (315–317). Similar immune activation of human viruses may occur following organ transplantation or blood transfusion.

Viruses can also act as triggers for aberrant host responses that may, in turn, cause clinical syndromes. Guillain-Barré syndrome, postinfectious encephalopathy, hemolytic-uremic syndromes, and Reye's syndrome have all been associated with antecedent virus infections (2,124). Frequently, other factors are also involved, as in Reye's syndrome where influenza B and varicella have been implicated, along with the use of salicylates (318,319).

### Virus: Immune Selection and Antigenic Variation

The complex interaction that takes place between the virus and host following infection affects the host as mentioned previously as well as the invading virus. Host responses may lead to antigenic variations of the virus.

Changes in antigenicity of surface glycoproteins of viruses is a well-recognized mechanism for escaping elimination by the immune system. This occurs in response to selective genetic pressure due to the presence of specific antibodies. This change in antigenecity is known as antigenic drift and has been described for a number of viruses. The most classical example is with influenza viruses (320). A gradual antigenic change takes place in the hemagglutinin (HA) and/or neuraminidase glycoproteins of the virus during major epidemics that result in variants that are different from the preceding strains of virus. The new variant is not neutralized by the antibodies generated against the original virus. This way the virus always has a susceptible host population.

Antigenic drift has been also described for equine infectious anemia (EIA) and visna virus of sheep (321,322). Both are nononcogenic retroviruses that cause progressive fatal illnesses. Horses infected with EIA virus develop neutralizing antibodies following the first episode of hemolytic anemia. New EIA variants develop, which cause subsequent episodes. These new variants are not responsive to antibodies existing against previous variants.

Recently, immune selection has been suggested as a mechanism for HIV persistence in AIDS patients, as with EIA and visna. A considerable genomic diversity among HIV isolates exists (323), which may assist the virus in evading the immune system contributing to persistence. Such antigenic variation is important, especially with regard to vaccine development, where it could be an obstacle for development of an efficacious, protective vaccine.

## ANTIVIRALS AND VACCINES

The variability and complexity of the virus/host interactions are apparent. Despite the progress in the development of antibiotics and chemotherapeutics for other microorganisms in the last half century, progress with antivirals has been limited. Early attempts at virus therapy were plagued by the problem that the agents employed not only affected viral replication, but host cell function. The effects of antivirals on the clinical course and disease patterns will be reviewed.

When interferon was discovered more than 30 years ago (52), it was thought it could become the penicillin drug against viruses. Although interferon has a broad spectrum of antiviral effect *in vitro,* clinical responses in humans have been more limited. Clinical studies, during which local administration of natural or recombinant interferon for prophylaxis and therapy of respiratory viral infections is used, have demonstrated reduction in the infection rate, duration, and severity of the illness with rhinoviruses and an antiviral effect with influenza A and corona viruses (324–327). With herpetic keratitis, both interferon-α or interferon-β have been shown effective in curing the disease but were more efficacious when administered with acyclovir (ACV). In addition, combination therapy was more effective than ACV alone (328, 329). In other small studies, interferon-α has had no effect on the clinical course of adenovirus conjunctivitis, CMV retinitis, and acute hemorrhagic conjunctivitis. For papilloma virus infections, interferon has been used in the treatment of condyloma acuminata, verruca vulgaris, and laryngeal papillomatosis (330–332). Local and systemic application as well as intralesional injection of interferon for condyloma acuminata significantly reduced the size of the outgrowths in some studies and cleared the lesion completely in some patients (330,333,334). Although interferon therapy was effective in some individuals with condyloma acuminata, it produced variable results with verruca valgaris (335). Some success was also reported with laryngeal papillomatosis; however, when interferon doses were decreased or discontinued, recurrence of the papillomas occurred (336, 337).

Interferons have also been used in a number of clinical trials for chronic hepatitis due to HBV. The HBV-DNA and DNA polymerase activity started diminishing shortly after therapy was initiated (338). Responses to human interferon-α were permanent in 17–43% (339–341) of the cases, and disease remissions were more likely to occur with longer courses of therapy. Permanent response was more likely to occur in patients with chronic active hepatitis compared to those with chronic persistent hepatitis and in those with low level of DNA polymerase compared to those with high level of this enzyme. However, controlled clinical trials of interferon alone have not revealed reproducible results in a significant number of patients as compared to placebo. Interferon therapy for management of non-A, non-B hepatitis is also being explored at several centers.

In AIDS, recombinant interferon-α therapy has been studied in a number of non-controlled trials, with variable responses (342–344). Other placebo controlled studies are now underway to evaluate therapeutic efficacy of interferons alone and in combination with chemotherapy in a number of centers across the United States.

With herpes simplex infections, ACV is the drug of choice in most instances. ACV is an acyclic nucleoside analogue of guanosine that is an effective inhibitor of viral DNA polymerase. With herpes encephalitis, it diminished the morbidity and mortality from the disease (345,346). With recurrent herpes genitalis, ACV enhances the recovery and healing of the lesions, but it does not affect the duration between episodes. Suppression therapy with ACV for recurrent herpes genitalis has been successful for up to 2 years and is recommended in severe cases where patients suffer more than six episodes a year (347). However, chronic ACV therapy for HSV-related diseases in patients with AIDS may select for resistant mutants, which result in low-grade chronic infections.

Amantadine and rimantadine are both equally efficacious for prophylaxis and therapy of influenza A virus, but not B (348). Administration of both drugs within 48 hr of infection leads to a significant improvement of the patient's illness with less fever and virus shedding, and better functional status when compared to placebo-treated patients. Ribavirin is an agent that has activity against lower respiratory infections caused by influenza A and B in adults and parainfluenza 3 in immunocompromised children (349) but has not been studied in placebo-controlled trials. The striking success with ribavirin is in the management of respiratory syncytial virus (RSV) infection in infants. Inhaled, ribavirin shortens the duration of disease and the severity of the illness, and reduces the pulmonary complications and mortality (350). Ribavirin is also used for treatment of Lassa fever (351) and has been reported to inhibit HIV replication *in vitro* (352).

Vidarabine (adenine arabinoside; ara-A) is a nucleoside analogue that is effective against herpesviruses. Its drawbacks are that it is insoluble and must be given intravenously in large amounts of fluid. ACV has replaced this compound in treatment of most herpesvirus infection. Vidarabine, however, remains the only drug proven to reduce mortality in neonatal herpes. Vidarabine, idoxuridine, and trifluorothymidine ointments are very efficient in treatment of herpetic keratitis and are still the drugs of choice for this ailment.

Azidothymidine (AZT) is a thymidine analog that is active *in vitro* and *in vivo* against a number of animal retroviruses including HIV. AZT is the only drug approved so far for the treatment of AIDS. In a double-blind placebo-controlled clinical trial that involved 282 patients, AZT appeared to prolong patients' survival. The patients generally gained weight, opportunistic infections were diminished, and Karnofsky scores of functional ability improved. Immunological parameters, including increased CD4 cells and development of skin test reactivity, also improved, and there were reductions in HIV p24 antigenemia (353,354). However, chronic administration of AZT is not without side effects and has been shown to cause macrocytic anemia, neutropenia, and pancytopenia (354,355). Although AZT inhibits viral replication, its effects on bone marrow may further the immune suppression of AIDS patients and, in the long run, would make them more vulnerable to fatal opportunistic infections.

Ganciclovir [dihydroxy propoxymethyl guanine (DHPG)], another acyclic nucleoside, has potent antiviral effects against CMV *in vitro*. In humans, uncontrolled studies have suggested beneficial effects on gastroenteritis and CMV retinitis in patients with AIDS. It appears less effective with CMV pneumonia but may produce some responses. This compound has a narrow margin of safety, producing irreversible testicular damage and transient neutropenia

(356,357). Ganciclovir changes the pattern of CMV disease from an acute destructive infection to a less severe chronic course, with relapsing episodes of infection.

Several other promising drugs and immune modulators are under study and included in clinical trials in many centers. It is clear that this is only the beginning and that there is still much to be done despite the significant progress in the past 10 years.

Understanding the mechanisms of host immunity to viral infections should also allow more effective manipulation of responsiveness. Discovery, characterization, purification, and commercial production of individual lymphokines such as interferons, interleukins, and transfer factors may result in reconstitution of defective responses and correction of acquired or congenital immune deficiencies. Once it is better understood how specific viruses induce immunological hyporesponsiveness, targeted approaches to prevention or reversal can be attempted. Similarly, the reduction of virus-induced immunopathology by pharmacologic means awaits a fuller understanding of the mechanisms involved. Certain agents, such as members of the interferon family, may act both as antivirals and as immunostimulants, providing synergistic effects.

Development of vaccines and vaccination programs have had their effect in changing disease patterns in the last half century. The best example is smallpox (358). Causing the disease that once frightened the entire world, the smallpox virus was eradicated from the globe in 1978, after a 10-year multinational campaign of education, vaccination, and containment of the disease. The last reported case was in 1977. Several factors contributed to the success of the effort to eradicate this agent. The nature of the biology and pathogenesis of this particular virus played the major role. First, humans are the only reservoir for smallpox; second, patients are not infectious before the eruption of rash; third, the virus does not persist in the body, i.e., no recurrences; and fourth, smallpox very rarely produced subclinical infections.

Another vaccine that gives solid protection to a viral disease is the yellow fever vaccine, which produces immunity and is recommended for those traveling to endemic areas. Live attenuated vaccines for polio, measles, mumps, and rubella are recommended for children. Since the introduction of the measles vaccines in the early 1960s, the incidence of the disease is declining both in the west as well as in developing countries. Severe cases are reported only among the nonvaccinated. Among the vaccinated, the disease is also reported but in a much milder form. However, individuals receiving killed vaccines are at risk of developing an atypical form of measles when exposed to the wild virus (359–363). In atypical measles, after 2 days of fever, patients experience a maculopapular rash that erupts on the extremities and spreads centripetally with edema of hands and feet, and is commonly accompanied by nodular pneumonitis with effusion. In spite of the severity of the disease, fatality is rare. Very rarely, this syndrome has been described for patients that received live attenuated virus (364,365). The killed vaccine was used between 1963 and 1967. The recipients of this vaccine are recommended for revaccination with the live attenuated vaccine in order to prevent typical and atypical measles (366,367).

A declining pattern was also apparent with poliomyelitis, with the number of cases of paralytic polio diminishing. With polio, there has been an age shift, with most of the paralytic cases being among adolescents and adults, due to a decline of specific serum antibodies.

Rabies vaccine is recommended when someone is bitten by a suspected infected dog or some other vector. If the vaccine regimen is started immediately, there is a good chance for patient survival. But once the signs and symptoms of rabies appear, the disease is usually fatal. Other vaccines that are also available are influenza vaccine, which can either prevent or influence the severity of the illness and is recommended for high-risk groups. Vaccines against HBV have been demonstrated effective and also are recommended for special risk groups.

Varicella is usually a mild disease in normal children, but infection of immunocompromised children and adults undergoes a more severe course. A live attenuated VZV vaccine has recently been described. It has been tested in the United States, Europe, and Japan, and appears to be efficacious among normal and immunocompromised children (368–371). The vaccine reduced the incidence of VZV among leukemia and lymphoma patients when compared with the unvaccinated controlled group. Chicken pox among the vaccinated children had a mild course when compared with the unvaccinated group (372). Long-term follow-up (7–10 years) of 106 vaccinated children showed long-term immunity to VZV (373). No cases of VZV were reported during that follow-up period. Despite the concerns about DNA virus vaccines and the role they may play in promoting virus-induced malignancies, particularly with viruses with proclavity for persistence, VZV is not known for its association with any type of cancer. This is in contrast to other members of the herpes virus group family that are known for their oncogenic potential and their association with malignancies.

Despite the progress that has been accomplished in the understanding and control of virus infections, much work is still needed. Although smallpox has been eliminated, AIDS has spread widely. The pathogenesis of viral infections require thorough investigation at each step of the infection, beginning at the site of initiation and ending at virus eradication or induction of latency. Each may reveal possible sites for intervention. The manner in which the virus replicates locally and disseminates to different sites, which particular host responses are induced and in what sequence, and how the virus modulates each response are necessary and legitimate questions for investigation. Therapeutic agents must be chosen with the knowledge of their pharmacokinetics relative to the target organs of virus replication. It does little good to treat a viral encephalitis with an agent that does not reach significant levels within the CNS. Also, effective levels of drug must be achieved at a time when active replication occurs. In a murine model of disseminated HSV infection, intravenous idoxuridine was effective in eliminating virus in organs where adequate levels were achieved, but not in the CNS, where uncontrolled virus replication resulted in the death of the animal (299).

The problem of latency remains a major impediment to curative therapy of many virus infections. Conceptual breakthroughs will be required in order to attack viral genome segments closely associated with cellular DNA. Thus, elimination of resident viral genomes such as HSV and VZV will remain elusive for the foreseeable future.

It is clear that we have entered an era of antiviral therapy, one that will produce major advances in the control of virus infections. The new era will also produce new problems requiring still newer solutions. Only with better understanding of the viruses involved, the host's responses, and the resultant virus/host interactions will we be able to anticipate problems to come and develop rational approaches to overcome them.

## ACKNOWLEDGMENT

We relied, in part, in writing this chapter on the text and tables of the chapter of the same name by Dr. Martin S. Hirsch in the previous edition of this volume.

## REFERENCES

1. Constantine DG. Rabies transmission by nonbite route. *Public Health Rep* 1962;77:287–9.
2. Corey L, Rubin RJ, Hattwick MAW, Noble

GR, Cassidy E. A nationwide outbreak of Reye's syndrome: its epidemiologic relationship to influenza. *Am J Med* 1976;61:615–25.
3. Winkler W. Airborne rabies virus isolation. *Bull Wild Dis Assoc* 1968;4:37–40.
4. Hirsch MS, Zisman B, Allison AC. Macrophages and age-dependent resistance to herpes simplex virus in mice. *J Immunol* 1970;104:1160–5.
5. Johnson RT. *Viral infections of the nervous system*. New York: Raven Press, 1982.
6. Lopez C, Ryshke R, Bennett M. Marrow-dependent cells depleted by 89Sr mediate genetic resistance to herpes simplex type 1 infection of mice. *Infect Immun* 1980;28:1028–32.
7. Mims CA. Aspects of the pathogenesis of virus diseases. *Bacteriol Res* 1964;28:30–71.
8. Mintz L, Drew WL, Hoo R, Finley TN. Age-dependent resistance of human alveolar macrophages to herpes simplex virus. *Infect Immun* 1980;28:417–20.
9. Mogensen SC. Role of macrophages in natural resistance to virus infections. *Microbiol Rev* 1979;43:1–26.
10. Bang FB, Warwick A. Mouse macrophages as host cells for mouse hepatitis and the genetic basis for their susceptibility. *Proc Natl Acad Sci USA* 1960;46:1065–75.
11. Haller O, Arnheiter M, Greser I, Lindenmann J. Genetically determined interferon-dependent resistance to influenza virus in mice. *J Exp Med* 1979;149:601–12.
12. CDC. Pneumocystis pneumonia—Los Angeles. *MMWR* 1981;30:250–2.
13. CDC. Kaposi's sarcoma and pneumocystis pneumonia among homosexual men, New York City and California. *MMWR* 1981;30:305–8.
14. Dover AS, Escobar JA, Duenas AL, Leal EC. Pneumonia associated with measles. *JAMA* 1975;234:612–4.
15. Gatmaitan BG, Chason JL, Lerner AM. Augmentation of the virulence of murine Coxsackie-virus B-3 myocardiopathy by exercise. *J Exp Med* 1970;131:1121–36.
16. Woodruff JF. The influence of quantitated post-weaning undernutrition on Coxsackie virus B3 infection of adult mice. II. Alteration of host defence mechanisms. *J Infect Dis* 1970; 121:164–81.
17. Djeu JY, Stocks N, Zoon K, Stanton GJ, Timonen T, Herberman RB. Positive self-regulation of cytotoxicity in human natural killer cells by production of interferon upon exposure to influenza and herpes viruses. *J Exp Med* 1982;156:1222–34.
18. Curran JW, Lawrence DN, Jaffe H, et al. Acquired immunodeficiency syndrome (AIDS) associated with transfusions. *N Engl J Med* 1984;310:69–75.
19. Centers for Disease Control. Human immunodeficiency virus infection transmitted from an organ donor screened for HIV antibody—North Carolina. *MMWR* 1987;36:306–8.
20. Betts RF, Freeman RB, Douglas RG Jr, Talley TE, Rundell B. Transmission of cytomegalovirus infection with renal allograft. *Kidney Int* 1975;8:387–94.
21. Ho M, Suwansirikul S, Dowling JN, Youngblood LA, Armstrong JA. The transplanted kidney as a source of cytomegalovirus infections. *N Engl J Med* 293:1109–12.
22. Tobin JO'H, Warrell MJ, Morris RJ. Cytomegalovirus infection and renal transplantation. *Lancet* 1979;1:926.
23. Marker SC, Howard RJ, Simmons RL, et al. Cytomegalovirus infection: a quantitative prospective study of 320 consecutive renal transplants. *Surgery* 1981;89:660–71.
24. Centers for Disease Control. Human-to-human transmission of rabies. *MMWR* 1981;30:473–4.
25. Centers for Disease Control. Update: Creutzfeldt-Jakob disease in a patient receiving a cadaveric dura mater graft. *MMWR* 1987;36:324–5.
26. Berry WR, Gottesfeld RL, Alter HJ, Vierling JM. Transmission of hepatitis B virus by artificial insemination. *JAMA* 1987;257:1079–81.
27. Stewart GJ, Cunningham AL, Driscoll GL, et al. Transmission of human T-cell lymphotropic virus type III (HTLV-III) by artificial insemination by donor. *Lancet* 1985;II:581–4.
28. Perreira L, Hoffman M, Gallo D, Cremer N. Monoclonal antibodies to human cytomegalovirus: three surface membrane proteins with unique immunological and electrophoretic properties specify cross-reactive determinants. *Infect Immun* 1982;36:924–32.
29. Yewdell JW, Gerhard W. Antigenic characterization of viruses by monocloncal antibodies. *Ann Rev Microbiol* 1981;35:185–206.
30. Pimmock NJ. Initial stages in infection with animal viruses. *J Gen Virol* 1982;59:1–22.
31. Co IS, Gaulton GN, Tominaga A, Homcy CJ, Fields BN, Greene MI. Structural similarities between the mammalian—adrenergic and reovirus type 3 receptors. *Proc Natl Acad Sci USA* 1985;82:5315–8.
32. Bowen DL, Lane HC, Fauci AS. Immunopathogenesis of the acquired immunodeficiency syndrome. *Ann Intern Med* 1985;103:704–9.
33. Dalgleish AG, Beverley PCL, Clapham PR, Crawford DH, Greaves MF, Weiss RA. The CD4 (T4) antigen is an essential component of the receptor for the AIDS retrovirus. *Nature* 1984;312:763–7.
34. Klatzmann D, Champagne E, Chamaret S, et al. T-lymphocyte T4 molecule behaves as the receptor for human retrovirus LAV. *Nature* 1984;312:767–8.
35. Lentz TL, Burrage TG, Smith AL, Crick J, Tignor GH. Is the acetylcholine receptor a rabies virus receptor? *Science* 1982;215:182–6.
36. Fingeroth JD, Weiss JJ, Teddler TF, Strominger JL, Biro A, Fearon DT. Epstein-Barr virus receptor of human B lymphocytes is the C3d receptor CR2. *Proc Natl Acad Sci USA* 1984;81:4510–4.
37. Nemerow GR, Wolfert R, McNaughton ME, Cooper NR. Identification and characterization of the Epstein-Barr virus receptor on human

B lymphocytes and its relationship to the C3d complement receptor (CR2). *J Virol* 1985;55:347–51.
38. Epstein MA, Achong BG. *The Epstein-Barr virus*. New York: Springer-Verlag, 1979.
39. Miller G. Biology of Epstein-Barr virus. In: Klein G, ed. *Viral oncology*. New York: Raven Press, 1980:712–38.
40. Carney WP, Hirsch MS. Mechanisms of immunosuppression in cytomegalovirus mononucleosis. II. Virus-monocyte interactions. *J Infect Dis* 1981;144:47–54.
41. Carney WP, Iacoviello V, Hirsch MS. Functional properties of T lymphocytes and their subsets in cytomegalovirus mononucleosis. *J Immunol* 1982;130:390–3.
42. Rinaldo CR Jr, Carney WP, Richter BS, Black PH, Hirsch MS. Mechanisms of immunosuppression in cytomegalovirus mononucleosis. *J Infect Dis* 1980;141:488–95.
43. Emmons RW, Oshiro LS, Johnson HN, Lennette EH. Intracrythrocyte location of Colorado tick fever virus. *J Gen Virol* 1972;17:185–95.
44. Murphy FA. Rabies pathogenesis: brief review. *Arch Virol* 1977;54:279–97.
45. Stevens JG. Latent herpes simplex virus and the nervous system. *Curr Top Microbiol Immunol* 1975;70:31–50.
46. Stevens JG, Cook ML. Maintenance of latent herpetic infection: an apparent role for antiviral IgG. *J Immunol* 1974;113:1685–93.
47. Allison AC. On the role of mononuclear phagocytes in immunity against viruses. *Prog Med Virol* 1973;18:15–31.
48. Morahan PS, Morse SS. Macrophage-virus interactions. In: Proffitt M, ed. *Virus-lymphocyte interactions: implications for disease*. New York: Elsevier, 1979:17–35.
49. Stohlman SA, Woodward JG, Frelinger JA. Macrophage antiviral activity: extrinsic versus intrinsic activity. *Infect Immun* 1982;36:672–7.
50. Kohase M, Henriksen-DeStefano D, May LT, Vicek J, Sehgal PB. Induction of beta$_2$-interferon by tumor necrosis factor, a homeostatic mechanism in the control of cell proliferation. *Cell* 1986;45:659.
51. Wong GHW, Krowka JF, Stites DP, Goeddel DV. *In vitro* anti-human immunodeficiency virus activities of tumor necrosis factor-α and interferon-γ. *J Virol* 1988;140:120–4.
52. Isaacs A, Lindenmann JI. The interferon. *Proc R Soc Lond* [*Biol*] 1957;147:258–67.
53. Strander H. *Report of the international workshop in interferon in the treatment of cancer.* New York: Sloan-Kettering Institute for Cancer Research, 1975:1–39.
54. Cantell K. Why is interferon not in clinical use today? In: Gresser I, ed. *Interferon, 1*. New York: Academic Press, 1979:2–28.
55. Stewart WE II, Lin LS. Antiviral activities of interferons. *Pharmacol Ther* 1979;6:443–512.
56. Baron S, Grossberg SE, Klimpel GR, et al. Immune and interferon systems. In: Galasso GJ, Merigan TC, Buchanan RA, eds. *Antiviral agents and viral diseases of man*. 2nd ed. New York: Raven Press, 1984:123–78.
57. Pestka S. Interferon from 1981 to 1986. *Meth Enzymol* 1986;119:3–4.
58. Carlin JM, Border EC. Interferons and their induction. In: Byrne GI, Turco J, eds. *Interferon and nonviral pathogens*. New York: Marcel Dekker, Inc., 1988:3–26.
59. Pestka S, Langer JA, Zoon KC, et al. Interferons and their actions. *Ann Rev Biochem* 1987;56:727–77.
60. Kirchner H. The interferon system as an integral part of the defense system against infections. *Antiviral Res* 1986;6:1–17.
61. Baron S, Stanton GJ, Fleischmann WR Jr, et al. Introduction: general considerations of the interferon system. In: Baron S, Dianzani F, Stanton GJ, et al., eds. *The interferon system: A current review to 1987*. Austin: University of Texas Press, 1987:1–17.
62. Rubinstein M, Rubinstein S, Familletti PC, et al. Human leukocyte interferon: production, purification to homogeneity, and initial characterization. *Proc Natl Acad Sci USA* 1979;76:640–4.
63. Nagata S, Mantei N, Weissmann C. The structure of one of the eight or more distinct chromosomal genes for human interferon-α. *Nature* 1980;287:401–8.
64. Goeddel DV, Leung DW, Dull TJ, et al. The structure of eight distinct cloned human leukocyte interferon cDNAs. *Nature* 1981;290:20–6.
65. Pestka S. Interferon standards and general abbreviations. *Meth Enzymol* 1986;119:14–23.
66. Wilson V, Jeffreys AJ, Barrie PA, et al. A comparison of vertebrate interferon gene families detected by hybridization with human interferon DNA. *J Mol Biol* 1983;166:457–75.
67. Goeddel DV, Yelverton E, Ullrich A, et al. Human leukocyte interferon produced by *E. coli* is biologically active. *Nature* 1980;287:411–6.
68. Brack C, Nagata S, Mantei N, et al. Molecular analysis of the human interferon-α gene family. *Gene* 1981;15:379–94.
69. Henco K, Brosius J, Fujisawa A, et al. Structural relationship of human interferon-α genes and pseudogenes. *J Mol Biol* 1985;185:227–60.
70. Hotta K, Collier KJ, Pestka S. Detection of a single base substitution between human leukocyte IFN-αA and -α2 genes with octadecyl deoxyoligonucleotide probes. *Meth Enzymol* 1986;119:481–5.
71. Rubinstein M, Rubinstein S, Familletti PC, et al. Human leukocyte interferon purified to homogeneity. *Science* 1978;202:1289–90.
72. Zoon KC, Miller D, ZurNedden D, et al. Human leukocyte-derived alpha interferons: Purification and amino-terminal-amino-acid sequence of two components. *J Interferon Res* 1982;2:253–60.
73. Kauppinen H-L, Hervonen S, Cantell K. Effect of purification procedures on the composition of human leukocyte interferon preparations. *Meth Enzymol* 1986;119:27–35.
74. Allen G, Fantes KH, Burke DC, et al. Analysis

and purification of human lymphoblastoid (Namalwa) interferon using a monoclonal antibody. *J Gen Virol* 1982;63:207–12.
75. Hobbs DS, Pestka S. Purification and characterization of interferons from a continuous myeloblastic cell line. *J Biol Chem* 1982;63:207–12.
76. Tanuguchi T, Mantei N, Schwarzstein M, et al. Human leukocyte and fibroblast interferons are structurally related. *Nature* 1980;285:547–9.
77. Zoon KC, Wetzel R. Comparative structures of mammalian interferons. *Handb Exp Pharmacol,* 1984;71:79–100.
78. DeChiara TM, Erlitz F, Tarnowski SJ. Procedures for *in vitro* DNA mutagenesis of human leukocyte interferon sequences. *Meth Enzymol* 1986;119:403–15.
79. Labdon JE, Gibson KD, Shun S, et al. Some species of human leukocyte interferon are glycosylated. *Arch Biochem Biophys* 1984; 232:422–6.
80. Thatcher DR, Panayotatos N. Purification of recombinant human IFN-α 1. *Meth Enzymol* 1986;119:166–77.
81. Staehellin T, Hobbs DS, Kung H-F, et al. Purification and characterization of recombinant human leukocyte interferon (IFLrA) with monoclonal antibodies. *J Biol Chem* 1981;256:9750–4.
82. Tarnowski SJ, Roy SK, Liptak RA, et al. Large-scale purification of recombinant human leukocyte interferons. *Meth Enzymol* 1986;119:153–65.
83. Wetzel R, Perry LJ, Estell DA, et al. Properties of a human interferon-α purified from *E. coli* extracts. *J Interferon Res* 1981;1:381–90.
84. Knight E Jr. Interferon. Purification and initial characterization from human diploid cells. *Proc Nat Acad Sci USA* 1976;73:520–3.
85. Sehgal PB, May LT. Human interferon-$\beta_2$. *J Interferon Res* 1987;7:521–7.
86. Lin LS, Yamamoto R, Drummond RJ. Purification of recombinant human interferon-β expressed in *Escherichia coli. Meth Enzymol* 1986;119:183–92.
87. Yip YK, Barrowclough BS, Urban C, et al. Purification of two subspecies of human gamma (immune) interferon. *Proc Natl Acad Sci USA* 1982;79:1820–4.
88. Braude IA. Purification of human interferon-γ to essential homogeneity and its biochemical characterization. *Biochemisty* 1984;23:5603–9.
89. Kung H-F, Pan Y-C E, Noschera J, et al. Purification of recombinant human immune interferon. *Meth Enzymol* 1986;119:204–10.
90. Arakawa T, Alton NK, Hsu Y-R. Preparations and characterization of recombinant DNA-derived human interferon-γ. *J Biol Chem* 1985;260:14435–9.
91. Rinderknecht E, O'Connor BH, Rodriguez H. Natural human interferon-γ: complete amino acid sequence and determination of sites of glycosylation. *J Biol Chem* 1984;259:6790–7.
92. Evinger M, Rubinstein M, Pestka S. Antiproliferative and antiviral activities of human leukocyte interferons. *Arch Biochem Biophys* 1981;210:319–29.
93. Eife R, Hahn T, DeTavera M, et al. A comparison of the antiproliferative and antiviral activities of alpha, beta, and gamma interferons: description of a unified assay for comparing both effects simultaneously. *J Immunol Methods* 1981;47:339–47.
94. Rehberg E, Kelder B, Hoal EG, et al. Specific molecular activities of recombinant and hybrid leukocyte interferons. *J Biol Chem* 1982;257:11497–502.
95. Epstein DA, Czarnieck CW, Jacobsen H, et al. A mouse cell line, which is unprotected by interferon against lytic virus infection, lacks ribonuclease F activity. *Eur J Biochem* 1981;118:9–15.
96. Sen GC, Herz RE. Differential antiviral effects of interferon in three murine cell lines. *J Virol* 1983;45:1017–27.
97. Weck PK, Qapperson S, Stebbing N, et al. Antiviral activities of hybrids of two major human leukocyte interferons. *Nucleic Acids Res* 1981;9:6153–66.
98. Ortaldo JR, Mantovani A, Hobbs D, et al. Effects of recombinant and hybrid recombinant human leukocyte interferon on cytotoxic activity of NK cells and monocytes. *Int J Cancer* 1983;31:285–9.
99. Ortaldo JR, Manson A, Rehberg E, et al. Effects of recombinant and hybrid recombinant human leukocyte interferons on cytotoxic activity of natural killer cells. *J Biol Chem* 1983;258:15011–5.
100. Ortaldo JR, Herberman RB, Harvey C, et al. A species of human alpha interferon that lacks the ability to boost the human natural killer activity. *Proc Natl Acad Sci USA* 1984;81:4926–9.
101. Greiner JW, Fisher PB, Pestka S, et al. Differential effects of recombinant human leukocyte interferons on cell surface antigen expression. *Cancer Res* 1986;46:4984–90.
102. Greiner JW, Hand PH, Noguchi P, et al. Enhanced expression of surface tumor-associated antigens on human breast and colon tumor cells after recombinant human leukocyte interferon-α treatment. *Cancer Res* 1984;3208–14.
103. Greiner JW, Scholom J, Pestka S, et al. Modulation of tumor associated antigen expression and shedding by recombinant human leukocyte and fibroblast interferons. *Pharmacol Ther* 1987;31:209–36.
104. Giacomini P, Aguzzi A, Pestka S, et al. Modulation by recombinant DNA leukocyte (α) and fibroblasts (β) interferons of the expression and shedding of HLA- and tumor-associated antigens by human melanoma cells. *J Immunol* 1985;133:1649–55.
105. Heron I, Hokland M, Berg K. Enhanced expression of $\beta_2$-microglobulin and HLA antigens on human lymphoid cells by interferon. *Proc Natl Acad Sci USA* 1978;75:6215–9.
106. Imai K, Ng A-K, Glassy MC, et al. Differential effect of interferon on the expression of tumor-

associated antigens and histocompatibility antigens on human melanoma cells: relationship to susceptibility to immune lysis mediated by monoclonal antibodies. *J Immunol* 1981;127:505–9.

107. Yoshie O, Aso H, Sakakibara A, et al. Differential effects of recombinant human interferon-α A/D on expression of three types of Fc receptors on murine macrophages *in vivo* and *in vitro*. *J Interferon Res* 1985;5:531–40.
108. Fleischmann WR Jr, Schwarz LA. Demonstration of potentiation of the antiviral and antitumor actions of interferon. *Meth Enzymol* 1981;79:432–40.
109. Balkwill FR. Smyth JF. Interferons in cancer therapy: a reappraisal. *Lancet* 1987;2:317–9.
110. Secher DS. Immunoradiometric assay of human leukocyte interferon using monoclonal antibody. *Nature* 1981;290:501–3.
111. Kelder B, Rashidbaigi A, Pestka S. A sandwich radioimmunoassay for human IFN-γ. *Meth Enzymol* 1986;119:582–7.
112. Steis RG, Smith JW, Urba WJ, et al. Resistance to recombinant interferon-α-2a in hairy-cell leukemia associated with neutralizing anti-interferon antibodies. *N Engl J Med* 1988;318:1409–13.
113. vonWussow P, Freund M, Block B, et al. Clinical significance of anti-IFN-α antibody titres during interferon therapy. *Lancet* 1987;2:635–6.
114. Grossberg SE, Jameson P, Sedmak JJ. Assay of interferon. In: Came P, Carter W, eds. *Interferons and their application, handbook of experimental pharmacology, vol. 71*. Berlin: Springer-Verlag, 1983:23–43.
115. NIH Workshop. Human antibodies to interferons: report of NIH workshop. *J Interferon Res* (in press).
116. Baglioni C, Branca AA, D'Alessandro SB, et al. Low interferon binding activity of two human cell lines which respond poorly to the antiviral and antiproliferative activity of interferon. *Virology* 1982;122:202–6.
117. Joshi AR, Sarkar FH, Gupta SL. Interferon receptors: cross-linking of human leukocyte interferon α-2 to its receptor on human cells. *J Biol Chem* 1982;257:13884–7.
118. Yonehara S, Yonehara-Takahashi M, Ishii A, et al. Different binding of human interferon-α-1 and -α-2 to its receptor on human and bovine cells. *J Biol Chem* 1983;258:9046–9.
119. Revel M, Bash D, Ruddle FH. Antibodies to a cell-surface component coded by human chromosome 21 inhibit action of interferon. *Nature* 1976;260:139–41.
120. Slate DL, Ruddle RH. Antibodies to chromosome 21 coded cell surface components can block response to human interferon. *Cytogenet Cell Genet* 1978;22:265–9.
121. Baron S, Blalock JE, Dianzani F, et al. Immune interferon: some properties and functions. *Ann NY Acad Sci* 1980;350:130–44.
122. Cheeseman SH, Rubin RH, Stewart JA, et al. Controlled clinical trial of prophylactic human-leukocyte interferon in renal transplantation. Effects on cytomegalovirus and herpes simplex virus infections. *N Engl J Med* 1979;300:1345–9.
123. Virelizier JL, Greser I. Roles of interferon in the pathogenesis of viral diseases of mice as demonstrated by the use of anti-interferon serum. V. Protective role in mouse hepatitis virus type 3 infection of susceptible and resistant strains of mice. *J Immunol* 1978;120:1616–9.
124. Glick TH, Ditchek NT, Salitsky S, Freimuth GH. Acute encephalopathy and hepatic dysfunction-associated with chickenpox in siblings. *Am J Dis Child* 1970;119:68–71.
125. Schellekens H, Weimar W, Cantell K, Stitz L. Antiviral effect of interferon *in vivo* may be mediated by the host. *Nature* 1979;278:742–6.
126. Kadish AS. Interferon as a mediator of human lymphocyte suppression. *J Exp Med* 1980;151:637–50.
127. Merigan TC. Host defenses against viral diseases. *N Engl J Med* 1974;290:323–8.
128. Neta R, Salvin SB. Interferons and lymphokines. In: Baron S, Dianzani F, Stanton GJ, eds. *The interferon system: a review to 1982. Texas Rep Biol Med* 1982;41:435–42.
129. National Institute of Allergy and Infectious Diseases. World Health Organization—U.S. National Center on Interferon. Interferon nomenclature. *Nature* 1980;286:110.
130. Dianzani F, Zucca M, Scupham A, Georgiades JA. Immune and virus induced interferons may activate cells by different depressional mechanisms. *Nature* 283:400–2.
131. Minato N, Reid L, Cantos H, Lengyel P, Bloom BR. Mode of regulation of natural killer cell activity by interferon. *J Exp Med* 1980;152:124–7.
132. Maluish AC, Conlon J, Ortaldo JR. Modulation of NK and monocyte activity in advanced cancer patients receiving interferon. In: Merigan TC, Friedman RM, eds. *Interferons*. New York: Academic Press, 1982:377–86.
133. Gresser I, Maury C, Tovery M, Morel-Maroger L, Pontillon F. Progressive glomerulonephritis in mice treated with interferon preparations at birth. *Nature* 1976;263:420.
134. Gresser I, Morel-Maroger L, Verroust P, Riviere Y, Guillon J. Anti-interferon globulin inhibits the development of glomerulonephritis in mice infected at birth with lymphocytic choriomeningitis virus. *Proc Natl Acad Sci USA* 1978;75:3413.
135. Jacobson S, Friedman RM, Pfau CJ. Interferon induction by lymphocytic choriomeningitis viruses correlates with maximum virulence. *J Gen Virol* 1981;57:275.
136. McIntosh K, Fishaut JM. Immunopathologic mechanisms in lower respiratory tract disease of infants due to respiratory syncytial virus. *Prog Med Virol* 1980;26:94.
137. Hooks JJ, Detrick B. The interferon system and disease. In: Pfeffer IM, ed. *Mechanisms of interferon action. Vol 2*. Boca Raton, FL: CRC, 1987:113.

138. Lopez C, Kirkpatrick D, Fitzgerald PA, et al. Studies of the cell lineage of the effector cells that spontaneously lyse HSV-1 infected fibroblasts [NK(HSV-1)]. *J Immunol* 1981;129:824–8.
139. Herberman RB. Natural killer (NK) cells and their possible roles in resistance against disease. *Clin Immunol Rev* 1981;1:1–65.
140. Fitzgerald PA, von Wussow P, Lopez C. Role of interferon in natural kill of HSV-1-infected fibroblasts. *J Immunol* 1982;129:819–23.
141. Hammer SM, Carney WP, Iacoviello VR, Lowe BR, Hirsch MS. Herpes simplex virus infection and human T-cell subpopulations. *Infect Immun* 1982;8:795–7.
142. Ching C, Lopez C. Natural killing of herpes simplex virus type 1 infected target cells. Normal human responses and influence of antiviral antibodies. *Infect Immun* 1979;26:49–56.
143. Welsh RM Jr, Kiessling RW. Natural killer cell response to lymphocytic choriomeningitis virus in beige mice. *Scand J Immunol* 1980;11:363–7.
144. Roder JC, Haliotis T, Klein M, et al. A new immunodeficiency disorder in humans involving NK cells. *Nature* 1980;284:553–5.
145. Quinnan GV Jr, Kirman N, Rook AH, et al. Cytotoxic T cells in cytomegalovirus infection. *N Engl J Med* 1982;307:6–13.
146. Cooper NR. Activation and regulation of the first complement component (C1). *Federation Proceedings* 1983;42:134–8.
147. Pangburn MK. Activation of complement via the alternative pathway. *Federation Proceedings* 1983;42:139–43.
148. Cooper NR. Humoral immunity to viruses. In: Fraenkel-Conrat H, Wagner RR, eds. *Comprehensive virology*. New York: Plenum Press, 1979:123.
149. Cooper NR, Jensen FC, Welsh Jr, RM, Oldstone MBA. Lysis of RNA tumor viruses by human serum: direct antibody independent triggering of the classical complement pathway. *J Exp Med* 1976;144:970–84.
150. Welsh RM Jr. Host cell modification of lymphocytic choriomeningitis virus and Newcastle disease virus altering viral inactivation by human complement. *J Immunol* 1977;118:348–54.
151. Mayes JT, Nemerow GR, Cooper NR. Alternative complement (C) pathway (AP) activation by Epstein-Barr virus (EBV) infected normal B lymphocytes. *Federation Proceedings* 1983;42:5530.
152. Hirsch RL, Winkelstein JA, Griffen DE. The role of complement in viral infections. *J Immunol* 1980;124:2507–10.
153. Nemerow GR, Jensen FC, Cooper NR. Neutralization of Epstein-Barr virus (EBV) by nonimmune human serum: role of cross-reacting antibody to herpes simplex virus (HSV-1) and complement (C). *J Clin Invest* 1982;70:1081–91.
154. Beebe DP, Schreiber RD, Cooper NR. Neutralization of influenza virus by normal human sera: mechanisms involving antibody and complement. *J Immunol* 1983;130:1317–22.
155. Allison AC. Interactions of antibodies, complement components and various cell types in immunity against viruses and pyogenic bacteria. *Transplant Rev* 1974;29:3–55.
156. Allison AC, Burns WH. Immunogenicity of animal viruses. In: Borek F, ed. *Immunogenicity*. Amsterdam: North-Holland, 1972:155–203.
157. Buns WH. Viral antigens. In: Notkins AL, ed. *Viral Immunology and immunopathology*. New York: Academic Press, 1975:43–56.
158. Wilfert CM, Buckley RH, Mohanakumar T, et al. Persistent and fatal central nervous system echovirus infections in patients with agammaglobulinemia. *N Engl J Med* 1977;296:1485–9.
159. Brunell PA, Ross A, Miller L, Kuo B. Prevention of varicella by zoster immune globulin. *N Engl J Med* 1981;280:1191–4.
160. Orenstein WA, Heyman DL, Ellis RJ, et al. Prophylaxis of varicella in high-risk children: dose response of zoster immune globulin. *J Pediatr* 1981;98:368–73.
161. Hirsch RL. The complement system: its importance in the host response to viral infection. *Microbiol Rev* 1982;46:71–85.
162. Sissons JGP, Oldstone MBA. Killing of virus-infected cells: the role of antiviral antibody and complement in limiting virus infection. *J Infect Dis* 1980;142:442–8.
163. Sissons JGP, Oldstone MBA, Schreiber RD. Antibody independent activation of the alternative complement pathway by measles virus infected cells. *Proc Natl Acad Sci USA* 1980;77:559–62.
164. Hicks JT, Ennis FA, Kim E, Verbonitz M. The importance of an intact complement pathway in recovery from a primary viral infection. Influenza in decomplemented and C5 deficient mice. *J Immunol* 1978;121:1437–44.
165. Hirsch RL, Griffin DE, Winkelstein JA. The role of complement in viral infections. II. The clearance of Sindbis virus from the blood stream and central nervous system of mice depleted of complement. *J Infect Dis* 1980;141:212–7.
166. Miller A, Morse HC, Winkelstein JA, Nathanson N. The role of antibody in recovery from experimental rabies. I. Effect of depletion of B and T cells. *J Immunol* 1978;121:321–6.
167. Drew WL, Miner RC, Ziegler JL, et al. Cytomegalovirus and Kaposi's sarcoma in young homosexual men. *Lancet* 1982;2:125–8.
168. Hirsch MS. Herpes group virus infections in the compromised host. In: Rubin RH, Young L, eds. *Clinical approach to infection in the immunocompromised host*. New York: Plenum, 1981:389–415.
169. Nahmias AJ, Griffith D, Salsbury C, Yoshida K. Thymic aplasia with lymphopenia, plasma cells, and normal immunoglobulins: relation to measles virus infection. *JAMA* 1967;201:729–34.
170. Siegal RP, Lopez C, Hammer GS, et al. Severe

acquired immunodeficiency in male homosexuals, manifested by chronic perianal ulcerative herpes simplex lesions. *N Engl J Med* 1981;305:1439–44.

171. Hirsch MS, Murphy FA. Effects of antilymphoid sera on viral infections. *Lancet* 1968;2:37–40.
172. Nahmias AJ, Hirsch MS, Kramer JM, Murphy FA. Effect of antithymocyte serum on herpesvirus hominis (type 1) infection in adult mice. *Proc Soc Exp Biol Med* 1969;132:696–8.
173. Blanden RV. Mechanisms of recovery from a generalized viral infection: mousepox. II. Passive transfer of recovery mechanisms with immune lymphoid cells. *J Exp Med* 1971; 133:1074–89.
174. Zinkernagal RM, Doherty PC. MHC restricted cytotoxic T cells: studies on the biological role of polymorphic major transplantation antigens determining T cell restriction specificity, function, and responsiveness. *Adv Immunol* 1979;27:51–177.
175. Stevens DA, Merigan TC. Interferon, antibody and other host factors in herpes zoster. *J Clin Invest* 1972;51:1170–8.
176. Kreth HW, Kress L, Kress HG, Ott HF, Eckert G. Demonstration of primary cytotoxic T cells in venous blood and cerebrospinal fluid of children with mumps meningitis. *J Immunol* 1982;128:2411–4.
177. Kreth HW, ter Meulen V, Eckert G. Demonstration of HLA restricted killer cells in patients with acute measles. *Med Microbiol Immunol* 1979;165:203–14.
178. McMichael A, Askonas B. Influenza virus specific cytotoxic T cells in man: induction and properties of the cytotoxic cell. *Eur J Immunol* 1978;8:705–10.
179. Schooley RT, Haynes BF, Grouse J, et al. Development of suppressor T-lymphocytes for Epstein-Barr virus-induced B-lymphocyte outgrowth during acute infectious mononucleosis. *Blood* 1981;57:510–7.
180. Shaw S, Biddison WE. HLA-linked genetic control of the specificity of human cytotoxic T-cell responses to influenza virus. *J Exp Med* 1979;149:565–75.
181. Sissons JGP, Oldstone MBA. Killing of virus-infected cells by cytotoxic lymphocytes. *J Infect Dis* 1980;142:114–9.
182. Thorley-Lawson DA, Chess L, Strominger JL. Suppression of *in vitro* Epstein-Barr virus infection. *J Exp Med* 1977;146:495–508.
183. Fenner F. Global eradication of smallpox. *Rev Infect Dis* 1982;4:916–22.
184. Wildy P, Gell PGH, Rhodes J, Newton A. Inhibition of herpes simplex virus multiplication by activated macrophages: a role for arginase. *Infect Immun* 1981;37:40–5.
185. Chapes SK, Tompkins WAF. Distribution of macrophage cytotoxic (MP) and macrophage helper (MP) functions on BSA discontinuous gradients. *J Reticuloendothel Soc* 1981;30:517–30.
186. Levin MJ, Rinaldo CR Jr, Leary PL, Zaia JA, Hirsch MS. Immune response to herpes virus antigens in adults with acute cytomegalovirus mononucleosis. *J Infect Dis* 1979;140:851–7.
187. Rinaldo CR Jr, Black PH, Hirsch MS. Virus-leukocyte interactions in cytomegalovirus mononucleosis. *J Infect Dis* 1977;136:667–8.
188. Bishop JM. Cancer genes come of age. *Cell* 1983;32:1018–20.
189. Rinaldo CR Jr, Stossel TP, Black PH, Hirsch MS. Leukocyte function during cytomegalovirus mononucleosis. *Clin Immunol Immunopathol* 1979;12:331–4.
190. Braun EW, Nankervis G. Cytomegalovirus viremia and bacteremia in renal allograft recipients. *N Engl J Med* 1978;299:1318–9.
191. Rubin RH, Cosimi AB, Tolkoff-Rubin NE, Russell PS, Hirsch MS. Infectious disease syndromes attributable to cytomegalovirus and their significance among renal transplant recipients. *Transplantation* 1977;24:458–64.
192. Schooley RT, Hirsch MS, Colvin RB, et al. Association of herpesgroup virus infections with T-lymphocyte subset alterations, glomerulopathy, and opportunistic infections following renal transplantation. *N Engl J Med* 1983;308:307–13.
193. Carney WP, Jacoviello VR, Hirsch MS, Starr SE, Fleisher G, Plotkin SA. T lymphocyte subsets and lymphocyte responses following immunization with cytomegalovirus vaccine. *J Infect Dis* 1983;147:158.
194. Carney WP, Rubin RH, Hoffman RA, Hansen WP, Healey K, Hirsch MS. Analysis of T lymphocyte subsets in cytomegalovirus mononucleosis. *J Immunol* 1981;126:2114–6.
195. Barré-Sinoussi F, Chermann JC, Rey F, et al. Isolation of a T-lymphotropic retrovirus from a patient at risk for acquired immune deficiency syndrome (AIDS). *Science* 1983;220:868–71.
196. Popovic M, Sarngadharan MG, Read E, Gallo RC. Detection, isolation, and continuous production of cytopathic retroviruses (HTLV-IUII) from patients with AIDS and pre-AIDS. *Science* 1984;224:497–500.
197. Gottlieb MS, Schroff R, Schanker HM, et al. Pneumocystis carinii pneumonia and mucosal candidiasis in previously healthy homosexual men: evidence of a new acquired cellular immunodeficiency. *N Engl J Med* 1981;305:1425–31.
198. Fauci AS. The human immunodeficiency virus: infectivity and mechanisms of pathogenesis. *Science* 1988;239:617–22.
199. Murray JL, Hersh EM, Reuben JM, et al. Abnormal lymphocyte response to exogenous interleukin-2 in homosexuals with acquired immune deficiency syndrome (AIDS) and AIDS related complex (ARC). *Clin Exp Immunol* 1985;60:25–30.
200. Prince HE, Kermani-Arab V, Fahey JL. Depressed interleukin-2 receptor expression in acquired immune deficiency and lymphadenopathy syndromes. *J Immunol* 1984;133:1313–7.

201. Ciobanu N, Welte K, Kruger G, et al. Defective T-cell response to PHA and mitogenic monoclonal antibodies in male homosexuals with acquired immunodeficiency syndrome and its *in vitro* correction by interleukin 2. *J Clin Immunol* 1983;3:332–40.
202. Kirkpatrick CH, Davis KC, Horsburgh CR Jr, Cohn DL, Penley K, Judson FN. Interleukin-2 production by persons with generalized lymphadenopathy syndrome or the acquired immune deficiency syndrome. *J Clin Immunol* 1985;5:31–7.
203. Nokta MA, Pollard RB. Differential reconstitution of zidovudine-induced inhibition of mitogenic responses by interleukin-2 in peripheral blood mononuclear cells from patients with the acquired immunodeficiency syndrome. *Antiviral Res* 1989;11:191–202.
204. Murray HW, Rubin BY, Masur H, Roberts RB. Impaired production of lymphokines and immune (gamma) interferon in the acquired immunodeficiency syndrome. *New Engl J Med* 1984;310:883–9.
205. Nokta MA, Pollard RB. Patterns of interferon-γ production by peripheral blood mononuclear cells from patients with acquired immunodeficiency syndrome (submitted).
206. Roberts HJ Jr. Different effects of influenza virus, respiratory syncytial virus, and Sendai virus on human lymphocytes and macrophages. *Infect Immun* 1982;35:1142–6.
207. Arneborn P, Biberfeld G. T lymphocyte subpopulations in relation to immunosuppression in measles and varicella. *Infect Immun* 1983; 39:29–37.
208. Veltri RW, Kikta VA, Wainwright WH, Sprinkle PM. Biologic and molecular characterization of the IgG serum blocking factor (SBF-IgG) isolated from sera of patients with EBV-induced infectious mononucleosis. *J Immunol* 1981;127:320–8.
209. Randrup A, Bro-Jorgensen K, Lokke, B. Lymphocytic choriomeningitis virus-induced immunosuppression: evidence for viral interference with T cell maturation. *Infect Immun* 1982;37:981–6.
210. Profitt MR, Hirsch MS, Gheridian B, McKenzie IFC, Black PH. Immunological mechanisms in the pathogenesis of virus-induced murine leukemia. I. Autoreactivity. *Int J Cancer* 1975;15:221–9.
211. Durack DT. Opportunistic infections and Kaposi's sarcoma in homosexual men. *N Engl J Med* 1981;305:1465–7.
212. Brinton MA, Nathanson N. Genetic determinants of virus susceptibility: epidemiologic implications of murine models. *Epidemiol Rev* 1981;3:115–39.
213. Darnell MB, Koprowski H. Genetically determined resistance to infection with group B arboviruses. II. Increased production of interfering particles in cell cultures from resistant mice. *J Infect Dis* 1974;129:248–56.
214. Haller O. Inborn resistance of mice to orthomyxoviruses. In: Haller O, ed. *Natural resistance to tumors and viruses*. Berlin: Springer-Verlag, 1981:25.
215. Teich N, Wyke J, Mak T, Bernstein A, Hardy W. Pathogenesis of retrovirus-induced disease. In: Weiss R, Teich N, Varmus H, Coffin J, eds. *Molecular biology of tumor viruses: RNA tumor viruses*. 2nd ed. New York: Cold Spring Harbor Laboratory, 1982:785.
216. Kumar V, Bennett M. Mechanisms of genetic resistance to Friend virus leukemia in mice. II. Resistance of mitogen-responsive lymphocytes mediated by marrow-dependent cells. *J Exp Med* 1976;143:713–27.
217. Oldstone MBA, Jensen F, Dixon FJ, Lampert PW. Pathogenesis of the slow disease of the central nervous system associated with wild mouse virus. II. Role of virus and host gene products. *Virology* 1980;107:180–93.
218. Lodmell DL. Genetic control of resistance to street rabies virus in mice. *J Exp Med* 1983;157:451–60.
219. Baringer JR. Herpes simplex infection of nervous tissue in animals and man. *Prog Med Virol* 1975;20:1–26.
220. Youssoufian H, Hammer SH, Hirsch MS, Mulder C. Methylation of the viral genome in an *in vitro* model of herpes simplex virus latency. *Proc Natl Acad Sci USA* 1981;79:2207–10.
221. Joseph BS, Oldstone MBA. Immunologic injury in measles virus infection: II. Suppression of immune injury through antigen modulation. *J Exp Med* 1975;142:864–76.
222. Oldstone MBA, Tishor A. Immunologic injury in measles virus infection. IV. Antigenic modulation and abrogation of lymphocyte lysis of virus-infected cells. *Clin Immunol Immunopathol* 1978:9:55–62.
223. Peterson PK, Balfour HH, Marker SC, et al. Cytomegalovirus disease in renal allograft recipients: a prospective study of the clinical features, risk factors, and impact on renal transplantation. *Medicine* 1980;59:283–300.
224. Marker SC, Howard RJ, Simmons RL, et al. Cytomegalovirus infection: a quantitative prospective study of 320 consecutive renal transplants. *Surgery* 1981;89:660–71.
225. Drummer SJ, Hardy A, Poorsattar A, Ho M. Early infections in kidney, heart, and liver transplant recipients on cyclosporine. *Transplantation* 1983;36:259–67.
226. Stover DE, White DA, Romano PA, et al. Spectrum of pulmonary diseases associated with the acquired immunodeficiency syndrome. *Am J Med* 1985;78:429–37.
227. Wallace JM, Hannah J. Cytomegalovirus pneumonitis in patients with AIDS. *Chest* 1985;9212:198–203.
228. Quinan GV Jr, Masur H, Rook AH, et al. Herpes virus infections in the acquired immune deficiency syndrome. *JAMA* 1984;252:72–76.
229. Nash G, Fligiel S. Pathologic features of the lung in the acquired immune deficiency syn-

drome (AIDS): an autopsy study of seventeen homosexual males. *Am J Clin Pathol* 1983;81:6–12.

230. ter Meulen V, Katz M, Muller D. Subacute sclerosing panencephalitis: a review. *Curr Top Microbiol Immunol* 1972;57:1–38.
231. Joseph BS, Oldstone MBA. Immunologic injury in measles virus infection. IV. Antigenic modulation and abrogation of lymphocyte lysis of virus-infected cells. *Clin Immunol Immunopathol* 1975;9:55–62.
232. Oldstone MBA, Tishon A. Immunologic injury in measles virus infection. IV. Antigenic modulation and abrogation of lymphocyte lysis of virus-infected cells. *Clin Immunol Immunopathol* 1978;9:55–62.
233. Wear DJ, Rapp F. Latent measles virus infection of the hamster central nervous system. *J Immunol* 1971;107:1593–8.
234. Albrecht P, Burnstein T, Klutch MJ, Hicks JT, Ennis FA. Subacute sclerosing panencephalitis: experimental infection in primates. *Science* 1977;195:64–6.
235. Rammohan KW, McFarland HF, McFarlin DE. Induction of subacute murine measles encephalitis by monoclonal antibody to virus haemagglutinin. *Nature* 1981;290:588–9.
236. Rammohan KW, McFarland HF, McFarlin DE. Subacute sclerosing panencephalitis after passive immunization and natural measles infection: role of antibody in persistence of measles virus. *Neurology* 1982;32:390–4.
237. Weller TH, Stoddard MB. Intranuclear inclusion bodies in cultures of human tissue inoculated with varicella vesicle fluid. *J Immunol* 1952;68:311–9.
238. School Epidemics Committee of Great Britain. *Epidemics in schools*. Medical Research Council, Special Report Series No. 227. London: His Majesty's Stationery Office, 1938.
239. Schmidt NJ, Lennette EH. Neutralizing antibody responses to varicella-zoster virus. *Infect Immun* 1975;12:606–13.
240. Lehmann-Grube F. *Lymphocytic choriomeningitis virus*. New York: Springer-Verlag, 1971.
241. Oldstone MBA, Dixon FJ. Immune complex disease in chronic viral infections. *J Exp Med* 1971;134:32–40.
242. Sergent JS, Lockshin MD, Christian CL, Gocke DJ. Vasculitis with hepatitis B antigenemia. *Medicine* 1976;55:1–18.
243. Gold E, Nankervis GA. Cytomegalovirus. In: Evans AS, ed. *Viral infections of humans*. New York and London: Plenum Medical Book Company, 1982:167–85.
244. Larke RPB, Wjeatley E, Saigal S, et al. Congenital cytomegalovirus infection in an urban Canadian community. *J Infect Dis* 1980;162:641–53.
245. Rowe WP, Hartleh JW, Cramblett MG, et al. Detection of human salivary gland virus in the mouth and urine of children. *Am J Hyg* 1958;67:57–65.
246. Stern H. Isolation of cytomegalovirus and clinical manifestations of infection at different ages. *Br Med J* 1968;1:665–9.
247. Levinsohn EM, Foy HM, Kenny GE, et al. Isolation of cytomegalovirus from a cohort of 100 infants throughout the first year of life. *Proc Soc Exp Biol Med* 1969;32:957–62.
248. Olson LC, Ketusinha R, Mansuwan P. Respiratory tract excretion of cytomegalovirus in Thai children. *J Pediatr* 1970;77:499–504.
249. Leinikki R, Heinonen K, Pettay O. Incidence of cytomegalovirus infections in early childhood. *Scand J Infect Dis* 1972;4:1–5.
250. Li F, Hanshaw JB. Cytomegalovirus among migrant children. *Am J Epidemiol* 1967;88:137–41.
251. Hirsch MS, Black PH. Activation of mammalian leukemia viruses. *Adv Virus Res* 1974;19:265–313.
252. Hirsch MS, Black PH, Tracy GS, Leibowitz S, Schwartz RS. Leukemia virus activation in chronic allogeneic disease. *Proc Natl Acad Sci USA* 1970;67:914–7.
253. Gajdusek DG. Unconventional viruses and the origin and disappearance of Kuru. *Science* 1977;197:943–59.
254. Kimberlin RH. Scrapie agent: prions or virinos? *Nature* 1982;297:107–8.
255. Prusiner SB. Novel proteinaceous infectious particles cause scrapie. *Science* 1982;216:136–44.
256. Ter Meulen V, Hall WW. Slow virus infections of the nervous system: virological, immunological and pathogenetic considerations. *J Gen Virol* 1978;41:1–15.
257. Narayan O, Penney JB Jr, Johnson RT, Herndon RM, Weiner LP. The etiology of progressive multifocal leukoencephalopathy: identification of virus in brains of 13 patients. *N Engl J Med* 1973;289:1278–82.
258. Gallo RC, Wong-Staal F. Retroviruses as etiologic agents of some animal and human leukemias and lymphomas and as tools for elucidating the molecular mechanism of leukemogenesis. *Blood* 1981;60:545–57.
259. Poiesz BJ, Ruscetti FW, Gazdar AF, Bunn PA, Minna JD, Gallo RC. Isolation of type-C retrovirus particles from cultured and fresh lymphocytes of a patient with cutaneous T cell-lymphoma. *Proc Natl Acad Sci USA* 1980;77: 7415–9.
260. Popovic M, Sarin PS, Robert-Gurroff M, et al. Isolation and transmission of human retrovirus (human T cell leukemia virus). *Science* 1982;219:856–9.
261. Snydman DR, Rudders RA, Daoust P, Sullivan JL, Evans AS. Infectious mononucleosis in an adult progressing to fatal immunoblastic lymphoma. *Ann Intern Med* 1982;96:737–42.
262. Desgranges C, Wolf H, de-Thé G, et al. Nasopharyngeal carcinoma. X. Presence of Epstein-Barr genomes in epithelial cells of tumors from high and medium risk areas. *Int J Cancer* 1975;16:7–15.
263. Desgranges C, Wolf H, Zur Hausen H, de-Thé

G. Further studies on the detection of the Epstein-Barr viral DNA on nasopharyngeal carcinoma biopsies from different parts of the world. In: de-Thé G, Epstein MA, Zur Hausen H, eds. *Oncogenesis and herpesviruses II, vol. 2*. IARC Scientific Publication No. 11. Lyon: IARC, 1975:191–3.
264. Alward WLM, McMahon BJ, Hall DB, Heyward WL, Francis DP, Bender TR. The long-term serological course of asymptomatic hepatitis B virus carriers and the development of primary hepatocellular carcinoma. *J Infect Dis* 1985;151:4.
265. Miller RH, Lee S-C, Liaw Y-F, Robinson WS. Hepatitis B viral DNA in infected human liver and in hepatocellular carcinoma. *J Infect Dis* 1985;151:6.
266. Zur Hausen H. Human papillomaviruses: why are some types carcinogenic? In: *Concepts in viral pathogenesis, vol. 2*. New York: Springer-Verlag, 1986:288–97.
267. Galloway DA, McDougall JK. The oncogenic potential of herpes simplex viruses: evidence for a hit-and-run mechanism. *Nature* 1983; 302:21–4.
268. Rapp F. Transformation by herpes simplex virus. In: Nahmias AS, Dowdle WR, Schinazi RF, eds. *The human herpesviruses*. New York: Elsevier, 1982:221–7.
269. Nelson JA, Fleckenstein B, Galloway DA, McDougall JK. Transformation of NIH 3T3 cells with cloned fragments of human cytomegalovirus strain AD 169. *J Virol* 1982;43:83–91.
270. Geder L, Lausch R, O'Neill F, Rapp F. Oncogenic transformation of human embryo lung cells by human cytomegalovirus. *Science* 1976; 192:1134–7.
271. Rapp F, Geder L, Murasko D, et al. Long-term persistence of cytomegalovirus genome in cultured human cells of prostatic origin. *J Virol* 1975;16:982–90.
272. Huang E-S, Roche JK. Cytomegalovirus DNA and adenocarcinoma of the colon: evidence for latent viral infection. *Lancet* 1978;1:957–60.
273. Croce CM, Nowell PC. Molecular basis of human B cell neoplasia. *Blood* 1985;65:1–7.
274. Leder P, Battey J, Lenoir G, et al. Translocations among antibody genes in human cancer. *Science* 1983;222:765.
275. Rabbitts TH, Foster A, Hamlyn P, Baer R. Effect of somatic mutation within translocated c-*myc* genes in Burkitt's lymphoma. *Nature* 1984;309:592.
276. Gilman AG. G proteins and dual control of adenylate cyclase. *Cell* 1984;36:577–9.
277. Shepherd GM. Olfactory transcution: welcome whiff of biochemistry. *Nature* 1985;316:214–5.
278. Doolittle RF, Hunkapiller MV, Hood LE, et al. Simian sarcoma virus *onc* gene, v-*sis*, is derived from the gene (or genes) encoding a platelet-derived growth factor. *Science* 1983;221:275–7.
279. Waterfield MD, Scrace GT, Whittle N, et al. Platelet-derived growth factor is structurally related to the putative transforming protein p28 of simian sarcoma virus. *Nature* 1983;304:35–9.
280. Downward J, Yarden Y, Mayes E, et al. Close similarity of epidermal growth factor receptor and v-*erbB* oncogene protein sequences. *Nature* 1984;307:521–7.
281. Sherr CJ, Rettenmier CW, Sacca R, Roussel MF, Look AT, Stanley ER. The c-*fms* proto-oncogene product is related to the receptor for the mononuclear phagocyte growth factor, CSF-1. *Cell* 1985;41:665–76.
282. Notkins AL, Rosenthal J, Johnson B. Rate-zonal centrifugation of herpes simplex virus-antibody complexes. *Virology* 1971;43:321–5.
283. Hirsch MS, Allison AC, Harvey JJ. Immune complexes in mice infected neonatally with Moloney leukaemogenic and murine sarcoma viruses. *Nature* 1969;223:739–40.
284. Almedia J, Waterson AP. Immune complexes in hepatitis. *Lancet* 1969;2:983–6.
285. Richardson WP, Colvin RB, Cheeseman SH, et al. Glomerular damage associated with cytomegalovirus: a cause of renal failure in allografts. *N Engl J Med* 1980;305:57–63.
286. Stagno S, Volanakis JE, Reynolds DW, Stroud R, Alfrod CA. Immune complexes in congenital and natal cytomegalovirus infections of man. *J Clin Invest* 1977;60:838–45.
287. Pardo V, Meneses R, Ossa L, Jaffe DJ, et al. AIDS-related glomerulopathy: Occurrence in specific risk groups. *Kidney Int* 1987;31:1167–73.
288. Alspaugh M, Henle G, Lennette E, Henle W. Elevated levels of antibodies to Epstein-Barr virus antigens in sera and synovial fluid of patients with rheumatoid arthritis. *J Clin Invest* 1981;67:1134–40.
289. Musiani M, Zerbani M, Ferri S, Plazzi M, Gentiliomi G, La Place M. Comparison of the immune response to Epstein-Barr virus and cytomegalovirus in sera and synovial fluids of patients with rheumatoid arthritis. *Ann Rheum Dis* 1987;46:837–42.
290. Stastny P. Association of the B cell alloantigen DRw4 with rheumatoid arthritis. *N Engl J Med* 1978;298:869–71.
291. Woodrow JC, Nichol FE, Zaphiropoulos G. DR antigens and rheumatoid arthritis: a study of two populations. *Br Med J* 1981;283:1287–8.
292. Roudier J, Rhodes G, Peterson J, Vaughan JH, Carson DA. The Epstein-Barr virus glycoprotein gp110, a molecular link between HLA DR4, HLA DR1, and rheumatoid arthritis. *Scand J Immunol* 1988;27:367–71.
293. Johnson TM, Duvic M, Rapini RP, Rios A. AIDS exacerbated psoriasis [Letter]. *N Engl J Med* 1985;313:1415.
294. Winchester R, Bernstein DH, Fischer HD, et al. The co-occurrence of Reiter's syndrome and acquired immunodeficiency. *Ann Intern Med* 1987;106:19–26.
295. Solinger AM, Adams LE, Friedman-Kjien AE, Hess EV. Acquired immune deficiency syn-

drome (AIDS) and autoimmunity—mutually exclusive entities? *J Clin Immunol* 1988;8:32–42.

296. Kopelman RG, Pazner-Zolla S. Association of human immunodeficiency virus infection and autoimmune phenomena. *Am J Med* 1988; 84:82–8.
297. Nathanson N, Monjan AA, Panitch HS, Johnson ED, Petersson G, Cole GA. Virus-induced cell-mediated immunopathological disease. In: Notkins AL, ed. *Viral immunology and immunopathology*. New York: Academic Press, 1975:357–91.
298. Pfau CJ, Valenti JK, Pevear DC, Hunt KD. Lymphocytic choriomeningitis virus killer T cells are lethal only in weakly disseminated murine infections. *J Exp Med* 1982;156:76–89.
299. Gilden DH, Cole GA, Nathanson N. Immunopathogenesis of acute central nervous system disease produced by lymphocytic choriomeningitis virus. II. Adaptive immunization of virus carriers. *J Exp Med* 1972;135:874–89.
300. Kirchner H, Kleinicke C, Northoff H. Replication of herpes simplex virus in human peripheral T lymphocytes. *J Gen Virol* 1977;37:647–9.
301. Naragi S, Jackson GG, Jonasson OM. Viremia with herpes simplex type I in adults. *Ann Intern Med* 1976;85:165–9.
302. Craig CP, Nahmias AJ. Different patterns of neurologic involvement with herpes simplex virus types 1 and 2: isolation of herpes simplex virus type 2 from the buffy coat of two adults with meningitis. *J Infect Dis* 1973;127:365–72.
303. Rinaldo CR Jr, Richter S, Black PH, Callery R, Chess L, Hirsch MS. Replication of herpes simplex virus and cytomegalovirus in human leukocytes. *J Immunol* 1978;120:123–36.
304. Joseph BS, Lampert PW, Oldstone MBA. Replication and persistence of measles virus in defined subpopulations of human lymphocytes. *J Virol* 1975;16:1638–49.
305. Chantler JK, Tingle AJ. Isolation of rubella virus from human lymphocytes after natural infection. *J Infect Dis* 1982;145:673–7.
306. Scott RM, Nisalak A, Cheamudon U, Seridhoranakul S, Nimmannitya S. Isolation of dengue viruses from peripheral blood leukocytes of patients with hemorrhagic fever. *J Infect Dis* 1980;141:1–6.
307. Andiman WA, Jacobson RI, Tucker G. Leukocyte-associated viremia with adenovirus type 2 in an infant with lower respiratory-tract disease. *N Engl J Med* 1977;297:100–1.
308. Fleisher B, Kreth HW. Mumps virus replication in human lymphoid cell lines and in peripheral blood lymphocytes: preference for T cells. *Infect Immun* 1981;35:25–31.
309. Daughaday CC, Brandt WE, McCown JM, Russell PK. Evidence for two mechanisms of dengue virus infection of adherent human monocytes: trypsin-sensitive virus receptors and trypsin-resistant immune complex receptors. *Infect Immun* 1981;32:469–73.
310. Rodgers B, Mims CA. Interaction of influenza virus with mouse macrophages. *Infect Immun* 1981;31:751–7.
311. Couch RB. The effects of influenza on host defenses. *J Infect Dis* 1981;144:284–91.
312. Lucas CJ, Ubels-Postma J, Galama JMD, Rezee A. Studies on the mechanism of measles virus-induced suppression of lymphocyte functions *in vitro*. *Cell Immunol* 1978;37:448–58.
313. Hirsch MS, Ellis DA, Kelly AP, et al. Activation of C-type viruses during skin graft rejection of the mouse. *Int J Cancer* 1975;15:493–502.
314. Hirsch MS, Phillips SM, Solnik C, Black PH, Schwartz RS, Carpenter CB. Activation of murine leukemia viruses by mixed lymphocyte reactions *in vitro*. *Proc Natl Acad Sci USA* 1972;69:1069–72.
315. Cheung KS, Lang DJ. Transmission and activation of cytomegalovirus with blood transfusions: a mouse model. *J Infect Dis* 1977; 135:841–5.
316. Olding LB, Jensen FC, Oldstone MBA. Pathogenesis of cytomegalovirus infection. I. Activation of virus from bone marrow-derived lymphocytes by *in vitro* allogeneic reaction. *J Exp Med* 1975;141:561–2.
317. Wu BC, Dowling JN, Armstrong JA, Ho M. Enhancement of mouse cytomegalovirus infection during host versus graft reaction. *Science* 1975;190:56–8.
318. Partin JS, Schubert WK, Partin JC, Hammond JG. Serum salicylate concentrations in Reye's disease—a study of 130 biopsy-proven cases. *Lancet* 1982;1:191–4.
319. Starko KM, Ray G, Dominguez LB, Stromberg WL, Woodal DF. Reye's syndrome and salicylate. *Pediatrics* 1980;66:859–64.
320. Webster RG, Laver WG, Air GM, Schild GC. Molecular mechanisms of variation in influenza viruses. *Nature* 1982;296:115–21.
321. Kono Y, Kobayashi K, Fukunaga Y. Antigenic drift of equine infectious anemia virus in chronically infected horses. *Archiv Virusforchung* 1973;41:1–10.
322. Narayan O, Griffin DE, Chase J. Antigenic shift of visna virus in persistently infected sheep. *Science* 1977;1975:376–8.
323. Saag MS, Hahn BH, Gibbons J, Li Y, et al. Extensive variation of human immunodeficiency virus type 1 *in vivo*. *Nature* 1988;334:440–4.
324. Greenberg SB, Hannon MW, Couch RB, et al. Prophylactic effect of low doses of human leukocyte interferon against infection with rhinovirus. *J Infect Dis* 1982;145:542.
325. Higgins PG, Al-Nakib W, Willman J, et al. Interferon-$\beta_{ser}$ as prophylaxis against experimental rhinovirus infection in volunteers. *J Interferon Res* 1986;6:153.
326. Solov'ev VD. The results of controlled observations on the prophylaxis of influenza with interferon. *Bull WHO* 1969;41:683.
327. Dolin R, Betts R, Treanor J, et al. Intranasally administered rIFN-$\alpha$ as prophylaxis against experimentally induced influenza in man [Ab-

stract]. In: *Proceedings of the 13th International Congress of Chemotherapy*. 1983.
328. DeKoning EWJ, van Bijsterveld OP, Cantell K. Combination therapy for dendritic keratitis with acyclovir and interferon-α. *Arch Ophthalmol* 1983;101:1866.
329. Vannini A, Cembrano S, Assetto V, et al. Interferon-β treatment of herpes simplex keratitis. *Ophthalmologica* 1986;192:6.
330. Vesterinen E, Meyer B, Purola E, et al. Treatment of vaginal flat condyloma with interferon cream. *Lancet* 1984;1:157.
331. Schouten TJ, Weimar W, Bos JH, et al. Treatment of juvenile laryngeal papillo-matosis with two types of interferon. *Laryngoscope* 1982;92:686.
332. Berman B, Davis-Reed L, Silverstein L, et al. Treatment of verrucae vulgaris with $\alpha_2$-interferon. *J Infect Dis* 1986;154:328.
333. Alawattegama AB, Kinghorn GR. Boweroid dysplasia in human papillomavirus-16 DNA positive flat condylomas during interferon-β treatment. (Letter) *Lancet* 1984;1:1468.
334. Scott GM, Csonka GW. Effect of injections of small doses of human fibroblast interferon into genital warts. A pilot study. *Br J Vener Dis* 1979;55:442.
335. Vance JC, Bart BJ, Hansen RC, et al. Intralesional recombinant alpha-2 interferon for the treatment of patients with condyloma acuminatum or verruca plantaris. *Arch Dermatol* 1986;122:272.
336. Haglund S, Lundquist P, Cantell K, et al. Interferon therapy in juvenile laryngeal papillomatosis. *Arch Otolaryngol* 1981;107:327.
337. Lundquist P-G, Haglund S, Carlsoo B, et al. Interferon therapy in juvenile laryngeal papillomatosis. *Otolaryngology* 1984;92:386.
338. Hoofnagle JH, Mullen KD, Peters M, et al. *Biology of the interferon system*. New York: Elsevier Science Publishers, 1985:493.
339. Carter WA, Dolen JG, Leong SS, et al. Interferon and hepatitis infection: current results and possible amplification of the therapeutic response. In: Kahn A, Hill NO, Dorn GL, eds. *Interferon: properties and clinical uses*. Dallas, Texas: Leland Fikes Foundation, 1988:693.
340. Omata M, Imazeki F, Yokosuka O, et al. Recombinant leukocyte A interferon treatment in patients with chronic hepatitis B virus infections: pharmacokinetics, tolerance, and biologic effects. *Gastroenterology* 1985;88:870.
341. Rizzetto M, Rosina F, Saracco G, et al. Treatment of chronic delta hepatitis with alpha-2 recombinant interferon. *J Hepatol* (in press).
342. Abrams DI, Volberding PA. Alpha interferon therapy of AIDS-associated Kaposi's sarcoma. AIDS Clinic, San Francisco General Hospital, California. *Semin Oncol* 1986;13:43.
343. Groopman JE, Gottlieb MS, Goodman J, et al. Recombinant alpha-2 interferon therapy for Kaposi's sarcoma associated with the acquired immunodeficiency syndrome. *Ann Intern Med* 1984;100:671.
344. Real FX, Krown SE, Krim M, et al. Treatment of Kaposi's sarcoma with recombinant leukocyte A interferon (rIFN-A). *Abstract Am Soc Chemother Oncol* 1984;1:55.
345. Whitley RJ, Alford CA, Hirsch MS, et al. Vidarabine versus acyclovir in herpes simplex encephalitis. *N Engl J Med* 1986;314:144–9.
346. Skoldenberg B, Forsgren M, Alestig K, et al. Acyclovir versus vidarabine in herpes simplex encephalitis. *Lancet* 1984;ii:707–11.
347. Mertz GJ. Diagnosis and treatment of genital herpes infections. *Infect Dis Clin N Am* 1987;1:341–66.
348. Tominack R, Hayden FG. Rimantadine hydrochloride and amantadine hydrochloride use in influenza A virus infections. *Infect Dis Clin N Am* 1987;1:459–78.
349. Knight V, Gilbert BE. Ribavirin aerosol treatment of influenza. *Infect Dis Clin N Am* 1987;1:441–58.
350. Rodriguez WJ, Parrott R. Ribavirin aerosol treatment of serious respiratory syncytial virus infection in infants. *Infect Dis Clin N Am* 1987;1:425–40.
351. McCormick JB, King IJ, Webb PA. Lassa fever: effective treatment with ribavirin. *N Eng J Med* 1986;314:20–6.
352. Hirsch MS, Kaplan JC. Treatment of human immunodeficiency virus infections. *Antimicrob Agents Chemother* 1987;31:839–43.
353. Mitsuya H, Weinhold KJ, Furman PA, St. Clair MH, et al. 3′-Azido-3′deoxythymidine (BWA509U): an antiviral agent that inhibits the infectivity and cytopathic effect of human T-lymphotropic virus type III/lymphadenopathy associate virus *in vitro*. *Proc Natl Acad Sci USA* 1985;82:7096–100.
354. Richman DD, Fischl MA, Grieco MH, et al. The toxicity of azidothymidine in the treatment of patients with AIDS and AIDS-related complex. A double-blind placebo-controlled trial. *N Engl J Med* 1987;317:192–7.
355. Gill PS, Rarick M, Brynes RK, Causey D, Loureiro C, Levine AM. Azidothymidine associated with bone marrow failure in the acquired immunodeficiency syndrome (AIDS). *Ann Intern Med* 1987;107:502–5.
356. Felsenstein D, Dimico D, Hirsch M, et al. Treatment of cytomegalovirus retinitis with 9-(2-hydroxy-l-(hydroxymethyl)propoxymethyl) guanine. *Ann Intern Med* 1985;103:377–80.
357. Erice A, Jordan C, Chace B, et al. Ganciclovir treatment of cytomegalovirus disease in transplant recipients and other immunocompromised hosts. *JAMA* 1987;257:3082–7.
358. Fenner F. Eradication and possible reintroduction of smallpox. In: *Concepts of viral pathogenesis*. New York: Springer-Verlag, 1986:339–44.
359. Krugman S, Katz SL, Gershon AA, Wilfert G. Measles. In: *Infectious diseases of children*. 8th ed. St. Louis: C.V. Mosby Co., 1985.
360. Cherry JD. Measles. In: Feigen RD, Cherry JD, eds. *Textbook of pediatric infectious dis-*

*eases*. 2nd ed. Philadelphia: W.B. Saunders Co., 1987.

361. McLean DM, Kettyls GDM, Hingston J, et al. Atypical measles following immunization with killed measles vaccine. *Can Med Assoc J* 1970;103:743–4.
362. Gokiert JG, Beamish WE. Altered reactivity to measles virus in previously vaccinated children. *Can Med Assoc J* 1970;203:724–7.
363. Buser F, Montagnon B. Severe illness in children exposed to natural measles after prior vaccination against the disease. *Scand J Infect Dis* 1970;2:157–260.
364. Linneman CC, Rotte TC, Schiff GM, Youtsey JL. A sero-epidemiologic study of a measles epidemic in a highly immunized population. *Am J Epidemiol* 1972;95:238–46.
365. Cherry JD, Feigen RD, Lobes LA, Shakelford PG. Atypical measles in children previously immunized with attenuated measles virus vaccines. *Pediatrics* 1972;50:712–7.
366. Krause PJ, Cherry JD, Naiditch MJ, Deseda-Tous J, Walbergh EJ. Revaccination of previous recipients of killed measles vaccine: clinical and immunologic studies. *J Pediatr* 1978;93:565–71.
367. Centers for Disease Control. Recommendations of the Immunization Practices Advisory Committee. Measles Prevention. *MMWR* 1987;36:409–18,423–25.
368. Takahashi M, Otsuka T, Okuno Y, Asano Y, Yazaki T, Isomura S. Live vaccine used to prevent the spread of varicella in children in hospital. *Lancet* 1974;2:1288.
369. Takahashi M, Asano Y, Kamiya H, Baba K, Yamanishi K. Active immunization for varicella-zoster virus. In: Nahmias AJ, Dowdle WR, Schinazi RE, eds. *Human herpes viruses*. New York: Elsevier, 1981:414.
370. Hattori A, Ihara T, Iwasa T, et al. Use of live varicella vaccine in children with acute leukemia or other malignancies. *Lancet* 1976;2:210.
371. Izawa T, Ihara T, Hattori A, et al. Application of a live varicella vaccine in children with acute leukemia or other malignant diseases. *Pediatrics* 1977;60:805.
372. Baba K, Yabuuchi H, Okumi H, Takahashi M. Studies with live varicella vaccine and inactivated skin test antigen: Protective effect of the vaccine and clinical application of the skin test. *Pediatrics* 1978;61:550.
373. Asaano Y, Nagai T, Miyata T, et al. Long-term protective immunity of recipients of the OKA strain of varicella vaccine. *Pediatrics* 1985;75:667.

*Antiviral Agents and Viral Diseases of Man, 3rd Edition*,
edited by G. J. Galasso, R. J. Whitley, and
T. C. Merigan, Raven Press, Ltd., New York © 1990.

# 3

# Preclinical Evaluation of Antiviral Agents: *In Vitro* and Animal Model Testing

Earl R. Kern

*Departments of Pediatrics, Comparative Medicine, and Microbiology, School of Medicine, University of Alabama at Birmingham, Birmingham, Alabama 35294*



In recent years, there has been renewed interest in the development of new drugs for the treatment of viral infections. This level of interest, which is at an all time high, was precipitated by four major developments: (a) the landmark studies with adenine arabinoside (ara-A, vidarabine, Vira-A), which first demonstrated that an antiviral could indeed alter the course of herpes encephalitis, neonatal herpes, and herpes zoster; (b) the development and licensure of acyclovir [Zovirax (ACV)] for treatment of severe herpes simplex virus (HSV) infections; (c) the appearance of a new fatal disease, acquired immunodeficiency syndromes (AIDS), which was subsequently shown to be caused by a retrovirus, human immunodeficiency virus (HIV); and (d) the rapid development and approval of azidothymidine [zidovudine (AZT)] for treatment of HIV infections.

The development of Vira-A and ACV was very important to the field of antiviral chemotherapy because it occurred at a time when the pharmaceutical industry had lost much of its interest and confidence that a drug for serious HSV infections could be developed. Although therapy for severe HSV infections is still not optimal, the development of these drugs sent a clear message to the antiviral research community that it was in fact possible to alter or modify the course of these diseases. The end result of these partial successes was that it stimulated new interest to develop antivirals that would be superior to ACV in treatment of HSV infections.

The highest level of stimulation in the history of the field of antiviral research came with the recognition of the disease syndromes caused by HIV. These infections not only resulted in a fatal disease but had a protracted clinical course spanning a number of years, allowing a reasonable amount of time for the use of a chemotherapeutic agent. The rapid development of AZT and the demonstration that this drug could ameliorate the symptoms of AIDS played a large role in renewing interest in the development of new and more effective antiviral agents. This renewed interest has motivated companies with historical interests in developing antivirals to increase their commitment, and literally hundreds of new companies have been formed and committed research and development resources to this area. The end result is that thousands of new compounds are being synthesized that require evaluation for antiviral activity. Similar numbers of old compounds that were developed for other reasons such as anticancer agents now are being retested for activity against HIV. The testing of all these compounds represents an immense effort in an attempt to select those few compounds that have sufficient antiviral activity and acceptable toxicity to be evaluated in clinical trials.

The purpose of this chapter is to provide some guidelines for preclinical testing and review some of the *in vitro* and *in vivo* systems that have successfully identified antiviral agents which eventually were shown to have significant activity against virus diseases of humans.

## TARGET VIRUSES FOR ANTIVIRAL THERAPY

There are numerous viral diseases of humans that are potential targets for the development of new or better antiviral therapies. Those that are considered to have the greatest priority at the present time as well as the current state of effective therapy are summarized here to point out the need for continued development of better antiviral agents. The clinical aspects of these and other viral infections and their specific therapies are considered in greater detail in other chapters of this volume.

### Herpesviruses

ACV has been reported to be more effective than Vira-A for the treatment of herpes encephalitis (1), and is equivalent to Vira-A for therapy of neonatal herpes (2). It significantly alters primary genital herpes and other HSV infections of the immunocompromised host (3–6), and is suppressive of recurrent genital herpes episodes (7,8). In spite of these successes, there is still no optimal therapy for any of the infections caused by HSV. Importantly, ACV has no demonstrated activity against HSV in its latent state (8–10), and resistant mutants have been identified recently (11), particularly in patients with AIDS (12) or those who receive intense, long-term, courses of therapy. For cytomegalovirus (CMV) infections, ganciclovir [dihydroxy propoxymethyl guanine (DHPG)] has been shown to reduce the severity of CMV retinitis, gastrointestinal disease, and, to a lesser extent, pneumonia, (13–17) in AIDS and organ or bone marrow transplant patients. However, at least for retinitis, when therapy is discontinued the beneficial effect is soon lost. Additionally, there is still a need for more effective treatment of CMV infections in organ and bone marrow transplant recipients. Although it has been recommended that DHPG be approved for treatment of CMV infections, its efficacy in many of these viral syndromes has not been adequately documented in controlled clinical trials. Foscarnet has also been reported to be effective for treatment of CMV infections (18,19); however, the clinical benefit of this drug has not been assessed in controlled clinical trials. For varicella-zoster virus (VZV) infections, both Vira-A and ACV have been shown to reduce the severity of disease (20–24). Nevertheless, better therapies are still needed, particularly for postherpetic neuralgia and outpatient therapy of zoster. There have only been two clinical trials conducted for Epstein-Barr virus (EBV) infection, and ACV was not effective (25,26). At the present time, there has not been serious disease entities identified for human herpesvirus type 6 (HHV-6) (27), and there has been only limited *in vitro* testing of antiviral agents against this virus (28).

### Respiratory Viruses

With the exception of the ongoing development of rimantadine, which is a less toxic analog of the approved drug, amantadine (29), and the continued evaluation of ribavirin (30), there has been no new developments in the treatment of influenza infections. This disease remains an important therapeutic target. In respiratory syncytial virus (RSV) infections, aerosolized ribavirin has been demonstrated to alter the clinical and virological course of this disease (31); however, this mode of therapy is not optimal. The prophylaxis or postexposure use of interferons administered by the intranasal route has resulted in a reduction of disease severity in the common cold caused by rhinoviruses (32); however, this mode of therapy has a number of inherent problems.

### Retroviruses

The use of AZT in patients infected with HIV has resulted in a reduction in the severity of the clinical symptoms (33,34); however, the drug has a number of serious side effects such as the development of anemia and neutropenia (34). Additionally, it was reported recently that AZT resistant mutants are emerging (35). Although the implications of the development of resistance to AZT are unknown at the present time, it is a point of considerable concern and suggests that additional chemotherapeutic agents are needed. AIDS, because mortality is a virtual certainty, has become the number one target for antiviral development. At the present time, there are numerous new modes of therapy undergoing preclinical and clinical evaluation.

### Hepadnaviruses

Hepadnaviruses, which include hepatitis B and non-A, non-B hepatitis (hepatitis C), are an important cause of disease, particularly in developing countries. Although some of the interferon studies have shown efficacy against hepatitis B and C (see Chapter 9), these viral infections continue to be important targets for development of antiviral agents. This area has been hampered seriously by the lack of *in vitro* test systems and readily available animal models.

### Papillomaviruses

The incidence of genital warts caused by human papilloma viruses (HPV) continues to increase, and these infections are caused by a number of different subtypes of HPV (36). There is currently no proven mode of therapy for these infections, and their importance as an antiviral target is enhanced by the implication that these viruses may be involved in cervical dysplasia (37). Developments in this area have also been hampered by the lack of *in vitro* and *in vivo* test systems.

There are a number of other viral infections of humans that warrant development of antiviral therapy, including members of the enterovirus, togavirus, arenavirus, and rotavirus groups. However, these viral infections have been given a reduced priority compared to the ones presented above and will not be considered further in this chapter.

## *IN VITRO* SUSCEPTIBILITY TESTING

The first step in determining the potential of a test compound is to use an initial or primary screen to identify whether the compound has some degree of antiviral activity. Since primary screening often involves the testing of large numbers of compounds, the assay system used should be as automated as possible in order to reduce human resources required and supply costs. The initial screen should be kept as simple as possible, using a single method, one virus isolate for each virus group and a single cell line, preferably of human origin. There are a number of assay systems that can be utilized for primary screening. Most of these can be adapted to 96-well culture dishes such that drug dilutions can be accomplished by an automated diluter, stains or substrates added, and end points read photometrically. The data obtained from enzyme-linked immunosorbent assay (ELISA) plate readers can then be fed into a computer and the results analyzed. Two basic types of assay systems are used depending on whether the particular virus replicates in tissue culture cells and produces some type of cellular destruction or morphological change [cytopathic effect (CPE)]. For those viruses that produce CPE, the most commonly used assay systems are those that measure inhibition of CPE, focus formation, or syncytial formation. Nucleic acid hybridization has recently become available for viruses such as CMV or VZV that may take a long time in culture to produce CPE, or for viruses such as EBV or even perhaps HBV that do not produce CPE in cell culture systems but do replicate their DNA. Using radiolabeled DNA probes, this technique can be used readily to quantify drug/virus interactions. Other assay systems that do not depend on complete viral replication with the production of CPE instead monitor the synthesis of specific gene products encoded by the virus. Examples of these assay systems include the detection and drug inhibition of the production of virus proteins such as P24 for HIV and enzymes such as thymidine kinase, DNA polymerases, or reverse transcriptase. A potential disadvantage of these latter systems is that they do not reflect a drug effect on complete viral replication that involves a number of events, but focus only on a single molecular target. Although this may be a more selective approach, these assay systems may miss compounds that exert their activity on other targets.

Once an antiviral compound has been identified in one of the primary screening assays, this activity needs to be verified in other test systems. For confirmation of antiviral activity, it is important, whenever possible, that assay systems involving complete viral replication and damage to the host cell should be used. Although CPE inhibition or focus formation inhibition can be used, the assay system of choice is either a plaque or yield reduction assay wherever applicable. These two assay systems provide the best quantitative measure of a drug's inhibitory potency. The selection of an appropriate test system for the initial screen and confirmation of antiviral activity will depend on a number of factors, including the particular virus of interest, the number of samples to be tested, and the capabilities of the testing laboratory. Many different types of assay systems have been developed, giving an investigator a wide choice of assay systems. The advantages and disadvantages of a number of these assay systems have been reviewed recently (38) and will not be covered in detail here. Some guidelines that should be considered for *in vitro* antiviral testing are summarized in Table 1.

If human cells are not utilized in the primary screen, then the activity of a new drug should be confirmed in cells of human origin. It is well documented that some compounds vary considerably in their activity when tested in cells from different species (39,40). Activity of a new drug should also be verified against additional virus strains, including fresh clinical isolates, since laboratory passaged strains may not be representative of the majority of isolates (41,42).

**TABLE 1.** *General principles for* in vitro *antiviral testing*

| |
|---|
| Human cells must be used if possible; cells from other species should also be used. |
| Representative virus strains, both lab and clinical isolates, should be utilized. |
| Virus pools and cell lines must be free of adventitious agents (mycoplasma). |
| All assays must include a reference drug as a positive control; negative controls also should be included. |
| Relative sensitivity of virus to drug should be determined by more than one assay method. |
| Sufficient concentrations of drug need to be tested in order to calculate an accurate end point. |
| $ED_{50}$ and $ED_{90}$ values should be calculated. |
| Drug toxicity should be assessed in both stationary and rapidly proliferating cells. |
| Effect of drug on uninfected cells should be expressed as the ID, and $ID_{50}$ and $ID_{90}$ values calculated. |
| The relationship between efficacy ($ED_{50}$) and toxicity ($ID_{50}$) is expressed as SI, SI = $ID_{50}/ED_{50}$. |

When appropriate, a new compound should also be tested against known drug-resistant mutants. This information provides both a comparison with the drug to which the virus became resistant and also preliminary information about the mechanism of action of the new compound. For all test systems used to determine antiviral activity of a new compound, it is necessary to use sufficient drug concentrations that span an appropriate dose range in order to calculate an accurate effective dose ($ED_{50}$, $ED_{90}$, etc.). This is usually accomplished by utilizing some form of linear regression analysis, and there are numerous computer software programs that can be used or adapted for this purpose. It is important that an accurate effective dose be obtained as this value will be used in conjunction with its toxicity [inhibitory dose ($ID_{50}$, $ID_{90}$)] for the calculation of a selectivity index (SI), SI = $ID_{50}/ED_{50}$, which provides information regarding the specificity of the antiviral activity. All assays should be repeated with enough replicate test wells to ensure the accuracy of these values.

### Herpesviruses

As an example of how the various assay systems can be utilized, a scheme for determining antiviral activity against herpesviruses is shown in Table 2. It is relatively

**TABLE 2.** *Schematic for determining* in vitro *activity and toxicity of antiviral drugs for herpesviruses*

| |
|---|
| Primary screening system, human cells |
| Antiviral |
| HSV-1 or HSV-2: semi-automated CPE, inhibition assay |
| CMV: DNA-DNA hybridization |
| VZV: DNA-DNA hybridization |
| EBV: superinfection of Raji cells with P3HR-1; early antigen production |
| Toxicity: visual inspection of treated cells in each assay system, generally stationary cells; cell proliferation, rapidly growing cells |
| Confirmatory assay systems, human cells |
| Antiviral |
| HSV-1 or HSV-2: plaque reduction assay or yield reduction assay |
| CMV: plaque reduction assay or yield reduction assay |
| VZV: plaque reduction assay or yield reduction assay |
| EBV: P3HR-1 infection of B-lymphocyte cell lines; early antigen production |
| Toxicity: radiolabeled precursor uptake into DNA, RNA, or protein |
| Additional studies |
| Antiviral: determine activity in additional cell lines from other species, i.e., mice, rabbits, guinea pigs, primates; test sensitivity of other virus strains and clinical isolates; determine sensitivity of drug resistant mutants |
| Toxicity: clonogenic assays; peripheral blood leukocytes and bone marrow cells |

easy to assess the activity of antiviral compounds against HSV since it rapidly produces CPE in a variety of mammalian cells. Assays used to determine inhibition of CPE lend themselves well to automation (43,44) and are a logical choice for screening systems. For confirmation of antiviral activity, either a plaque reduction (45,46) or yield inhibition assay (46) is generally used. In addition to these classical methods, DNA hybridization (47) and ELISA assays (48) have also been used to quantify antiviral activity. The assay of choice is an individual one, depending on personal choice and laboratory capabilities. All the assay systems appear to have a similar level of sensitivity as long as the conditions of the assay—multiplicity of infection, time of harvest, etc.—are controlled rigidly. CMV strains are generally slow growing, and although they will form plaques in cell cultures, growth is usually not sufficiently rapid or lytic to use CPE inhibition assays for detection of antiviral activity. Thus, the assay systems of choice currently are the plaque reduction or yield reduction assay (49,50). Since these assays are time consuming and labor intensive, there is a need for more rapid assay systems to measure antiviral activity. A DNA hybridization assay has been described (51), and a test kit is available commercially (Diagnostic Hybrids, Athens, OH). Assays for determining antiviral activity against VZV strains have many of the same problems as those for CMV. Additionally, the use of plaque assay techniques is complicated by the fact that cell free virus stocks can not be maintained and cell-associated virus pools must be used, which results in some difficulty in standardizing the multiplicity of infection. Although a standard plaque assay is still used by many investigators (52,53), there have been recent efforts to develop alternative assay systems such as ELISA (54) and DNA hybridization (55). For use in assessing antiviral activity against VZV, a commercial kit for DNA hybridization of VZV is also available commercially from Diagnostic Hybrids.

The evaluation of antiviral agents against EBV represents a unique set of problems compared with HSV, CMV, or VZV, in that there is no system in which the infecting virus produces any detectable cytopathology. EBV is a lymphotropic virus and is present as a latent infection in B cells of most adults. EBV-containing cell lines have been established and are classified as producers or nonproducers depending on whether or not a few cells in the culture go into a productive virus cycle. Most are nonproducers and do not express antigens that are associated with production of infectious progeny virus. Nonproducer cells express a nuclear antigen called Epstein-Barr nuclear antigen (EBNA). Antigens detectable in producer cells or cells superinfected by EBV are early antigens (EA), viral capsid antigen (VCA), and membrane antigen (MA). A few continuous cell lines have been established from Burkitt's lymphomas that contain no detectable EBV genomes. These cell lines also respond to primary infection with EBV by expressing EBV-specified EA. Three basic assay systems have been utilized to evaluate the activity of antiviral agents against EBV replication: (a) a high virus producer cell line (P3HR-1), which can be treated with drug and monitored for the production of viral genomic copies, EA, VCA, and MA, which are indicators of EBV DNA replication (56–59); (b) superinfection with P3HR-1 virus of nonproducer cell lines that contain a large number of resident EBV genomes (Raji) (60, 61); and (c) superinfection of nonproducer transformed cell lines that contain few or no detectable resident genomes (Ramos). The end point used in the latter two assay systems is detection of EA using specific monoclonal antibodies in an immunofluorescence (IF) assay (60,61). Using one or more of these assay systems, a number of antiviral agents including phosphonoacetic acid (PAA), phosphonoformic acid (PFA), Vira-A, ACV, E-5-(2-bromovinyl)-2′-deoxyuridine (BVDU), 9-(1,3-dihydroxy-2-propoxymethyl) guanine (DHPG) and the fluorinated nucleoside analogs, 2′-

fluoro-5-iodo-arabinosyl-cytosine (FIAC) and 2′-fluoro-5-methyl-arabinosyl-uracil (FMAU) have been shown to inhibit EBV replication *in vitro* (62); however, only ACV has been evaluated in clinical studies.

### Respiratory Viruses

In general, wild-type or clinical isolates of influenza virus do not grow well in cell cultures, and, therefore, CPE inhibition or plaque reduction assays are not always applicable for use in antiviral testing against these viruses. In these cases, a hemadsorption (HAd) assay can be utilized (63). When a virus isolate has been adapted to grow in cell cultures, CPE or plaque reduction assays can be used (64); these, generally, are more easily performed, and the results are less subjective than those obtained in the HAd assay. For determination of antiviral activity against RSV, the CPE inhibition assay (65,66) works very well. Yield inhibition can also be determined simply by harvesting the supernatant fluids from wells or tubes and titrating for RSV. Many rhinovirus strains will also form plaques or produce CPE in cell cultures, and these assays are generally used to determine antiviral activity against these viruses (67–69).

### Retroviruses

The major emphasis in recent years has been the development of new antiviral agents for HIV. This high level of interest has generated numerous compounds, and a variety of assay methods using various T-cell or macrophage-derived cell lines have been developed to determine activity *in vitro*. The initial assays that were utilized monitored the viability of infected cells or the production of viral enzymes (reverse transcriptase) or viral proteins (p24) in cells that were permissive for HIV but that did not adhere to plastic plates (70–76). Subsequently, cells were adhered to plastic and CPE inhibition, and plaque reduction assays developed (77–80). These assays were then adapted to semiautomated screening systems in which cell viability was determined by the addition of vital stains or tetrazolium reagent (81,82) and read on a spectrophotometer or ELISA reader (83,84). The XTT assay described by Weislow et al. (84) offers a particular safety advantage in that a soluble Formazan product is produced, thus minimizing the number of manipulations involving infected materials that are required. These assays have been automated to the point that 20,000–40,000 potential antiviral compounds per year can be screened for anti-HIV activity (84).

### Hepadnaviruses

The determination of antiviral activity against Hepatitis B virus (HBV) is an especially difficult task since the virus does not grow in any cell culture system. In attempts to develop *in vitro* systems for the study of HBV replication and the interaction between virus and host cells, human cell lines derived from human hepatocellular carcinomas or hepatoblastomas have been transfected with HBV DNA. These cells then produce HBV DNA and complete virions, and express surface and core antigens (85–87). At the present time, the use of these systems for determining antiviral activity has not been reported; however, they should be useful for this purpose since they are somewhat analogous to the EBV producer cell lines that are used for determination of antiviral activity. Duck HBV (DHBV) and woodchuck hepatitis virus (WHV) are closely related to human HBV, and duck or woodchuck hepatocytes infected with their respective virus provide *in vitro* systems in which antiviral activity against hepadnaviruses can be assessed (88–94). The importance of these systems is further emphasized because WHV infection of woodchucks and DHBV infection of Pekin ducks currently serve as the available animal model systems for evaluating antiviral activity. These experimental infections will be discussed in more detail in the animal model section.

### Papillomaviruses

At the present time, there are no *in vitro* assay systems available for evaluating antiviral agents against papillomaviruses. It is anticipated, however, that the use of new molecular biology techniques, such as those applied to HBV, will soon yield *in vitro* models.

### Toxicity Evaluation

In addition to determination of antiviral activity in cell culture systems, it is of equal importance to assess the toxicity of a potential new compound. This information is not only necessary for comparing drugs and in making decisions regarding the future pursuit of the compound, it also provides data back to the chemist to assess structure/activity relationships. Information regarding the efficacy and toxicity of a compound can aid in the design of new compounds or modification of existing ones to obtain maximum antiviral activity with a minimum of toxicity.

Valuable information regarding the toxicity of antiviral compounds to tissue culture cells can be obtained by observing drug-treated, uninfected cultures in the screening and confirmation assays used for assessing antiviral activity. In general, the ability of drug-treated cells to take up a vital stain such as neutral red (44) or the use of other methods such as trypan blue exclusion (95,96) and the reduction of tetrazolium salts (84,97,98) can provide a quantitative estimate of toxicity in drug-treated, uninfected cells along with antiviral activity. In most cases, these assay systems use confluent cell monolayers so only an effect on stationary cells is obtained in these systems. To determine the toxicity on rapidly growing cells, cell proliferation or growth curve studies need to be performed (49,99). Cells are seeded into 6-well culture dishes or 25 $cm^2$ tissue culture flasks at a concentration that will result in approximately 25% confluency in 24 hr. Various concentrations of the antiviral drug are added to replicate cultures and incubated for about 72 hr or until a 1–2 log increase in the number of cells in the control culture is obtained. The cells from each group are then trypsinized and counted. Drug-treated cultures are compared with untreated control cultures, and an inhibitory dose ($ID_{50}$, $ID_{90}$, etc.) is calculated using the same regression analysis method used to determine $ED_{50}$. Another measure of cell toxicity is to treat cells with antiviral drug and then add radiolabeled precursors ([$^3$H]-thymidine, [$^3$H]-uridine, or [$^3$H]-amino-acids) and measure incorporation into DNA, RNA, or protein. Again, by comparing drug-treated with untreated control cultures, an inhibitory dose can be calculated. Not surprisingly, most antiviral compounds have considerably greater toxicity for proliferating cells than stationary or contact-inhibited cells. Although these methods provide valuable information regarding toxicity of antiviral drugs in tissue culture cells, these results may not be predictive of *in vivo* toxicity. It has been reported that clonogenic assays using peripheral blood mononuclear cells or bone marrow progenitor cells (100,101) may be more predictive of potential toxicity in humans than the tissue culture assays. Further *in vitro* toxicity tests that need to be conducted on a promising compound include mutagenesis and genetic toxicity, etc. (102).

## EVALUATION IN ANIMAL MODEL INFECTIONS

The importance of experimental viral infections in animal models for the development and evaluation of new antiviral agents prior to their use in humans should not be underemphasized. Although tissue culture systems are of great value in determining if a new drug has activity against a particular virus, these systems should not be used as indicators or predictors of activity in humans. Only where suitable animal models are not available should a compound be taken from tissue culture directly into human trials. Although one can legitimately argue that most, if not all, animal model infections are not identical to the human disease, it can be demonstrated that a compound does in fact have activity in an *in vivo* system, and early indications of its antiviral activity, tissue distribution, metabolic disposition, pharmacokinetics, and acute toxicity can be realized. Importantly, all of these parameters of drug pharmacodynamics can be correlated with inhibition of viral replication in target organs. Additionally, our understanding of the pathogenesis of many viral infections, the response of the host to infection, and the interaction among the viral infection, the host's immune response, and a therapeutic agent has been enhanced greatly through the use of animal model systems.

When selecting or developing an animal model for determining efficacy of an antiviral, one should utilize systems that best simulate the corresponding human disease. Some of the factors that need to be considered when selecting an animal model have recently been reviewed by Field (103). It is obvious that there is currently no experimental viral infection that meets all of the properties of an ideal animal model. The most common animals used are rodents, and these differ from humans by most criteria. Chimpanzees or other nonhuman primates, however, cannot be used as models for most viral diseases due to their lack of availability, cost, space requirements, and the inability to experimentally infect these animals with many human viruses. An additional problem is that many human viruses such as CMV, VZV, HBV, HPV, and HIV are species specific and generally do not cause disease in animals. In these cases, an animal virus counterpart must be used in order to perform antiviral evaluations in animal models. There are also significant differences in drug metabolism and pharmacokinetics between humans and most animal species that must be considered when extrapolating results obtained in animal models to the design of initial clinical trials.

Although we do not have ideal animal models, there are numerous examples of good experimental viral infections in animals that can be used to evaluate new antiviral agents. In order to obtain the best information regarding the predictability of an animal model system for efficacy of a new compound, a number of guidelines for using animal models should be considered. These are listed in Table 3. The use of as many of these guidelines as possible will result in an accumulation of data that should allow one to make predictions regarding the efficacy of a compound in humans. Once human trials are completed, the data obtained should then be compared with those acquired in the animal system to help establish the predictability of the animal model. It is not the intent of this chapter to review all the animal model infections, but to focus on those used most commonly and to highlight those that have demonstrated predictability for human disease. Those diseases where new animal models have been developed recently in response to the need for *in vivo* systems to evaluate new compounds for their activity against hepatitis viruses, papillomaviruses, and particularly against retroviruses will also be described.

### Herpesvirus Infections

The herpesviruses, and particularly HSV, are the etiologic agents of a wide variety of diseases in humans. It is important that new antiviral agents be tested in animal models that simulate each of those disease states in humans. A summary of some of the animal models of HSV infections is shown in Table 4. Some specific examples of these animal models will be used to illustrate how they

**TABLE 3.** *Guidelines for animal model testing*

| |
|---|
| The most appropriate animal species should be used. |
| Drug should be evaluated in more than one species. |
| Age of animal should be considered. |
| Sensitivity of virus to drug should be known in cells from same species. |
| Animals should be free of adventitious agents. |
| Use the human virus with minimum alteration through adaptation, if possible. |
| Use natural animal pathogen that is closely related to human virus. |
| Use animal virus that produces infection similar to that seen in humans. |
| The natural route of infection with similar inoculum size should be utilized when feasible. |
| Virus infection should be varied—route, inoculum, size. |
| An infectivity or mortality rate of 80–95% should be used. |
| The course of infection and pathogenesis should be similar to that in human disease. |
| Pathogenesis of viral infection and effect of drug on pathogenesis should be defined. |
| The host response should be similar to that seen in humans. |
| Effect of drug on immune system should be determined. |
| Route of drug administration should be similar to that used for human disease. |
| Drug administration must be varied—route, dose and time of initiation—so that a maximum tolerated dose and a minimum ED can be determined. |
| Time of initiation of drug treatment should be varied to correlate with use in humans. |
| Drug pharmacodynamics, metabolism, and toxicity must be determined and should be similar to that observed in humans. |
| The end points used for evaluation of efficacy are the same as used in human trials. |
| Mortality is generally not a sensitive end point; determine effect of treatment on virus replication in target organs. |
| Results from animal models must be compared with human trials. |
| Predictability of animal model needs to be established. |

can be used to determine efficacy of antiviral agents. In addition, since animal models for HSV infections have been the most widely used, the predictability for most of these infections can be established.

The use of mice inoculated intranasally with HSV-1 as a model for herpes encephalitis was initially described by De Clercq and Luczak (104) and has been used extensively in our laboratory for evaluation of antiviral agents directed against this disease. The pathogenesis of this experimental infection is shown in Fig. 1. After HSV-1 inoculation, the virus travels from the nasopharynx via olfactory and trigeminal nerve tracts to the brain, resulting in death from an acute encephalitis. In this model, treatment with Vira-A initiated within 24–48 hr after infection results in significant protection (105). The protection against mortality observed with Vira-A treatment also correlated with alteration of HSV-1 replication in target organs, particularly in the CNS. As shown in Fig. 1, therapy with 250 mg/kg of Vira-A twice daily for 7 days initiated 48 hr after viral inoculation reduced considerably the virus titers in olfactory lobes, cerebral cortex, cerebrum, diencephalon, and the pons-medulla when compared with placebo-treated mice. Treatment also reduced viral replication in spleen but had only a marginal effect in lung. In clinical trials of HSV-1 encephalitis, treatment with Vira-A also resulted in significant reduction in mortality (106,107). In this animal model infection, treatment with ACV was considerably more effective than Vira-A in preventing mortality (105). Concentrations as low as 15 mg/kg significantly reduced mortality when therapy was begun 72 hr after infection, a time when virus is replicating in the CNS (Fig. 1). A comparison between Vira-A and ACV treatment on the pathogenesis of HSV-1 encephalitis in mice is also depicted in Fig. 1. In all target organs, virus titers in ACV-treated animals were lower than placebo-treated animals. In the cerebellum, dien-

**TABLE 4.** *Animal models for herpesvirus infections*

| Virus | Animal | Disease | Measure of efficacy |
|---|---|---|---|
| HSV-1 | Mice | Encephalitis | Mortality, pathogenesis |
| | Rabbits | Encephalitis | Mortality, pathogenesis |
| | Rabbits | Eye disease | Lesion severity, virus titers |
| | Guinea pigs | Skin lesions | Lesion severity, virus titers |
| | Guinea pigs | Genital herpes | Lesion severity, virus titers |
| HSV-2 | Mice | Disseminated neonatal herpes, encephalitis | Mortality, pathogenesis |
| | Mice, guinea pigs | Genital herpes | Lesion severity, virus titers, recurrences |
| CMV | | | |
| MCMV | Mice | Generalized, acute, chronic | Mortality, pathogenesis |
| GPCMV | Guinea pigs | Generalized, acute, chronic | Pathogenesis, histopathology |
| VZV | Guinea pigs | Viremia, rash, nasal shedding | Virus isolation, seroconversion |
| | Rabbits | Rash, lesions | Virus isolation |
| SVV | Monkeys | Disseminated with skin lesions | Mortality, rash, virus titers, blood chemistry |

cephalon, and pons-medulla, ACV treatment was superior to Vira-A in reducing the magnitude of viral replication and promoted a more rapid clearance of HSV-1 in these tissues. ACV therapy was also more effective than Vira-A in reducing viral replication in lung tissue. Based on these experimental data, it was predicted that ACV would be more effective than Vira-A in treatment of HSV-1 encephalitis in humans. Subsequent clinical trials confirmed observations from the animal model studies as ACV was shown to be significantly more effective than Vira-A (1).

Mice inoculated intranasally with HSV-2 appear to be a good model for disseminated neonatal herpes. After viral inoculation, replication of virus is initially detectable in lung with subsequent dissemination to visceral organs. Virus is also transmitted concomitantly by neural routes from the nasopharynx to olfactory lobe, cerebellum–brain stem, cerebrum, and spinal cord (108). This animal model provides a severe test of antiviral efficacy, and treatment with Vira-A failed to provide any protection against mortality; however, there was some alteration of virus replication in brain, lung, liver, and spleen (105,108–110). This is a complex model infection involving both CNS and non-CNS tissues and historically has not responded well to most antiviral agents. In placebo-controlled clinical trials, however, Vira-A did reduce mortality (111), but many survivors had permanent neurological sequelae (112). Parenteral treatment with ACV in the murine model was very effective in reducing mortality when therapy was initiated 48–96 hr after infection (105,113), and also reduced viral replication in target organs significantly (114). In recently completed clinical trials in which Vira-A and ACV were compared for efficacy against neonatal herpes, the two agents were judged to be comparable (2). We have reported previously (113) that oral administration of ACV is considerably more effective than parenteral therapy in the mouse model, but this mode of treatment has not been utilized for therapy of this human disease. The experimental infection, therefore, accurately predicted efficacy for treatment of human disease with Vira-A or ACV but apparently failed to de-

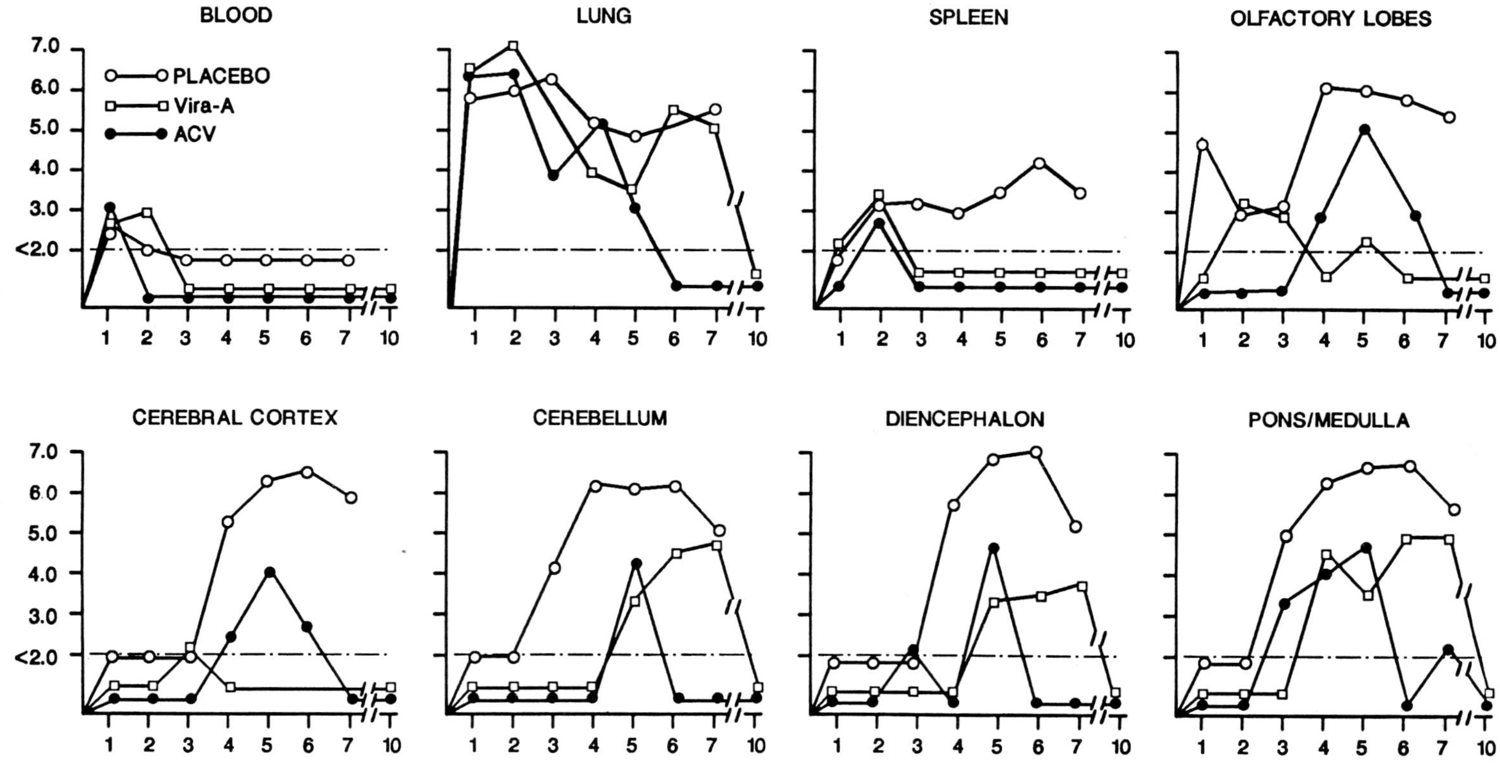


**FIG. 1.** Effect of treatment with Vira-A or ACV on the pathogenesis of an HSV-1 encephalitis in mice. Animals were inoculated intranasally and treated IP with 250 mg/kg of Vira-A or 30 mg/kg of ACV. Treatment was initiated 48 hr after viral inoculation and continued twice daily for 7 days.

termine which of the two drugs would be most active. It should be stressed, however, that disseminated HSV-2 infections of mice and humans are complex and that the animal model may not accurately represent the pathogenesis of human disease.

The rabbit model for herpetic eye disease was the first experimental animal system that demonstrated predictability for antiviral efficacy in humans. The effectiveness of iododeoxyuridine (IUDR) (115, 116), Vira-A (117,118), trifluorothymidine (TFT) (119,120), and ACV (121,122) was first determined in the rabbit model and subsequently confirmed in HSV-1 infections of the eye in humans. Since IUDR, Vira-A, and TFT are all approved for use in HSV ocular disease in humans and ACV is at least equally effective, there has been no recent progress in this area and, therefore, will not be considered further.

Cutaneous infections of guinea pigs with HSV-1 appears to be a model for skin and oral infections caused by this virus in humans, and may be a predictive model for herpes labialis (123). When the animals are inoculated according to the procedure originally described by Hubler et al. (124), the skin infection is characterized by rapid development of discreet 3–5-mm diameter vesicular lesions. The lesions then crust and heal completely by 10–12 days. The lesions and pattern of healing are similar to human cutaneous HSV disease (123,125). The primary advantage of this model is that animals do not develop zosteriform lesions or die of neurological disease, commonly seen in mouse models of cutaneous HSV-1 infections. One of the disadvantages of the model is that recurrent skin lesions do not develop spontaneously nor have they been induced successfully (123). Although a variety of antiviral compounds has been tested in this model infection, there are few compounds that have been shown to be efficacious in humans. Comparative data in the guinea pig and humans using topical or oral administration of ACV continues to be accumulated; however, at this time, the predictive value of the model has not been established. There are however, some reasonable correlations with ACV cream and PFA cream (123,126,127). A major advantage of this animal model system is that it lends itself well to studying skin penetration of antiviral drugs both *in vitro* and *in vivo*, and is especially useful for determining the best formulation for topical therapy (128). This type of system becomes extremely valuable for the formulation of new topical antiviral preparations.

Genital HSV infections continue to be a major health problem worldwide. Although the use of ACV has contributed greatly to the management of primary and recurrent disease, there is still a need for additional modes of therapy for the prevention or treatment of these infections. As pointed out previously, it is important that animal model infections utilized for evaluation of new antiviral compounds be selected that most closely represent the target disease in humans. A number of animal species including mice, hamsters, guinea pigs, rabbits, and nonhuman primates have been utilized as model infections for genital herpes. In our laboratory, mice and guinea pigs inoculated intravaginally with HSV have been used as models of genital herpes (9). As with all experimental infections, there are advantages and disadvantages to these two experimental systems. The size and cost of mice make them particularly useful for use in initial screening experiments and to determine optimal dosage and treatment regimens against vaginal virus replication (129,130). A number of antiviral agents including Vira-A, PAA, PFA, and ACV have been tested in this model infection, and the results agree with those obtained in clinical studies (42, 130–133). However, since mice inoculated with HSV by the intravaginal route generally die of acute encephalomyelitis, and neither develop typical lesions on external genital skin, nor exhibit spontaneous recurrent lesions, the model does not accurately reflect all aspects of the disease in humans.

The pathogenesis of primary and recurrent genital HSV-2 infection of guinea pigs is summarized in Table 5. The advantages of the guinea pig as a model for genital HSV infection include the following: (a) animals are susceptible to infection with HSV-2 or HSV-1; (b) initial viral replication occurs in the vaginal tract; (c) natural external lesions develop on the external genital skin; (d) there is low mortality; (e) all surviving animals become latently infected; and (f) spontaneous recurrent lesions appear on the external genital skin. The main disadvantages of the guinea pig model are cost, space requirements, and the need for additional care. Both the mouse and guinea pig models have been used for evaluation of a large number of potential antiviral agents, and efficacy in the two models has essentially been identical. Since genital HSV-2 infection in the guinea pig results in the development of external lesions similar to those seen in humans and has spontaneous recurrent lesions, this model most closely simulates disease in humans (9,134–137). The natural history of primary and recurrent HSV infection in the guinea pig, the measures of efficacy utilized for evaluation of antivirals, and the effectiveness of a number of antiviral agents in this model have been reported previously (9,133, 136,138,139), and will be reviewed only briefly to illustrate the similarity to the human disease. The clinical and virological course of this infection is also summarized in Table 5. Intravaginal inoculation of guinea pigs with HSV-2 results in a primary infection characterized by viral replication in the vaginal tract, followed by the development of vesicular lesions on the external genital skin similar to those seen in human disease (140). After recovery from the primary infection, spontaneous recurrent lesions appear at the site of initial primary lesions. Unlike recurrent genital herpes in humans, the recurrent lesions in guinea pigs remain small, do not spread, last only 1–3 days, and recur at a frequency of approximately one episode per week; generally lesions do not contain infectious virus, but viral antigens can be detected. Nevertheless, the genital HSV-2 infection of guinea

**TABLE 5.** *Pathogenesis of genital HSV-2 infection in guinea pigs*

Primary infection, virologic course
- After intravaginal inoculation with HSV-2, virus replicates to high titers in the vaginal tract; less so in cervix and uterus.
- Virus invades into sensory nerves within 24–36 hr and ascends to involve the dorsal root ganglia and spinal cord by day 2–3.
- From the dorsal root ganglia and/or spinal cord, HSV descends back down nerves to the external genital skin and produces lesions by day 3–4.
- HSV replication within the spinal cord may cause paralysis; virus transmitted up the cord to the brain may cause encephalitis and death.
- No evidence for viremia or involvement of visceral organs.
- All infected animals have latent infections in dorsal root ganglia.

Primary infection, clinical course
- External genital lesions—onset day 3–4, peak severity day 6–7, healing by day 15–20.
- Urinary retention in most—onset day 5–10, resolution by day 10–15.
- Hind limb paralysis in 20–30%—onset day 7–10, resolution in survivors by day 15–20.
- Deaths infrequent (10–30%)—occur between day 9 and 15.

Recurrent disease, clinical and virologic course
- All infected animals have spontaneous recurrences.
- External erythematous or vesicular lesions.
- Most lesions persist for approximately 2 days.
- Animals average approximately one recurrent episode per week.
- Virus can be isolated from only a small percentage of lesions; however, HSV antigen can be detected in lesion biopsies.
- Asymptomatic shedding of HSV in cervicovaginal tract.

pigs appears to be the model that most closely resembles primary and recurrent disease in humans.

The ultimate test of any animal model system is its predictability for human disease. Until the past few years, there has not been sufficient experience in testing antiviral agents in both animal models and humans to establish the predictability of a model system for genital HSV-2 infections. The large body of information that has been collected using ACV now allows one to make comparisons of efficacy in the genital HSV-2 infections of guinea pigs with those reported in clinical trials. These comparisons, using a number of measures of efficacy, are summarized in Table 6. Topical treatment (intravaginal and external) during primary infection with 5% ACV significantly reduced viral replication in the vaginal tract, prevented or reduced the severity of external lesion development, and markedly reduced systemic clinical symptoms such as paralysis and urinary retention (9,133). Subsequent recurrence rates, however, were not altered. Similar results have been observed in patients treated topically for primary or recurrent genital HSV infection (3,141). During primary disease, oral or parenteral administration of ACV effectively reduced lesion severity, virus shedding, and clinical symptoms in both guinea pigs (133,138) and humans (4,5). Subsequent recurrence rates were not altered in the guinea pig (9) and generally are unchanged in humans (4,5,142). With long-term follow-up, there are suggestions from one study that treatment during primary infection may have an effect on the frequency of recurrent episodes (142), but this observation has not been confirmed in other studies (143). When oral therapy with ACV is initiated during recurrent disease, the frequency and severity of the episodes are reduced significantly in the guinea pig infection (9) and markedly altered in human disease during the period of treatment (7,8). After cessation of therapy, however, the frequency of recurrences returns to pretreatment levels in both the guinea pig and humans. Thus, the data collected to date using topical or oral administration of ACV in the guinea pig and humans indicate that the genital HSV-2 infection of guinea pigs is predictive for the outcome of antiviral therapy of genital herpes in humans (Table 6).

The experimental animal systems for CMV and VZV are also listed in Table 4. CMV is the causative agent of a variety of clinical syndromes in the fetus, neonate, and, particularly, patients who are immunosuppressed for organ transplantation, during chemotherapy for malignancies (144), or as a result of another infection such as HIV (13–15). Due to the strict species specificity of human CMV, it is not possible to test potential antiviral agents against this virus in experimental animals.

**TABLE 6.** *Predictability of the guinea pig model for treatment of genital HSV infection in humans*

| | Topical ACV | | Oral ACV | |
|---|---|---|---|---|
| | Guinea pig | Humans | Guinea pig | Humans |
| Primary infection | | | | |
| Reduce lesion severity | Yes | Yes | Yes | Yes |
| Reduce virus shedding | Yes | Yes | Yes | Yes |
| Reduce clinical symptoms | Yes | Yes | Yes | Yes |
| Reduce recurrence rates | No | No | No | No |
| Recurrent disease | | | | |
| Reduce frequency during treatment | No | No | Yes | Yes |
| Reduce severity during treatment | No | No | Yes | Yes |
| Reduce frequency after treatment | No | No | No | No |

There are a number of natural CMV infections in various animal species; however, the two experimental systems that have been utilized for antiviral evaluation are murine CMV (MCMV) and guinea pig CMV (GPCMV). Inoculation of mice with MCMV provides a model infection that shares many characteristics with the human disease. Both acute lethal and chronic nonlethal MCMV infections have been used in our laboratory to determine efficacy of antivirals (145). After intraperitoneal (IP) inoculation of 3-week-old Swiss Webster female mice with $1 \times 10^6$ pfu of MCMV, 90–100% of animals die with a mean day of death of 5–6 days. With an inoculum of $1 \times 10^5$ pfu, all animals survive. With either inoculum, high titers of virus are present in lung, liver, spleen, kidney, and blood within 24 hr and in salivary gland by 48–72 hr. In the nonlethal infection, persistent viral replication occurs in lung, liver, kidney, and spleen for at least 20–30 days and in salivary glands for months. In Balb/c mice infected with MCMV, immunosuppression with cyclophosphamide produces a severe interstitial pneumonitis (146,147). The MCMV infection, therefore, involves many of the same target organs as HCMV. When guinea pigs are inoculated with GPCMV, virus can be isolated from the blood, lung, liver, kidney, urine, and salivary glands. This model infection has many of the clinical syndromes seen in humans including transplacental transmission of virus, mononucleosis, interstitial pneumonia, and transmission of virus by blood transfusion (148). It has been difficult to establish which, if either, of these two animal models is predictive of antiviral efficacy for human CMV infection since, until recently, there has been no effective therapy in either the animal models or humans.

The acyclic nucleoside analogue of ACV, DHPG, is a highly effective inhibitor of human CMV replication in tissue culture cells and is approximately 50 times as active against this virus as ACV. To determine the predictability of the murine model for HCMV infections, the sensitivity of MCMV to DHPG in tissue culture cells was determined and compared with the results for human CMV. The results of numerous experiments indicated that MCMV was inhibited by 3.0–9.0 μM of DHPG using a 50% plaque-reduction assay in MEF cells, whereas approximately 1.0–3.0 μM of DHPG is required to inhibit human strains of CMV in human fibroblast cells. These data indicate that both murine and human strains of CMV are equally susceptible to DHPG and support the validity of using the murine infection as a model for human CMV infections. This MCMV infection has been utilized for evaluation of antiviral drugs such as Vira-A, ACV, PFA, and DHPG. In these experiments, Vira-A was ineffective (149), whereas ACV was extremely effective in reducing mortality and altering viral replication in lung, liver, spleen, and kidney (145,150,151). The predictability of ACV could not be established for HCMV infection, however, because HCMV is relatively insensitive to this drug (152). In the animal model, PFA reduced mortality if initiated by 24 hr postinfection (42,151), and clinical trials are still in progress, with promising results being reported (14). Treatment of an MCMV infection with DHPG has been highly effective in preventing mortality even when drug is initiated as late as 48 hr postinfection (50,105,153). DHPG treatment of MCMV-infected mice results in significant alteration of viral titers in blood, lung, liver, spleen, and kidney (Fig. 2). Viral clearance was also more rapid in these organs from treated animals. In salivary gland, a site of persistent infection in these animals, there was a 2-day delay in virus replication, and virus titers were consistently lower for the first 15 days. Both MCMV and HCMV are sensitive to DHPG *in vitro,* and the results from the animal model experiments suggested that this compound may be an excellent candidate for treatment of CMV infections in humans.

The $ED_{50}$ of DHPG against GPCMV has

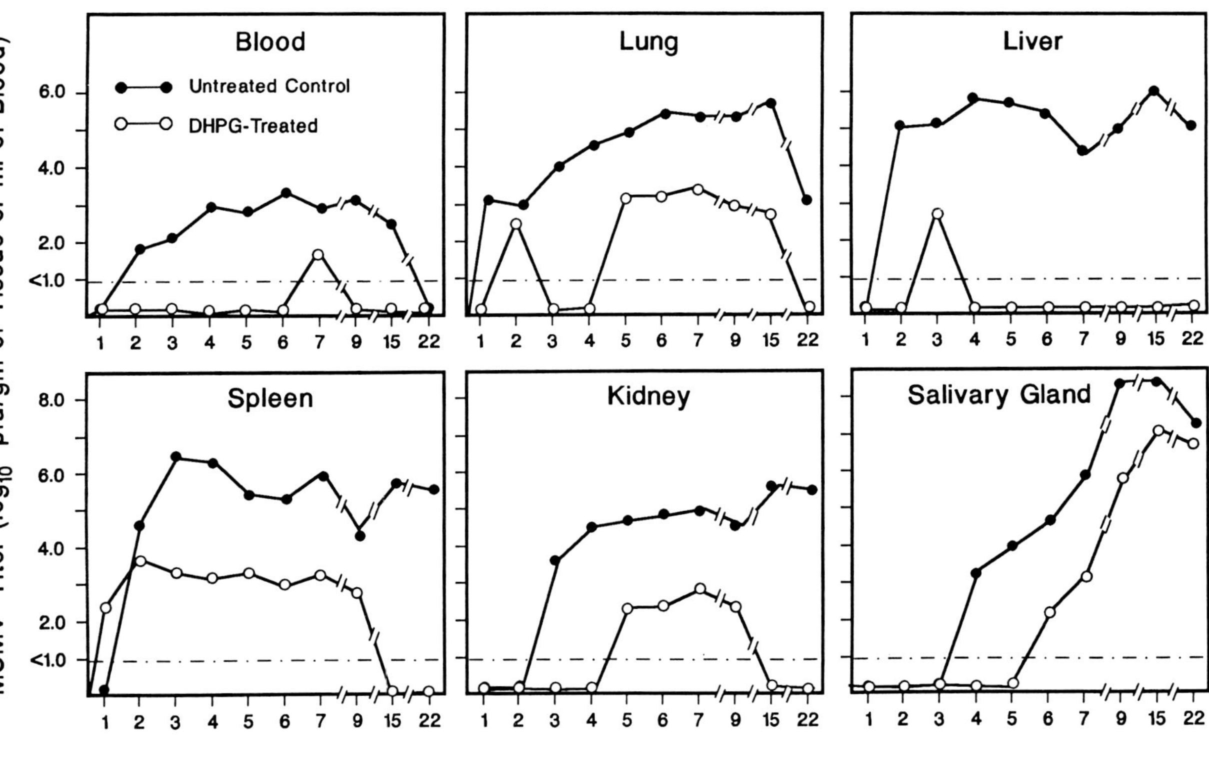


**FIG. 2.** Effect of treatment with DHPG on a chronic MCMV infection in mice. IP treatment with 40 mg/kg was begun 24 hr after infection and continued twice daily for 14 days.

been reported to be 71 μM in tissue culture cells (154), indicating that GPCMV is considerably less susceptible to DHPG than either murine or human CMV. When guinea pigs were inoculated IP with GPCMV and treated twice daily for 7 days with 25 mg/kg of DHPG, virus titers in the lung were higher in drug-treated animals than in those treated with placebo. There were no significant differences in the severity of histopathologic lesions in the lung, liver, and spleen between drug and placebo-treated animals; however, DHPG-treated animals had fewer lesions in kidney and salivary glands than those treated with placebo, and virus titers in salivary gland were also lower in DHPG-treated animals (154). These data indicate that DHPG had only minimal activity against GPCMV both in tissue culture and in the animal model, but also supported the use of DHPG for treatment of HCMV infections.

Although DHPG has not yet been approved for general use, it has been used extensively to treat human CMV infections on a compassionate use basis. Since there has not been any double-blind, placebo-controlled studies conducted regarding the efficacy of DHPG against HCMV infections, its effectiveness has not been established. However, there are numerous reports attesting to its activity in retinitis, (13,14) gastrointestinal disease (13,15), and pneumonia due to CMV (13,16). The effect of DHPG treatment for CMV-induced pneumonia, however, has been less pronounced (16) than for the other diseases. In one study designed to determine the effect of DHPG therapy on CMV replication in lung tissue, there was a dramatic 4–6 log decrease in viral titers after therapy with DHPG (155). The results obtained in the clinical studies, particularly those that did virus cultures, correlated well with the data obtained in the murine model. There is not as good a correlation with the guinea pig model, presumably due to the lack of *in vitro* susceptibility of GPCMV to DHPG. Based on the limited amount of data available, it would appear that the mouse model, at least for DHPG, is more predictive of antiviral efficacy for human CMV than is the guinea pig model.

VZV infections in the immunocompromised host continues to be a problem of great magnitude. Due to the species specificity of VZV, there is currently no established animal model for evaluating antiviral drugs against this virus. It has been reported that weanling guinea pigs are susceptible to VZV that has been adapted in fetal guinea pig cells (156). After intranasal or subcutaneous inoculation, the virus replicates in the nasopharynx, viremia can be detected, specific humoral antibodies are produced, and animal-to-animal transmission has been documented. Models for ocular and disseminated VZV have also been developed recently using the guinea pig (157) and the rabbit (158). Since these model infections have not yet been utilized for antiviral studies, their suitability is unknown at the present time. The models should certainly aid in enhancing our understanding of the pathophysiology and the role of the immune system in VZV infections. They may also provide a system for investigating the mechanism of latent infections.

A model for VZV that does not use the human virus is simian varicella virus (SVV) infection of monkeys. After intratracheal inoculation, the animals develop fever and viremia followed by a disseminated infection with skin rash (159). A large number of antiviral agents have been tested in this animal model including Vira-A, ACV, and BVDU. These agents have also been evaluated in placebo-controlled human studies. When African green monkeys were infected with SVV and treated intravenously (IV) with 15 mg/kg of Vira-A per day for 10 days beginning 48 hr after infection, no significant differences in viremia, rash, or serum transaminase levels were observed between treated and control animals (160). ACV treatment of African green monkeys at 10 mg/kg IV twice daily for 10 days also had no effect on clinical symptoms, development of rash, or viremia (161). In contrast, ACV administration at 100 mg/kg intramuscularly (IM) effectively prevented or reduced viremia, appearance of rash, and elevated transaminases (162). The difference in the two ACV studies appeared to be due to achievement of sufficient plasma levels of ACV when the higher dose was given by the IM route. The best therapeutic effect in this model infection was obtained with BVDU (163). Oral, IM or IV administration of 10 mg/kg/day prevented the development of viremia and the appearance of rash and anorexia. Administration of BVDU as late as 6 days after infection effectively modified the course of disease.

In immunocompromised patients, both ACV and Vira-A have been reported to prevent the development of visceral disease in immunocompromised children with varicella and reduce dissemination of herpes zoster (20–23). In a study comparing the two drugs, it was shown that ACV was significantly more effective than Vira-A treatment for VZV infections in severely immunocompromised patients (24). In other studies, BVDU has also been reported to be effective in treatment of varicella or VZV infections of immunocompromised subjects (164). Although the experimental SVV infection of African green monkeys did not accurately predict efficacy of Vira-A in humans, it was predictive of efficacy for ACV and BVDU. The model is also of great value in determining drug pharmacokinetics, metabolism, and toxicity prior to use in humans.

Another herpesvirus for which there is no animal model available is EBV. It was reported recently that guinea pigs infected with guinea pig herpes-like virus (GPHLV) and then immunosuppressed undergo a lymphocytosis and lymphoid hyperplasia similar to that seen in chronic EBV syndrome (165). This model will need additional characterization, and a better understanding of the clinical syndrome is necessary before its usefulness can be established.

### Respiratory Virus Infections

There have been few antiviral agents developed in recent years that have activity against respiratory infections in either experimental animals or humans. Consequently, there are few comparative data on which to judge the predictability of the animal model infections. The experimental animal infections that have been most widely used for evaluating antiviral agents are listed in Table 7. A wide range of animal species including mice, cotton rats, ferrets, hamsters, guinea pigs,dogs, pigs, and nonhuman primates have been used; however, those most commonly used for evaluation of antiviral agents have been mice and ferrets and, more recently, cotton rats. Mice are not particularly susceptible to infection with influenza virus unless the virus is adapted by passage through mouse lung. Ferrets are highly susceptible to human influenza viruses without adaptation and develop symptoms similar to those seen in humans. One main disadvantage to the use of

**TABLE 7.** *Animal models for respiratory virus infections*

| Virus | Animal | Disease | Measure of efficacy |
|---|---|---|---|
| Influenza A or B | Mice | Respiratory | Mortality, virus titers in lung |
| | Cotton rat | Respiratory | Mortality, virus titers, histopathology |
| | Ferret | Respiratory | Mortality, virus titers, histopathology |
| RSV | Cotton rat | Respiratory | Virus titers, histopathology |
| | Hamster | Respiratory | Virus titers, histopathology |

ferrets as an animal model for antiviral studies is their size and cost. Amantadine, which is approved for both prophylaxis and treatment of influenza A virus infection, has reasonably good activity in mice depending on virus strain, inoculum size, route of challenge, dosage, time, and route of drug administration (166,167). In contrast to the results in most other animals or humans, amantadine treatment is not effective in ferrets (168), which suggests that this may not be the most predictable model. In experimental infections of mice, rimantidine is as active if not more so than amantadine (169). In human disease, amantadine appears to be slightly more active, but may also produce more side effects (29,170). Ribavirin also has been shown to have activity against influenza virus infections of mice, cotton rats, ferrets, hamsters, and squirrel monkeys (171,172); in human studies, aerosolized ribavirin has been reported to alter clinical symptoms and reduce shedding of influenza virus from the respiratory tract (30). Based on the limited studies that have been performed in animals and human diseases, it appears that the mouse and the cotton rat may be predictable models for determining efficacy in influenza virus infections.

RSV is the causative agent of severe bronchiolitis in infants and young children. Mice, hamsters, cotton rats, ferrets, and nonhuman primates infected with RSV have been utilized as models for this disease. The cotton rat appears to be the current animal of choice for antiviral studies directed against RSV. After intranasal inoculation of cotton rats, RSV replicates to high titer in the nose and lungs, with lower titers found in the trachea (173). In this model, ribavirin delivered by aerosol decreased RSV titers in lung 10–50-fold (174). In a trial of RSV infection of infants with lower respiratory tract disease, aerosolized ribavirin significantly increased improvement of clinical severity scores; at the end of therapy, treated infants had lower virus titers in nasal wash samples than placebo recipients (31). These and other clinical studies with RSV support the predictability of the cotton rat as a model.

Rhinoviruses are the most widespread cause of the common cold syndrome in humans. Although there have been reports of mouse models for rhinovirus infections using highly adapted virus, there is currently no accepted animal model for these infections.

### Retrovirus Infections

The emergence of AIDS and the subsequent isolation of HIV as the etiologic agent of this disease have intensified the search for animal models of human retrovirus infections. The experimental animal systems that are currently being investigated are summarized in Table 8. The chimpanzee was the first animal to be successfully infected with HIV; viremia was readily and consistently demonstrated and seroconversion occurred (175–177). Although many of the animals have a persistent infection, an AIDS-like disease has not developed (178). A transient lymphadenopathy syndrome or alterations in T4 or T8 cells have been reported but are an unusual occurrence. Due to the shortage of chimpanzees, it is unlikely that this animal model will be available for use in widespread testing of antiviral agents, but animals that have already been infected could be used (179). In an attempt to develop a model in other nonhuman primates using the human virus, Letvin et al. (180) inoculated two baboons and two rhesus monkeys with HIV-2, a virus that appears to be more closely related to simian immunodeficiency virus (SIV) than to HIV-1. No significant disease was observed in either the baboon or the rhesus monkeys. However, virus isolation and seroconversion occurred in both inoculated baboons but not in the rhesus monkeys. In another study in which HIV-2 was inoculated into ten rhesus monkeys (181), one developed clinical symptoms and nine

**TABLE 8.** *Animal models for retrovirus infections*

| Virus | Animal | Disease | Measure of efficacy |
|---|---|---|---|
| HIV | Chimpanzee | Viremia, lymphadenopathy, no immunodeficiency | Virus isolation, seroconversion |
| | Baboons | Viremia, seroconversion | Virus isolation |
| | Rabbits | Viremia, splenomegaly | Virus isolation, seroconversion, splenomegaly |
| | Transgenic mice | Viremia, lymphadenopathy, splenomegaly | Virus isolation, seroconversion, pathogenesis |
| | SCID-hu mice | Viral replication | Virus isolation |
| SIV | Rhesus macaques | Viremia, lymphadenopathy, immunodeficiency syndrome, persistent infection, encephalitis | Virus isolation, seroconversion, pathogenesis |
| Lentiviruses | Sheep, goats | Virus replication, pneumonia, encephalitis, persistent infection | Virus isolation, seroconversion, pathogenesis |
| FeLV | Cats | Viremia, lymphadenopathy, immunodeficiency | Virus isolation, seroconversion, pathogenesis |
| MuLV Rauscher | Mice | Viremia, erythroleukemia, splenomegaly | Virus isolation, splenomegaly, mortality |
| LP-BM5 | | Immunosuppression, lymphadenopathy, immunodeficiency | Splenomegaly, mortality |
| Friend | | Splenomegaly | Splenomegaly, mortality |
| Cas-Br-E | | Paralysis | Mortality, paralysis |

of 10 animals had either evidence of viral replication and/or seroconversion. The differences observed in rhesus monkeys in the two studies may have been due to variation between HIV-2 strains or the fact that in the second study the virus had been adapted in cell culture prior to inoculation of animals. At the present time, infection of nonhuman primates with HIV has not resulted in an appropriate animal model for evaluating antiviral agents. It has been reported recently that inoculation of rabbits with HIV results in an infection characterized by viremia, pulmonary lymphocytic infiltrate, and enlargement of spleen or thymus (182). More details regarding this experimental model are needed before an assessment of its usefulness can be made. Since rodents are refractory to infection with HIV, an alternative approach has been to construct transgenic mice that carry HIV proviral DNA (183). When mated with nontransgenic mice, the progeny developed clinical disease characterized by epidermal hyperplasia, lymphadenopathy, splenomegaly, pulmonary lymphoid infiltrates, and growth retardation. Importantly, infectious HIV was recovered from the skin, lymph nodes, and spleen of affected animals. These types of animals, if large enough numbers can be produced, will provide extremely valuable information regarding the pathogenesis of HIV infection and probably can be used to evaluate various modes of antiviral chemotherapy. In another novel approach, severe combined immunodeficient (SCID) mice that had received human fetal thymic or lymph node implants were inoculated with a cloned HIV isolate (184). There was subsequent evidence of viral replication and spread within the human lymphoid tissue. The utility of this model for evaluation of antiviral agents is also unknown at this time.

Since there is currently no readily available animal model for HIV-induced immunodeficiency disease, experimental nonhuman retrovirus systems will have to be utilized for initial determination of antiviral efficacy *in vivo*. Animal model infections using simian, ovine, caprine, feline, and murine retroviruses all have potential for use in antiviral research. There are obvious advantages and disadvantages of each of the model systems, and variables such as sensitivity of the virus to an antiviral *in vitro,* relatedness of the virus to HIV, similarity of the animal disease to AIDS in humans, interaction of the virus with components of the immune system, and the availability of animals and appropriate biological containment facilities must all be considered when selecting an animal model for HIV infections.

SIV was first isolated from rhesus macaques (185) and subsequently from African green monkeys (186), mangabeys (187), pit-tailed macaques (188), and other nonhuman primates. A number of these virus isolates have been analyzed and found to be antigenically related to HIV. Other similarities between HIV and SIV include (a) tropism for cells bearing CD4 antigen, which can be cytopathic in these cells; (b) characteristic morphology typical of the lentivirus family; (c) an overall sequence homology of approximately 75%; and (d) an AIDS-like disease produced by the viruses in their respective host (189,190). The inoculation of rhesus macaques with SIV results in an AIDS-like disease with a high final mortality. Most animals have a typical immunodeficiency syndrome including (a) lymphadenopathy, diarrhea, and wasting; (b) the occurrence of multiple opportunistic infections; (c) immune system abnormalities including a decrease in peripheral blood T4 lymphocytes and mitogen-induced proliferative responses; (d) persistent infections, an antibody response, and recovery of SIV on multiple occasions; and (e) in many of the animals, an encephalitis similar to that often seen in human HIV infections (189–195). The rhesus macaque, therefore, is susceptible to infection with a variety of SIV isolates and undergoes a disease process that shares many similarities to human AIDS. The use of this model will greatly enhance our understanding of the pathogenesis of HIV infections in humans and may suggest new approaches to the prevention or therapy of human disease. The model is well suited for use as the final preclinical testing stage of promising antiviral agents. The limitations of the model remain cost, availability, and facilities. Given the number of reported therapies that are currently undergoing some phase of preclinical evaluation, it is clear that nonhuman primates cannot be used for early-stage testing of these therapeutic agents and that other animal models will need to be developed.

Other lentivirus infections that have been proposed as model infections include Maedi-visna virus of sheep (196), caprine arthritis encephalitis virus in goats (197), equine infectious anemia (EIA) virus of horses (198), and bovine immunodeficiency virus in cattle (199). Although none of these natural viral diseases of animals results in a true immunodeficiency disease, the viruses share many similarities to HIV and the various diseases all have some of the clinical features of AIDS in humans (200). Since these viruses are closely related to HIV, there is much interest from a safety standpoint in the use of these viruses to determine *in vitro* antiviral activity directed against HIV (201). The relevance of the use of these animal model systems for determining antiviral activity against HIV infections is currently unknown.

Feline leukemia virus (FeLV) is a natural pathogen of pet cats that causes neoplastic and nonneoplastic diseases and immunosuppression in animals that become persistently infected. Certain variants of FeLV have been isolated that cause severe immunodeficiency disease characterized by persistent viremia, weight loss, lymphoid hyperplasia, lymphoid depletion, suppression of immune function, opportunistic infections, and death (202–205). This syndrome, referred to as "feline AIDS," shares many features with those seen in human AIDS (206,207). This experimental infection of cats is an excellent model in a small, readily available animal and has been used for the evaluation of a number of antiviral agents including AZT and 2′,3′-dideoxycytidine (ddc) (208–210). In the above studies with AZT, results indicated that the time drug was initiated in relation to the time of infection was a critical determinant for outcome of therapy. If treatment was initiated 1 hr after infection, viral replication was inhibited and viremia never developed. In contrast, when initiation of therapy was delayed until 28 days after infection, levels of viremia were lower during treatment but rebounded when therapy was discontinued. Similar observations were made with ddc. These results in the FeLV model correlate fairly well with those obtained in the treatment of human AIDS (211) and validate the use of this model infection. One main advantage of this model is that specific pathogen-free animals are readily available and, when compared with nonhuman primates, are relatively inexpensive.

The murine retroviruses have little in common with HIV, and no murine lentivirus has been described. There is a very strong need, however, for small animals that are models of HIV infections to screen antiviral agents *in vivo*. The replication cycle of the murine leukemia viruses (MuLV) involve many of the same replicative functions that are common to all retroviruses including the reverse transcriptase, protease, and integrase. There is no one murine system that simulates the human disease; however, various systems do produce one or more of the HIV-induced syndromes such as persistent viremia, immunosuppression, splenomegaly, lymphoproliferative disease, infection of the CNS, transplacental and perinatal infection, and an immunodeficiency syndrome. Rauscher leukemia virus produces an erythroleukemia and splenomegaly (212). The LP-BM5 strain of MuLV causes a lymphoproliferation, immunosuppression, a loss in T lymphocyte mitogen responses, progressive lymphadenopathy, and a profound immunodeficiency, and increases susceptibility to opportunistic infections (213–215). The Cas-Br-E variant causes CNS disease (216) and may be a model for therapy of the AIDS dementia complex seen in HIV infections (217). Transgenic mice carrying moloney murine leukemia virus have been used as a model for *in utero* and perinatal infections (218).

In order to use the MuLV models for testing antiviral compounds directed against HIV, three criteria that should be met have been proposed by Ruprecht (219): (a) a potential inhibitor is targeted against a retroviral function common to both HIV as well as the murine test virus; (b) *in vitro* inhibition of HIV and the murine test virus is comparable; and (c) the pharmacokinetics of potential inhibitors are similar in humans and mice. These guidelines, of course, should apply to the use of all animal model infections that do not use the human virus. AZT and a few other antiviral agents have been tested in essentially all the systems described previously, and AZT had activity in all the experimental models (218–223) indicating that the MuLV infections can be used for screening of antiretrovirus compounds, provided appropriate precautions are taken when interpreting the results or when extrapolating the data to other model systems and to HIV infections in humans.

Although there are no proven and predictable animal models for HIV, there are many choices ranging in species from the mouse to the cat, and, finally, to nonhuman primates. The problem at hand is which model should be used, in what sequence. At the present time, a logical sequence is to use the murine models for screening of *in vivo* activity (for one reason, they use less drug) and then test promising compounds in cats or nonhuman primates. Only if a logical testing sequence is developed will the large burden of evaluating numerous antiretroviral compounds in animal models and humans be accomplished in an efficient and effective manner.

### Hepadnavirus Infections

HBV exhibits strong species and tissue specificity, and attempts to establish a model infection in laboratory animals have been unsuccessful. The one animal that has been shown to be susceptible to infection with HBV is the chimpanzee (224,225) (Table 9). These animals regularly develop an antigenemia, and some go on to be chronic carriers of surface antigen (226). It has also been demonstrated recently that HBV DNA can be detected in peripheral blood lymphocytes (227) similar to what has been observed in human HBV infections (228). The animals do not, however, develop cirrhosis or hepatomas (229). Chimpanzees infected with HBV have been used in the past as a model for evaluating the efficacy of antiviral therapy in humans (230). However, given the shortage and cost of these animals and their use as a model for HIV infection, this is no longer a viable use for these valuable and expensive animals. A recent approach to the development of animal models for studying HBV infection has been the production of transgenic mice containing integrated copies of cloned HBV genome. Some of the progeny of these animals became chronic carriers and produced surface antigen (231–234). In another approach, nude mice injected intrahepatically with HBV DNA also became chronic carriers, produced HBV surface and e antigen, produced antibody to HBV gene products, and many developed chronic hepatitis. There was no evidence of viral replication, however (235). The utility of using these two mouse models of HBV infection to evaluate antiviral activity remains to be determined; however, valuable information regarding viral replication and pathogenesis of HBV will certainly be forthcoming in future years.

Since there is currently no usable animal model for determining antiviral activity to HBV, efforts have been directed in developing experimental models using other hepadnaviruses that share many of the features of HBV infections. These are naturally occurring infections of woodchucks, Pekin ducks, and the ground squirrel (Table 9). Of the three models, the WHV system may have the greatest potential for antiviral studies since it appears to most closely simulate HBV-induced liver disease, including the development of hepatocellular carcinoma (236,237). Animals are available commercially or can be bred in captivity and have been used in the evaluation of at least one candidate antiviral (94). DHBV is less

**TABLE 9.** *Animal models for hepadnavirus and papillomavirus infections*

| Virus | Animal | Disease | Measure of efficacy |
|---|---|---|---|
| Hepadnaviruses | | | |
| HBV | Chimpanzee | Antigenemia, persistent infections | Viremia |
| | Transgenic mice | Antigenemia, chronic carriers, hepatitis | Viremia, pathogenesis |
| WHV | Woodchucks | Viremia, persistent infections, hepatocellular carcinoma | DNA polymerase |
| DHBV | Pekin ducks | Viremia, persistent infections, hepatomas | DNA polymerase |
| GSHV | Ground squirrels | Viremia, persistent infections | DNA polymerase |
| Papillomaviruses | | | |
| HPV-11 | Xenographs in nude mice | Graft, transformation | Xenograft growth, histopathology |
| Shope papilloma | Rabbits | Warts | Size and severity |
| Bovine papilloma | Cattle | Warts | Size and severity |

closely related to HBV than the viruses of woodchucks or ground squirrels (238), but the virus can produce hepatocellular carcinoma (239) and integrated DHBV DNA has been identified in duck hepatocytes in a manner similar to HBV and WHV (240). Advantages of this model system include its availability, low cost, the establishment of chronic infections (241), and the fact that tissue culture assay systems can be established. The model has been used for evaluation of a number of antiviral compounds including Foscarnet, ACV, and Suramin (242,243). The ground squirrel hepatitis virus (GSHV) system also involves a persistent infection and the probable development of hepatocellular carcinoma (244); the primary drawback of the model is its lack of availability. Ground squirrels are not available commercially, do not breed in captivity, and have a limited geographic distribution, which severely limits, if not rules out completely, their use as a model for HBV. There has been one limited trial comparing the effectiveness of adenine arabinoside monophosphate (ara-AMP) and DHPG in locally trapped animals with persistent GSHV (245). Of the three animal virus model infections for HBV, only the woodchuck and the duck are viable systems at the present time. As these models get more widespread use, a wealth of information regarding potential antiviral therapies for HBV will be forthcoming.

### Papillomavirus Infections

HPVs also exhibit extreme species and tissue specificity and do not infect laboratory animals. Therefore, alternative models have been used (Table 9). One novel system has been developed in which human foreskin xenografts infected with HPV-11 are placed under the renal capsule of nude mice (246). The grafts form cysts under the renal capsule, and morphological transformation identical to that seen in biopsies from cervical cancer has been observed. Only recently has this system been utilized for determining efficacy of an antiviral agent, and it was demonstrated that the growth of the transformed xenograft could be suppressed (J.W. Kreider, unpublished observations). A model using a nonhuman virus, the Shope papilloma of rabbits, has been well described (247) and has been available for many years. With the renewed interest in HPV as a sexually transmitted disease and as a cause of cervical carcinoma, it is anticipated that this model will surely be used extensively in evaluating antivirals for potential activity against HPV.

### Pharmacokinetic and Metabolism Studies

In order to interpret antiviral efficacy data obtained in animal models correctly and extrapolate this information to the design of clinical trials, it is necessary to understand the pharmacokinetic and pharmacodynamic profiles of the investigational drug in experimental animals. Variables such as drug adsorption, whether adsorption be by oral, topical, or parenteral administration; the organ or tissue distribution of the drug; and metabolism and excretion of the drug and/or its metabolites all must be considered in assessing the potential for use of a new drug in humans (248). These data are also important for estimating dosages, route of treatment, and dosing schedules for efficacy trials as well as for assessing toxicity in animals and humans.

The pharmacologic profile of a new drug should be determined in multiple species, which should include one nonhuman primate. Animals most commonly used for these studies have been mice, rats, dogs, and rhesus monkeys. There are many variables that must be considered when determining the pharmacokinetics of an investigational drug including (a) peak or maximum plasma levels; (b) time necessary to reach maximum levels; (c) area under the plasma concentration-time curve; (d) the elimination or terminal phase plasma half-life; (e) tissue distribution; (f) volume of distribution; (g) urinary excretion; (h) total body clearance; (i) bioavailability if the drug is administered other than intravenous; (j) binding of drug to plasma proteins; and (k) a material balance study using radiolabeled drug. It is well documented that there are many differences in the pharmacokinetics and metabolic disposition of antiviral drugs such as Vira-A and ACV among various animal species and between animals and humans (249–254). Although there may be variability in the pharmacodynamics of a drug between animals and humans, the purpose of the preclinical studies is to develop a broad-based understanding of the adsorption, pharmacokinetic, metabolic, and excretion profiles, so this information can be used to design toxicological studies in animals and Phase I clinical trials.

### Toxicity

Prior to the filing of an Investigational New Drug application to begin Phase I clinical trials, it is necessary to establish the safety of a new drug. The guidelines for toxicity testing have been formulated by the Food and Drug Administration (FDA) and are tailored to each specific drug investigation. An overview of these basic requirements has been published recently by a private firm (255), and are summarized here only as general guidelines.

#### *Acute*

The purpose of acute toxicity studies is to determine the short-term effects of a single dose of drug or multiple doses given over 24 hr or a shorter amount of time. Drug should be administered to various species (i.e., 2 rodent and 1 nonrodent) by various routes using wide dosage ranges including ones far beyond that expected to be used in efficacy studies. The animals are observed for 1 week, and information that should be gained from these studies include (a) acute toxic dose, or preferably, a rising dose tolerance study; (b) a therapeutic index where efficacy in the same species is available; (c) age, sex, and species differences; (d) effects on physical and behavioral characteristics; and (e) pharmacokinetic and metabolic disposition as a measure of drug adsorption and distribution.

#### *Subacute*

The length of treatment to determine subacute toxicity is variable but usually ranges from a minimum of 30 days to as long as 90 days. These studies are usually performed using once daily dosing in one rodent and one nonrodent species. Multiple doses need to be used including a high dose known to be toxic. Information that needs to be collected during this phase includes (a) any physical or behavioral modification, (b) hematology and clinical chemistry profiles to assess liver and kidney function, and (c) results of histopathologic examination of key organs and tissues. The purpose of these studies is to determine the distribution of the drug and identify any target organ toxicity.

#### *Chronic*

Chronic studies are required when a drug is anticipated to be used chronically or intermittently over a prolonged period of time. The time frame for this phase of testing can span a period of 1–2 years depending on the drug's intended use. Again, these tests are usually conducted in at least two species of animals, and similar information to that described for subacute testing needs to be collected. If topical administration is anticipated, dermal and ocular toxicity also needs to be assessed.

### *Carcinogenicity*

Carcinogenicity studies are required for any drug that is intended for use in a large population. They usually require 2 years and are often done in parallel with chronic testing. The aim of these studies is to determine if the new drug induces tumor formation or cellular neoplasms. Carcinogenic assessment involves sacrifice of animals at interim time periods as well as at the end of lifetime dosing. Complete clinical and pathological evaluations are needed.

### *Teratology and Reproductive Fertility*

Tests for the effect of drug treatment on reproductive processes are required for any drug that is to be used in women that have child-bearing potential. Studies need to be conducted to determine if drug treatment has any effect during numerous stages of the reproductive process. These include male and female fertility, zygote implantation, embryo toxicity, fetal death, the birth process, and any effects on the neonate, lactation, and general care of the young. Reproductive fertility studies are conducted by mating drug-treated males and females, and examining the offspring. The reproductive performance of this generation is assessed, and often the $F_2$ generation is also evaluated.

### *Neonatal*

Evaluation of therapeutic agents for use in newborn infants is particularly rigorous and requires that single and multiple dose effects be determined in various stages of neonatal life. Examination at intervals as well as at the terminal stage should include effect on body weight and development, gross examination, and histopathologic, clinical chemistry, and hematological examinations.

### *Genetic*

There is a battery of *in vitro* and *in vivo* tests designed to determine if a drug has the ability to induce mutagenesis or chromosome damage. Some of the *in vitro* assays include the Ames test and cultured mammalian cells such as mouse lymphoma cells, chinese hamster ovary cells, or human lymphocytes. Cultures are exposed to high concentrations of drug and then evaluated for specific mutagenic effects or chromosome abnormalities. For *in vivo* studies, animals are treated with various concentrations of drug and their chromosomes examined for any drug-induced abnormalities.

Detailed descriptions regarding the preclinical toxicology of antiviral agents, particularly ACV, currently being used in humans have been published (256–260), and the reader is referred to these studies for specific details about the toxicity of these agents.

## SUMMARY

There are many excellent cell culture assays and animal model infections for HSV and to a lesser extent for CMV, VZV, influenza, and RSV. The predictability of many of the animal models for antiviral activity against these viruses causing human disease has been established. The current problem is that many of the viral infections in humans that have the greatest need for an effective antiviral agent such as those caused by HIV, CMV, VZV, EBV, HBV, and HPV exhibit strong species and tissue specificity and do not cause productive infections in experimental animals. For these viral infections, there is a need to continue the development of natural animal infections that closely resemble the corresponding disease in humans. For HIV infections, where there is a wide range of animal models available, it is important that the predictability of these various models be determined. The development of new *in vitro* and *in vivo* models for HIV, HBV, and HPV using transfection or other novel approaches using molecular biology techniques to circumvent species specificity needs to be pursued until the feasibility of using these model systems for determination of antiviral activity can be evaluated and their predictability established. It is anticipated that in the next few years a wealth of information using these experimental systems to evaluate classical as well as novel approaches to antiviral therapy will be obtained.

## ACKNOWLEDGMENT

I thank Rita Smith for typing the manuscript. This work was supported in part by Public Health Service Contracts N01-AI-62518 and N01-AI-82518 from the Antiviral Substances Program, Antiviral Research Branch, National Institute of Allergy and Infectious Diseases, National Institutes of Health, Bethesda, MD.

## REFERENCES

1. Whitley RJ, Alford CA, Hirsch MS, et al. Vidarabine versus acyclovir therapy in herpes simplex encephalitis. *N Engl J Med* 1986;314:144–9.
2. Whitley RJ, Arvin A, Prober C, et al. Vidarabine versus acyclovir therapy of neonatal herpes simplex virus infection (submitted).
3. Corey L, Nahmias AJ, Guinan ME, et al. A trial of topical acyclovir in genital herpes simplex virus infections. *N Engl J Med* 1982;306: 1313–9.
4. Bryson YJ, Dillon M, Lovett M, et al. Treatment of first episodes of genital herpes simplex virus infection with oral acyclovir. A randomized double-blind controlled trial in normal subjects. *N Engl J Med* 1983;308:916–21.
5. Corey L, Fife KH, Benedetti JK, et al. Intravenous acyclovir for the treatment of primary genital herpes. *Ann Intern Med* 1983;98: 914–21.
6. Straus SE, Smith HA, Brickman C, et al. Acyclovir for chronic mucocutaneous herpes simplex virus infection in immunosuppressed patients. *Ann Intern Med* 1982;96:270–7.
7. Reichman RC, Badger GJ, Mertz GJ, et al. Treatment of recurrent genital herpes simplex infections with oral acyclovir. *JAMA* 1984; 251:2103–7.
8. Douglas JM, Critchlow C, Benedetti J, et al. A double-blind study of oral acyclovir for suppression of recurrences of genital herpes simplex virus infection. *N Engl J Med* 1984;310:1551–6.
9. Kern ER. Treatment of genital herpes simplex virus infections in guinea pigs. In: Rapp F, ed. *Herpesvirus*. New York: Alan R. Liss, Inc., 1984:617–36.
10. Mertz GJ, Critchlow CW, Benedetti J, et al. Double-blind placebo-controlled trial of oral acyclovir in first-episode genital herpes simplex virus infection. *JAMA* 1984;252:1147–51.
11. Straus SE, Takiff HE, Seidlin M, et al. Suppression of frequently recurring genital herpes. A placebo-controlled double-blind trial of oral acyclovir. *N Engl J Med* 1984;310: 1545–50.
12. Erlich KS, Mills J, Chatis P, et al. Acyclovir-resistant herpes simplex virus infections in patients with the acquired immunodeficiency syndrome. *N Engl J Med* 1989;320:293–6.
13. Buhles WC, Mastre BJ, Tinker AJ, Strand V, Koretz SH, and the Syntex Collaborative Ganciclovir Treatment Study Group. Ganciclovir treatment of life-or sight threatening cytomegalovirus Infection: experience in 314 immunocompromised patients. *Rev Infect Dis* 1988;10:(suppl)S495–506.
14. Mills J, Jacobson MA, O'Donnell JJ, Cederberg D, Holland GN. Treatment of cytomegalovirus retinitis in patients with AIDS. *Rev Infect Dis* 1988;10(suppl):S522–31.
15. Dieterich DT, Chachoua A, Lafleur F, Worrell C. Ganciclovir treatment of gastrointestinal infections caused by cytomegalovirus in patients with AIDS. *Rev Infect Dis* 1988; 10:(suppl)S532–7.
16. Crumpacker C, Marlowe S, Zhang JL, Abrams S, Watkins P, and the ganciclovir bone marrow transplant treatment group. *Rev Infect Dis* 1988;10(suppl):S538–46.
17. Winston DJ, Ho WG, Bartoni K, et al. Ganciclovir therapy for cytomegalovirus infections in recipients of bone marrow transplants and other immunosuppressed patients. *Rev Infect Dis* 1988;10(suppl):S547–53.
18. Walmsley SL, Chew E, Read SE, et al. Treatment of cytomegalovirus retinitis with trisodium phosphonoformate hexahydrate (Foscarnet). *J Infect Dis* 1988;157:569–72.
19. Oberg B, Behrnetz S, Eriksson B, et al. Clinical use of Foscarnet (phosphonoformate). In: De Clercq E, ed. *Clinical use of antiviral drugs*. Boston: Martinus Nijhoff, 1988:223–40.
20. Whitley RJ, Hilty M, Haines R, et al. Vidarabine therapy of varicella in immunocompromised patients. *J Pediatr* 1982;101:125–31.
21. Whitley RJ, Soong S-J, Dolin R, et al. Early vidarabine therapy to control the complications of herpes zoster in immunocompromised patients. *N Engl J Med* 1982;307:971–5.

22. Prober CG, Kirk LE, Keeney RE. Acyclovir therapy of chickenpox in immunosuppressed children—a collaborative study. *J Pediatr* 1982;101:622–5.
23. Balfour HH Jr, Bean B, Laskin OL, et al. Acyclovir halts progression of herpes zoster in immunocompromised patients. *N Engl J Med* 1983;308:1448–53.
24. Shepp DH, Dandliker PS, Meyers JD. Treatment of varicella-zoster virus infection in severely immunocompromised patients. A randomized comparison of acyclovir and vidarabine. *N Engl J Med* 1986;314:208–12.
25. Andersson J, Britton S, Ernberg I, et al. Effect of acyclovir on infectious mononucleosis: a double-blind, placebo-controlled study. *J Infect Dis* 1986;153:283–90.
26. Straus S, Dale JK, Armstrong G, Preble O, Lawley T, Henle W. Acyclovir (ACV) treatment of a chronic fatigue syndrome with unusual EBV serologic profiles: lack of efficacy in a controlled trial. *Clin Res* 1987;35:618A.
27. Lopez C, Pellet P, Stewart J, et al. Characteristics of human herpesvirus-6. *J Infect Dis* 1988;157:1271–3.
28. Streicher HZ, Hung CL, Ablashi DV, et al. *In vitro* inhibition of human herpesvirus-6 by phosphonoformate. *J Virol Methods* 1988;21:301–4.
29. Dolin R. Rimantadine and amantadine in the prophylaxis and therapy of influenza A. In: De Clercq E, ed. *Clinical use of antiviral drugs*. Boston: Martinus Nijhoff, 1988:277–87.
30. Knight V, Gilbert BE. Ribavirin aerosol treatment of influenza. In: Knight V, Gilbert BE, eds. *Infectious disease clinics of North America*. Philadelphia: W.B. Saunders Co, 1987:441–57.
31. Hall CB, McBride JT, Gala CL, Hildreth SW, Schnabel KC. Ribavirin treatment of respiratory syncytial viral infection in infants with underlying cardiopulmonary disease. *JAMA* 1985;254:3047–51.
32. Hayden FG. Use of interferons for prevention and treatment of respiratory viral infections. In: Mills J, Corey L, eds. *Antiviral chemotherapy: new directions for clinical applications and research*. New York: Elsevier, 1986:28–39.
33. Fischl MA, Richman DD, Grieco MH, et al. The efficacy of azidothymidine (AZT) in the treatment of patients with AIDS and AIDS-related complex. A double-blind, placebo-controlled trial. *N Engl J Med* 1987;317:185–91.
34. Richman DD, Fischl MA, Grieco MH, et al. The toxicity of azidothymidine (AZT) in the treatment of patients with AIDS and AIDS-related complex. A double-blind, placebo-controlled trial. *N Engl J Med* 1987;317:192–7.
35. Larder BA, Darby G, Richman DD. HIV with reduced sensitivity to Zidovudine (AZT) isolated during prolonged therapy. *Science* 1989;243:1731–4.
36. Kiviat NB, Koutsky LA, Pravonen JA, et al. Prevalence of genital papillomavirus infections among women attending a college student health clinic or a sexually transmitted disease clinic. *J Infect Dis* 1989;159:293–302.
37. Koss LG. Carcinogenesis in the uterine cervix and human papillomaviruses infection. In: Syrjanen K, Gissman L, Koss LG, eds. *Papillomaviruses and human disease*, New York: Springer-Verlag, 1987:235–67.
38. Newton A. Tissue culture methods for assessing antivirals and their harmful effects. In: Field HJ, ed. *Antiviral agents: the development and assessment of antiviral chemotherapy, vol. I*, Boca Raton: CRC Press, 1988:23–66.
39. De Clercq E. Comparative efficacy of antiherpes drugs in different cell lines. *Antimicrob Agents Chemother* 1982;21:661–3.
40. Kern ER, Overall JC Jr, Glasgow LA. *Herpesvirus hominis* infection in newborn mice: Comparison of the therapeutic efficacy of 1-*B*-D-arabinofuranosylcytosine and 9-*B*-D-arabinofuranosylandenine. *Antimicrob Agents Chemother* 1975;7:587–95.
41. De Clercq E, Descamps J, Verheist G, et al. Comparative efficacy of antiherpes drugs against different strains of herpes simplex virus. *J Infect Dis* 1980;141:563–74.
42. Kern ER, Glasgow LA, Overall JC Jr, Reno JM, Boezi JA. Treatment of experimental herpesvirus infections with phosphonoformate and some comparisons with phosphonoacetate. *Antimicrob Agents Chemother* 1978;14:817–23.
43. McLaren C, Ellis MN, Hunter GA. A colorimetric assay for the measurement of the sensitivity of herpes simplex viruses to antiviral agents. *Antiviral Res* 1983;3:223–34.
44. Moran DM, Kern ER, Overall JC Jr. Synergism between recombinant human interferon and nucleoside antiviral agents against herpes simplex virus: examination with an automated microtiter plate assay. *J Infect Dis* 1985;151:1116–22.
45. Kern ER, Overall JC Jr, Glasgow LA. *Herpesvirus hominis* infection in newborn mice. I. An experimental model and therapy with iododeoxyuridine. *J Infect Dis* 1973;128:290–9.
46. Collins P, Bauer DJ. Relative potencies of antiherpes compounds. In: Herrmann EC Jr, ed. *Third Conference on Antiviral Substances*, 3rd ed, New York: The New York Academy of Sciences, 1976:49–59.
47. Swierkosz EM, Scholl DR, Brown JL, Jollick JD, Gleaves CA. Improved DNA hybridization method for detection of acyclovir-resistant herpes simplex virus. *Antimicrob Agents Chemother* 1987;31:1465–9.
48. Rabalais GP, Levin MJ, Berkowitz FE. Rapid herpes simplex virus susceptibility testing using an enzyme-linked immunosorbent assay performed *in situ* on fixed virus-infected monolayers. *Antimicrob Agents Chemother* 1987;31:946–8.
49. Turk SR, Shipman C Jr, Nassiri R, et al. Pyrrolo[2,3-d]pyrimidine nucleosides as inhibitors of human cytomegalovirus. *Antimicrob Agents Chemother* 1987;31:544–50.
50. Freitas VR, Smee DF, Chernow M, Boehme R, Matthews TR. Activity of 9-(1,3-dihydroxy-2-

propoxymethyl) guanine compared with that of acyclovir against human, monkey, and rodent cytomegaloviruses. *Antimicrob Agents Chemother* 1985;28:240–5.

51. Dankner WM, Spector SA. Determination of antiviral activity of ganciclovir (DHPG) and antiretroviral agents against human cytomegalovirus (HCMV) using a novel DNA-DNA hybridization assay [Abstract]. *Antiviral Res* 1988;9:114.
52. Bryson YJ, Connor JD. *In vitro* susceptibility of varicella zoster virus to adenine arabinoside and hypoxanthine arabinoside. *Antimicrob Agents Chemother* 1976;9:540–3.
53. Biron KK, Elion GB. Effect of acyclovir combined with other antiherpetic agents on varicella zoster virus *in vitro*. Symposium on acyclovir. *Am J Med* 1982;73:54–7.
54. Berkowitz FE, Levin MJ. Use of an enzyme-linked immunosorbent assay performed directly on fixed infected cell monolayers for evaluating drugs against varicella-zoster virus. *Antimicrob Agents Chemother* 1985;28:207–10.
55. Stanberry LR, Myers MG. Evaluation of varicella-zoster antiviral drugs by a nucleic acid hybridization assay. *Antiviral Res* 1988;9:367–77.
56. Margalith M, Manor D, Usieli V, Goldblum N. Phosphonoformate inhibits synthesis of Epstein-Barr virus (EBV) capsid antigen and transformation of human cord blood lymphocytes by EBV. *Virology* 1980;102:226–30.
57. Lin J-C, De Clercq E, Pagano JS. Novel acyclic adenosine analogs inhibit Epstein-Barr virus replication. *Antimicrob Agents Chemother* 1987;31:1431–3.
58. Lin J-C, Machida H. Comparison of two bromovinyl nucleoside analogs, 1-*B*-D-arabinofuranosyl-E-5-(2-bromovinyl) uracil and E-5-(2-bromovinyl)-2′-deoxyuridine, with acyclovir in inhibition of Epstein-Barr virus replication. *Antimicrob Agents Chemother* 1988;32:1068–72.
59. Lin J-C, Zhang Z-X, Smith MC, Biron K, Pagano JS. Anti-human immunodeficiency virus agent 3′-azido-3-deoxythymidine inhibits replication of Epstein-Barr virus. *Antimicrob Agents Chemother* 1988;32:265–7.
60. Lidin BIM, Lamon EW, Cloud G, Soong S-J. Complementation between infecting Epstein-Barr virus and intrinsic viral genomes in human lymphoid cell lines. *Intervirology* 1982;18:66–75.
61. Lidin BIM, Lamon EW. Effects of DNA synthesis inhibitors on early antigen expression following primary infection or superinfection by Epstein-Barr virus. *Arch Virol* 1983;77:13–25.
62. Pagano JS. Nucleoside analogs for Epstein-Barr virus infections. In: Mills J, Corey L, eds. *Antiviral chemotherapy: new directions for clinical application and research*. New York: Elsevier, 1986:184–9.
63. Finter NB. Methods for screening *in vitro* and *in vivo* for agents active against myxoviruses. *Ann NY Acad Sci*. 1970;173:131–8.
64. Babiker HA, Rott R. Plaque formation by influenza viruses in monolayers of chicken kidney cells. *J Gen Virol* 1968;3:285–7.
65. Kawana F, Shigeta S, Hosoya M, Suzuki H, De Clercq E. Inhibitory effects of antiviral compounds on respiratory syncytial virus replication *in vitro*. *Antimicrob Agents Chemother* 1987;31:1225–30.
66. Wyde PR, Gilbert BE, Ambrose NW. Comparison of the antirespiratory syncytial virus activity and toxicity of papaverine hydrochloride and pyrazofurin *in vitro* and *in vivo*. *Antiviral Res* 1989;11:15–26.
67. Otto MJ, Fox MP, Fancher MJ, Kuhrt MF, Diana GD, McKinlay MA. *In vitro* activity of WIN 51711, a new broad-spectrum antipicornavirus drug. *Antimicrob Agents Chemother* 1985;27:883–6.
68. Ahmad ALM, Dowsett AB, Tyrrell DAJ. Studies of rhinovirus resistant to an antiviral chalcone. *Antiviral Res* 1987;8:27–39.
69. Conti C, Orsi N, Stein ML. Effect of isoflavans and isoflavenes on rhinovirus 1B and its replication in HeLa cells. *Antiviral Res* 1988;10:117–27.
70. Mitsuya H, Weinhold KJ, Furman PA, et al. 3′-Azido-3′-deoxythymidine (BW A509U): an antiviral agent that inhibits the infectivity and cytopathic effect of human T-lymphotropic virus type III/lymphadenopathy-associated virus *in vitro*. *Proc Natl Acad Sci USA* 1985;82:7096–100.
71. Mitsuya H, Broder S. Inhibition of the *in vitro* infectivity and cytopathic effect of human T-lymphotrophic virus type III/lymphadenopathy-associated virus (HTLV-III/LAV) by 2′, 3′-dideoxynucleosides. *Proc Natl Acad Sci* 1986;83:1911–5.
72. Popovic M, Sarngadharan MG, Read E, Gallo RC. Detection, isolation, and continuous production of cytopathic retroviruses (HTLV-III) from patients with AIDS and pre-AIDS. *Science* 1984;224:497–500.
73. Vrang L, Bazin H, Remaud G, Chattopadhyaya J, Oberg B. Inhibition of the reverse transcriptase from HIV by 3′-azido-3′-deoxythymidine triphosphate and its threo analogue. *Antiviral Res* 1987;7:139–49.
74. Schinazi RF, Eriksson BFH, Hughes SH. Comparison of inhibitory activities of various antiretroviral agents against particle-derived and recombinant human immunodeficiency virus type 1 reverse transcriptases. *Antimicrob Agents Chemother* 1989;33:115–7.
75. Veronese FD, Sarngadharan MG, Rahman R, et al. Monoclonal antibodies specific for p24, the major core protein of human T-cell leukemia virus type III. *Proc Natl Acad Sci USA* 1985;82:5199–202.
76. Pauwels R. Balzarini J, Schols D, et al. Phosphonylmethoxyethyl purine derivatives, a new class of anti-human immunodeficiency vi-

rus agents. *Antimicrob Agents Chemother* 1988;32:1025–30.
77. Harada S, Koyanagi Y, Yamamoto N. Infection of HTLV-III/LAV in HTLV-I-carrying cells MT-2 and MT-4 and application in a plaque assay. *Science* 1985;229:563–6.
78. Nakashima H, Matsui T, Harada S, et al. Inhibition of replication and cytopathic effect of human T cell lymphotropic virus type III/lymphadenopathy-associated virus by 3′-azido-3′-deoxythymidine *in vitro*. *Antimicrob Agents Chemother* 1986;30:933–7.
79. Ito M, Nakashima H, Baba M, et al. Inhibitory effect of glycyrrhizin on the *in vitro* infectivity and cytopathic activity of the human immunodeficiency virus [HIV(HTLV-III/LAV)]. *Antiviral Res* 1987;7;127–37.
80. Hamamoto Y, Nakashima H, Matsui T, Matsuda A, Ueda T, Yamamoto N. Inhibitory effect of 2′,3′-didehydro-2′,3′dideoxynucleosides on infectivity, cytopathic effects, and replication of human immunodeficiency virus. *Antimicrob Agents Chemother* 1987;31:907–10.
81. Montefiore DC, Robinson WE, Schuffman SS, et al. Evaluation of antiviral drugs and neutralizing antibodies to human immunodeficiency virus by a rapid and sensitive microtiter infection assay. *J Clin Microbiol* 1988;26:231–5.
82. Pauwels R, Balzarini J, Baba M, et al. Rapid and automated tetrazolium-based colorimetric assay for the detection of anti-HIV compounds. *J Virol Methods* 1988;20:309–21.
83. Vince R, Hau M, Brownell J, et al. Potent and selective activity of a new carbocyclic nucleoside analog (Carbovir: NSC 614846) against human immunodeficiency virus *in vitro*. *Biochem Biophys Res Commun* 1988;156:1046–53.
84. Weislow OS, Kiser R, Fine DL, Bader J, Shoemaker RH, Boyd MR. New soluble-formazan assay for HIV-1 cytopathic effects: application to high-flux screening of synthetic and natural products for AIDS-antiviral activity. *J Natl Can Inst* 1989;81:577–86.
85. Sureau C, Romet-Lemonne J-L, Mullins, JI, Essex M. Production of hepatitis B virus by a differentiated human hepatoma cell line after transfection with cloned circular HBV DNA. *Cell* 1986;47:37–47.
86. Sells MA, Chen M-L, Acs G. Production of hepatitis B virus particles in Hep G2 cells transfected with cloned hepatitis B virus DNA. *Proc Natl Acad Sci USA* 1987;84:1005–9.
87. Yaginuma K. Shirakata Y, Kobayashi M, Soike K. Hepatitis B virus (HBV) particles are produced in a cell culture system by transient expression of transfected HBV DNA. *Proc Natl Acad Sci USA* 1987;84:2678–82.
88. Tuttleman JS, Pugh JC, Summers JW. *In vitro* experimental infection of primary duck hepatocyte cultures with duck hepatitis B virus. *J Virol* 1986;58:17–25.
89. Tao P-Z, Lofgren B, Lake-Bakaar D, Johansson NG, Datema R, Oberg B. Inhibition of human hepatitis B virus DNA polymerase and duck hepatitis B virus DNA polymerase by triphosphates of thymidine analogs and pharmacokinetic properties of the corresponding nucleosides. *J Med Virol* 1988;26:353–62.
90. Petcu DJ, Aldrich CE, Coates L, Taylor JM, Mason WS. Suramin inhibits *in vitro* infection by duck hepatitis B virus, Rous sarcoma virus, and hepatitis delta virus. *Virology* 1988; 167:385–92.
91. Suzuki S, Lee B, Luo W, Tovell D, Robins MJ, Tyrrell DLJ. Inhibition of duck hepatitis B virus replication by purine 2′,3′-dideoxynucleosides. *Biochem Biophys Res Commun* 1988;156:1144–51.
92. Fourel I, Hantz O, Cova L, Allaudeen HS, Trepo C. Main properties of duck hepatitis B virus DNA polymerase: comparison with the human and woodchuck hepatitis B virus DNA polymerases. *Antiviral Res* 1987;8:189–99.
93. Korba BE, Cote PJ, Gerin JL. Mitogen-induced replication of woodchuck hepatitis virus in cultured peripheral blood lymphocytes. *Science* 1988;241:1213–6.
94. Venkateswaran PS, Millman I, Blumberg BS. Effects of an extract from *Phyllanthus niruri* on hepatitis B and woodchuck hepatitis viruses: *in vitro* and *in vivo* studies. *Proc Natl Acad Sci USA* 1987;84:274–8.
95. Phillips HJ. Dye exclusion tests for cell viability. In: Kruse PF Jr, Patterson MK Jr, eds. *Tissue culture: methods and applications*, New York: Academic Press, 1973:406–8.
96. Freshney RI. *Culture of animal cells. A manual of basic techniques*. 2nd ed. New York: Alan R. Liss, Inc., 1987:245–56.
97. Mosmann T. Rapid colorimetric assay for cellular growth and survival: application to proliferation and cytotoxicity assays. *J Immunol Methods* 1983;55–63.
98. Scudiero DA, Shoemaker RH, Paull KD, et al. Evaluation of a soluble tetrazolium/formazan assay for cell growth and drug sensitivity in culture using human and other tumor cell lines. *Cancer Res* 1988;48:4827–33.
99. Freshney RI. *Culture of animal cells. A manual of basic techniques*. 2nd ed. New York: Alan R. Liss, Inc., 1987:227–44.
100. Sommadossi J-P, Carlisle R, Schinazi RF, Zhou Z. Uridine reverses the toxicity of 3′-azido-3′-deoxythymidine in normal human granulocyte-macrophage progenitor cells *in vitro* without impairment of antiretroviral activity. *Antimicrob Agents Chemother* 1988;32:997–1001.
101. Sommadossi J-P, Carlisle R. Toxicity of 3′-azido-3′deoxythymidine and 9-(1,3-dihydroxy-2-propoxymethyl) guanine for normal human hematopoietic progenitor cells *in vitro*. *Antimicrob Agents Chemother* 1987;31:452–4.
102. Esber EC, Nelson RC, Browder NJ. Safety assessment of antiviral drugs. In: De Clercq E, Walker RT, eds. *Antiviral drug development. A multidisciplinary approach*. New York: Plenum Press, 1988:261–73.
103. Field HJ. Animal models in the evaluation of

antiviral chemotherapy. In: Field HJ, ed. *Antiviral agents: the development and assessment of antiviral chemotherapy, vol. I.* Boca Raton: CRC Press, Inc., 1988:67–84.

104. De Clercq E, Luczak M. Intranasal challenge of mice with herpes simplex virus: an experimental model for evaluation of the efficacy of antiviral drugs. *J Infect Dis* 1976; 133(suppl):A226–36.
105. Kern ER. Animal models as assay systems for the development of antivirals. In: De Clercq E, Walker RT, eds. *Antiviral drug development. A multidisciplinary approach.* New York: Plenum Press, 1988:149–72.
106. Whitley RJ, Soong S-J, Dolin R, et al. Adenine arabinoside therapy of biopsy-proved herpes simplex encephalitis. *N Engl J Med* 1977;297:289–94.
107. Whitley RJ, Soong S-J, Hirsch MS, et al. Herpes simplex encephalitis. Vidarabine therapy and diagnostic problems. *N Engl J Med* 1981;304:313–8.
108. Kern ER, Richards JT, Overall JC Jr, Glasgow LA. Alteration of mortality and pathogenesis of three experimental *Herpesvirus hominis* infections of mice with adenine arabinoside 5′-monophosphate, adenine arabinoside, and phosphonoacetic acid. *Antimicrob Agents Chemother* 1978;13:53–60.
109. Kern ER, Overall JC Jr, Glasgow LA. *Herpesvirus hominis* infection in newborn mice: comparison of the therapeutic efficacy of 1-*B*-D-arabinofuranosylcytosine ad 9-*B*-D-arabinofuranosyladenine. *Antimicrob Agents Chemother* 1975;7:587–95.
110. Overall JC Jr, Kern ER, Glasgow LA. Treatment of *Herpesvirus hominis* type 2 infections in mice with adenine arabinoside. In: Pavan-Langston D, Buchanan RA, Alford CA Jr, eds. *Adenine arabinoside: an antiviral agent.* New York: Raven Press, 1975:95–110.
111. Whitley RJ, Nahmias AJ, Soong S-J, Galasso GG, Fleming CL, Alford CA. Vidarabine therapy of neonatal herpes simplex virus infections. *Pediatrics* 1980;66:495–501.
112. Whitley RJ, Yeager A, Kartus P, et al. Neonatal herpes simplex virus infection. Follow-up evaluation of vidarabine therapy. *Pediatrics* 1983;72:778–85.
113. Kern ER, Richards JT, Glasgow LA, Overall, JC Jr, De Miranda P. Optimal treatment of herpes simplex virus encephalitis in mice with oral acyclovir. Symposium on acyclovir. *Am J Med* 1982;73:125–31.
114. Kern ER, Richards JT, Overall JC Jr. Acyclovir treatment of disseminated herpes simplex virus type 2 infection in weanling mice: alteration of mortality and pathogenesis. *Antiviral Res* 1986;6:189–95.
115. Kaufman HE. Clinical cure of herpes simplex keratitis by 5-iodo-2′-deoxyuridine. *Proc Soc Exp Biol Med* 1962;109:251–2.
116. Kaufman HE, Martola F, Dohlman C. The use of 5-iodo-2′-deoxyuridine (IDU) in the treatment of herpes simplex keratitis. *Arch Ophthalmol* 1962;68:235–9.
117. Pavan-Langston D, Langston RHS, Geary PA. Idoxuridine, adenine arabinoside, and hypoxanthine arabinoside in the prophylaxis and therapy of experimental ocular herpes simplex. In: Pavan-Langston D, Buchanan RA, Alford CA Jr, eds. *Adenine arabinoside: an antiviral agent.* New York: Raven Press, 1975:337–44.
118. Pavan-Langston D, Dohlman CH. A double-blind clinical study of adenine arabinoside therapy of viral keratoconjunctivitis. *Am J Ophthalmol* 1972;74:81–8.
119. Kaufman HE, Heidelberger C. Therapeutic antiviral action of 5-trifluoromethyl-2′-deoxyuridine. *Science* 1964;145:585–6.
120. Wellings PC, Awdry PN, Bors FH, Jones BA, Brown DC, Kaufman HE. Clinical evaluation of trifluorothymidine in the treatment of herpes simplex corneal ulcers. *Am J Ophthalmol* 1972;73;932–42.
121. Trousdale MD, Nesburn AB. Evaluation of the herpetic activity of acyclovir in rabbits. Symposium on acyclovir. *Am J Med* 1982;73:155–60.
122. Laibson PR, Pavan-Langston D, Yeakley WR, Lass J. Acyclovir and vidarabine for the treatment of herpes simplex keratitis. Symposium on acyclovir. *Am J Med* 1982;73:281–5.
123. Spruance SL, McKeough MB. Evaluation of antiviral treatments for recurrent herpes simplex labialis in the dorsal cutaneous guinea pig model. *Antiviral Res* 1988;9:295–313.
124. Hubler WR, Felber TD, Troll D, Jarratt M. Guinea pig model for cutaneous herpes simplex virus infection. *J Invest Dermatol* 1974;62: 92–5.
125. Schaefer TW, Lieberman M, Everitt J, Came P. Cutaneous herpes simplex virus infection as a model for antiviral chemotherapy. *Ann NY Acad Sci* 1977;284:624–31.
126. Spruance SL, Freeman DJ, Sheth NV. Comparison of topical foscarnet, acyclovir (ACV) and ACV ointment in the treatment of experimental cutaneous herpes simplex virus (HSV) infection. *Antimicrob Agents Chemother* 1986;30:196–8.
127. Spruance SL. Treatment of herpes simplex labialis. In: De Clercq E, ed. *Clinical use of antiviral drugs.* Boston: Martinus Nijhoff, 1988:67–86.
128. Spruance SL, McKeough MB, Cardinal JR. Penetration of guinea pig skin by acyclovir in different vehicles and correlation with the efficacy of topical therapy of experimental cutaneous herpes simplex virus infection. *Antimicrob Agents Chemother* 1984;25:10–5.
129. Overall JC Jr, Kern ER, Schlitzer RL, Friedman SB, Glasgow LA. Genital *Herpesvirus hominis* infection in mice. I. Development of an experimental model. *Infect Immun* 1975;11:476–80.
130. Kern ER, Richards JT, Overall JC Jr, Glasgow LA. Genital *Herpesvirus hominis* infection in

mice. II. Treatment with phosphonoacetic acid, adenine arabinoside, and adenine arabinoside 5′-monophosphate. *J Infect Dis* 1977;135:557–67.

131. Kern ER, Richard JT, Overall JC Jr, Glasgow LA. A comparison of phosphonoacetic acid and phosphonoformic acid activity in genital herpes simplex virus type 1 and type 2 infections of mice. *Antiviral Res* 1981;1:225–35.
132. Kern ER, Richards JT, Overall JC Jr, Glasgow LA. Acyclovir treatment of experimental genital herpes simplex virus infections. I. Topical therapy of type 2 and type 1 infections of mice. *Antiviral Res* 1983;3:253–67.
133. Kern ER. Acyclovir treatment of experimental genital herpes simplex virus infections. Symposium on acyclovir. *Am J Med* 1982;73:100–8.
134. Stanberry LR, Kern ER, Richards JT, Abbott TA, Overall JC Jr. Genital herpes in guinea pigs: pathogenesis of the primary infection and description of recurrent disease. *J Infect Dis* 1982;146:397–404.
135. Stanberry LR, Kern ER, Richards JT, Overall JC Jr. Recurrent genital herpes simplex virus infection in guinea pigs. *Intervirology* 1985;24:226–31.
136. Hsiung GD, Mayo DR, Lucia HL, Landry ML. Genital herpes: pathogenesis and chemotherapy in the guinea pig model. *Rev Infect Dis* 1984;6:33–50.
137. Overall JC Jr. Herpes simplex virus latency and reactivation: human disease/animal model correlations. In: Rapp F, ed. *Herpesvirus*, New York: Alan R. Liss, Inc., 1984:145–58.
138. Pronovost AD, Lucia HL, Dann PR, Hsiung GD. Effect of acyclovir on genital herpes in guinea pigs. *J Infect Dis* 1982;145:904–8.
139. Fraser-Smith EB, Smee DF, Matthews TR. Efficacy of the acyclic nucleoside 9-(1,3-dihydroxy-2-propoxymethyl) guanine against primary and recrudescent genital herpes simplex virus type 2 infections in guinea pigs. *Antimicrob Agents Chemother* 1983;24:883–8.
140. Corey L, Adams HG, Brown ZA, Holmes KK. Genital herpes simplex virus infections: clinical manifestations, course, and complications. *Ann Intern Med* 1983;98:958–72.
141. Reichman RC, Badger GJ, Guinan ME, et al. Topically administered acyclovir in the treatment of recurrent herpes simplex genitalis: a controlled trial. *J Infect Dis* 1983;147:336–40.
142. Bryson YJ, Dillon M, Lovett M, Bernstein D, Garrantty E, Sayre J. Treatment of first episode genital HSV with oral acyclovir: long term follow-up of recurrences. A preliminary report. *Scand J Infect Dis* 1985;47(suppl):70–5.
143. Mertz GJ, Critchlow CW, Benedetti J, et al. Double-blind placebo controlled trial of oral acyclovir for first episode genital herpes. *JAMA* 1984;252:1147–51.
144. Ho M. *Cytomegalovirus, biology and infection*. New York: Plenum Medical Book Co., 1982.
145. Glasgow LA, Richards JT, Kern ER. Effect of acyclovir treatment on acute and chronic murine cytomegalovirus infection. Symposium on acyclovir. *Am J Med* 1982;73:132–7.
146. Shanley JD, Pesanti EL, Nugent KM. The pathogenesis of pneumonitis due to murine cytomegalovirus. *J Infect Dis* 1982;146:388–96.
147. Shanley JD, Pesanti EL. The relation of viral replication to interstitial pneumonitis in murine cytomegalovirus lung infection. *J Infect Dis* 1985;151:454–8.
148. Bia FJ, Griffith BP, Fong CKY, Hsiung GD. Cytomegalovirus infections in the guinea pig: experimental models for human disease. *Rev Infect Dis* 1983;5:177–95.
149. Overall JC Jr, Kern ER, Glasgow LA, Effective antiviral chemotherapy in cytomegalovirus infection of mice. *J Infect Dis* 1976; 133(suppl):A237–44.
150. Wingard JR, Bender WJ, Saral R, Burns WH. Efficacy of acyclovir against mouse cytomegalovirus *in vivo*. *Antimicrob Agents Chemother* 1981;20:275–8.
151. Debs RJ, Montgomery AB, Baunette EN, DeBruin M, Shanley JD. Aerosol administration of antiviral agents to treat lung infection due to murine cytomegalovirus. *J Infect Dis* 1988;157:327–31.
152. Lang DJ, Cheung K-S. Effectiveness of acycloguanosine and trifluorothymidine as inhibitors of cytomegalovirus infection *in vitro*. Symposium on acyclovir. *Am J Med* 1982;73:49–53.
153. Shanley JD, Morningstar J, Jordan C. Inhibition of murine cytomegalovirus lung infection and interstitial pneumonitis by acyclovir and 9-(1,3-dihydroxy-2-propoxymethyl) guanine. *Antimicrob Agents Chemother* 1985;28:172–5.
154. Fong CKY, Cohen SD, McCormick S, Hsiung GD. Antiviral effect of 9-(1,3-dihydroxy-2-propoxymethyl) guanine against cytomegalovirus infection in a guinea pig model. *Antiviral Res* 1987;7:11–23.
155. Shepp DH, Dandliker PS, de Miranda P, et al. Activity of 9-[2-hydroxy-1-(hydroxymethyl) ethoxymethyl] guanine in the treatment of cytomegalovirus pneumonia. *Ann Intern Med* 1985;103:368–73.
156. Myers MG, Duer HL, Hausler CK. Experimental infection of guinea pigs with varicella-zoster virus. *J Infect Dis* 1980;142:414–20.
157. Pavan-Langston D, Dunkel EC. Varicella zoster virus ocular infection in guinea pigs: a model. *Arch Ophthalmol* (in press).
158. Dunkel EC, Siegel MI, Rong BL, Pavan-Langston D. Systemic and ocular spread of VZV infection after intranasal inoculation. *Abstracts of the Association of Research in Vision and Ophthalmology* 1989;30:213.
159. Felsenfeld AD, Schmidt NJ. Antigenic relationships among several simian varicella-like viruses and varicella-zoster virus. *Infect Immun* 1977;15:807–12.
160. Soike KF, Felsenfeld AD, Gibson S, Gerone PJ. Ineffectiveness of adenine arabinoside and adenine arabinoside 5-monophosphate in

simian varicella infection. *Antimicrob Agents Chemother* 1980;18:142–7.
161. Soike KF, Felsenfeld AD, Gerone PJ. Acyclovir treatment of experimental simian varicella infection of monkeys. *Antimicrob Agents Chemother* 1981;20:291–7.
162. Soike KF, Gerone PJ. Acyclovir in the treatment of simian varicella virus infection of the African Green monkey. Symposium on Acyclovir. *Am J Med* 1982;73:112–7.
163. Soike KF, Gibson S, Gerone PJ. Inhibition of simian varicella virus infection of African Green monkeys by (E)-5-(2-bromovinyl)-2′-deoxyuridine (BVDU). *Antiviral Res* 1981; 1:325–37.
164. Benoit Y, Laureys G, Delbeke M-J, De Clercq E. Oral BVDU treatment of varicella in children with cancer. *J Pediatr* 1985;143:198–202.
165. Nagy-Oltvai Z, Jennings TA, Brady TG, Lucia HL, Armstrong, JA, Hsiung GD. Effect of cyclosporin A immunosuppression on primary lymphotropic herpesvirus infection in the guinea pig. Intervirology 1987;28:105–9.
166. Grunert RR, McGahen JW, Davis WL. The *in vivo* antiviral activity of 1-adamantanamine (amantadine). 1. Prophylactic and therapeutic activity against influenza viruses. *Virology* 1965;26:262–9.
167. Walker JS, Stephen EL, Spertzel RO. Small particle aerosols of antiviral compounds in treatment of type A influenza pneumonia in mice. *J Infect Dis* 1976;133(suppl):A140–4.
168. Potter CW, Oxford JS. Animal models of influenza virus infection as applied to the investigation of antiviral compounds. In: Oxford JS, ed, *Chemoprophylaxis and virus infections of the respiratory tract*. Cleveland: CRC Press, 1977:1–55.
169. Schulman JL. Effect of 1-amantanamine hydrochloride (amantadine HC1) and methyl-1-adamatanethylamine hydrochloride (rimantadine HC1) on transmission of influenza virus infection in mice. *Proc Soc Exp Biol Med* 1968;128:1173–8.
170. Tominack RL, Hayden FG. Rimantadine hydrochloride and amantadine hydrochloride use in influenza A virus infections. In: Knight V, Gilbert BE, eds. *Infectious disease clinics of North America*. Philadelphia: WB Saunders Co., 1987:459–78.
171. Hayden FG. Animal models of influenza virus infection for evaluation of antiviral agents. In: Zak O, Sande MA, eds. *Experimental models in antimicrobial chemotherapy, vol. 3*. New York: Academic Press, 1986:353–71.
172. Wyde PR, Wilson SZ, Gilbert BE, Smith RHA. Protection of mice from lethal influenza virus infection with high dose–short duration ribavirin aerosol. *Antimicrob Agents Chemother* 1986;30:942–4.
173. Prince GA, Jenson AB, Horswood RL, Camargo E, Chanock RM. The pathogenesis of respiratory syncytial virus infection in cotton rats. *Am J Pathol* 1978;93:771–83.
174. Wyde PR, Wilson SZ, Petrella R, Gilbert BE. Efficacy of high dose–short duration ribavirin aerosol in the treatment of respiratory syncytial virus infected cotton rats and influenza B virus infected mice. *Antiviral Res* 1987;7:211–20.
175. Alter HJ, Eichberg JW, Masur H, et al. Transmission of HTLV-III infection from human plasma to chimpanzees: an animal model for AIDS. *Science* 1984;226:549–52.
176. Francis DP, Feorino PM, Broderson JR, et al. Infection of Chimpanzees with lymphadenopathy-associated virus. *Lancet* 1984;ii:1276–7.
177. Gajdusek DC, Gibbs CJ Jr, Rodgers-Johnson P, et al. Infection of Chimpanzees by human T-lymphotropic retroviruses in brain and other tissues from AIDS patients. *Lancet* 1985;i: 55–6.
178. Fultz PN, McClure HM, Swenson RB, et al. Persistent infection of chimpanzees with human T-lymphotropic virus type III/lymphadenopathy associated virus: a potential model for acquired immunodeficiency syndrome. *J Virol* 1986;58:116–24.
179. Fultz PN, McClure HM, Swenson RB, Anderson DC. HIV infection of chimpanzees as a model for testing chemotherapeutics. *Intervirology* 1989;30(suppl):51–8.
180. Letvin NL, Daniel MD, Sehgal PK, et al. Infection of baboons with human immunodeficiency virus-2 (HIV-2) *J Infect Dis* 1987; 156:406–7.
181. Dormont D, Livartowski J, Chamaret S, et al. HIV-2 in rhesus monkeys: serological, virological and clinical results. *Intervirology* 1989;30(suppl):59–65.
182. Kindt TJ, Kulaga H, Truckenmiller ME, Recker D, Folks TM. In: *Abstracts of the Fifth International Conference on AIDS. Montreal Canada. June 4–9, 1989*. 1989:598. Ottawa, Ont:Intl Dev Res Ctr.
183. Leonard JM, Abramczuk JW, Pezen DS, et al. Development of disease and virus recovery in transgenic mice containing HIV proviral DNA. *Science* 1988;242:1665–70.
184. Namikawa R, Kaneshima H, Lieberman M, Weissman L, McCune JM. Infection of the SCID-hu mouse by HIV-1. *Science* 1988; 242:1684–6.
185. Daniel MD, Letvin NL, King NW, et al. Isolation of T-cell tropic HTLV-III-like retrovirus from Macaques. *Science* 1985;228:1201–4.
186. Otha Y, Masuda T, Tsujimoto H, et al. Isolation of simian immunodeficiency virus from African green monkeys and seroepidemiological survey of the virus in various non-human primates. *Int J Cancer* 1988;41:115–22.
187. Fultz PN, McClure HM, Anderson DC, Swenson RB, Anand R, Srinivasan A. Isolation of a T-lymphotropic retrovirus from naturally infected sooty mangabey monkeys (cercocebus Atys) *Proc Natl Acad Sci USA* 1986;83:5286–90.
188. Benveniste RE, Arthur LO, Tsai C-C, et al. Isolation of a lentivirus from a macaque with lymphoma: comparison with HTLV-III/LAV and other viruses. *J Virol* 1986;60:483–90.

189. Desrosiers RC, Letvin NL. Animal models for acquired immunodeficiency syndrome. *Rev Infect Dis* 1987;9:438–46.
190. Desrosiers RC. Simian immunodeficiency viruses. *Ann Rev Microbiol* 1988;42:607–25.
191. Letvin NL, Daniel MD, Sehgal PK, et al. Induction of AIDS-like disease in macaque monkeys with T-cell tropic retrovirus STLV-III. *Science* 1985;230:71–74.
192. Daniel MD, Letvin NL, Sehgal PK, et al. Long-term persistent infection of macaque monkeys with the simian immunodeficiency virus. *J Gen Virol* 1987;68:3183–9.
193. Zhang, J-Y, Martin LN, Watson EA, et al. Simian immunodeficiency virus/delta-induced immunodeficiency disease in rhesus monkeys: relation of antibody response and antigenemia. *J Infect Dis* 1988;158:1277–86.
194. Benveniste RE, Morton WR, Clark EA, et al. Inoculation of baboons and macaques with simian immunodeficiency virus/Mne, a primate lentivirus closely related to human immunodeficiency virus type 2. *J Virol* 1988;62:2091–101.
195. Herchenroder O, Stahl-Hennig C, Luke W, et al. Experimental infection of rhesus monkeys with SIV isolated from African green monkeys. *Intervirology* 1989;30(suppl):66–72.
196. Petursson G, Palsson PA, Georgsson G. Maedi-visna in sheep: host-virus interactions and utilization as a model. *Intervirology* 1989: 30(suppl):36–44.
197. Straub OC. Caprine arthritis encephalitis—a model for AIDS? *Intervirology* 1989: 30(suppl):45–50.
198. McGuire TC. Pathogenesis of equine infectious anemia. In: Salzman LA, ed. *Animal models of retrovirus infection and their relationships to AIDS*. Orlando: Academic Press, Inc., 1986:295–300.
199. Van Der Maaten MJ. Pathogenesis of bovine retrovirus infection. In: Salzman LA, ed. *Animal models of retrovirus infection and their relationship to AIDS*. Orlando: Academic Press, Inc., 1986:213–22.
200. Haase AT. Pathogenesis of lentivirus infections. *Nature* 1986;322:130–6.
201. Frank KB, McKernan PA, Smith RA, Smee D. Visna virus as an *in vitro* model for human immunodeficiency virus and inhibition by ribavirin, phosphonoformate, and 2′3′-dideoxynucleosides. *Antimicrob Agents Chemother* 1987;31:1369–74.
202. Mullins JI, Chen CS, Hoover EA. Disease-specific and tissue-specific production of unintegrated feline leukemia virus variant DNA in feline AIDS. *Nature* 1986;319:333–6.
203. Pedersen NC, Ho EW, Brown ML, Yamamoto JK. Isolation of a T-lymphotropic virus from domestic cats with an immunodeficiency-like syndrome. *Science* 1987;235:790–3.
204. Overbaugh J, Donahue PR, Quackenbush SL, Hoover EA, Mullins JI. Molecular cloning of a feline leukemia virus that induces fatal immunodeficiency disease in cats. *Science* 1988; 239:906–10.
205. Hoover EA, Mullins JI, Quackenbush SL, Gasper PW. Experimental transmission and pathogenesis of immunodeficiency syndrome in cats. *Blood* 1987;70:1880–92.
206. Hoover EA, Mullins JI, Quackenbush SL, Gasper PW. Pathogenesis of feline retrovirus-induced cytopathic diseases: acquired immunodeficiency syndrome and aplastic anemia. In: Salzman LA, ed. *Animal models of retrovirus infection and their relationship to AIDS*. Orlando: Academic Press, Inc., 1986:59–74.
207. Hardy WD Jr. Feline acquired immunodeficiency syndrome: a feline retrovirus-induced syndrome of pet cats. In: Salzman LA, ed. *Animal models of retrovirus infection and their relationship to AIDS*. Orlando: Academic Press, Inc., 1986:75–93.
208. Tavares L, Roneker C, Johnston K, Nusinoff-Lehrman S, de Noronha F. 3′-Azido-3′-deoxythymidine in feline leukemia virus-infected cats: a model for therapy and prophylaxis of AIDS. *Cancer Res* 1987;47:3190–4.
209. Hoover EA, Zeidner NS, Perigo NA, et al. Feline leukemia virus-induced immunodeficiency syndrome in cats as a model for evaluation of antiretroviral therapy. *Intervirology* 1989; 30(suppl):12–25.
210. Tavares L, Roneker C, Postie L, de Noronha F. Testing of nucleoside analogues in cats infected with feline leukemia virus: a model. *Intervirology* 1989;30(suppl):26–35.
211. Yarchoan R, Broder S. Development of antiretroviral therapy for the acquired immunodeficiency syndrome and related disorders. *N Engl J Med* 1987;316:557–64.
212. Rauscher FJ. A virus-induced disease of mice characterized by erythrocytopoiesis and lymphoid leukemia. *JNCI* 1962;29:515–32.
213. Mosier DE, Yetter RA, Morse HC III. Retroviral induction of acute lymphoproliferative disease and profound immunosuppression in adult C57BL/6 mice. *J Exp Med* 1985;161:766–84.
214. Mosier DE, Yetter RA, Morse HC III. Functional T lymphocytes are required for a murine retrovirus-induced immunodeficiency disease (MAIDS). *J Exp Med* 1987;165:1737–42.
215. Yetter RA, Buller ML, Lee JS, et al. CD4+ T cells are required for development of a murine retrovirus-induced immunodeficiency syndrome (MAIDS). *J Exp Med* 1988;168:623–35.
216. Gardner MB, Henderson BE, Officer JE, et al. A spontaneous lower motor neuron disease apparently caused by indigenous type-C RNA virus in wild mice. *JNCI* 1973;51:1243–9.
217. Price RW, Brew B, Sidtis J, Rosenblum M, Scheck AC, Cleary P. The brain in AIDS: Central nervous system HIV-1 infection and AIDS dementia complex. *Science* 1988;239:586–92.
218. Sharpe AH, Hunter JJ, Ruprecht RM, Jaenisch R. Maternal transmission of retroviral disease: transgenic mice as a rapid test system for evaluating perinatal and transplacental antiretroviral therapy. *Proc Natl Acad Sci USA* 1988;85:9792–6.

219. Ruprecht RM. Murine models for antiretroviral therapy. *Intervirology* 1989;30(suppl):2–11.
220. Ruprecht RM, O'Brien LG, Rossoni LD, Nusinoff-Lehrman S. Suppression of mouse viraemia and retroviral disease by 3′-azido-3′-deoxythymidine. *Nature* 1986;323:467–9.
221. Ruprecht RM, Rossoni LD, Haseltine WA, Broder S. Suppression of retroviral propagation and disease by suramin in murine systems. *Proc Natl Acad Sci USA* 1985;82:7733–7.
222. Gangemi JD, Cozens RM, De Clercq E, Balzarini J, Hochkeppel H-K. 9-(2-Phosphonylmethoxyethyl) adenine (PMEA) in the treatment of murine acquired immunodeficiency disease (MAIDS) and opportunistic herpes simplex virus infections (submitted).
223. Fraser-Smith EB, Pecyk RA, Matthews TR. Friend leukemia virus murine model for evaluation of anti-retroviral drugs *Antimicrob Agents Chemother* (In press).
224. Maynard J, Berquist K, Krushak D, Purcell R. Experimental infection of chimpanzees with the virus of hepatitis B. *Nature* 1972;237:514–5.
225. Barker L, Chisari F, McGrath P. Transmission of viral hepatitis, type B, to chimpanzees. *J Infect Dis* 1973;127:648–62.
226. Barker L, Maynard J, Purcell R. Viral hepatitis, type B, in experimental animals. *Am J Med Sci* 1975;270:189–96.
227. Korba BE, Wells F, Tennant BC, Yoakum GH, Purcell RH, Gerin JL. Hepadnavirus infection of peripheral blood lymphocytes *in vivo:* woodchuck and chimpanzee models of viral hepatitis. *J Virol* 1986;58:1–8
228. Laure F, Zagury D, Saimot AG, Gallo RC, Hahn BH, Brechot C. Hepatitis B virus DNA sequences in lymphoid cells from patients with AIDS and AIDS-related complex. *Science* 1985;229:561–3.
229. Ganem D. Animal models of hepatitis B virus infections. In: Zak O, Sande MA, eds. *Experimental models in antimicrobial chemotherapy, vol. 1.* Orlando: Academic Press, 1986;259–73.
230. Scullard G, Greenberg H, Smith J, Gregory P, Merigan T, Robinson W. Antiviral treatment of chronic hepatitis B virus infections: infectious virus cannot be detected in patient serum after permanent responses to treatment. *Hepatology* 1982;2:39–49.
231. Chisari FV, Pinkert CA, Milich DR, et al. A transgenic mouse model of the chronic hepatitis B surface antigen carrier state. *Science* 1985;230:1157–60.
232. Babinet C, Farza H, Morello D, Hadchouel M, Pourcel C. Specific expression of hepatitis B surface antigen (HBsAG) in transgenic mice.*Science* 1985;230:1160–3.
233. Chisari FV, Filippi P, Buras J, et al. Structural and pathological effects of synthesis of hepatitis B virus large envelope polypeptide in transgenic mice. *Proc Natl Acad Sci USA* 1987;84:6909–13.
234. Burk RD, DeLoia JA, Elawady MK, Gearhart JD. Tissue preferential expression of the hepatitis B virus (HBV) surface antigen gene in two lines of HBV transgenic mice. *J Virol* 1988;62:649–54.
235. Feitelson MA, DeTolla LJ, Zhou X-D. A chronic carrierlike state is established in nude mice injected with cloned hepatitis B virus DNA. *J Virol* 1988;62:1408–15.
236. Popper H, Shih JW-K, Gerin JL, et al. Woodchuck hepatitis and hepatocellular carcinoma: correlation of histologic with virologic observations. *Hepatology* 1981;1:91–8.
237. Popper H, Roth L, Purcell RH, Tennant BC, Gerin JL. Hepatocarcinogenicity of the woodchuck hepatitis virus. *Proc Natl Acad Sci USA* 1987;84:866–70.
238. Mason W, Seal G, Summers J. Virus of Pekin ducks with structural and biological relatedness to human hepatitis B virus. *J Virol* 1980;36:829–36.
239. Omata M, Uchiumi K, Ito Y, et al. Duck hepatitis B virus and liver disease. *Gastroenterology* 1983;85:260–7.
240. Imazeki F, Yaginuma K, Omata M, Okuda K, Kobayashi M, Koike K. Integrated structures of duck hepatitis B virus DNA in hepatocellular carcinoma. *J Virol* 1988;62:861–5.
241. O'Connell AP, Urban MK, London WT. Naturally occurring infection of Pekin duck embryos by duck hepatitis B virus. *Proc Natl Acad Sci USA* 1983;80:1703–6.
242. Sherker AH, Hirota K, Omata M, Okuda K. Foscarnet decreases serum and liver duck hepatitis B virus DNA in chronically infected ducks. *Gastroenterology* 1986;91:818–24.
243. Zuckerman AJ. Screening of antiviral drugs for hepadnavirus infection in Pekin ducks: a review. *J Virol Methods* 1987;17:119–26.
244. Marion PL, Van Davelaar MJ, Knight SS, et al. Hepatocellular carcinoma in ground squirrels persistently infected with ground squirrel hepatitis virus. *Proc Natl Acad Sci USA* 1986;83:4543–6.
245. Smee DF, Knight SS, Duke AE, Robinson WS, Matthews TR, Marion PL. Activities of arabinosyladenine monophosphate and 9-(1,3-dihydroxy-2-propoxymethyl)guanine against ground squirrel hepatitis virus *in vivo* as determined by reduction in serum virion-associated DNA polymerase. *Antimicrob Agents Chemother* 1985;27:277–9.
246. Kreider JW, Howett MK, Wolfe SA, et al. Morphological transformation *in vivo* of human uterine cervix with papillomavirus from condylomata acuminata. *Nature* 1985;317:639–41.
247. Kreider JW, Bartlett GL. The Shope papilloma-carcinoma complex of rabbits: a model system of neoplastic progression and spontaneous regression. *Adv Cancer Res* 1981;35:81–110.
248. Prusoff WH, Lin T-S. Experimental aspects of antiviral pharmacology. In: De Clercq E, Walker RT, eds. *Antiviral drug development. A multidisciplinary approach.* New York: Plenum Press, 1988:173–202.
249. Glazko AJ, Chang T, Drach JC, et al. Species

differences in the metabolic disposition of adenine arabinoside. In: Pavan-Langston D, Buchanan RA, Alford CA Jr, eds. *Adenine arabinoside: an antiviral agent,* New York: Raven Press, 1975:111–33.

250. De Miranda P, Krasny HC, Page DA, Elion GB. Species differences in the disposition of acyclovir. Symposium on acyclovir. *Am J Med* 1982;73:31–5.
251. Good SS, De Miranda P. Metabolic disposition of acyclovir in the guinea pig, rabbit, and monkey. Symposium on acyclovir. *Am J Med* 1982;73:91–5.
252. Krasny HC, De Miranda P, Blum MR, Elion GB. Pharmacokinetics and bioavailability of acyclovir in the dog. *J Pharmacol Exp Ther* 1981;216:281–8.
253. De Miranda P, Good SS, Krasny HC, Connor JD, Laskin OL, Lietman PS. Metabolic fate of radioactive acyclovir in humans. Symposium on acyclovir. *Am J Med* 1982;73:215–20.
254. Laskin OL, Longstreth JA, Saral R, De Miranda P, Keeney R, Lietman PS. Pharmacokinetics and tolerance of acyclovir, a new antiherpesvirus agent, in humans. *Antimicrob Agents Chemother* 1982:21:393–8.
255. Parexel International Corporation, Mathieu MP, Murphy WJ, eds. *New drug development: a regulatory overview.* Washington: OMEC International, Inc., 1987:19–27
256. Kurtz SM. Toxicology of adenine arabinoside. In: Pavan-Langston D, Buchanan RA, Alford CA Jr, eds. *Adenine arabinoside: an antiviral agent.* New York: Raven Press, 1975;145–57.
257. Tucker WE Jr. Preclinical toxicology profile of acyclovir: an overview. Symposium on acyclovir. *Am J Med* 1982;73:27–30.
258. Szczech GM. The toxicity of nucleoside analogues. In: Mills J, Corey L, eds. *Antiviral chemotherapy. New directions for clinical application and research,* New York: Elsevier, 1986:205–25.
259. Dayan AD, Anderson D. Toxicity of antiviral compounds. In: Field HJ, ed. *Antiviral agents: the development and assessment of antiviral chemotherapy, vol. I,* Boca Raton: CRC Press, Inc., 1988:111–26.
260. Canonico PG; Kende M. Huggins JW. The toxicology and pharmacology of ribavirin in experimental animals. In: Smith RA, Knight V, Smith JAD, eds. *Clinical application of Ribavirin.* Orlando: Academic Press, Inc., 1984:65–92.

*Antiviral Agents and Viral Diseases of Man, 3rd Edition,*
edited by G. J. Galasso, R. J. Whitley, and
T. C. Merigan, Raven Press, Ltd., New York © 1990.

# 4

# Clinical Drug Development: Human Pharmacology, Safety, and Tolerance Trials

Oscar L. Laskin

*Department of Clinical Pharmacology, Merck, Sharp & Dohme Research Laboratories, Rahway, New Jersey 07065; and Department of Medicine and Clinical Pharmacology, Cornell University Medical College, New York, New York 10021*



The development of effective chemotherapy against viral diseases has long lagged behind other areas of antiinfective chemotherapy. Some of the reasons for this have included the following: First, until relatively recently, many scientists believed that it would not be possible to develop antiviral agents that would have selective toxicity against viruses and still be safe in humans. This was based on the mistaken belief that since viruses require host cells for viral replication, any agent that was capable of inhibiting viral replication would also be extremely toxic to the uninfected cell. Second, until relatively recently, there had been a lack of fundamental knowledge concerning viral replication and the infectious cycle. Without this knowledge, viral specific events could not be identified that could then serve for targets for therapeutic attack. Third, during the past decade, facilities for clinical virology were inadequate or absent in most hospitals. Fourth, many physicians were inexperienced and had a lack of training in understanding the techniques available for the specific identification of viral diseases. Fifth, and finally, the spectrum of activity of most antiviral agents are narrow, but the clinical presentation of viral syndromes are often nonspecific. Different viruses can cause identical syndromes, and the same virus may manifest clinical illness in many different ways. Therefore, it is difficult, if not impossible, to accurately identify the specific etiologic virus based entirely on clinical grounds.

In general, for antiviral chemotherapy to be effective, treatment must be instituted early. Many of the techniques for viral isolation in the past were slow and required days to weeks to make a specific diagnosis. Only by coupling the ability to rapidly identify the causative virus with effective and safe antiviral agents can optimal treatment be achieved. We are only now entering a period of time when there has been development of sensitive and rapid diagnostic tests for the specific identification of viral

**TABLE 1.** *Outline for the development of an antiviral agent*

- PRECLINICAL DATA AS IT RELATES TO CLINICAL STUDIES
  - *In vitro*
    - Potency
    - Cellular toxicity
    - *In vitro* therapeutic index
    - Intracellular metabolism
  - *In vivo* animal studies
    - Toxicity
    - Efficacy
    - Therapeutic index
- PHASE I CLINICAL TRIALS
  - Single-dose/multiple-dose studies in healthy volunteers/patients
    - Pharmacokinetics
    - Pharmacodynamics (usually in patients)
      - Viral challenge in subjects or antiviral effect in patients
      - Immunologic parameters
      - Biochemical end points
      - Clinical end points in either challenge studies or in patients
    - Tolerance/safety
  - Radioactive labeled drug trials
  - Trials in patients where the major organ of elimination is diseased
    - Renal insufficiency
    - Liver disease
    - Diseases likely to have an adverse effect on the pharmacokinetics or pharmacodynamics of an agent
  - Miscellaneous
    - Bioavailability studies of different formulations (IM, PO, SQ)
    - Drug/drug interactions
    - Studies in populations with various physiological states (as warranted)
      - Neonate or infant
      - Children
      - Elderly
      - Pregnancy or postpartum
- PHASE II STUDIES
  - Dose-ranging studies
  - Open and control trials to establish preliminary efficacy and safety data; parameter assessed may include the following
    - Virology
    - Immunology
    - Biochemical end points
    - Clinical end points
    - Toxicity
    - Concentration response relationship
- DESIGN OF PHASE III TRIALS
  - Definitive trials, numbers greater than 100
  - Usually double-blind, controlled, randomized
  - Frequently multiple centers
  - Dose and dose interval selected based on Phase I–II data
  - Usually clinical trials address numerous potential indications
  - At lease two definitive trials for each indication
- POST-NDA STUDIES
  - Phase III–like trials for additional indications
  - Postmarketing surveillance (Phase IV)
  - Adverse drug reporting (Phase IV)

IM, intramuscular; PO, oral; SQ, subcutaneous.

illness. With the advent and recognition of an epidemic and fatal disease caused by the human retrovirus, human immunodeficiency virus (HIV), there has been a great amount of effort and resources focused on antiviral drug development.

The purpose of this chapter is to present an overview (Table 1) of a generalized approach to antiviral drug development with an emphasis on the Phase I–II clinical pharmacology studies necessary to design Phase III trials. Since the agents in this class will be developed for diseases as trivial as the common cold, where essentially no significant side effects can be tolerated, to infections that are as serious and life-threatening as herpes simplex virus (HSV) encephalitis, acquired immune deficiency syndromes (AIDS), and cytomegalovirus (CMV) pneumonitis in immunocompromised patients, the generic approach of this chapter will need to be tailored to the specific investigational agent. Since, inherently, the design of Phase III trials needs to be based on specific knowledge of the properties of the agent and its indications, these trials are not really amendable to a generic approach. Therefore, this chapter will emphasize the Phase I–IIA trials, which are necessary to define the therapeutic window or appropriate dosage regimes that will be used to proceed into clinical trials to establish efficacy and safety. For the purpose of this chapter, clinical pharmacology trials, which will encompass Phases I to early Phase II (Phase IIA), will be defined as those trials that (a) evaluate the safety, tolerability, pharmacodynamics, and pharmacokinetics in healthy volunteers and/or patients; (b) demonstrate biological activity; (c) establish the dose range to be used in late Phase II and III trials; (d) provide a preliminary assessment of the efficacy of the drug in selected patient populations; and (e) evaluate pharmacodynamic and kinetic interactions of the drug with other specific drugs. Late Phase II (Phase IIB) and Phase III trials are defined as those studies necessary to demonstrate definitive effectiveness for each particular indication, to establish the safety or toxicity for a long term and/or repeated intermittent use, and to evaluate any further drug interactions. Whenever possible, it is imperative that the utmost effort be made to ensure that these trials be conducted in a prospective, double-blinded, randomized, and controlled fashion. The control group should be the standard therapy in practice for that indication at that time. If there are no pharmacological modalities that have been shown to be effective for a particular indication, then it is not only ethical but essential that the control group be a placebo. This is especially important in viral chemotherapy where the natural history of viral diseases are frequently not well documented and extremely variable in their clinical manifestations and duration. There are numerous examples where the lack of a control group led one to disastrous conclusions until properly controlled trials were conducted [e.g., iododeoxyuridine and cytosine arabinoside (ara-C) for HSV encephalitis, ara-C for herpes zoster].

## PRECLINICAL REQUIREMENTS

Before one can initiate studies in humans with a new chemical entity, a significant amount of preclinical information is required. These include *in vitro* data as well as *in vivo* animal studies. The purpose of the preclinical studies are to elucidate the main pharmacological activity of the drug and to provide the rationale for development of this compound in humans. These studies are necessary to demonstrate *in vitro* and *in vivo* activity against the viruses in question, to define the spectrum of activity of the compound, to determine the mechanism of action and the mechanism by which resistance is likely to occur, to have a general understanding of the pharmacokinetics likely to be seen in humans, and to establish the toxicological profile of the drug.

*In vitro* testing should be completed in order to assess the spectrum of its antiviral activity and to determine potency (the effective dose 50% and/or 90%) and the *in vitro* therapeutic index as compared to appropriate positive and negative controls. Too often in the past a great emphasis had been placed on the potency of antiviral drugs. Usually when a new antiviral drug is considered, the concentration required to inhibit a specific virus, usually a 50% inhibitory or effective dose ($ID_{50}$ or $ED_{50}$, respectively) is compared with the inhibitory concentration of another agent. This by itself is usually not very important. Potency only determines the amount of drug that needs to be given. What limits the amount that can be given is its toxicity. For example, if a drug is five times less potent but 10 times less toxic, then it has a better margin of safety or therapeutic index than the more potent one.

In tissue culture, this concept has been termed the "*in vitro* therapeutic index." After all, what is important is the ratio of the concentration that is toxic to uninfected host cells compared to the concentration of drug that inhibits virus replication (i.e., cytotoxic dose to viral inhibitory dose). The larger the therapeutic index, the greater the clinical potential for the antiviral agent. For example, both ara-C and acyclovir (ACV) have equal potency against HSV ($ID_{50}$ of approximately 0.1–0.2 μM); however, the cytotoxic concentration of ara-C is approximately 0.1 μM, whereas ACV inhibits cellular growth at concentrations in excess of 300 μM (1). Thus, although both agents are equally potent against HSV, ara-C has an *in vitro* therapeutic index of 1, whereas acyclovir has a therapeutic index of greater than 3,000. This difference is reflected *in vivo* and may have predicted why ara-C–treated patients did worse than placebo in clinical trials, whereas ACV has been found to be therapeutically active against infections due to herpes viruses while having minimal toxicity.

If possible, the mechanism of therapeutic action and the mechanism by which viral resistance to the drug develops should be elucidated. Frequently, the mechanism by which a drug exerts its antiviral activity is discovered by studying viral strains that are resistant to the agent.

Pharmacology studies in various species of animals should be performed. Ideally, this should include at least one nonhuman primate species. Also included in the preclinical package is a material balance study using radiolabeled drug. The development of a specific and sensitive assay is important and if at all possible should be developed before going into humans. The assay can be radioimmunoassay, high-pressure liquid chromatography (HPLC), gas chromatography, or microbiological. Disposition, pharmacokinetics, and toxicity will allow one to choose an appropriate initial study dose in the clinical pharmacology trials. Formal preclinical toxicology studies will need to be conducted. In these toxicology studies, the drug is given to at least two species of animals (at least one being in a nonrodent species) for a duration of 1–3 months. The antiviral drug is administered by the same route and with the same formulation as that intended for use in humans. The importance of the preclinical toxicology is to identify which organ systems are most likely to be the most sensitive to the toxic effects of the agent. In clinical testing, these will be areas where particular and special attention will be focused. Finally, the drug must be in a pharmaceutical formulation that is acceptable for human use. For example, it should be free of potentially toxic impurities, stable in its stored state, relatively soluble, etc.

The reader is referred to Chapter 3 for more specific information regarding preclinical testing.

## CLINICAL DEVELOPMENT PLAN

Although the clinical development of a new drug entity is artificially separated into several phases (Table 1), these phases are not discrete and one phase does not necessarily start when another phase ends. In fact, it is the rule rather than the exception that these phases overlap. For example, one may be doing a Phase I study in hemodialysis patients while Phase III trials are ongoing. However, it is convenient to refer to various aspects of clinical development as phases, and perhaps a better division of the drug development process is to actually split the pre New Drug Application (NDA) into two major phases: Phases I–IIA and Phases IIB–III. The emphasis of this chapter will be on Phases I–IIA (clinical pharmacology studies). These represent studies that explored the pharmacokinetics and tolerance or safety of new drug entities. In addition, in the IIA trials, biological effect and some early efficacy and safety data are collected. In general, a study in this phase usually consists of fewer than 100 patients, especially in Phase I trials. In Phase IIB and III, one is primarily interested in the definitive trials that demonstrate that the drug is efficacious and sufficiently safe for various indications. By sufficiently safe, one is referring to the risk/benefit ratio.

Depending on the underlying disease and the availability of alternative therapy, the degree of toxicity or adverse effects that one is willing to accept will vary. For example, the amount of toxicity that is acceptable for the treatment of upper respiratory infections (i.e., the common cold) is very small, and, essentially, the drug must be free of any serious toxicity. Agents of this class would have to be as safe or safer than penicillin. On the other hand, in the treatment of HSV encephalitis or symptomatic HIV disease, significant toxicity would be tolerated if the overall effect was beneficial. For example, zidovudine (azidothymidine; AZT) causes significant bone marrow toxicity in approximately 40% of patients (2). However, because of the seriousness and the high morbidity and mortality of untreated disease and the absence of any other effective alternative therapy, the risk to benefit ratio is clearly in favor of treating patients with this agent (3). Similarly, use of ganciclovir for the treatment of CMV retinitis is also justified (4,5). As mentioned previously, the degree of toxicity that one is willing to tolerate is also dependent on alternative therapies. For example, although ganciclovir would probably be efficacious for life-threatening HSV infections, its use is not justified (because of its toxicity) since alternative therapy with ACV has been shown to be safe and effective (6). Therefore, the approach to the development of an antiviral drug to treat rhinoviruses and the development of an agent to treat CMV infections in immunocompromised patients or symptomatic HIV disease will differ greatly. In fact, a promising agent for use against HIV disease will probably have its drug development program, prior to submission of the NDA, greatly abbreviated. For example, AZT was approved before its Phase III trials were completed. The Phase III Program for AZT occurred after the drug was licensed for marketing in the United States. In the information that follows, one must remember that this is a generic approach that will need to be individualized and modified with respect to the agent that is being developed.

## CLINICAL PHARMACOLOGY PROGRAM: PHASE I–IIA TRIALS

The initiation of Phase I trials for a promising antiviral drug represents the first time that a new chemical entity is being administered to a human. Of utmost concern is human tolerability. However, one is also interested in assessing pharmacokinetics, pharmacodynamics, duration of biological effect, and the effect of disease (renal, cardiac, and/or hepatic failure) on the kinetics or dynamics of the new antiviral agent. The main goal of the clinical pharmacology program is to allow one to select a rational dosage range to be used in Phase II–III trials in order to demonstrate that the antiviral agent is effective and has an acceptable risk to benefit ratio. An acceptable risk to benefit ratio will depend on the degree of toxicity, the seriousness of the indication, and the availability of alternative therapy. For example, an agent that is designed to provide prophylaxis or even treatment against mild infections caused by respiratory viruses ("common cold") must be essentially free of any significant toxicity. On the other hand, agents that are effective in treating symptomatic infections caused by HIV or to treat CMV disease in AIDS and/or organ transplant recipients can have significant toxicity. An effective agent for influenza would be of little use if it had a toxicologic profile similar to ganciclovir or zidovudine.

### Subject Selection

It is customary to recruit normal volunteers for Phase I trials. Usually they are men rather than women so that concerns regarding tetratogenicity and embryotoxicity are minimized. They are usually between the ages of 18 years (the age of legal consent) and 40–50 years. They are excluded if they are on current medications and/or if they have significant diseases, especially those that affect the organs of elimination. They are excluded if they use illicit

**TABLE 2.** *An example of incremental single/multiple-dose trial of hypothetical anti-HIV agent*

Objectives
- To determine safety and MTD
- To determine dose and dose interval for the multiple dose study based on dose-response and pharmacodynamics
- To determine the disposition in humans

Design
- Double-blind, placebo-controlled, single dose. Each group will contain 10 patients (eight on drug, two on placebo). Each group will be given increasing doses of drug until MTD is reached or a plateau is reached on the dose-response curve with regard to effect and duration of effect.

Patient number
- Anticipated to be 50–60 patients

Patients
- HIV infected with P-24 antigenemia[a]

First study duration
- Single dose, with at least 2-week follow-up

Second study duration
- Multiple dose, usually for at least five half-lives of the drug (usually 5–14 days)

[a]Severity of disease will be based on the toxicologic profile of drug. A drug with a clean profile can be used in asymptomatic patients, and an agent with a high risk of toxicity will require patients to have advanced symptomatic disease.

MTD, maximum tolerated dose.

**TABLE 3.** *An example of a Phase I–IIA multiple-dose ranging trial of hypothetical anti-HIV agent*

Dose ranging
- Incremental multiple dose

Objectives
- To determine safety and MTD of multiple dose
- To determine dose-response and pharmacodynamics
- Determine short-term biological efficacy
- Determine dose necessary for long-term trials

Design
- Double-blind, placebo-controlled, multiple dose; anticipated no more than three different regimens tested, with each group having 20 patients (15 on drug and five on placebo)
- Total study will be as follows
  - Treatment A, n = 15
  - Treatment B, n = 15
  - Treatment C, n = 15
  - Control, n = 15
- Parameters to be followed as per Table 4

Dose/dose interval
- Determined by first trial results

Duration
- 6–12 weeks

Patients
- HIV-infected patients[a]

Patient number
- 60 patients

[a]See Table 2.

drugs and/or if they consume excessive amounts of alcoholic beverages. They are expected to have no clinical or laboratory abnormality. However, with some antiviral agents that are being developed for serious and/or life-threatening indications and where preclinical toxicity or previous experience with the class of agents indicate a significant risk of adverse effects in humans, it may be necessary for patients to be included. Examples are ganciclovir and zidovudine where initial Phase I studies were performed in CMV-infected or in symptomatic HIV-infected patients, respectively. In addition, sometimes a patient population must be employed when the aims of the study include investigating pharmacodynamic parameters that can only be studied in patients, such as antiviral effect and recovery of immunological defects (e.g., P-24 antigenemia, CD4 cells number, recovery of immune cell function in HIV-infected patients), as outlined in Tables 2–4.

However, since one of the primary functions of Phase I trials is to assess tolerance, the population selected should be one that is as healthy as possible. This is because it is often difficult to distinguish whether an adverse event is caused by the drug under study or the underlying disease. For example, if rhinitis and nasal stuffiness occurred in a patient being treated for a respiratory virus infection with an intranasal preparation, one might assume that this adverse event is due to the viral infection. However, intranasally administered interferon can cause rhinitis and nasal stuffiness in healthy volunteers (7), and, therefore, this adverse effect may have been masked if

**TABLE 4.** *Parameters examined in Phase I–IIA trials for a hypothetical anti-HIV agent*

DISPOSITION
- Pharmacokinetics
- Concentrations in various biological fluids:
  - Saliva
  - Vaginal secretions
  - Semen
  - Urine
  - Red blood cells and lymphocytes
  - CSF (when available)
  - Autopsy specimens (when available)

PHARMACODYNAMICS
- Virology
  - HIV culture (performed once a week)
  - P-24 antigenemia (once a week)
  - Polymerase chain reaction assay (once a week)
- Immunologic
  - CD4 lymphocyte count (once a week)
  - CD4/CD8 ratio, total lymphocyte count (once a week)
  - Mitogen- and antigen-induced lymphocytic proliferation studies (once a week)
  - Mitogen- and antigen-induced $\gamma$-interferon production in lymphocytes (once a week)
  - Delayed hypersensitivity conversions (every 2 weeks)
- Clinical assessment
  - Global response
  - Weight change
  - Physical exam
  - Performance score
  - Subjective response
  - Number and severity of any opportunistic infections and AIDS-related tumors

TOLERANCE
- Queries regarding adverse events, physical exam
- Standard battery of laboratory monitoring tests
  - Hematologic
    - CBC, differential, platelets, reticulocyte counts. Bone marrows when available for clinical indications. Transfusion requirements.
  - Hepatic
    - Liver function enzymes
  - Renal
    - Creatinine, creatinine clearance, blood urea nitrogen (BUN)
  - Electrolytes
  - CNS and peripheral nervous system work-up as indicated by clinical situation

studies were performed only in patients. On the other hand, if one was to administer a new antiviral agent to patients with advanced symptomatic HIV infections, then it is likely that even in a relatively small number of patients, serious adverse events would be seen, such as neutropenia, anemia, neuropathy, renal dysfunction, etc. These serious and potentially life-threatening adverse events may be incorrectly attributed to the agent, even though they frequently occur in patients with AIDS. Alternatively, serious adverse effects of the drug may wrongly be ascribed to the patient's disease state.

Because clinically it is often difficult to assess the relationship between an adverse event that would have occurred even if the drug was not given and an adverse effect caused by the drug, it is imperative to employ an appropriate control group even in Phase I trials. In Phase I trials, the control agent is usually placebo. Occasionally, in ill patients, an active control agent is employed. In this case, the control agent should be whatever is considered standard therapy for a particular disease.

## Design

To assess tolerability, a dose-ranging schedule is usually employed in which patients or volunteers are exposed to increasing drug doses, usually until a maximal tolerated dose is reached. Table 1 provides an outline of the specific clinical pharmacology studies that are frequently conducted as part of the Phase I program for an antiinfective agent. Tables 2 and 3 provide examples of single- and multiple-dose Phase I–IIA trials, respectively, for a hypothetical agent for HIV disease, in which patients are the study population. Table 4 provides the parameters that are being assessed in these studies.

Clinical pharmacology studies frequently include the following:

1. Incremental single-dose trials are used where the main objective is to establish the tolerance of single doses of the antiviral agent. If possible, pharmacokinetics and

dynamics are determined. Kinetics require that a sensitive and specific assay be available. Usually, pharmacodynamics of antiviral agents can only be assessed if the study population is virally infected patients. However, it is possible to study *ex vivo* effects of some antiviral drugs such as interferon. For example, Barouki et al. (8) investigated the pharmacodynamics of interferon in healthy volunteers by measuring the 2′,5′-oligoadenylate synthetase activity of blood mononuclear cells and the inability to infect them *ex vivo* with vesicular stomatitis virus.

The choice for the initial dose is often difficult. The initial starting dose is usually based on preclinical data. This is based roughly on a dose that should provide concentrations that are the same order of magnitude as that found to inhibit the virus *in vitro*. However, in order to protect the patient by allowing for species difference in drug effect, the starting dose is usually 1–2% (on a mg/kg basis) of the highest dose that did not produce any significant toxicity in animals (no effect level for toxicity). However, there are other ways to determine a starting dose, and the amount of risk one is willing to assume is in part based on the seriousness and expected outcome without treatment. An example of a study for HIV disease where the toxicity of the drug is such that a healthy subject cannot be used is outlined in Tables 2 and 4.

2. Incremental multiple-dose trials are also conducted, and as the name implies, either drug or placebo is given repeatedly, usually for 5–14 days. The duration of drug administration is such that steady state conditions are reached. The time to steady state can be approximated from the terminal phase half-life calculated from the single dose studies. The time to 90% of steady state concentrations is 3.3 half-lives, and the time to steady state is approximately 5 half-lives. For example, a drug like ACV with a half-life of 2–3 hr will reach steady state condition within the first day, whereas a drug like ribavirin with a terminal half-life on the order of days may continue to accumulate for longer than a week. These studies should be conducted in a double-blinded, controlled fashion. If an assay is available, then frequent blood and urine samples for kinetic analysis should be obtained on the first dose, the last dose, and usually at some intermediate dose. In addition, a trough (predose) blood sample obtained every day or so provides information regarding accumulation and time to achieve steady state conditions. Frequently, there are approximately eight to 10 patients per dose group, with three to four of these receiving placebo (an example of such a study for a hypothetical anti-HIV drug is outlined in Tables 2 and 4). The dose and dose interval will be selected based on information obtained from the single-dose study. Usually, the dose interval is based on the terminal phase half-life.

3. If feasible, the distribution, metabolites and material balance of a drug is determined using single-dose radiolabeled trials. This study is important to determine the fate of the drug and to find all possible metabolites as well as to account for the entire dose administered.

4. Bioavailability studies are done if the formulation is delivered by a route other than by intravenous (IV) infusion and if an IV formulation is available. This is accomplished by administering both an IV dose and a dose by the intended route of administration to the same subject usually in a cross-over fashion with an adequate washout period between doses.

5. Clinical pharmacokinetics and tolerance studies are conducted in patients with varying degrees of renal dysfunction. These studies are especially important if the major route of elimination of the drug or any active metabolites is by renal excretion. These studies are performed in patients with mild, moderate, and severe renal insufficiency. In addition, Phase I trials are conducted in patients with end-stage renal

disease, both in the interdialysis period as well as during hemodialysis in order to assess the hemadialyzibility of the compound. These studies allow recommendations for dose modification, if necessary, in patients with various degree of renal dysfunction.

6. Studies of clinical pharmacokinetics in patients with hepatic dysfunction are important with agents that have appreciable metabolism. Unfortunately, there are no reliable parameters of hepatic function analogous to that of serum creatinine or creatinine clearance for assessing renal dysfunction. In addition, hepatic damage affects different metabolic pathways to varying degrees. For example, oxidative pathways are more sensitive to hepatic damage than are glucuronide conjugation. These studies can determine the degree of caution that is warranted when the antiviral agent is administered to patients with hepatic disease.

7. In Phase I trials in special age groups, the pharmacokinetics, dynamics, and tolerance of the antiviral drug may differ with respect to age. In general, the elimination of drugs from the body in children older than 6 months of age is similar to adults when normalized to body surface area. In neonates, especially when they are born prematurely, the liver and kidneys are immature and hepatic and renal function are markedly decreased from that of adult even when normalized to body surface area. By 6 months of age, hepatic and renal functions reach full maturation. In infants older than 6 months of age and children, the clearance of drugs is more proportional to body surface area than weight. Since the ratio of body surface area to weight is greater in small children, we tend to underdose children if we adjust pediatric doses by extrapolating on a linear mg/kg basis from adults. Rowland and Tozer (9) provides the following nonlinear relationship of extrapolating the child dose from the adult dose, using weight rather than body surface area:

$$\text{Child's dose} = \left[\frac{\text{wt of child (kg)}}{70\text{ kg}}\right]^{0.7} \times \text{AMD}$$

where AMD = adult maintenance dose

This equation can be used in children older than 6 months of age. Other reasons for difference in activity or toxicity in some patients may be the breakdown in the blood-brain and blood–cerebrospinal fluid (CSF) barrier and alterations in CSF transport systems in various diseases or age groups.

If the antiviral agent is likely to be used in the elderly (e.g., ACV for herpes zoster in otherwise healthy adults), then studies in this group (older than 65 years of age) will need to be conducted. This is necessary because many physiologic changes occur with age so that as a group the elderly respond differently to many drugs as compared to young adults. There are both pharmacokinetic and pharmacodynamic differences that occur with aging. The reasons we need to individualize therapy in the elderly is based on several factors. First, the elderly tend to have a decrease in body size and, therefore, a decrease in their volume of distribution. Thus, if a standard adult dose (not normalized to body size) is given, the elderly, on the average, will have a higher plasma drug concentration than the average young adult. This can be avoided by normalizing their dose to their body weight (i.e., dosing on a mg/kg basis). Second, the rate of metabolism is slower in the elderly as a group. On the average, the elderly metabolizes drugs one-half to two-thirds as fast as the young adult. Similarly, renal function decreases with aging so that the elderly have a decreased creatinine clearance. However, the elderly also have a decrease in creatinine production. Thus, as people age, their creatinine clearances decrease to approximately one-half of that of young adults, whereas their serum creatinine tends to remain normal ($\leq$1.5 mg/dl). When doing studies, it is better to estimate renal function by estimated or measured creatinine clearances rather than just relying on serum creatinine. In other words, it is always important to interpret the serum creatinine with respect to the patient's age, sex, and weight as shown in the equation below (10):

Creatinine clearance for males

$$= \frac{[140 - \text{age (yrs)}] \times \text{weight (kg)}}{72 \times \text{serum creatinine (mg/dl)}}$$

Creatinine clearance for females

$$= 0.85\left[\frac{[140 - \text{age (yrs)}] \times \text{weight (kg)}}{72 \times \text{serum creatinine (mg/dl)}}\right]$$

This equation is just one of many equations that are used to estimate creatinine clearances from serum creatinine. Actually, if possible, more direct measures of glomerular filtration rate (GFR) [such as inulin or [$^{51}$Cr-ethylenediamine tetraacetic acid (EDTA) clearances] are preferred. In addition to these kinetic differences, the elderly may have a change in tissue sensitivity to certain drugs and, therefore, respond differently than the young to the same plasma drug concentration. For example, the elderly appear to have a marked increase in sensitivity to the CNS effects of various drugs, such as sedative-hypnotics. This sensitivity is not related to kinetic differences.

8. If the drug is being targeted for women who are either pregnant or postpartum, additional studies will be necessary. There are major physiological changes that occur during pregnancy that may affect the pharmacokinetics of a drug. In addition, if the drug is administered postpartum, then one will be concerned with distribution and elimination of the drug in breast milk.

9. Drug/drug interaction studies are also conducted as part of the Phase I–IIA program. The dose-response relationships of drugs depend on absorption, distribution, protein binding, elimination, and tissue sensitivity. Drugs, food, environmental factors, and smoking may alter the dose-response of the investigational drug by affecting the pharmacokinetics or pharmacodynamics of the agent being studied. There are hundreds of potential drug interactions. Fortunately, there are relatively few interactions that actually do result in clinically significant effects. These interactions can be either pharmacokinetic or pharmacodynamic in character. Pharmacokinetic interactions include the effect of food on the absorption of an oral formulation. Bioavailability of an oral formulation would be determined in the fed and fasted state. These studies may allow one to rationally decide whether an agent should be taken before or after meals. Drugs that are highly protein bound may be affected by other drugs that have a strong affinity for the same protein binding sites and, therefore, will compete for these sites. Therefore, if the investigational agent is tightly protein bound (greater than 90%), then a concern regarding a potential interaction with such agents as phenylbutazone, phenytoin, or warfarin are warranted. If the investigational agent is found to be metabolized, then there are many drugs that may either induce or inhibit the enzyme systems involved with the metabolism of other drugs. The consequences of hepatic enzyme alterations depends on the drug's margin of safety, route of elimination, and the dose administered. Drugs such as phenytoin and phenobarbitol, which induce the enzymes involved with the metabolism of an antiviral agent, will tend to lower drug concentrations and may result in subtherapeutic concentrations. Drugs that inhibit hepatic enzymes, such as allopurinol, isoniazid, cimetidine, or chloramphenicol, may result in enhanced toxicity because of higher than anticipated plasma concentrations. Alternatively, if the major route of elimination of the compound is by renal tubular secretion, then other agents that are also renally secreted by the same secretory pathway may have a major pharmacokinetic interaction. If the antiviral drug is secreted and is an anionic compound, then it will probably be secreted by the renal tu-

bular organic acid transport system, and other drugs that are organic acids may similarly be secreted and compete for the same system. For example, probenecid, penicillin, and methotrexate are all compounds that are secreted by the organic acid transport system and may interact with such a compound. This may result in higher levels of either or both compounds and may result in an enhanced effect for either compound. For example, an interaction between an antiviral drug and methotrexate may result in both the methotrexate and the antiviral drug concentrations to increase. The increase in the antiviral drug may be clinically unimportant, but the effect of the methotrexate may be enhanced and result in increased toxicity. Frequently, when one is interested in whether there is significant renal organic acid secretion of an investigational antiviral drug, one looks at the interaction between probenecid and the antiviral agent being studied. If the antiviral is a cationic or basic compound and may be excreted by renal tubular secretion, then one would look at the interaction with either quinine or quinidine, which are both secreted by the organic base transport system in the kidney. The interaction of zidovudine and probenecid is an example of a clinically significant interaction where both the metabolism and renal tubular secretion of zidovudine are affected.

In addition to pharmacokinetic interactions, there are also pharmacodynamic interactions where two compounds may have additive or synergistic adverse effects. For example, if two compounds both caused bone marrow suppression, their combined use may result in a greater suppression than either agent by itself. For example, both zidovudine and ganciclovir result in significant bone marrow suppression; the resulting neutropenia that results from the combined administration of the two preclude their concomitant use.

Although the separation between Phase I and IIA studies at times may be blurred, basically Phase IIA studies address efficacy and safety for the first time in patients. Usually small numbers of patients are employed in these trials, and they are monitored in great details. These studies, which include dose-ranging trials, allow one to make a rational choice of the dose to be used in Phase IIB–III trials in order to establish definitive efficacy and safety. In dose-ranging studies, the dose-response relationship for a particular agent is established. This is done by looking at various parameters of efficacy and toxicity at varying doses. These studies establish in humans the therapeutic index and the therapeutic window. The therapeutic window is that range of doses that results in a therapeutic effect with acceptable tolerance. Table 3 outlines a dose-ranging multiple-dose trial for a hypothetical anti-HIV agent. The main objective of this trial is to determine the optimal dose regimen or regimens necessary for testing in the long-term trials. This trial will assess safety, disposition, pharmacodynamics, and short-term biological efficacy with various dose regimens. The dose to be utilized in the study will be determined from the results of the single dose trial or, if available, a previous multiple dose trial. One possible scenario would be to give doses of three-fourths the maximum tolerated dose (MTD), one-half MTD, and one-fourth MTD at an interval determined by the single-dose study. Examples of some of the parameters for efficacy and toxicity that may be assessed in the Phase IIA dose-ranging study for an antiviral drug with activity against HIV in patients with AIDS-related complex or AIDS is provided in Table 4. As you can see, at varying doses, one assesses the antiviral effect, the effect on immunological factors, and clinical response. Phase IIA trials would also try to establish the rational dose interval as well as the appropriate population to initiate the definitive clinical trials. In general, the interval between doses depends on the half-life of the drug, the margin of safety, and the route of administration. The therapeutic index is a very important determinant of the dosing interval because it determines the therapeutic window and, therefore, the degree of permissible fluctuation in drug concentration. If the dosage interval is less than or equal to the half-life of a drug, the calculated maintenance dose will produce plasma concentrations that will fluctuate by 50% or less during the dosing interval. The plasma level will initially be above the average plasma concentration and then fall below the average plasma concentration in the second half of the dosing interval. If the interval is several half-lives of the drug, then the difference between peak and trough concentrations may be greater than 10-fold. If drugs are given at a dose interval four- to five-fold greater than their half-life, then all the drug is eliminated before the next dose. Each new dose essentially acts as a loading dose. On the other hand, if a drug has a long terminal half-life and the drug is given several times a day, then drug accumulation would be expected to occur. In this situation, if one needs to rapidly attain steady state, then a loading dose would be necessary, followed by a maintenance dose. This has been found to be the situation with ribavirin, which has a terminal-phase half-life on the order of days (11,12). However, as explained in the next section, for many antiviral drugs, plasma half-life may not be as critical as the intracellular pharmacology.

### Special Considerations with Regard to Antiviral Drugs

Many of the antiviral drugs that are nucleoside analogues are, in fact, prodrugs. Drugs like ACV, vidarabine, ganciclovir, zidovudine, and the dideoxynucleoside analogues are active only once metabolized intracellularly to their phosphorylated forms. The active form is usually the triphosphate, which then acts as a substrate and/or inhibitor of the viral nucleic acid polymerase. In some instances, these incorporated antiviral nucleotides are chain terminating and prevent further DNA or RNA elongation. In addition, there are situations where the monophosphate appears to be active. Once these compounds are phosphorylated inside the cell, they become polar and become trapped intracellularly. Therefore, it is the intracellular concentrations of these phosphorylated nucleotides that determines the drug's antiviral activity. The termination of the antiviral effect is probably related to the rate of intracellular degradation of the active metabolite. Frequently, this termination is due to phosphatases, which convert the active nucleotides to its parent form, which can then be released from the cell into the plasma, where it is eliminated from the body. Therefore, although it is the plasma half-life that usually correlates with the duration of antibacterial activity of antibiotics, with most antiviral nucleosides the termination of antiviral effect probably correlates better with the intracellular elimination half-life of the active form of the drug. Usually, this is the half-life of the nucleotide triphosphate. This may mean that even if a drug has a very short plasma half-life, it may exert a prolonged antiviral effect if the half-life of the active compound is very long. For example, ganciclovir has a plasma half-life of 2 to 4 hr in patients with normal renal function (4,5), but the intracellular half-life of ganciclovir triphosphate is approximately 1 day (13,14). This may explain why once daily dosing of ganciclovir is adequate for suppressive therapy for CMV infections in immunocompromised patients (4). ACV, on the other hand, has a plasma half-life of 2 to 3 hr, (6) but ACV triphosphate half-life is only approximately 1 to 2 hr (15). This may explain why once daily administration is inadequate in preventing relapses of HSV infection in immunocompromised patients. The interval initially chosen for dosing zidovudine (every 4 hr) was based on its plasma half-life of 1.1 hr (16). Because the intracellular half-life of zidovudine triphosphate is approximately 3 hr (17), it may be possible to increase the dose interval for the drug to every 6 to 8 hr, or even to 12 hr. Ultimately, the optimal dose and dose interval for any antiviral drug for various indications will need to be determined in properly conducted clinical trials.

The development of biological agents will require special attention. Almost all drug development has been with simple organic compounds, and procedures for their development are well known. However, most biologic agents are not simple organic compounds but complex polypeptides [e.g., monoclonal antibodies, genetically engineered molecules containing portions of the CD4 receptors attached to cellular toxin like *Pseudomonas* exotoxin (18), antibodies with toxins attached, various lymphokines]. Therefore, the development of biologically compounds will need to be defined. For example, the concept of a half-life may be irrelevant. Interferon has a plasma half-life of several hours, but interferon induces an antiviral state that appears to persist for several days (8). This area may represent one of the greatest challenges for drug development in the decade of the 1990s.

## PHASE IIB–III TRIALS

Phase IIB–III trials are usually large-scale trials to establish the comparative safety and efficacy of the new agent with the currently accepted best method. In the case of antiviral drug development, this may be a placebo. Based on the previous Phase I–IIA trials, a rational choice of one or two different regimens are selected and tested during each trial. It is during this phase that the large-scale, definitive trials are conducted to demonstrated efficacy and safety. These trials are usually multicenter, collaborative efforts. Usually, at least two controlled trials demonstrating efficacy are conducted for each desired indication. It is during Phase III that the full scope of the indications and range of dosage regimes are defined. For example, Phase III testing of ACV defined the drug's efficacy for varicella-zoster virus (VZV) infections at a dosage that was greater than that for HSV infections in general. In addition, the various indications and dosage ranges for the suppression and treatment of HSV disease in various population and with various clinical manifestations were defined for ACV during this phase. At the end of Phase III testing, an NDA and/or a marketing authorization application (MAA) are submitted to the appropriate regulatory agencies in the countries where the drug is to be licensed. In the development of drugs for the treatment of infections in patients with HIV disease, these guidelines are being abbreviated so that it is possible to license a drug much more quickly than has been conventionally the case. For example, zidovudine was licensed while it was still in Phase II.

After the drug is marketed, post-NDA trials that involve continued safety monitoring and postmarketing surveillance are conducted (Phase IV). In addition, new indications and new formulation may be studied. These trials are conducted in a fashion similar to those principles already described for Phases I–III.

## CONCLUSIONS

The purpose of this chapter was to provide some insight and a format for the development of antiviral agents. Since antiviral drug development is still in its infancy, refinement in the development of these agents will evolve with time. In the past, there was a temptation to develop antiviral drugs similar to antibacterial agents or along the vein of antineoplastics agents. This has been less than satisfactory since antiviral drugs require their own individual development since they are neither antibacterial nor antineoplastics agents. Unfortunately, the reason antiviral drugs have been developed in many cases similar to anticancer agents is probably because the initial cer agents is probably because the initial candidates were in fact cytotoxic agents that may have had a slight preference for virally infected cells. These agents included such toxic compounds as iododeoxyuridine, ara-C, and trifluorothymidine. Even an effective agent like vidarabine suffered from a very narrow margin of safety and an extremely short half-life of several minutes. This made it difficult to try to administer this agent in a rational and convenient way. In addition, the intracellular site of action and the complexities of the intracellular metabolism with respect to both activation and degradation of the active form of many antiviral drugs make the development of these compounds much more difficult than that of a third-generation cephalosporin.

As we learn more about viral processes, such as the infectious cycle and latency, new targets for therapeutic attack will be identified. Misconception sometimes hinders development. It is unfortunate that many people state that some viruses like herpes cannot be eradicated because of latency. This is not too dissimilar from those who said in the 1970s that effective and safe antiviral drug therapy was not possible. Very little is known about the process that has been termed "latency." However, as more is uncovered, it is obvious that latency is not a dormant state where no virally medicated processes are being expressed, but is an active state. Once latency is better understood, then there may be the ability to develop agents that affect this interaction between viral and mammalian nucleic acid in a therapeutically positive way. Although those who say that herpes will never be able to be eradicated may be right, if we accept this opinion then it will most certainly be correct. Finally, as the ability to rapidly identify viral infections becomes more readily available, the need for effective and safe viral chemotherapy will assume an even greater importance. Only by coupling rapid viral diagnosis with effective viral chemotherapy coupled with knowledge of the pharmacokinetics, pharmacodynamics, and intracellular pharmacology can we hope to develop optimal dose strategies for the treatment of viral illnesses.

## REFERENCES

1. Hayden FG, Laskin OL, Douglas RG. Susceptibility testing of viruses and pharmacodynamics of antiviral agents. In: Lorian V, ed. *Antibiotics in laboratory medicine*. Baltimore: Williams and Wilkins, 1986.
2. Richman DD, Fischl MA, Grieco MH, et al. The toxicity of azidothymidine (AZT) in the treatment of patients with AIDS and AIDS-related complex. A double-blind, placebo-controlled trial. *N Engl J Med* 1987;317:192–7.
3. Fischl MA, Richman DD, Grieco MH, et al. The efficacy of azidothymidine (AZT) in the treatment of patients with AIDS and AIDS-related complex. A double-blind, placebo-controlled trial. *N Engl J Med* 1987;317:185–191.
4. Laskin OL, Cederberg DM, Mills J, et al. Ganciclovir for the treatment and suppression of serious infections caused by cytomegalovirus. *Am J Med* 1987;83:201–7.
5. Laskin OL, Stahl-Bayliss CM, Kalman CM, Rosecan LR. Use of ganciclovir to treat serious cytomegalovirus infections in patients with AIDS. *J Infect Dis* 1987;155:323–7.
6. Laskin OL. Acyclovir. Pharmacology and clinical experience. *Arch Intern Med* 1984;144: 1241–6.
7. Hayden FG, Mills SE, Johns ME. Human tolerance and histopathologic effects of long-term administration of intranasal interferon-α2. *J Infect Dis* 1983;148:914–21.
8. Barouki FM, Witter FR, Griffin DE, et al. Time course of interferon levels, antiviral state, 2′,5′-oligoadenylate synthetase and side effects in healthy men. *J Interferon Res* 1987;7:29–39.
9. Rowland M, Tozer TN. *Clinical pharmacokinetics: concepts and applications*. 2nd ed. Philadelphia: Lea and Febiger, 1989.
10. Cockcroft DW, Gault MK. Prediction of creatinine clearance from serum creatinine. *Nephron* 1976;16:34–41.
11. Laskin OL, Longstreth JA, Hart CC, et al. Ribavirin disposition in high risk patients for acquired immunodeficiency syndrome. *Clin Pharmacol Ther* 1987;41:546–55.
12. Roberts RB, Laskin OL, Laurence J, et al. Ribavirin pharmacodynamics in high-risk patients for acquired immunodeficiency syndrome. *Clin Pharmacol Ther* 1987;42:365–73.
13. Biron KK, Stanat SC, Sorrell JB, et al. Metabolic activation of the nucleoside analog 9 - [(2 - hydroxy - 1 - (hydroxymethyl)ethoxy) methyl]guanine in human diploid fibroblasts infected with human cytomegalovirus. *Proc Natl Acad Sci USA* 1985;82:2473–7.
14. Smee DF, Boehme R, Chernow M, Binko BP, Matthews TR. Intracellular metabolism and en-

zymatic phosphorylation of 9-(1,3-dihydroxy-2-propoxymethyl)guanine and acyclovir in herpes simplex virus-infected and uninfected cells. *Biochem Pharmacol* 1985;34:1049–56.

15. Elion GB. Mechanism of action and selectivity of acyclovir. *Am J Med* 1982;73:7–13.
16. Blum MR, Liao SHT, Good SS, de Miranda P. Pharmacokinetics and bioavailability of zidovudine in humans. *Am J Med* 1988;85:189–94.
17. Furman PA, Fyfe JA, St. Clair MH, et al. Phosphorylation of 3′-azido-3′-deoxythymidine and selective interaction of the 5′-triphosphate with human immunodeficiency virus reverse transcriptase. *Proc Natl Acad Sci USA* 1986;83:8333–7.
18. Chaudhary VK, Mizukami T, Fuerst TR, et al. Selective killing of HIV-infected cells by recombinant human CD4-Pseudomonas exotoxin hybrid protein. *Nature* 1988;335:369–72.

*Antiviral Agents and Viral Diseases of Man, 3rd Edition*, edited by G. J. Galasso, R. J. Whitley, and T. C. Merigan, Raven Press, Ltd., New York © 1990.

# 5

# Laboratory Diagnosis of Viral Infections

Robert H. Yolken

*Eudowood Division of Infectious Diseases, Department of Pediatrics, Johns Hopkins University School of Medicine, Baltimore, Maryland 21205*



Enhanced prospects for treatment and prophylaxis of viral infections with antiviral agents have created an increasing need for rapid laboratory diagnosis of viral infections. The narrow activity of some of the antivirals emphasizes the need for specific, as well as rapid, identification of the infecting virus. There is also a need for methods of viral quantification suitable for the monitoring of the response to antiviral chemotherapy. The development of additional antiviral agents will undoubtedly increase the need for specific, accurate, and practical methods for the diagnosis and monitoring of viral infections.

In the past, clinical microbiology laboratories have often relied on reference laboratories for confirmation and identification of viral isolates, but now they are required increasingly to provide the methodology and expertise for definitive diagnosis of a wide range of viral infections. Numerous developments in recent years have helped to place diagnostic virology within the scope of activities of clinical microbiology laboratories. Immunoassays of improved sensitivity, specificity, and efficiency have been developed; basic test procedures have been carefully standardized; well-characterized reference viruses and antisera have been made available through the National Institutes of Health, the World Health Organization, and commercial sources. Furthermore, there has been steady improvement in the scope and quality of commercially available antisera and conjugates. Finally, the techniques of nucleic acid hybridization and other molecular procedures are being applied to viral diagnosis.

Many of the traditional isolation and serological procedures for viral diagnosis could provide only a retrospective indication of the viral etiologic agent involved and, thus, were of limited value for immediate clinical management of the patient. However, newer methods often can provide results in time to allow successful intervention in treatment of patients or in controlling the spread of viral diseases.

An ideal assay system for the diagnosis of viral infections would be capable of the detection of all pathogenic viruses early in the course of infection. Unfortunately, there is no single system that approaches this ideal. There are a number of limitations that are faced by all assay systems which have been used for viral detection. The most important limitations derive from the fact that viral pathogens are capable of initiating disease at stages in which the concentration of viable virus is very low. At this stage of infection, the concentration of viral antigen or nucleic acid in blood or other accessible body sites is extremely small. Furthermore, the amount of virus can diminish later in the course of infection, when the level of viral replication is diminished but when the patient is still displaying manifestations of illness and is still capable of transmitting the virus to other susceptible individuals. The level of virus that can be detected later in the course of infection is further decreased by the generation of antiviral immunoglobulins and the complexing of viral antigens to circulating antibodies (1). The occurrence of viral latency further complicates the task of viral diagnosis since it can be difficult, if not impossible, to detect viral antigens or viable virions once the virus has become integrated into the host nucleic acid. In this regard, viral diagnosis by means of nucleic acid detection offers an important theoretical advantage since viral nucleotides incorporated into the host chromosome can be detected by complementary base pairing at latency stages, during which viral sequences are being transcribed and no viral antigens are being produced (2,3).

These considerations play an important role in the evaluation and interpretation of assays for the diagnosis of viral infections. For example, an assay for the detection of viral antigens can be very efficient at a stage in which the amount of antigen produced is relatively large, such as at the height of rotavirus diarrhea or during the chronic infection stage of hepatitis B. On the other hand, it is possible that the same assays will prove to be less efficient during the early or late stages of viral infection, during which time the amount of antigen available for binding to labeled antibody is reduced. These factors often make it difficult to compare different assay systems, especially when different formats are utilized (i.e., nucleic acid hybridization versus antigenic assays). These considerations also can make it difficult for the clinician or investigator to interpret assay evaluations that are presented in the literature (4,5). The suitability of the assays for clinical diagnosis and for epidemiological studies thus depend greatly on the clinical situation encountered and the diagnostic needs of the clinician or investigator.

Generally, the most important aspects of a diagnostic system are related to assay sensitivity. Although there are many factors that determine the sensitivity of immunoassay systems, the most important ones are based on the affinity characteristics of the antiviral immunoreagents utilized in the assay. We have found that the theoretical limitation of the assays is based on the affinity of the antibodies for the target antigen and the affinity of the antibodies for cross-reacting materials. We have found that the theoretical sensitivity of assays utilizing antibodies with affinities of $10^{-10}$ moles/liter is in the order of $10^{-12}$ moles/liter (6). This corresponds to the detection of an antigen with a molecular weight of 100,000 daltons at a level of $10^{-7}$gm/liter or $10^{-10}$ gm/ml. Although this level of sensitivity compares quite favorably with assays for the detection of defined bioactive peptides and hormones, it should be noted that a single molecule of influenza virus weights approximately $10^{-16}$ gm. Although immunoassays can thus be expected to detect the presence of viral antigens in some situations, it is unlikely that assays making use of immunological reagents will be capable of the direct detection of all viral antigens early or late in the course of infection. Thus, a negative result with currently available assays must be interpreted in the context of assay sensitivity, the clinical state of the infected individual, and the natural history of the underlying viral infection.

Viral cultivation methods have the advantage over available "rapid diagnostic" technology in that lower levels of viruses are detectable following replication in susceptible cell lines. However, in the case of many viruses, the time required for growth and identification is too long to be of use to the clinician. In addition, many agents of medical interest are somewhat fastidious and selective in their growth parameters, making cultivation difficult without the use of large numbers of specialized cell lines. On the other hand, the generation of increased amounts of virus by means of cultivation can markedly improve the ability of immunoassays or hybridization assays to detect the target antigen. Thus, rather than being mutually exclusive, cultivation and "rapid diagnostic" procedures can be used together to provide for the earliest and most accurate diagnosis.

Another factor that must be taken into consideration in the evaluation of viral diagnostic assays is the specificity of the detector reactions. It should be noted that viral antigens and nucleic acids coexist *in vivo* with a large excess of extraneous cellular and bacterial proteins. Many of these proteins are capable of nonspecific binding to immunoglobulins and other components of immunoassay systems. It is, thus, imperative that assay systems be devised which do not yield false-positive results in the presence of materials such as those capable of binding labeled immunoglobulins. Fortunately, a number of methods exist for the quenching of nonspecific reactions and for the quantitative identification of false-positive results (see below). In the case of hybridization reactions, formats must be utilized that will not display cross-reactions with nonviral sequences homologous to the probe or to the vector (such as a bacterial plasmid) utilized for probe generation (7).

In light of these considerations, it is extremely important that new assays be evaluated under a range of clinical and laboratory conditions. Multicenter evaluations are particularly informative since they allow for the determination of assay performance under a range of laboratory conditions and degrees of user expertise. The careful evaluation of new diagnostic techniques is a crucial component of the application of immunological and molecular biological to the detection and study of human infections.

## DIAGNOSTIC METHODS

The three basic approaches to laboratory diagnosis of viral infection are (a) direct examination of the specimen for virus viral antigen or viral nucleic acids; (b) isolation and identification of virus from clinical materials; and (c) serological diagnosis based on demonstrating a significant increase in viral antibody over the course of the patient's illness.

Whatever approaches are selected for viral diagnosis, the reliability of the examination will depend to a large extent on the quality of the specimens tested. In collecting material for direct examination or virus isolation, it is important to obtain specimens as early as possible in the course of the illness, when virus is being excreted at relatively high levels and has not yet been bound by antibody. The volume of the sample should be sufficient to permit direct examination, if feasible, as well as virus isolation attempts and storage of some of the specimen for retesting. It is also important to select the most appropriate specimens for the disease suspected, i.e., those from the sites at which virus is most likely to be present, based upon the pathogenesis of the disease. If nasopharyngeal or rectal swabs, or lesion specimens, are collected into a holding medium, the medium should contain protein (known to be free from viral inhibitors or antibody) to protect against loss of viral infectivity. Ideally, specimens should be inoculated into host systems as soon as possible after collection. They may be held at 4°C if they are to be tested within 24 hr, or should be kept frozen at −70°C for longer periods. It is well recognized that freezing and thawing of specimens reduce virus recovery rates. More detailed information on appropriate specimens, and their collection and handling is available in other sources (8–11).

## DIRECT EXAMINATION OF CLINICAL MATERIALS FOR VIRUS

Methods that permit direct detection of virus or viral antigen in the clinical specimen can avoid the need for cultivation of the virus and, thus, are the most rapid and economical for viral diagnosis. In addition, they permit diagnosis of infections with agents that cannot be cultivated by standard procedures, e.g., hepatitis viruses and certain human gastroenteritis agents, and they may permit virus detection in specimens in which the virus is no longer viable.

Valuable as they may be for rapid viral diagnosis, direct examination methods are limited by the small size of viruses, their close association with host materials, and by the low levels and short duration of virus shedding at body sites accessible for specimen collection. Direct methods are restricted to those agents for which suitable diagnostic reagents are available and by the number of tests permitted by the volume of specimen. Since it is feasible to test each specimen against only a few reagents in direct immunoassays, it is necessary to have some idea of the viral agent(s) that might possibly be involved. Antigenic examination obviously is not applicable to detection of viruses in large groups with multiple immunotypes and no common antigens. Whenever possible, clinical specimens should also be inoculated into appropriate host systems as a backup to direct examination.

### Electron Microscopy

Direct electron microscopy (EM) for viral detection in clinical materials is feasible only in situations where virus is present in the specimen at high concentrations and is sufficiently free from background debris to permit detection and definitive recognition to the virus morphology. EM on vesicular lesion specimens is particularly useful for identifying members of the herpesvirus and poxvirus groups, and it can be used on scabs and lesion fluids, which are unsatisfactory for virus isolation or immunofluorescence (IF) staining. EM is also valuable for identification, on morphological grounds, of certain viruses that cannot be cultivated or that require special host systems, such as human papilloma, molluscum contagiousum, and Orf viruses. Probably the widest use of direct EM has been in the diagnosis of human rotavirus infection. These viruses were first discovered by EM examination of epithelial cells of duodenal mucosa (12), but were soon found to be present in sufficient concentration and to have a morphology distinctive enough to be demonstrable in fecal extracts (13,14). Other noncultivable human enteric viruses such as certain adenoviruses, caliciviruses, astroviruses, and coronaviruses may also be demonstrated by EM on fecal specimens (14); however, the role of these agents in human disease is not yet defined.

The basic technique for EM examination of clinical specimens for viral particles consists of negative staining with phosphotungstic acid (PTA) prior to examination

(15,16). For successful detection of virus by this method, it must generally be present in the specimen at a concentration of $1 \times 10^6$ particles/ml. Sensitivity can be increased by the use of the pseudoreplica technique, in which the specimen is added to an agarose surface and the virus is subsequently collected onto a Formvar film. This serves to concentrate the virus in the specimen as the fluid and interfering substances such as salts are absorbed into the agarose. In one report, this technique permitted detection of human cytomegalovirus (CMV) in urine specimens with particle concentrations as low as $1 \times 10^4$/ml (17). Sensitivity of EM for virus detection has also been increased by using high-speed centrifugation to pellet virus directly onto the specimen grid (18).

EM for viral diagnosis has the advantage of speed and relative simplicity. The ability to see a virus directly and identify its characteristic morphology ensures high specificity of results. Also, a single EM examination has the potential for detecting a wide range of viral agents, in contrast to immunoassays, which employ highly specific antibody probes. This latter advantage is well illustrated by the recent recognition by EM of viruses morphologically identical to human and animal rotaviruses but which are antigenically different and would not be detectable by immunoassays using conventional rotavirus antisera (19).

Disadvantages of EM include the requirements for an expensive instrument and highly trained personnel, and the low volume of specimens that can be handled. In addition, electron microscopes are subject to mechanical failure, especially when they are used by multiple individuals. Also, EM can identify viruses only as to their major groups, but cannot differentiate between members of the same morphologic group or family.

## Immunoassays for Direct Virus Detection

Immunoassays for detection of viruses in clinical specimens are based on mixing the specimen with specific viral antibodies, and then demonstrating an immunological reaction between these antibodies and viral antigen in the specimen. This approach permits detection and identification of the virus in a single step. Immunoassays are potentially more sensitive than direct EM for virus detection because the antibodies amplify the viral content of the specimen, either by aggregation or through labels or "tags" on the antibodies that enhance their ability to be detected when complexed with virus in the specimen. The labels can be a fluorescent marker, an enzyme, or a radioisotope. These methods require specific and high-titered viral antisera, and they are restricted in scope since it is feasible to apply only a limited number of antibody probes to a specimen.

### *Immunoelectron Microscopy*

Immunoelectron microscopy (IEM) provides a means for direct observation of the reactions between viruses and their specific antibodies. After the specimen is reacted with antibodies, it is negatively stained and then examined by EM for the presence of immune aggregates. Reaction of virus with specific antibodies not only aggregates and concentrates the particles, enhancing the possibility of detection by EM, but also provides a specific identification of the virus if the antisera employed are well characterized and appropriate negative control sera are used. IEM permitted the initial recognition of the agents of acute infectious nonbacterial gastroenteritis and hepatitis A (13,20), despite the fact that they could not be cultivated. These agents generally cannot be detected by IEM without the use of antibody for concentration.

The range of agents detectable by IEM can be extended by using commercial pools of human $\gamma$ globulin as a source of antibodies against a variety of different agents likely to be encountered. Obviously, this permits morphological, but not specific immunological identification of agents.

Solid-phase modifications of IEM have been developed in which virus is trapped by specific antibodies coating the grid (21), or that use grids coated with staphylococcal protein A followed by antibodies (22). Serological coating of grids in these ways can eliminate the need for concentrations of specimens for IEM. Another modified IEM technique consists of trapping viral particles on an antibody coated grid and then using a second application of antibody to coat or "decorate" the virus, thus facilitating its detection and identification (23).

Although IEM is simple in principle, interpretation requires considerable experience. Problems and pitfalls are discussed in a review by Kapikian et al. (20).

### *Immuno-fluorescence (IF) Staining*

IF staining, based on the use of antibodies labeled with fluorescence isothiocyanate (FITC), is the immunoassay that has had the widest application in diagnostic virology. Reactivity of the labeled antibodies with virus in the specimen is demonstrated by microscopic examination using ultraviolet light. The preparation, characterization, and requirements of satisfactory reagents, the necessary controls, and the clinical applications of IF staining in diagnostic virology are discussed elsewhere (8,24–26).

For direct IF staining, viral antibody is labeled with FITC, and the conjugate is applied to the specimen to be examined for the presence of viral antigen. Although this method has the drawbacks of needing a specific antibody conjugate for each viral agent to be sought and of requiring high-titered antisera for conjugation, it has certain advantages over the indirect method for virus detection in clinical specimens. These include greater specificity and freedom from background staining, and fewer manipulations and reagents.

For indirect IF staining, smears of cells or tissues are treated with unlabeled viral antiserum, and homologous antibodies combine with virus in the specimen. After washing to remove other serum proteins, the preparation is treated with fluorescein-labeled antibodies directed against the animal species in which the virus antiserum was prepared. The unlabeled virus antibodies complexed with virus in the specimen then act as antigen, which binds the labeled antispecies antibodies. This technique is somewhat more sensitive than the direct procedure because the layer of antibody globulin built up around the virus increases the surface area from attachment of the labeled antibodies. Also, it requires labeled antibodies only against certain animal species, and not against individual viruses. However, the introduction of additional reagents into the system may result in reduced specificity as compared with direct IF. Indirect IF staining also requires more controls and manipulations.

Human sera should not be used as a source of antibodies for virus detection by indirect IF since they contain antibodies to a variety of human viruses, and one cannot be certain which of these are reacting with the unknown virus. Another drawback to the use of human serum in indirect IF staining for detection of viral antigen in human tissues is the fact that certain viruses, e.g., measles in brain tissue or respiratory syncytial in nasopharyngeal cells, may be complexed with antibody from the patient's serum, and the labeled antihuman globulins will combine with these virus/immunoglobulin complexes independently of specific viral antibodies in the intermediate serum, thereby possibly giving a false identification of the infecting virus. It is particularly important in using indirect IF staining for virus detection to control the specificity of the reaction by examining the specimen against the conjugate alone in the absence of intermediate viral antiserum.

The anticomplement immunofluorescent (ACIF) procedures uses unlabeled viral antisera to bind to virus in the specimen, followed by complement and, then, labeled antibodies to the C3 component of complement. This technique requires only a single labeled reagent (anti-C3) but may show reduced specificity because of the greater number of reactants in the system. The ACIF shows high sensitivity for detection of certain human herpesvirus antigens. A major advantage is the fact that, since complement attaches only to antigen/antibody complexes, the ACIF procedure avoids staining of the receptors for crystallizable fragment of immunoglobulin (Fc) produced by herpesvirus-infected cells. These receptors bind immunoglobulin G (IgG) of all specificities and cause confusing nonspecific cytoplasmic staining.

IF staining (or any immunoassay) for direct detection of virus in clinical materials can be applied successfully only to specimens that contain large numbers of virus-infected cells and are free from debris or contaminating microorganisms that might cause nonspecific reactivity. The most satisfactory specimens for IF examination for respiratory viruses are collected by suction of secretions from the nasopharynx; the cells are washed free of mucus before they are examined (8). In performing IF examinations on vesicular lesion specimens, it is important to prepare smears of epithelial cells collected from the base of the lesion; vesicular fluids or crusts are not suitable (8,25).

The IF procedure has the built-in safeguard of demonstrating typical patterns of staining morphology in virus-infected cells, and it is only by detecting stained antigen at intracellular sites that a positive reading can be made.

IF staining is used on a routine basis in many laboratories for direct detection of rabies virus in animal and human tissues; to detect herpes simplex virus (HSV) in brain biopsy or autopsy specimens and in corneal scrapings; to demonstrate measles virus antigen in brain tissues from cases of subacute sclerosing panencephalitis; to detect Colorado tick fever virus in blood clots from human cases; and to demonstrate HSV, varicella-zoster virus (VZV), and vaccinia virus antigens in cellular scrapings from vesicular lesions (8.25). Various workers have shown the feasibility of using IF procedures to demonstrate antigens of influenza viruses (25,27,28), parainfluenza viruses (28–30), respiratory syncytial virus (RSV) (8,28,31,32), adenoviruses (8,28), and measles virus (33) in nasal or throat exudates. Although IF staining may not be as sensitive as virus isolation for some respiratory virus infections, when properly performed it can provide a more rapid diagnosis in a large proportion of cases.

An important advantage of IF staining over virus isolation is the fact that it can sometimes demonstrate viral antigen, e.g., respiratory syncytial, measles, and VZV, in specimens taken late in the course of illness when infectious virus is no longer present, either as a result of liability of infectivity or complexing of the virus with antibody (8,33–35).

The demonstration that trypsin treatment can make formalin-fixed paraffin-embedded tissue sections suitable for IF staining (36,37) has been an important advance, which permits the use of IF staining in situations where fresh or frozen tissue is not available. Also, fixed, embedded tissues give better preservation of morphological detail for correlation of antigen distribution with histopathology.

### *Enzyme Immunoassays*

Enzyme immunoassay (EIA) methods for detecting viral antigens are similar in principle to IF staining, but they are based on labeling antibodies with an enzyme rather than fluorescein. Horseradish peroxidase and alkaline phosphatase are the enzyme labels most commonly employed, although β-galactosidase and β-lactemase can also be utilized (38). The labeled antibodies bound to virus or virus/antibody complexes are detected by the addition of a substrate on which the enzyme acts to produce a colored, fluorescent, or luminescent product. Theoretically, EIA should be more sensitive than IF staining, since the enzyme label can have a continuous action on the substrate, producing increasing amounts of reaction product, and thus amplifying the initial reaction at the site where virus is present in the specimen. In the few direct comparative studies that have been reported to date on IF and EIA for virus detection, sensitivity of EIA has been the same as or only slightly greater than that of IF procedures (39–41). However, solid-phase EIA techniques have the advantage that they can be performed by less experienced personnel in a reproducible manner. In addition, since EIA techniques can measure soluble antigens, intact cells are not required and the assay can be performed on a wide range of clinical samples. EIA procedures can also be quantitated, allowing for their use to follow the course of a disease or the effectiveness of chemotherapeutic interventions.

The EIA systems for virus detection may be categorized into those in which the substrate gives an insoluble reaction product that is detected by microscopic examination and those that yield substrate giving a soluble reaction product that is colored, fluorescent, or luminescent.

### *Immunoperoxidase Staining*

The technique of immunoperoxidase (IP) staining uses horseradish peroxidase as the enzyme label, and the substrate contains hydrogen peroxide and a reagent that is oxidized to give a colored insoluble precipitate at the site of the peroxidase activity.

IP staining has been applied to virus detection in the same manner as IF staining using direct or, more commonly, indirect procedures (42,43). A modification of IP staining, reported to give greater sensitivity by virtue of producing a larger reaction site, is the peroxidase/antiperoxidase (PAP) method (44). This procedure employs two antibodies, one against the viral antigen and the other against peroxidase, both of which are produced in the same species, e.g., rabbit. These are bridged together in the reaction by antibodies produced against that species in another species, e.g, goat. In practice, the material to be examined for viral antigen is treated first with the antiviral serum (rabbit) followed by the bridging antibodies (goat anti-rabbit immune globulins), and then with the antiperoxidase serum (rabbit) coupled to peroxidase. To this is added the substrate. The PAP method may give less background staining than is seen with other IP procedures.

Advantages of IP staining over IF procedures are the potential for greater sensitivity, the fact that then an ordinary light microscope can be used, and that permanent preparations can be made. Disadvantages include the need for a few more manipulations and the fact that some of the earlier substrates used were subsequently shown to be mutagenic. However, nonmutagenic substrates can be substituted satisfactorily (45). Undesirable background or nonspecific reactivity can occur in both IF and IP systems. IF staining is beset with problems of autofluorescence and nonspecific staining, whereas IP staining is hampered by the fact that certain types of tissues, particularly blood cells, have endogenous peroxidase activity that causes nonspecific reactivity. However, methods have been described that inactivate endogenous peroxidase activity without destroying viral antigen (46,47). Another approach is differential staining of endogenous peroxidase (48) so that it can be distinguished from specific staining of viral antigen.

IP staining for direct detection of virus in clinical materials has had the greatest use in detecting HSV antigen in brain and lesion materials (39,42,43,46). As is the case with IF staining, positive IP results must be based on the demonstration of typical intracellular staining morphology of the viral antigen. More comparative studies still need to be done using IP and IF methods on the same clinical specimens for detection of a wider range of viruses to provide a valid evaluation of the actual advantages of one method over the other in terms of sensitivity, specificity, and ease of performance.

### *EIA Employing Substrates Giving Soluble Reaction Products*

The past few years have seen considerable interest and activity in the development of solid-phase EIA procedures for virus detection that employ substrates giving soluble reaction products (6,49). This category of tests has sometimes been referred to as "enzyme-linked immunosorbent assays" (ELISA). The colored, fluorescent, or luminescent reaction product can be quantitated by appropriate instrumentation, or detected visually in the case of colored or fluorescent products. Fluorogenic and chemiluminescent substrates produce reaction products that can be detected at lower concentrations than colored products, and tests using these substrates have shown greater sensitivity than those using color-producing substrates (49–51). However, it should be recognized that the major limiting factor in the sensitivity of any immunoassay for virus detection is the quality of the initial virus/antibody reaction. Again, either direct or indirect systems can be used for virus detection by these immunoassays.

In direct procedures, viral antibody is immobilized onto a solid phase such as polyvinyl or polystyrene microtiter plates or polystyrene beads (Fig. 1). The test specimen is added, and virus present is bound to the "capture" antibodies and retained on the solid phase. After washing, bound virus is detected through the addition of enzyme-labeled "detector" virus antibody, followed by substrate. The indirect system (Fig. 2) uses unlabeled "detector" virus antibody, and this must be from an animal species different from that in which the "capture" antibody was produced. This is followed by enzyme-labeled antibodies directed against the species in which the "detector" viral antibodies were produced. The indirect procedure may have greater sensitivity than the direct (52), due to an increased surface area of reactants to bind the labeled reagent. It also has the advantage of requiring only antispecies-labeled immunoglobulins, but the requirement for viral antisera prepared in two different animal species may present problems for some agents. The direct procedure using fewer reagents may show greater specificity.

However, these test systems have the potential for nonspecific reactivity, which can result from a number of causes and can give misleading results. Immune reagents that are not adequately specific may react with other immune reagents in the test systems or with nonviral material in the specimen. Improper washing between steps can result in nonspecific binding of reagents or in cross-contamination between specimens; suction washing devices and the use of Tween 20 in the washing fluids help to overcome this problem. Nonspecific binding of viral antibodies to bacteria or bacterial products in the specimen may also cause false-positive reactions (13,53,54).

Fortunately, the quantitative nature of the assay allows for the facile performance of control reactions to document assay specificity. In the case of reactions performed in microtiter plates, the most effective control reactions involve the coating of wells with nonimmune serum in place of the antiviral antibody (Fig. 3). In the case of monoclonal antibodies, a monoclonal antibody directed at an irrelevant antigen can be utilized. The sample is simultaneously assayed in both antibody and control wells under the same conditions. In this assay format, a specific reaction is manifested by greater reactivity in wells coated with the antiviral antibody, whereas nonspecific reactions are manifested by the generation of excessive signal in the control wells.

Another approach is the use of a "blocking" or inhibition test in which the specimen is treated in parallel with a viral antiserum and with a known negative serum before it is added to the test system. The blocking viral antiserum must be a different one from the antiserum used in the test

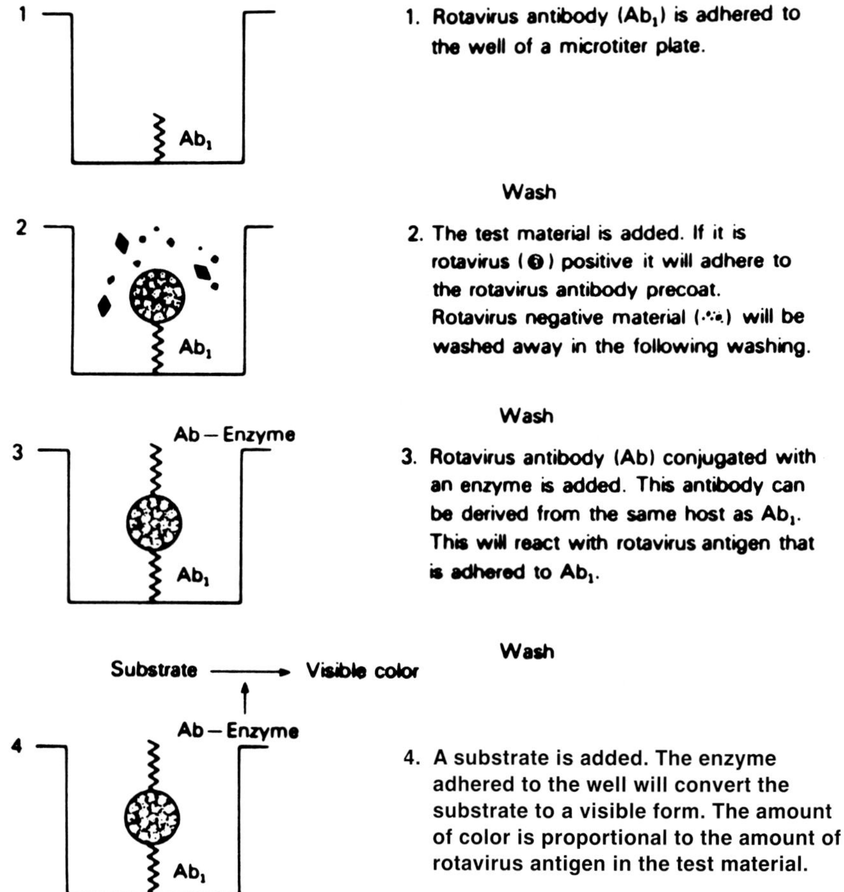


**FIG. 1.** Direct enzyme immunoassay for viral detection. (Modified from ref. 6.) A washing step is performed between each incubation.

proper. The blocking antiserum should inhibit reactivity of the specimen by more than 50% as compared to inhibition by the negative serum.

These EIA's have had the greatest use and success in detection of certain noncultivable agents such as rotaviruses (13,55), noncultivable enteric adenoviruses (56), hepatitis B surface antigen (57,58), and HSV antigen (59). These viruses or antigens occur at remarkably high concentrations in clinical specimens, relatively free from host material, and thus lend themselves well to detection by the immunoassays. Commercially available EIA systems for rotavirus detection have shown approximately 90% or greater correlation with sensitive EM or IEM methods (18,53,54), and commercial EIA's for hepatitis B surface antigen have been approximately as sensitive as RIA methods (57).

The EIA systems have also been applied successfully, although not as extensively, to direct detection of certain respiratory viruses in clinical specimens. Sensitivity as compared to cell culture isolation has ranged roughly from 60% to 80% (60–65). Success for virus detection appears to be largely dependent on obtaining adequate samples of nasopharyngeal secre-

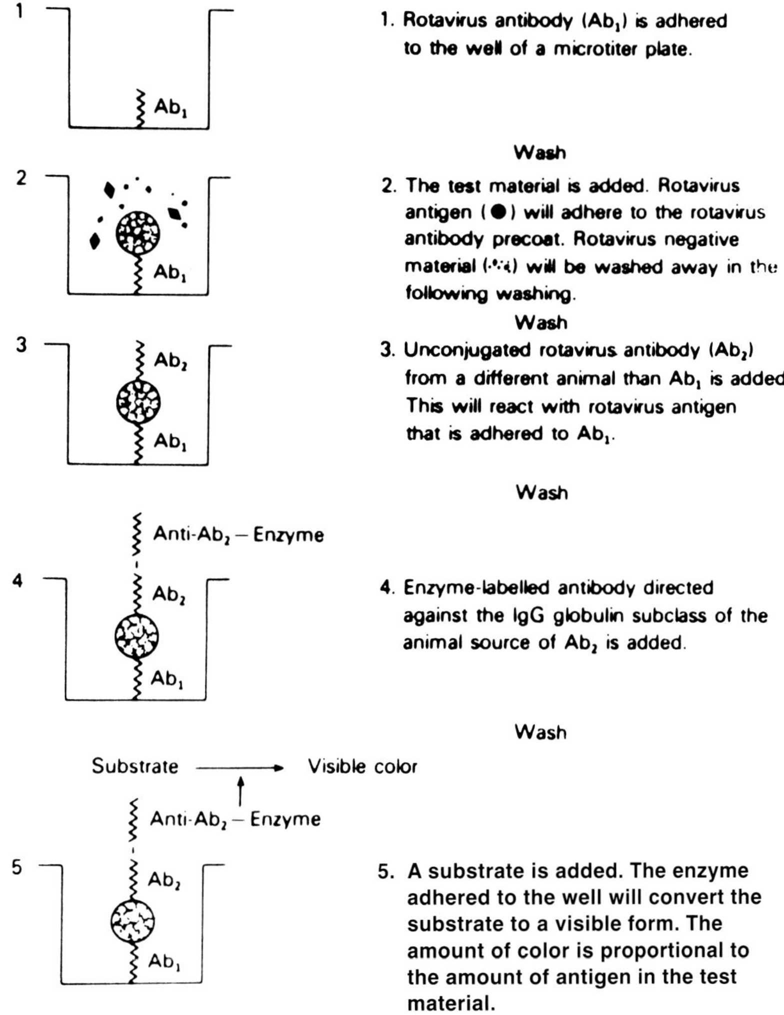


**FIG. 2.** Indirect enzyme immunoassay for viral detection. (Modified from ref. 6.) A washing step is performed between each incubation.

tions (40,41,61) and on effective disruption of mucus in the specimens by treatment with N-acetyl cystine (61,65) or by sonication (40,41). These EIA methods offer considerable promise for rapid and accurate respiratory virus detection in a high proportion of positive specimens, but they need to be further evaluated for their reliability and practicality in clinical settings.

EIAs based on chemiluminescence have been developed for direct virus detection (50,51). Horseradish peroxidase is used as the enzyme label, and this catalyzes the oxidation of isoluminol by hydrogen peroxide, producing chemically excited aminophthalate, from which emitted light is measured. The procedure detected HSV antigen in 88% of vesicular lesion specimens that were positive by cell culture isolation (51), and in a small series of specimens the immunoassay was comparable to cell culture isolation for detection of human CMV (50).

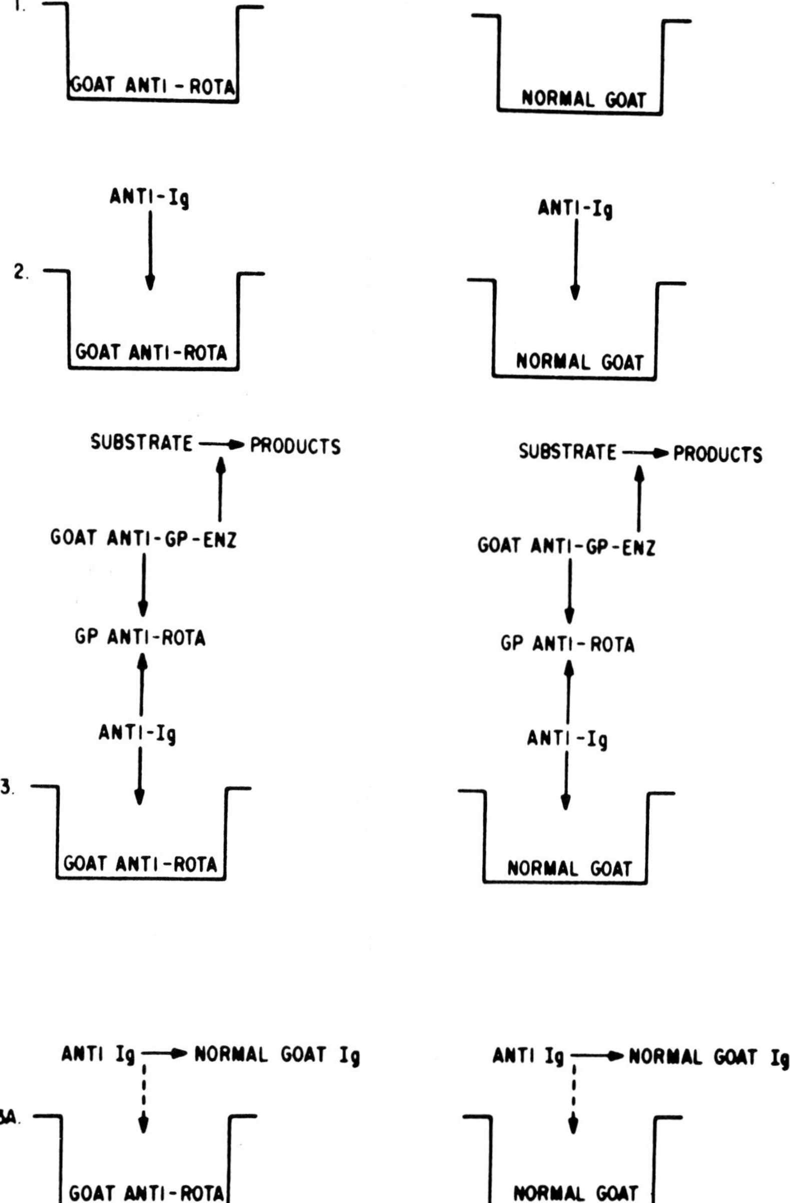


**FIG. 3.** Nonspecific reactions in enzyme immunoassays. **1:** Alternate rows of microtiter plates are coated with goat anti-rotavirus Ig and an equal concentration of Ig from the serum of a goat without demonstrable anti-rotavirus antibody. **2:** The specimen is added to both wells. If a nonspecific anti-immunoglobulin is present it will bind to both the goat anti-rotavirus Ig and the normal goat Ig. **3:** This anti-Ig will react with the subsequent antisera leading to a reaction in both wells. If rotavirus is also present, there will be an increased reaction in the well coated with the goat anti-rotavirus Ig. If rotavirus is not present, the reaction will be equal in both wells. Since most anti-immunoglobulins are of the IgM class, the cross-reactivity can be eliminated by the pre-treatment of the specimen with a mild reducing agent. **3A:** The effect of anti-Ig is reduced by the addition of normal goat serum to the specimen. If the concentration of added serum is substantially greater than that bound to the well, the anti-Ig will not bind and will be removed in the subsequent washing steps. (From ref. 6.)

### *Avidin/Biotin Immunoassays*

Immunoassays based on the strong interaction between avidin, a protein in egg white, and biotin, a coenzyme, are coming into use for virus detection (49,66,67). Antibody is linked to biotin, and, after this complex had reacted with virus or virus/antibody in a solid phase, avidin with a fluorescein or enzyme label is added. Another system consists of adding unlabeled avidin after the biotin/antibody complex, followed by enzyme-labeled biotin. These systems have high binding affinity due to the multiple linking of biotin to the antibody molecule and the multiple attachment of avidin to biotin. An additional feature that contributes to sensitivity is the fact that avidin and biotin are low-molecular-weight markers that avoid the steric hindrance that may be encountered in labeling antibodies directly with large enzyme molecules, which can obscure specific antibody binding sites. Also, biotinylation allows for the simplified labeling of large numbers of different antibodies under controlled conditions. This allows for the efficient evaluation of labeled reagents prior to final reagent selection and use in a clinical laboratory.

### *Radioimmunoassays*

Labeling antibodies with radioisotopes provides a highly sensitive probe for detection of viral antigens. Iodine-125 ($^{125}$I) is the radiolabel generally used, and tests can be performed by a direct method in which viral antibody labeled with the $^{125}$I is added to the specimen, or by an indirect procedure in which unlabeled viral antibody coupled with virus in the specimen is detected through the use of radiolabeled antispecies globulin (68,69). Most radioimmunoassays (RIAs) for viral antigen are conducted in a solid-phase system in which virus or capture antibodies are fixed to a plastic or glass surface. Binding of detector and antibodies by a virus-positive specimen is demonstrated by counting the radioactivity of the specimen in a $\gamma$ counter after completion of the reaction and demonstrating a significant increase in radioactivity over that of negative controls.

RIA has been most widely used for assay of marker antigens for hepatitis B virus (HBV), since it is important to use tests of the highest possible sensitivity to detect potentially infectious blood products or infected individuals. The sensitivity of RIA is also an asset in assaying hepatitis A virus (HAV) (70) and the viruses of acute infectious nonbacterial gastroenteritis (13,14). These agents cannot be cultivated by standard procedures and are present at relatively low concentrations in fecal specimens, making it difficult to detect them by simpler less sensitive methods.

The sensitivity levels of individual immunoassay systems vary depending upon the nature of the immunoreagents. However, in most cases the sensitivity levels of RIAs for the detection of viral antigens are similar to the levels attainable by enzyme immunoassays utilizing similar reagents. Enzyme immunoassays offer a number of advantages over RIAs in terms of the avoidance of hazardous radiation and the stability and reproducibility of reagents. It can, thus, be expected that most new solid-phase immunoassays for the detection of viral antigens will utilize enzymes or other nonisotopic labels and that existing RIAs will eventually be converted to nonisotopic formats.

### *Particle Agglutination*

Particle agglutination assays have been devised for the detection of a number of protein and polysaccharide antigens. Particle agglutination assays generally involve the use of latex or other particles labeled with antibody. Although antibodies can be bound to particles by means of passive absorption, the linkage of antibody to the solid-phase surface by covalent means generally results in the formation of a more stable reagent. The availability of a wide range of particles substituted with carboxyl or amino group suitable for reaction with bifunctional reagents such as carbodiamide or glutaraldehyde allows for the covalent linkage of virtually any antibody species (71,72).

Although there are a number of ways in which particles can be utilized for the detection of protein antigens, most assays make use of simple reaction protocols. In these formats, antibody-coated particles are cross-linked by reaction with polymeric antigens present in the sample. This cross-linkage can be observed by simple inspection or measured by means of suitable instrumentation.

Particle agglutination assays offer a number of potential advantages that make them enticing for use as viral diagnostic assays. For example, the large surface area and mobility of particles as compared to fixed solid phase surfaces allows for rapid antigen/antibody interactions and favorable reaction kinetics. Furthermore, the simple nature of the reaction formats minimizes the need for washing steps and sample manipulations, thus allowing for the completion of reactions and the interpretation of results in comparatively short periods of time (often less than 30 min).

Despite these attractive advantages, particles agglutination assays present a number of problems for use in the viral diagnostic laboratory. First, a problem is related to the fact that the assays are often less sensitive than analogous assays performed in enzyme immunoassay or RIA formats. Second, there are many materials in clinical samples that can nonspecifically agglutinate latex beads, thus leading to false-positive reactions. Although control reactions can be performed, the qualitative nature of the reactions makes interpretation difficult. Third, particle agglutination assays performed in simple formats rely on subjective determinations of flocculation. Such determinations can be unreliable if performed by inexperienced readers, especially if low concentrations of antigen are present. These limitations can be overcome by the use of instrumentation for the quantitation of the agglutination assays. However, the use of such instrumentation adds greatly to the cost and complexity of the particle reactions.

Particle agglutination reactions have been widely used for the detection of bacterial antigens, especially polymeric polysaccharides (71,73) in human body fluids. However, they have been less widely used for the detection of viral protein antigens, largely due to the limitations outlined above. Particle assays have been most widely used for the detection of rotavirus antigens in stool samples (74). The success of the assays in this area is undoubtedly related to the fact that many children with symptomatic rotavirus gastroenteritis shed large amounts of viral antigens and can thus be diagnosed by these methods. One comparative study (75) found that rotaviruses could be detected by latex agglutination assays early in the course of infection. However, after 3–4 days, antigen was not detectable in many samples by the particle assays despite the fact that antigen could be detected by means of solid-phase immunoassay procedures and by analysis of the RNA viral genomes. Thus, particle agglutination assays might be very useful for the rapid diagnosis of infection early in the course of disease when the antigen load is large. More sensitive assays are required for diagnosis at times when the antigen load is lower but when diagnosis is still required for patient analysis or for the prevention of disease transmission. It is likely that similar relative sensitivities will be found for the detection of other viral antigens by particle assay systems. Recently, there has been interest in improving the sensitivity of particle assays by using centrifugation solid-phase formats (76) and by the coupling of particles with enzymes, fluorescein, or other high-energy markers. The development of assays that retain the simplicity and rapidity of particle agglutination assays but which offer enhanced sensitivity and objectivity might represent a major advance in the field of viral diagnostics.

### Nucleic Acid Hybridization

In the past, virtually all direct detection techniques for the identification of viral infections made use of antigen/antibody interactions. Recently, techniques involving nucleic acid hybridization have been applied to the direct detection of viral nucleic acids in human body fluids (4,49). Nucleic acid hybridization procedures offer a number of potential advantages for rapid viral diagnosis. Nucleic acid hybridization reactions are not limited by the same affinity constraints inherent in antigen/antibody interactions. The reactive unit of hybridization reactions is the single purine or pyrimidine nucleotide with a molecular weight of approximately 600 daltons. This is substantially smaller than the antigen-binding fragment (Fab) portion of the immunoglobulin molecule, which is the active unit of antigen antibody interactions (approximately 75,000 daltons). Thus, for molecules of equivalent sizes, nucleic acid interactions would be expected to generate more hydrogen bonds and thus have more favorable free energy levels and more rapid kinetics than equivalent reactions involving antibody molecules.

Hybridization reactions display additional traits that make them attractive for use in rapid diagnosis. For example, advances in cloning techniques and in the synthesis of nucleotides allow for the practical generation of large amounts of defined probes. Since the probe can be accurately analyzed as to concentration and nucleotide sequence, standardization among laboratories can be accomplished in an effective manner. Also, the chemical stability of nucleic acids might allow for long-term storage of reagents under a variety of conditions. In addition, the stability of nucleic acids allows them to be extracted from immune complexes, intracellular sites, and other locations that might preclude detection by means of immunoassay procedures or other protein interactions. Furthermore, since the nucleotide sequence of many pathogens is known, it is possible to develop nucleic acid probes with defined degrees of specificity in a fairly rapid manner. This is particularly useful in the case of newly discovered pathogens for which the nucleotide sequence is known, but for which specific antigens have not been identified. In these cases, hybridization assays can be developed and evaluated without the need to cultivate the agent in high titer or to develop methods for viral purification. Hybridization procedures also have the advantage that they can detect nucleic acids which are not being transcribed into proteins, and hybridization reactions can thus detect latent viral infections. Similarly, nucleic acid probes can be targeted to markers of pathogenicity or type specificity so that definitive determinations can be made despite the occurrence of antigenic cross-reactivities.

Despite these advantages, there are a number of problems inherent in the use of nucleic acid hybridization for the diagnosis of viral infections. For example, one problem related to the use of nucleic acid hybridization assays for clinical diagnosis is that many published procedures make use of radioactively labeled probes. The assays claiming the highest degree of sensitivity often use nucleotide labeled with the β-emitter phosphorus-32 ($^{32}P$) to a high specific activity. Although numerous methods have been devised to label nucleotides with biotin, enzymes, or other nonisotopic probes, these assays have generally displayed lower degrees of sensitivity than equivalent assays making use of radioisotopes (77). This situation contrasts with that of immunological detection systems, where assays making use of enzymatic markers can generally attain levels of sensitivity that are equivalent to those achievable with assays utilizing antibodies labeled with radioactive isotopes such as $^{125}I$. This phenomenon is probably explained by the fact that large numbers of $^{32}P$ molecules can be inserted into nucleic acids without alteration of nucleotide reassociation kinetics, whereas only limited numbers of radioactive molecules can be inserted into antibodies and other protein molecules without alteration in biological function.

An additional problem with the application of hybridization assays for viral diagnosis is related to the fact that free viral nucleic acids are rapidly degraded by nucleases present in many body sites unless the nucleic acids are located inside the viral capsid or bound to specific proteins. Stability *in vivo* is particularly a problem in the case of single-stranded RNA species. Since nucleic acids located inside of viral capsids or bound to proteins cannot anneal with complementary nucleotides, viral nucleic acids must be extracted from virions before analysis. This requires the performance of multiple extraction and separation procedures. This situation contrasts to that of immunoassays, where relatively stable antigens can be shed into blood and other body fluids and can thus be detected without extensive processing. The fact that these extractions often require the use of phenol or other highly toxic chemicals further complicates the performance of hybridization procedures in the clinical laboratory, especially when large numbers of samples have to be tested. The need for extraction is particularly evident when standard "dot blot" formats are utilized. Since these procedures involve the direct application of extracted nucleic acids to a solid phase consisting of nitrocellulose or similar substance, the presence of extraneous proteins or nucleic acids can competitively inhibit binding of viral nucleic acids and thus limit assay sensitivity. The use of reaction formats that involve the interactions of nucleic acids in liquid phase or make use of more specific methods for binding to the solid phase surface can avoid this problem (78), These formats might thus be particularly applicable for use in the detection of viral nucleic acids in crude clinical samples.

Most of the isotopic and nonisotopic assays published to date rely on the subjective visualization of bands or spots to determine assay end points. Although such determinations can be useful in research settings, they do not allow for the facile performance of control reactions and can be difficult to apply in an accurate manner to the detection of nucleic acids from crude clinical samples. The development of nonisotopic methods for the sensitive, quantitative measurement of nucleic acids would represent a major advance in this regard.

Hybridization assays for the detection of viruses in clinical samples have been devised for the detection of a wide range of DNA and RNA viruses. Hybridization techniques using specimens blotted onto nitrocellulose filters have been applied to the detection of HSV types 1 and 2 in cell extracts (79) and clinical samples (80–82), detection of Epstein-Barr virus (EBV) in lymphocytes (83), detection of hepatitis B DNA in serum (84,85), identification of human CMV in urine specimens (86), detection of adenoviruses in respiratory (11) and gastrointestinal specimens (87,88), and the detection of rotaviruses in fecal samples (89) for the detection of papillomaviruses (90) and rabies viruses (91).

However, although hybridization assays have been widely utilized in research laboratories for the study of viral function, epidemiology, and pathogenesis, they have attained less usage for clinical diagnosis. In most cases, hybridization assays making use of radioactive isotopes have attained degrees of sensitivity approximately equivalent to that of immunoassays for the detection of the same pathogen. (R. Yolken, unpublished observations). Hybridization assays using nonisotopic probes have generally displayed lower levels of sensitivity. Thus, although they are widely used in virological research and have a great deal of promise for diagnostic virology, hybridization assays will have to be improved before they will be available for widespread diagnostic analyses.

An additional problem with hybridization assays is related to nonspecific reactions that occur between irrelevant nucleic acids in the clinical sample and sequences present in the vector utilized for probe generation. Since many of these vectors are derived from *Escherichia coli,* labeled vector sequences can hybridize with nucleotide sequences present in bacterial plasmids present in human body fluids or introduced into sterile specimens by bacterial contamination, thus leading to false-positive reactions (7). We have also found that the use of RNA probes generated by promoters and RNA polymerase (i.e., SP6 or pGEM plasmid systems) can also display nonspecific binding, presumably due to a small amount of transcription past the termination codons. It is, thus, preferable that probes be excised from the vector by means of restriction endonuclease digestion and that they be carefully separated from plasmid by means of gel purification or equivalent separation techniques. The nonspecific activity can often, but not always, be detected by performing a control reaction involving the measurement of the binding of labeled probe to vector that does not contain the probe insert (7). It should be noted that several separation procedures are often required in order to remove trace amounts of vector sequences, which can result in nonspecific signal following hybridization. Nonspecific reactions can also occur due to nonspecific interactions involving linker molecules that are utilized to ligate the probe to the vector, especially when the linkers utilize polynucleotides.

These problems can be largely avoided by the use of probes generated by the synthesis of oligonucleotides rather than by cloning procedures; however, the use of short oligonucleotide probes often results in the loss of assay sensitivity. The development of vectors that do not share homology with human bacterial or genomic sequences would represent a major development in the application of hybridization to practical viral diagnosis.

Recently, it has been reported that substantially greater degrees of sensitivity can be achieved by the magnification of sample nucleic acid by means of repeated reactions with specific primers and DNA polymerase. The repeated cycling of these reactions in a polymerase chain reaction (PCR) format results in a substantial amplification of target nucleic acid with a corresponding increase in assay sensitivity. The use of the thermostabile *Taq* DNA polymerase allows for the performance of repeated polymerase reactions at elevated temperatures without the need to add additional reagents at each step (92). PCR has been applied to the detection of nucleic acids from a number of viruses, including HIV-1, HTLV-I HTLV-II, CMV, EBV, hepatitis B virus, parvoviruses, and rhinoviruses. However, PCR techniques have not as yet been applied for the diagnosis of viral infections under clinical laboratory conditions (93).

PCR formats offer a number of advantages in terms of extreme sensitivity. However, current PCR formats have some limitations in terms of viral diagnosis. The efficient performance of the polymerase chain reactions requires the careful extraction of nucleic acids from clinical samples. Also, there are currently no practical, nonisotopic methods for the quantitation of the nucleic acids generated by the repeated polymerase reactions. In addition, the specificity of the reactions has not been documented, especially when performed under reaction conditions likely to be found in clinical laboratories. In light of the magnifying nature of the assay, it is likely that nonspecific reactions will occur unless extreme care is taken to avoid nonspecific base-pairing reactions. The current formats are limited to the measurement of DNA, thus making them difficult to apply for the detection of RNA viruses. Although, in theory, viral RNA can be converted to complementary DNA (cDNA) by reaction with promoters and the enzyme reverse transcriptase, the need to perform this step might markedly increase the cost and complexity of the assay system. Despite these limitations, the principle of enzymatic magnification of small samples has a great deal of potential for viral diagnosis. The practical application of these systems for viral diagnosis might represent an important achievement in the ability to diagnose viral infections and to study the epidemiology and pathophysiology of viral infections in humans.

## ISOLATION AND IDENTIFICATION OF VIRUSES FROM CLINICAL SPECIMENS

Although rapid identification of viruses in clinical materials often can be accomplished by the direct procedures described in the preceding section, there are obvious limitations to these approaches, including the narrow focus, the requirement for clinical materials containing large amounts of virus or antigen, and the scarcity of adequately sensitive and specific immune reagents. Thus, isolation and identification are required to provide an adequate range of viral diagnostic capabilities, as well as to back up and confirm many of the direct approaches. As antiviral therapy comes into wider use, it appears likely that resistant viral strains will emerge, and it will be essential to have patients' viral isolates available for sensitivity testing.

For those agents that can be propagated in standard laboratory host systems, isolation is generally more sensitive than direct examination for virus detection, since small amounts of virus in the specimen are amplified by replication in a susceptible host. Also, virus grown in culture is freed from contaminating host materials such as mucus and antibodies, which might interfere with virus identification in the original specimen.

Some earlier workers took the view that simply indicating the recovery of a cytopathic or hemadsorbing agent from a patient, together with a presumptive impression as to the broad category to which it might belong, was sufficient information to transmit to the physician and that further identification was unwarranted or should be done by a reference laboratory. An early identification of a viral isolate certainly is important, and should be reported if definitive identification cannot be made by an immunoassay within a few hours. However, it becomes increasingly apparent that specific viral identification is highly relevant from a clinical standard and should be accomplished as rapidly as possible. Definitive virus identification assumes particular importance in the rational use of antiviral agents because of the narrow specificity of some of the agents. Looking to the future, one can envision a need for rapid and specific tests to determine whether the isolate produces the specific viral enzymes through which the agents exert their pharmacological effect (94). Additionally, specific viral identification aids in the management of viral infections or exposures in pregnancy, can provide a rational approach to controlling the spread of hospital-acquired or epidemic viral infections, and can be of prognostic value, as in distinguishing between meningoencephalitis due to HSV and that due to an echovirus. In the long run, specific viral identification educates the physician to develop an awareness of the clinical manifestations of certain viral infections. Virus identification also ensures that the isolate is a human virus, rather than acytopathic or hemadsorbing contaminant from the laboratory host system. Furthermore, the availability of the practical assays for the specific detection of viral antigens and nucleic acids described above allows for the accurate identification of viruses cultivated in *in vitro* systems. The use of assay systems for the detection of specific viruses is discussed below.

### Selection of Appropriate Host System

Most clinical laboratories rely solely on cell culture host systems for virus isolation.

However, reference laboratories may be required to have available additional host systems that will permit recovery of a wider spectrum of human viruses, e.g., suckling mice for isolation of alphaviruses, flaviviruses, bunyaviruses, and group A coxsackieviruses, and embryonated eggs for isolation of influenza viruses at the beginning of the disease season, when there is the possibility that strains may have emerged for which cell cultures are not adequately sensitive.

The basic cell culture systems that have been employed for many years in this laboratory for virus isolation attempts are primary rhesus of cynomologus monkey kidney (MK) cells, together with a human fetal diploid (HFD) cell line; diploid fetal kidney cells are used for virus isolation attempts on enteric specimens of vesicular lesion specimens, and diploid fetal lung cells are used for respiratory specimens. In addition, if rubella is suspected, the RK-13 line of rabbit kidney cells and the BS-C-1 line of grivet monkey kidney cells are used. If human CMV is suspected, human fetal diploid fibroblast cells (lung) are employed, but with prolonged incubation. Human rhabdomyosarcoma cells may be used as an alternate to suckling mice in suspected group A coxsackievirus infections. Preparation, inoculation, and maintenance of these cell culture systems are described elsewhere (95).

Because of the serious shortage and high cost of rhesus MK cells, most laboratories have been forced to substitute primary African green (grivet) or cynomologus MK cells. The range of viruses cultivatable by these cells is similar to that of rhesus MK cells, although greater problems may be encountered with contaminating simian viruses. Efforts have been made to conserve MK cells through the use of the Madin-Darby canine kidney cell line with trypsin in the maintenance medium for isolation of respiratory viruses; although this host system is sensitive for isolation of influenza A and B viruses, it is not adequate for parainfluenza virus isolation (29,96).

Culturing viable cells from biopsy or autopsy specimens is a more sensitive method for virus recovery than is inoculation of tissue homogenates into cell cultures, and this approach might be considered whenever fresh, unfrozen tissue is available. This can be done by establishing cell cultures from the minced or trypsinized tissue specimen, by cocultivating cells from the tissue specimen with cells that are permissive for the virus being sought, or by fusing cells cultivated from the tissue specimen with those of a permissive cell line. These procedures are described in other sources (95).

To minimize the risk of cross-contamination of isolates, medium should not be changed on cell cultures after they have been inoculated with clinical materials, except in special circumstances such as CMV isolation. Most primary and diploid cell cultures can be maintained for 14 days without a medium change.

The quality assurance measures that should be taken to ensure maximum sensitivity and reliability of various host systems for virus isolation are discussed elsewhere (11).

### Basic Approaches to Virus Isolation and Identification

Comprehensive information on the selection processing and inoculation of various clinical specimens into host systems for recovery of viruses is given in other sources (9,10), together with detailed methods for the various identification procedures. We are concerned here with the basic approaches to virus recovery and identification that permit the most efficient, reliable, and rapid identification of viral isolates.

Tables 1 and 2 show the basic steps that can be employed for the recovery and identification of viruses from respiratory and enteric specimens, respectively. The scheme shown in Table 1 is also applicable to vesicular lesion materials, urine, and biopsy or autopsy specimens. If CMV infec-

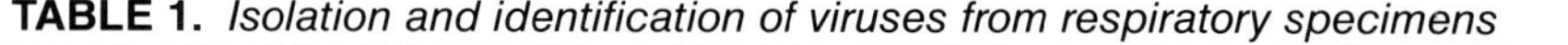

**TABLE 1.** *Isolation and identification of viruses from respiratory specimens*

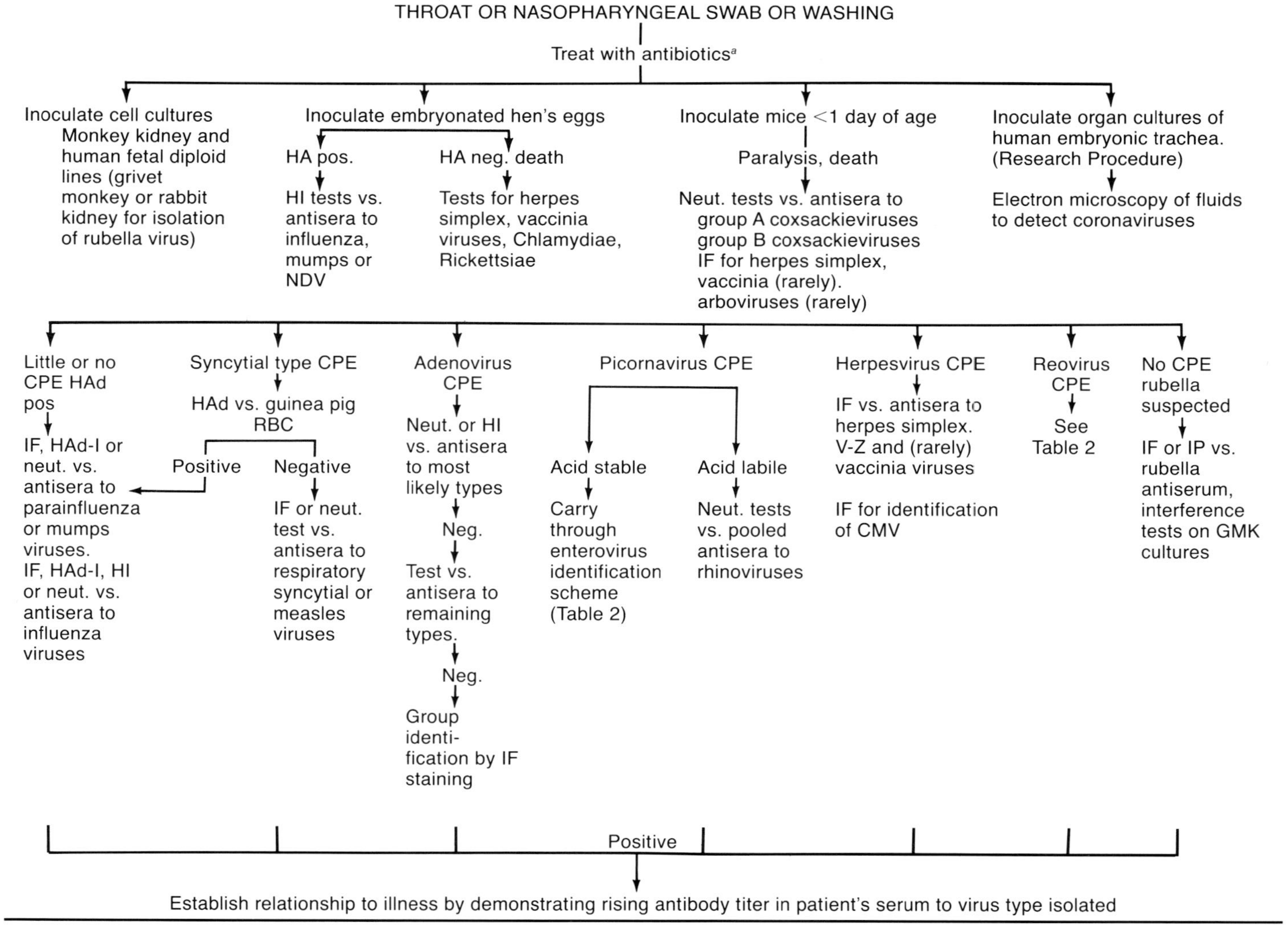

THROAT OR NASOPHARYNGEAL SWAB OR WASHING

↓

Treat with antibiotics[a]

↓

- Inoculate cell cultures
  - Monkey kidney and human fetal diploid lines (grivet monkey or rabbit kidney for isolation of rubella virus)
- Inoculate embryonated hen's eggs
  - HA pos. → HI tests vs. antisera to influenza, mumps or NDV
  - HA neg. death → Tests for herpes simplex, vaccinia viruses, Chlamydiae, Rickettsiae
- Inoculate mice <1 day of age
  - Paralysis, death → Neut. tests vs. antisera to group A coxsackieviruses group B coxsackieviruses IF for herpes simplex, vaccinia (rarely). arboviruses (rarely)
- Inoculate organ cultures of human embryonic trachea. (Research Procedure)
  - → Electron microscopy of fluids to detect coronaviruses

↓

- Little or no CPE HAd pos → IF, HAd-I or neut. vs. antisera to parainfluenza or mumps viruses. IF, HAd-I, HI or neut. vs. antisera to influenza viruses
- Syncytial type CPE → HAd vs. guinea pig RBC
  - Positive → (IF, HAd-I or neut. vs. antisera to parainfluenza or mumps viruses)
  - Negative → IF or neut. test vs. antisera to respiratory syncytial or measles viruses
- Adenovirus CPE → Neut. or HI vs. antisera to most likely types → Neg. → Test vs. antisera to remaining types. → Neg. → Group identification by IF staining
- Picornavirus CPE
  - Acid stable → Carry through enterovirus identification scheme (Table 2)
  - Acid labile → Neut. tests vs. pooled antisera to rhinoviruses
- Herpesvirus CPE → IF vs. antisera to herpes simplex. V-Z and (rarely) vaccinia viruses
  - IF for identification of CMV
- Reovirus CPE → See Table 2
- No CPE rubella suspected → IF or IP vs. rubella antiserum, interference tests on GMK cultures

Positive

↓

Establish relationship to illness by demonstrating rising antibody titer in patient's serum to virus type isolated

[a]Omit if chlamydial or rickettsial infection is suspected.
IF, immunofluorescence; IP, immunoperoxidase: either procedure would be applicable.
HA, hemagglutination; HI, hemagglutination inhibition; HAd, hemadsorption; HAd-I, hemadsorption inhibition.

**TABLE 2.** *Isolation and identification of cultivable enteric viruses*

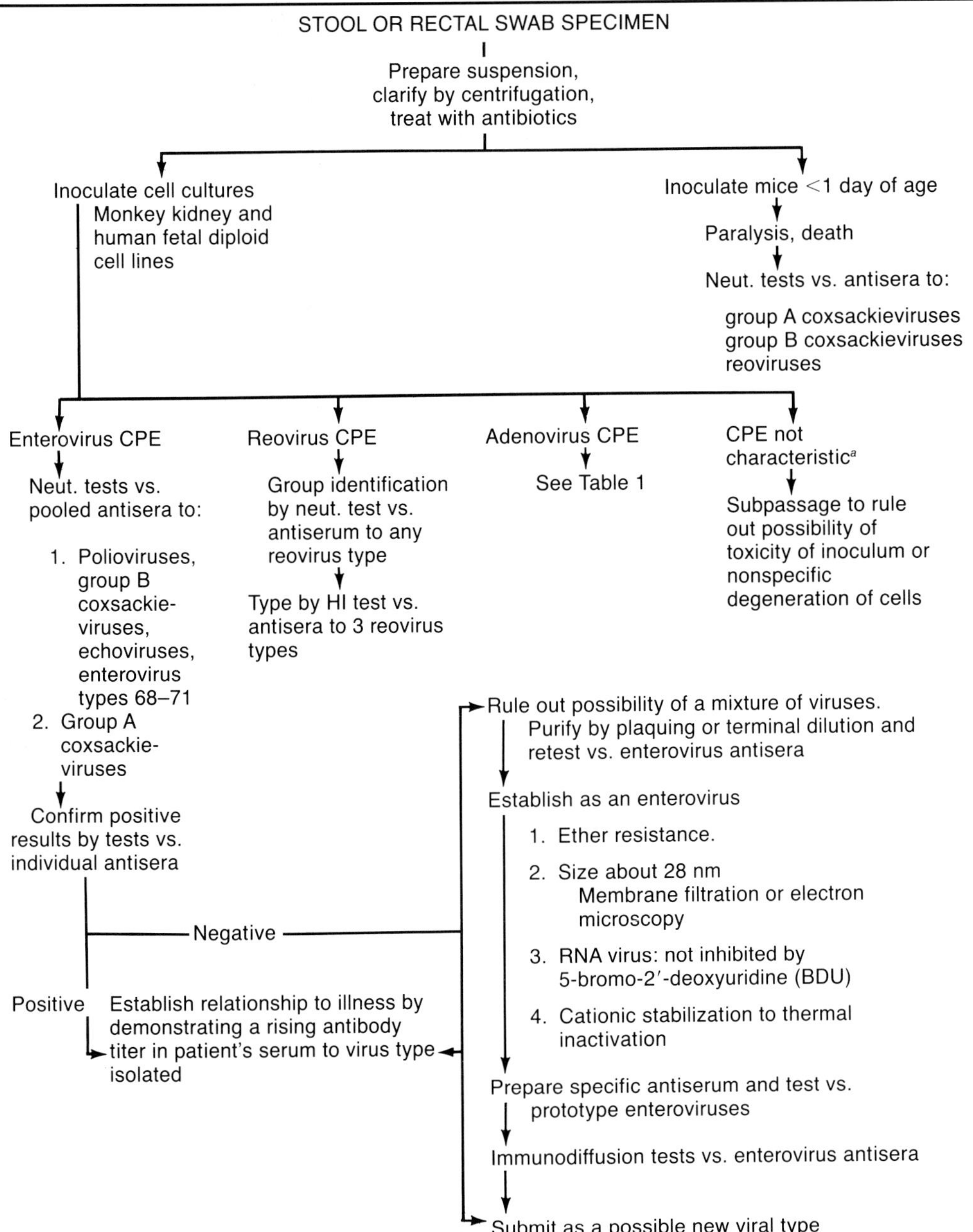


[a]Toxin neutralization test on original stool specimen if CPE is characteristic of that produced by *Cl. difficile* toxin.

tion is suspected, the inoculated human fibroblast cell cultures are observed for up to 60 days. Isolates from vesicular lesions are tested against immune reagents for HSV and VZV, and vaccinia in rare instances. In most cases, only cell culture systems are employed, but in the situations discussed above, and in fatal cases, it may be appropriate to use mouse or embryonated egg host systems.

The speed and efficiency of virus identification are expedited greatly if the microbiologist is able to recognize an early characteristic effect of the virus on the host system; this provides a clue as to the major group to which the isolate may belong and thus guides the selection of the most suitable immunological method for identification. The type of cytopathic effect (CPE) that the isolate produces in cell cultures is the most useful clue, and an experienced observer generally, but not invariably, can recognize CPE characteristics of the major virus groups. However, this skill is acquired only through long and continuous experience based on reading of actual diagnostic runs, as opposed to cultures inoculated with laboratory strains of viruses. Photographs are generally of little value in training personnel to recognize characteristic viral CPE by microscopic observation. Virus-infected cell cultures with 10% formaldehyde are more useful for this purpose. A positive hemadsorption reaction with guinea pig erythrocytes gives a presumptive identification of an orthomyxovirus or a paramyxovirus, and leads to testing against immune reagents to these viruses.

Determining the physical and chemical properties of a viral isolate such as size, either sensitivity, and nucleic acid content generally is not a useful early step in virus identification, since these procedures require considerable time and effort and give little significant information beyond that obtained from the CPE or hemadsorption reaction. An exception is the determination of acid liability to distinguish rhinoviruses from enterovirus recovered from the respiratory tract.

## Immunological Methods for Virus Identification

### *Immunoassays*

The increasing applications of some of the immunoassays described in the previous section for the more rapid identification of viruses isolated in cell cultures or other laboratory host systems have constituted major advances in viral diagnosis. These assays can be more successful on viral isolates than on the original specimen due to the increased content of virus and reduction of interfering host materials. With these techniques, an isolate can be specifically identified within a few hours after the CPE or hemadsorbing activity has provided a clue as to its possible identity. This has made virus isolation and identification a much more rewarding undertaking for clinical microbiology laboratories.

IF staining has been used routinely in various laboratories for rapid identification of isolates of HSV, VZV, CMV, vaccinia, rubella, RSV, parainfluenza, measles, Colorado tick fever, Western and Eastern equine encephalitis, and lymphocytic choriomeningitis viruses (LCMV), as well as for group-specific identification of influenza A and B and adenovirus isolates (8,25,35). Good success has been reported in the use of IP procedures to speed the identification of cell culture isolates of HSV, CMV, paramyxoviruses, rubella virus, and VZV (42,43). The use of monoclonal antibodies with the high specificity should extend the usefulness of these immunoassays for more discriminating identification of viral isolates, e.g., for rapid strain-specific identification or influenza viruses (97), and for efficient typing of HSV (98) and dengue virus isolates (99).

If only a single or a few viral agents are being sought by the inoculation of cell cultures with clinical specimens, immunoassays can be used to screen the cultures for a specific viral antigen even before the agent has demonstrated a CPE or hemadsorption (HAd). Thus, it may be possible to identify a specific virus within 24 hr after cell culture inoculation. This approach has been used for diagnosis of respiratory virus infections in outbreaks where the predominant agent was known (100) and for detection of HSV (67).

The principle of viral identification following a brief period of cultivation is exemplified by the use of "shell Vial" and similar techniques for the detection of CMV and herpesviruses. These methods involve the inoculation of cells in a single unit vial and the subsequent examination of the cells for antigens by means of microscopic immunofluorescence using labeled antibodies directed at viral antigens. In some systems, the initial infection of the cells is accelerated by the centrifugation of the sample in the vial prior to incubation. In most cases, viral antigen will be detectable by IF prior to the development of visible CPE, and the specific nature of the staining procedure will allow for the identification of the infecting virus. This method thus combines some of the benefits of cultivation and IF assay systems and allows for the detection of most strains of CMV and HSV in fewer than 3 days. Disadvantages of the system are that it is somewhat expensive and the processing of large numbers of samples is somewhat tedious. However, it is likely that the system can be adapted for measurement by means of enzyme immunoassay or other procedures suitable for large-scale, objective testing.

IEM procedures have been used for identification of viral isolates (101) and would appear to have the greatest advantage for identification of isolates in large groups with multiple immunotypes, such as enteroviruses, which conventionally require neutralization tests for identification of adventitious agents such as mycoplasmas and contaminating viruses that may be encountered in the course of virus isolation of routine virus cultivation.

### *Neutralization Tests*

Neutralization tests are based on the ability of viral antibodies to combine with virus and render it noninfectious. These are the most specific of conventional methods for virus identification and have been the standards against which other identification methods have been evaluated. However, the marked specificity of the neutralization reaction may be a disadvantage, since field strains within a viral immunotype may vary antigenically to the extent that they are not identifiable by neutralization tests with protype antisera, and tests of broader reactivity may be required (102,103).

The major drawback of the neutralization test for virus identification is the fact that results generally are not available for at least a week or even longer, for some viruses that replicate slowly. At present, however, neutralization test are the only ones feasible for routine type-specific identification of picornaviruses and adenoviruses. The performance of neutralization assays can be facilitated by the incorporation of antigen detection assays into the reaction protocol. For example, the ability of a reference serum to inhibit viral replication can be specifically monitored by measuring the concentration of viral antigens generated in the presence and absence of the antibody. These determinations, which can be more accurate than ones making use of the prevention of cytopathic effect, are particularly useful for determining viral serotypes and for distinguishing closely related strains of viruses.

Neutralization tests for identification of viruses in large groups can be facilitated greatly by the use of immune serum pool schemes (95,102), in which a type-specific antiserum is incorporated into one, two, or three pools, and identification is made by demonstrating neutralization in the pool or pools sharing common type-specific antiserum. Results obtained with antiserum pools should be confirmed by tests against the individual antiserum that showed a positive reaction in the pools.

### *Hemadsorption Inhibition and Hemagglutation Inhibition*

Orthomyxovirus and paramyxovirus isolates may produce little or no CPE, but the surfaces of these viruses have hemagglutinins (HAs) (sites that combine with erythrocytes of certain species) that permit their identification by HAd or hemagglutation procedures. In HAd systems, virus budding from the surface of infected cells is detected by its ability to adsorb erythrocytes onto the infected cell cultures. Virus can be identified by neutralization tests in which cell cultures inoculated with serum-virus mixtures are treated with guinea pig erythrocytes at the end of the incubation period; absence of hemadsorption is taken as evidence of virus neutralization. Identification can be accomplished more rapidly by hemadsorption inhibition (HAd-I) or hemagglutation inhibition (HI) 104) if the isolate produces a sufficiently high titer of HAs in the infected fluids or cell sheets. For HAd-I tests, cell cultures inoculated with the viral isolate are incubated until representative cultures show a HAd reaction; other infected cultures are treated with various myxovirus virus antisera, incubated for a short time, and then examined for their ability to adsorb guinea pig erythrocytes. Identification is based on the ability of one of the antisera to inhibit the HAd reaction. This method requires antisera with higher titers than those suitable for use in neutralization or HI tests. HI tests are performed in tubes or microtiter cups and are based on the ability of a specific viral antiserum to inhibit macroscopic agglutination of test erythrocytes by the viral isolate (104).

## Problems and Pitfalls in the Isolation and Identification of Viruses

Difficulty may be encountered in determining whether an effect observed in a host cell system inoculated with a clinical specimen is actually due to a virus. Confusion can result from cytotoxicity of the inoculum, nonspecific degeneration of host cells, or nonspecific HAd caused by aging of cell cultures. Also, cell cultures may be contaminatcd with morphologically dissimilar cells that grow in discrete foci resembling a viral CPE (e.g., contamination of fibroblast cultures with epithelial cells); these may be transferred to new cultures by subpassage of the specimen, thus compounding the confusion.

Subpassage and titration of first-passage material usually indicates whether a replicating agent is present, and subpassage usually results in a more rapid and typical viral CPE. However, toxicity of some specimens, including that due to *Clostridum difficile* toxin, which is present in some fecal specimens (105), may require three passages to be diluted out. One useful way to distinguish between toxicity and viral CPE is to make a reading 2–3 hr after inoculation, which is too early for a viral CPE to have occurred but sufficient time for a toxic effect to be exerted. The application of antigen assays as discussed above can also be used to distinguish viral replication from nonspecific cellular distinction.

The question may arise as to whether a replicating agent in an inoculated cell culture actually originated from the test specimen or as a contaminant. If the agent is not identifiable by antisera to the most likely human viruses, the latter possibility should be considered. Hemadsorbing agents that are not identifiable as human orthomyxoviruses or paramyxoviruses should be tested against antiserum to SV-5, and reference laboratories should also have antiserum to SV-41, a less common simian hemadsorbing virus. Other common contaminating simian viruses are SV-40, which can be identified readily by IF staining, and simian CMV, which can be distinguished from human CMV by its ability to grow in MK cells. The possibility of a simian virus contaminant should be considered regardless of the passage history of the isolate. Simian viruses can be introduced into human cell cultures by using the same pipette to inoculate MK and human cell cultures or by cross-contamination from MK cells being handled in the same laboratory. Simian and human cell cultures should always be prepared, inoculated, and handled separately. Mycoplasma contaminants originating either from the cell culture system or the clinical specimen can produce CPE or HAd. These may be identified by culturing the isolate on mycoplasma medium, or noncultivable mycoplasma contaminants can be detected by a DNA staining method (106), nucleic acid hybridization, (73) or EM.

It is very important to retain a portion of original specimen, and this should be the unprocessed material rather than the inoculum used for the original isolation. This permits reisolation attempts on specimens giving equivocal results or yielding unusual isolates, and aids in confirming the human origin of viruses recovered.

Field strains of enteroviruses, rhinoviruses, or adenoviruses may differ antigenically from the prototype virus to the extent that they are not neutralized effectively by prototype antiserum. Identification sometimes can be accomplished by using tests of broader reactivity than neutralization, such as complement fixation, immunodiffusion, or IF, but may require preparing antiserum to the variant strain and performing cross-neutralization tests with the prototype virus (102,103).

Failure of prototype immune sera to neutralize picornavirus isolates is often due simply to aggregation of the virus rather than to antigenic variation. Therefore, virus dispersed by deoxycholate or chloroform treatment (107) should be tried in neutralization tests before it is assumed that the isolate is an antigenic variant. Enterovirus isolates sometimes may be neutralized more efficiently in one host cell system than another, regardless of whether untreated or monodispersed virus is used (103), and this probably relates to the differing abilities of cell types to reactivate virus/antibody complexes (108). Performing neutralization tests in different host cell systems may be a useful approach to the identification of problem enterovirus isolates.

Human sera are unreliable for virus identification, particularly in neutralization tests, because they contain antibodies to a wide variety of human viruses, which easily can result in misidentification of viral isolates.

### Viral Monoclonal Antibodies

The reliability of any immunological method for virus detection or identification depends to a large extent on the quality of the immune reagents employed. In the past, inconsistencies in quality and supply of viral antisera have been major deterrents to the development and standardization of viral diagnostic procedures in clinical and microbiology laboratories. However, these problems should be overcome in the near future through the availability of monoclonal antibodies (109–111) to a wide variety of viral agents. The marked specificity of these antibodies avoids previous problems with antibodies to host or other extraneous antigens in viral immune reagents, and also permits more precise characterization of isolates. The narrow specificity of monoclonal antibodies for individual viral determinants could be a drawback for routine viral identification if the determinant were not present in all field strains or if it constituted only a minor portion of the virus-specific proteins. However, this can be overcome by the use of pools of monoclonal antibodies to different viral determinants, and particularly to those determinants that are shown to be highly conserved among clinical isolates (98,112).

The ability to store antibody-producing hybridomas in the frozen state ensures a virtually unlimited and consistent supply of viral antibodies, and the extremely high-titered antibody preparations that can be derived by using the hybridoma cells to produce immune ascitic fluids in mice should solve problems previously encountered with low-titered standard viral antisera, which frequently were unsuitable for labeling for use in immunoassays.

## Viral Genome Analysis

The immunological methods described above for virus identification are directed primarily against viral proteins and are of limited value for detecting subtle differences between viral strains of the same immunotype. More definitive information on similarities or dissimilarities between viral strains can be obtained by genome analysis, and various techniques are now available for "fingerprinting" viral DNA or RNA genomes (113). These procedures have been extremely useful in epidemiological studies for defining relationships between viral isolates from different individuals or outbreaks, and in studies on evolutionary changes that have occurred in certain viruses. Although the methods are not feasible at present for routine use in clinical microbiology laboratories, they are within the scope of activities of reference laboratories and large medical center laboratories, and there is increasing interest on the part of the medical community in applying these highly discriminating techniques to epidemiological studies and disease surveillance.

### *Restriction Enzyme Analysis of DNA Viral Genomes*

For this procedure, the viral DNA is treated with various restriction enzymes that cleave the DNA at specific sites. The segments are then separated by slab gel electrophoresis, and, after staining with ethidium bromide, the electroporetic patterns of fragments from different virus strains are compared. Strains that are unrelated epidemiologically show different gel patterns. These procedures have been useful in identifying sources of HSV infection in newborns, unusual clusters of HSV infections, and recurrent genital HSV infections (114). Genomic analyses can also be utilized to distinguish HSV types 1 and 2 (HSV-1, HSV-2). Restriction enzyme analysis has been used to distinguish between reactivated CMV infections and superinfections with new CMV strains, and also to study the genetic stability of CMV strains transmitted from mothers to their offspring (115). Vaccine and wild strains of VZV have been differentiated by restriction enzyme analysis (116).

### *Oligonucleotide "Fingerprinting" of RNA Viral Genomes*

This technique involves extracting radiolabeled viral RNA with phenol, digesting it with ribonuclease T1 (which cleaves the RNA at guanosine residues to produce fragments of varying lengths), and then separating the fragments by two-dimensional gel electrophoresis. Autoradiography of the two-dimensional gel gives a pattern of oligonucleotides referred to as a "fingerprint" or map, which is specific for the RNA of a given viral strain. Genetic relatedness of dissimilarity between strains is determined by comparing the presence or absence of the various oligonucleotide spots in the fingerprint. This method has been used to study antigenic drift and recombination of influenza viruses and to define origins of influenza virus strains circulating in different outbreaks (117,118). Oligonucleotide fingerprinting has been shown to be a more definitive method than standard marker tests for determining epidemiological relationships between poliovirus strains, and has been useful in tracing the origins of outbreaks and individual cases of paralytic poliomyelitis (119,120). This approach has also been particularly useful for defining relationships among various strains of alphaviruses, flaviviruses, bunyaviruses, and arenaviruses (121).

### *Analysis of Rotavirus RNA Genomes*

The rotavirus genome is a double-stranded RNA consisting of 11 segments, and when the viral RNA is electrophoresed these segments show characteristic migration patterns. Comparison of the electrophoretic patterns of rotavirus RNAs can detect differences among strains of human and animal origin finer than can be demonstrated by antigenic analysis (122,123), and this approach should contribute much to our future understanding of the epidemiology of rotavirus infections. RNA analysis also allows for the detection of antigenically distinct, non–group-A rotaviruses, which cannot be detected by currently available immunoassay systems (124). Genome analysis of rotaviruses has also permitted identification of the gene segments that code for the viral proteins with specific antigenic or biological functions (125,126).

## SEROLOGICAL DIAGNOSIS

Serodiagnosis of viral infection is based on demonstrating a significant increase in the antibody titer to a given virus over the course of the patient's illness. This requires the testing, in parallel, of an acute-phase serum collected as early as possible after onset of illness, together with a convalescent-phase serum taken at least 14 days later. Generally, little or no diagnostic significance can be attached to an elevated antibody titer in a single specimen, although high titers to agents rarely encountered in the population, e.g., LCMV, or of antibodies that decline rapidly after infection, such as those to the soluble antigens of influenza or mumps viruses, may be suggestive of recent or current infection in individuals with compatible clinical syndromes. However extreme caution should be exercised in making an interpretation of "presumptive positive" based on an elevated antibody titer, since titers of antibody demonstrated in a given serum may vary widely depending on the type and amount of antigen used and the testing system employed. Further, few laboratories have sufficient baseline data on non-ill individuals or those with other infections to permit designation of titers that could be considered indicative of current or recent infection. Because of the wide individual variation in decay of viral antibodies after natural infections, diagnostic significance rarely can be attached to a four-fold or greater decline in antibody titer between paired serum specimens.

Because of the delay in obtaining a convalescent-phase serum specimen, serologic diagnosis is retrospective, which limits its usefulness in many clinical situations. However, this approach is more economical than virus isolation, and serodiagnosis is often required for diagnosis of infections where virus rarely can be isolated or antigen detected, such as nonfatal arbovirus infections, or for certain respiratory viral infections where virus excretion is of short duration. Also, antibody assays on single-serum specimens are needed for determining the immunity status of individuals at high risk for rubella, mumps, hepatitis B, or VZV infection, or for determination of CMV antibody status in donors and recipients of organs for transplantation, or of blood for transfusion to newborns.

### Standard Serological Procedures

The conventional methods for serodiagnosis of viral infections include neutralization, HI, complement fixation (CF), indirect IF staining, and (to a much lesser extent) passive hemagglutination (PHA). Each of these procedures has its advantages and limitations, and none is uniformly applicable to all of the common viral infections of humans.

The neutralization test is based on the reaction of antibody with virus to render it noninfectious for a susceptible host. Major limitations are the requirements for expensive living host systems and the time required to obtain results; sensitivity and specificity are advantages. Neutralizing antibody is of long duration, and its presence is often, but not always, associated with immunity.

The HI test is based on the fact that many viruses have the capacity to agglutinate erythrocytes of certain species (hemagglutination), but combination of the virus with specific antibody prevents this reaction. Thus, viral antibody can be assayed by demonstrating ability of the test serum to inhibit agglutination of red blood cells (RBC) by a standard dose of viral antigen. The chief drawback to this system is the fact that nonantibody serum components may also inhibit hemagglutination, and these must be removed or inactivated before a valid antibody assay can be performed. Also, not all viruses agglutinate RBC. Advantages are the economy of an *in vitro* system, and sensitivity and specificity approximating those of the neutralization test.

The CF test has been the most widely used *in vitro* method for serodiagnosis of viral infections because of its versatility, broad reactivity, and effectiveness in detecting antibody titer rises. However, it is relatively insensitive, particularly for detecting antibody of long duration, and requires high concentrations of antigen. Reliable CF antigens are not available for all important human viruses. Also, valid results cannot be obtained on anticomplementary sera or those containing antibodies against host components.

Indirect IF or IP techniques are more cumbersome than other *in vitro* viral antibody assays that do not require microscopic reading, and are generally reserved for those infections for which other adequately sensitive and specific *in vitro* tests are not available, such as EBV infections and arenavirus infections. Solid-phase indirect IF systems that utilize instrument readings have been developed for viral antibody assays (127).

Erythrocytes can be made to adsorb viral antigens to their surfaces by treatment with tannic acid, glutaraldehyde, or chromic chloride, and these can be used in PHA tests for assay of viral antibodies. PHA tests are useful *in vitro* systems for viruses that do not hemagglutinate RBC directly—e.g., human herpesvirus and HBV. The tests are simple and relatively sensitive, and can detect viral antibody of the IgM class. Improved methods for stabilization storage of antigen-coated RBC have made the procedures more practical for routine use (128,129). Disadvantages are the requirement for purified antigens in some cases and occasional nonspecific agglutination of RBC by the test sera.

### Newer Methods for Assay of Viral Antibodies

In recent years, various newer methods for detection of viral antibodies have been described that offer advantages over conventional serological methods in terms of economy, sensitivity, specificity, or rapidity with which results can be obtained. After adequate evaluation, some of these are being put into routine use in clinical microbiology laboratories.

### *Single Radial Diffusion*

Single radial diffusion (SRD) is a technique in which virus, either intact or disrupted, is immobilized in an agarose gel and test serum samples are placed in wells cut in the gel. Antibody diffuses radially and produces an immunoprecipitate around the well. Conversely, antigen can be assayed by diffusing from wells in a gel containing antibody. The size of the resulting zone of immunoprecipitate is directly proportional to the concentration of antibody or antigen in the test sample. Single radial diffusion is sensitive for measuring significant antibody increases between acute- and convalescent-phase sera in natural viral infections and immunized individuals (130), and is being applied increasingly to determination of antigen content of influenza (131) and poliovirus (132) vaccines. Advantages of the technique are simplicity, lack of interference by nonspecific inhibitors in serum, and stability of reagents. However, high concentrations of antigen are required in gels used to measure antibody, and purified or partially purified antigens may be required.

### *Hemolysis-in-Gel*

For hemolysis-in-gel (HIG), RBC coated with viral antigen are immobilized in a gel. Test serum placed in wells in the gel diffuses radially, and in the presence of complement, specific antibodies lyse the viral antigen-coated RBC, producing a zone of hemolysis, the size of which is related to the antibody content of the serum. Advantages are simplicity, sensitivity comparable to that of HI or neutralization tests, lack of interference by nonspecific serum inhibitors, and lack of a requirement for purified antigen. This is a relatively simple procedure for determination of rubella immunity status (133) and for large-scale assay of antibodies to various arboviruses (134). HIG has shown greater specificity than HI for determination of certain togavirus antibodies (135). The gels are not as stable as those for SRD tests, but the development of methods for storage of antigen-coated RBC in the frozen state (136) should increase practicality of the procedure. The test has not been reliable for detection of IgM antibodies to most of the viruses tested.

### *Immune Adherence Hemagglutination*

Immune adherence hemagglutination (IAHA) is a complement-mediated reaction in which the attachment of complement to an antigen/antibody complex activates the third component of complement so that it adheres to receptors on human RBC and produces hemagglutination. This technique demonstrates higher antigen and antibody titers than are demonstrable by CF, and has been applied to detection of antibodies for a variety of viral agents (137). The IAHA results are obtained within 2–3 hr, and the balance between concentrations of test reagents is not as critical as in CF. Prozone reactions may occur in regions of antigen or antibody excess, necessitating the examination of a range of specimen dilations. Human RBCs from different individuals vary in their suitability for the reaction, requiring the selection of appropriate donors. Also, specifically processed microtiter plates are required. Other drawbacks are that some soluble viral antigens are not reactive in IAHA (138) and that the tests may detect viral IgM antibody or early IgG antibody of low avidity (139).

### *Radioimmunoassays*

Solid-phase indirect RIAs, in which antigen in the form of virus-infected cells, lysates of infected cells, or purified virus is immobilized onto plastic microtiter plates or beads, have shown high sensitivity for detection of viral antibody (68,69). Although efforts generally have been made to substitute EIA procedures for RIA in viral antibody assays, the high sensitivity of RIA may make this a more satisfactory approach for detecting low levels of viral antibody fluids such as cerebrospinal fluids (CSFs) (140) or other secretions and excretions. RIA is also useful for detecting viral antibodies in eluates from virus-infected tissues (141,142) and thus can be a useful tool for indirectly identifying the presence of virus in tissues from certain chronic diseases.

### *Enzyme Immunoassays*

Solid-phase indirect EIAs, commonly referred to as "ELISA," have been widely applied in recent years to assay of viral antibodies. They have become standard and routine procedures for viral serology for a number of viral agents. Viral antigens are immobilized onto a solid phase (bead, microtiter cup, or plastic paddle), test sera are added, and after incubation followed by thorough washing, antibodies coupled with the test antigen are detected through the addition of an enzyme-labeled antispecies immune globulin, followed by the appropriate substrate. Results can be read visually, or more sensitively by spectrophotometer or fluorimeter. This system is most suitable for assay of viral antibodies of the IgG class; viral IgM and probably IgA and IgE antibodies are detected more reliably by the "capture" system described below.

Advantages of these EIA tests are their versatility, sensitivity, objectivity in terms of instrument readings, adaptability to automation, lack of interference by nonspecific inhibitors in test sera, and stability and safety of the labeled antibodies. In practice, they have shown greater ability than conventional serological procedures to demonstrate seroconversion or significant antibody titer rises (143–145). The use of purified viral subunit antigens can increase the specificity and diagnostic value of EIAs for example, to detect subtype-specific antibody titer rises to HI or H3 HAs of influenza A viruses (146) or type-specific antibody responses to HSV (147). The use of EIA for the measurement of antibodies to human retroviruses is discussed in chapter 15.

The EIA systems for assay of viral antibodies are now becoming available from commercial sources. In evaluating these kits, researchers have found that results have generally been in agreement with those of standard assay procedures, but some problems have been encountered in obtaining reproducible results on sera containing low levels of antibody (148). This has resulted in setting higher levels for positive readings and establishing an equivocal range of results, which requires the performance of another type of backup antibody assay.

There has been increasing recognition of the need to test each serum against control antigen prepared from uninfected cells or tissues in the same manner as the viral antigen (149). This provides a specificity control on each test serum more appropriate than can be obtained by comparing the serum's antiviral activity with that of negative sera or other background controls.

In evaluating new EIA systems, it has become apparent that results obtained are not linearly proportional to antibody titers and that the antibody in a test serum cannot be accurately quantitated from results on a single concentration of the serum (106,143, 150). This is related to variations in specificities, affinities, and immunoglobulin classes in the antibody responses of different individuals to a viral infection (151).

### *Latex Agglutination Tests*

A test for rubella antibody that utilizes latex particles coated with rubella antigen has been developed recently (152). A drop of the undiluted or diluted test serum is mixed with a drop of the antigen preparation, and a positive agglutination reaction is demonstrable within a few minutes. For the most part, this test has shown a sensitivity for rubella antibody detection or for demonstration of seroconversion similar to those of HI and neutralization (152,153). In one evaluation, it showed a rather high rate of false negative results in sera having low titers by EIA (152). Sera with high levels of rubella antibody may give a prozone reaction when tested undiluted (153), and for this reason it may be desirable to examine diluted, as well as undiluted, sera. The test is not affected by nonspecific inhibitors of rubella hemagglutination, and preliminary evidence suggests that it may be able to detect IgM as well as IgG viral antibody (153). Because of its simplicity, rapidity, and economy, this test system probably will be extended for assay of antibodies to a wider range of viral agents.

### Class-Specific Viral Antibody Determinations

In some instances, the speed or specificity of viral serodiagnosis may be improved by the assay of viral antibodies in specific classes of immunoglobulins, particularly IgM. In postnatal viral infections, IgM antibodies characteristically appear within 7–10 days after infection, and generally persist at detectable levels for somewhere between 3 and 6 months. Thus, the presence of viral IgM antibody implies a current or recent infection with the agent, and this offers the possibility of making a rapid diagnosis by demonstrating viral IgM in a single, acute-phase serum specimen. Since maternal IgM antibody does not cross the placenta, virus-specific IgM in the newborn can be assumed to be a result of congenital infection, and viral IgM assays can provide a more rapid diagnosis than can be achieved by demonstrating persistence of antibody in a later specimen taken from the infant at a time when maternal antibody would have disappeared. In some alphavirus and flavivirus infections, IgM antibody responses may show narrower specificity than IgG antibody responses, which show broad cross-reactivity between members of the same group, and assays for virus-specific IgM antibodies may improve the specificity of serodiagnosis.

In the past, viral IgM antibody assays have sometimes shown low sensitivity or specificity, resulting from various features of the assay systems (154,155). When viral antigen is immobilized on the solid phase, as in indirect IF, EIA, and RIA systems, viral IgG antibodies can reduce sensitivity by competing with IgM antibodies for antigen. Further, if rheumatoid factor (RF) of the IgM class is present in the serum, this can give false-positive results by reacting with viral IgG antibody coupled with the viral antigen, and then binding the labeled anti-IgM reagent (156,157). Assays have been described based on adsorbing test sera with staphylococcal protein A to remove most IgG antibodies and then assaying for residual antibody, presumed to be IgM. However, these are now recognized to be unreliable due to residual IgA antibodies and IgG antibodies of subclass 3, which might give false positive results (158). Poor specificity and inconsistencies in supply of commercially available anti-$\mu$ chain reagents have also hindered development of reliable viral IgM antibody assays.

Viral IgM assay systems in which antibodies to human IgM are used as "capture" antibodies on a solid phase (159,160) have overcome some of these problems and are the current methods of choice. When test serum is added, IgM is selectively retained on the solid phase, whereas IgG and other serum components are removed by washing. Viral antigen is added next and is bound to homologous IgM antibodies if they were present in the test serum. Enzyme-labeled or radiolabeled antibody of the viral antigen is added next and is retained if the antigen has been bound to virus-specific IgM from the test serum. Advantages are that whole serum can be examined and competing IgG antibodies are removed from the system. Sensitivity of the test depends on the proportion of virus-specific IgM in the test serum; this is particularly high in sera of congenitally infected newborns and CSFs, making the capture system highly suitable for examining these types of specimens. The system is not as satisfactory for viral IgG antibody assays, since antibodies to a given virus constitute a relatively low proportion of the total IgG. The competition between IgM of various specificities for solid-phase binding sites appears not to decrease sensitivity as compared to that of tests using viral antigen in solid phase (161). RF of the IgM class is bound to the solid phase, along with IgM of other specificities, and has the potential for causing false-positive reactions. This can result from RF being complexed with virus-specific IgG, which binds the viral antigen, or from RF binding directly to the labeled antiviral IgG. The latter is a particular problem if human IgG is used as a source of viral antibody. False-positive reactions due to RF have been avoided by diluting test sera and the conjugate in aggregated IgG or antibody-negative human serum to bind and saturate RF (160), or by using labeled F $(ab')_2$ fragments of viral antibody, which lack the Fc portion to which RF binds (159). Testing sera against an uninfected control antigen as well as viral antigen permits detection of false-positive reactions due to RF or other factors and prevents misinterpretation of results (49).

Capture systems for assays of viral IgM antibody have also been described that use enzyme-labeled viral antigens rather than viral antibodies (162–164). Advantages are fewer steps in the procedure and elimination of labeled IgG with which RF might react.

Other modifications of capture viral IgM assays have been based on using RBC to detect binding of viral hemagglutinins by specific IgM retained on the solid phase; these have been applied to IgM antibody assays for rubella virus (165,166) and orthoand paramyxoviruses (167,168). Advantages are the lack of a requirement for a labeled antiviral reagent and the fact that results can be read macroscopically. However, some of the systems have required a very precise balance between antigen and RBC concentrations in order to obtain the desired HI or HAd reactions indicative of positive results (165,167,168). Systems in which an excess of HA is used and unreacted antigen is removed before the addition of RBC would appear to be the most reliable and practical (166).

Monoclonal antibodies to human IgM have been produced for use as capture antibodies in assay of viral IgM (169), and the availability of reagents of this source should overcome previously encountered problems with specificity and supply of anti-μ chain reagents.

As information accumulates about IgM antibody responses in viral infections, it becomes apparent that results of viral IgM antibody assays must be interpreted with caution. It is now recognized that IgM antibody responses cannot distinguish primary from secondary viral infections, as they have been shown to occur in reactivated herpesvirus infections (170–172) and in reimmunization with live rubella (173) or poliovirus (174) vaccines. Also, the occasional prolonged persistence of IgM antibody to rubella, arboviruses, and human herpesviruses, as well as the heterotypic IgM antibody responses that occur in some herpesvirus infection emphasize the importance of interpreting viral IgM assays in light of clinical and epidemiological details of each case, and together with results of other virological and serological tests wherever possible.

Serum IgA viral antibody responses have been studied less extensively than have IgM responses. In congenital rubella or CMV infections, there appears to be no virus-specific IgA antibody detectable in the serum, and in postnatal viral infections serum IgA antibodies develop simultaneously with IgM and IgG antibodies. Although there have been some suggestions that the presence of viral IgA antibody can be taken as evidence of an active infection, studies using sensitive detection methods have shown that persistence of viral IgA antibody after infection is highly variable, ranging from weeks to years, and the presence of IgA antibody in a single serum specimen cannot be taken as evidence of a current or recent viral infection (175,176). However, a notable example of the diagnostic and prognostic significance of serum viral IgA antibodies is that of IgA antibodies to EBV capsid antigen; these are present in 100% of patients with nasopharyngeal carcinoma, and changes in antibody levels are related to changes in tumor activity (177).

Assay of serum and secretory viral IgA antibodies may prove to be of value in determining the quality of immunity produced in response to viral vaccines, as it appears that vaccines that fail to elicit serum or secretory IgA antibody may not produce as solid immunity as do vaccines that stimulate these antibodies. Stimulation of secretory virus-specific IgA appears to be particularly important in inducing immunity to certain respiratory viruses (178).

There has also been some interest in the measurement of antiviral antibodies of the IgE class. Studies have documented that the local production of antibodies of this class to respiratory viruses is associated with allergic-type symptoms, a finding that is consistent with the known biological properties of IgE antibodies (179). It has also been reported that IgE antibodies do not cross the placenta and thus might be useful for the diagnosis of prenatal and perinatal infections. One study found that the measurement of antiviral IgE in a solid phase capture format was more efficient for the detection of congenital CMV than the measurement of IgM antibodies (180). The value of IgE measurements for the diagnosis of this and other viral infections should be the subject of additional investigations.

IgG subclasses have also been used to monitor the course of viral infections. These assays are performed in a manner analogous to that described for the measurement of the immunoglobulin classes except that labeled antibodies specific for IgG subclasses $IgG_1$–$IgG_4$ are utilized in place of the class-specific antibodies. The recent availability of monoclonal and polyclonal antibodies specific for the immunoglobulin subclasses has made such assays practical for many laboratories. The subclass response to a number of viral agents has been studied, including HSV (181), CMV (182), EBV (183), VZV (184), influenza viruses (185), and a number of other viral agents (186). Although there are some differences in the responses to individual viruses, the majority of the antiviral antibodies measured are to the $IgG_1$ and $IgG_3$ classes of antibodies. Although antibodies to $IgG_4$ subclass occur, they are usually in lower titer. Antibodies of the $IgG_2$ class are rarely produced in significant quantities in response to viral infections, whereas they are generated in response to infection with bacteria and fungi. The fact that antiviral $IgG_3$ antibodies arise earlier than $IgG_1$ antibodies has suggested that the measurement of immunoglobulin subclasses might be useful in determining the time course of viral infections (184,187). However, little direct data are available concerning this hypothesis. Current limitations on the application of immunoglobulin subclass measurement for viral diagnosis include the lack of standard antisubclass antibodies and the lack of defined positive and negative control specimens. The availability of such reagents should allow for the more widespread application of immunoglobulin subclass measurement and for the determination of the role of such measurements in the clinical virology.

## SAFETY OF VIRAL ANTIGENS

As clinical microbiology laboratories adopt viral antibody assay procedures, the infectivity of the antigens becomes an important consideration. Many laboratories are not equipped for or experienced in handling infectious viral materials, and some of the new automated or semiautomated methods tend to produce aerosols that are potentially hazardous if infectious antigens are used.

It has been clearly demonstrated over the years that viral antigens prepared by standard methods may retain infectivity, and inactivating agents such as heat, formalin, ultraviolet light, and β-propiolactone have been used with varying success as regards preservation of antigenic activity. An important advance has been the use of psoralen derivatives irradiated with long wavelength ultraviolet light to render viral serological antigens noninfectious (188). The advantage of this method is that it inactivates virus by damaging the nucleic acid, rather than the protein coat responsible for antigenic activity. Psoralen inactivation has been used for preparation of a wide variety of viral serological antigen, including those for highly hazardous agents, and reactivity of these antigens has been identical to that of uninactivated ones (188).

## CONCLUSION

As indicated in the above discussion, there are a wide range of methodologies that have been applied to the diagnosis of viral infections. As might be surmised from the number of different methods, there is no one system that is ideal for the detection of viral infections. Some of the diversity of diagnostic methods derives from the inherent heterogeneity of the biophysical and biochemical properties of pathogenic viruses. In addition, incomplete understanding of the factors that determine cell tropism makes it difficult to derive general principles for the cultivation of viruses. Similarly, a more complete understanding of the determinants of the host immune response to viral infections would facilitate the development of widely applicable assay systems for serological diagnosis. It is highly likely that the development of additional information related to the protein structure, genomic constitution, and immunogenicity of pathogenic viruses will lead to the more accurate application of available diagnostic assays. It is also likely that technical advances in the fields of antibody measurement, protein analysis, and genomic magnification combined with an increased understanding of the viruses themselves will result in the development of new diagnostic assays with greater degrees of specificity, sensitivity, and clinical application. The availability of these assays after careful evaluation should lead not only to the improved management of patients with viral infections, but to the facilitated usage of antiviral chemotherapy and to the development of improved methods for the prevention and treatment of viral infections.

## ACKNOWLEDGMENT

This work was supported by contract number N01-AI-52579 from the National Institutes of Health. Much of this material is derived from material presented in the chapter of the same name by Dr. Natalie J. Schmidt (deceased) in the previous edition of this volume.

## REFERENCES

1. Losonsky G, Johnson J, Winkelstein JA, Yolken RH. Oral administration of human serum immunoglobulin in immunodeficient patients with viral gastroenteritis: a pharmacokinetic and functional analyses. *J Clin Invest* 1985;76:2362–7.
2. Smith T, Jakobsen J, Gaub J, Helweg-Larsen S. Clinical and electrophysiological studies of human immunodeficiency virus-seropositive men without AIDS. *Ann Neurol* 1988;23:295–7.
3. Stephanopoulos DE, Kappes JC. Enhanced in vitro reactivation by herpes simplex virus type 2 from latently infected guinea-pig neural tissues by 5-azacytidine. *J Gen Virol* 1988;69:1079–83.

4. Viscidi RP, Yolken RH. Molecular diagnosis of infectious diseases by nucleic acid hybridization. *Mol Cell Probes* 1987;1:3–14.
5. Yolken RH. Nucleic acids or immunoglobulins: which are the molecular probes of the future. *Mol Cell Probes* 1988;2:87–96.
6. Yolken RH. Enzyme immunoassays for the detection of infectious antigens in body fluids: current limitations and future prospects. *Rev Infect Dis* 1982;4:35–68.
7. Ambinder RF, Charache P, Staal S, et al. The vector homology problem in diagnostic nucleic acid hybridization of clinical specimens. *J Clin Microbiol* 1986;24:16–20.
8. Gardner PS, McQuillin J. *Rapid Virus diagnosis: application of immunofluorescence*. 2nd ed. London: Butterworth, 1980.
9. Lennette EH, Balows A, Hausler WJ Jr, Truant JP, eds. *Manual of clinical microbiology*. 3rd ed. Washington, D.C.: American Society for Microbiology, 1980.
10. Lennette EH, Schmidt NJ, eds. *Diagnostic procedures for viral, rickettsial and chlamydial infection*. 5th ed. Washington, D.C.: American Public Health Association, 1979.
11. Schmidt NJ, Hamparian VV, Sather GE, Wong YW. Quality assurance practices for virology laboratories. In: Inhorn SL, ed. *Quality assurance practices in health laboratories*. Washington, D.C.: American Public Health Association, 1979:1096–144.
12. Bishop RF, Davidson GP, Holmes IH, Ruck BJ. Virus particles in epithelial cells of duodenal mucosa from children with acute nonbacterial gastroenteritis. *Lancet* 1973;2:1281–3.
13. Kapikian AZ, Yolken RH, Greenberg HB, et al. Gastroenteritis viruses. In: Lennette EH, Schmidt NJ, eds. *Diagnostic procedures for viral, rickettsial and chlamydial infections*. 5th ed. Washington, D.C.: American Public Health Association, 1979:927–95.
14. Tyrrell DAJ, Kapikian AZ, eds. *Viral infections of the gastrointestinal tract*. New York: Marcel Dekker, 1980.
15. Almeida JD. Practical aspects of diagnostic electron microscopy. *Yale J Biol Med* 1980; 53:5–18.
16. Field AM. Diagnostic virology using electron microscopic techniques. In: Lauffer MA, Bang FB, Maramorosch K, Smith KM, eds. *Advances in virus research, vol. 27*. New York: Academic Press, 1982:2–69.
17. Lee FK, Nahmias AJ, Stagno S. Rapid diagnosis of cytomegalovirus infection in infants by electron microscopy. *N Engl J Med* 1978;299:1266–70.
18. Hammond GW, Hazelton PR, Chuang I, Klisko B. Improved detection of viruses by electron microscopy after direct ultracentrifuge preparation of specimens. *J Clin Microbiol* 1981; 14:210–21.
19. Rodger SM, Bishop RF, Holmes IH. Detection of a rotavirus-like agent associated with diarrhea in an infant. *J Clin Microbiol* 1982;16: 724–6.
20. Kapikian AZ, Dienstag JL, Purcell RH. Immune electron microscopy as a method for the detection, identification, and characterization of agents not cultivable as an in vitro system. In: Rose NR, Friedman H, eds. *Manual of clinical immunology*. 2nd ed. Washington, D.C.: American Society for Microbiology, 1980: 70–83.
21. Derrick KS. Immuno-specific grids for electron microscopy of plant viruses. *Phytopathology* 1972;62:753–4.
22. Nicolaieff A, Obert G, Van Regenmortel MHV. Detection of rotavirus by serological trapping on antibody-coated electron microscope grids. *J Clin Microbiol* 1980;12:101–4.
23. Giraldo G, Beth E, Lee J, deHarven E, Chernesky M. Solid-phase immune electron microscopy-double antibody technique for rapid detection of papovaviruses. *J Clin Microbiol* 1982;15:517–21.
24. Cherry WB. Immunofluorescence techniques. In: Lennette EH, Balows A, Hausler WJ Jr, Triant JP, ed. *Manual of clinical microbiology*. 3rd ed. Washington, D.C.: American Society for Microbiology, 1980:501–8.
25. Emmons RW, Riggs JL. Application of immunofluorescence to diagnosis of viral infections. In: Maramorosch K, Koprowski H, eds. *Methods of virology, vol. 6*. New York: Academic Press, 1977:1–28.
26. Nakamura RM. Fluorescent antibody methods: quality assurance procedures. In: Nakamura RM, Dito WR, Tucker III ES, eds. *Immunoassays in the clinical laboratory*. New York: Alan R. Liss, 1979:150–72.
27. Diasy JA, Lief FS, Friedman HM. Rapid diagnosis of influenza A infection by direct immunofluorescence of nasopharyngeal aspirates in adults. *J Clin Microbiol* 1979;9:688–92.
28. Minnich L, Ray CG. Comparison of direct immunofluorescent staining of clinical specimens for respiratory virus antigens with conventional isolation techniques. *J Clin Microbiol* 1980;12:391–4.
29. Frank AL, Couch RB, Griffis CA, Baxter BD. Comparison of different tissue cultures for isolation and quantitation of influenza and parainfluenza viruses. *J Clin Microbiol* 1979;10: 32–6.
30. Wong DT, Welliver RC, Riddlesberger KR, Sun MS, Ogra PL. Rapid diagnosis of parainfluenza virus infections in children. *J Clin Microbiol* 1982;16:164–7.
31. Fulton RE, Middleton PJ. Comparison of immunofluorescence and isolation techniques in the diagnosis of respiratory viral infections of children. *Infect Immun* 1974;10:92–101.
32. Orstavik I, Grandien M, Halonen P, et al. Rapid immunofluorescence diagnosis of respiratory syncytial virus infections among children in European countries. *Lancet* 1980;ii:32.
33. Fulton RE, Middleton PJ. Immunofluorescence in diagnosis of measles infections in children. *J Pediatr* 1975;86:17–22.
34. Drew WL, Mintz L. Rapid diagnosis of vari-

cella-zoster virus infection by direct immunofluorescence. *Am J Clin Pathol* 1980;73: 699–701.

35. Schmidt NJ, Gallo D, Devlin V, Woodie JD, Emmons RW. Direct immunofluorescence staining for detection of herpes simplex and varicella-zoster virus antigens in vesicular lesions and certain tissue specimens. *J Clin Microbiol* 1980;12:651–5.
36. Rowse-Eagle D, Watson HD, Tignor GH. Improved methods for trypsin digestion of paraplast sections before immunofluorescence staining. *J Clin Microbiol* 1981;13:996–7.
37. Swoveland PT, Johnson KP. Enhancement of fluorescent antibody staining of viral antigens in formalin-fixed tissues by trypsin digestion. *J Infect Dis* 1979;140:758–64.
38. Avrameas S, Ternynck T, Guesdon JL. Coupling of enzymes to antibodies and antigens. *Scand J Immunol* 1978;8:7–23.
39. Mosely RC, Corey L, Benjamin D, Winter C, Remington ML. Comparison of viral isolation, direct immunofluorescence, and indirect immunoperoxidase techniques for detection of genital herpes simplex virus infection. *J Clin Microbiol* 1981;13:913–8.
40. Sarkkinen HK, Halonen PE, Arstila PP, Salmi AA. Detection of respiratory syncytial, parainfluenza type 2, and adenovirus antigens by radioimmunoassay on nasopharyngeal specimens from children with acute respiratory disease. *J Clin Microbiol* 1981;13:258–65.
41. Sarkkinen HK, Halonen PE, Salmi AA. Type-specific detection of parainfluenza viruses by enzyme-immunoassay and radioimmunoassay in nasopharyngeal specimens of patients with acute respiratory disease. *J Gen Virol* 1981; 56:49–57.
42. Benjamin DF. Immunoenzymatic methods. In: Lennette EH, Schmidt NJ, eds. *Diagnostic procedures for viral, rickettsial and chlamydial infection*. 5th ed. Washington, D.C.: American Public Health Association, 1979.
43. Kurstak E, Tijssen P, Kurstak C, Morisset R. Progress in the application of new immunoenzymatic methods in virology. *Ann NY Acad Sci* 1975;254:369–84.
44. Sternberg LA. The unlabeled antibody peroxidase-antiperoxidase (PAP) method. In: Weir J, ed. *Immunochemistry*. 2nd ed. New York: John Wiley & Sons, 1979:104–69.
45. Elias JM. A rapid, sensitive myeloperoxidase stain using 4-chloro-1-naphthol. *Am J Clin Pathol* 1980;7:797–9.
46. Pearson NS, Fleagle G, Docherty JJ. Detection of herpes simplex virus infection of female genitalia by the peroxidase-antiperoxidase method alone or in conjunction with the Papanicolaou stain. *J Clin Microbiol* 1979;10:737–46.
47. Wirahadiredja RMS. Immunoperoxidase technique used for the detection of Herpes suis infection in pigs. In: Feldman G, Druet P, Bignon J, Avrameas S, eds. *First International Symposium on Immunoenzymatic Techniques, INSERM Symposium No. 2*. Amsterdam: North Holland, 1976:461–4.
48. Robinson G, Dawson I. Immunochemical studies of the endocrine cells of the gastrointestinal tract. I. The use and value of peroxidase-conjugated antibody techniques for the localization of gastrin-containing cells in the human pyloric antrum. *Histochem J* 1975;7:321–33.
49. Yolken RH. Enzymatic assays for the diagnosis of infectious diseases. In: Falkow S, Kingsbury D, eds. Rapid detection and identification of infectious agents. Orlando: Academic Press, 1985;19–32.
50. Pronovost AD, Baumgarten A, Andiman WA. Chemiluminescent immunoenzymatic assay for rapid diagnosis of viral infections. *J Clin-Microbiol* 1982;16:345–9.
51. Pronovost AD, Baumgarten A, Hsiung GD. Sensitive chemiluminescent enzyme-linked immunosorbent assay or quantification of human immunoglobulin G and detection of herpes simplex virus. *J Clin Microbiol* 1981;13:97–101.
52. Yolken RH, Stopa PJ. Comparison of seven enzyme immunoassay systems for measurement of cytomegalovirus. *J Clin Microbiol* 1980;11:546–51.
53. Rubenstein AS, Miller MF. Comparison of an enzyme immunoassay with electron microscopic procedures for detecting rotavirus. *J Clin Microbiol* 1982;15:938–44.
54. Brandt CD, Kim HW, Rodriguez WJ, et al. Comparison of direct electron microscopy, immune electron microscopy, and rotavirus enzyme-linked immunosorbent assay for detection of gastroenteritis viruses in children. *J Clin Microbiol* 1981;13:976–81.
55. Yolken RH, Stopa PJ. Enzyme-linked fluorescence assay: ultrasensitive and solid-phase assay for detection of human rotavirus. *J Clin Microbiol* 1979;10:317–21.
56. Johansson ME, Uhnoo I, Kidd AH, Madeley CR, Wadell G. Direct identification of enteric adenovirus, a candidate new serotype, associated with gastroenteritis. *J Clin Microbiol* 1980;12:95–100.
57. Mushawar IK, Dienstag JL, Polesky HF, McGrath LC, Decker RH, Overby LR. Interpretation of various serological profiles of hepatitis B virus infection. *Am J Clin Pathol* 1981;76:773–7.
58. Wolters G, Kuijpers L, Kacaki J, Schuurs A. Solid phase enzyme-immunoassay for detection of hepatitis B surface antigen. *J Clin Pathol* 1976;29:873–9.
59. van Ulsen J, Dumas AM, Wagenvoort JH, van Zuuren A, van Joost T, Stolz E. Evaluation of an enzyme immunoassay for detection of herpes simplex virus antigen in genital lesions. *Eur J Clin Microbiol* 1987;6:410–3.
60. Berg RA, Rennard SI, Murphy BR, Yolken RH, Dolin R, Strauss SW. New enzyme immunoassays for measurement of influenza A/Victoria/3/75 virus in nasal washes. *Lancet* 1980;ii: 851–3.

61. Chao RK, Fishaut M, Schwartzman JD, McIntosh K. Detection of respiratory syncytial virus in nasal secretions from infants by enzyme-linked immunosorbent assay. *J Infect Dis* 1979;139:483–6.
62. Harmon MW, Pawlik KM. Enzyme immunoassay for direct detection of influenza type A and adenovirus antigens in clinical specimens. *J Clin Microbiol* 1982;15:5–11.
63. Harmon MW, Russo LL, Wilson SZ. Sensitive enzyme immunoassay with β-D-galactosidase-Fab conjugate for detection of type A influenza virus antigen in clinical specimens. *J Clin Microbiol* 1983;17:305–11.
64. Hendry RM, McIntosh K. Enzyme-linked immunosorbent assay for detection of respiratory syncytial virus infection: development and description. *J Clin Microbiol* 1982;16:324–8.
65. McIntosh K, Hendry M, Fahnestock ML, Pierik LY. Enzyme-linked immunosorbent assay for detection of respiratory syncytial virus infection: application to clinical samples. *J Clin Microbiol* 1982;16:329–33.
66. Guesdon JL, Ternynck T, Avrameas S. The use of avidin-biotin interaction immunoenzymatic techniques. *J Histochem Cytochem* 1979;27:1131–9.
67. Nerurkar LS, Jacob AJ, Madden DL, Sever JL. Detection of genital herpes simplex infection with a tissue culture–FA technique using biotin-avidin. *J Clin Microbiol* 1983;17:149–54.
68. Forghani B. Radioimmunoassay. In: Lennette EH, Schmidt NJ, eds. *Diagnostic procedures for viral, rickettsial and chlamydial infections*. Washington, D.C.: American Public Health Association, 1979:171–89.
69. Halonen P, Meurman O. Radioimmunoassay in diagnostic virology. In: Howard CR, ed. *New developments in practical virology*. New York: Alan R. Liss, 1982:83–124.
70. Purcell RH, Wong DC, Moritsugu Y, Dienstag JL, Routenberg JA, Boggs JD. A microtiter solid-phase radioimmunoassay for hepatitis A antigen and antibody. *J Immunol* 1976;116: 349–56.
71. Ballard TL, Roe MH, Wheeler RC, Todd JK, Glode MP. Comparison of three latex agglutination kits and counter immunoelectrophoresis for the detection of bacterial antigens in a pediatric population. *Pediatr Infect Dis J* 1987;6:630–4.
72. Kaldor J, Asznowicz R, Dwyer B. Serotyping of *Streptococcus pneumoniae* by latex agglutination. *Pathology* 1988;20:45–7.
73. Santha M, Burg K, Rasko I, Stipkovits L. A species-specific DNA probe for the detection of *Mycoplasma gallesepticum*. *Infect Immun* 1987;55:2857–9.
74. Prey MU, Lorelle CA, Taff TA, et al. Evaluation of three commercially available rotavirus detection methods for neonatal specimens. *Am J Clin Pathol* 1988;89:675–8.
75. Miotti PG, Eiden J, Yolken RH. Comparative efficiency of commercial immunoassays for the diagnosis of rotavirus gastroenteritis during the course of infection. *J Clin Microbiol* 1985;22:693–8.
76. Miotti PG, Viscidi RP, Eiden J, Cerny E, Yolken RH. Centrifugation augmented solid phase immunoassay (CASPIA): a practical and sensitive assay for the rapid diagnosis of infectious diseases. *J Infect Dis* 1986;154:301–8.
77. Viscidi RP, Connelly CJ, Yolken RH. Novel chemical method for the preparation of nucleic acids for non-isotopic hybridization. *J Clin Microbiol* 1986;23:311–7.
78. Viscidi RP, O'Meara C, Farzadegan H, Yolken R. Monoclonal solution hybridization assay for detection of human immunodeficiency virus nucleic acids. *J Clin Microbiol* 1989;27:120–5.
79. Stalhandski P, Pettersson U. Identification of DNA viruses by membrane filter hybridization. *J Clin Microbiol* 1982;15:744–7.
80. Swierkosz EM, Scholl DR, Brown JL, Jolleck JD, Gleaves CA. Improved DNA hybridization method for detection of acyclovir-resistant herpes simplex virus. *Antimicrob Agents Chemother* 1987;31:1465–9.
81. Sauerbrei A, Wutgler P, Farber I, Brechacek B, Swoboda R, Macheleidt S. Comparative detection of herpesviruses in tissue specimens by *in situ* hybridization and immunofluorescence. *Acta Virol (Praha)* 1986;30:213–9.
82. Schuster V, Matz B, Wiegand H, Polack A, Corsten B, Neumann-Haefelin D. Nucleic acid hybridization for detection of herpes viruses in clinical specimens. *J Med Virol* 1986;19:277–86.
83. Brandsma J, Miller G. Nucleic acid spot hybridization: rapid quantitative screening of lymphoid cell lines for Epstein-Barr viral DNA. *Proc Natl Acad. Sci. USA* 1980;77:6851–5.
84. Berninger M, Hammer M, Hoyer B, Gerin JL. An assay for the detection of the DNA genome of hepatitis B virus in serum. *J Med Virol* 1982;9:57–68.
85. Urdea MS, Running JA, Horn T, Clyne J, Ku LL, Warner BD. A novel method for the rapid detection of specific nucleotide sequences in crude biological samples without blotting or radioactivity; application to the analysis of hepatitis B virus in human serum. *Gene* 1987;61:253–64.
86. Chou S, Merigan TC. Rapid detection and quantitation of human cytomegalovirus in urine via DNA hybridization. *N Engl J Med* 1983;308:921–5.
87. Virtanen M, Laaksonen M, Soderlund H, Palva A, Halonen P, Marjut R. Novel test for rapid viral diagnosis: detection of adenovirus in nasopharyngeal mucus aspirates by means of nucleic-acid sandwich hybridization. *Lancet* 1983;1:381–3.
88. Neumann R, Genersch E, Eggers HJ. Detection of adenovirus nucleic acid sequences in human tonsils in the absence of infectious virus. *Virus Res* 1987;7:93–7.
89. Eiden JJ, Sato S, Yolken RH. Specificity of dot

hybridization in assay in the presence of rRNA for detection of rotaviruse in clinical specimens. *J Clin Microbiol* 1987;25:1809–11.
90. Wilbur DC, Reichman RC, Stoler MH. Detection of infection by human papillomavirus in genital condylomata. A comparison study using immunocytochemistry and in situ nucleic acid hybridization. *Am J Clin Pathol* 1988;4:505–10.
91. Ermine A, Tordo N, Tsiang H. Rapid diagnosis of rabies infection by means of a dot hybridization assay. *Mol Cell Probes* 1988;2:75–82.
92. Liang W, Johnson JP. Rapid plasmid insert amplification with polymerase chain reaction. *Nucleic Acids Res* 1988;16:3579.
93. Yolken RH, Coutlee F, Viscidi RP. New prospects for the diagnosis of viral infections. *Yale J Biol Med* 1989;62:131–139.
94. Tenser RB, Jones JC, Ressel SJ, Fralish FA. Thymidine plaque autoradiography of thymidine kinase-positive and thymidine kinase-negative herpesviruses. *J Clin Microbiol* 1983; 17:122–7.
95. Schmidt NJ. Cell culture technics for diagnostic virology. In: Lennette EH, Schmidt NJ, eds. *Diagnostic procedures for viral, rickettsial and chlamydial infections*. 5th ed. Washington, D.C.: American Public Health Association, 1979;65–139.
96. Meguro H, Bryant JD, Torrence AE, Wright PF. Canine kidney cell line for isolation of respiratory viruses. *J Clin Microbiol.* 1979;9: 175–9.
97. Schmidt NJ, Ota M, Gallo D, Fox VL. Monoclonal antibodies for rapid, stain-specific identification of influenza virus isolates. *J Clin Microbiol* 1982;16:763–5.
98. Pereira L, Dondero DV, Gallo D, Devlin V, Woodie JD. Serological analysis of herpes simplex virus types 1 and 2 with monoclonal antibodies. *Infect Immun* 1982;35:363–7.
99. Henchal EA, Gentry MK, McCown JM, Brandt WE. Dengue virus-specific and flavivirus group determinants identified with monoclonal antibodies by indirect immunofluorescence. *Am J Trop Med Hyg* 1982;31:830–6.
100. Hers JEP, van der Kuip L, Masurel N. Rapid diagnosis of respiratory virus infection in infected tissue cultures. *Ann NY Acad Sci* 1971;177:70–7.
101. Doane FW. Virus morphology as an aid for rapid diagnosis. *Yale J Biol Med* 1980;53: 19–25.
102. Melnick JL, Wenner HA, Phillips CA. Enteroviruses. In: Lennette EH, Schmidt NJ, eds. *Diagnostic procedures for viral, rickettsial and chlamydial infections*. 5th ed. Washington, D.C.: American Public Health Association, 1979:471–534.
103. Schmidt NJ, Lennette EH, Ho HH. An apparently new enterovirus isolated from patients with disease of the central nervous system. *J Infect Dis* 1974;129:304–9.
104. Dowdle WR, Kendal AP, Noble GR. Influenza viruses. In: Lennette EH, Schmidt NJ, eds. *Diagnostic procedures for viral, rickettsial and chlamydial infections*. 5th ed. Washington, D.C.: American Public Health Association, 1979:585–609.
105. Schmidt NJ, Ho HH, Dondero ME. Clostridium difficile toxins as a confounding factor in enterovirus isolation. *J Clin Microbiol* 1980;12:796–8.
106. Chen RR. In situ detection of mycoplasma contamination in cell cultures by fluorescent Hoechst 33258 stain. *Exp Cell Res* 1977; 104:255–62.
107. Kapsenberger JG, Ras A, Korte J. Improvement of enterovirus neutralization by treatment with sodium deoxycholate or chloroform. *Intervirology* 1979;12:329–34.
108. Mandel B. Interaction of viruses with neutralizing antibodies. In: Frankel-Conrat H, Wagner RR, eds. *Comprehensive virology, vol. 15, virus-host interactions. Immunity to viruses.* New York: Plenum Press. 1979:37–121.
109. Fazekas de St. Groth S, Scheidegger D. Production of monoclonal antibodies: strategy and tactics. *J Immunol Methods* 1980;35:1–21.
110. Goding JW. Antibody production by hybridomas. *J Immunol Methods*. 1980;39:285–308.
111. Kennett RH, McKearn TJ, Bechtol KB, eds. *Monoclonal antibodies hybridomas: a new dimension in biological analyses*. New York: Plenum Press, 1980.
112. Pereira L, Hoffman M, Gallo D, Cremer N. Monoclonal antibodies to human cytomegalovirus: three surface membrane proteins with unique immunological and electrophoretic properties specify cross-reactive determinants. *Infect Immun* 1982;36:924–32.
113. Palese P, Roizman B, eds. Genetic variation of viruses. *Ann NY Acad Sci* 1980;354.
114. Buckman TG, Simpson T, Nosal D, Roizman B, Nahmias AJ. The structure of herpes simplex virus DNA and its application to molecular epidemiology. *Ann NY Acad Sci* 1980;354:29–90.
115. Huang ES, Huong SM, Tegtmeier GE, Alford C. Cytomegalovirus: genetic variation of viral genomes. *Ann NY Acad Sci* 1980;354:332–46.
116. Mishra L, Dahner DE, Wellinghoff WJ, Gelb LD. Physical maps of varicella-zoster virus DNA derived with 11 restriction enzymes. *J Virol* 1984;50:615–8.
117. Nakajima S, Nakajima K, Takeuchi Y, Sugiura A. Influenza surveillance based on oligonucleotide mapping of RNA of HINI viruses present in Japan, 1978–1979. *J Infect Dis* 1980;142:492–502.
118. Young JF, Palese P. Evolution of human influenza A viruses in nature: recombination contributes to genetic variation of HINI strains. *Proc Natl Acad Sci USA* 1979;76:6547–51.
119. Minor PH. Comparative biochemical studies of type 3 poliovirus. *J Virol* 1980;34:73–84.
120. Nottay BK, Kew OM, Hatch MH, Heyward

JT, Obijeski JF. Molecular variation of type 1 vaccine-related and wild polioviruses during replication in humans. *Virology* 1981;108: 405–23.

121. Clewey JP, Bishop DHL. Oligonucleotide fingerprinting of viral genomes. In: Howard CR, ed. *New developments in practical virology.* New York: Alan R. Liss, 1982;231–77.
122. Kalica AR, Wyatt RG, Kapikian AZ. Detection of differences among human and animal rotaviruses using analysis of viral RNA. *J Am Vet Med Assoc* 1978;173:531–7.
123. Rodger SM, Bishop RF, Birch C, McLean B, Holmes IH. Molecular epidemiology of human rotaviruses in Melbourne, Australia, from 1973 to 1979, as determined by electrophoresis of genome ribonucleic acid. *J Clin Microbiol* 1981;13:272–8.
124. Eiden J, Vonderfecht S, Theil K, Torres-Medina A, Yolken RH. Antigenically distinct rotaviruses: genetic and antigenic relatedness of human and animal strains. *J Infect Dis* 1986;154:972–82.
125. Dyall-Smith ML, Holmes IH. Genecoding assignments of rotavirus double-stranded RNA segments 10 and 11. *J Virol* 1981;38:1099–103.
126. Kalica AR, Greenberg HB, Wyatt RG, et al. Genes of human (strain W[a]) and bovine (strain UK) rotaviruses that code for neutralization and subgroup antigens. *Virology* 1981;112: 385–90.
127. Cremer NE, Hagens SJ, Cossen C. Comparison of the hemagglutination inhibition test and an indirect fluorescent-antibody test for detection of antibody to rubella virus in human sera. *J Clin Microbiol* 1980;11:746–7.
128. Cabau N, Crainic R, Duros C, et al. Freeze-dried erythrocytes for an indirect hemagglutination test for detection of cytomegalovirus antibodies. *J Clin Microbiol* 1981;13:1026–30.
129. Yeager AS. Improved indirect hemagglutination tests for cytomegalovirus using human O erythrocytes in lysine. *J Clin Microbiol* 1979;10:64–8.
130. Norrby E, Grandien M, Orvell C. New tests for characterization of mumps virus antibodies: haemolysis-inhibition, single radial immunodiffusion with immobilized virions and mixed hemadsorption. *J Clin Microbiol* 1977;5:346–52.
131. Williams MS, Mayner RE, Daniel NJ, et al. New developments in the measurement of the hemagglutinin content of influenza virus vaccines by single-radial-immunodiffusion. *J Biol Stand* 1980;8:289–96.
132. Schild GC, Wood JM, Minor PH, Dandawate CN, Magrath DI. Immunoassay of poliovirus antigens by single-radial-diffusion: development and characteristics of a sensitive autoradiographic zone size enhancement (ZE) technique. *J Gen Virol* 1980;51:157–70.
133. Neumann PW, Weber JM. Single radial hemolysis test for rubella immunity and recent infection. *J Clin Microbiol* 1983;17:28–34.
134. Duca M, Duca E, Ionescu T, Abdalla H. Single radial haemolysis for the assay of antibodies to some haemagglutinating arboviruses. *Bull WHO* 1979;57:937–42.
135. Vaananen P. The use of red cells with fused Semliki Forest virus envelope proteins in antibody determinations by hemolysis in gel. *J Virol Methods* 1982;4:117–26.
136. Wesslen L. Hemolysis-in-gel (HIG) test for antibodies to influenza A, measles and mumps using liquid nitrogen freezed erythrocytes coupled with the respective viral antigens. *J Immunol Methods* 1978;24:1–8.
137. Lennette ET. Applications of immune adherence hemagglutination assay to diagnostic serology. In: Lennett D, Spector S, Thompson K, eds. *Diagnosis of viral infections: the role of the clinical laboratory.* Baltimore: University Park Pess, 1979;73–83.
138. Inouye S, Matsuno S, Hasegawa A, Miyamura K, Kono R, Rosen L. Serotyping of dengue viruses by an immune adherence hemagglutination test. *Am J Trop Med Hyg* 1980;29:1389–93.
139. Inouye S, Matsuno S, Kono R. Differences in antibody reactivity between complement fixation and immune adherence hemagglutination tests with virus antigens. *J Clin Microbiol* 1981;14:241–6.
140. Forghani B, Cremer NE, Johnson KP, Fein G, Likosky WH. Comprehensive viral immunology of multiple sclerosis. III. Analysis of CSF antibodies by radioimmunoassay. *Arch Neurol* 1980;37:616–9.
141. Forghani B, Schmidt NJ, Lennette EH. Radioimmunoassay of measles virus antigen and antibody in SSPE brain tissue. *Proc Soc Exp Biol Med* 1978;157:268–72.
142. Smith KO, Gehle WD, Saford BA. Evidence for chronic viral infections in human arteries. *Proc Soc Exp Biol Med* 1974;147:357–60.
143. Cremer NE, Cossen CK, Hanson CV, Shell GR. Evaluation and reporting of enzyme immunoassay determinations of antibody to herpes simplex virus in sera and cerebrospinal fluid. *J Clin Microbiol* 1982;15:815–23.
144. Richardson LS, Yolken RH, Belshe RB, Camargo E, Kim HW, Chanock RM. Enzyme-linked immunosorbent assay for measurement of serological response to respiratory syncytial virus infection. *Infect Immun* 1978;20:660–4.
145. Sever JL, Madden DL, eds. Symposium, enzyme-linked immunosorbent assay (ELISA) for infectious agents. National Institutes of Health, Bethesda, Md., 9–10 Sept 1976. *J Infect Dis* 1977;136(suppl):257–340.
146. Murphy BR, Phelan MA, Nelson DL, et al. Hemagglutinin-specific enzyme-linked immunosorbent assay for antibodies to influenza A and B viruses. *J Clin Microbiol* 1981;13: 554–60.
147. Vestergaard BF, Grauballe PC. Isolation of the major herpes simplex virus type (HSV-I)-specific glycoprotein by hydroxylapatite chromatography and its use in enzyme-linked

immunosorbent assay for titration of human HSV-I-specific antibodies. *J Clin Microbiol* 1979;10:772–7.
148. Castellano GA, Madden DL, Hazzard GT, et al. Evaluation of commercially available diagnostic test kits for rubella. *J Infect Dis* 1981;143:578–84.
149. Forghani B, Schmidt NJ. Antigen requirements, sensitivity, and specificity of enzyme immunoassays for measles and rubella viral antibodies. *J Clin Microbiol* 1979;9:657–64.
150. Shekarchi IC, Sever JL, Tzan N, Ley A, Ward LC, Madden D. Comparison of hemagglutination inhibition test and enzyme-linked immunosorbent assay for detecting antibody to rubella virus. *J Clin Microbiol* 1981;13:850–4.
151. deSavigny D, Voller A. The communication of ELISA data from laboratory to clinician. *J Immunoassay* 1980;1:105–28.
152. Sever JL, Tzan NR, Shekarchi IC, Madden DL. Rapid latex agglutination test for rubella antibody. *J Clin Microbiol* 1983;17:52–4.
153. Meegan JM, Evans B, Horstmann DM. Comparison of the latex agglutination test with the hemagglutination inhibition test, enzyme-linked immunosorbent assay, and neutralization test for detection of antibodies to rubella virus. *J Clin Microbiol* 1982;16:644–9.
154. Chantler S, Diment JA. Current status of specific IgM antibody assays. In: Voller A, Bartlett A, Bidwell D, eds. *Immunoassays for the 80's*. Baltimore: University Park Press, 1981;417–30.
155. Schmidt NJ. Application of class-specific antibody assays to viral serodiagnosis. *Clin Immunol Newsletter* 1980;1:1–5.
156. Shirodaira PV, Fraser KB, Stanford F. Secondary fluorescent staining of virus antigens by rheumatoid factor and fluorescein-conjugated anti-IgM. *Ann Rheum Dis* 1973;32:53–7.
157. Vejtorp M. The interference of IgM rheumatoid factor in enzyme-linked immunosorbent assays of rubella IgM and IgG antibodies. *J Virol Methods* 1980;1:1–9.
158. Beck OE. Distribution of virus antibody activity among human IgG subclasses. *Clin Exp Immunol*. 1981;43:626–32.
159. Duermeyer W, Wieland F, van der Veen J. A new principle for the detection of specific IgM antibodies applied in an ELISA for hepatitis A. *J Med Virol* 1979;4:25–32.
160. Gerlich WH, Luer W. Selective detection of IgM antibody against core antigen of the hepatitis B virus by a modified enzyme immune assay. *J Med Virol* 1979;4:227–38.
161. Roggendorf M, Frosner GG, Deinhardt F, and Scheid R. Comparison of solid phase test systems for demonstrating antibodies against hepatitis A virus (anti-HAV) of the IgM class. *J Med Virol* 1980;5:47–62.
162. Schmidtz H. Detection of immunoglobulin M antibody to Epstein-Barr virus by use of an enzyme-labeled antigen. *J Clin Microbiol* 1982;16:361–6.
163. Schmitz H, von Deimling U, Flehmig B. Detection of IgM antibodies to cytomegalovirus (CMV) using an enzyme-labeled antigen (EIA). *J Gen Virol* 1980;50:59–68.
164. van Loon AM, Heessen FWA, van der Logt JTM, van der Veen J. Direct enzyme-linked immunosorbent assay that uses peroxidase-labeled antigen for determination of immunoglobulin M antibody to cytomegalovirus. *J Clin Microbiol* 1981;13:416–22.
165. Krech U, Wilhelm JA. A solid-phase immunosorbent technique for the rapid detection of rubella IgM by haemagglutination inhibition. *J Gen Virol* 1979;44:281–6.
166. Sexton SA, Hodgson J, Morgan-Capner P. The detection of rubella-specific IgM by an immunosorbent assay with solid-phase attachment of red cells (SPARC). *J Hyg (Camb)* 1982;88:453–61.
167. Denoyel GA, Gaspar A, Peyramond D. A solid-phase reverse immunosorbent test (SPRIST) for the demonstration of specific-mumps virus IgM-class antibody *Arch Virol* 1982;71:349–52.
168. van der Logt JTM, Heessen FWA, van Loon AM, van der Veen J. Hamadsorption immunosorbent technique for determination of mumps immunoglobulin M antibody. *J Clin Microbiol* 1982;15:82–6.
169. Forghani B, Myoraku CK, Schmidt NJ. Production of monoclonal antibodies to human IgM for assay of viral IgM antibodies. *J Virol Methods* 1982;5:317–27.
170. Arvin AM, Koropchak CM. Immunoglobulins M and G to varicella-zoster measured by solid-phase radioimmunoassays: antibody responses to varicella and herpes zoster infections. *J Clin Microbiol* 1980;12:367–74.
171. Joncas JH, Granger-Julien M, Gervais F. Improved Epstein-Barr virus immunoglobulin M antibody test. *J Clin Microbiol* 1975;1:192–5.
172. Schmitz H, Kampa D, Doerr HW, et al. IgM antibodies to cytomegalovirus during pregnancy. *Arch Virol* 1977;53:177–84.
173. Harcourt GC, Best JM, Banatvala JE. Rubella-specific serum and nasopharyngeal antibodies in volunteers with naturally acquired and vaccine-induced immunity after intranasal challenge. *J Infect Dis* 1980;142:145–55.
174. Ogra PL, Karzon DT, Righthand F, MacGilliray M. Immunization with live and inactivated poliovaccine and natural infections. *N Engl J Med* 1986;279:893–900.
175. Halonen P, Bennich H, Torfason E, et al. Solid-phase radioimmunoassay of serum immunoglobulin A antibodies to respiratory syncytial virus and adenovirus. *J Clin Microbiol* 1979;10:192–7.
176. Halonen P, Meurman O, Matikainen M. IgA antibody response in acute rubella determined by solid-phase radioimmunoassay. *J Hyg (Lond)* 1979;83:69–75.
177. Henle G, Henle W. Epstein-Barr virus-specific IgA serum antibodies as an outstanding feature of nasopharyngeal carcinoma. *Int J Cancer* 1976;17:1–7.

178. Dayton DH, Small PA, Chanock RM, Kaufman HE, Tomasi TB Jr, eds. *The secretory immunologic system*. Washington, D.C.: U.S. Department of Health, Education and Welfare, Public Health Services, National Institutes of Health, 1971.
179. Welliver RC, Ogra PL. Respiratory syncytial virus-specific IgE antibody responses at the mucosal surface: predictive value for recurrent wheezing and suppression by ribavirin therapy. *Adv Exp Med Biol* 1987;216B:1701–8.
180. Nielson SL, Srensen I, Andersen HK. Kinetics of specific immunoglobulins M, E, A, and G in congenital, primary, and secondary cytomegalovirus infection studied by antibody-capture enzyme-linked immunosorbent assay. *J Clin Microbiol* 1988;26:654–61.
181. Coleman RM, Williams SC, Black CM, Nahmias AJ, Phillips DJ, Reimer CB. IgG subclass antibodies to herpes simplex virus. *J Infect Dis* 1985;151:929–36.
182. Sundqvist V-A, Linde A, Wahren B. Virus-specific immunoglobulin G subclasses in herpes simplex and varicella-zoster virus infections. *J Clin Microbiol* 1984;20:94–8.
183. Linde A, Anderson J, Lundgren G, Wahren B. Subclass reactivity to Epstein-Barr virus capsid antigen and reactivated EBV infections. *J Med Virol* 1987;21:109–21.
184. Asano Y, Hiroishi Y, Itakura N, et al. Immunoglobulin subclass antibodies to varicella-zoster virus. *Pediatrics* 1987;80:933–6.
185. Julkunen I, Hovi T, Seppala I, Makela O. Immunoglobulin G subclass antibody responses in influenza A and parainfluenza type 1 virus infections. *Clin Exp Immunol* 1985;60:130–8.
186. Skvaril F. IgG subclasses in viral infections. *Monogr Allergy* 1986;19:134–43.
187. Doerr HW, Rentschler M, Scheifler G. Serologic detection of active infections with human herpes viruses (CMV, EBV, HSV, VZV): diagnostic potential of IgA class and IgG subclass-specific antibodies. *Infection* 1987;15:93–8.
188. Hanson CV. Inactivation of viruses for use as vaccines and immunodiagnostic reagent. In: de la Maza LM, ed. *Medical virology*. 2nd ed. New York: Elsevier Biomedical, 1983:45–79.

*Antiviral Agents and Viral Diseases of Man, 3rd Edition,* edited by G. J. Galasso, R. J. Whitley, and T. C. Merigan, Raven Press, Ltd., New York © 1990.

# 6

# Major Ocular Viral Infections

Deborah Pavan-Langston

*Eye Research Institute, Massachusetts Eye and Ear Infirmary, and Department of Ophthalmology, Harvard Medical School, Boston, Massachusetts 02114*



The list of viruses that may affect the anterior segment of the eye is protean, including such RNA viruses as enterovirus, rubella, influenza, and mumps and such DNA viruses as adenovirus, herpes simplex (HSV), varicella zoster (VZV), and Epstein-Barr virus (EBV). The RNA organisms generally cause a mild to moderate self-limited punctate keratitis and watery follicular conjunctivitis for which therapy is purely supportive (1). Congenital rubella may also involve the entire eye (2), causing severe keratitis, glaucoma, and chorioretinitis; it is discussed elsewhere in this book.

Many, but not all, of the organisms that most seriously affect the eyes anteriorly or posteriorly are amenable to therapy. These are the DNA viruses HSV, VZV, cytomegalovirus (CMV), EBV, and adenovirus, and the RNA virus of acute hemorrhagic conjuctivitis (AHC) and the human immunodeficiency (HIV) virus. Of less concern, at least in the postsmallpox era, are the pox viruses. The ocular conditions caused by infection with the above named DNA viruses and the RNA agents of AHC and AIDS are the primary focus of discussion in this chapter.

## ANTIVIRAL DRUGS

Five antiviral agents have proven efficacy for ocular viral infections: idoxuridine (IDU), vidarabine (ara-A), trifluridine ($F_3T$), acyclovir (ACV), and ganciclovir (DHPG). IDU, $F_3T$, and ara-A are commercially available (Table 1) for topical therapy of herpes simplex keratitis. Ara-A and ACV also are used systemically for therapy of herpetic encephalitis, mucocutaneous herpes, and neonatal herpes (see Chapter 8) (3–6). ACV may be used topically for herpes simplex keratitis and systemically for herpes zoster ophthalmicus but is not yet FDA approved for either use (7–9). Ganciclovir (Cytovene) is currently under investigation for efficacy in CMV retinitis (10–12). A sixth drug, azidothymidine (AZT) (Zidovudine) is also under study for systemic treatment of acquired immune deficiency syndrome (AIDS), but to date only one study on ocular effects has been reported (13–18).

IDU, $F_3T$, and ara-A are activated by either cellular or viral thymidine kinases. Although this makes them extremely effective as antiviral agents, it also adds to their toxicity in that they may be activated, although to a lesser extent, in noninfected cells. IDU and $F_3T$ work by means of incorporation as thymidine analogs into viral DNA and by viral enzyme inhibition. Ara-A has been reported to inhibit DNA polymerase and to be incorporated to a small extent into viral and host DNA (3–6,19,20).

The recommended frequency of use and concentration in eyes with active herpes simplex infection is indicated in Table 1. The overall cure rate for IDU is 76%; ara-A, $F_3T$, and ACV each have levels of efficacy approximating 90–95%, and all appear more effective therapeutically than IDU when concomitant steroids are in use (4–6,21–24). Adverse side effects include lacrimal punctal occlusion, superficial punctate keratitis (SPK), follicular conjunctivitis, and true allergic blepharodermatitis. All but ACV interfere to some extent with corneal wound healing. Dosages for ACV in herpes zoster and for DHPG in CMV retinitis are discussed in their respective sections on clinical disease.

ACV is a second-generation antiviral agent that, like the European drugs bromovinyldeoxyuridine (BVDU) and ethyldeoxyuridine (EDU), is specifically activated by herpesvirus-induced thymidine kinase, thereby effectively bypassing all noninfected normal cells (25,26). Viral thymidine kinase initiates phosphorylation of the drug; subsequently, host cell kinases lead to production of the active triphosphate form. These triphosphate derivatives are inhibitory for herpetic DNA polymerase more than for cellular polymerase, thus conferring specificity for virus. ACV has been found to be essentially a nontoxic drug both topically and systemically (7–9,21,23,27). BVDU and EDU are not under investigation in the United States. Antiviral drugs are discussed in greater detail in other chapters of this volume.

DHPG has a 30-fold greater anti-CMV activity than ACV. It is a purine analog differing from ACV only in the addition of a 3′ methoxyl group to the acyclic side chain. The triphosphate metabolite of DHPG com-

**TABLE 1.** *Commercially available ocular herpes antiviral drugs*

| Drug (commercial name) | Concentration (%) | Usual dosage in acute infection |
|---|---|---|
| IDU ointment (Stoxil) | 0.5 | 5 times daily for 14 days |
| IDU drops (Stoxil, Herplex, Dendrid) | 0.1 | Hourly by day, every 2 hr by night for 14 days |
| Ara-A ointment (Vira A) | 3.0 | 5 times daily for 14–21 days |
| $F_3T$ drops (Viroptic) | 1.0 | Every 1–2 hr by day (total of 9 drops) for 14 days |

ACV 3% ointment (Zovirax) is available by compassionate plea from Burroughs Wellcome Co., Research Triangle Park, NC. Apply 5 times daily for 14–21 days.

petitively inhibits viral DNA polymerase in a manner similar to the action of ACV. Unfortunately, the drug is more toxic to bone marrow than is ACV. Currently, it is the only drug with activity against CMV in current clinical use (10–13).

The nucleoside analog AZT (Zidovudine, Retrovir) inhibits HIV infectivity *in vitro*. The ocular pharmacodynamics of this drug are poorly understood, but it is known to cross the blood-brain barrier with beneficial effects in some patients with AIDS-associated neurological disease (15). It may also be effective in AIDS-related iridocyclitis (14). Foscarnet sodium, a newer investigational drug, appears to hold promise similar to that of AZT. It is discussed with other antivirals under CMV retinitis (28).

Another antiviral of some interest is interferon. Endogenous interferon production has proven ineffective, and human leukocyte interferon produced in tissue culture is expensive and impractical (29). Of potential use, however, is cloned human leukocyte interferon obtained by recombinant DNA technology in *Escherichia coli*. Smolin et al. (30) reported that both natural and *E. coli*–derived interferon-α applied topically at $0.5 \times 10^6$ U/day were equally and significantly effective in therapy of experimental herpetic keratitis in rabbits. Additionally, $F_3T$ or ACV has been combined with human interferon-α to treat herpetic keratitis successfully, the combined therapy being better than either agent alone (31).

Adenoviral keratitis has also been found to be responsive to topical interferon therapy. Romano et al. (32) reported that topical leukocyte interferon reduced the duration of disease from an average of 27 to 6.5 days and reduced the incidence of keratitis to 10% from 57% compared to controls. Similar favorable results using human leukocyte interferon in adenoviral epidemic keratoconjunctivitis have been reported by Ikic et al. (33).

Although topical interferon is not yet available commercially, the promise of recombinant DNA technology makes this "natural drug" one of great interest for future studies in a variety of ocular viral diseases.

## CORTICOSTEROID THERAPY: PROS AND CONS

Corticosteroids adversely affect immunologically competent lymphocytes and inhibit white-cell amoeboid migration and release of cellular digestive enzymes (34,35). The administration of topical or systemic steroids results in the local inhibition of antibody-forming lymphocytes in the cornea and uveal tract. As there is no effect on the number of lymphocytes in the draining lymph nodes or on circulating antibody response, however, the host is still capable of immune reaction once the inflammation-inhibiting steroids are removed (36). High titers of corneal viral antigen gain access to deeper tissues and subsequently generate an antibody complex reaction (37).

Corticosteroids commonly used in inflammatory ocular disease include topical dexamethasone, prednisolone, and fluoromethalone. These steroids also inhibit the formation of both mucopolysaccharides and collagen, substances critical to the integrity of the corneal structure. One alternative to corticosteroids, medroxyprogesterone acetate (Provera), results in the suppression of collagenase, a destructive enzyme often released in corneal inflammatory states (38). The use of this medication was correlated clinically and histologically (in an experimental model) with a marked reduction in white cell infiltrate and stromal neovascularization without interference with wound healing. Infectious epithelial disease was enhanced but could be counteracted by concomitant antiviral therapy. Medroxyprogesterone acetate at 1% was felt to have an antiinflammatory efficacy equivalent to 0.12% prednisolone. It appears to be a safer steroid for use in any case threatened by corneal thinning or melting.

In favor of steroid use in the eye, then, are significant inhibition of (a) cellular infiltration, (b) release of toxic hydrolytic enzymes, (c) scar tissue formation, and (d) neovascularization. On the negative side are (a) suppression of the normal inflammatory response allowing spread of potentially superficial viral infection, (b) possible corneal addiction to steroids through build-up of leukocyte-attracting antigen, the reaction to which must be constantly suppressed, (c) enhancing the risk of opportunistic bacterial or fungal infection through suppression of the immune defense system, (d) inhibition of collagen synthesis in healing ulcers, and (e) the well-known side effects of steroid glaucoma and cataract.

Once a patient is committed to topical steroid therapy, it may be difficult to withdraw treatment. Abrupt cessation may result in rebound inflammation. A useful rule of thumb in tapering therapy is never to reduce the dosage more than one-half the current level. The lower the dosage, the longer the patient should be maintained at that level, often for several weeks or months.

## DIAGNOSTIC TESTS

Scrapings taken with a sterile platinum spatula from skin lesions, corneal ulcers, or inflamed conjunctiva may greatly assist diagnosis when stained with Giemsa and examined under the microscope. The cellular inflammatory reaction characteristic of viral infection is a monocytic white cell infiltrate. In addition, herpetic infections are characterized by epithelial cells that show ballooning degeneration. For both herpes zoster and simplex, there may be typical eosinophilic viral inclusion bodies of Lipshutz or Cowdry in the nuclei. In severe inflammatory reaction, the monocytic response may be overwhelmed by an acute outpouring of polymorphonuclear leukocytes. In pox infections, epithelial cells often contain diagnostic eosinophilic inclusion bodies of Guanieri in the cytoplasm. Scrapings from eyes infected with adenovirus reveal no viral inclusion bodies in the epithelium but will have a characteristic monocytic cell reaction (1).

Office diagnostic kits are now available for HSV. The Herpchek (DuPont) system is highly specific for HSV types 1 or 2 (HSV-1, HSV-2) of the eye or skin. This immunoassay test does not cross-react with other ocular pathogens, including herpes zoster, and involves only a swabbing of the infected area with a sterile cotton-tip applicator. The applicator is sent to a nearby laboratory or mailed in the accompanying folder; the results are returned to the physician frequently by return mail or by telephone in 4 hr if the laboratory is local. This test is 99% reliable in active infection (39).

Definitive diagnosis is also possible through viral cultures. HSV and vaccinia grow on almost any tissue monolayer such as human embryonic kidney, rabbit kidney, or chick or mouse embryo. Herpes varicella-zoster and adenovirus, however, are more fastidious and require cells of human origin. The recovery rate from an acutely infected herpetic or vaccinia lesion is approximately 70% if antiviral drugs have not been used recently. Adenovirus or zoster are recovered approximately 45% of the time if cultures are taken within 3–4 days of onset of disease. Culture requirements and recovery rates as well as immune diagnostic tests for CMV and AIDS virus are discussed in the pertinent sections in this chapter and elsewhere in this volume.

Primary viral infection may be differentiated from a recurrent infection by evaluation of acute and convalescent sera. A clotted blood sample is drawn during the acute phase, and a second sample 2 to 4 weeks later. Both samples may be sent to a state laboratory or many private or university hospitals with a request for antibody level against the suspected agent. Absence of antibodies in the first sample and their appearance in the second indicate a recent infection (1).

## HERPES SIMPLEX OCULAR DISEASE

With almost 500,000 cases of herpes simplex ophthalmic disease diagnosed yearly in the United States, physicians are justifiably concerned about the appropriate therapy for this often baffling infection and primary infectious cause of corneal blindness in this country (40). To understand the advantages and disadvantages of the many drugs used in treating ocular herpes, it is necessary to understand not only the effects of the drugs themselves but the various forms and pathogenesis of this multifaceted disease (41–44).

### Epidemiology

The epidemiology of ocular herpes simplex is not well understood in comparison to that of extraocular herpes infections. Nonetheless, information from the latter appears applicable to the ocular disease.

Humans are the only natural reservoir of HSV, with sources of infection being children with primary disease, adults with recurrent disease, and healthy asymptomatic carriers of any age. By the age of 5, up to 60% of all children will have been infected with HSV-1, usually through the oral route (45–47). This, however, allows virus access to the trigeminal ganglion, which also feeds the ocular structures. Transmission of the virus is usually by direct oral contact or salivary droplets. Most ocular herpes viral disease appears to be due to recrudescence of latent trigeminal ganglion infection, with subsequent appearance of the virus in the eye rather than, or along with, an eruption of cold sores around the nose or mouth. Recent studies indicate that the cornea itself may also serve as a site of latent virus capable of reactivation (48–53).

In a study on the epidemiologic characteristics of ocular herpes, a review of 141 patients with infectious epithelial keratitis indicated that there was an overall predominance of men in those over 40 years of age. Of 65 patients who suffered more than one episode, 34% had a mean recurrence rate of one or more episodes per year and 68% had a recurrent rate of one or more episodes every 2 years (54). The highest incidence of recurrences occurred during the cold-weather months of November through February and correlated with increased incidence of viral respiratory infections. In another epidemiologic study of ocular HSV infection in 119 patients, the recurrence rates were 24% of patients having a recurrence within 1 year and 33% within 2 years (55). A positive correlation was found between short intervals between past attacks and short intervals between future recurrences. Although the incidence of HSV-1 versus HSV-2 in the eye is not known, the latter is thought to be rare, with the exception of infants contracting ocular herpes during passage through an infected birth canal.

### Clinical Disease

Ocular herpes may be classified into two general groups: primary and recurrent.

#### *Primary Herpes*

Primary disease is an acute keratoconjunctivitis with or without skin involvement in the nonimmune host. It is caused by infectious HSV. Although approximately 60% of all children will have had a primary infection by age 5, only 1–6% of that group will suffer overt clinical disease; the remainder undergo subclinical infection (45,46). All 100% then become viral carriers, with the agent residing in a latent state (48,49,52).

Clinically, overt disease begins 3–9 days after exposure to an infected carrier and usually manifests as intense vesiculitis of the lids, conjunctival follicular disease occasionally with pseudomembranes, and nonsuppurative preauricular adenopathy (Fig. 1). In the immunologically competent host, the vesicular eruption of the skin remains fairly localized and is a self-limited disease that resolves entirely without scarring and often without specific therapy.

Corneal disease following primary HSV infection is frequently atypical. Initially there may be diffuse punctate staining converting within 24 hr to multiple diffuse microdendrites, or there may be serpiginous ulcers without clearcut branching effect covering the entire cornea (Fig. 2).

Specific therapy may be outlined as follows (see Table 1):

(a) If there is no corneal ulceration, prophylactic antiviral ointment should be applied to the eyes three times a day until skin lesions resolve.

(b) If there is corneal ulceration, simple corneal debridement with a sterile cotton-tip applicator after anesthetic drops, followed by antiviral ointment or drops for 14–21 days should be undertaken. The drug is then stopped or tapered over a several-day period.

(c) A Cartella shield or hand restraints may be used with young children.

(d) Topical betadine gel may be applied to badly ulcerated skin, avoiding the eyes; otherwise, no therapy is necessary except warm saline soaks and general good hygiene.

(e) Topical antibiotics should be used twice a day if the cornea is ulcerated.

(f) Cycloplegics (e.g., 1% cyclopentolate) twice a day are indicated if iritis is present (rare in primary disease).

### *Recurrent Herpes*

#### *Latency*

Within the first 1–2 days of primary infection, the virus travels by retrograde axoplasmic flow to the sensory (trigeminal) ganglia, ciliary ganglia, mesencephalic nucleus of the brain stem, and, in some cases, to the sympathetic ganglia where it enters a latent or dormant state (48–50,52,56,57). There is also growing evidence that the cor-

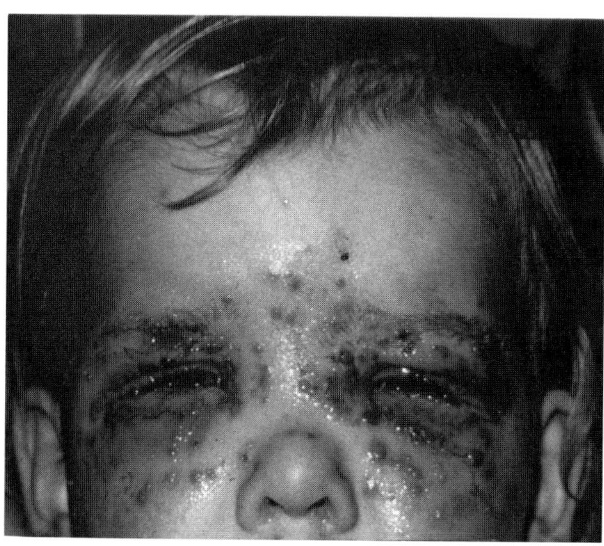

**FIG. 1.** Resolving primary HSV infection of periorbital skin, conjunctiva, and cornea. (From Pavan-Langston, ref. 199, with permission.)

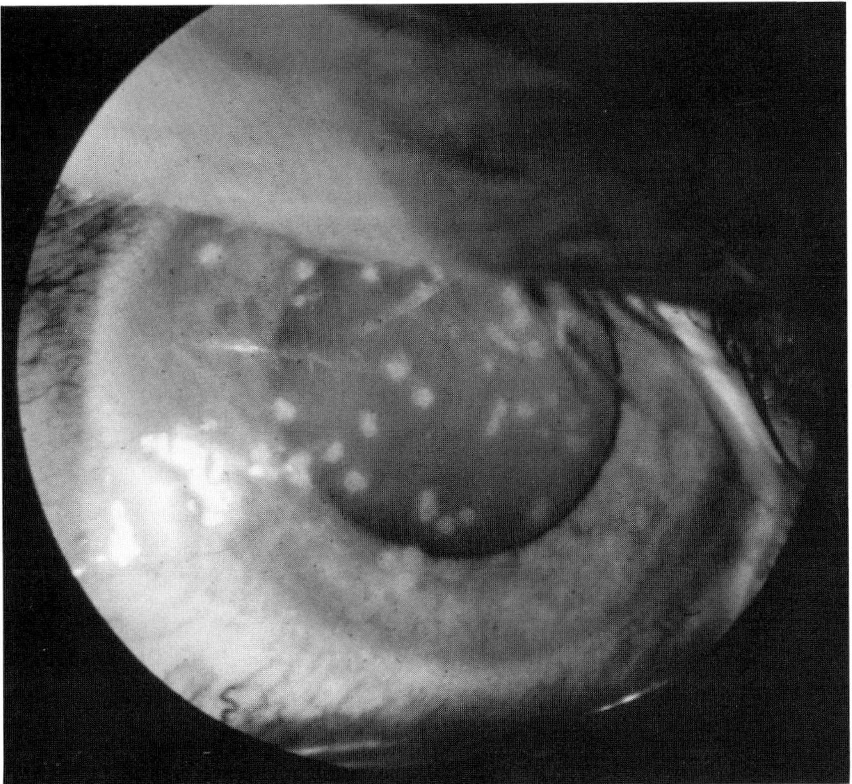

**FIG. 2.** Primary herpes simplex of cornea with diffuse microdendritic ulcers.

nea itself may serve as a nonneuronal site of latency and, like the neuronal sites, serve as a source of future infectious virus during reactivation (51,58–61) (see section on Stromal Herpes). Whether latency is a static or smoldering but dynamic state is not established for the eye model. Current data indicate that at least the ICP0 or junctional region of the viral genome is retained in the latent state and that an antisense RNA (viral RNA transcribed from the DNA strand opposite the ICP0 region) may be required for either maintenance of latency or prevention of reactivation (50,53,62). Both animal and human studies indicate that reactivation, namely switching from latent to infectious virus production, results in a switch from production of antisense RNA to sense RNA (transcribed from the ICP0 region on the viral DNA). Subsequently, a cascade of events leads to production of viral polypeptides and, ultimately, to infectious progeny virions.

Data on the nature of different viral strains indicate that some are more likely to cause repeated and severe disease with stromal deposition of much viral glycoprotein, an immune reaction stimulant, and others rarely cause recurrences and, therefore, little if any disease after the primary infection (41,61,63,64).

### *Clinical Disease*

Recurrent herpes, then, is a disease of the previously infected host, who, unless severely immunosuppressed, has both cellular and humoral immunity. The disease may occur as any one of or a combination of the following: (a) epithelial infectious ulcers; (b) epithelial trophic ulcers; (c) stromal disease, either antigen/antibody-complement–mediated (AAC) or lymphocyte-mediated; (d) combined epithelial and stromal disease; and (e) iridocyclitis.

The mechanisms of recurrence are not fully understood. Various forms of physical and emotional stress appear to play a role in viral reactivation. Although it is known that topical and systemic corticosteroids may predispose to severe herpetic infections, it has been established that these drugs do not increase the incidence of ocular recurrences but do increase the severity in the event of "spontaneous" recurrence. Systemic epinephrine appears to be more at fault as an inciting agent in experimental animal model studies (65).

*Epithelial Infectious Ulcers.* Dendritic (branching), dendrogeographic, or geographic ulcerations of the cornea are caused by live virus. Van Horn et al. (66) have reported little inflammatory cell reaction (polymorphonuclear leukocytes but no B-lymphocytes) in an experimental model of this disease but many free viruses lying in intra- and extracellular locations, particularly in the basal epithelium.

Patients usually present complaining of tearing, irritation, photophobia, and, occasionally, blurred vision. Since the ocular infection occasionally presents as conjunctivitis alone, the history should include previous corneal ulcers, iritis, nasal or oral cold sores, genital ulceration, recent use of topical or systemic steroids or immunosuppressive drugs, and immunological deficiency states (malignancy, organ transplants, chronic eczema, AIDS).

Clinically, dendritic keratitis is herpes simplex until proved otherwise. Herpes zoster and some healing corneal abrasions may also cause dendritic or dendritiform ulcers. respectively. Corneal sensation is often decreased early in infection and may be permanently impaired, particularly in chronic forms of keratitis. The corneal le-

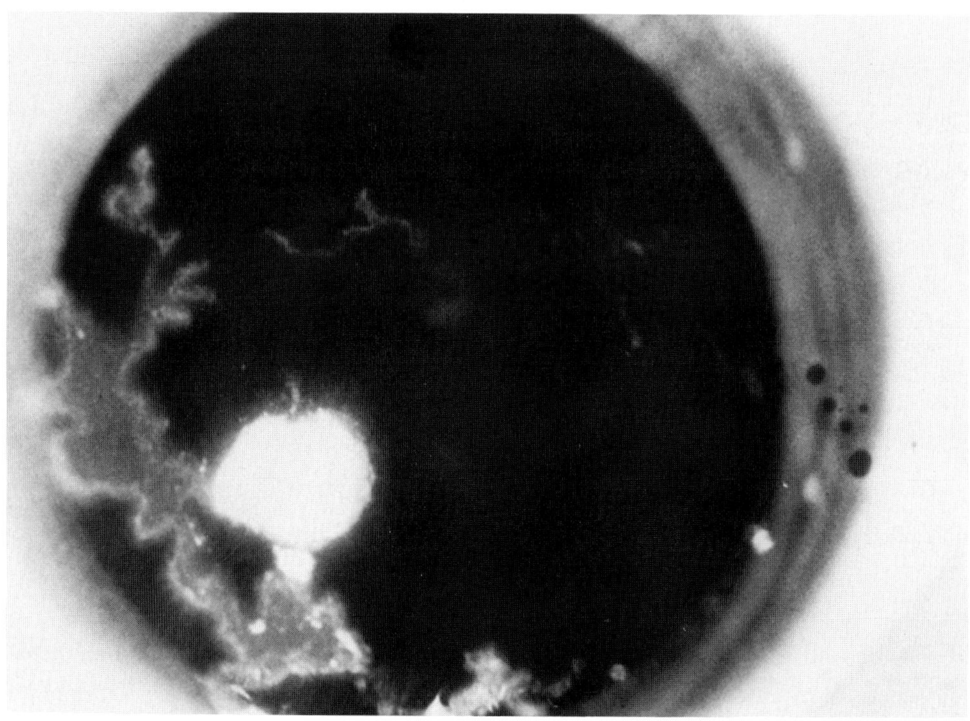

**FIG. 3.** HSV dendrogeographic and dendritic ulcers of cornea.

sions frequently form branching dendritic figures—large, small, single, or multiple (Fig. 3). They also may expand into map-like geographic ulcers and present to the physician in any of these patterns (Fig. 4). The mechanism for the branching formation has never been adequately explained. Relation to the neuronal distribution has generally been refuted, and current evidence suggests that it may simply be related to the virus pattern of linear spread by contiguous cell-to-cell movement (66,67). If the lesion comes within 2 mm of the limbus, it will be much more resistant to treatment than is a central herpetic infection, and it will be predisposed to chronic trophic ulceration. The reasons for this are unknown.

In milder epithelial keratitis, stromal involvement is usually absent or relatively mild and confined to the superficial layers. However, there may be considerable edema and iritis associated with the superficial disease. In these eyes, stromal scarring or true disciform reaction is more likely. This may be obviated by gentle debridement (preferably without chemicals) of the involved epithelium with a sterile cotton-tip applicator prior to instituting chemotherapy. This removes much of the inciting antigen.

The therapy of infectious epithelial herpes is as follows: (a) gentle debridement of involved epithelium with a sterile cotton-tip applicator, (b) antiviral ointment or drops for 14–21 days (Table 1), (c) topical antibiotics while ulcers are present, and (d) cycloplegics (e.g., 1% cyclopentolate three times a day) if needed for iritis.

With antiviral chemotherapy arresting virus replication until the infected cells slough from the eye or with debridement alone, the infectious epithelial disease can be effectively resolved approximately 90% of the time without complication or need for an antiinflammatory drug.

*Epithelial Trophic (Metaherpetic) Ulcers.* After the infectious keratitis has passed,

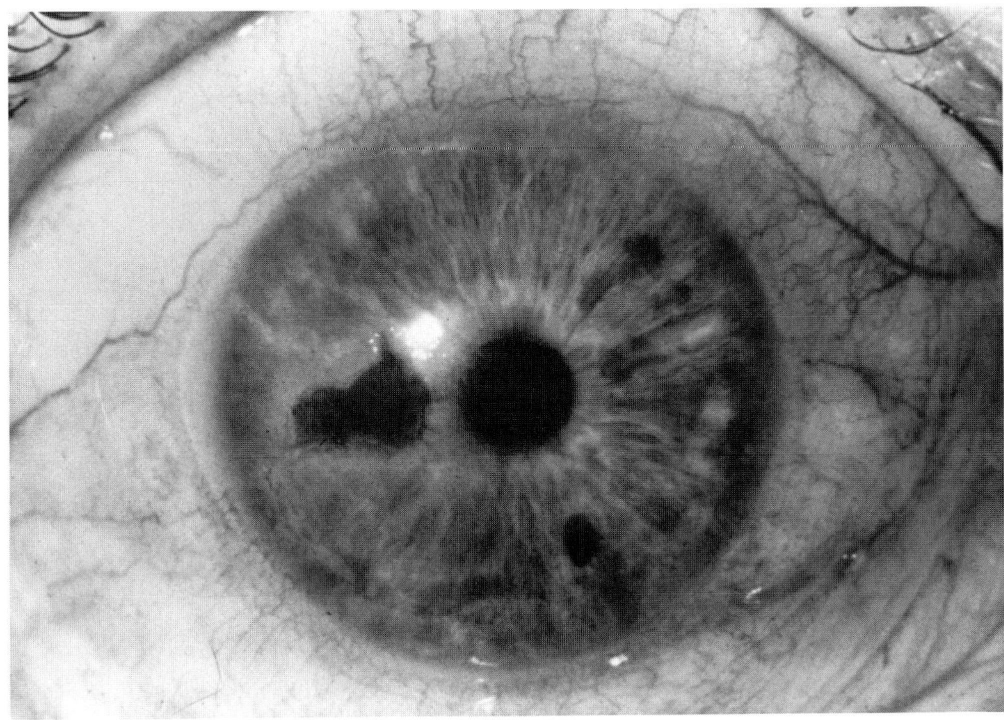

**FIG. 4.** HSV geographic ulcer. Note discrete edges stained with fluorescein and rose bengal.

the corneal epithelium occasionally ulcerates again in a few days or weeks to form a nondescript ovoid ulcer. This is known as postinfectious or metaherpetic trophic keratitis. Metaherpetic ulcers are secondary to residual mechanical corneal damage that occurred during the infectious stage. Corneal epithelial cells do not inter-digitate with their basement membrane but simply lie on top, attached only by electron-dense hemidesmosomes. If the basement membrane is damaged during the infection, healing is slow, occurring over a 12–15-week period; adequate healing of the overlying epithelium thus is retarded (68,69).

A trophic ulcer must be distinguished clinically from an actively infected geographic ulcer. The former has a gray, thickened border formed by the piling up of epithelial cells unable to move across the ulcer base; active geographic ulcers have discrete, flat edges that may change in configuration as the ulcer spreads (Fig. 5).

Multiplying virus does not cause the trophic form of disease, so there is no need for antiviral therapy. Similarly, cauterization will worsen the condition by further damaging the basement membrane. Scraping off all corneal epithelium results in regrowth of the epithelium up to the borders of the metaherpetic ulcer, but the cells are usually still unable to adhere to the damaged ulcer base.

Perhaps the greatest danger posed by trophic ulceration comes with persistence of the defect over a period of several weeks or months. Collagenolytic activity with subsequent stromal thinning (melting) and perforation becomes more likely the longer the ulcer is present. This is particularly true in males and if the ulcer is located centrally away from peripheral neovascularization, which scars but also heals (68).

Because of the mechanical nature of the problem, treatment is aimed at protecting the damaged basement membrane by copi-

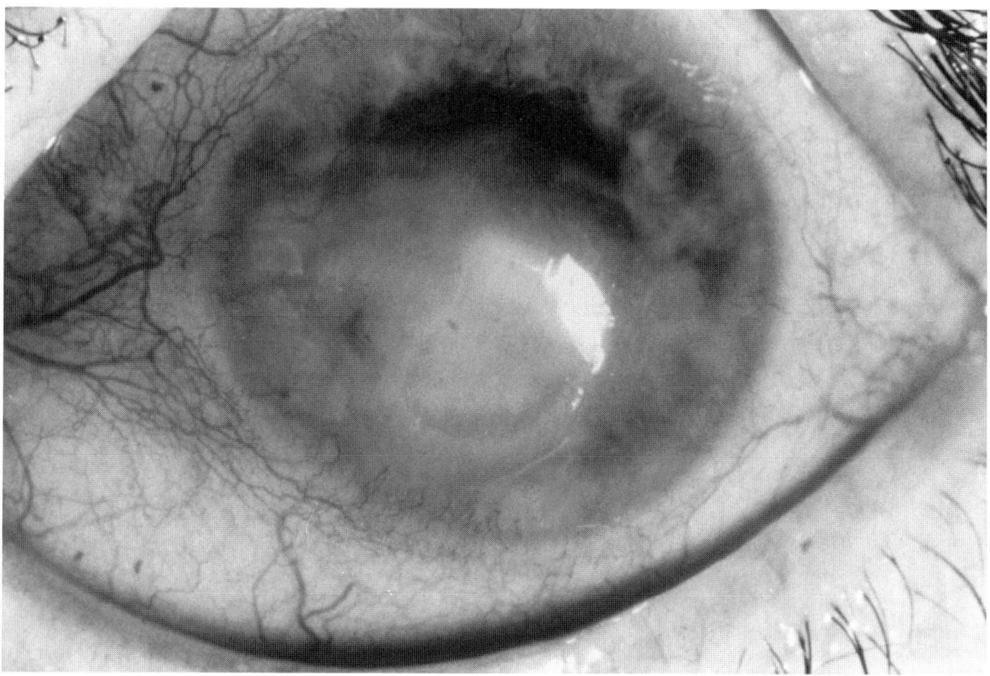

**FIG. 5.** Necrotic white HSV interstitial keratitis with neovascularization and trophic ulceration with characteristic rolled, thickened edge.

ous lubrication with artificial tears and ointments, patching, soft contact lens, or, occasionally, conjunctival flap or transplant. In the absence of underlying stromal inflammatory disease that may interfere with basement membrane healing, there is usually no call for antiinflammatory steroid therapy (to be discussed further).

Use of therapeutic soft contact lenses such as the Bausch & Lomb plano T, 0-4, or Sauflon lens has greatly increased the frequency and rapidity with which these ulcers may be healed (41,43,70). The lenses are thought to work by splinting and protecting the cornea from abrasive lid action, and by keeping the ulcer well lubricated through slowing tear-film evaporation. They may be worn for just a few weeks, if healing is rapid, or for many months, if it is slow. They should be removed, cleaned, and resterilized if deposits build up.

If healing is successful, topical lubrication with bland ophthalmic ointment or artificial tears should be continued for 2–3 months to prevent lid action from rubbing the newly healed epithelium off the still-fragile ulcer base. If healing does not occur and thinning becomes apparent, the use of cyanoacrylate tissue adhesive (Histoacryl) has frequently forestalled emergency surgery on an eye with an impending perforation or progressive melt. As the adhesive is not yet approved by the Food and Drug Administration (FDA) for use in the eye, informed consent should be obtained from the patient before use (41,43,71). Adhesive therapy of corneal ulcers is currently under study for review by the FDA Orphan Drug Committee.

In the face of a threatened perforation and the decision to use adhesive having been made, the epithelium should be gently debrided from the ulcer edge and base, the area to be glued carefully dried with Weck-cel sponges, and the polyethylene applicator tube containing liquid tissue adhesive gently touched in concentric circles to the edge of the ulcer, working toward the center until the area is entirely covered. Sterile saline may then be dripped on the eye at the end of the procedure to hasten polymerization. A soft therapeutic contact lens is then applied for continuous wear to protect the lids from irritation by the rough surface of the glue (Fig. 6). Antibiotic drops are instilled twice a day, and any steroid drops warranted for inflammation may be used with safety greater than in the presence of an open ulcer. Normally, the ulcer will heal with continued therapy, and new epithelium will ultimately dislodge the adhesive leaving a scarred but intact eye amenable to surgery, if needed, to restore vision.

The therapy of trophic (metaherpetic) ulceration is as follows:

(a) A therapeutic soft contact lens should be worn continuously around the clock, with twice-a-day administration of antibiotic drops. If no lens is immediately available, intermittent 48-hr pressure patching may be used, with antibiotic ointment.

(b) Artificial tears should be instilled 4–5 times a day while the lens is in and for 2–3 months after removal.

(c) A mild steroid (0.12% prednisolone) may be used 1–4 times a day every day as needed (only if significant stromal edema is present); 1% medroxyprogesterone (made in hospital pharmacy) is safer if the cornea is thinning.

(d) Cycloplegics (e.g., 1% cyclopentolate or atropine) should be used if iritis is present.

(e) Consider antiviral drops 5 times a day as prophylactic cover if steroid equivalent of 1% prednisolone is used more than twice a day or there is propensity to recurrent infection.

(f) For active stromal melting or thinning, consider cyanoacrylate glue (Histoacryl surgical adhesive; not FDA approved for ocular use) to seal ulcer, and cover with therapeutic soft lens.

*Stromal Disease.* This disease is commonly divided into two categories, both

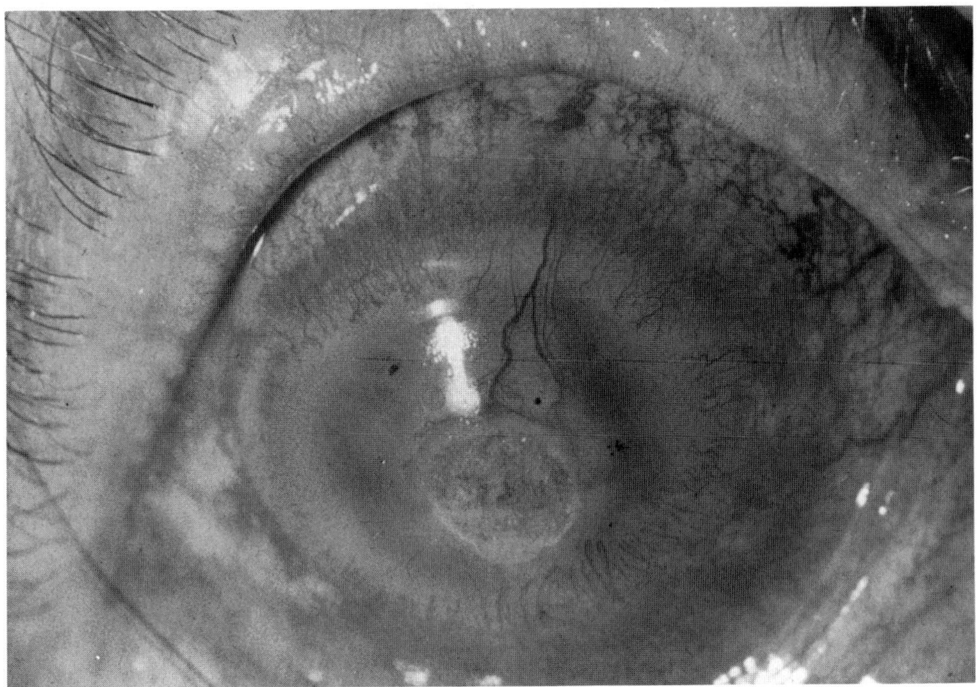

**FIG. 6.** HSV stromal disciform edema with neovascularization and melting (thinning) ulcer filled with cyanoacrylate tissue adhesive under therapeutic soft contact lens.

immune in nature: AAC and lymphocyte-mediated (disciform) (41,43,44,72–75). They will be discussed below as immune entities, but there is increasing evidence that the cornea itself may be a site of latent herpetic infection (51,58–60). The viral genome is apparently retained, actively transcribes RNA, and potentially serves as the source of new viral antigen, which may in turn stimulate the immune disease. These events may be entirely independent of reactivation of the virus in the trigeminal or other ganglia. Intact virus particles have been demonstrated in the stroma of patients by electron microscopy and by tissue cocultivation but not in cell-free cultures. Additionally, Pavan-Langston et al. (51) and others (59,60) have demonstrated retention of herpetic DNA and RNA in all layers of the cornea for at least 90 days postinfection, well into the latency period.

AAC-mediated keratitis includes interstitial keratitis, immune rings, and vasculitis. AAC disease presents as (a) a necrotic blotchy, cheesy-white interstitial keratitis (IK), (b) immune rings (Wessley), or (c) limbal vasculitis (local Arthus) (41,43, 72,75). These may lie under ulcers or appear independently. It is important, and occasionally difficult, to distinguish IK from secondary bacterial or fungal infections. Interstitial keratitis is much more indolent than these latter two, however, and may be associated with the presence of intact virus in the stroma (76). In IK, after several weeks of smoldering, dense leashes of deep neovascularization begins to move in as if in pursuit of the infiltrates (Fig. 5). Immune rings and limbal vasculitis do not incite significant neovascularization, but immune rings and IK tend to scar despite treatment (Figs. 7 and 8). In the absence of steroid therapy, antiviral drugs do not appear indicated.

If the infiltrates do not involve the visual axis, there is often little indication for ste-

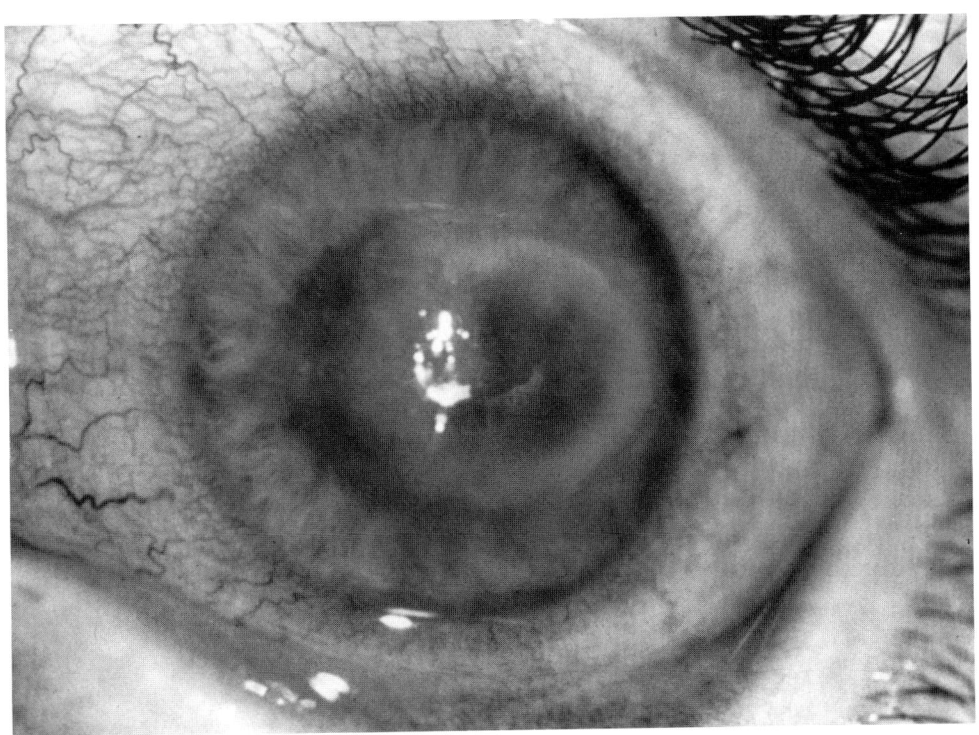

**FIG. 7.** HSV stromal immune ring (Wessley ring).

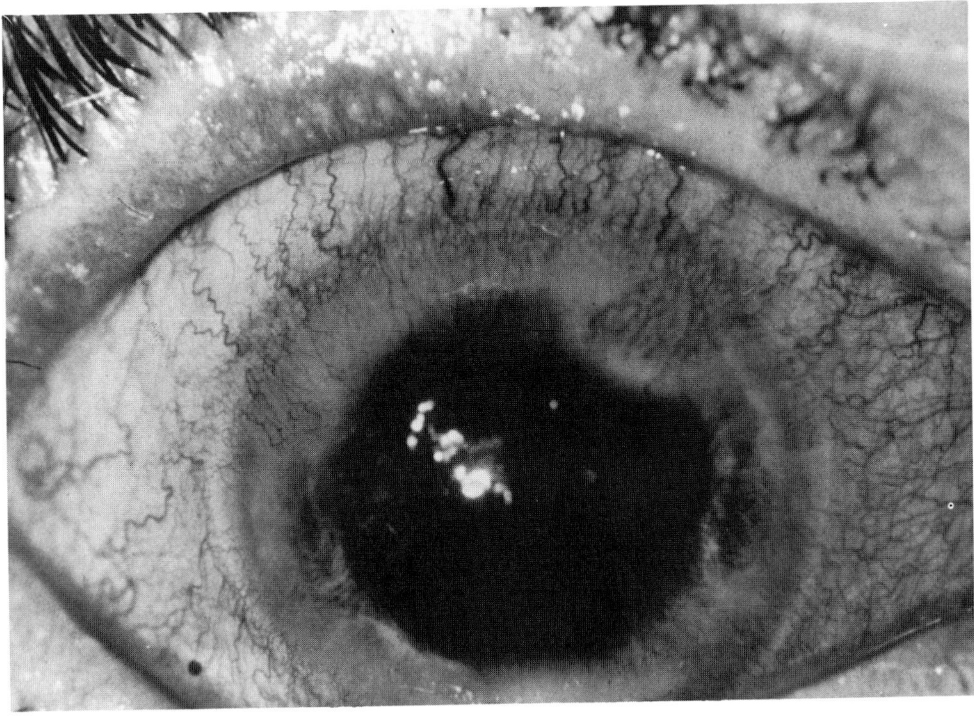

**FIG. 8.** HSV limbal vasculitis. (From Pavan-Langston, ref. 199, with permission.)

roid therapy. The process usually resolves spontaneously in weeks to months with some, but often mild to moderate, scarring. Neovascularization regresses to become barely visible ghost vessels. An overlying irregular astigmatism will often improve with time. Therapeutically, a general guideline is that if steroids have never been used in a particular eye with herpetic AAC disease, one should try to carry the patient through the course of disease without starting them. Unfortunately, this often is not possible.

The exact cause of disciform keratitis is not completely understood. Currently, it is felt that immune changes from the original viral invasion mediate this form of keratitis, although subclinical ganglionic reactivation with migration to the cornea or end organ reactivation of retained genome may also play key roles. Antigenic alteration of the surface membrane of corneal cellular elements such that the body sees them as "foreign" and the antigenically active residue of viral particles may serve as immune stimulants against which the host elicits inflammatory response. This is a delayed type of hypersensitivity reaction characterized by sensitized lymphocytes, plasma cells, and, ultimately, macrophages and polymorphonuclear cells (72,73,76).

In its most benign form, disciform keratitis is characterized clinically by focal, disc-shaped (hence the name) stromal edema without necrosis or neovascularization (Fig. 9). There may be keratitic precipitates made up of lymphocytes and plasma cells clinging to the endothelium just in the area of disciform edema or true endotheliitis. The fact that iritis may be absent even in a moderate case suggests that the keratitic precipitates are especially attracted to focal corneal antigen (77,78).

In moderate disciform disease, more diffuse edema and folds in Descemet's membrane are frequently seen, indicating that

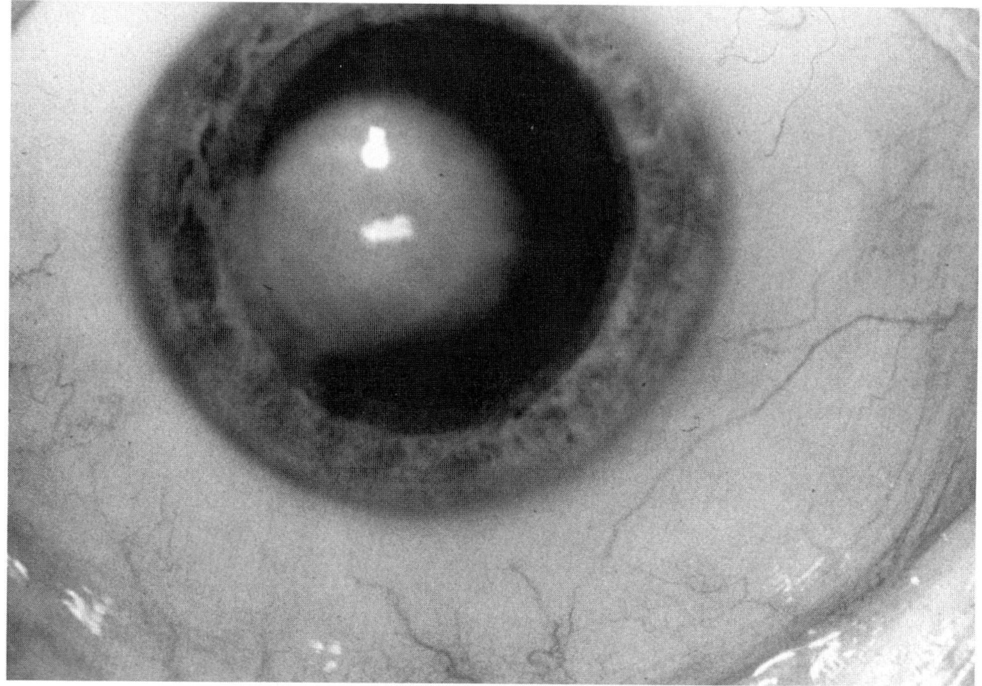

**FIG. 9.** Moderate stromal disciform keratitis of visual axis. Epithelium is intact and relatively healthy.

the endothelium is compromised by the toxic inflammatory reaction and that fluid is entering the cornea in abnormally great amounts. Vessels are frequently present. The most severe forms of disciform keratitis produce the greatest destructive effects of an uncontrolled inflammatory reaction in the cornea. There is diffuse edema and frequently an ulcerating bullous keratopathy with necrotic stromal thinning, melting, neovascularization, and severe iritis. Patches of white interstitial keratitis may be seen scattered in these corneas.

Essentially the same rules apply to the treatment of disciform keratitis as to AAC disease. If a patient has never been on steroids and the disease is mild, every effort should be made to avoid their introduction into the therapeutic regimen. Since the disease is immune in etiology, there is probably no role for antivirals except as prophylaxis against potential spontaneous reactivation of epithelial infection. Patients are kept more comfortable with cycloplegics as there is usually a mild iridocyclitis. Artificial tears and dark glasses may also help to carry the patient through a difficult period until the reaction subsides, usually with little or no scarring.

It is the eye with moderate or severe disciform or AAC keratitis, or both, that needs the antiinflammatory, antiscarring, antineovascular effects of the steroids. In the face of a notable antigen/antibody reaction of the stroma with all its associated immune cellular invasion and release of lysosomal enzymes, the neighboring endothelium may be irreversibly damaged if not protected by steroids. Additionally, if allowed to run unchecked, the inflammatory reaction will cause increased scarring and promote deep neovascularization, which not only compromises the potential success of a future graft but also gives circulating lymphocytes and humoral antibodies direct access to the deeper and central areas of the cornea (79–81).

Therapy again is aimed at using the minimum dose of steroid that will control the reaction, followed by a gradual but not abrupt taper and, if possible, cessation. A typical regimen is to decrease progressively the strength and frequency of steroid dosage, e.g., starting with 1% prednisolone every 3 hr for severe disease or less often for moderate inflammation and working down in a stepwise fashion over several weeks to several months. For example, prednisolone 1% every 3 hr tapered to every 6 hr to three times a day, each step for 1–3 weeks, then twice a day to once a day over a several-week period. If the reaction is controlled, ⅛% prednisolone four times a day is substituted for 1% once a day. Then taper to ⅛% three times a day, to two times a day, to once a day, staying at each level for 2–4 weeks. Then to every other day, every three days, to cessation if possible. Less severe disease would warrant starting at lower levels of steroid therapy.

Too abrupt cessation of steroids will result in recrudescence of immune disease, and the dosage of steroid will have to be increased temporarily. Occasional patients will never be able to discontinue steroids completely without relapse and may have to be maintained on "homeopathic" doses daily or once or twice weekly. Until the patient is down to twice daily medication or less at the equivalent of 1.0% prednisolone, a prophylactic antiviral ointment three times a day or drop 5–6 times a day and antibiotics every day should be used unless there is toxic or allergic reaction. Cycloplegics, if used for iritis, may be discontinued when the anterior chamber is clear as the daytime photophobia may be quite uncomfortable.

The treatment of herpetic stromal disease may be summarized as follows:

(a) Nothing need be done if the disease is mild and not in the visual axis.

(b) Cycloplegics as needed for iritis (e.g., cyclopentolate).

(c) Steroids should be used if necessary, ranging from 0.1% dexamethasone or 1%

prednisolone every 3 hr, for severe disease, to prednisolone 0.12% once or twice a day for milder disease (regimen adjusted accordingly). Antibiotic ointment daily prophylaxis at higher steroid doses (see below).

(d) Prophylactic antiviral ointment three times a day or drops five times a day if steroids are used more than twice a day at doses greater than 1% prednisolone equivalent in eyes predisposed to recurrent infection.

(e) If the epithelium is ulcerated, topical steroids should be reduced or stopped. Use of 1% medroxyprogesterone is a safer topical drop (see section on adjunct corticosteroids and trophic ulcers).

If the inflammatory process begins to reactivate after a dose reduction, steroids should be increased to the previous level for a longer period of time and attempts at taper should be started again as the process ultimately resolves. The currently available antivirals have no proven effect on the stromal keratitis per se. Keratoplasty should be deferred until the eye has been quiet on little or no steroid treatment for several months. Viral interstitial keratitis is the most likely form of ocular herpes to recur in a new graft (81).

*Combined Epithelial and Stromal Disease.* Occasionally a patient will present with a combination of disciform disease and a viral-infected epithelial ulcer or a noninfected trophic healing defect. In the former case, gentle debridement and antiviral therapy should be started at least a day or two prior to starting steroids. If the ulcer progresses in the face of topical steroid therapy, the frequency or strength of dosage should be reduced until the ulcer is under control and healing. Systemic steroids are of little use in corneal disease alone, as negligible tissue titers are attained. If disciform keratitis with trophic ulceration presents or if the originally infected ulcer becomes trophic in nature, healing will be aided by controlling underlying stromal edema with steroids and the application of a therapeutic soft contact lens (see section on trophic ulcers).

*Iridocyclitis.* Recurrent iridocyclitis and, on occasion, panuveitis may be caused by HSV (77,82–84). The intraocular inflammation may occur prior to any known infection or without concomitant active keratitis. It frequently accompanies active keratitis, however, and may be due to specific involvement with the virus or may be secondary to the irritative effects of the keratitis. Uveitis in an eye with previously known herpetic keratitis should be considered herpetic until proven otherwise by examination or laboratory tests.

The exact etiology of this uveitis is not clear. Intact virus particles are known to be present in the aqueous humor in a few cases and, in one case, in a retrocorneal membrane (83–85). There is also an immune inflammatory component.

Treatment is nonspecific. Topical antivirals do not penetrate in sufficient therapeutic titers, and systemic ACV is equivocal at best (3,5,86). Suppression of the inflammatory reaction is still the best therapy available, albeit far from ideal. Again, if a patient has never been on steroids, every effort should be made to avoid their introduction. Cycloplegic mydriatics may help a patient avoid structural alteration of the iris and lens. If, however, the reaction is persistent and more than mildly symptomatic, aqueous cell and flare reaction threatens iris-lens synechia formation, or the patient has been controlled only with steroids previously, one should reinstitute topical steroids using a regimen similar to those described in the treatment of disciform keratitis. The starting dose and frequency of steroid administration should be compatible with the relative severity of disease, and prophylactic antivirals and antibiotics should be used accordingly along with the usual cycloplegic mydriatics.

The therapy of herpetic uveitis is as follows:

(a) Cycloplegics (e.g., scopolamine or cyclopentolate) should be given once to three times a day.

(b) Topical steroids are managed as under stromal disease.

(c) If the cornea has ulcerated or is thinning, topical steroids should be reduced or stopped, and prednisone 20–30 mg by mouth may be given twice a day for 7–14 days, then tapered off over 10 days. Use of 1% medroxyprogesterone is a safer drop in the presence of ulceration (see section on adjunct corticosteroids and trophic ulcers).

(d) Antiviral ointment three times a day or drops five times a day and antibiotics daily should be given while topical steroids are used more often than twice per day (1% prednisolone equivalent).

(e) Carbonic anhydrase inhibitors and/or epinephrine or β blockers should be given if secondary glaucoma is present.

(f) There is currently no proven efficacy of the use of systemic antivirals in this condition.

Patients may develop toxic or allergic reactions to topical antivirals. These inflammatory responses should not be confused with worsening of disease, and an alternative antiviral agent should be substituted (Fig. 10).

*Retinitis.* Although rare, both HSV-1 and HSV-2 may cause a chorioretinitis. In the neonate, HSV infection is commonly acquired during passage through an infected birth canal and can be associated with central nervous system infection. Anterior segment findings in these infants may include the symptoms of photophobia and tearing and the signs of conjunctivitis, corneal ulceration, iritis, and cataract. Acute signs in the posterior segment in the neonate are disseminated choroidal hemorrhages with choroidal and intraretinal exudates, fine vitreous haze, retinal edema with narrowing of the arterioles, and secondary obstruction (83,87–90). Similar findings may be noted in the more severely immunocompromised adult patient such as those with organ transplants, blood dyscrasia, neoplasia, or, now, with increasing frequency, AIDS. In milder cases, small focal yellow-white retinal infiltrates may be seen with or without optic nerve involvement. Histopathologic examination reveals retinal necrosis with inflammatory cell infiltrate and intranuclear inclusions in the retina. The differential diagnosis in both neonate and immunosuppressed adult includes toxoplasmosis, cytomegalic inclusion disease (CMV), rubella (neonate), and syphilis.

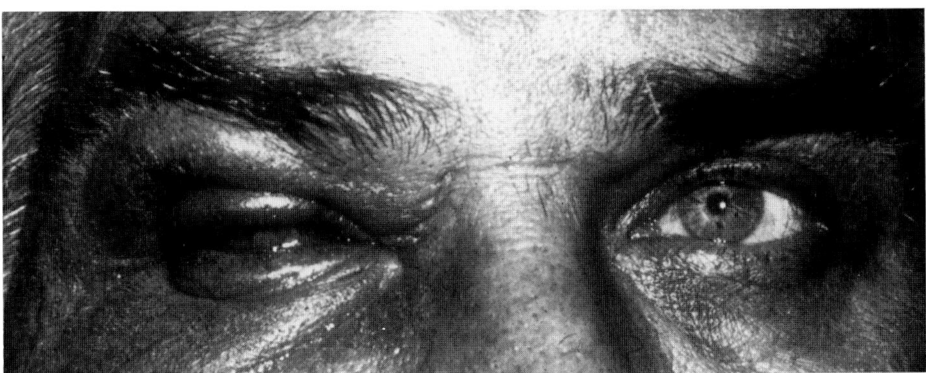

**FIG. 10.** Antiviral drug toxic-allergic medicamentosa; not to be confused with acute or chronic viral infection.

As specific and rapid diagnosis is essential to any attempt at preserving ocular integrity and useful visual acuity, laboratory tests tend to be more confirmatory than acute diagnostic. Acute and convalescent sera are useful, but evaluation may take weeks to complete. Elevated local antibody production in the aqueous as assayed by enzyme-linked immunosorbent assay (ELISA) is useful if available. Other diagnostic tests are discussed earlier in this chapter, but initiation of therapy must be very early to be effective and, therefore, based largely on clinical suspicion.

Therapy at this time is primarily confined to systemic acyclovir which appears to be specific for both herpes type 1 and type 2 with few systemic side effects. Dosage is 5 mg/kg intravenously every 8 hr for 5–10 days (86,91–93). Systemic prednisone may also be useful in controlling the inflammatory reaction in conjunction with antiviral therapy. However, prednisone should probably not be used in severely immunocompromised patients but only in those in whom some cell-mediated immunity is still preserved.

### Surgical Intervention

With the advent of more judicious use of steroids, antiviral drugs, therapeutic soft lenses, and cyanoacrylate tissue adhesive, urgent surgery on the herpetic eye has become progressively less frequent. The conjunctival flap or transplant is now reserved to resolve acute disease in inflamed, ulcerated, thinning corneas that cannot be controlled with the other available therapeutic measures mentioned above (94,95). Penetrating grafts placed in acutely inflamed eyes almost certainly have poor postoperative courses. Similarly, partial tarsorrhaphy may be used as adjunctive therapy to a therapeutic lens with an aim toward protecting and healing recalcitrant or unhealthy surface epithelium. Lamellar keratoplasty has had an unsuccessful record but is currently being used again with increasing frequency and success in cases with scarring confined to the anterior 50% of the stroma (79–81).

In the significantly scarred or chronically inflamed but clinically uninfected eye, penetrating keratoplasty is increasingly the procedure of choice in many herpetic patients. The improved medical management and surgical techniques now justify this surgery not simply to restore vision in a relatively quiet eye but also to remove viral antigenic material lodged in the cornea and inciting repeated immune inflammatory episodes significantly disrupting the patient's normal daily life.

Langston et al. (80) evaluated factors leading to a clear graft success rate greater than 85% in herpetic eyes and noted that this success was related to the following factors: (a) reduced or absent inflammation, (b) minimal deep neovascularization, (c) use of 10-0 or finer nylon suture, and (d) use of very high doses of topical steroids in the immediate postoperative period followed by tapering over the ensuing 3 months. Recurrence of dendritic disease in the graft averaged 15% within 2 years regardless of the level of steroid use. Postoperative complications such as wound synechia, graft rejection, and secondary glaucoma were significantly lower in the high steroid dosage groups.

Cohen et al. (79) also reported a success rate greater than 85% but found no correlation between preoperative vascularization and rejection. There was also no greater incidence of recurrent dendritic keratitis in the grafts (19%) when steroids were used without prophylactic antivirals. This agreed with the study of Fine and Cignetti (96) in which no antivirals were given and indicated that the use of antivirals in the study by Langston et al. (80) may not have been necessary. Of note is the finding by Cohen et al. (79) that 32% of herpetic eyes undergoing rejection and under treatment for that rejection developed infectious epithelial herpetic ulceration. This suggested that antiviral prophylaxis is unnecessary except in those cases in which allograft rejection is occurring and is under treatment.

## CMV

### Congenital Infection

CMV is the most common virus known to be transmitted *in utero;* the incidence of infection is up to 2.2% of all live births. Ocular manifestations include chorioretinitis and optic atrophy and are a sign of systemic CMV infection (11). Of the infected children who do not manifest clinical disease at birth, 5–15% will go on to develop late complications of this disease. Cell-mediated immunity (CMI) is impaired specifically with respect to the CMV virus; the impairment resolves over several years along with disappearance of virus from urine and saliva (97,98). This is discussed in greater detail elsewhere in this volume.

In severe cases of symptomatic congenital CMV infection, ocular involvement may range from very mild with just a few patchy peripheral retinal infiltrates or vasculitis to total bilateral retinal necrosis in which few islands of retinal tissue remain intact. Congenital retinal involvement may be either peripheral or central, at the posterior pole or all inclusive (panretinitis). In cases involving only the peripheral retina, the clinical findings are small foci of retinal inflammation with overlying peripheral vitreous haze resembling the fog bank of peripheral uveitis. With resolution of these lesions the underlying pigment epithelium becomes clumped and mottled, the retina atrophic, and the overlying vitreous hazy to clear (99,100).

More frequently the posterior pole of the eye is affected in infants, and these lesions may be identical to those found with congenital toxoplasmosis. This includes intense necrotizing retinochoroiditis located only in the macula and which may resolve to a hyperplastic pigmented macular scar, or there may be multiple focal lesions that resolve into many small, round, pigmented chorioretinal scars or result in total destruction of the retina.

### Acquired Adult Infection and CMV in AIDS

There are six means of acquiring infection with CMV: transplacentally, during birth through an infected canal, fomite transmission, droplet infection, sexual contact, and contaminated blood transfusion. As a result of the ease with which this virus is spread, more than 80% of the population 35 years or older has positive complement fixation titers to CMV. In healthy adults, latent infection may be found in multiple organ systems, but not in the central nervous system and, therefore, not in the retina (100). However, CMV infection in the immunosuppressed adult may result in florid findings involving virtually any organ system including the eye. Prior to the advent of the AIDS epidemic, active CMV infection was largely seen in immunosuppressed patients such as those with neoplastic, autoimmune disease, or blood dyscrasia or those under treatment after organ transplantation. The number of patients at risk for CMV retinitis is increasing rapidly, not only because of the growing number of transplant patients and use of immunosuppressive drugs in general but, more urgently, because of the rapid spread of the AIDS epidemic. CMV is now the most common opportunistic ocular infection in AIDS, occurring in 15 to 40% of all patients. Untreated, it progresses rapidly to blindness (11,101).

The clinical findings of ocular CMV in patients with neoplastic or iatrogenic immunosuppression are similar to those seen in AIDS patients but tend to be not so uniformly progressive although potentially the cause of serious visual loss (11,102–104). The clinical appearance of CMV retinitis varies according to its intraocular location.

Typically involvement of the posterior pole is that of a dense, patchy white retinal necrosis developing most frequently along the vascular arcades. Pepose (103) and Holland (105) noted that CMV retinitis is consistently preceded by the appearance of cotton wool spots (microinfarctions) (Fig. 11). As AIDS patients frequently have elevated levels of circulating immune complexes, it is postulated that the deposition of these complexes results in microvascular lesions with subsequent ischemia, stasis of axoplasmic flow, and subsequent cotton wool spot formation. CMV viremia through such vessels in AIDS patients may lead to retinal infection via the damaged vascular endothelium and explain the association of precedent cotton wool spots with subsequent CMV focal retinitis. Along with the areas of retinal necrosis there may be associated areas of retinal hemorrhage either along the leading edge or within the area of retinitis.

Peripheral retinal CMV infection tends to be a more granular, white retinitis that is less intense and may or may not have associated retinal hemorrhages. The prospective study by Henderly et al. (11) of 109 AIDS or ARC (AIDS-related complex) patients indicated that CMV retinitis may be manifested early in that setting. Fifteen of 82 AIDS patients and three of 27 ARC patients presented with CMV retinitis (11). Four patients had CMV retinitis as an initial manifestation of AIDS and two of these presented without evidence of other opportunistic infection or Kaposi's sarcoma. This report is in contrast to earlier, nonprospective studies by Holland (105) that CMV retinitis presents only late in the disease and carries a poor prognosis for both vision and survival. In several earlier studies survival

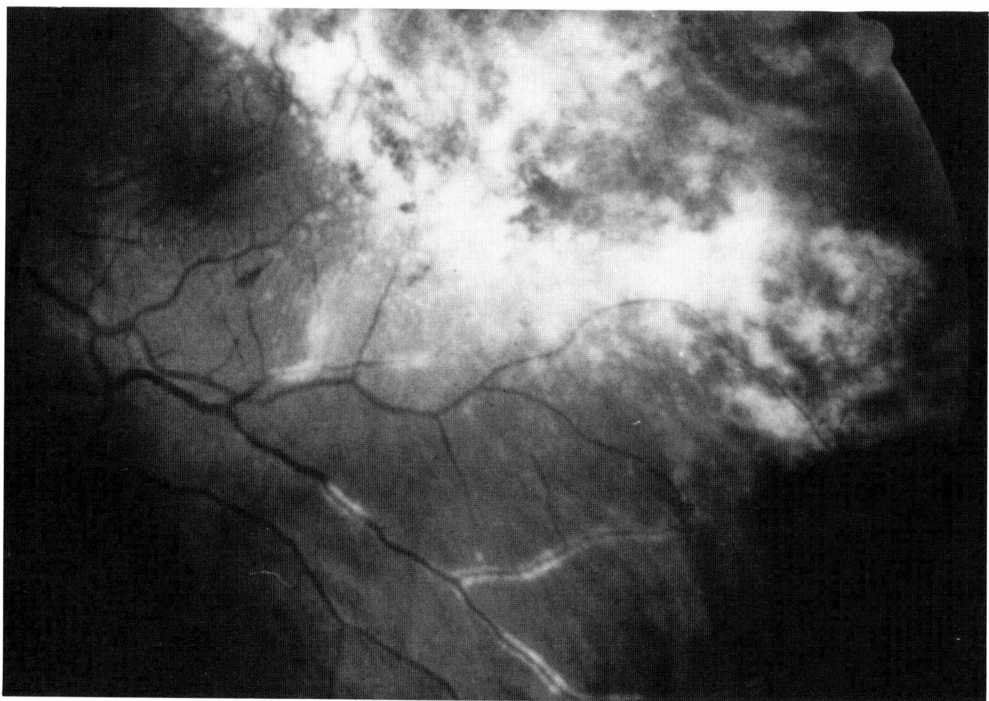

**FIG. 11.** CMV retinitis in AIDS patient characterized by intraretinal hemorrhaging and confluent cotton wool spots superiorly and vasculitis inferiorly. (Courtesy of Dr. D. J. D'Amico, Massachusetts Eye and Ear Infirmary, Boston, Massachusetts.)

ranged from six weeks to four months after the diagnosis of CMV retinitis. As will be noted under treatment, these figures have now changed (101–104,106).

Although the disease is similar in AIDS patients and in those immunosuppressed from other causes, there is one distinction in that non-AIDS patients have an essentially uninflamed CMV retinopathy. Granulocyte function appears to be intact in AIDS patients in contrast to infants, organ recipients, and patients with neoplasia who do have impaired granulocyte function and are unable to mount the acute inflammatory response seen in the AIDS patient with CMV retinitis. As a result the amount of vitreous haze noted in the non-AIDS patient is significantly less than that in the AIDS counterpart (103,104).

There is some dispute as to which retinal layers are involved with CMV virus. Pepose et al. (104) reported that CMV involves all layers of the retina with the exception of the endothelial cells as these cells appear incapable of supporting a productive infection. In contrast, Grossniklaus et al. (107) have reported CMV inclusions in all layers of the involved retinas including the retinal pigment epithelium, and in the glial cells of an infected optic nerve in an AIDS patient with CMV retinitis and optic neuritis (104–107).

### Therapy of CMV Retinitis

Treatment of CMV infection of any type is still highly unsatisfactory. Although ACV, an inhibitor of CMV DNA polymerase, has been reported as significantly effective when used prophylactically to reduce risk of CMV infection in seropositive patients undergoing allogeneic bone marrow transplantation and significantly improving their survival, this drug has largely been abandoned in favor of its analog, didehydroxy propoxymethyl guanine, or DHPG (ganciclovir) (10–12,102,104,108,109).

Palestine et al. (102) studied eight patients with CMV retinitis; two were iatrogenically immunosuppressed, six had AIDS. All had characteristic retinitis and blood and urine cultures positive for CMV. Therapy with DHPG consisted of 5 mg/kg body weight intravenously twice a day for 3 weeks unless the neutrophil count dropped to less than 500/mm$^3$. Some patients were treated up to four weeks because of continued improvement. Of the 14 eyes with retinitis, eight showed greater than 90% resolution, and four had partial improvement. When therapy was discontinued in the chemotherapy-induced immunosuppressed patients, they remained in ocular remission for at least several months. Unfortunately, the six AIDS patients suffered relapses within 5 weeks after discontinuation of therapy. Blood and urine cultures for CMV were negative during the periods of treatment but became positive again after therapy was stopped in all AIDS patients and remained negative in the iatrogenically immunosuppressed patients. When relapses in the retinitis occurred, they were both at the edges of healed lesions and in regions of previously uninvolved retina. The rapidity of recurrence in AIDS patients as opposed to the non-AIDS group indicates both the greater severity of immunosuppression in the former group and that in both groups the virus is suppressed by drug but not eliminated. There appeared to be a good response rate in patients with CMV retinitis who were retreated with DHPG after relapse.

The larger study by Henderly et al. (11) reported a prospective study of 109 patients with AIDS or ARC. Of the 23 patients with retinitis (15 developed this in the prospective phase of the study), 11 were unilaterally affected. Of 35 eyes with retinitis, 51% were peripherally affected only, 9% posterior pole only, and approximately 40% diffuse involving both the periphery and posterior pole. Nine patients had other systemic involvement. Treatment with DHPG was set at 2.5 mg/kg every 8 hr for 10 days intravenously and then maintenance dosage of 5 mg/kg/day for 5 days per week. Recurrences of retinitis were treated with reinduction dose similar to the initial dosing above and subsequent maintenance on 5 mg/kg/day 7 days per week.

The retinitis regressed in all patients after initiating DHPG therapy, but 57% had recurrence, seven of these recurring while on maintenance therapy and seven after discontinuation of ganciclovir. Recurrence occurred within 10–21 days after discontinuing treatment. Neutropenia directly attributable to DHPG occurred in only two patients.

Clinically resolution of the retinitis was similar to that seen when non-AIDS immunosuppressed patients have reversals of their immune defect and subsequently resolve the CMV retinitis. In effect, the retinitis became more patchy with ultimate regression of the white area of necrosis leaving behind areas of atrophic, thinned retina with ghost vessels and underlying retinal pigment epithelial (RPE) atrophy or hyperplasia. The hemorrhages also regressed but more slowly than the retinitis.

The life span of patients in this study was significantly extended; two patients lived longer than 1 year after the diagnosis of CMV retinitis. This is in contrast to earlier figures noted above. The average survival in patients treated with ganciclovir for CMV retinitis was greater than 6 months. Additionally, patients reported a subjective improvement in the quality of life, increased feeling of well being, and the ability to resume many normal activities of daily life.

Recently, Ussery et al. (110) reported the successful suppression of AIDS-asociated CMV retinitis in 11 of 14 patients receiving intravitreal injections of 200 μg of DHPG (110). All patients were severely myelosuppressed, obviating continued intravenous DHPG (five patients), or had progressive retinitis despite maximum tolerable doses of intravenous DHPG (six patients). Nine of the 14 eyes required repeat injections due to reactivation of disease. There was no discernible local or systemic drug toxicity. Intravitreal injection of this drug may offer an alternative therapy to intravenous DHPG or serve as useful concomitant therapy with systemic administration but must at this time be considered an experimental procedure. See page 227 for late FDA action.

Le Hoang et al. (28) also reported data on a newer investigational drug, foscarnet sodium. Studies in the United States have only recently begun, but data from Europe show that the drug may be as effective as AZT, with approximately 80% of patients achieving stability or improvement of their CMV retinitis. The drug is thought to have a direct antiviral effect on the HIV as well.

Dosage used in current clinical trials is 60 mg/kg body weight three times daily for 2–3 weeks before starting maintenance dosage once daily; optimal dosage is yet to be ascertained. Although the drug is not myelosuppressive, it is nephrotoxic and therefore should not be used in patients with renal failure. Creatinine levels must be monitored in all patients on the drug.

In brief, although CMV retinitis is on the rise both because of the AIDS epidemic and the increasing use of immunosuppressive drugs for other illnesses, therapy is far from satisfactory. Reducing or eliminating the cause of iatrogenic immunosuppression is one approach that has proved effective in a significant number of patients in the past, and the advent of DHPG provides at least a holding action for many patients but is certainly not a cure for this illness. In addition, animal studies have demonstrated a dose-dependent toxicity that included inhibition of spermatogenesis and testicular atrophy, gastrointestinal reactions such as vomiting, diarrhea, and mucosal necrosis, obstructive nephropathy, and bone marrow suppression. In clinical use, only reversible neutropenia has necessitated discontinuation of DHPG therapy, however (108). Nonetheless, results are sufficiently encouraging to continue investigation into this drug, AZT, and foscarnet and to expand where possible other approaches to CMV retinitis as well as to AIDS.

## VARICELLA-ZOSTER OPHTHALMICUS

### Varicella

The most common clinical manifestation of the varicella virus is chicken pox; approximately 2.8 million cases occur annually in the United States (111,112). Rarely in the course of chicken pox, vesicular lesions will appear on the conjunctiva. These are usually unilateral, small papular phlyctenular lesions that erupt along the lid margins or most commonly at the corneal limbus. They may resolve without problems or may become pustular or punched out, dark-red painful ulcers with swollen margins with secondary reaction in the eye. In some cases, the cornea may become involved with a superficial punctate keratitis or branching dendritic keratitis. Rarely, a fibrinous iridocyclitis may develop and destroy useful vision in the eye. Occasionally, the keratitis will not develop until several months after the original illness and in these cases the keratitis is caused by an immune reaction (113–115).

Treatment is essentially good hygiene, topical antibiotics, and mydriatics, if necessary. Ara-A or IDU ointment five times daily may be of some benefit.

### Herpes Zoster Ophthalmicus

In the United States, approximately 20% of the herpes zoster cases each year involve the eye [herpes zoster ophthalmicus (HZO)]. Approximately 50–72% of patients with periocular zoster will have involvement of the ocular structures themselves and develop chronic disease with moderate to severe degrees of visual loss. The aging process and depressed immune responses greatly enhance the risk of developing zoster. Disturbance of cell mediated immunity is a critical factor with resulting increasing incidence of zoster due to increasing immunosuppressed patients due both to the AIDS epidemic and to increasing iatrogenic immunosuppression in organ transplant, neoplasia and blood dyscrasia patients (116–121).

#### *Pathogenesis*

Zoster infections of the eye may occur by one of two mechanisms: (a) reactivation in the trigeminal sensory ganglion of virus persisting there in latency after the primary attack of chicken pox or (b) reintroduction of exogenous virus through direct or indirect contact with either a chicken pox or zoster patient. The incubation period for endogenous zoster is not known, but in those cases following exposure to chicken pox, incubation varied between a few days to 2 weeks (122). The illness may begin with headache, malaise, fever, and chills, preceded or followed by neuralgic pain. In 2–3 days, hot, flushed hyperesthesia and edema of the dermatome(s) develops and then erupt(s) with a single or multiple crops of clear vesicles from which virus may be cultured for approximately 3 days. The vesicles then become turbid and yellow and, unlike herpes simplex, form deep eschars that may leave behind permanent telltale pitted scars over the dermatome (Figs. 12 and 13).

The acute inflammatory period lasts 8–14 days, but the skin ulceration may take many weeks to heal and result in the equivalent of third-degree burns, with total lid retraction or ptosis and sloughing of lashes and tissues (116,121).

#### *Neuronal Relationships*

The dermatomes most commonly affected are the thoracic, followed in frequency by the cranial, the cervical, and, oc-

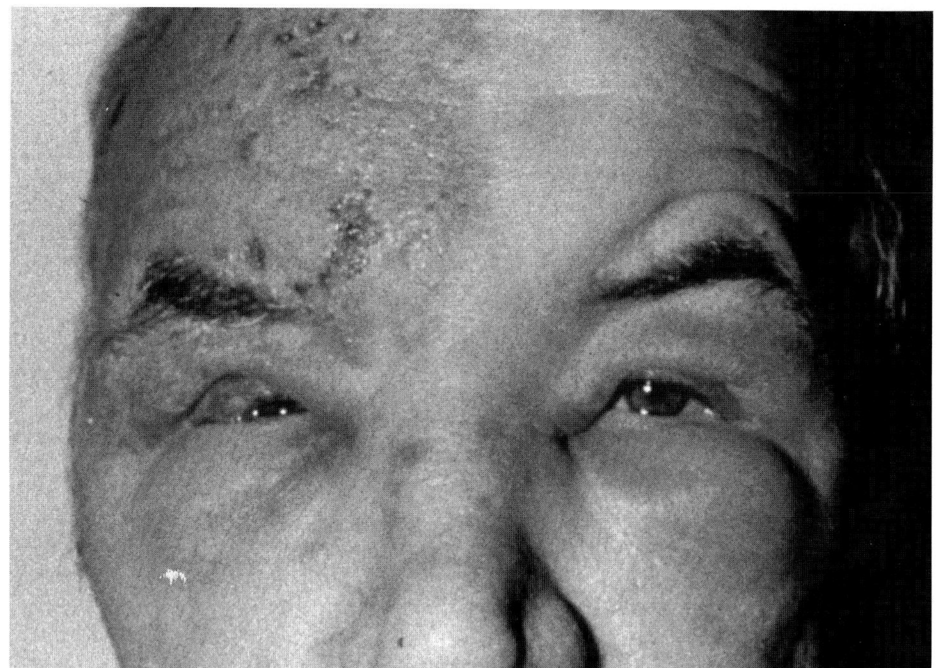

**FIG. 12.** Herpes zoster virus eruption involving the frontal branch dermatome of cranial nerve VII with sympathetic edema of contralateral lids.

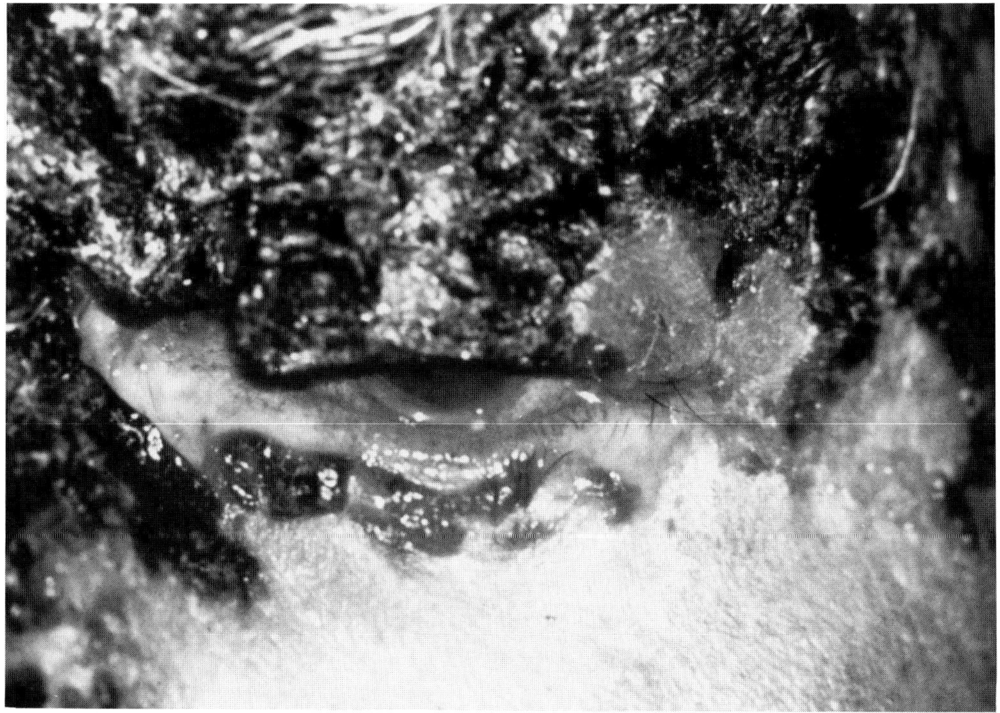

**FIG. 13.** Herpes zoster virus hemorrhagic scarring with loss of lashes and equivalent of third-degree skin burns and partial lid sloughing.

casionally, the lumbar or sacral. When the first or ophthalmic division of the fifth sensory cranial nerve (trigeminal ganglion) is involved, herpes zoster ophthalmicus usually results. Occasionally the second or maxillary division will be involved as well, and very rarely the mandibular.

The frontal nerve is the most frequently affected; via its supraorbital and supratrochlear branches, it innervates the upper lid, forehead, and some superior conjunctiva. The main sensory nerve to the eyeball is the nasociliary branch. This nerve divides in the posterior orbit into the infratrochlear, which supplies the lacrimal sac, the conjunctiva, the skin of both lids, and the root of the nose. The nasal nerve, however, supplies the most critical structures of all (Fig. 14). Along the sympathetic branches from the ciliary ganglion it innervates the sclera, cornea, iris, ciliary body, and choroid via the long and short ciliary nerves (as well as the less critical but diagnostically helpful tip of the nose (Hutchinson's sign) via the nasal nerve proper. It is by direct neural connection to the many structures of the eye, both external and internal, and by direct spread through the orbital tissues to other cranial and to autonomic nerves that the zoster virus is able to cause such a wide variety and severity of disease. These include cicatricial lid retraction, paralytic ptosis, conjunctivitis, scleritis, keratitis, iridocyclitis, retinitis (hemorrhagic vasculitis with or without retinal detachment), choroiditis, optic neuritis and

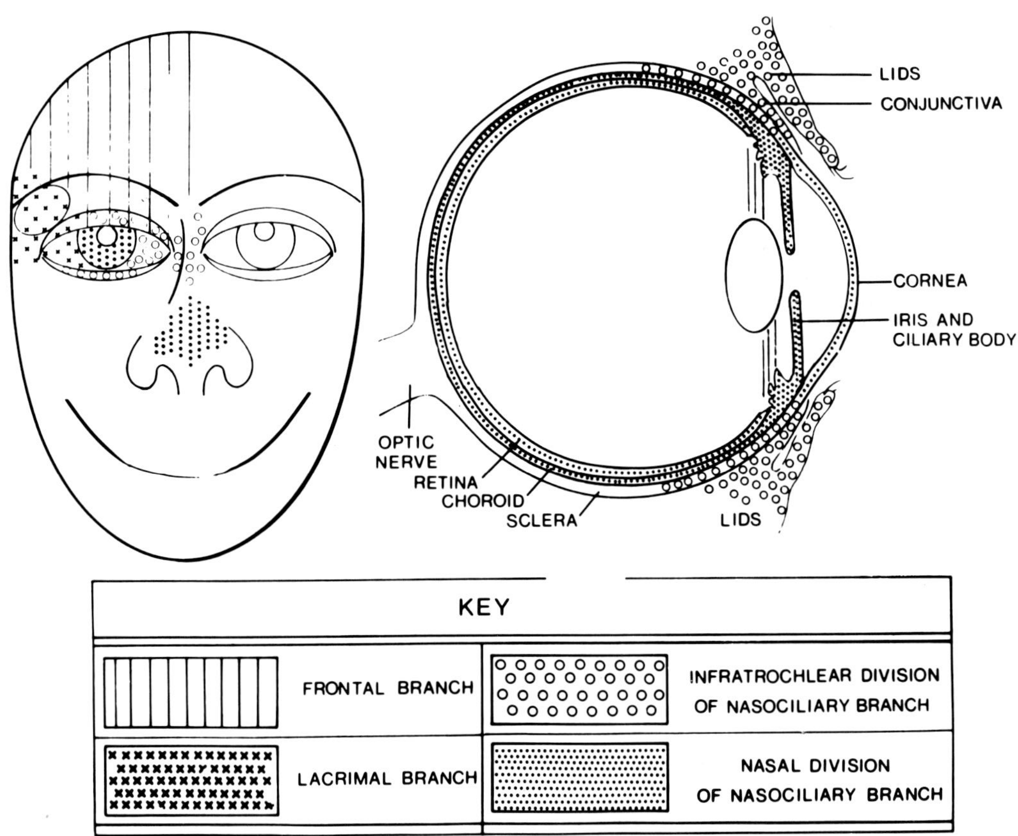


**FIG. 14.** Neuronal relations of the 1st division of the trigeminal nerve (CR VII). (From Pavan-Langston, ref. 199, with permission.)

atrophy, retrobulbar neuritis, Argyll Robertson pupil, exophthalmos, partial or complete third-nerve palsy, isolated pupillary paralysis, fourth- and sixth-nerve palsies, acute and chronic glaucoma, and even sympathetic ophthalmia (116,121,123).

## Clinical Disease

### Conjunctivitis and Scleritis

Conjunctival involvement is common and may be watery hyperemia with petechial hemorrhages, follicular conjunctivitis with regional adenopathy, or severe necrotizing membranous inflammation. Scleritis may be diffuse, associated with keratitis or iritis, or appear as focal elevated tender nodules during the acute disease or 2–3 months after the cutaneous eruption has cleared. As these resolve, scleral thinning and staphyloma formation are not unusual. One striking complication of HZO is the development of perilimbal ischemia, which may be 360°, resulting in anterior segment ischemic necrosis (Fig. 15). This may come years after the initial insult, may be due to vasculitis, and appears responsive to systemic steroid therapy.

### Keratitis

The keratitis that occurs in approximately 66% of all patients with HZO causes marked decrease in corneal sensation, may assume many forms, and even may precede or follow by several weeks the neuralgia or other skin lesions. It may be a fine or coarse punctate epithelial keratitis with or without stromal edema, giving the cornea a groundglass appearance. More frequently, there will be actual group vesicle formation

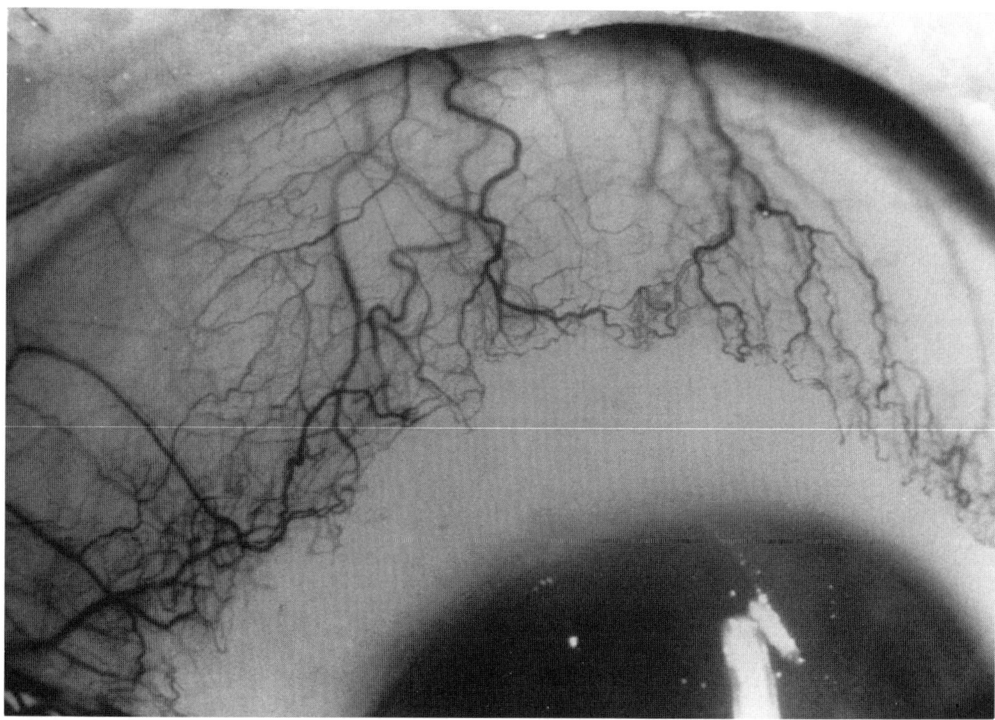

**FIG. 15.** Severe herpes zoster episcleritis with occlusion of all perilimbal vessels resulting in anterior ischemic necrosis and corneal ulceration.

with ulceration that is dendritic in pattern and easily mistaken for herpes simplex keratitis (124). Zoster has been isolated from these dendritic lesions by Pavan-Langston and McCulley (125) (Fig. 16). They described two lesions as Medusa-like in pattern and a third zoster dendrite as gray and linear, appearing to be "painted on" the surface of the cornea. The dendrites cleared rapidly on idoxuridine or steroid therapy, leaving mild anterior stromal nebulae. Piebenga and Laibson (126) described similar lesions in 13 patients and noted that they seemed to be gray, heaped up, superficial, plaque-like formations that were coarser than simplex dendrites, lacking in terminal bulbs, and staining poorly with fluorescein. The authors were not able to culture zoster virus from these dendrites, but negative serum antibodies for herpes simplex and florid zosteriform dermal involvement strongly supported the diagnosis of zoster dendritic keratitis.

Rarely chronic serpiginous ulceration may occur; in particularly devastating disease, the entire corneal epithelial surface may slough. The stroma in these severe cases is usually diffusely cloudy and edematous and epithelial healing quite slow. Corneal thinning and perforation may supervene in situations where neither epithelium nor vascularized pannus moves across to cover the corneal surface.

Stromal keratitis, disciform or diffuse, may occur in conjunction with or entirely independent of any epithelial disease. This edematous interstitial inflammation may smolder for months and induce neovascularization unless controlled with topical steroids (Fig. 17). It is indistinguishable from simplex stromal keratitis in clinical appearance and probably represents an immune response similar to that seen with chronic simplex, but this is not established with certainty (43,116,121,123,127).

Neuroparalytic ulceration similar to that seen after trigeminal-nerve ablation may develop slowly without any spontaneous cicatrization—in which case corneal thinning and perforation may ensue—or with dense

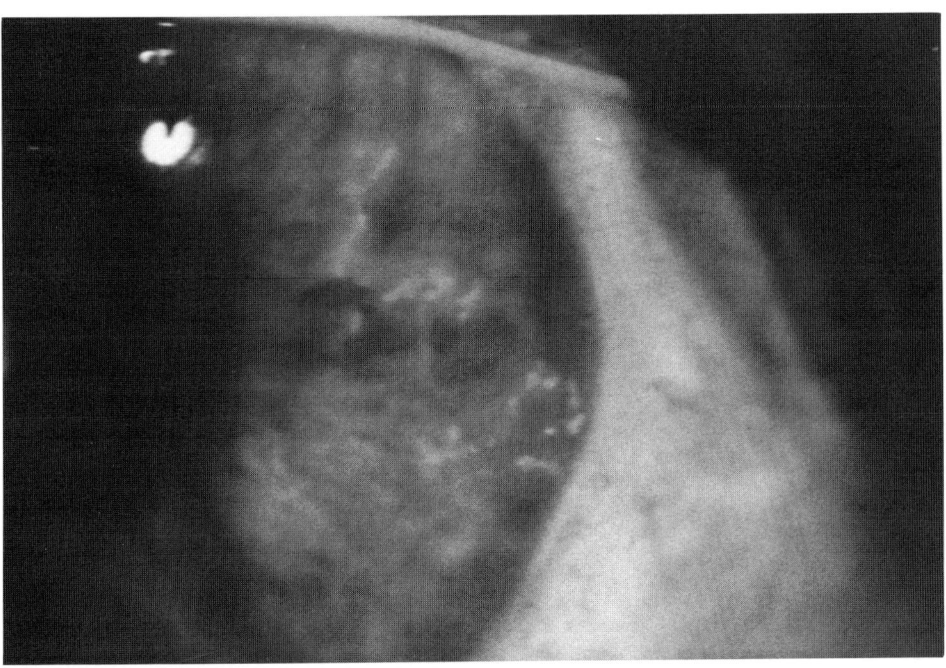

**FIG. 16.** Herpes zoster virus linear dendritic ulcerations.

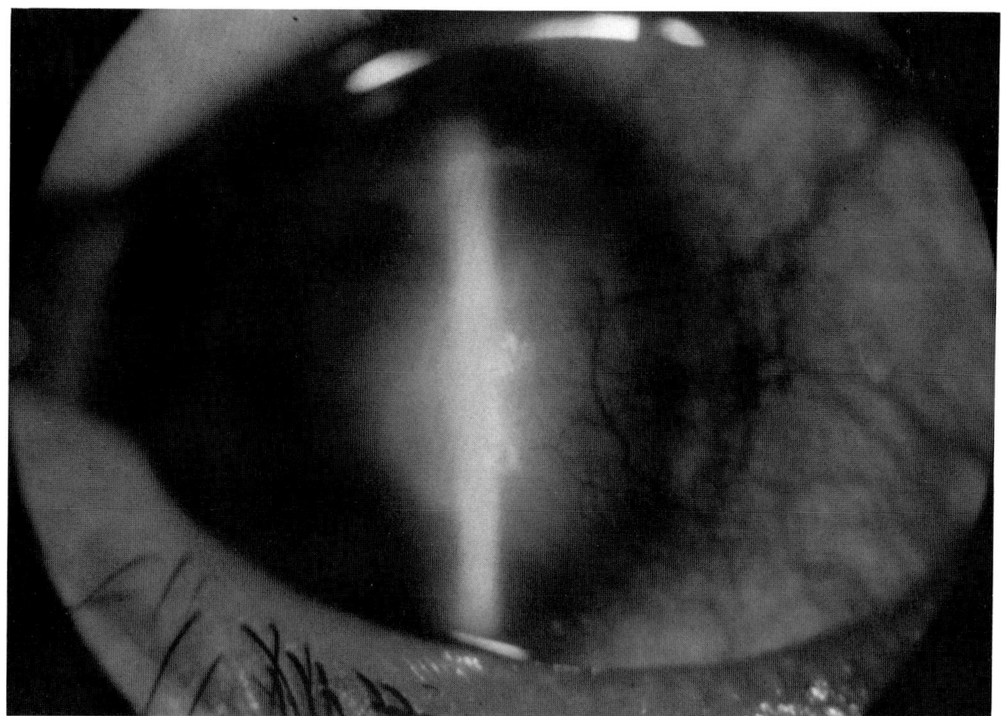

**FIG. 17.** Herpes zoster combined viral interstitial and disciform keratitis with dense neovascularization. Cornea is anesthetic.

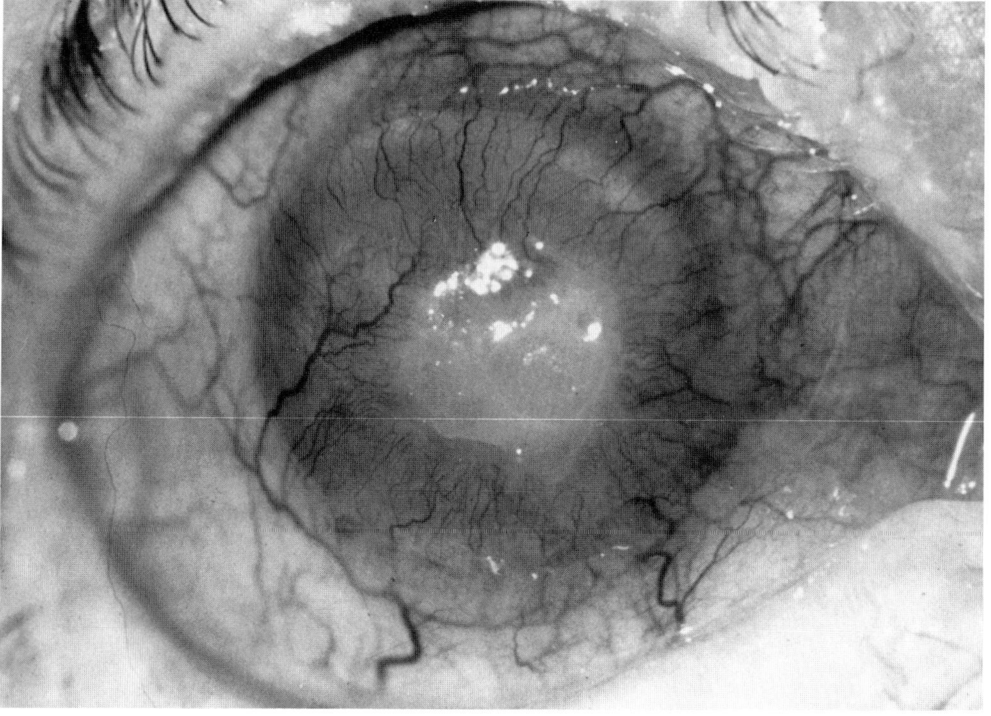

**FIG. 18.** Herpes zoster virus neurotrophic keratopathy with neovascular pannus moving to cover trophic central ulceration.

**TABLE 2.** *Incidence of anterior segment findings in HZO*[a]

| Finding | Incidence (%) |
|---|---|
| Punctate keratitis | 51 |
| Pseudodendrites | 51 |
| Anterior stromal infiltrates | 41 |
| Keratouveitis-endotheliitis | 34 |
| Neurotrophic keratitis | 25 |
| Delayed mucous plaques (pseudodendrites) | 13 |
| Exposure keratitis | 11 |
| Disciform keratitis | 10 |
| Serpiginous ulceration | 7 |
| Scleral keratitis | 1 |
| Delayed limbal vasculitis | <1 |

[a]Adapted from Liesgang, ref. 200.

neovascular pannus, which heals but also severely scars the cornea (Fig. 18). Persistent epithelial defects that threaten to thin or those that have actually started to thin may heal under soft contact lens therapy. Very thin lenses, because of their oxygen permeability, are usually most successful. Any vascularization occurring under the lens should probably be allowed to progress, as it may aid in healing the defect. As these neuresthetic corneas are poor surgical risks, it is unlikely that a future keratoplasty would be planned. Paralysis of the sensory root is not invariably accompanied by neurotrophic disease, however, and patients with markedly anesthetic corneas may maintain clear stroma and epithelium. Table 2 summarizes the study by Liesgang reporting the incidence of various corneal complications of HZO in 94 patients (127).

### *Iridocyclitis*

Other than the cornea, the anterior uveal tract is the most frequently affected ocular structure. Involvement may occur late or early in the disease and independent of corneal activity. The iridocyclitis may be characterized by photophobia, ciliary flush, miosis, intense ocular pain, decreased vision, fine keratic precipitates, iris edema and hyperemia, and anterior peripheral and posterior synechiae secondary to a fibrinous exudate.

Histopathologically, the unique characteristic of zoster ophthalmicus is a plasma cell-lymphocyte infiltration of the posterior ciliary nerves and vessels, particularly in the retrobulbar tissue and uveal structures. Zoster iritis differs from simplex iritis in that the former is chiefly a vasculitis whereas the latter is primarily a diffuse lymphocytic infiltrate of iris stroma. The usual iris focal or sector atrophy seen in herpes zoster is the result of the localized ischemic necrosis similar to that seen after acute angle closure glaucoma or excessive diathermy and muscle detachment in retinal surgery (Fig. 19). Hypopyon, hemorrhage into the anterior chamber, sympathetic ophthalmia, and phthisis bulbi may all result from a severe zoster vasculitis and ischemia (121,123,128).

### *Glaucoma*

The marked decrease in intraocular pressure often seen with zoster is probably the result of massive necrosis of the pars plicata of the ciliary body, which caused decreased aqueous production. This may be more than counterbalanced, however, by impairment of outflow facility through clogging of the trabecular meshwork by pigment and cellular debris, acute trabeculitis, or angle closure by synechia formation. In the event of any or all of these, the intraocular pressure may be low, normal, or elevated (121,123,127,128).

### *Herpes Zoster Retinitis and Optic Neuritis*

Zoster retinitis, optic neuritis, and retrobulbar neuritis are rare but may appear during acute disease or weeks to months after the initial dermatologic disease. In a study by Tunis and Tapert (129), 25% of neuritis patients had associated cranial nerve palsies. Clinically, posterior retinal involvement is characterized by severe patchy vas-

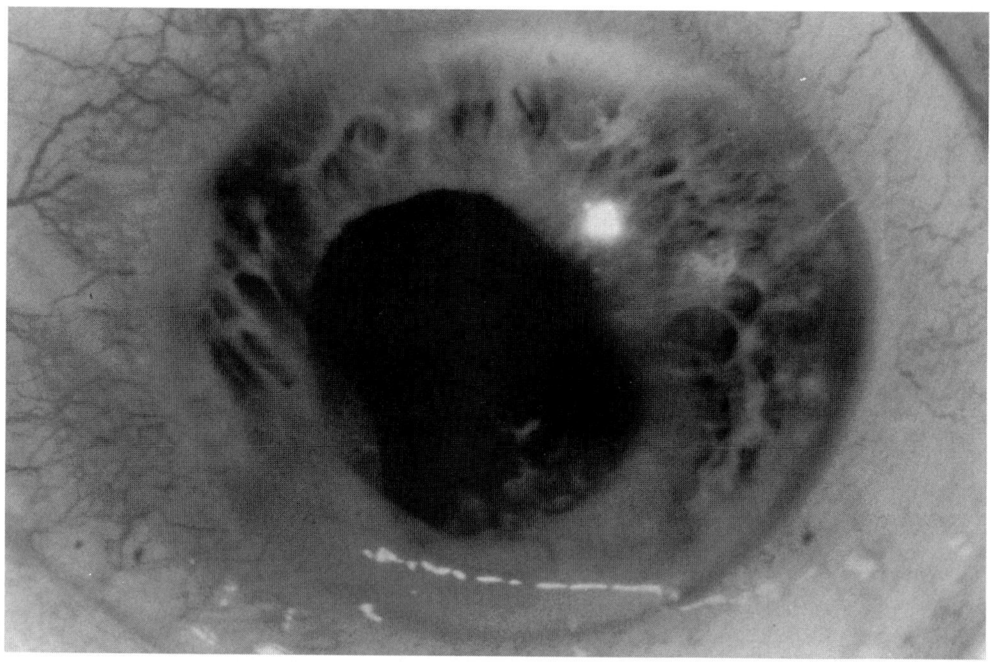

**FIG. 19.** Chronic herpes zoster keratouveitis with iris and pupillary sphincter atrophy and distortion. Lymphocytic keratic precipitates are seen on corneal endothelium inferiorly.

culitis which may lead to focal necrosis. Combined vasculitis and perineuritic reactions block vascular supply to the posterior structures resulting in severe inflammation and damage. A combined mechanism of active viral destruction of retinal and vascular tissues is recognized in combination with retinal endothelial damage and damage to the choriocapillaris through immune complex deposition and obstruction of the fine vessels. Histopathologic studies reveal lymphocytic infiltration in the endoneurium and perineurium of the ciliary nerves, periarteritis, and retinal perivasculitis. Granulomatous choroiditis and arteritis have also been reported (123,130–133). The recently described syndrome acute retinal necrosis (ARN) may be a variant of zoster retinitis as this virus had frequently been noted in association with ARN, unlike CMV or HSV. ARN is responsive to the same therapy given to known zoster retinitis patients (134–137).

The therapy of acute zoster retinitis currently presented in the literature is ACV 500 mg/m$^2$ intravenously every 8 hr for 7 days and is best given within 3 days of onset of the rash. For late onset of zoster, retinitis experience is limited with no established protocol. It would seem reasonable to institute dosage somewhere between that noted above in standard zoster and that for ARN. Therapy of ARN is empirical at ACV dosages of 500 mg/m$^2$ every 8 hr intravenously for 7 days (136). Lesions have resolved with this treatment modality. Low doses of aspirin may be reasonably used as a mild anticoagulant. There is no established therapy for optic neuritis, but systemic steroids may have a role (see therapy summary for doses) (129). The use of ACV in zoster retinitis or ARN has not been approved by the FDA, but the drug is currently under FDA review for therapy of varicella/zoster infections.

During the healing phase, vitreous traction, subretinal fluid accumulation, and retinal detachment are not uncommon. For this reason, pars plana vitrectomy, scleral buckling procedures, laser coagulation, and silicone oil injection may all have a place in the long-term management of this very difficult condition (132,133).

### *HZO Neuralgia*

The acute neuritis experienced by patients during the early phases of the illness is attributed to swelling of the trigeminal nerve in association with a lymphocytic infiltrate as well as the pain of inflammatory reaction in and around the eye itself. Postherpetic neuralgia is seen in approximately 17% of patients and appears to be secondary to inflammatory scarring of nerves (123,128,138–140). Milder cases will resolve spontaneously within 2–4 weeks and moderate ones over several months to 1–2 years but often with residual dysesthesia in the area of the dermatome. Severe postherpetic neuralgia fortunately is rare but may to some extent be permanent and incapacitating. Children and young adults may have acute neuralgic pain but do not develop the chronic incapacitating long-term neuralgia seen in older patients or the immunocompromised. It is because of the risk of long-term pain secondary to scarring of the nerves that systemic steroids may still maintain a place in the therapy of selected patients. Although steroids appear to reduce the incidence of postherpetic neuralgia, the issue is still controversial (122,138,139,141). Trials with systemic ACV, although effective in ocular disease, have had no effect on postherpetic neuralgia (7,8). Management of both neuralgia and ocular zoster are discussed below.

## *Medical Treatment of HZO*

### *Antiviral Drugs*

There is currently no evidence to suggest that HZO is clinically responsive to the commercially available topical antiviral medications despite susceptibility *in vitro*. McGill et al. (142–144) reported several studies indicating that topical 5% ACV five times daily was highly effective in resolving epithelial keratitis and preventing recurrences in comparison to 63% of controlled patients receiving topical steroids. Additionally, the combination of ACV and steroids was less effective than ACV alone. There was no significant difference in resolution of stromal keratitis, scleritis, iritis, or secondary glaucoma among any groups, ACV alone or ACV-steroid. While encouraging, these data are yet to be confirmed in other medical centers. Similarly, BVDU has been reported effective both topically and systemically in HZO, but potential mutagenesis had precluded the clinical trial of this drug in the United States (26).

Of greater interest and immediate use is systemic ACV in therapy of herpes zoster. Shepp et al. (145) reported that intravenous ACV is significantly better than ara-A in therapy of zoster infections in immunocompromised patients presenting within 72 hr of onset of disease. Two of the 22 patients had cranial involvement; both received ACV. ACV dosage of 500 mg/m$^2$ body surface area every 8 hr as a 1-hr infusion compared to ara-A dosage of 10 mg/kg body weight as a single 12-hr infusion for 7 days resulted in significantly shortened periods of positive virus cultures, new lesion formation, duration of pain and fever, pustulation, crusting, and healing of all lesions. Toxicity in ACV-treated patients was minimal with hematologic changes frequent but not necessitating change in treatment. Three of 11 patients had an increase in creatinine levels, which may, in fact, have been due to concomitant cyclosporine therapy. Cobo et al. (7,8) studied oral ACV in a masked, controlled clinical trial in 55 immunocompetent patients with acute HZO given either placebo or ACV 600 mg by mouth five times daily for 10 days. In comparison to controls, those patients treated within 72 hr of onset had a prompt resolution of skin rash and virus shedding and a marked reduction in incidence of episcleritis, keratitis, and iritis. Systemic and local toxicity was insignificant. Unfortunately, long-term follow-up indicated no beneficial effect on postherpetic neuralgia. Nonetheless, because of the favorable results in these studies, the current literature recommends that patients with acute zoster ophthalmicus be given ACV 600 mg by mouth five times a day for maximum control and resolution of this illness in both immunocompetent and immunocompromised patients. Use of systemic ACV in therapy of herpes zoster is currently under FDA review for approval.

In comparison to systemic antivirals, then, the role of topical antivirals appears reserved for those patients presenting with dendritic keratitis in whom the differentiation from herpes simplex is not absolutely clear. If the diagnosis is secure (and this may be ascertained by the Herpchek test; see section on diagnostic tests above) and in the absence of commercially available topical ACV, there appears to be little or no indication for topical antivirals in the management of HZO.

### *Corticosteroids*

Reports by Pavan-Langston and McCulley (125) and by Piebenga and Laibson (126) of the successful treatment of zoster dendritic keratitis with topical steroids alone would suggest that these drugs have a beneficial effect on anterior segment zoster and that topical antivirals may not be indicated. In 1967, Berghaust and Westerby (146) recorded 45 cases of HZO treated with topical steroids and antibiotics. There was a marked reduction in corneal infiltrates and anterior uveitis in this group in comparison to 25 nonsteroid controls and no adverse side effects.

The point of greatest contention at present is whether steroids should be administered systemically. In general, the literature pertinent to the use of systemic steroids in this disease is favorable. In 1970, Scheie (121) reported a study of 87 patients with HZO treated with topical steroids and intravenous adrenocorticotropic hormone (ACTH) or systemic corticosteroids. He found this regimen to be more effective in rapid control of pain and in reducing the incidence and severity of keratitis, uveitis, and secondary glaucoma. No patient disseminated the infection; postherpetic neuralgia developed in 16 patients and recurrent steroid-sensitive keratitis in four.

All these data compared favorably with those of Carter and Royds (141), who used prednisone in HZO to reduce edema and scarring but did not succeed in reducing the incidence of postherpetic neuralgia, possibly because of relatively low doses of drug.

However, in 1964, Elliott (147) reported the treatment of zoster with high doses of prednisone. Sixteen patients (11 with truncal, two with geniculate, and three with ophthalmic disease) were begun on 60 mg/day from 1 to 10 days after the onset of the rash. In comparison to the 10 control patients, the pain lasted only 3½ days, as opposed to 3½ weeks. There were no cases of postherpetic neuralgia in the treated group, as opposed to two cases in the controls. Dissemination of the disease did not occur. Furthermore, Elliott (147) noted that the earlier treatment was started the better, preferably within 2 weeks of onset. Beginning therapy after the sixth week was ineffective, presumably because scarring around the nerves had already taken place. In addition, the use of low doses of steroids was of no value; i.e., 15 mg of prednisone was as effective as no treatment at all.

In one masked controlled study by Keczkes and Basheer (139) on the effect of systemic steroid on postherpetic neuralgia, 40 otherwise healthy herpes zoster patients treated with 40 mg prednisone by mouth daily tapered over 4 weeks did significantly better than a control series treated with carbamazepine. Of the control group, 65% developed postherpetic neuralgia lasting up to 2 years, with only 15% of the prednisone group developing neuralgia which lasted only up to 6 months. There was no dissemination of disease.

Contrary to these findings, Esmann et al. (138) reported that high-dose oral prednisolone even in combination with oral ACV does not prevent postherpetic neuralgia. Seventy-eight patients, 60 years or older, with acute herpes zoster infections of less than 4 days duration, were treated prospectively in a double-blind masked study receiving either 225 mg prednisolone or calcium lactate over a 10-day period plus acyclovir 300 mg by mouth five times daily for 7 days. Twelve of these patients had HZO. Although the steroids relieved the acute pain during the first 3 days of treatment, the long-term results were not significantly different among treatment groups. At 6 months, approximately 23% of both placebo- and steroid-treated patients had persistent neuralgia. Of the 78 patients entering the study, 29% of the trigeminal patients but only 22% of the nontrigeminal patients still suffered pain. In many patients, the onset of pain did not develop until 1–2 weeks after entry into the study, and there was no difference between treatment groups.

Also aligned against the proponents of systemic steroids are those who cite the work of Merselis et al. (148), who reported 17 cases of dissemination of zoster while the patients were on steroids. A closer look at his figures, however, reveals that 11 of these patients had immunologically crippling disease, such as leukemia and lymphoma; of these, four died of zoster. Of the six patients with no underlying illness, only two had received any steroids. These six basically healthy patients all underwent an illness similar to chicken pox and recovered without sequelae.

With the spread of the AIDS epidemic and the fact that zoster ophthalmicus is an early presenting sign of this syndrome, there will be an ever-increasing need to evaluate immunocompetence and restrict the use of steroids in those patients manifesting immunodeficiency of whatever cause (120,149).

### *Cimetidine*

Cimetidine (Tagamet) is currently marketed for therapy of gastrointestinal ulcers, but in two small studies it has been useful in the relief of discomfort, edema, and erythema of acute early HZO. The mechanism of action is postulated as both a histamine blockade ($H_2$ receptors) and an immunomodulating effect in the form of augmented human lymphocyte blastogenesis and inhibition of suppressor T cells (150,151). It is of note that ranitidine, a close relative of cimetidine, is not bound by receptor sites on human lymphocytes as is cimetidine (152).

In two open studies, cimetidine 300–400 mg by mouth four times daily for 7 days resulted in rapid relief of pain, itching, and erythema and resolution of vesicles if given within 72 hr of onset of disease or before ulceration of the vesicles. The drug was effective in both immunocompromised and immunocompetent patients. A third control study reported no significant effect of the drug on these parameters, but dosage was lower and follow-up of patients less complete (150,151,153). Further controlled studies to ascertain the efficacy of cimetidine are needed.

### *Levodopa*

Levodopa has been investigated in a double-masked study on the effects of relief of acute and intermediate term zoster neuralgia (154). Therapy involved 100 mg levodopa three times a day with meals and 25 mg benserazide (a peripheral decarboxylase inhibitor) or placebo for 10 days. There was a marked decrease in pain after 3 days of treatment and total cessation of pain and sleep disturbance in the treated group by the end of the treatment. There was also a marked reduction in herpetic neuralgia at 2 months in the treated group compared to the untreated, but numbers were too small for statistical significance. The major side effect of nausea and vomiting could be avoided by titrating up to full dosage over 3–4 days. The mechanism by which this drug works is not known, but it is postulated that it interferes with brain peptides such as the endorphins via its action on the dopaminergic neurons.

### *Surgical Intervention*

Surgical intervention for HZO is most common for exposure keratopathy of the anesthetic cornea. If lid structures are basically intact but closure is incomplete because of scarring, a lateral tarsorrhaphy will frequently suffice to protect the globe. If lid tissue has been lost, plastic reconstruction involving the swinging of flaps may be required. Such procedures are often difficult because the remaining tissues are friable and hold sutures poorly.

Additional indications for lateral tarsorrhaphy are the anesthetic eye which may not be exposed but which, because of loss of innervation, manifests gray unhealthy epithelium with impending breakdown (Fig. 20). It is *not* advisable to use therapeutic soft contact lenses in these eyes as the lens itself may induce epithelial breakdown in an eye which may have remained intact had tarsorrhaphy alone with artificial tear lubricants been used.

If the epithelium does break and corneal thinning ensues, sealing the defect with sterile cyanoacrylate tissue adhesive as described under trophic ulcer in herpes simplex keratitis will frequently suffice to allow healing and ultimate dislodging of the adhesive. An alternative but more extensive surgical procedure involves the pulling down of a conjunctival flap or conjunctival transplant (95,96).

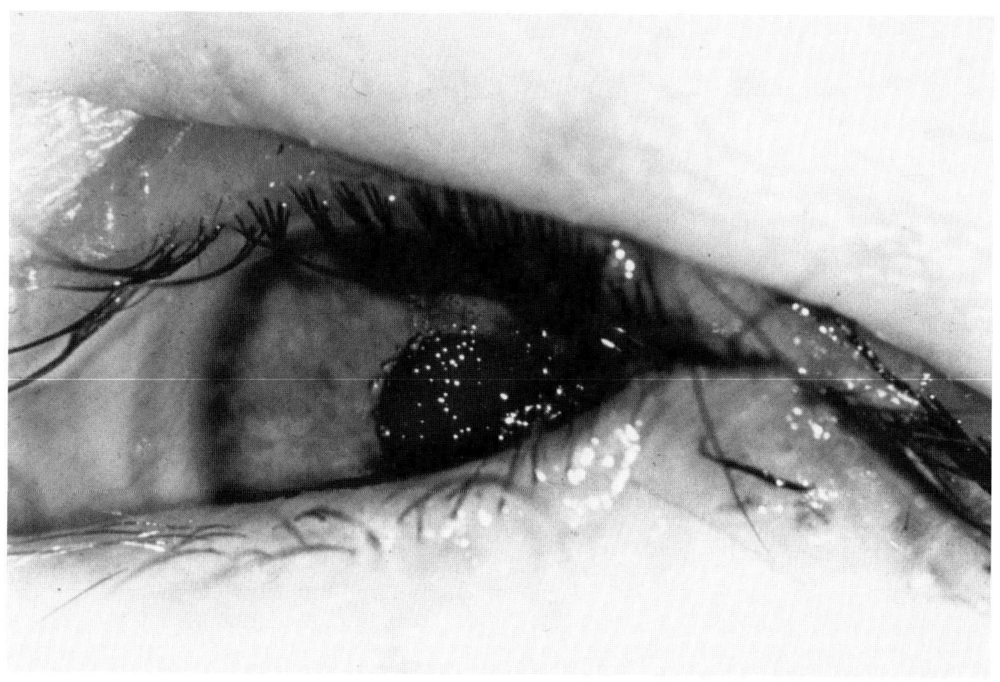

**FIG. 20.** Lateral tarsorrhaphy to protect herpes zoster-induced anesthetic cornea from ulcerating.

Corneal transplantation has a limited place in HZO. As the majority of these eyes are anesthetic, the corneas heal poorly and the transplanted eye is prone to melting and superinfection. A scarred cornea that has retained a reasonable amount of sensation may be considered a candidate for such a surgical procedure, however. If possible, other elective major surgical procedures such as cataract extraction should not be attempted for 2–3 years after the disease has become quiescent. The longer surgery is deferred on these eyes, the better. Should surgical intervention become necessary for removal of a dangerous mature cataract before the 3-year period or while the eye is inflamed, the pars plana approach may be more advisable.

### *Summary of Therapeutic Approaches to HZO*

The following therapeutic guidelines are currently recommended in management of HZO:

(a) Acute inflammatory disease
- (i) Mild or no pain or ocular involvement: warm compresses to keep involved skin clean and minimize scarring.
- (ii) For moderate to severe corneal disciform disease with intact epithelium or for iritis: topical steroids (1/8% prednisolone two to four times a day up to 0.1% dexamethasone in the same frequency, as warranted by disease). Taper over several weeks.
- (iii) Antiviral ointment or drops if topical steroids are used during the acute ulcerative phase when there is a question that herpes simplex may be mimicking zoster.
- (iv) Topical antibiotic during use of topical steroids or if ulcer is present.
- (v) Cycloplegics as needed for iritis.
- (vi) Acyclovir (Zovirax) 200 mg, three tablets by mouth, five times daily for 10 days preferably starting within 72 hr of onset of disease in immunocompetent patients. Intravenous ACV 500 mg/m$^2$ body surface area every 8 hr over 1-hr infusion for 7 days in immunocompromised patients. (ACV is under FDA review for use in zoster infections.)
- (vii) Cimetidine, 300 mg by mouth four times a day for 14 days starting within 72 hr of onset of disease. (Not FDA approved for zoster infections.)
- (viii) Artificial tears and ointment for unstable tear film or exposure keratitis.
- (ix) Nonnarcotic or narcotic analgesics for neuralgia on days 1 through 7–10 for significant neuralgia. If no resolution of pain at this time, consider instituting systemic steroid in the immunologically competent patient. Dosage described in the literature is prednisone 20 mg by mouth three times a day for 7 days, then 15 mg twice a day for 7 days, then 15 mg daily for 7 days, and continue mydriatics, cycloplegics, and topical steroids as needed. Monitor frequently for disseminated infection with internist or dermatologist. Systemic steroids are not FDA approved for this condition.

(b) Long-term or chronic problems
- (i) Therapeutic soft contact lenses, cyanoacrylate glue (not FDA approved for use in corneal ulcers), partial tarsorrhaphy, conjunctival flap or transplant, as described for exposure or corneal thinning.
- (ii) Nonnarcotic analgesics for mild to moderate neuralgia or discomfort. Consider trigeminal block or ablation for severe incapacitating neuralgia of several months duration per neurosurgical opinion.

## EBV OCULAR INFECTIONS

The EBV, a ubiquitous member of the herpesvirus family, is the etiologic agent of infectious mononucleosis and strongly associated with African Burkitt's lymphoma and nasopharyngeal carcinoma. The virus has an affinity for B lymphocytes, transforming them *in vitro* into lymphoblasts capable of continuous cultivation (155). Ophthalmic manifestations of EBV infection may involve the external eye, choroid, and retina, or neurological structures of the visual system (155–158).

The most common anterior segment finding is a follicular conjunctivitis, usually unilateral, and occurring in up to 38% of mononucleosis patients. Epithelial keratitis may be punctate or mimic herpes simplex as multiple microdendritic ulcers. The EBV virus has been cultured from conjunctival and tear film samples from such a patient with microdendrites (158). Stromal keratitis may be manifested by development of coin-shaped nummular deposits, discrete multifocal pleomorphic or ring-shaped granular anterior opacities separated by clear stroma, or full-thickness, soft, blotchy infiltrates.

The uveal tract may also be involved as manifested by an acute iritis responsive to topical steroids or a relcalcitrant chronic smoldering focal or pan chorioretinitis with development of secondary cataract and macular edema. It is not uncommon for the inflammatory disease to develop several months after onset of acute mononucleosis.

Neurologic lesions affecting the eye include optic neuritis, papilledema, convergence insufficiency, and extraocular muscle paresis. These all may resolve without treatment (157).

Appropriate therapy for ocular EBV infections is still ill defined, and many manifestations such as conjunctivitis and epithelial keratitis self-resolve. Intraocular inflammation may or may not respond well to topical or systemic steroids, or both in combination. Wong et al. (158) reported three cases of chronic EBV systemic infection with ocular manifestations ranging from keratitis and iritis responsive to 1% prednisolone drops four times a day over a 3-week period to severe panuveitis recalcitrant to topical and systemic steroids. In one patient, prednisone was discontinued, and oral ACV 600 mg by mouth five times daily was instituted without great success over a 10-month period despite concomitant topical and systemic steroids. At that time topical 3% ACV ointment four times a day was added to the systemic ACV regimen. Over the ensuing 5 months of combined topical and systemic ACV and steroids, there was marked clearing of the ocular inflammatory disease.

Whether ACV has a role in therapy of ocular EBV infection is still undetermined. Although the organism lacks a virus-specific thymidine kinase, EBV DNA polymerase is sensitive to the drug. Topical application of ACV in rabbit eyes, however, results in aqueous and vitreous drug levels that are subtherapeutic for EBV, and subconjunctival injection produces only transiently adequate levels (159). Clearly, much work remains in developing effective therapy for this potentially severe ocular infection.

## AIDS

### Virus and Immune Alterations

AIDS is a transmissible viral infection of the cellular immune system characterized by multiple recurring, often severe opportunistic infections with or without neoplasms or neuropsychiatric disorders, usually in relatively young people in previous good health (160–165). The etiologic agent is the human immunodeficiency virus HIV-1. Patients may be culture- or antibody-positive. The agent and general disease manifestations are discussed further in other chapters of this volume.

Striking immunologic abnormalities occur in the infected T-helper lymphocyte population. This includes reduced lymphokine production, inhibition of mitogen and antigen response, depressed clonal expansion, and decreased ability to assist B lymphocytes in immunoglobulin production. The ocular disease seen in AIDS is probably related to the finding that B lymphocytes in AIDS patients are polyclonally activated and spontaneously secrete antibody. This results in elevated total serum immunoglobulin levels, primarily immunoglobulin G (IgG) and IgA, and results in circulating immune complexes. These B lymphocytes do not, however, respond to the normal signals for proliferation and differentiation, and do not usually respond to common immunizations or new antigens. Monocytes also appear refractory to normal signals and lose their chemotactic migratory abilities as well as their ability to kill certain target cells and to secrete interleukin I. Natural killer cell immune surveillance and virus-specific T cytotoxic lymphocyte function are also impaired. This progressive decline of the immune function results in the eye being subject to multiple opportunistic infections not seen prior to this epidemic as well as to unusual malignancies normally held in check by an intact immune surveillance system (101,103, 104,166,167).

### Ophthalmic Manifestations

The ocular findings in AIDS patients have both prognostic and diagnostic significance. Ocular signs include keratitis, conjunctivitis, Kaposi's sarcoma, retinal cotton wool spots, retinal hemorrhages, Roth spots, microaneurysms, ischemic maculopathy, retinal periphlebitis, and papilledema. Etiologic agents in opportunistic infectious retinitis include HSV, VZV, CMV, cryptococcus, toxoplasma, *Candida*, and *Mycobacterium avium-intracellulare* choroidal granulomas. AIDS patients with ocular manifestations are often significantly more immunosuppressed than those without eye findings (102–104,107,168).

#### *Anterior Segment Findings*

Involvement of the anterior segment of the eye is less common but includes ocular herpes, herpes-like ulcerations, diffuse keratitis, and Kaposi's sarcoma (105,106). The ocular herpes seen in AIDS patients is similar to that described earlier in this chapter, and management is the same. In addition, some cases of severe bilateral keratitis similar to herpetic geographic ulceration have been reported in AIDS patients. Immunofluorescence (IF) studies at autopsy, however, failed to reveal any HSV antigen, thus raising the question as to whether this was truly herpetic or secondary to invasion by HIV. HZO has also been reported as a presenting symptom in previously undiagnosed AIDS patients (120,149). The disease is similar to that noted earlier in the section on herpes zoster, and management is described there.

The keratitis seen in AIDS patients other than that described above may simply be a diffuse punctate keratitis that is transient and may be associated with a marked anterior iritis requiring intensive topical steroid therapy. Conjunctivitis seen in AIDS patients is nonspecific with diffuse hyperemia of the eyes, irritation, and tearing. This is transient in nature. HIV-1 has been isolated from the tears, conjunctiva, and corneal epithelium of AIDS patients. This poses an epidemiologic concern not only in that the eye may be an as yet unproven source of infectious virus but also in the implications for corneal transplantation. Eye banks now screen all potential donors for HIV-1, but, as noted below, screening tests are not completely reliable (169–171).

Kaposi's sarcoma occurs in approximately 9% of AIDS patients and may involve the eyelid or conjunctiva (106). The conjunctival involvement occurs in about 10% of AIDS patients and is most frequently found in the inferior cul-de-sac. It will be missed without retraction of the lower lid on examination. Sarcoma of the lid presents as a bright red subconjunctival mass which may appear to be a subconjunctival hemorrhage. These masses may be focal nodules or diffuse infiltrative lesions.

Sarcoma therapy includes local cryotherapy, radiotherapy, and local excision. There is no well-established treatment mode for this local ocular manifestation of the tumor because of the high mortality rate in these patients who invariably have numerous other systemic problems.

### *Fundus Disease*

HIV vasculopathy frequently presents as cotton wool spots that appear as white, fluffy, nerve fiber layer opacities secondary to ischemia-induced axoplasmic stasis (103,172). They are the most common ocular finding in AIDS patients and tend to be transient, often resolving over a several-week period. Similar but unrelated lesions may be seen in hypertension, diabetes, systemic lupus erythematosus, anemia, and leukemia. Fluorescein angiography of these eyes shows areas of capillary nonperfusion, and histopathology reveals thickened and occluded capillaries with microaneurysms characteristic of a retinal vasculopathy that may produce extensive retinal ischemia. Perivasculitis of retinal vessels not associated with CMV has also been noted in AIDS patients. Immunofluorescence studies indicate that AIDS viral antigen is present within retinal endothelial cells and neuroretinal cells at all layers. One case has been reported in which a particle morphologically similar to HIV was demonstrated by electron microscopy in the retina of a patient with AIDS and CMV retinitis (173), and Cantrill et al. (166) have isolated HIV from iris, retina, and vitreous. Pepose et al. (103,104) has found double and triple infections of the retina with HIV-1, HSV, and CMV. It is felt that the retinal microvasculopathy seen in AIDS patients is related to vascular damage from the immune complex deposition. As inflammatory cells are not seen in areas of cotton wool spot formation, however, the mechanism of damage is unknown (103,104).

A variety of other retinal findings in AIDS patients have been reported (103) (Fig. 11). These include retinal hemorrhage in areas without CMV infection (40%), CMV retinitis (34%) often with associated retinal detachment, Roth spots (white spots with red centers thought to be embolic) (23%), retinal microaneurysms (20%), papilledema (14%), cryptococcal chorioretinitis (6%), *Mycobacterium avium-intracellulare* in retinal and choroidal granulomas (6%), ischemic maculopathy (6%), and herpes simplex retinitis (3%). Ocular infection with *Candida* and toxoplasmosis have also been reported and are thought to be more associated with intravenous drug abusers than with patients who have acquired AIDS sexually (103,104,120). CMV, the most common viral retinitis in these patients, is discussed more extensively under that category.

### *Therapy*

At present there is no means of curing the patient infected with AIDS virus. The antiviral drug AZT has been found to inhibit viral replication and prolong survival in patients diagnosed as having *Pneumocystis carinii* pneumonia (15,16). AZT is taken orally and crosses the blood-brain barrier, thus making it useful in AIDS-induced neurological disease and implying that the blood-eye barrier, which is similar, may also be crossed (174). Unfortunately, it may cause significant bone marrow suppression, particularly of red blood cell precursors, but does reverse HIV-induced thrombocytopenia.

Farrell et al. (14) have recently reported

a case of chronic iridocyclitis and anterior vitritis poorly responsive to high-dose topical and systemic steroids in a drug abuser with known HIV infection. Eleven weeks after initiation of steroid therapy, aqueous humor was tapped for culture, and therapy with oral AZT 100 mg four times a day was initiated. Steroids were tapered. Aqueous humor culture supernatants contained 220 pg HIV p 24 antigen/ml. After 10 days of AZT therapy, the intraocular disease had markedly diminished, and the AZT dosage was increased to 200 mg every 4 hr for two additional weeks with no resulting hematologic toxicity. At this time, visual acuity had improved from 20/200 to 20/20, and the inflammation was essentially resolved. Although it may be postulated that resolution of the iridocyclitis was due to a general improvement in the patient's immune status, it was felt that the beneficial results of AZT were due directly to antiviral effect as neither the absolute T-cell counts nor the helper/suppression ratios changed during the therapeutic period.

Perhaps the greatest step forward in the therapy of AIDS has been in the use of DHPG in the management of CMV infection. This is discussed under the section on CMV retinitis. Neither systemic ACV nor ara-A have been found effective against AIDS virus. In addition, ACV and AZT have an adverse interaction inducing deep somnolence in patients taking this drug combination (13).

Unfortunately, because of the mechanisms of disease in the eye, whether circulating immune complex-mediated or opportunistic infection, ocular disease in the AIDS patient has a very poor prognosis for the eye as well as for the patient. Those patients presenting with cytomegalovirus retinitis, for example, are often dead within 4 months of presentation of disease unless treated with DHPG. Those with circulating immune complexes do not survive much longer as this complex formation becomes clinically significant only in the very late stages of disease. Our current best hopes for control of disease are through preventive measures in lieu of effective therapy in the near future (10,11,15,103,104).

## ADENOVIRAL INFECTION

The adenoviruses constitute a group of some 35 morphologically similar but serologically distinct DNA viruses that share a common group complement fixing antigen. They are highly stable, ether-resistant organisms measuring 80–120 mm (175,176).

The virus is ubiquitous throughout the world and tends to cause infections of the upper respiratory tract and outer eye. Numerous syndromes are associated with the adenoviruses, but only two are of prime concern in relation to the eye, pharyngoconjunctival fever (PCF) and epidemic keratoconjunctivitis (EKC). Both are highly contagious for 8–12 days.

### PCF

PCF is usually attributed to adenovirus types 3 and 7 but has been associated with a number of other types (adenovirus types 1, 4–6, and 14), being isolated from conjunctiva, nasopharynx, and feces (175,176). It is an acute and highly infectious illness characterized by fever, pharyngitis, and a nonpurulent follicular conjunctivitis often associated with slightly tender preauricular adenopathy. It is seen predominantly in young and institutionalized people, and epidemics occur within families, schools, and military organizations. After an incubation period of 5–8 days, the patient experiences the sudden or gradual onset of fever, which may range from 100°F to 104°F and last up to 10 days. Associated with the fever are malaise, myalgia, and often gastrointestinal disturbances. The pharyngitis is not very painful and is typically a reddened posterior oropharynx covered with glassy follicules with nontender cervix lymphadenopathy.

The chief source of discomfort is the conjunctivitis. It is bilateral, starting in one or both eyes as an itchy, boggy hyperemia with watery discharge. Lymphoid follicles are present and predominate in the lower fornix, making this area somewhat tender to palpation.

A few days after the onset of symptoms a punctate keratitis may appear. This begins as small epithelial dots that stain with fluorescein, and progresses to combined epithelial and subepithelial focal whitish lesions and finally to nonstaining subepithelial infiltrates, which are thought to be antigen/antibody complexes. These are usually scattered in little clumps around the central cornea. The entire illness is generally acute and transient and resolves over a few days to 3 weeks, although the subepithelial infiltrates may last for several months. The patients may spread infectious virus from their mouths and eyes during the first 8–10 days. After this time it becomes more difficult to culture the virus, and one must rely primarily on serologic testing to prove the diagnosis.

No specific treatment has yet been developed. Vaccine prophylaxis is as effective as the immunity after natural infection. This approach, however, is practical more for military use than for the general population. Ara-A and IDU are ineffective (4). Mild topical steroids may offer some comfort by reducing local inflammation but should be used as described below. Other than that, bed rest, aspirin, fluids, and good hygiene are the only therapeutic answers for this short-lived but distressing illness (175,176).

### Epidemic Keratoconjunctivitis

The more serious of the adenoviral illnesses, in relation to the eye, is epidemic keratoconjunctivitis (175–179). This entity is generally associated with adenoviruses types 8 and 19, but a similar clinical picture, without tendency to epidemic, has been produced by other adenovirus types such as 1–3, 7, 9, 10, and 11. Epidemics have been reported sporadically, usually from hospitals, industrial plants, schools, and among families, and most recently type 19 in Philadelphia and Nashville (180,181). The United States seems to be more susceptible to epidemics than the Far Eastern countries, where subclinical infection is more common. In this country only 5% of the adult population have protective antibodies against the virus, in contrast to 30% in Japan and 60% in Taiwan (182).

The disease generally attacks young adults during the fall and winter months. It is unilateral in 66% of the cases and produces few to no systemic symptoms, unlike PCF, which is usually bilateral and associated with fever and sore throat. The incubation period is about 8 days, at which time the lids swell and may become black and blue as if traumatized. The eye becomes very hyperemic, with glassy conjunctival chemosis often starting medially but spreading diffusely. There is a mild foreign-body sensation and watery tearing but not much discomfort. In 75% of the patients, lymphoid follicles develop on the palpebral and bulbar conjunctiva simultaneous with the appearance of a tender preauricular, and occasionally submaxillary and cervical, adenopathy. In those in whom the disease goes on to bilaterality, the second eye becomes involved at about this time but generally much less severely than the first, probably due to partial immune protection at the host (Fig. 21).

The conjunctival involvement may become so severe as to develop extensive pseudomembranes or true membranes, which are friable and may bleed, or symblepharon may scar lid to eye (Fig. 22). The discharge even with this event, however, is still remarkably watery and clear, and the patients are only moderately uncomfortable. Pain comes with development of keratitis, which occurs in approximately 80% of patients and begins around the eighth day, heralded by marked discomfort, pho-

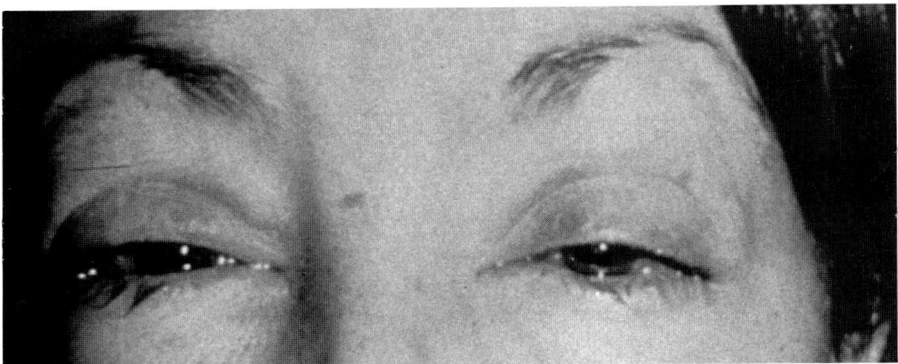

**FIG. 21.** Acute bilateral adenoviral keratoconjunctivitis with characteristic "bleary-eyed" appearance of patient.

tophobia, lacrimation, and blepharospasm. These symptoms persist until the acute keratitis subsides, usually for a week or two, by which time the conjunctivitis has also subsided.

The keratitic disease is typically divided into four stages (177,179). The first stage is the diffuse fine superficial epithelial punctate keratitis, which moves quickly to become a staining focal punctate white epithe-

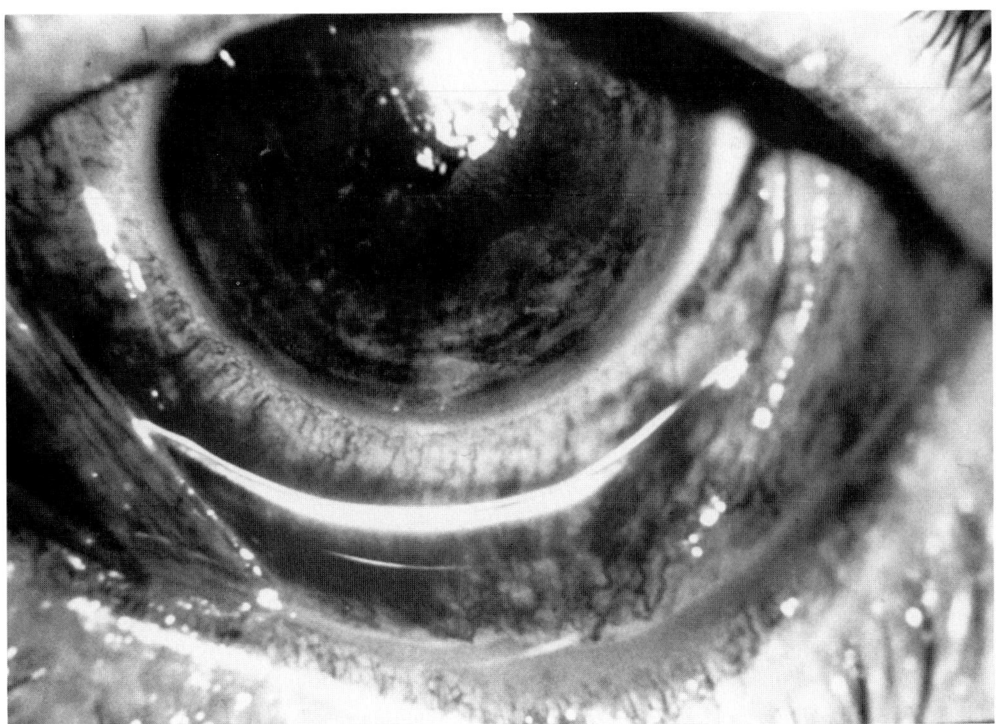

**FIG. 22.** Same patient as in Fig. 21, showing severe adenoviral keratoconjunctivitis with early symblepharon scarring between lid and bulbar conjunctiva.

lial keratitis. Within 24–48 hr these lesions become combined epithelial and subepithelial, and over the next few days become entirely subepithelial white macular lesions that no longer stain with fluorescein (Fig. 23). The keratitis typically involves the central cornea in clumps or rows of macular opacities, but it may reach the periphery. Occasionally the lesions coalesce to form scallop-edged nummular opacities up to 1.5 mm in diameter. In severe cases, geographic epithelial ulceration mimicking herpes simplex may occur (177,178).

Cytological studies have shown the stromal lesions to be clumps of mononuclear cells and polymorphonuclear leukocytes, with degenerative changes in the epithelium, Bowman's membrane, and anterior stroma. The epithelial lesions are thought to be caused by viral infection and the stromal opacities by the antigen/antibody reaction. Very rarely there may be an anterior chamber reaction, but there is no tendency for iris synechia formation in this disease.

During the acute keratitis visual acuity may be reduced from 20/20 to 20/100, which, along with pain, is most distressing to the patient. In general the patient may be reassured, however, that this will improve markedly over the ensuing weeks as the symptoms resolve. The conjunctivitis usually resolves during the second week, but the keratitis may persist for 2–3 months. Rarely, both may persist for 2–3 years. During this time the eye may be slightly red and photophobic, and there may be occasional relapses, but no true infectious recurrences have been reported. Cicatricial conjunctivitis sicca with symblepharon formation may occur rarely. In Dawson's study, 25% of his patients were left with more than 10 subepithelial opacities, which persisted for more than several months (177). Hogan and

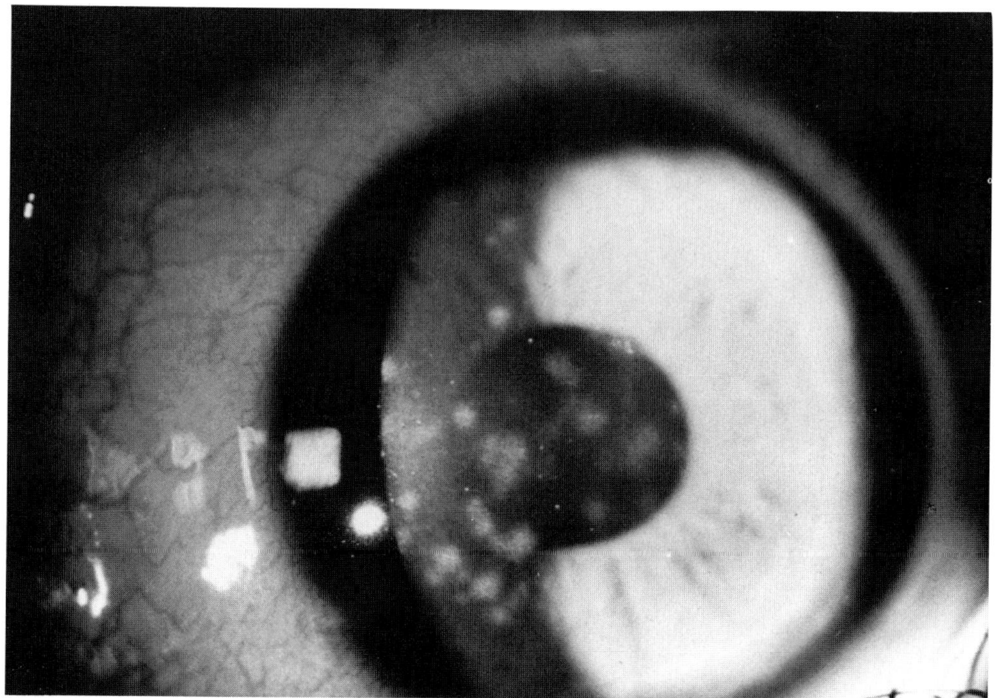

**FIG. 23.** Nonstaining, chronic subepithelial adenoviral corneal stromal infiltrates characteristic of both EKC and PCF.

Crawford's (183) study in 1942 revealed that one could predict the patients who would have severe prolonged keratitis; they were the ones with bilateral involvement who had bilateral onset simultaneously or almost simultaneously. Infectious virus can be recovered up to 8–10 days after the onset of symptoms from approximately 40% of patients. Subsequently, diagnosis must be based on the acute and convalescent serum antibody titers.

As in PCF, treatment is nonspecific and largely supportive. Laboratory tests have indicated that the adenovirus is sensitive to idoxuridine, but clinical studies have not borne this out. EKC treated with IDU or placebo showed no difference in clinical course or outcome (184). Pavan-Langston and Dohlman (4) and Waring et al. (185) have also found vidarabine of little or no use therapeutically. Topical steroids have been advocated by some authors as the treatment of choice for this disease as they do afford some relief to the patient by reducing local edema, inflammatory reaction and the corneal infiltrates. They have no beneficial therapeutic effect on the ultimate clinical outcome. Laibson et al. (178) have shown that the subepithelial infiltrates recur when steroids are discontinued and that only time will resolve their presence.

The therapy of adenoviral keratoconjunctivitis is as follows and generally palliative:

(a) Antivirals are ineffective, except for the preliminary results with interferon (32,33).

(b) Mild topical steroid relieves symptoms and infiltrates temporarily; reserve for more severe cases only (once to three times a day for 1–2 weeks).

(c) Cycloplegics should be used as needed for iritis.

(d) Local antibiotic should be applied.

(e) Ice packs and dark glasses are relieving.

(f) Prophylaxis by physician should be as follows: tonofilm on tonometers and hygiene (wash hands after each patient).

Perhaps one of the most important aspects of this disease for the ophthalmologist is that this epidemic disease is often preventable. A significant number of outbreaks have been traced to ophthalmologists' offices, specifically to the use of a tonometer on an infected patient and then on other patients without interim cleaning (180). To avoid these problems it is recommended that one use a disposable tonofilm cover on the tonometer to preserve the sterility of the instrument if glaucoma testing absolutely must be done during the acute disease. Similarly, careful washing of hands is the key to prevention, because the virus spreads easily from eye to hand to another eye. These measures are especially important during times of known adenovirus epidemics. Ignoring personal hygiene may result in an overload of unhappy patients who can blame their disease on defective medical technique.

## POXVIRUSES

The poxviruses, which include smallpox (variola), vaccinia, and molluscum contagiosum, are a group of large DNA viruses that share a common group antigen. They have a primary affinity for the skin (44,186).

### Molluscum Contagiosum

Molluscum contagiosum causes multiple, umbilicated, wartlike growths along the lid margins (186). The shedding of virus into the tear film results in a serous follicular conjunctivitis and punctate keratitis. Untreated patients may develop vascularized pannus formation of the cornea. Therapy is surgical with removal of the growths by excision, chemical cauterization, or cryotherapy.

### Variola and Vaccinia

Ocular complications in smallpox, a disease now extinct, were not very common but could be devastating (44,187). During the clinical course of the disease, an exanthematous watery conjunctivitis developed around the fifth day. It was usually mild and cleared without complication. In a few cases, however, actual pustules appeared, usually on the bulbar conjunctiva. These were painful with tremendous inflammatory reaction and purulent discharge, and often extended onto the cornea causing inflammation and scarring.

Ocular vaccinia, an organism still used in some laboratory studies, is a derivative of variola and may produce similar disease. Lesions may involve the lids, conjunctiva, and the cornea, the most dangerous being corneal involvement (44,188–191). Patients afflicted with ocular vaccinia may be divided into two categories: the unvaccinated who have primary involvement of the eye, and those who formed some but low antibody titers in response to vaccination. The first group usually suffers the most serious lesions, 30–50% developing keratitis. In the second group, only 10% develop keratitis, and the lid lesions may heal without scarring. The lids are the most common site of autoinoculation because of their very thin skin. Infection of the conjunctiva or cornea are generally but not always secondary to transmission from lid lesions.

In a nonimmune patient, there is an incubation period of approximately 3 days, at which time redness and swelling of the lids increase rapidly, pustules appear, and the eye completely closes as orbital cellulitis develops. The cellulitis is mediated by virus toxin acting on the vascular endothelium in and about the orbit. The viral vascular toxin is rapidly neutralized by passively administered immune globulin. The pre- and postauricular nodes are swollen and tender, and there is extensive ulceration of the lids and conjunctiva. The lids may be covered by punched-out ulcers coated with a necrotic membrane. The acute inflammation lasts for about 10–14 days and then heals with varying amounts of scarring.

Corneal complications, which occur in approximately 30% of cases, are much more serious, ranging from a mild superficial punctate keratitis to a blinding disciform or necrotizing stromal keratitis that may perforate. Virus may be seen developing in the epithelial cells both within and outside the Guarnieri's bodies. Beneath these epithelial gray areas develop yellow opacities in the superficial stroma, ranging from tiny punctate lesions to corneal abscesses of considerable size. At a later stage, deep stromal involvement may appear or suddenly worsen when the epithelium is recovering. This may occur 2–3 months after the original infection. Live virus cannot be isolated from this area of diffuse stromal edema and opacification, and it seems probable that although the initial acute epithelial or stromal lesions are due to a direct viral infection, the later stromal involvements are toxic or immunologic sequelae. This stromal reaction may clear completely or persist as a corneal nebula that may seriously impair vision. In severe active or chronic cases, a corneal transplant may be necessary.

The therapy of ocular vaccinia is as follows (4,190,192–194):

(a) Hyperimmune VIG (VIG, from the American Red Cross), 0.3 ml/lb, or 0.5 ml/kg body weight should be given intramuscularly; repeat in 48 hr if no improvement.

(b) Topical vaccinia immune globulin (100 mg/ml) should be used every 2 hr.

(c) Topical ara-A ointment or trifluridine drops should be given every 4 hr for 7 days minimum; IDU ointment four times a day can be used as a secondary alternative, though it is not FDA approved for this use.

(d) Systemic and topical antibiotic should be used.

(e) Topical steroid for disciform keratitis should be used if epithelium is healed or full antiviral therapy has been in use at least 4 days with favorable clinical response.

(f) Dilate pupil; cleanse eye.

### Acute Hemorrhagic Conjunctivitis

Acute hemorrhagic conjunctivitis (AHC) is a highly contagious ocular infection caused by the enteroviruses, members of the picornavirus family. The enteroviruses include several well-known organisms: poliovirus, Coxsackie A and B, and the echoviruses. The specific enterovirus that most commonly causes the conjunctivitis is type 70 (EV70), but reports from the Far East indicate that other picornaviruses not cross-reacting with antibody against known enteroviruses may also induce the disease (195–197).

AHC may be distinguished from other infections of the external eye both by its proclivity for widespread epidemic proportions and its clinical presentation. It may afflict tens of millions of people in densely populated humid areas of the Far East to several hundred people in Western countries in any given epidemic (198). Epidemics may recur.

The incubation period is 1–2 days, followed by the sudden onset of ocular foreign-body sensation, which may be extremely painful, itching, photophobia, profuse watery discharge, and lid edema. Progression of disease is very rapid over the ensuing 24 hr, with development of pink conjunctival chemosis (edema) and characteristic subconjunctival petechial hemorrhages that appear like concentric ridges encircling the corneal limbus. There is an associated superficial punctate keratitis and preauricular adenopathy, and the entire clinical picture may initially be confused with acute adenoviral keratoconjunctivitis. Systemic symptoms may or may not be present and are described as malaise, myalgia, and upper respiratory tract symptoms similar to influenza. Rarely, there may be a radiculomyelitis.

Fortunately, the disease resolves spontaneously within 2–4 days and is completely gone by 10 days after onset. Antibiotics and steroids have no established effect on the illness. Treatment is, therefore, purely supportive, with bedrest, analgesics, and cool compresses over the closed eyes.

## SUMMARY

Of all the organs of the body, the eye is perhaps the most amenable to new diagnostic and therapeutic technologies. Ocular herpes was the model in which the first effective antiviral, IDU, was evaluated. The eye remains the premier testing ground for many drugs under evaluation today in both experimental and human clinical studies. With the evolution of more specific topical and systemic antiviral agents and the multiple viral infections manifested by ocular disease of the anterior and posterior segment, the prospects for development of effective therapy pertinent to both this and other organ systems remain highly promising in the foreseeable future.

*Added in proof:* The FDA approved (June, 1989) ganciclovir (DHPG) for therapy of CMV retinitis at a dosage of 5 mg/kg intravenously over 1 hr every 12 hr for 14–21 days.

## REFERENCES


1. Fedukowicz HB. *External infections of the eye: bacterial, viral and mycotic*. 2nd ed. New York: Appleton-Century-Crofts, 1978:191–220.
2. Duke-Elder S. The myxoviruses. In: *System of ophthalmology, vol. VIII*. London: Henry Kimpton, 1965:367–71.
3. Pavan-Langston D, Buchanan RA. Vidarabine therapy of simple and IDU-complicated herpetic keratitis. *Trans Am Acad Ophthalmol Otolaryngol* 1976;81:OP813–25.
4. Pavan-Langston D, Dohlman CH. A double-blind clinical study of adenine arabinoside therapy of viral keratoconjunctivitis. *Am J Ophthalmol* 1972;74:81–8.
5. Pavan-Langston D, Dohlman CH, Geary P, Sulzewski D. Intraocular penetration of Ara-A and IDU—therapeutic implications in clinical herpetic uveitis. *Trans Am Acad Ophthalmol Otolaryngol* 1973;77:OP455–66.

6. Pavan-Langston D, Foster CS. Trifluorothymidine and idoxuridine therapy of ocular herpes. *Am J Ophthalmol* 1977;84:818–25.
7. Cobo M, Lass JH, Liesegang TJ, Jones DB, Foulks GN. Oral acyclovir in the therapy of acute herpes zoster ophthalmicus. *Ophthalmology* 1984;91(suppl 2):80.
8. Cobo LM, Foulks GN, Liesegang T, et al. Oral acyclovir in the therapy of acute herpes zoster ophthalmicus: an interim report. *Ophthalmology* 1985;92:1574–83.
9. Pavan-Langston D, Lass J, Hettinger M, Udell I. Acyclovir and vidarabine in the treatment of ulcerative herpes simplex keratitis. *Am J Ophthalmol* 1981;92:829–35.
10. Bach MC, Hedstram PS. CMV retinitis treated with ganciclovir [9(1,3-dihydroxy-2-propoxymethyl) guanine] in patients with AIDS. *Ann Ophthalmol* 1987;19:369–75.
11. Henderley DE, Freeman WR, Causey DM, Rao NA. Cytomegalovirus retinitis and response to therapy with ganciclovir. *Ophthalmology* 1987;94:425–34.
12. Robinson MA, Streeten BW, Hampton GR, Siebold EC, Taylor-Findlay C. Treatment of cytomegalovirus optic neuritis with dihydroxy propoxymethyl guanine. *Am J Ophthalmol* 1986;102:533–4.
13. Bach MC. Possible drug interaction during therapy with azidothymidine and acyclovir for AIDS. *N Engl J Med* 1987;316:547.
14. Farrell PL, Heinemann M-H, Roberts CW, Polsky B, Gold JWM, Mamelok A. Response of human immunodeficiency virus-associated uveitis to zidovudine. *Am J Ophthalmol* 1988;106:7–10.
15. Fischl MA, Richman DD, Grieco MH, et al. The efficacy of azidothymidine (AZT) in the treatment of patients with AIDS and AIDS-related complex: A double-blind, placebo controlled trial. *N Engl J Med* 1987;317:185–91.
16. Harris PJ, Caceres CA. Azidothymidine in the treatment of AIDS. [Letter]. *N Engl J Med* 1988;318:250.
17. Hymes KB, Greene JB, Karpatkin S. The effect of azidothymidine on HIV-related thrombocytopenia. *N Engl J Med* 1988;318:516–7.
18. Richman DD, Fischl MA, Grieco MH, Gottlieb MS, Voldberding PA, Laskin OL, et al. The toxicity of azidothymidine (AZT) in the treatment of patients with AIDS and AIDS related complex: a double-blind, placebo-controlled trial. *N Engl J Med* 1987;317:192–7.
19. Pavan-Langston D, Dunkel EC. Principles of antiviral chemotherapy. In: Duane TD, ed. *Biomedical foundations of ophthalmology, vol. 2*. Philadelphia: Harper & Row, 1986: chapter [illegible]9.
20. Prusoff WH, Ward DC. Nucleoside analogs with antiviral activity. *Biochem Pharmacol* 1976;25:1233–9.
21. Collum LMT, Benedict-Smith A, Hillary IB. Randomised double-blind trial of acyclovir and idoxuridine in dendritic corneal ulceration. *Br J Ophthalmol* 1980;64:766–9.
22. Coster DJ, McKinnon JR, McGill JI, Jones B, Fraunfelder FC. Clinical evaluation of adenine arabinoside and trifluorothymidine in the treatment of corneal ulcers caused by herpes simplex virus. *J Infect Dis* 1976;133(suppl):A173–7.
23. Coster DJ, Wilhelmus KR, Michaud R, Jones BR. A comparison of acyclovir and idoxuridine as treatment for ulcerative herpetic keratitis. *Br J Ophthalmol* 1980;64:763–5.
24. Pavan-Langston D. Clinical evaluation of adenine arabinoside and idoxuridine in the treatment of ocular herpes simplex. *Am J Ophthalmol* 1975;80:495–502.
25. Elze K. Ten years of clinical experience with ethyldeoxyuridine. In: Gauri KK, ed. *Antiherpesvirus chemotherapy: experimental and clinical aspects. (Advances in ophthalmology, vol 38).* New York: S. Karger, 1979:134–9.
26. Maudgal PC, De Clercq E, Missotten L. Efficacy of bromovinyldeoxyuridine in the treatment of herpes simplex virus and varicella-zoster virus eye infections. *Antiviral Res* 1984;4:281–91.
27. Laibson PR, Pavan-Langston D, Yeakley WR, Lass J. Acyclovir and vidarabine for the treatment of herpes simplex keratitis. *Am J Med* 1982;73(1A):281–5.
28. Le Hoang P, Girard B, Saraux H, et al. Foscarnet in the treatment of cytomegalovirus retinitis in AIDS patients. *Ophthalmology* 1988;95(acad suppl):22.
29. Jones BR, Coster DJ, Falcon MG, Cantell K. Topical therapy of ulcerative herpetic keratitis with human interferon. *Lancet* 1976;2:128–9.
30. Smolin G, Stebbing N, Friedlaender M, Friedlaender R, Okumoto M. Natural and cloned human leukocyte interferon in herpesvirus infections of rabbit eyes. *Arch Ophthalmol* 1982;100:481–3.
31. Sundmacher R, Cantell K, Neumann-Haefelin D. Combination therapy of dendritic keratitis with trifluorothymidine and interferon. *Lancet* 1978;2:687.
32. Romano M, Revel M, Guarari-Rotman D, Blumenthal M, Stein R. Use of human fibroblast-derived (beta) interferon in the treatment of epidemic adenovirus keratoconjunctivitis. *J Interferon Res* 1980;1:95–100.
33. Ikic D, Cupak K, Trajer D, Soos D, et al. Therapy and prevention of epidemic keratoconjunctivitis with human leukocyte interferon. In: *Proceedings of the Symposium on the Clinical Use of Interferon*. Zagreb: Yugoslavian Academy of Science and Arts, 1975;189–194.
34. Lundin M, Schelin U. The effect of steroids on the histology and ultrastructure of lymphoid tissue. I. Acute thymic involution. *Pathol Europ* 1966;1:15–28.
35. Makman MH, Nakagawa S, White A. Studies of the mode of action of adrenal steroids on lymphocytes. *Recent Prog Horm Res* 1967;23:195–227.
36. Meyer RF, Smolin G, Hall JM, Okumoto M. Effect of local corticosteroids on antibody-

forming cells in the eye and draining lymph nodes. *Invest Ophthalmol* 1975;14:138–44.
37. Henson D, Helmsen R, Becker KE, Strano AJ, Sullivan M, Harris D. Ultrastructural localization of herpes simplex virus antigens on rabbit corneal cells using sheep antihuman IgG antihorse ferritin hybrid antibodies. *Invest Ophthalmol* 1974;13:819–27.
38. Lass JH, Berman MB, Campbell RC, Pavan-Langston D, Gage J. Treatment of experimental herpetic interstitial keratitis with medroxyprogesterone. *Arch Ophthalmol* 1980;98:520–7.
39. Dunkel EC, Pavan-Langston D, Fitzpatrick K, Cukor G. Rapid detection of herpes simplex virus (HSV) antigen in human ocular infections. *Curr Eye Res* 1988;7:661–6.
40. Annual Summary 1980. Reported morbidity and mortality in the United States. *Morbidity and Mortality Weekly Report* 1981;29:1.
41. Hyndiuk RA, Glasser D. Herpes simplex keratitis. In: Tabbara KF, Hyndiuk RA, eds. *Infections of the eye*. Boston: Little, Brown, 1986:343–68.
42. Kimura E. Herpes simplex keratitis. In: Allen HF, ed. *Symposium of the New Orleans Academy of Ophthalmology*. St. Louis: C.V. Mosby, 1963:124–136.
43. Pavan-Langston D. Viral diseases: herpetic infections. In: Smolin G, Thoft RA, eds. *The cornea: scientific foundations and clinical practice*. 2nd ed. Boston: Little, Brown, 1987: 240–66.
44. Pavan-Langston D. Ocular viral diseases. In: Galasso GJ, Merigan TC, Buchanan RA, eds. *Antiviral agents and viral diseases of man*. 2nd ed. New York: Raven Press, 1984:207–45.
45. Buddingh GJ, Schrum DI, Lanier JC, Guidry DJ. Studies of the natural history of herpes simplex infections. *Pediatrics* 1953;11:595–609.
46. Nahmias AJ, Roizman B. Infection with herpes-simplex viruses 1 and 2. Part 3. *N Engl J Med* 1973;289:781–9.
47. Smith IW, Peutherer JF, MacCallum FO. The incidence of Herpesvirus hominis antibody in the population. *J Hyg (Camb)* 1967;65:395–408.
48. Baringer JR, Swoveland P. Recovery of herpes-simplex virus from human trigeminal ganglions. *N Engl J Med* 1973;288:648–50.
49. Bastian FO, Rabson AS, Yee CL, Tralka TS. Herpesvirus hominis: isolation from human trigeminal ganglion. *Science* 1972;178:306–7.
50. Croen KD, Ostrove JM, Dragovic LJ, Smialek JE, Straus SE. Latent herpes simplex virus in human trigeminal ganglia: Detection of an immediate early gene "anti-sense" transcript by *in situ* hybridization. *N Engl J Med* 1987;317:1427–32.
51. Pavan-Langston D, Rong BL, Dunkel EC. Extraneuronal herpetic latency: animal and human corneal studies. *Acta Ophthalmol* 1989; (in press).
52. Stevens JG. Latent infections by herpes simplex virus in experimental animals. *Surv Ophthalmol* 1976;21:175–7.
53. Stevens JG, Wagner EK, Devi-Rao GB, Cook ML, Feldman LT. RNA complementary to a herpesvirus α gene mRNA is prominent in latently infected neurons. *Science* 1987;235: 1056–9.
54. Bell DM, Holman RC, Pavan-Langston D. Herpes simplex keratitis: epidemiologic aspects. *Ann Ophthalmol* 1982;14:421–4.
55. Shuster JJ, Kaufman HE, Nesburn AB. Statistical analysis of the rate of recurrence of herpesvirus ocular epithelial disease. *Am J Ophthalmol* 1981;91:328–31.
56. Openshaw H, Asher LV, Wohlenberg C, Sekizawa T, Notkins AL. Acute and latent infection of sensory ganglia with herpes simplex virus: immune control and virus reactivation. *J Gen Virol* 1979;44:205–15.
57. Stevens JG, Cook ML. Latent herpes simplex virus in sensory ganglia. *Perspect Virol* 1971;8:171.
58. Abghari SZ, Stulting RD. Recovery of herpes simplex virus from ocular tissues of latently infected mice. *Invest Ophthalmol Vis Sci* 1988;29:239–43.
59. Rong BL, Kenyon KR, Bean KM, Pavan-Langston D, Dunkel EC. Direct detection of the HSV-1 genome in the human cornea by slot blot hybridization (Submitted).
60. Sabbaga EMH, Pavan-Langston D, Bean KM, Dunkel EC. Detection of HSV nucleic acid sequences in the cornea during acute and latent ocular disease. *Exp Eye Res* 1988;47:545–53.
61. Varnell ED, Centifanto-Fitzgerald YM, Kaufman HE. Herpesvirus infection and its effect on virulent superinfection, ganglionic colonization, and shedding. *Invest Ophthalmol Vis Sci* 1981;20(ARVO suppl):137.
62. Gordon YJ. RNA complementary to the ICP0 region retained in human trigeminal ganglia during HSV latency. In: Piatigorsky J, Shinohara T, Zelenka P, eds. *Molecular Biology of the Eye*. New York: Alan R. Liss, 1989:382.
63. Hubbard A, Centifanto-Fitzgerald Y. Variability among HSV-1 strains and its importance in disease. Proceedings of the Ninth International Herpesvirus Workshop, Seattle, Washington, 1984;108.
64. Kaufman HE, Centifanto-Fitzgerald YM, Varnell ED. Herpes simplex keratitis. *Ophthalmology* 1983;90:700–6.
65. Kibrick S, Takahashi GH, Leibowitz HM, Laibson PR. Local corticosteroid therapy and reactivation of herpetic keratitis. *Arch Ophthalmol* 1971;86:694–8.
66. Van Horn DL, Edelhauser HF, Schultz RO. Experimental herpes simplex keratitis: early alterations of corneal epithelium and stroma. *Arch Ophthalmol* 1970;84:67–75.
67. Baum J. Morphogenesis of the dendritic figure in herpes simplex keratitis: a negative study. *Am J Ophthalmol* 1970;70:722–4.
68. Cavanagh HD. Herpetic ocular disease: therapy of persistent epithelial defects. *Int Ophthalmol Clin* 1975;15(4):67–88.
69. Kaufman HE. Epithelial erosion syndrome:

metaherpetic keratitis. *Am J Ophthalmol* 1964;57:983–7.
70. Kaufman HE, Uotila MH, Gasset AR, Wood TO, Ellison ED. The medical uses of soft contact lenses. *Trans Am Acad Ophthalmol Otolaryngol* 1971;75:361–73.
71. Refojo MF, Dohlman CH, Koliopoulos J. Adhesives in ophthalmology: a review. *Surv Ophthalmol* 1971;15:217–36.
72. Jones BR, Falcon MG, Williams HP, Coster DJ. Objectives in therapy of herpetic eye disease. *Trans Ophthalmol Soc UK* 1977;97:305–13.
73. Meyers RL, Chitjian PA. Immunology of herpesvirus infection: immunity to herpes simplex virus in eye infections. *Surv Ophthalmol* 1976;21:194–204.
74. Meyers RL, Pettit TH. Corneal immune response to herpes simplex virus antigens. *J Immunol* 1973;110:1575–90.
75. Meyers-Elliott RH, Pettit TH, Maxwell WA. Viral antigens in the immune ring of herpes simplex stromal keratitis. *Arch Ophthalmol* 1980;98:897–904.
76. Dawson C, Togni B, Moore TE Jr. Structural changes in chronic herpetic keratitis: studied by light and electron microscopy. *Arch Ophthalmol* 1968;79:740–7.
77. Sundmacher R. A clinico-virologic classification of herpetic anterior segment disease with special reference to intraocular herpes. In: Sundmacher R, ed. *Herpetic Eye Disease: International Symposium*. New York: Springer-Verlag, 1981:203–10.
78. Sutcliffe E, Baum J. Acute idiopathic corneal endotheliitis. *Ophthalmology* 1984;91:1161–5.
79. Cohen EJ, Laibson PR, Arentsen JJ. Corneal transplantation for herpes simplex keratitis. *Am J Ophthalmol* 1983;95:645–50.
80. Langston RHS, Pavan-Langston D, Dohlman CH. Penetrating keratoplasty for herpetic keratitis: prognostic and therapeutic determinants. *Trans Am Acad Ophthalmol Otolaryngol* 1975;79:577–583.
81. Weiss N, Jones BR. Problems of corneal grafting in herpetic keratitis. *Ciba Found Symp* 1973;15:220–41.
82. Abelson MB, Pavan-Langston D. Viral uveitis. *Int Ophthalmol Clin* 1977;17(3):109–20.
83. Pavan-Langston D, Brockhurst RJ. Herpes simplex panuveitis: a clinical report. *Arch Ophthalmol* 1969;81:783–7.
84. Sundmacher R, Neumann-Haefelin D. Herpes simplex virus isolation from the aqueous of patients suffering from focal iritis, endotheliitis, and prolonged disciform keratitis with glaucoma. *Klin Monatsbl Augenheilkd* 1979;175:488–501.
85. Collin HB, Abelson MB. Herpes simplex virus in human cornea, retrocorneal fibrous membrane, and vitreous. *Arch Ophthalmol* 1976;94:1726–9.
86. Schwab IR. Oral acyclovir in the management of herpes simplex ocular infections. *Ophthalmology* 1988;95:423–30.
87. Hagler WS, Walters PV, Nahmias AJ. Ocular involvement in neonatal herpes simplex virus infection. *Arch Ophthalmol* 1969;82:169–76.
88. Johnson BL, Wisotzkey HM. Neuroretinitis associated with herpes simplex encephalitis in an adult. *Am J Ophthalmol* 1977;83:481–9.
89. Minckler DS, McLean EB, Shaw CM, Hendrickson A. *Herpesvirus hominis* encephalitis and retinitis. *Arch Ophthalmol* 1976;94:89–95.
90. Partamian LG, Morse PH, Klein HZ. Herpes simplex type 1 retinitis in an adult with systemic herpes zoster. *Am J Ophthalmol* 1981;92:215–20.
91. Selby PJ, Powles RL, Janeson B, Kay HE, Watson JG, Thornton R, et al. Parenteral acyclovir therapy for herpes virus infections in man. *Lancet* 1979;2:1267–70.
92. Straus SE, Smith HA, Brickman C, de Miranda P, McLaren C, Keeney RE. Acyclovir for chronic mucocutaneous herpes simplex virus infection in immunosuppressed patients. *Ann Intern Med* 1982;96:270–7.
93. Wade JC, Newton B, McLaren C, Flournay N, Keeney RE, Meyers JD. Intravenous acyclovir to treat mucocutaneous herpes simplex virus infection after marrow transplantation: a double-blind trial. *Ann Intern Med* 1982;96:265–9.
94. Gundersen T. Conjunctival flaps in the treatment of corneal disease with reference to a new technique of application. *Arch Ophthalmol* 1958;60:880–8.
95. Thoft RA. Conjunctival transplantation. *Arch Ophthalmol* 1977;95:1425–7.
96. Fine M, Cignetti FE. Penetrating keratoplasty in herpes simplex keratitis. *Arch Ophthalmol* 1977;95:613–6.
97. Stagno S, Whitley RJ. Herpesvirus infections of pregnancy. Part I: Cytomegalovirus and Epstein-Barr virus infections. *N Engl J Med* 1985;313:1270–4.
98. Okabe M, Chiba S, Tamura T, Chiba Y, Nakao T. Longitudinal studies of cytomegalovirus-specific cell mediated immunity in congenitally infected infants. *Infect Immun* 1983;41:128–31.
99. Lonn LI. Neonatal cytomegalic inclusion disease chorioretinitis. *Arch Ophthalmol* 1972;88:434–8.
100. Nicholson DH. Cytomegalovirus infection of the retina. *Int Ophthalmol Clin* 1975;15(4):151–62.
101. Pollard RB, Egbert PR, Gallagher JG, Merigan TC. Cytomegalovirus retinitis in immunosuppressed hosts. I. Natural history and effects of treatment with adenine arabinoside. *Ann Intern Med* 1980;93:655–64.
102. Palestine A, Rodrigues MM, Macher AM, et al. Ophthalmic involvement in acquired immunodeficiency syndrome. *Ophthalmology* 1984;91:1092–9.
103. Pepose JS, Holland GN, Nestor MS, Cochran AJ, Foos RY. Acquired immune deficiency syndrome: pathogenic mechanisms of ocular disease. *Ophthalmology* 1985;92:472–84.

104. Pepose JS, Newman C, Bach MC, et al. Pathologic features of cytomegalovirus retinopathy after treatment with the antiviral agent ganciclovir. *Ophthalmology* 1987;94:414–24.
105. Holland GN. Ocular manifestations of the acquired immune deficiency syndrome. *Int Ophthalmol Clin* 1985;25(2):179–87.
106. Holland GN, Gottlieb MS, Yee RD, Schanker HM, Pettit TH. Ocular disorders associated with a new severe acquired cellular immune deficiency syndrome. *Am J Ophthalmol* 1982;93:393–402.
107. Grossniklaus HE, Frank KE, Tomsak RL. Cytomegalovirus retinitis and optic neuritis in acquired immune deficiency syndrome: report of a case. *Ophthalmology* 1987;94:1601–4.
108. Masur H, Lane H, Palestine A, et al. Effect of 9-(1,3-dihydroxy-2-propoxymethyl) guanine on serious cytomegalovirus disease in eight immunosuppressed homosexual men. *Ann Int Med* 1986;104:41–4.
109. Meyers JD, Reed EC, Shepp DH, et al. Acyclovir for prevention of cytomegalovirus infection and disease after allogeneic marrow transplantation. *N Engl J Med* 1988;318:70–5.
110. Ussery FM III, Gibson SR, Conklin RH, Piot DF, Stool EW, Conklin AJ. Intravitreal ganciclovir in the treatment of AIDS-associated cytomegalovirus retinitis. *Ophthalmology* 1988; 95:640–8.
111. Fleisher G, Henry W, McSorley M, Arbeter A, Plotkin S. Life threatening complications of varicella. *Am J Dis Child* 1981;135:896–9.
112. Preblud SR. Age-specific risks of varicella complications. *Pediatrics* 1981;68:14–7.
113. Edwards TS. Ophthalmic complications from varicella. *J Pediatr Ophthalmol* 1965;2:37–40.
114. Nesburn AB, Borit A, Pentelei-Molnar J, Lazaro R. Varicella dendritic keratitis. *Invest Ophthalmol* 1974;13:764–70.
115. Strachman J. Uveitis associated with chicken pox. *J Pediatr* 1955;46:327–8.
116. Edgerton AE. Herpes zoster ophthalmicus: report of cases and review of literature. *Arch Ophthalmol* 1945;34:40–62,114–53.
117. Hope-Simpson RE. The nature of herpes zoster: a long-term study and a new hypothesis. *Proc Roy Soc Med* 1965;58:9–20.
118. Miller AE. Selective decline in cellular immune response to varicella-zoster in the elderly. *Neurology* 1980;30:582–7.
119. Ragozzino MW, Melton LJ 3rd, Kurland LT, Chu CP, Perry HO. Population-based study of herpes zoster and its sequelae. *Medicine* 1982;61:310–6.
120. Sandor EV, Millman A, Croxson S, Mildvan D. Herpes zoster ophthalmicus in patients at risk for the acquired immune deficiency syndrome (AIDS). *Am J Ophthalmol* 1986;101:153–5.
121. Scheie HG. Herpes zoster ophthalmicus. *Trans Ophthalmol Soc UK* 1970;90:899–930.
122. Thomas M, Robertson W. Dermal transmission of a virus as a cause of shingles. *Lancet* 1968;2:1349–50.
123. Liesegang TJ. The varicella-zoster virus: systemic and ocular features. *J Am Acad Dermatol* 1984;11:165–91.
124. Forrest WM, Kaufman HE. Zosteriform herpes simplex. *Am J Ophthalmol* 1976;81:86–8.
125. Pavan-Langston D, McCulley JP. Herpes zoster dendritic keratitis. *Arch Ophthalmol* 1973;89:25–9.
126. Piebenga LW, Laibson PR. Dendritic lesions in herpes zoster ophthalmicus. *Arch Ophthalmol* 1973;90:268–73.
127. Liesegang T. Corneal complications from herpes zoster ophthalmicus. *Ophthalmology* 1985;92:316–24.
128. Naumann G, Gass JDM, Font RL. Histopathology of herpes zoster ophthalmicus. *Am J Ophthalmol* 1968;65:533–41.
129. Tunis SW, Tapert MJ. Acute retrobulbar neuritis complicating herpes zoster ophthalmicus. *Ann Ophthalmol* 1987;19:453–60.
130. Ruppenthal M. Changes of the central nervous system in herpes zoster. *Acta Neuropathol (Berl)* 1980;52:59–68.
131. Weller TH. Varicella and herpes zoster: changing concepts of the natural history, control, and importance of a not-so-benign virus (part 1). *N Engl J Med* 1983;309:1362–8.
132. Wilson F II. Varicella and herpes zoster ophthalmicus. In: Tabbara KF, Hyndiuk RA, eds. *Infections of the eye.* Boston: Little, Brown, 1986:369–86.
133. Womack LW, Liesegang TJ. Complications of herpes zoster ophthalmicus. *Arch Ophthalmol* 1983;101:42–5.
134. Culbertson WW, Blumenkranz MS, Haimes H, Gass DM, Mitchell KB, Norton EWD. The acute retinal necrosis syndrome. Part 2: Histopathology and etiology. *Ophthalmology* 1982;89:1317–25.
135. Culbertson WW, Clarkson JG, Blumenkranz M, Lewis ML. Acute retinal necrosis. *Am J Ophthalmol* 1983;96:683–5.
136. Hirst LW, Beyer TL, Waters D, Fleischman J. Successful management of acute retinal necrosis with intravenous acyclovir. *Ann Ophthalmol* 1987;19:445–8.
137. Sternberg P Jr, Knox DL, Finkelstein D, Green WR, Murphy RP, Patz A. Acute retinal necrosis syndrome. *Retina* 1982;2:145–51.
138. Esmann V, Geil JP, Kroon S, et al. Prednisolone does not prevent post-herpetic neuralgia. *Lancet* 1987;2:126–9.
139. Keczkes K, Basheer AM. Do corticosteroids prevent post-herpetic neuralgia? *Br J Dermatol* 1980;102:551–5.
140. Sklar SH, Blue WT, Alexander EJ, Bodian CA. Herpes zoster, treatment and prevention of neuralgia with adenosine monophosphate. *JAMA* 1985;253:1427–30.
141. Carter A, Royds J. Systemic steroids in herpes zoster. *Br Med J* 1957;2:746–51.
142. McGill J, Chapman C. A comparison of topical acyclovir with steroids in the treatment of herpes zoster keratouveitis. *Br J Ophthalmol* 1983;67:746–50.

143. McGill J, Chapman C, Copplestone A, Maharasingam M. A review of acyclovir treatment of ocular herpes zoster and skin infections. *J Antimicrob Chemother* 1983;12(suppl B):45–9.
144. McGill J, MacDonald DR, Fall C, McKendrick GD, Copplestone A. Intravenous acyclovir in acute herpes zoster infection. *J Infect* 1983;6:157–61.
145. Shepp DH, Dandliker PS, Meyers JD. Treatment of varicella-zoster infection in severely immunocompromised patients. *N Engl J Med* 1986;314:208–12.
146. Bergaust B, Westby RK. Zoster ophthalmicus: local treatment with cortisone. *Acta Ophthalmol* 1967;45:787–93.
147. Elliott RA. Treatment of herpes zoster with high doses of prednisone. *Lancet* 1964;2:610–8.
148. Merselis J, Kaye D, Hook E. Disseminated herpes zoster. *Arch Intern Med* 1961;113:679–84.
149. Cole EL, Meisler DM, Calabrese LH, Holland GN, Mondino BJ, Conant MA. Herpes zoster ophthalmicus and AIDS. *Arch Ophthalmol* 1984;102:1027–9.
150. Mavligit GM, Talpaz M. Cimetidine for herpes zoster. *N Engl J Med* 1984;310:318–9.
151. van der Spuy S, Levy DW, Levin W. Cimetidine in the treatment of herpesvirus infections. *S Afr Med J* 1980;58:112–6.
152. Burtin C, Scheinmann P, Fray A, Lespinats G, Noirot C, Paupe J. Ranitidine versus cimetidine. *N Engl J Med* 1984;310:1603.
153. Levy DW, Banerjee AK, Glenny HP. Cimetidine in the treatment of herpes zoster. *J R Coll Physicians Lond* 1985;19:96–8.
154. Kernbaum S, Hauchecorne J. Administration of levodopa for relief of herpes zoster pain. *JAMA* 1981;246:132–4.
155. Aaberg TM, O'Brien WJ. Expanding ophthalmologic recognition of Epstein-Barr virus infections. *Am J Ophthalmol* 1987;104:420–3.
156. Raymond LA, Wilson CA, Linneman CC Jr, Ward MA, Bernstein DI, Love DC. Punctate outer retinitis in acute Epstein-Barr virus infection. *Am J Ophthalmol* 1987;104:424–6.
157. Tanner OR. Ocular manifestations of infectious mononucleosis. *Arch Ophthalmol* 1952;51:229–41.
158. Wong KW, D'Amico DJ, Hedges TR III, Soong HK, Schooley RT, Kenyon KR. Ocular involvement associated with chronic Epstein-Barr virus disease. *Arch Ophthalmol* 1987;105:788–92.
159. Schulman J, Peyman GA, Fiscella R, Greenberg D, Horton MB, De Miranda P. Intraocular acyclovir levels after subconjunctival and topical administration. *Br J Ophthalmol* 1986;70:138–40.
160. Bowen DL, Lane HC, Fauci AS. Immunopathogenesis of the acquired immunodeficiency syndrome. *Ann Intern Med* 1985;103:704–9.
161. Broder S. Pathogenic human retroviruses. *N Engl J Med* 1988;318:243–5.
162. Centers For Disease Control. Revision of the CDC Surveillance Case Definition for AIDS. *Morbidity and Mortality Weekly Report* 1987;36:1S.
163. Centers for Disease Control. Provisional Public Health Service Interagency Recommendations for Screening Donated Blood and Plasma for Antibody to the Virus Causing AIDS. *Morbidity and Mortality Weekly Report* 1985;43:1–4.
164. Fauci AS. Immunologic abnormalities in the acquired immunodeficiency syndrome (AIDS). *Clin Res* 1984;32:491–9.
165. Redfield RR, Markham PD, Salahuddin SZ, Wright DC, Sarngadharan MG, Gallo RC. Heterosexually acquired HTLV-III/LAV disease (AIDS-related complex and AIDS): epidemiologic evidence for female-to-male transmission. *JAMA* 1985;254:2094–6.
166. Pomerantz RJ, Kuritzkes DR, De La Monte SM, et al. Infection of the retina by human immunodeficiency virus type 1. *N Engl J Med* 1987;317:1643–7.
167. Sherertz RJ. Acquired immune deficiency syndrome: a perspective for the medical practitioner. *Med Clin North Am* 1985;69:637–55.
168. Rosenberg PR, Uliss AE, Friedland GH, Harris CA, Small CB, Klein RS. Acquired immune deficiency syndrome: ophthalmic manifestations in ambulatory patients. *Ophthalmology* 1983;90:874–8.
169. Hoff R, Berardi VP, Weiblen BJ, Mahoney-Trout L, Mitchell ML, Grady GF. Seroprevalence of human immunodeficiency virus among childbearing women. *N Engl J Med* 1988;318:525–30.
170. O'Day DM. The risk posed by HTLV-III-infected corneal donor tissue. *Am J Ophthalmol* 1986;101:246–7.
171. Salahuddin SZ, Palestine AG, Heck E, et al. Isolation of the human T-cell leukemia/lymphotropic virus type III from the cornea. *Am J Ophthalmol* 1986;101:149–52.
172. Friedman AH. The retinal lesions of the acquired immune deficiency syndrome. *Trans Am Ophthalmol Soc* 1984;82:447–91.
173. Cantrill HL, Erice A, Ussery F. Recovery of HIV from ocular tissues of patients with AIDS. *Ophthalmology* 1987;94(suppl):70–5.
174. Yarchoan R, Berg G, Brouwers P, et al. Response of human-immunodeficiency-virus associated neurological disease to 3′-azido-3′-deoxythymidine. *Lancet* 1987;1:132–5.
175. Duke-Elder S. The adenoviruses. In: *System of ophthalmology, vol VIII*. London: Henry Kimpton, 1965:348–58.
176. Vastine DW. Adenoviruses and miscellaneous viral infections. In: Smolin G, Thoft RA, eds. *The cornea: scientific foundations and clinical practice*. 2nd ed. Boston: Little, Brown, 1987:267–85.
177. Dawson CR, Hanna MA, Wood TR, Despain R. Adenovirus type 8 keratoconjunctivitis in the United States. III. Epidemiologic, clinical, and microbiologic features. *Am J Ophthalmol* 1970;69:473–80.

178. Laibson PR, Dhiri S, Oconer J, Ortolan G. Corneal infiltrates in epidemic keratoconjunctivitis: response to double-blind corticosteroid therapy. *Arch Ophthalmol* 1970;84:36–40.
179. Murrah WF. Epidemic keratoconjunctivitis. *Ann Ophthalmol* 1988;20:36–8.
180. Laibson PR, Ortolan G, Dupré-Strachan S. Community and hospital outbreak of epidemic keratoconjunctivitis. *Arch Ophthalmol* 1968; 80:467–73.
181. O'Day DM, Guyer B, Hierholzer JC, Rosing KJ, Schaffner W. Clinical and laboratory evaluation of epidemic keratoconjunctivitis due to adenovirus types 8 and 19. *Am J Ophthalmol* 1976;81:207–15.
182. Inoue S. Diagnosis of adenovirus infection by use of fluorescent antibody technique. *Acta Soc Ophthalmol Jpn* 1968;72:728–41.
183. Hogan M, Crawford T. Adenoviral keratitis. *Am J Ophthalmol* 1942;25:1059–63.
184. Hecht SD, Hanna L, Sery TW, Jawetz E. Treatment of epidemic keratoconjunctivitis with idoxuridine (IUDR). *Arch Ophthalmol* 1965;73:49–54.
185. Waring GO III, Satz J, Laibson PR, Joseph N. Use of vidarabine in epidemic keratoconjunctivitis due to adenovirus types 3, 7, 8 and 19. *Am J Ophthalmol* 1976;82:781–5.
186. North RD. Presumptive viral keratoconjunctivitis, mononucleosis, and the oncogenic viruses. *Int Ophthalmol Clin* 1975;15(4):211–27.
187. Koplan JP, Hicks JW. Smallpox and vaccinia in the United States—1972. *J Infect Dis* 1974;129:224–6.
188. Francois J, De Molder E, Gildemyn H. Ocular vaccinia. *Acta Ophthalmol* 1967;45:25–31.
189. Jawetz E, Melnick JL, Adelberg EA. Vaccinia virus. In: Vaughn D, Cook R, Asbury T, eds. *Medical microbiology*. Los Altos, California: Lange, 1972:103–10.
190. Jones BR, Galbraith JEK, Al-Hussaini MK. Vaccinial keratitis treated with interferon. *Lancet* 1962;1:875–9.
191. Rennie AGR, Cant JS, Foulds WS. Ocular vaccinia. *Lancet* 1974;2:273–5.
192. Ellis PP, Winograd LA. Ocular vaccinia: a specific treatment. *Arch Ophthalmol* 1962;68: 600–9.
193. Hyndiuk RA, Okumoto M, Damiano RA, Valenton M, Smolin G. Treatment of vaccinial keratitis with vidarabine. *Arch Ophthalmol* 1976;94:1363–4.
194. Hyndiuk RA, Seideman S, Leibsohn JM. Treatment of vaccinial keratitis with trifluorothymidine. *Arch Ophthalmol* 1976;94:1785–6.
195. Baum J. Discussion of Mitsui Y et al., Hemorrhagic conjunctivitis: a new type of epidemic viral keratoconjunctivitis. *Surv Ophthalmol* 1973;17:489–90.
196. Mitsui Y, Kajima M, Matsumura K, Shiota H. Hemorrhagic conjunctivitis: a new type of epidemic viral keratoconjunctivitis. *Jpn J Ophthalmol* 1972;16:33–40.
197. Patriaca PA, Onorato IM, Sklar VEF, et al. Acute hemorrhagic conjunctivitis: investigation of a large-scale community outbreak in Dade County, Florida. *JAMA* 1983;249: 1283–9.
198. Whitcher JP, Schmidt NJ, Malbrouk R, et al. Acute hemorrhagic conjunctivitis in Tunisia. *Arch Ophthalmol* 1975;94:51–5.
199. Pavan-Langston D. Diagnosis and management of herpes simplex ocular infection. *Int Ophthalmol Clin* 1975;15(4):19–35.

*Antiviral Agents and Viral Diseases of Man, 3rd Edition,*
edited by G. J. Galasso, R. J. Whitley, and
T. C. Merigan, Raven Press, Ltd., New York © 1990.

# 7

# Varicella-Zoster Virus Infections

Richard J. Whitley

*Departments of Pediatrics and Microbiology, The University of Alabama at Birmingham Medical Center, School of Medicine, Birmingham, Alabama 35294*



Varicella-zoster virus (VZV) causes two clinically distinct diseases. Varicella, or more commonly chicken pox, is the primary infection, resulting from exposure of a susceptible individual to this virus. Varicella, a ubiquitous, extremely contagious, and for the most part benign illness, is characterized by a generalized exanthematous rash and occurs in epidemics. Recurrent infection results in the localized phenomenon of herpes zoster, or shingles, a common infection among the elderly.

VZV remains on the short list of pathogenic viral agents for which a vaccine is not licensed, although a promising one is currently being evaluated. Regardless, VZV infections are of medical significance. In 1974, chicken pox resulted in at least 1 million physician visits, and nearly half of these individuals required a second office appointment. Herpes zoster during the same year accounted for over 1.75 million physician visits, and nearly three-quarters of these patients required subsequent follow-up medical care. With the development of increasingly aggressive treatment modalities for children and adults with malignancies and the recognition that an increasing number of other diseases benefit from long-term immunosuppression, the frequency of severe and life-threatening VZV infections is likely to increase. Although an effective vaccine for prevention of these infections is not yet licensed in the United States, one has been successfully utilized in the research setting and may be routinely available in the near future (1).

## HISTORY

Although shingles has been recognized since ancient times as a unique clinical entity because of the dermatomal vesicular rash, varicella was often confused with smallpox. The two diseases were differentiated by the clinical descriptions of Heberbed in 1867, as reviewed by Gordon (2). In 1975, 100 years later, Steiner (3) successfully demonstrated the transmissibility of VZV by inoculation of vesicular fluid from an individual suffering from chicken pox to "volunteers" who subsequently developed the same disease. The infectious nature of VZV was further elucidated by von Bokay (4,5) who reported the occurrence of chicken pox in individuals who had close contact with others suffering from herpes zoster and also defined the incubation period for chicken pox. In addition to close contact, the inoculation of vesicular fluid from patients suffering from herpes zoster into susceptible individuals resulted in chicken pox (6,7). Clinical reports, such as that of the School Epidemics Committee of Great Britain in 1938 (8), confirmed the infectivity of VZV. In 1943, Garland (9) suggested that zoster was the consequence of reactivation of latent VZV, as reported for herpes simplex virus (HSV) infections. As this clinical relationship between chicken pox and herpes zoster was being defined, the histopathology of skin lesions, particularly the intranuclear inclusions and multinucleated giant cells, was described (10,11).

The first propagation of VZV in tissue culture was reported by Weller in 1952, leading to the universal acceptance that both chicken pox and herpes zoster were caused by VZV (12). No differences were identified between the viral agents isolated from patients with these two clinical entities from either a biologic or an immunologic standpoint (12–16). Recently, restriction endonuclease analyses of VZV DNA have been applied to the study of the DNA structure and to the epidemiology of VZV infections (17–20). Unless epidemiologically related, VZV isolates differ from one another (19), although minor variations will occur after serial passage *in vitro* (21). Chicken pox and herpes zoster VZV isolates from the same patient have been proven identical when examined by restriction enzyme analyses. These recent observations should allow for further advances in epidemiologic and natural history investigations.

## CHARACTERISTICS OF VZV

### Molecular Configuration

VZV, being a member of the family *Herpetoviridae* (genus herpesvirus), shares structural characteristics with other members of this family. The virus has icosahedral symmetry, containing centrally located double-stranded DNA with a surrounding envelope. The complete virion is approximately 150–200 nm in diameter, and the capsid measures approximately 90–95 nm in diameter (22,23). It has a lipid-containing envelope with glycoprotein spikes (24). Enveloped virions are infectious.

Radiolabeled VZV DNA has been purified and characterization studies performed (24–26). The molecular weight of VZV DNA approximates $100 \times 10^6$ dl (26). Cesium-chloride-purified VZV DNA has a density of approximately 1.703–1.709 g/cm$^3$ after ultracentrification (26–28). Analysis of VZV DNA reveals a lower guanosine and cytosine composition when compared with that of other human herpesviruses (28,29). It contains 125,000 base pairs, and the genome is organized similar to other herpesjviruses. There are unique long ($U_l$)—105kb—and unique short ($U_s$)—5.2 kb—regions of the genome (30). Each unique sequence contains terminal repeat sequences. The $U_s$ region can invert upon itself and result in two isomeric forms (31–34).

Five VZV glycoproteins have been identified: gp I, gp II, gp III, gp IV, and gp V. Viral infectivity can be neutralized by monoclonal antibodies directed against gp I, gp II, and gp III, as recently reviewed (35). These glycoproteins have been the subject of intense investigative interest as they represent the primary markers for both humoral and cell-mediated immunity.

## *In Vitro* Replication

VZV can be isolated in a variety of continuous and discontinuous cell culture systems of human and simian origin. Cellular cytopathic effect (CPE) begins as a focal process with subsequent cell-to-cell spread, as displayed in Fig. 1. Approximately 8–10 hr after infection, virus-specific immunofluorescence (IF) can be detected in cells adjacent to the initial focus of infection. This parallels the microscopic observation of radial extension of cytopathology (36,37). Electron microscopic (EM) studies show the appearance of immature viral particles within 12 hr of the onset of infection. Subsequently, as with HSV, the capsids acquire their envelope at the nuclear membrane, being released into the perinuclear space where large vacuoles are formed (22,38).

## Pathology

The histopathologic findings in human infection resulting from VZV, whether varicella or herpes zoster, are virtually identical. Vesicles involve the corium and dermis. As viral replication progresses, the epithelial cells undergo degenerative changes characterized by ballooning, with the subsequent appearance of multinucleated giant cells and prominent eosinophilic intranuclear inclusions (4,39). These intranuclear inclusions have been labeled as Cowdry type A intranuclear inclusions indicative of

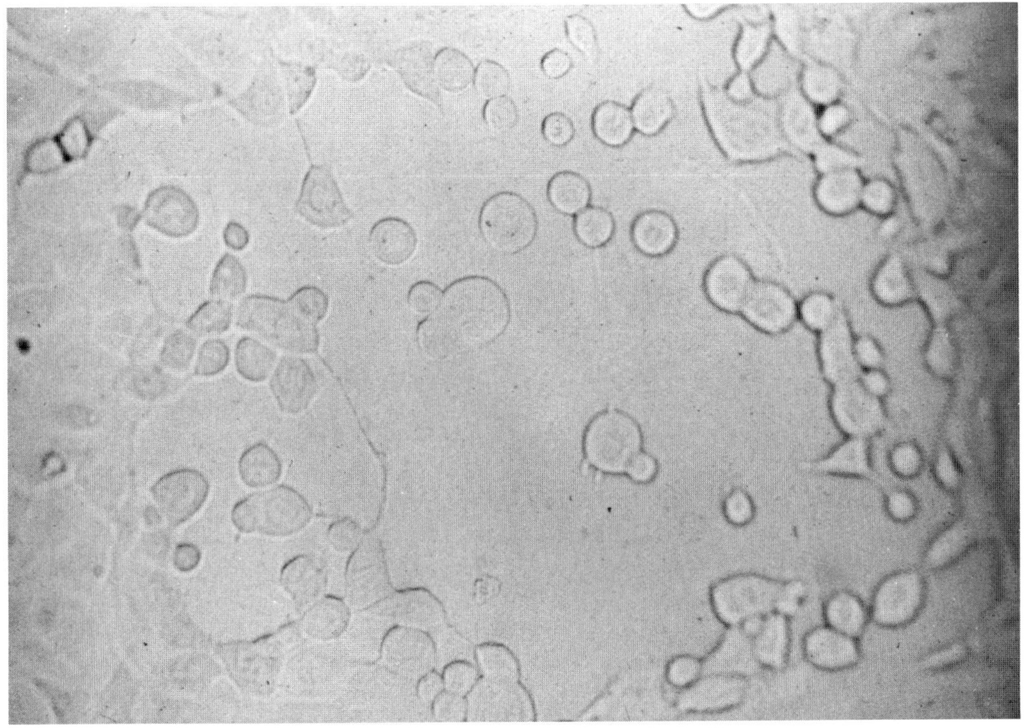

**FIG. 1.** Cytopathic effect of varicella-zoster virus.

herpesvirus infections (40). Under unusual circumstances (disease in severely immunocompromised hosts), necrosis and hemorrhage may appear in the dermis. As the vesicle evolves, the collected fluid becomes cloudy with the appearance of leukocytes, degenerated cells, and fibrin. Ultimately, the vesicles either rupture or gradually become reabsorbed.

## EPIDEMIOLOGY

### Chicken Pox

Humans are the only known reservoir for VZV. Chicken pox follows exposure of a susceptible or seronegative individual to VZV, being a primary infection. Although it is assumed that the virus is spread by the respiratory route and replicates in the nasopharynx or upper respiratory tract, retrieval of virus from individuals incubating VZV has been uncommon. Varicella is endemic in the population at large; however, it becomes epidemic among susceptible individuals during seasonal periods, namely, late winter and early spring (8,41). Overall, chicken pox is a disease of childhood, with 90% of the cases occurring in children younger than 10 years of age, involving both sexes equally and individuals of all races. Only an additional 3% of individuals over the age of 15 are considered susceptible to VZV infection. Typically, the virus is introduced in susceptible school age or preschool children. In a study by Wells and Holla (42), 61 of 67 (91%) susceptible school age children in kindergarten to grade 4 contracted chicken pox during an outbreak. Intimate contact appears to be the key determinant for transmission as evident from infectivity data for household versus societal contacts, where the attack rates were 61% and 12%, respectively (41). Higher household attack rates have been reported by other investigators, approaching 91–96% for susceptible individuals (43,44). These latter attack rates are the most accurate.

Limited data suggest that chicken pox occurs at a higher frequency in adults resident in tropical regions than in other geographic areas. Stokes (45) noted a higher incidence of chicken pox among soldiers during World War II, where the incidence was 1.41 and 2.27 per 1,000 individuals annually. This contrasts with data from the United States during a similar period of time when the rates were approximately one-half (44). It was suggested that the population densities in the tropical countries might influence disease incidence. Socioeconomic factors do not appear to influence the incidence of varicella in the population.

The incubation period of chicken pox, namely, the time interval between exposure of a susceptible person to an infected individual—the index case—and the development of a vesicular rash, is generally regarded as 14–15 days (2,43), with a range of 10–20 days. Slightly over 95% of patients will develop chicken pox between 11 and 20 days following exposure (46). Of children who developed chicken pox, 52% do so on days 13, 14, or 15 following exposure to the index case.

The most accurate data regarding the frequency of secondary attack have been derived from prospective studies examining the prevention of chicken pox through utilization of immune serum products. Rose (46) defined a secondary attack rate of 87% in siblings within the household following introduction of the primary case of varicella. He subsequently identified an attack rate of 71% among siblings who escaped infection on exposure to the primary household index case. Supportive data have come from prospective practice evaluations performed in a semirural community by Hope-Simpson (43). In these studies, attack rates after exposure to an index case among susceptible children aged 0–15 years were 61% in the population at large, as compared to a 68% attack rate among hospitalized individuals. Hospital infectivity studies where infected patients were transferred from the floor or discharged prior to the development of the eruption are most helpful. Children were clearly infectious in the preeruptive stage, approximately 48 hr prior to the onset of a vesicular rash. They remained infectious throughout the period of vesicle formation (generally 4–5 days) until the old vesicles were well pustulated, if not completely crusted (2,47). It should be stressed that the hospital environment is recognized as a site where transmission of VZV infection can occur (48,49). Susceptible hospital employees or patients can acquire chicken pox under such circumstances, particularly when airflow between rooms is not controlled.

### Herpes Zoster

Following initial infection, it is presumed that VZV will establish latency within the dorsal root ganglia and remain so until an appropriate stimulus leads to its reactivation. Histopathologic and molecular biologic examination of the nerve root following infection with VZV demonstrates characteristics indicative of infection. In those individuals who die after recent herpes zoster, a histopathologic examination of the dorsal root ganglia reveals satellitosis, lymphocytic infiltration, and degeneration of the ganglia cells (50–52). Intranuclear inclusion can be found within the ganglia cells. Although it is possible to demonstrate the presence of VZV by electron microscopy, it is not possible to isolate this virus in cultures from the explanted dorsal root ganglia, although viral RNA transcripts have been reported (53,54). In contrast to recurrent labial or genital HSV infections, reactivation of VZV is a much less common event, implying different mechanisms for the establishment and reactivation of these viruses.

Shingles is a disease that occurs in individuals seropositive for VZV or, more specifically, individuals who have suffered prior chicken pox. The standard serologic tools that have been employed historically—namely, detection of complement-fixing antibodies—have been limited by late appearance and early decay of antibodies such that their persistence was found in only approximately 35–40% of individuals with past infection. Thus, the clinical manifestations of disease have been the basis for defining the incidence of infection (55).

Because herpes zoster is a sporadic disease, reactivation appears dependent on a balance between virus and host factors, specifically the host immune system. In contrast to chicken pox, shingles is a disease that occurs for the most part in older individuals, although there are obvious exceptions. Herpes zoster is endemic with no evidence of epidemicity. There appears to be neither demographic differences nor seasonal predisposition in the occurrence of herpes zoster. Similarly, there is no influence of sex, race, or occupation on the incidence of disease.

Although it has been postulated that herpes zoster can lead to the acquisition of shingles in close contacts to the index case, this presumption cannot be substantiated by factual observation. Clearly, herpes zoster can lead to chicken pox, yet the reverse is not apparent.

The most extensive epidemiologic studies of shingles have been performed by McGregor (56) and Hope-Simpson (57). From the studies of Hope-Simpson (57), herpes zoster occurred at an overall annual rate of 3.4 cases per 1,000 persons. The lowest incidence of disease was in individuals younger than 10 years of age where this rate was 0.74 per 1,000 per annum. This rate increased to 5.09 per 1,000 per annum for the sixth through eighth decades of life, and then to over 10 for the ninth decade of life. Eight individuals (4%) suffered a second episode of infection, and one patient had a third episode of disease. For the population of 2,400 patients followed by McGregor (58), the annualized rate was 4.8 per 1,000 (58). McGregor (58) found 75% of those individuals who developed shingles were over 45 years of age.

Herpes zoster can occur early in life, within the first 2 years, in children born to women who had chicken pox during pregnancy (59). These cases likely reflect *in utero* chicken pox with reactivation early in life.

## VARICELLA

### Clinical Manifestations

In most children, the onset of chicken pox begins with rash, low-grade fever, and malaise. A few children will develop the latter symptoms 1 or 2 days prior to the onset of the exanthem. For the most part, chicken pox in the immunocompetent child is a benign illness associated with lassitude and fever of 100–103°F of only 3–5 days' duration. Constitutional symptoms that develop after the onset of rash include pruritus, anorexia, and listlessness. These symptoms gradually resolve as the illness abates. The appearance of the lesions is highly suggestive of the diagnosis. Appearing as small erythematous macules on the trunk and the face, the lesions spread centripetally to involve other areas of the body. The lesions initially contain clear vesicular fluid but over a very short period of time pustulate and scab. Most lesions are small, having an erythematous base with a diameter from 5 mm to as large as 12–13 mm. The lesions can be round or oval, with central umbilication occurring as healing progresses. Examples of the characteristic lesions are shown in Fig. 2, as well as the subsequent events of healing. The lesions themselves have often been referred to as "dew-drop-like" during the early stages of formation. If they do not rupture within a few hours, the contents will become purulent and subsequently will crust. The rash usually remains more severe centrally and on the proximal extremities, often being absent from the lower or distal extremities. Successive crops of lesions generally appear over a period of 2–4 days. Thus, early in the disease, the hallmark of the infection is the appearance of lesions at all stages of development (namely, vesiculation, pustulation, and scabbing), especially when the illness is at its peak. The lesions can also be found on the mucosa of the oropharynx and even the vagina; however, these sites are less common in overall involvement. The crusts completely fall off within 1–2 weeks after the onset, leaving a slightly depressed area of skin.

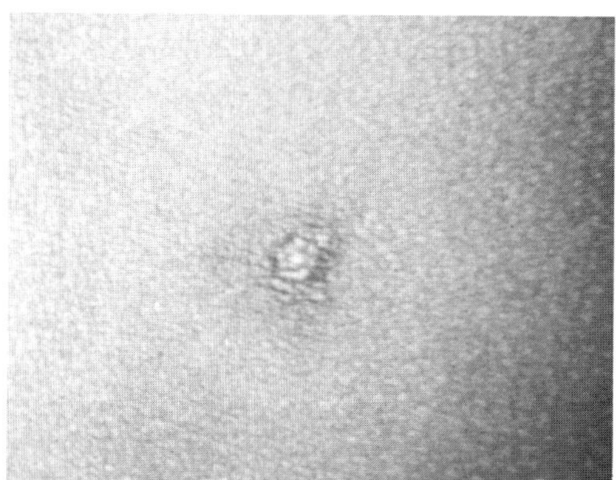

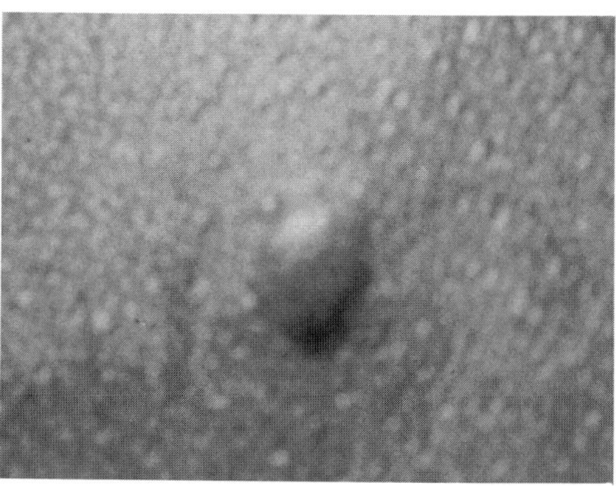

**FIG. 2. Left:** Vesicle on patient with chickenpox. **Right:** Coalesced vesicle on patient with chickenpox.

The severity of the skin lesions varies dramatically from individual to individual, ranging from a complete absence to almost total involvement of the skin. Vesicle counts have been reported to vary between 12 and 2,000 (mean of 258) (60,61). Younger children tend to have fewer vesicles as compared to older children. Lesions tend to be more severe in areas of trauma, as a consequence of intense pruritus or in the diaper region.

In most normal children, there are few gastrointestinal symptoms; however, protracted vomiting occurring late in the course of varicella should suggest the diagnosis of Reye's syndrome.

### Clinical Diagnosis

Today, the differential diagnosis of varicella is less confusing than it was 20 or 30 years ago. Smallpox and disseminated vaccinia were confused with varicella because of their similar cutaneous lesions. With the worldwide eradication of smallpox and the discontinuation of vaccination, these disease entities no longer confuse the clinical diagnosis. In general, the characteristic skin rash with evidence of lesions in all stages of development, associated pruritus, and low-grade fever are sufficient to establish a clinical diagnosis of chicken pox. The epidemiologic history of exposure to an index case with chicken pox in the same classroom or home or to individuals with herpes zoster will further reinforce the presumptive clinical diagnosis.

Impetigo and varicella can be confused clinically. Impetigo is usually caused by the group β-hemolytic streptococcus (*Streptococcus pyogenes*). Following an abrasion of the skin and inoculation of the bacteria at the site of the skin break, small vesicles can appear in the surrounding area. There generally are no systemic signs of disease unless the skin infection is associated with progressive cellulitis or secondary bacteremia. Unroofing of the lesions and careful gram staining of a scraping of the base of the lesion should reveal evidence of Gram-positive cocci in chains, indicative of streptococcus, or Gram-positive cocci in clusters, suggestive of staphylococcus, a less common cause of vesicular skin lesions. The treatment for these diseases are distinctly different from that used in the management of chicken pox and would require the administration of an appropriate antibiotic as predicted upon bacterial culture data.

In a small number of cases, disseminated vesicular lesions can be caused by HSV. In these children, disseminated HSV infection usually is the consequence of an underlying skin disease such as atopic dermatitis or eczema. In this situation, unequivocal diagnosis can only be confirmed by isolation of the offending pathogen in tissue culture. Recently, it has been recognized that disseminated vesiculopapular lesions can be the consequence of enterovirus infections, particularly those caused by the group A Coxsackie virus. These rashes are commonly morbilliform or hemorrhagic in nature rather than vesicular or vesiculopustular. Generally, these diseases occur during the warm months and are associated with lesions of the oropharynx, palms, and soles. This latter finding is most helpful in distinguishing enteroviral disease from varicella.

### Spectrum of Illness

#### *Central Nervous System Disease*

The most common extracutaneous site of involvement by VZV is the central nervous system (CNS), usually resulting in acute cerebellar ataxia. It is estimated to occur in one in 4,000 cases (62,63). This is a generally benign complication of VZV infection and does not require hospitalization. In addition, aseptic meningitis, encephalitis, transverse myelitis, and Reye's syndrome can also occur (64,65). Cerebellar ataxia appears approximately 1 week after the onset of the exanthem, although it may occur prior to and as late as 21 days after the onset of the eruption. An extensive review of 120 cases demonstrated that ataxia, vomiting, altered speech, fever, vertigo, and tremor were all common on physical examination. The most prominent clinical finding was ataxia with minimal, if any, evidence of meningeal irritation. Lymphocytes are present in the cerebrospinal fluid (CSF), and the CSF protein may be elevated. Ataxia generally persists for only 1 week; however, in a small percentage of patients it may persist for 2–4 weeks (66).

Encephalitis is another manifestation of CNS involvement caused by varicella, occurring in 0.1–0.2% of patients (65,67). Underwood's (66) review of 134 cases characterized the illness by depression in the level of consciousness with progressive headache, vomiting, altered thought patterns, fever, and frequent seizures. The CSF findings were pertinent for lymphocytosis and proteinosis. With findings of overt encephalitis, the expected duration of disease is at least 2 weeks. In some patients, there is progressive neurologic deterioration and resultant death, with mortality rates as high as 20% in the elderly. It is essential to distinguish progressive encephalitis from Reye's syndrome (65,66).

Other manifestations of neurologic involvement include polyradiculitis and myelitis. The association of varicella with Guillain-Barre is well documented in the literature (68).

Parenthetically, no form of therapy other than excellent supportive care is available for managing patients with CNS involvement. Frequently, these individuals will require intensive care for support of intravascular volume, ventilation, and control of cerebral edema. There is no indication that antiviral medications, immune serum products, or antibiotics are useful in altering the manifestations of CNS involvement. The encephalitic manifestations are associated with significant mortality, varying between 5% and 20%, and morbidity, approximately 15% of survivors (61,66).

### *Varicella Pneumonitis*

An equally serious complication of varicella is the appearance of pneumonitis (69). This complication appears to be more common in adults than children (70), occurring in approximately one in 400 cases. Three to 5 days into the course of illness, progressive tachypnea and cough appear (71). Respiratory distress may increase rapidly, probably as a consequence of hemorrhagic necrosis of the lung. As shown in Fig. 3, the chest roentgenogram demonstrates diffuse nodular infiltrates of the lung (72). Prospective studies of military personnel found roentgenographic abnormalities in nearly 16% of enlisted men who developed varicella, yet only one-quarter of these individuals had evidence of cough (69). Only 10% of those with radiographic abnormalities developed evidence of tachypnea, indicating that asymptomatic pneumonitis may exist more commonly than initially predicted. The normal child rarely develops pneumonitis (71).

### *Secondary Bacterial Infections*

*Streptococcus pyogenes* and *Staphylococcus aureus* can cause secondary bacterial infections in patients with chicken pox. Pruritus is common in children with varicella; thus, inoculation of bacteria directly into scratched skin is common. Gram stain of the lesions should help clarify the etiology of pustular lesions that appear beyond the normal time course of varicella and will allow for rational intervention with antimicrobial therapy. In the preantibiotic era, bacterial complications of chicken pox were common, occurring in 5.2% of the patient population (73,74). Extracutaneous sites of bacterial infection developed, including otitis media, sinusitis, meningitis, osteomyelitis, and bacterial pneumonia. In

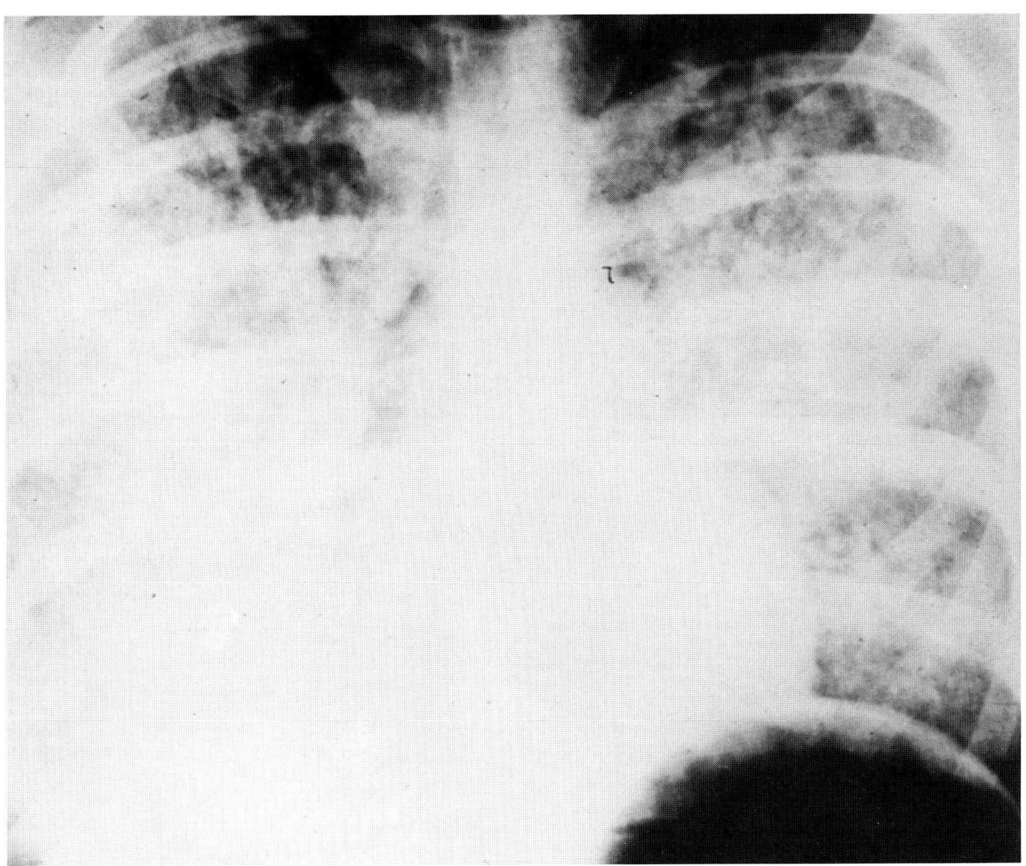

**FIG. 3.** Varicella pneumonitis.

the antibiotic era, these complications have posed less of a problem. Improved hygiene, daily bathing, and utilization of astringent soaps have helped further decrease the frequency of cutaneous skin infections.

### *Reye's Syndrome*

Varicella has been associated epidemiologically with Reye's syndrome (75,76). The syndrome begins with vomiting in the latter stages of varicella infection, followed by restlessness, irritability, and progressive decrease in level of consciousness, all associated with progressive cerebral edema. Encephalopathy is associated with elevated serum levels of ammonia, bleeding diatheses, hyperglycemia, and elevated transaminase levels (77). Management of patients with Reye's syndrome is directed at correcting the altered physiology rather than attacking replication of VZV, which is often no longer present. The recent association between Reye's syndrome and aspirin administration should be stressed. Acetaminophen administration should be used for alleviation of fever in these patients.

### *Other Complications*

A variety of other complications have been reported in patients suffering from varicella (78). These include bleeding diatheses (79), arthritis (80), appendicitis (81), and acute glomerulonephritis (82), among other less common clinical manifestations.

## Laboratory Diagnosis

### *Virus Isolation*

Confirmation of the diagnosis is possible only through isolation of virus in susceptible tissue culture lines or the demonstration of seroconversion by antibody assessment. A rapid diagnostic impression can be obtained by scraping the base of the lesions in an attempt to demonstrate intranuclear inclusion bodies and multinucleated giant cells by Tzanck smear. These changes are not pathognomonic for VZV infection and require differentiation from other herpesvirus infections, specifically HSV. The ideal diagnostic confirmation is isolation of VZV from clinical specimens. It is important to emphasize that bedside collection and inoculation of specimens are imperative for recovery of virus in tissue culture. Vesicles should be aspirated with a tuberculin syringe containing viral transport media at the bedside and inoculated directly into susceptible cell lines. Cell lines suitable for isolation of VZV include either human embryonic skin-muscle tissue or foreskin fibroblasts. Although cytopathic effects can appear within 48–72 hr, it is more likely for them to appear approximately 7–10 days after inoculation of clinical specimens into the tissue. The description of the cytopathology has been noted previously. Unequivocal confirmation of the CPE can be achieved by neutralization with antibody in a complement-dependent neutralization assay or through fluorescent staining of the cell sheet.

### *Serologic Confirmation*

Serologic assessment of patients with VZV infections has focused historically on utilization of the complement-fixing (CF) antibody assay, although other approaches have included indirect IF, fluorescent antibody to VZV membrane antigen (FAMA), complement-dependent neutralization, immune adherence hemagglutination (IAHA), enzyme-linked immunoabsorbance assay (ELISA), and radioimmunoassay (RIA). The CF assay has been replaced by more sensitive antibody detection procedures that utilize antigens prepared in alternative fashions (83–86).

Sensitive routinely applied antibody assays include the FAMA, IAHA, and ELISA. The development of the FAMA assay provided a particularly sensitive antibody detection procedure, allowing for the demonstration of prompt seroconversion with eightfold or higher rises in patients who developed herpes zoster or chicken pox (87). The FAMA antibodies appear earlier and, when compared to other antibodies, persist much longer. Moreover, individuals who suffered from distant past VZV infections had persistence of antibodies. The application of this test has been widespread, including its utilization in clinical trials of zoster immune globulin in order to assess patient immunity at the time of passive immunization and for monitoring host response in VZV vaccine trials.

A more cumbersome assay, but one which is biologically relevant for the detection of antibodies to VZV, is a neutralization assay. Classically, neutralizing antibodies have been utilized to advantage to determine status of immunity to a variety of viral infections. However, because of VZV's lack of production of cell-free virus, the development of a neutralization assay has been particularly difficult. Early efforts (88) have been replaced by the development of a sensitive plaque reduction assay utilizing the principle of complement enhancement (89). Concordance does exist between complement-enhanced neutralizing tests and the FAMA assays; however, the necessity of maintaining live tissue and the inherent requirement of several days for the performance of the neutralization assay preclude its routine clinical usefulness (89,90).

An IAHA assay has similarly been adapted for assessing serologic status as related to VZV infection (91). This assay compares favorably with FAMA for sensitivity and specificity. When sera from patients with either chicken pox or herpes zoster were tested simultaneously by these methods, antibodies resulting from subclinical infections were detectable in the serum of patients slightly more often by the FAMA assay than by the IAHA assay. Thus, the FAMA test is perhaps superior to the IAHA for determination of humoral immune status.

An ELISA for VZV infections has been developed (92). Utilizing contemporary technology for rapid identification of antibodies to VZV, this assay has a high concordance with complement-dependent neutralizing antibody assays and requires significantly less time to perform (67). Comparative studies will need to define whether this method may prove to be an acceptable substitute for the popular FAMA assay. The reader is referred to the detailed discussion of each of these assays and their practical applicability for diagnostic purposes in an excellent review (16).

Recently, research efforts have focused on defining host responses to specified polypeptides, particularly the glycoproteins, as well as immunoglobulin subclass responses (93,94). These studies are currently being performed to understand disease pathogenesis (95), identify risk factors for severe disease, and provide insight into the antigenic composition of vaccines.

### Perinatal Varicella

Chicken pox has been reported in the newborn child. This is not a common occurrence, since 90–95% of the population has preexisting antibodies to VZV, and, therefore, the risk of infection during pregnancy is small. Two routes of infection for the fetus are apparent. First, transplacental infection following maternal viremia can be associated with *in utero* chicken pox. The fetus *in utero* will manifest chicken pox approximately 2 days following the onset of maternal disease (96). Second, there may be direct contact with infected genital secretions if the maternal rash involves the vaginal mucosa.

The consequence of chicken pox on the developing fetus *in utero,* specifically the incidence of fetal wastage and malformation, is unclear. The first case report suggesting an association between varicella and birth defects appeared in 1947 with a description of an infant having multiple congenital abnormalities who was born to a mother who developed varicella during the eighth week of gestation (97). A review has summarized the congenital malformations associated with chicken pox and correlated their appearance to the time of acquisition of infection (98). For the most part, newborns suffered from cicatricial skin scarring, often overlying hypoplastic limbs with hypo- or hyperplastic digits. Most of the infants described with this syndrome have had evidence of encephalitis and significant motor retardation. Eye abnormalities, including combinations of chorioretinitis, microphthalmia, and cataracts, are common. The majority of these infants died during early infancy. It is clear that most of these children had infection during the first trimester, especially prior to 15 weeks. Nevertheless, the total number of babies suffering from these manifestations remains small, as reiterated in a more recent and detailed report (59). In a prospective investigation performed of 1,500 women during pregnancy, 150 women were detected to have varicella. In this group of women, there was no increase in fetal deaths or abortions when compared with appropriate controls. Two children had stigmata that suggested congenital disease (99).

Chicken pox that occurs later in gestation has been recognized to have different risks for the developing fetus or newborn. If infection of the mother occurs during the second or early third trimester of gestation, *in utero* fetal infection results in clearing of the virus prior to delivery, probably controlled in part by transplacental antibodies (100). Some children who had *in utero* disease develop herpes zoster during early infancy (101). The recognition of shingles early in infancy in the absence of postnatal chicken pox has been reported (102,103). An uncomplicated clinical course is the rule rather than the exception.

A more life-threatening situation occurs in infants who develop varicella within the first 10 days of life; these newborns are considered to have congenital varicella (104–108) and probably acquired infection by the placental route. Infection of the fetus may well have been initiated prior to the accumulation of transplacental VZV antibodies; therefore, the consequences of infection can be extreme. However, if a vesicular rash is present at the time of birth, it is likely that the disease has been ameliorated by transplacental maternal antibodies. Thus, it is only those children whose mothers have not had an adequate opportunity to elicit a humoral immune response that appear to be at greatest risk for visceral dissemination. Specifically, those infants born to mothers whose rash develops within 4 days of delivery have the greatest propensity for developing severe disease. As a consequence, vesicles will appear in the newborn child between approximately 5 and 10 days of life, given the average 14-day incubation period. When infants are born under such conditions, the mortality rate may be as high as 30%. These children have progressive disease involving visceral organs, especially the lung. The outcome in these children has been summarized by Brunell (109). He further described the possible beneficial effects of transplacental maternal antibody (100). It must be remembered that the maternal infection does not invariably cause fetal disease. Furthermore, susceptible newborns or their postpartum mothers, when exposed to VZV in the community, may develop chicken pox that may not be of great severity.

No data support the efficacy of immune serum globulin administered to the exposed susceptible pregnant woman, although intravenous immune globulin has been given. Recommendations for the woman who develops chicken pox early in gestation cannot be made because of the lack of information regarding the routine outcome of all pregnancies. On the other hand, infants born to mothers with evidence of varicella that begins less than 4 days prior to delivery are known to be a risk for severe and life-threatening complications. This group of newborns should receive zoster immune globulin. If vesicular lesions are present at the time of birth, isolation would be of value in limiting the potential spread of infection in the newborn nursery.

### Varicella in the Immunocompromised Host

Chicken pox in the immunocompromised child or adult is associated with significant morbidity and mortality. Clearly, disease takes on proportions not evident in the normal host. The largest historical survey of chicken pox in children with lymphoproliferative malignancies and solid tumors was performed by Feldman (110). He reported that children not receiving chemotherapy for induction or relapse infrequently develop progressive chicken pox; yet, or those children receiving cancer chemotherapy, approximately one-third had progressive disease with involvement of multiple organs (including the lungs, liver, and CNS). The majority of these children—20% of all those who acquired chicken pox—developed pneumonitis within the first week of illness. Visceral organ involvement is probably the consequence of viremia (111). It was within this group that the largest number of deaths occurred. It was concluded that if chemotherapy was terminated 5 days prior to the onset of disease, progression to severe illness was decreased. More recently, the severity of chicken pox has been documented in bone marrow transplant recipients (112). Observations of other investigators, particularly in those studies performed in asthmatic children receiving prednisone in dosages up to 15 mg/

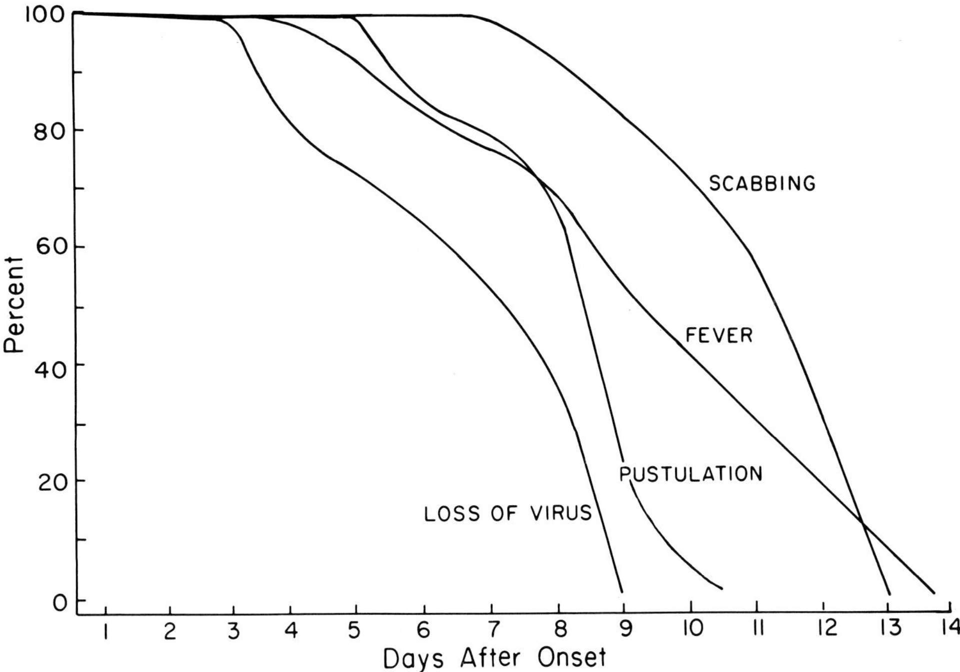


**FIG. 4.** Events of healing in chickenpox.

day, do not support increased risk in this particular subpopulation of patients (113).

Other studies have elaborated the natural history of chicken pox in the immunocompromised host and focus on the parallel between prolonged lesion formation and active viremia. The rash of chicken pox in the immunocompromised host begins centrally and spreads peripherally as it does in the normal host; however, in this situation the lesions tend to be larger and more numerous. Often, the lesions have hemorrhagic bases with large purpuric spots appearing. The natural events of healing are displayed in Fig. 4. New lesions continue to form for a period of approximately 10 days. Fever persists as long as 10–14 days in untreated patients (114). Complete scabbing and resolution of disease in the immunocompromised host with varicella appear prolonged by approximately twofold when compared to the normal host.

Immunocompromised children have been prospectively evaluated for the appearance of complications when they received no modality of therapy. Of 48 children, 13 (27%) developed evidence of life-threatening disease and eight died (17%) (115–117). These data are summarized in Table 1 along with the effects of treatment, which will be discussed below. Individuals with lymphoproliferative malignancies requiring chemotherapy appeared to be at greatest risk for progressive visceral involvement and death.

## Clinical Management of Varicella

### *Prevention*

As with other infectious diseases, prophylaxis can take one of two possible forms: either immunization or prevention with immune serum products. For the normal host, prophylaxis and treatment are of no special importance since the disease is generally benign. Thus, medical manage-

**TABLE 1.** *Therapy for chicken pox in immunocompromised patients*[a]

| Demographics | Vidarabine ($N$ = 19) | Leukocyte interferon ($N$ = 23) | ACV ($N$ = 8) | Placebo ($N$ = 48) |
|---|---|---|---|---|
| ALL or AML | 12 (63%) | 18 (78%) | 6 (75%) | 37 (77%) |
| Disease duration (days ± SE) | 1.7 ± 0.8 | 1.61 ± 0.50 | 2.2 ± 1.6 | 1.94 ± 1.08 |
| Healing, time to lesion cessation (days ± SE) | 3.8 ± 1.1 | 3.8 ± 1.89 | NR | 5.45 ± 2.16 |
| Visceral complications | | | | |
| Postenrollment pneumonia | 1 (5%) | 3 (13%) | 0 | 13 (27%) |
| Encephalitis | 0 | 0 | 0 | 3 (6%) |
| Hepatitis | 0 | 5 (22%) | 0 | 9 (19%) |
| Overall | 0 | 8 (35%) | 0 | 25 (52%) |
| Mortality | 0 | 2 (9%) | 0 | 8 (17%) |

[a]Data from refs. 12, 125, and 168.
ALL, acute lymphoblastic; AML, acute myelocytic leukemia; NR, not reported.

ment simply involves preventing avoidable complications. These include secondary bacterial infection of the skin, which can be averted by meticulous care of the skin lesions and by measures to decrease the pruritus. The pruritus can be significantly lessened with topical dressings of calamine lotion or by the oral administration of Benadryl or Atarax at appropriate dosages. Furthermore, maintaining closely cropped fingernails will prevent excoriation of the skin and associated secondary infection. Administration of antipyretics should be approached with care in the child suffering from chicken pox because of the association between aspirin derivatives and the development of Reye's syndrome.

Because the immunocompromised child is at risk for developing progressive varicella, two potential modalities of prevention are immune prophylaxis and vaccination. Ross (60) has studied the effect of serum γ globulin (at varying dosages) in 242 children exposed to chicken pox but given γ globulin within 72 hr. The results were compared to data derived from 209 children who served as unimmunized controls. At the higher dosages of γ globulin, the total vesicle count was significantly decreased. Children who formed less than 20 lesions accounted for approximately 40% of the globulin recipients, compared to only 1% of those in the control group (60).

This observation of the beneficial effect of serum globulin on the natural history of chicken pox, when added to the knowledge that herpes zoster and varicella were caused by the same virus, led to a field trial designed to assess the value of high-titered immune globulin for disease prevention (118). This globulin product has become known as zoster immune globulin (ZIG) and is derived from adults suffering from recent herpes zoster. In subsequent placebo-controlled studies of six families, the recipients of ZIG failed to develop chicken pox, whereas the controls acquired disease (118). Thus, ZIG appeared to prevent infection when given to healthy children shortly after exposure.

This study led to trials performed in immunocompromised children at high risk for complications from chicken pox (119). Safety and tolerance studies performed following the administration of 5 ml ZIG to high-risk household contacts of children with chicken pox demonstrated both ameliorative and protective effects (120,121). The administration of ZIG did not unequivocally prevent disease but simply modified the disease course (122). Its utilization has become increasingly widespread.

For true effectiveness, ZIG must be administered within 72 hr of contact and only to individuals at extremely high risk. It is available for individuals with underlying diseases of leukemia or lymphoma, congenital or acquired immunodeficiency, active immunosuppressive therapy, or the newborn of a mother with chicken pox who developed disease within 4 days of delivery. For purposes of ZIG administration, close exposure is defined as either a household contact, indoor contact of greater than 1 hr with a playmate, or a hospital contact on the same ward. There should be no prior history of chicken pox, and the age of the patient should be less than 15 years (123). ZIG can be obtained for immunodeficient children through the local Red Cross offices and hospital pharmacies. The administration of intravenous globulin products will result in plasma antibody levels equated with protection, but these products have not yet been formally tested for these indications (124).

### *Vaccination*

Vaccine development is discussed in detail in Chapter 19. Only recently has a live attenuated vaccine been developed for prevention of chicken pox in high-risk groups, particularly through the efforts of Takahashi et al. (125,126). This vaccine is being developed for prevention of chicken pox in the normal host as well (127). Although licensed in Japan, this vaccine remains experimental in the United States (128). Studies performed to date indicate a high probability of protection following vaccination. Results from these trials have been summarized (125,129,130). The effects of vaccination on the transmissibility of VZV in a children's hospital ward have been studied. The patients on this ward suffered from nephrotic syndrome, nephritis, bacterial meningitis, and hepatitis. With vaccination, side effects were minimal (minimal rash 10–14 days after vaccination) (126). Transmission was prevented within a high-risk group. Follow-up clinical and antibody responses indicated persistence of protection (131).

Trials performed in immunocompromised children have determined protective efficacy of this attenuated VZV vaccine. Vaccine recipients seroconverted, but approximately 8% developed a mild rash 10–14 days after immunization (132). Follow-up of vaccine recipients 2 years after immunization demonstrated persistence of immunity in 50 of 51 original vaccinees (133). These landmark studies were performed in immunocompromised children who no longer received chemotherapy. Further studies have been conducted in children whose chemotherapy has not been suspended. In this subgroup of patients, the incidence of side effects and the appearance of rash suggestive of varicella occur frequently, indicating a degree of concern for the status of chemotherapy at the time of immunization (134). It appears that the vaccine is protective but not without risk. An unknown entity at this time is whether the administration of vaccine will change the subsequent natural history of herpes zoster or predispose the immunocompromised child to severe forms of herpes zoster, as are encountered in other immunosuppressed patients. This problem has not yet emerged in detailed follow-up studies. Thus, the OKA strain developed by Takahashi et al. in Japan has been studied extensively in both the normal and leukemic child (133,134,136). Parenthetically, the vaccine strain of VZV can be distinguished from wild-type virus isolates (135).

In immunocompromised children, serologic evidence of host response following vaccination has been achieved in between 89% and 100% of vaccinated individuals (21) in well over 1,000 patients. Antibody response to vaccine differs from natural infection (136). Vaccine induced rash, however, is not uncommon occurring at a low of 6% to as high as 47%. Those factors that are most likely to be predictive of the appearance of rash are the extent of immunosuppression. Specifically, for children with acute lymphoblastic leukemia, the likelihood of rash is as high as 40–50%. The subsequent occurrence of varicella after community exposure is decreased, averaging 8–16%. The occurrence of herpes zoster following vaccination does not seem to pose a major risk (137,138).

Similar studies have been performed in normal children, with total numbers well in excess of 1,000 individuals, as recently reviewed (35). In these studies, antibody responses were higher than in the immunocompromised host, varying between 94% and 100% (127,139,140). Vaccine-induced rash was far less common in these individuals, occurring at a frequency of 0.5% to approximately 19% overall, with subsequent appearance of varicella following community exposure averaging between 1% and 5%. Theoretically, this vaccine might be useful for boosting immunity in older individuals as a mechanism to prevent herpes zoster infection; however, this hypothesis remains to be tested.

Some concern exists regarding the universal administration of this vaccine to the normal host. If universal vaccination was to be employed, it would be important to determine whether such a procedure would change the epidemiology of VZV infections, allowing for a larger number of cases of either chicken pox or herpes zoster during early adulthood, at which time the infection might be more severe. This has not been the case in vaccine studies done in the immunocompromised host to date.

### *Other Observations*

A discussion of prevention of chicken pox must recognize that the hospital environment can be a setting for transmission of infection to individuals at greater risk (susceptible adult health care workers or immunocompromised patients). Thus, patients with chicken pox who require hospitalization must be isolated to avoid cases of hospital acquired disease. Ideally, isolation requires negative airflow ventilation.

### *Antiviral Treatment*

Because of the recognized complications of varicella, several experimental antiviral treatments have been attempted in immunocompromised subjects. Historically, the first of the therapeutic trials employed cytosine arabinoside (ara-C), a drug that failed because of a low therapeutic index (ratio of efficacy to toxicity) (141–145).

The data from three successful antiviral trials of chicken pox are summarized in Table 1. The first successful antiviral chemotherapeutic for the management of chicken pox in the immunocompromised host was the drug vidarabine (adenine arabinoside). In controlled investigations of 34 immunocompromised patients performed by the National Institute of Allergy and Infectious Diseases (NIAID) Collaborative Antiviral Study Group, a dosage of 10 mg/kg/day resulted in treated patients ceasing to form new lesions and defervescing more rapidly than the placebo counterparts (114). Importantly, the treated patients had a significantly lower incidence of life-threatening complications, 53% in placebo versus 5% in drug recipients, $p < 0.01$ (Fischer exact test) (114). Thus, when therapy is instituted within 72 hr of the onset of chicken pox in the immunocompromised host, outcome is beneficially influenced (114). Neurologic toxicity has been reported in children treated with vidarabine for chicken pox (146).

A similar study model was employed for the evaluation of acyclovir (ACV) (116). In this trial, therapy had no effect on cutaneous healing or fever; however, the administration of ACV did decrease the development of pneumonitis from 45% to 0%. No significant toxicity was reported. In spite of the lack of large-scale controlled studies, the safety of ACV and its efficacy for other VZV infections have led to its preferential use in this disease.

ACV has been studied in adults with chicken pox who were considered to have normal immune systems. This clinical trial suggested the value of therapy (147).

Interferons are a series of naturally occurring low molecular weight glycoproteins that, among other functions, act as a host defense to viral infection. High titers of interferon have been found in vesicle fluid from patients with varicella at the termination of illness, suggesting that interferon may play a role in the control of this disease (148). High dosages of interferon have been shown to decrease the frequency of visceral complications and prevent progressive disease in children with varicella (115,149). The dosage of interferon used in these studies was $30 \times 10^6$ IU administered intramuscularly daily for 5 days. These interferons were produced by Dr. Kari Cantell from leukocytes harvested and challenged for interferon production (see Chapter 2). To date, no published studies have reported evaluations of recombinant DNA interferons alone or in combination with antiviral agents for the management of varicella in high-risk populations.

## HERPES ZOSTER

### Clinical Manifestations

As noted earlier, herpes zoster is the consequence of reactivation of latent VZV. It is characterized by excruciating pain—in most adults, localized within the dermatome of the vesicular eruption. The vesicular rash is unilateral in involvement in most patients, as shown in Fig. 5. The dermatomes most usually involved are form T3 through L4 (57,150). Involvement of cervical and facial dermatomes can have special complications. If the opthalmic branch of the trigeminal nerve is involved, zoster ophthalmicus is a common complication, as discussed in Chapter 7. With involvement of the ophthalmic branch, it is not at all unusual to have lesions on the forehead as well as the tip of the nose. Lesions of other branches of the trigeminal nerve (the maxillary branch or the mandibular branch) can result in intraoral involvement, with lesions of the palate, tonsilar fossa, floor of the mouth, and the tongue. A Ramsey-Hunt syndrome will occur if the geniculate ganglion is involved, with skin manifestations of the ear as shown in Fig. 6.

No known factors are responsible for the precipitation of the events of herpes zoster. If herpes zoster does occur in the child, the course is generally benign and not associated with progressive pain or discomfort. In the adult, systemic manifestations, particularly acute neuritis and postherpetic neuralgia, can be debilitating. The onset of disease is heralded by pain within the dermatome that may precede by approximately 24–48 hr the appearance of an erythematous rash prior to the onset of vesicular lesions. In the normal host, these lesions remain few in number and progress for a period of approximately 3–5 days before pustulating and scabbing. The total duration of disease is generally between 7 and 10 days; however, it may take as long as 3–4 weeks before the skin returns to normal.

### Clinical Diagnosis

Unilateral vesicular lesions in a dermatomal pattern lead the clinician to suspect a diagnosis of shingles. The diagnosis can be confirmed by isolation of virus from the involved lesions. Again, the optimal method for retrieval of virus is bedside inoculation of aspirated vesicular fluid into susceptible tissue culture. It has been reported that HSV and Coxsackie virus infections can masquerade as dermatomal vesicular lesions. In such situations, diagnostic viral cultures remain the best method for determining the etiology of the infection. The utilization of lesion scrapings and staining by Tzanck smear to demonstrate the presence of intranuclear inclusions and multinucleated giant cells will be of help in

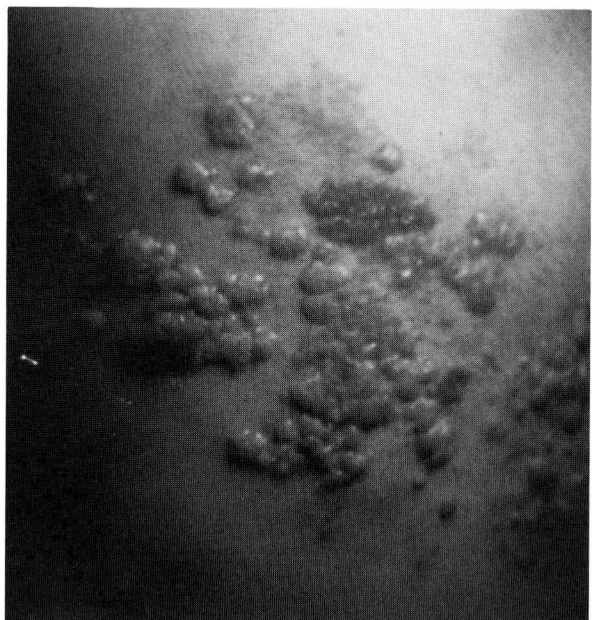

**FIG. 5. Left:** Localized herpes zoster. **Below:** Cluster of lesions from patients with herpes zoster.

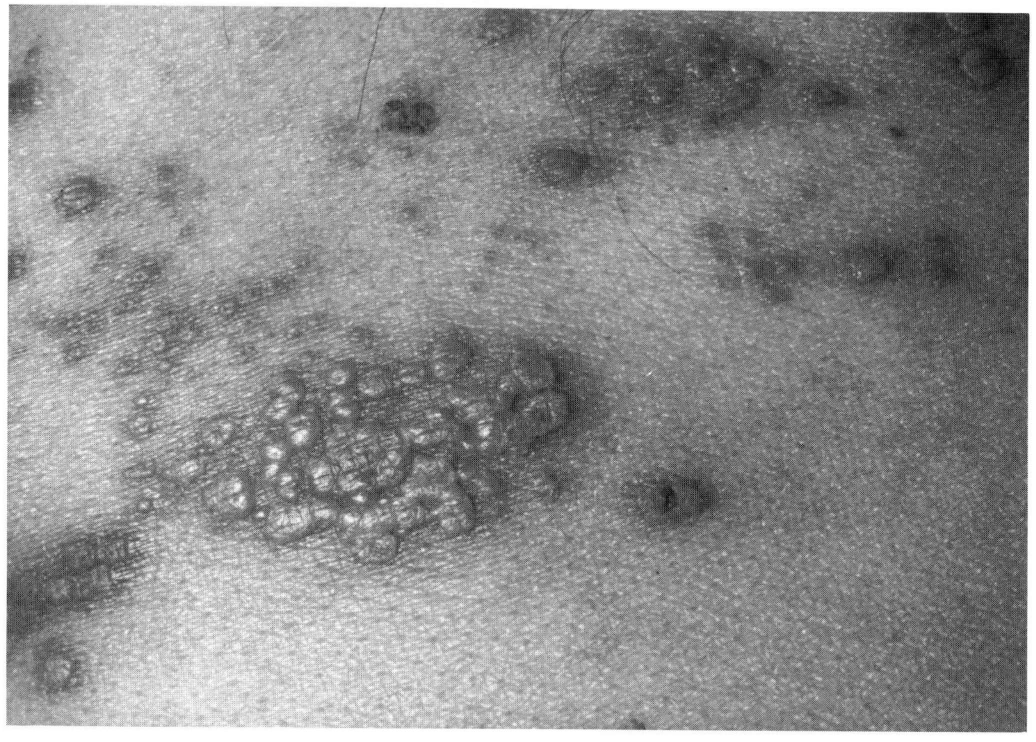

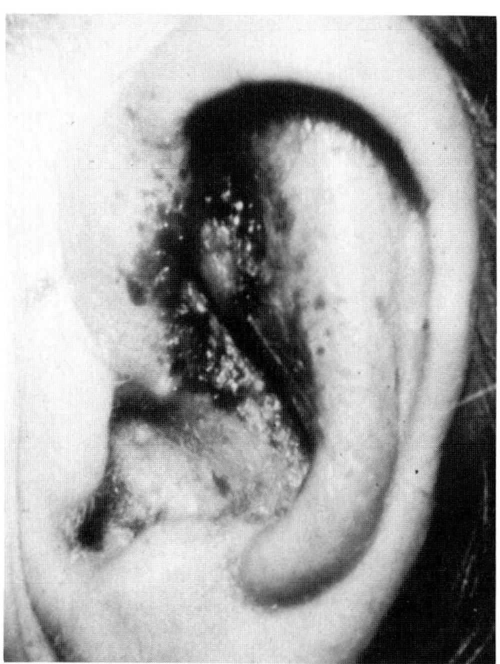

**FIG. 6.** Herpes zoster lesions of ear in the Ramsey-Hunt syndrome.

establishing a presumptive diagnosis of herpesvirus infection, as discussed.

## Spectrum of Illness

### *Pain*

The most debilitating complication of zoster both in the immunocompromised host and the normal individual is its association with acute neuritis and postherpetic neuralgia. Although postherpetic neuralgia is extremely uncommon in young individuals, at least 50% of afflicted patients over the age of 60 will have persistent pain. The mean duration of pain is variable, but it generally lasts for less than 6 months in most patients. Approximately 5–10% of patients return to the physician, with recurrent complaints persisting 6 months after the onset of infection (57). The incidence of this complication has prompted a variety of treatment regimens, ranging from long-term administration of narcotic analgesics to attempts at altering the acute pain course with hopes of having an impact on the subsequent appearance of postherpetic neuralgia (steroids, Elavil, prolixin, etc.). These modalities of management will be discussed under treatment.

### *CNS Involvement*

Involvement of the CNS in the presence of herpes zoster is probably more common than recognized (151). Invariably, patients who undergo CSF examination for other reasons during episodes of shingles are found to have evidence of pleocytosis without proteinosis. These patients are without signs of meningeal irritation and infrequently complain of headaches. Asymptomatic meningoencephalitis is common in these patients. The onset begins with headache, fever, photophobia, meningeal irritation, and vomiting. Progressive alteration in level of consciousness with or without seizures has been reported in patients who develop encephalitis. Importantly, a rare manifestation of herpes zoster infections of the CNS is granulomatous arteritis (152,153). This particular syndrome can be diagnosed by cerebral arteriography and is associated clinically with contralateral hemiparesis. It usually follows zoster ophthalmicus (154), as reviewed (26).

Classically, VZV involves dorsal root ganglia. Motor paralysis can occur and is the consequence of involvement of the anterior horn cells in a manner similar to that encountered with polio. Patients with involvement of the anterior horn cells are particularly prone to excruciating pain. Other neuromuscular disorders associated with herpes zoster include transverse myelitis (155) and myositis (46,71). The latter has been associated with electromyographic changes indicative of true motor paralysis. The Ramsey-Hunt syndrome represents involvement of the facial nerve resulting in lesions of the external auditory canal or the tympanic membrane. This may be associated with facial paralysis and almost always with auditory symptoms.

### *Zoster Ophthalmicus*

Involvement of the ophthalmic branch of the fifth cranial nerve, seen in approximately 7% of all cases of herpes zoster, results in zoster ophthalmicus. Inflammation can lead to cicatricial lid retraction, ptosis, conjunctivitis, scleritis, uveitis, chorioretinitis, and even blindness.

### *Unusual Manifestations*

Other complications following herpes zoster generally occur in the presence of disseminated disease, with resulting pneumonitis, gangrene of the involved dermatomal, or hepatitis; these complications are usually seen only in immunocompromised hosts. Myositis has been reported (156).

## Herpes Zoster in the Immunocompromised Host

As noted for varicella infections of the immunocompromised host, herpes zoster poses particular challenges for the clinician in the presence of an underlying malignancy. Disease is exaggerated with prolonged vesicle formation and time to total scabbing. As displayed in Fig. 7, the median time to total cessation of new vesicle formation, pustulation, and scabbing in a group of 59 untreated immunocompromised patients was 8, 9, and 18 days, respectively. Thus, the natural history is extended by approximately 1 week. Patients at greatest risk for developing herpes zoster are individuals suffering from Hodgkin's disease and non-Hodgkin's lymphoma. At our institution, the annualized incidence of herpes zoster following newly diagnosed lymphoproliferative malignancies is 15% per year. This particular patient population represents a subgroup at increased risk for complications. In part, the high risk of complications is paralleled by impaired cell-mediated immunity (157,158). Lymphocyte reactivity (transformation assays) is decreased in patients with lymphoproliferative malignancies, being an indirect indicator of impaired host response (158,159). It has been presumed that individuals who developed zoster but appeared healthy were at risk for cancer; yet, this cannot be substantiated (160).

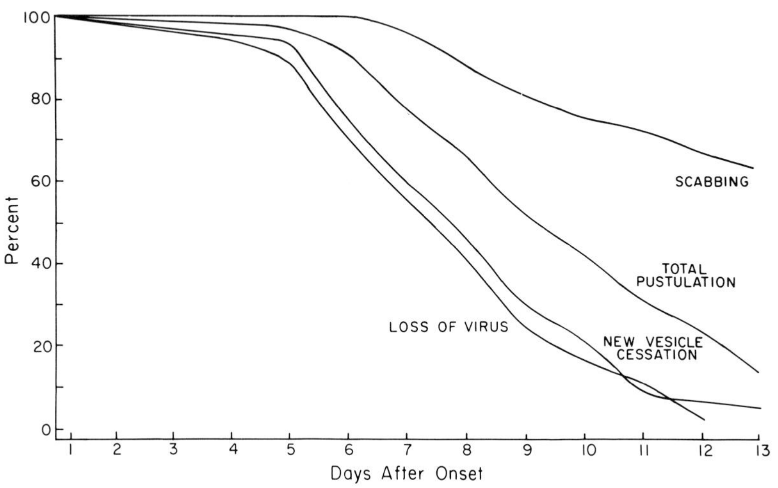


**FIG. 7.** Cutaneous resolution of herpes zoster in the immunocompromised host.

Clearly, the major problem encountered with herpes zoster in the immunocompromised host is the risk for cutaneous dissemination and visceral involvement. Those patients at greatest risk are individuals who have lymphoproliferative malignancies. Logistic regression analyses demonstrated that patients with Hodgkin's disease, non-Hodgkin's lymphoma, leukemia, and oat-cell carcinoma of the lung had a 40% risk of cutaneous dissemination following the development of localized herpes zoster (117). Furthermore, there was a direct correlation between cutaneous dissemination and the appearance of visceral complications. No other factor, including preceding and concurrent corticosteroid and cytotoxic therapy, age, sex, or duration of disease, predicted visceral complications other than the underlying malignancy. These findings segregate a subset of patients for whom early institution of antiviral therapy will be mandatory.

Over the past several years, herpes zoster has been documented in male homosexuals, intravenous drug abusers, and others with human immunodeficiency virus (HIV) infections. Although disease frequency is higher, visceral complications are uncommon.

## Clinical Management

### *Supportive Care*

There is no specific therapy for herpes zoster in the normal host. The optimal approach is supportive care with appropriate administration of analgesics for control of pain. Cleansing of the lesions and frequent Burrow's solution soaks to the involved surface area are soothing and help to prevent secondary bacterial infection. With severe neuritis, it has been suggested that Elavil (amitriptyline hydrochloride) and Prolixin (fluphenazine hydrochloride), alone or in combination, are useful for amelioration of acute neuritis and may decrease the frequency of postherpetic neuralgia. In addition, administration of steroids has been reported to be useful in small controlled studies (161,162). Utilization of orally administered steroids may, however, delay healing in the primary dermatome (117). One recent large study concluded that pain was not beneficially influenced by the administration of corticosteroids (163). Severe unrelenting pain may necessitate nerve blocks.

### *Antiviral Therapy*

Specific therapeutic measures have been developed for treatment of herpes zoster in the immunocompromised host. Obviously, the high-risk patient with lymphoproliferative malignancy has the greatest need for parenteral antiviral therapy. At the present, although three medications have been shown useful, only two therapies are of relevance. These therapeutic trials are summarized in Table 2. In two studies, vidarabine has been shown to accelerate the events of cutaneous healing, namely cessation of new vesicle formation, time to total pustulation, and scabbing (Fig. 8) (117,164,165). Furthermore, therapy within 72 hr of onset prevents progression of lesion formation within the dermatome and allows gradual regression of the disease in the area involved. The most important advantage of administration of vidarabine to immunocompromised patients is the reduction of visceral complications from a frequency overall of 19% to 5%. Of the 58 placebo recipients with herpes zoster, 11 had significant complications that included encephalitis (three patients, 5%), hepatitis (three patients), and uveitis leading to blindness (three patients). These complications were significantly reduced in the drug recipients (117). Thus, early vidarabine therapy administered within 72 hr of lesion formation is effective in preventing complications and accelerating healing. Benefit can be achieved at a dosage of 10 mg/kg/day administered in

**TABLE 2.** *Therapeutic trials of antivirals for herpes zoster in immunocompromised hosts*

| | *N* | Days of new lesion formation | Dissemination/ progression of cutaneous disease | Visceral disease | Resolution of postherpetic neuralgia |
|---|---|---|---|---|---|
| Interferon (106) | | | | | |
| Drug | 45 | $p < 0.01$ | $p < 0.025$ | 1/45 | 27/29 |
| Placebo | 45 | | | 6/45 | 21/29 |
| | | | | ($p < 0.05$) | ($p = 0.05$) |
| Vidarabine (164,166) | | | | | |
| Drug | 47 | $p = 0.004$ | CNE | CNE | CNE |
| Placebo | 40 | | | | |
| Drug | 63 | $p = 0.002$ | 5 (8%) | 3 (5%) | 35 (56%) |
| Placebo | 58 | | 14 (24%) | 11 (19%) | 10 (17%) |
| | | | $p = 0.014$ | $p = 0.015$ | $p = 0.047$ |
| ACV (16) | | | | | |
| Drug | 52 | NS | 9/28 | 0/52 | |
| Placebo | 42 | | 15/24 | 4/42 | NS |
| | | | NS | ($p = 0.04$) | |
| ACV versus vidarabine (136) | | | | | |
| Drug | 11 | $p = 0.03$ | $p = 0.016$ | 0 | NS |
| Placebo | 11 | | | 0 | |

CNE, could not evaluate; NS, not significant.

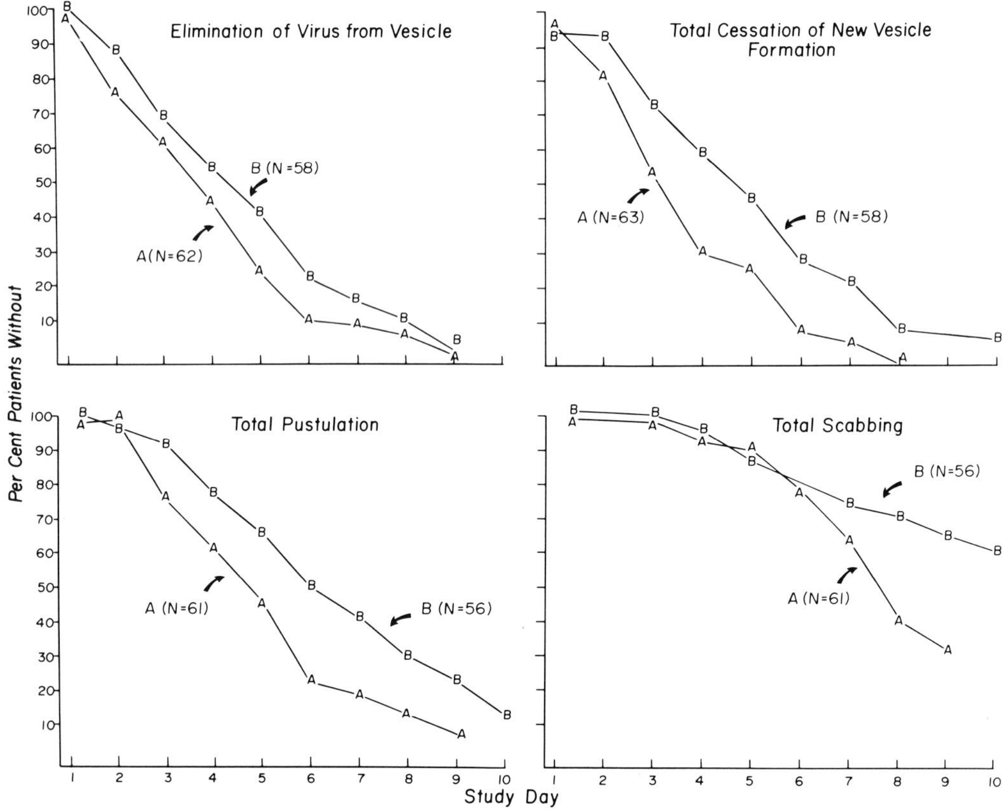


**FIG. 8.** Beneficial effects on acceleration of cutaneous healing with vidarabine administration. *A,* vidarabine recipients; *B,* placebo recipients.

standard intravenous solutions at a concentration of 0.5 mg/ml over 12 hr for 5 days.

Vidarabine treatment requires hospitalization and intravenous drug administration over prolonged periods of time, being given over 12 hr because of poor solubility. Thus, therapy has a degree of risk for nosocomial infection. Furthermore, many immunocompromised patients will heal spontaneously. Hopefully, the development of antiviral medications that are orally bioavailable will obviate the need for hospitalization of these patients. There is no evidence to suggest that either ZIG or zoster immune plasma is useful.

A second therapeutic modality, but which is not clinically useful at this time, is the administration of interferon. It has been employed successfully in a dose-escalating study of 90 patients with herpes zoster and an underlying malignancy (166). In this study, administration of interferon at a dosage of 1–2 × $10^6$ IU/kg intramuscularly resulted in decreased vesicle formation in the primary dermatome and a lowered frequency of cutaneous dissemination. The interferon-treated patients did not show a significant decrease in total healing time, but they did have significant amelioration of postherpetic neuralgia. Toxicity included fever, malaise, myalgia, and depressed leukocyte counts. The usefulness of leukocyte interferon for treatment of herpes zoster infections in the immunocompromised host may be expanded with the availability of recombinant-DNA–produced interferon.

A third treatment modality is the administration of intravenous ACV at dosages of 500 mg/m$^2$ every 8 hr for 7–10 days. Intravenous ACV therapy results in plasma levels of medication that exceed the 50% inhibitory dose ($ID_{50}$) of VZV; however, oral administration of medication does not result in similar plasma concentrations (167). Two studies, one placebo controlled and the other a comparative trial with vidarabine, indicate that progressive disease is slowed in the immunocompromised host (168,169). In bone marrow transplant recipients, ACV therapy was superior to vidarabine treatment. In this latter study, all events of cutaneous healing and disease progression were statistically significantly improved with ACV therapy (169). Furthermore, a small comparative study of these two medications for disseminated zoster also suggested superiority of ACV therapy (170). Thus, intravenous ACV therapy has become the choice for patients at high risk for progressive disease.

Other treatment modalities have been explored for the management of herpes zoster in the immunocompromised host such as transfer factor (171,172). The value of any of these therapies for patients with acquired immune deficiency syndromes (AIDS) remains to be established.

Recently, several trials have reported the outcome of patients receiving oral (173–175)—400–800 mg five times daily—or intravenous ACV (58,176,177) for localized zoster in the normal host. Therapy accelerated (but variably so) the duration of lesion formation and time to healing but appears to have little effect on postherpetic neuralgia. The data are currently too inconclusive to ascribe enough clinical benefit to warrant the routine use of this drug as a therapeutic at this time. Hopefully, ongoing trials will help clarify these issues.

## CONCLUSION

This chapter has summarized the state of knowledge of VZV infections in humans. As members of the medical community, we are cognizant of the benign nature of chicken pox in children but its propensity toward more severe illness in adults. The same age parallel is appropriate for herpes zoster. With advancing age, both varicella and herpes zoster take on more serious ramifications. If we introduce the variable of immunosuppression upon the expression of VZV infections, an even greater propensity to life-threatening illness is encountered. Individuals who develop herpes zoster while immunocompromised are at risk for the life-threatening complications of varicella pneumonitis, whereas the older individual, immunocompromised or not, may suffer from severe neuritis as well as postherpetic neuralgia.

Currently, antiviral treatment regimens are available only for the immunocompromised host. To date, successful and practical therapeutic approaches have involved the utilization of ACV and vidarabine for the management of disease. Evaluations of orally administered ACV for management of herpes zoster in the immunocompromised and normal host continue. Ideally, prevention of VZV infections is most desirable, and vaccine trials are being completed worldwide.

## ACKNOWLEDGMENT

Studies performed by the author and reported in this chapter were supported by contracts NO1-AI-62554 and 62532 from the Development and Applications Branch of the National Institute of Allergy and Infectious Diseases, a grant from the National Institutes of Health (NIH) Division of Research Resources (RR-032), and a grant from the state of Alabama.

## REFERENCES

1. Davis DJ. Measurements of the prevalence of viral infections. *J Infect Dis* 1976;133:A3.
2. Gordon JE, Meader FM. The period of infectivity and serum prevention of chickenpox. *JAMA* 1929;93:2013.
3. Steiner P. Zur inokulation der varicellen. *Wien Med Wochenschr* 1875;25:306.
4. Bokay J. Das auftreten der schafblattern unter besonderen umstanden. *Ungar Arch Med* 1892; 1:159.
5. von Bokay J. Uber den atiologischen zusammenhang der varizellen mit gewissen fallen von herpes zoster. *Wien Klin Wochenschr* 1909; 22:1323.
6. Bruusgaard E. The natural relation between zoster and varicella. *Br J Dermatol* 1932;44:1.
7. Kundratiz K. Experimentelle ubertragungen von herpes zoster auf menschen und die beziehungen von herpes zoster zu varicellen. *A Kinderheilkd* 1925;39:379.
8. School Epidemics Committee of Great Britain. *Epidemics in schools. Medical Research Council, special report series, no. 227*. London: His Majesty's Stationery Office, 1938.
9. Garland J. Varicella following exposure to herpes zoster. *N Engl J Med* 1943;228:336.
10. Lipschutz B. Untersuchungen uber die atiologie der krankheiten der herpesgruppe (herpes zoster, herpes genitalis, herpes febrilis). *Arch Dermatol Syph* 1921;136:428.
11. Tyzzer EE. The histology of the skin lesions in varicella. *Philippine J Sci* 1906;1:349.
12. Weller TH. The progagation *in vitro* of agents producing inclusion bodies derived from varicella and herpes zoster. *Proc Soc Exp Biol Med* 1953;83:340.
13. Weller TH. Varicella and herpes zoster. In: Lennette EH, Schmidt NJ, eds. *Diagnostic procedures for viral, rickettsial, and chlamydial infections*. Washington, D.C.: American Public Health Association, 1970:375.
14. Weller TH, Coons AH. Fluorescent antibody studies with agents of varicella and herpes zoster propagated *in vitro*. *Proc Soc Exp Biol Med* 1954;86:789.
15. Weller TH, Stoddard MB. Intranuclear inclusion bodies in cultures of human tissue inoculated with varicella vesicle fluid. *J Immunol* 1952;68:311.
16. Weller TH, Witton HM. The etiologic agents of varicella and herpes zoster: serologic studies with the viruses as propagated *in vitro*. *J Exp Med* 1958;108:869–90.
17. Oakes JE, Iltis JP, Hyman R, Rapp F. Analyses by restriction enzyme cleavage of human varicella-zoster virus DNAs. *Virology* 1977;82:353.
18. Stow ND, Davison AJ, Identification of a varicella-zoster virus origin of DNA replication and its activation by herpes simplex virus type I gene products. *J Gen Virol* 1986;67:1617–23.
19. Straus SE, Hays J, Smith H, Owens J. Genome differences among varicella-zoster virus isolates. *J Gen Virol* 1983;64:1031.
20. Straus SE, Reinhold W, Smith HA, et al. Endonuclease analysis of viral DNA from varicella and subsequent zoster infection in the same patient. *N Engl J Med* 1984;311:1362–4.
21. Zernik HJ, Morton DH, Stanton GW, Neff BJ. Restriction endonuclease analysis of the DNA from varicella-zoster virus: stability of the DNA after passage *in vitro*. *J Gen Virol* 1981;55:207.
22. Achong BC, Meurisse EV. Observations on the fine structure and replication of varicella virus in cultivated human amnion cells. *J Gen Virol* 1968;3:305.
23. Almeida JD, Howatson AF, Williams MG. Morphology of varicella (chickenpox) virus. *Virology* 1962;16:353.
24. Straus SE, Aulakh H, Ruyechan WT, et al. Structure of varicella-zoster virus DNA. *J Virol* 1981;40:516.
25. Hyman R. Structure and function of the vari-

cella-zoster virus genome. In: Nahmias AJ, Dosdle WR, Schinizai RF, eds. *The human herpesviruses*. New York: Elsevier, 1981:63.
26. Iltis JP, Oakes JE, Hyman RW, Rapp F. Comparison of the DNA's of varicella-zoster viruses isolated from clinical cases of varicella and herpes zoster. *Virology* 1977;82:345.
27. Dumas AM, Geelen JL, Mares W, Van Der Noordaa J. Infectivity and molecular weight of varicella-zoster virus DNA. *J Gen Virol* 1980; 47:233–5.
28. Ludwig H, Haines HG, Biswal N, Benyesh-Melnick M. The characterization of varicella-zoster virus DNA. *J Gen Virol* 1972;14:111.
29. Plummer G, Goodheart CR, Henso D, Bowling DP. A comparative study of the DNA density and behavior in tissue cultures of fourteen different herpesviruses. *Virology* 1969;39:134.
30. Dumas AM, Geelen JL, Westrate MW, Wertheim P, Van Der Noordaa J. Xba, Pst, BglII restriction enzyme maps of the two orientations of the varicella-zoster virus genome. *J Virol* 1981;39:390–400.
31. Davison AJ, Edson CM, Ellis RW, et al. New common nomenclature for glycoprotein genes of varicella-zoster virus and their glycosylated products. *J Virol* 1986;57:1195–7.
32. Davison AJ, McGeoch DJ. Evolutionary comparisons of the S segments in the genomes of herpes simplex virus type I and varicella-zoster virus. *J Gen Virol* 1986;67:597–611.
33. Davison AJ, Scott JE. The complete DNA sequence of varicella-zoster virus. *J Gen Virol* 1986;67:1759–816.
34. Ecker JR, Hyman RW. Varicella zoster virus DNA exists as two isomers. *Proc Natl Acad Sci USA* 1982;79:156–60.
35. Straus SE, et al. Varicella-zoster virus infections. *Ann Intern Med* 1988;108:221–37.
36. Rapp F, Vanderslice D. Spread of zoster virus in human embryonic lung cells and the inhibitory effect of idoxyuridine. *Virology* 1964;22:321.
37. Vaczi L, Geder L, Koller M, Jeney E. Influence of temperature on the multiplication of varicella virus. *Acta Microbiol Hung* 1963; 10:109.
38. Grose C, Perrotta DM, Burnell PA, Smith GC. Cell-free varicella-zoster virus in cultured human melanoma cells. *J Gen Virol* 1979;43:15.
39. Cheatham WJ, Weller TH, Dolan TF Jr, Dower JC. Varicella, report of two fatal cases with necropsy, virus isolation and serologic studies. *Am J Pathol* 1956;2:1015.
40. Cowdry EV. The problem of intranuclear inclusions in virus diseases. *Arch Pathol* 1934;18:527.
41. Gordon JE. Chickenpox: an epidemiologic review. *Am J Med Sci* 1962;244:362.
42. Wells MW, Holla WA. Ventilation in the flow of measles and chicken pox through a community. *JAMA* 1950;142:1337.
43. Hope-Simpson RE. Infectiousness of communicable diseases in the household (measles, chickenpox, and mumps). *Lancet* 1952;2:549.
44. Yorke JA, London WP. Recurrent outbreaks of measles, chickenpox, and mumps. Systematic differences in contact rates and stochastic effects. *Am J Epidemiol* 1973;98:469.
45. Stokes J Jr. Chicken pox. In: *Preventive medicine in World War II, vol. IV: communicable diseases transmitted chiefly through respiratory and alimentary tracts*. Washington, D.C.: Department of Army, 1958:55.
46. Rubin D, Fusfeld RD. Muscle paralysis in herpes zoster. *Calif Med* 1965;103:261.
47. Evans P. An epidemic of chickenpox. *Lancet* 1940;2:339.
48. Gustafson TL, Lavely GB, Brawner ER Jr, Hutcheson RH Jr, Wright PF, Schaffner W. An outbreak of airborne nosocomial varicella. *Pediatrics* 1982;70:550–6.
49. Leclair JM, Zaia JA, Levin MJ, Congdon RG, Goldmann DA. Airborne transmission of chickenpox in a hospital. 1980;302:450–3.
50. Bastain FO, Rabson AS, Yee CL, Tralka TS. Herpesvirus varicellae: isolated from human dorsal root ganglia. *Arch Pathol* 1974;97:331.
51. Esiri MM, Tomlinson AH. Herpes zoster: demonstration of virus in trigeminal nerve and ganglion by immunofluorescence and electron microscopy. *J Neurol Sci* 1972;15:35.
52. Ghatak NR, Zimmerman HM. Spinal ganglion in herpes zoster. *Arch Pathol* 1973;95:411.
53. Gilden DH, Vafai A, Shturam Y, Becker Y, Devlin M, Wellish M. Varicella-zoster virus DNA in human sensory ganglia. *Nature* 1983; 306:478–80.
54. Hyman RW, Ecker JR, Tenser RB. Varicella-zoster virus RNA in human trigeminal ganglia. *Lancet* 1983;2:184–6.
55. Wentworth BB, Alexander ER. Seroepidemiology of infections due to members of herpesvirus group. *Am J Epidemiol* 1971;94:496.
56. McGregor RM. Herpes zoster, chickenpox, and cancer in general practice. *Br Med J* 1957;1:84.
57. Hope-Simpson RE. The nature of herpes zoster: a long-term study and a new hypothesis. *Proc R Soc Med* 1965;58:9.
58. McGill J, MacDonald DR, Fall C, McKendrick GD, Copplestone A. Intravenous acyclovir in acute herpes zoster infection. *J Infect* 1983; 6:157–61.
59. Paryani SG, Arvin AM. Intrauterine infection with varicella-zoster virus after maternal varicella. *N Engl J Med* 1986;314:1542–6.
60. Ross AH. Modification of chickenpox in family contacts by administration of gamma globulin. *N Engl J Med* 1962;267:369.
61. Preblud SR, Orenstein WA, Bart KJ. Varicella: clinical manifestations, epidemiology, and health impact in children. *Pediatr Infect Dis* 1984; 3:505–9.
62. Fleisher G, Henry W, McSorley M, Arbeter A, Plotkin S. Life threatening complications of varicella. *Am J Dis Child* 1981;135:896–9.
63. Preblud SR. Varicella: complications and costs. *Pediatrics* 1986;78:728–35.
64. Goldston AS, Millichap JG, Miller RH. Cerebellar ataxia with pre-eruptive varicella. *Am J Dis Child* 1963;106:111.

65. Johnson R, Milbourn PE. Central nervous system manifestations of chickenpox. *Can Med Assoc J* 1970;102:831.
66. Underwood EA. The neurological complications of varicella: a clinical and epidemiological study. *Br J Child Dis* 1935;32:83,177,241.
67. Forghani B, Schmidt NJ, Dennis J. Antibody assays for varicella-zoster virus: comparison of enzyme immunoassay with neutralization, immune adherence hemagglutination, and complement fixation. *J Clin Microbiol* 1978;8:545.
68. Miller HG, Stanton JB, Gibbons JL. Parainfectious encephalomyelitis and related syndromes. *Q J Med* 1956;25:428.
69. Weber DM, Pellecchia JA. Varicella pneumonia. *JAMA* 1965;192:572.
70. Krugman S, Goodrich CH, Ward R. Primary varicella pneumonia. *N Engl J Med* 1957; 257:843.
71. Nisenbaum C, Wallis K, Herczeg E. Varicella pneumonia in children. *Helv Paediatr Acta* 1969;24:212.
72. Triebwasser JH, Harris RE, Bryant RE, Rhoades ER. Varicella pneumonia in adults: report of seven cases and a review of literature. *Medicine* 1967; 46:409.
73. Bullowa JGM, Wishik SM. Complications of varicella. Their occurrence among 2534 patients. *Am J Dis Child* 1935;49:923.
74. Wishik SM, Bullowa JGM. Complications of varicella. Surface complications. *Am J Dis Child* 1935;49:927.
75. Linnemann CC, Shea L, Partin JC, Shubert WK, Schiff GM. Reye's syndrome: epidemiologic and viral studies, 1963–1974. *Am J Epidemiol* 1975;101:517.
76. Reye RD, Morgan G, Baral J. Encephalopathy and fatty degeneration of the viscera. A disease entity in childhood. *Lancet* 1963;2:749.
77. Hilty MD, Romshe CA, Delamater PV. Reye's syndrome and hyperamino-acidemia. *J Pediatr* 1974;84:362.
78. Guess HA, Broughton DD, Melton LJ III, Kurland LT. Population-based studies of varicella complications. *Pediatrics* 1987;78:723–7.
79. Charkes ND. Purpuric chickenpox: report of a case review of the literature, and classification by clinical features. *Ann Intern Med* 1961;54:745.
80. Ward JR, Bishop B. Varicella arthritis. *JAMA* 1970;212:1954.
81. Alagna G. Histopathologishe veranderungen der Tonsille und der schleimhaut der esten luftwege bei masern. *Arch Laryngol Rhinol* 1911;25:527.
82. Minkowitz S, Wenk R, Friedman E, Yuceoglu A, Berkovitch S. Acute glomerulonephritis associated with varicella infection. *Am J Med* 1968;44:489.
83. Brunell PA, Casey HL. Crude tissue culture antigen for determination of varicella-zoster complement fixing antibody. *Public Health Rep* 1964;79:839.
84. Gold E, Godek G. Complement-fixation studies with a varicella zoster antigen. *J Immunol* 1965;95:692.
85. Taylor-Robinson D, Downie AW. Chickenpox and herpes zoster. I. Complement fixation studies. *Br J Pathol* 1959;40:398.
86. Tomlinson AH, MacCallum RO. The incidence of complement-fixing antibody to varicella-zoster virus in hospital patients and blood donors. *J Hyg (Camb)* 1970;68:1229.
87. Williams V, Gershon A, Brunell PA. Serologic response to varicella-zoster membrane antigens measured by indirect immunofluorescence. *J Infect Dis* 1974;130:669.
88. Caunt AE, Shae DG. Neutralization tests with varicella-zoster virus. *J Hyg (Camb)* 1969;67:343.
89. Yoshino K, Taniguchi S. Evaluation of the demonstration of complement-requiring neutralizing antibody as a means for early diagnosis of herpes virus infections. *J Immunol* 1966;96:196.
90. Grose S, Edmond BJ, Brunell PA. Complement-enhanced neutralizing antibody response to varicella-zoster virus. *J Infect Dis* 1979; 139:432.
91. Kalter ZG, Steinberg S, Gershon AA. Immune adherence hemagglutination: further observations on demonstration of antibody to varicella-zoster virus. *J Infect Dis* 1977;135: 1010.
92. Shehab ZM, Burnell PA. Enzyme-linked immunosorbent assay for determining susceptibility to varicella. *J Infect Dis* 1983;148: 472–6.
93. Arvin AM, Kinney-Thomas E, Shiriver K, et al. Immunity to varicella-zoster viral glycoproteins, gpI (gp 90/58) and gp III (gp 118), and to a nonglycosylated protein, p 170. *J Infect Dis* 1986;154:422–9.
94. Wittek AE, Arvin AM, Koropchak CM. Serum immunoglobulin A antibody to varicella-zoster virus in subjects with primary varicella and herpes zoster infections and in immune subjects. *J Clin Microbiol* 1983;18:1146–9.
95. Arvin AM, Koropchai CM, Williams BR, Grumet FC, Foung SK. Early immune response in healthy and immunocompromised subjects with primary varicella-zoster virus infection. *J Infect Dis* 1986;154:422–9.
96. Middelkamp JN. Varicella in newborn twins. *J Pediatr* 1953;43:573.
97. Laforet EG, Lynch DL. Multiple congenital defects following maternal varicella. *N Engl J Med* 1974;236:534.
98. Williamson AP. The varicella-zoster virus in the etiology of severe congenital defects. *Clin Pediatr* 1975;14:553.
99. Siegel M. Congenital malformations following chickenpox, measles, mumps, and hepatitis. Results of a cohort study. *JAMA* 1973;26: 1521–4.
100. Brunell PA. Placental transfer of varicella zoster antibody. *Pediatrics* 1966;38:1034.
101. Lomer D. Herpes zoster bei einem 4 tage alten kinde. *Zentralbil Gynakol* 1889;13:778.
102. Brunell PA, Miller LH, Lovejoy F. Zoster in children. *Am J Dis Child* 1968;115:432.

103. Kouvalainen K, Salmi A, Salmi TT. Infantile herpes zoster. *Scand J Infect Dis* 1972;4:91.
104. Hubbard TW. Varicella occurring in an infant twenty-four hours after birth. *Br Med J* 1878;1:822.
105. Hyatt HH. Report of a case in a five day old infant and review of the literature. *J Natl Med Assoc* 1967;59:32.
106. Joel L. Varicella in Sydney. *Med J Aust* 1966;2:728.
107. Preblud SR, Bregman DJ, Vernon LL. Deaths from varicella in infants. *Pediatr Infect Dis* 1985;4:503–7.
108. Pridham FC. Chickenpox during intrauterine life. *Br Med J* 1913;1:1054.
109. Brunell PA. Varicella-zoster infections in pregnancy. *JAMA* 1967;199:93.
110. Feldman S, Hughes WT, Daniel CB. Varicella in children with cancer: seventy-seven cases. *Pediatrics* 1975;56:388.
111. Feldman S, Epp E. Isolation of varicella-zoster virus from blood. *J Pediatr* 1976;88:265.
112. Locksley RM, Flournoy N, Sullivan KM, Meyers JD. Infection with varicella-zoster virus after marrow transplantation. *J Infect Dis* 1985;152:1172–81.
113. Falliers DJ, Ellis EF. Corticosteroids and varicella: six year experience in an asthmatic population. *Arch Dis Child* 1965;40:593.
114. Whitley RJ, Soong SJ, Dolin R, et al. Early vidarabine therapy to control the complications of herpes zoster in immunosuppressed patients. *N Engl J Med* 1982;307:971.
115. Arvin AM, Kushner JH, Feldman S, Buchner RL, Hammond D, Merigan TC. Human leukocyte interferon for treatment of varicella in children with cancer. *N Engl J Med* 1982; 306:761.
116. Prober DG, Kirk LE, Keeney RE. Acyclovir therapy of chicken pox in immunosuppressed children—a collaborative study. *J Pediatr* 1982;101:622.
117. Whitley RJ, Hilty M, Haynes R, et al. Vidarabine therapy of varicella in immunosuppressed patients. *J Pediatr* 1982;1:125.
118. Brunell PA, Ross A, Miller L, Kuo B. Prevention of varicella by zoster immune globulin. *N Engl J Med* 1969;280:1191.
119. Zaia JA, Levin MJ, Preblud SR, et al. Evaluation of varicella-zoster immune globulin: protection of immunosuppressed children after household exposure to varicella. *J Infect Dis* 1983;147:737–43.
120. Brunell PA, Gershon AA, Hughes WT, Riley HD, Smith J. Prevention of varicella in high-risk children: a collaborative study. *Pediatrics* 1972;50:718.
121. Brunell PA, Gershon AA. Passive immunization against varicella-zoster infections and other modes of therapy. *J Infect Dis* 1973; 127:415.
122. Gershon AA, Steinberg S, Brunell PA. Zoster immune globulin. A further assessment. *N Engl J Med* 1974;290:243.
123. American Academy of Pediatrics. *Report of the Committee on Infectious Diseases*. 18th ed. Elk Grove Village, IL: American Academy of Pediatrics, 1982:285.
124. Paryani SG, Arvin AA, Koropshak CM. Varicella zoster antibody titers after the administration of intravenous immune serum globulin or varicella zoster immune globulin. *Am J Med* 1984;76:124–7.
125. Takahashi M, Okuno Y, Otsuka T, et al. Development of a liver attenuated varicella vaccine. *Biken J* 1975;18:25.
126. Takahashi M, Otsuka T, Okuno Y, Asano Y, Yazaki T, Isomura S. Live vaccine used to prevent the spread of varicella: in children in hospital. *Lancet* 1974;2:1288.
127. Arbeter AM, Starr SE, Preblud ST, et al. Varicella vaccine trials in healthy children: a summary of comparative and follow-up studies. *Am J Dis Child* 1984;138:434–8.
128. Preblud SR, Orenstein WA, Koplan JP, Bart KJ, Hinman AR. A benefit-cost analysis of a childhood varicella vaccination programme. *Postgrad Med J* 1985;61(suppl 4):17–22.
129. Gershon AA, Steinberg, SP, Gelb LA, et al. Live attenuated varicella vaccine: efficacy for children with leukemia in remission. *JAMA* 1984;252:355–62.
130. Gershon AA, Steinberg SP, Gelb L. Live attenuated varicella vaccine use in immunocompromised children and adults. *Pediatrics* 1986;78:757–62.
131. Asano Y, Takahashi M. Clinical and serologic testing of a live varicella vaccine and two year follow-up for immunity of the vaccinated children. *Pediatrics* 1977;60:810.
132. Izawa T, Ihara T, Hattori A, et al. Application of a live varicella vaccine in children with acute leukemia or other malignant diseases. *Pediatrics* 1977;60:805.
133. Asano Y, Nakayama H, Yazaki T, et al. Protection against varicella in family contacts by immediate inoculation with live varicella vaccine. *Pediatrics* 1977;59:3.
134. Ha K, Baba K, Ikeda T, Nishida M, Yabuuchi H, Takahashi M. Application of live varicella vaccine to children with acute leukemia or other malignancies without suspension of anticancer therapy. *Pediatrics* 1980;65: 346.
135. Martin JJ, Dohner DE, Wellinghoff WJ, Gelb KD. Restriction endonuclease analysis of varicella-zoster vaccine virus and wild-type DNAs. *J Med Virol* 1982;9:69–76.
136. Bogger D, Goren S, Baba K, Hurley P, Yabuuchi H, Takahashi M. Antibody response to varicella-zoster virus after natural or vaccine-induced infection. *J Infect Dis* 1982;146(2): 260–5.
137. Brunell PA, Talyor-Wiedeman J. Risk of herpes zoster in children with leukemia: varicella vaccine compared with history of chickenpox. *Pediatrics* 1977;77(1):53–6.
138. Gelb LK, Dohner DE, Gershon AA, et al. Molecular epidemiology of live, attenuated varicella virus vaccine in children with leu-

kemia and in normal adults. *J Infect Dis* 1987;155:633–40.
139. Arbeter AM, Starr SE, Plotkin SA. Varicella vaccine studies in healthy children and adults. *Pediatrics* 1986;78:748–56.
140. Arbeter AM, Baker L, Starr SE, Levine BL, Books E, Plotkin SA. Combination measles, mumps, rubella and varicella vaccine. *Pediatrics* 1986;78:742–7.
141. Barrett FF, Wexler ML, Douglas RG. Treatment of progressive varicella with cytarabine. *Tex Med* 1972;68:65.
142. Chow AW, Forester JH, Ryniuk W. Cytosine arabinoside therapy for herpesvirus infections. *Antimicrob Agents Chemother* 1971;1970:214.
143. Hall TC, Wilfert C, Jaffe N, et al. Treatment of varicella-zoster with cytosine arabinoside. *Trans Assoc Am Physicians* 1969;82:201.
144. Prager D, Bruder M, Sawitsky A. Disseminated varicella in a patient with acute myelogenous leukemia: treatment with cytosine arabinoside. *J Pediatr* 1971;78:321.
145. Stevens DA, Merigan TC. Uncertain roles of cytosine arabinoside in varicella infection of compromised hosts. *J Pediatr* 1972;81:562.
146. Feldman S, Robertson PK, Lott L, Thornton D. Neurotoxicity due to adenine arabinoside therapy during varicella-zoster virus infections in immunocompromised children. *J Infect Dis* 1986;87:630–3.
147. Al-Nakib W, Al-Kandari S, El-Khalik DM, El-Shirbiny AM. A randomized controlled study of intravenous acyclovir (Zovirax) against placebo in adults with chickenpox. *J Infection* 1983;6:49–56.
148. Stevens DA, Merigan TC. Interferon, antibody, and other host factors, in herpes zoster. *J Clin Invest* 1972;51:1170.
149. Arvin A, Feldman S, Merigan TC. Human leukocyte interferon in the treatment of varicella in children with cancer: a preliminary controlled trial. *Antimicrob Agents Chemother* 1978;13:605.
150. Mazur MH, Dolin R. Herpes zoster at the NIH: a 20 year experience. *Am J Med* 1978;65:738–44.
151. Jemsek J, Greenberg S, Taber L, Harvey D, Gershon A, Couch RB. Herpes zoster associated encephalitis: clinicopathologic report of 12 cases and review of the literature. *Am J Med* 1983;62:81.
152. Hilt DC, Buchholz D, Krumholz A, Weiss H, Wolinsky JS. Herpes zoster ophthalmicus and delayed contralateral hemiparesis caused by cerebral angiitis: diagnosis and management approaches. *Ann Neurol* 1983;14:543–53.
153. Rosenblum WI, Hadfield MD. Granulomatous angiitis of the nervous system in cases of herpes zoster and lymphosarcoma. *Neurology (Minneapolis)* 1972;22:348.
154. Acers TE. Herpes zoster ophthalmicus with contralateral hemiplegia. *Arch Ophthalmol* 1964; 71:371.
155. Hogan EL, Krigman MR. Herpes zoster myelitis. *Arch Neurol* 1973;29:309.
156. Norris FH, Dramov B, Calder CD, Hohnson SG. Virus-like particles in myositis accompanying herpes zoster. *Arch Neurol* 1969;21:25.
157. Ruckeschel JC, Schimpff SC, Smyth AC, Mardiney MR. Herpes zoster and impaired cell-associated immunity to the varicella zoster virus in patients with Hodgkin's disease. *Am J Med* 1977;62:77.
158. Russell AS, Maini RA, Bailey M, Dumonde DC. Cell-mediated immunity to varicella-zoster antigen in acute herpes zoster (shingles). *Clin Exp Immunol* 1972;14:181.
159. Jordan GW, Merigan TC. Cell-mediated immunity to varicella-zoster virus: *in vitro* lymphocyte responses. *J Infect Dis* 1974;130:495.
160. Ragozzino MW, Melton LJ, Kurland LT, Chu CP, Perry HO. Risk of cancer after herpes zoster: a population based study. *N Engl J Med* 1982;307:93.
161. Eaglstein WH, Katz R, Brown JA. The effects of early corticosteroid therapy on the skin eruption and pain of herpes zoster. *JAMA* 1970;211:1681.
162. Elliott FA. Treatment of herpes zoster with high doses of prednisone. *Lancet* 1964;2:610–1.
163. Esmann V, Kroon S, Peterslund NA, et al. Prednisolone does not prevent post-herpetic neuralgia. *Lancet* 1987;2:126–9.
164. Ch'ien LT, Whitley RJ, Alford CA, Galasso GJ. Adenine arabinoside for therapy of herpes zoster in immunosuppressed patients: preliminary results of a collaborative study. *J Infect Dis* 1976;133:A184.
165. Whitley RJ, Chien LT, Dolin R, Galasso GJ, Alford CA Jr, and the Collaborative Antiviral Study Group. Adenine arabinoside therapy of herpes zoster in the immunosuppressed. *N Engl J Med* 1976;294:1193.
166. Merigan TC, Rand KH, Pollard RB. Human leukocyte interferon for the treatment of herpes zoster in patients with cancer. *N Engl J Med* 1978;298:981.
167. Biron KK, Elion GB. In vitro susceptibility of varicella-zoster virus to acyclovir. *Antimicrob Agents Chemother* 1980;18:443–7.
168. Balfour HH, Bean B, Laskin O, et al. Acyclovir halts progression of herpes zoster in immunocompromised patients. *N Engl J Med* 1983; 308:1448–53.
169. Shepp D, Dandliker PS, Meyers JD. Treatment of varicella-zoster virus in severely immunocompromised patients: a randomized comparison of acyclovir and vidarabine. *N Engl J Med* 1987;314:208–21.
170. Vild'e JL, Bricaire F, Leport C, Renaudie M, Burn-V'ezinet F. Comparative trial of acyclovir and vidarabine in disseminated varicella-zoster virus infections in immunocompromised patients. *J Med Virol* 1986;20:127–34.
171. Bowden RA, Siegel MS, Steele RW, Day LM, Meyers JD. Immunologic and clinical responses to varicella-zoster virus-specific transfer factor following marrow transplantation. *J Infect Dis* 1985;152:1324–7.

172. Steele RW, Myers MG, Vincent MM. Transfer factor for the prevention of varicella-zoster infection in childhood leukemia. *N Engl J Med* 1980;303:355.
173. Cobo LM, Foulks GN, Liesegang T, et al. Oral acyclovir in the treatment of acute herpes zoster ophthalimicus. *Ophthalmology* 1986;93:763–70.
174. Essman V, Ipens J, Peterslund NA, Seyer-Hansen K, Shonheyder H, Henning J. Therapy of acute herpes zoster with acyclovir in the nonimmunocompromised host. *Am J Med* 1982;73:320.
175. McKendrick MW, McGill JI, White JE, Wood MJ. Oral acyclovir in acute herpes zoster. *Br Med J* 1986;293:1529–32.
176. Bean B, Braun C, Balfour HH Jr. Acyclovir therapy for acute herpes zoster. *Lancet* 1982; 2:118–21.
177. Peterslund NA, Seyer-Hansen K, Ipen J, Esmann V, Schonheyder H, Juhl H. Acyclovir in herpes zoster. *Lancet* 1981;2:827–30.

*Antiviral Agents and Viral Diseases of Man, 3rd Edition,*
edited by G. J. Galasso, R. J. Whitley, and
T. C. Merigan, Raven Press, Ltd., New York © 1990.

# 8

# Herpes Simplex Virus

Gregory J. Mertz

*Division of Infectious Diseases, Department of Medicine, University of New Mexico School of Medicine, Albuquerque, New Mexico 87131*



In the past 20 years, there has been substantial progress in our understanding of the pathogenesis and natural history of mucocutaneous herpes simplex virus (HSV) infections. Effective antiviral therapy has been developed and has enjoyed wide clinical acceptance (1). During the same period, there has been a 16-fold increase in the number of visits to clinicians for genital herpes infections (2). Although changes in sexual practices in the past 5 years have led to a dramatic reduction in the transmission of sexually transmitted diseases including human immunodeficiency virus (HIV) infection among homosexual men (3), there is little evidence that similar changes are occurring among heterosexual men and women (4). Finally, both the acquired immunodeficiency syndrome (AIDS) epidemic and development of aggressive chemotherapy for malignancies have increased numbers and broadened the clinical spectrum of mucocutaneous HSV infections in the immunocompromised host (5–7). This section will review the pathogenesis, epidemiology, and natural history of mucocutaneous HSV infections and suggest approaches to diagnosis and management.

## THE VIRUS

Members of the human herpes virus group include HSV types 1 and 2 (HSV-1, HSV-2), varicella-zoster virus (VZV), Epstein-Barr virus (EBV), cytomegalovirus (CMV), and the newly recognized human herpes virus-6 (HHV-6). HSV-1 and HSV-2 contain a viral genome with linear, double-stranded DNA large enough to code for more than 60 gene products (8). There is approximately 50% base sequence homology between HSV-1 and HSV-2, whereas different strains of the same type differ by approximately 5–8% (8–10). Restriction endonuclease analysis of viral DNA can be employed to differentiate the two types and to identify different strains of the same type (9,10).

Viral DNA and DNA-binding proteins are packaged in an icosahedral capsid with 162 capsomeres. Between the capsid and the envelope are a number of proteins, and within the envelope are five or six glycoproteins that allow attachment and penetration into the cell (11). The glycoproteins contain both type-common and type-specific antigens; strain-specific antigens have not been identified. HSV-1 and HSV-2 may be differentiated by monoclonal antibodies and by restriction endonuclease analysis, the former being faster, less expensive, and easily applied in clinical virology laboratories (12). Serologic tests such as western blot analysis and immunodot testing can now reliably differentiate between the antibody response to type-specific HSV-1 and HSV-2 glycoproteins (10,13–15), but antibody responses to different strains of the same type cannot be differentiated. Thus, restriction endonuclease analysis of viral DNA is the only method available for strain differentiation.

### Viral Replication and Latency

HSV can infect a wide range of hosts and cells in cell culture, suggesting that cell-surface receptors are widely distributed (16,17). After attachment to the cell surface, fusion occurs between the viral envelope and cell membrane, followed by entry of the nucleocapsid into the cytoplasm. Viral DNA is released from the nucleocapsid and then migrates to the nucleus where expression of viral genes and DNA replication occur. Viral glycoproteins are found in both the nuclear membrane and cell surface. The nucleocapsid is assembled in the nucleus of the cell, and the envelope surrounds the nucleocapsid as it buds through the nuclear membrane. Virions are then transported to the cell surface through the endoplasmic reticulum and the Golgi apparatus (8,11).

HSV infection results in viral replication and cell death in most susceptible cell lines. However, a process known as "latent infection" may occur in cells such as neurons in sensory and autonomic ganglia. In latent infection, virus can rarely be isolated directly from infected cells, but virus may be isolated when permissive cell lines are cocultivated with latently infected neural cells (18–20). The state of DNA in latently infected cells is unclear, although there is evidence that some transcription occurs and some evidence that DNA may be present in episomes or may be integrated into the genome of the neuron (8,21–23).

### Transmission and Pathogenesis

Although intact skin is not susceptible to infection, contact of virus with mucosa or abraded skin may lead to infection of the epidermis and dermis. Infection spreads to contiguous cells and to sensory and autonomic nerve endings, and either virus or, more likely, the nucleocapsids are transported inside the axons to nerve cell bodies in sensory and autonomic ganglia (24). At this stage, active viral replication occurs in ganglia and is followed by centrifugal migration of virions to other mucosal and skin surfaces. This process, which is supported by experimental studies in animals, probably explains the large affected surface areas and crops of new lesion formation distant from the initial crop of vesicles that often characterize initial episodes (8,25,26).

Infected cells show ballooning and degeneration of cell nuclei, often with eosinophilic nuclear inclusions (Chowdry type A). Vesicles that form in the epithelium contain inflammatory cells (polymorphonuclear cells followed by mononuclear cells), multinucleated giant cells, and cells with virus-induced changes, as described above.

Following the initial infection, active viral replication ceases in the skin and in sensory and autonomic ganglia. As indicated earlier, the state of viral DNA in latently infected neurons is not known. Although some evidence suggests that viral replication continues at a very low level, most data suggest that the genome is present in a nonreplicative, static state. In the former theory, virions would migrate to the skin at more or less a constant rate, and recurrences would be triggered by local factors allowing productive infection to occur in the skin or mucous membranes. In the latter, more commonly held theory, viral DNA in neurons, usually in a nonreplicative state, would intermittently be stimulated to cause productive infection in the ganglia, followed by centrifugal migration of virions to the skin where productive infection of the mucosa or skin would occur (18,24).

Reinfection with the same virus strain has been demonstrated in humans, and multiple strains of the same type have occasionally been isolated from patients (27,28). However, reinfection appears to be exceedingly rare, especially in immunocompetent patients, and virtually all recurrent episodes represent reactivation of latent virus rather than reinfection (29).

Although the exact mechanisms responsible for triggering reactivation remain unclear, recurrent episodes can be triggered in humans and in animal models by exposure to ultraviolet light, by trauma to sensory or autonomic ganglia, or following immunosuppression, particularly involving cell-mediated immunity (5,7,19,30,31).

In humans, both virus type and site of infection influence the frequency of viral reactivation. Corey et al. (26) reported that more than 80% of patients have recurrences within 12 months of first-episode genital HSV-2 infection compared to 55% after first episode genital HSV-1 infection, and the median number of episodes in the first year is four and one, respectively. Lafferty et al. (32) recently reported that the mean number of recurrences after first-episode oral or genital HSV-1 or HSV-2 infection was 0.33 per month for genital HSV-2, 0.12 per month for oral-labial HSV-1, 0.02 per month for genital HSV-1, and 0.001 per month for oral-labial HSV-2 infection, respectively. These data suggest that factors responsible for severity of infections and the frequency of recurrences are complex and may include external triggers, local and systemic immune responses, and virus type or strain.

### Immune Response

The immunological response to infection is an important factor in determining the severity and duration of first episode and recurrent disease, frequency of recurrences, and risk of complications such as dissemination (7,33–38). Although animal models suggest that both cellular and antibody-mediated immune responses may be important, cellular responses appear to play the more important role (33,34,36). Patients with defects in cell-mediated immune responses tend to have more severe infections than patients with defects in humoral immunity. Cells active in cell-mediated immune responses to HSV infection include macrophages, natural killer (NK) cells, and T cells (33,35,39). Lymphokines produced by these cells are also important both through direct antiviral effects of lymphokines such as interferons and through effects on other effector cells (40). Viral antigens responsible for stimulating protective cellular immune responses have not been clearly defined.

Both viral glycoproteins (B, C, D, E, and G) and nonglycosylated proteins stimulate antibody responses, and antibodies to the glycoproteins have been shown to mediate both viral neutralization and antibody-dependent cell-mediated cytotoxicity of HSV-infected target cells (11,41).

In normal adults, it has not been possible to identify immunologic markers to differentiate persons with frequent from infrequent recurrences of oral or genital herpes. Patients with frequent recurrences tend to have higher antibody titers, presumably secondary to repeated antigenic stimulation (8,42). Thus, there is no rationale for administration of γ globulin to patients with frequently recurrent genital or oral herpes. Similarly, no consistent abnormalities have been demonstrated in lymphocyte transformation, lymphokine production, or lymphocyte cytotoxicity in patients with oral or genital HSV episodes (37,43–49).

There is no evidence that prior infection with other herpes viruses such as VZV, CMV, or EBV influences the course of HSV infection. However, in persons with prior infection with HSV-1, protective immune responses to type-common antigens decrease the risk of acquisition of HSV-2 infection (G. J. Mertz, unpublished observations), modify the course of initial HSV-2 infection (26,42), and decrease the frequency of long-term recurrences of HSV-2 (50). Finally, serologic differentiation of dual infection with HSV-1 and HSV-2 from infection with HSV-1 or HSV-2 alone is technically difficult because of antibody responses to type common antigens.

## EPIDEMIOLOGY

Estimates regarding the incidence and prevalence of HSV infections have been generated by a variety of means including visits to clinicians for symptomatic illness, serologic surveys, viral cultures, and examination of sensory and autonomic ganglia at autopsy (2,19–21,51–55). Each of these methods has limitations. Viral culture is sensitive in the presence of viral shedding, but viral shedding is usually intermittent. HSV infections are not reportable illnesses, and the majority of HSV infections are asymptomatic or unrecognized (10,15,51,56,57). Thus, studies based on reports of clinical illness grossly underestimate prevalence. Serologic assays are sensitive but until recently have lacked specificity in differentiating dual infection from infection with HSV-1 or HSV-2 alone (13–15). In addition, serologic studies cannot determine the anatomic site of infection and, unless seroconversion is documented, cannot determine the time of acquisition of infection (10,15,56).

Despite these limitations, several clear trends have become evident in recent decades, particularly in middle and upper socioeconomic groups in Western countries. In these groups, there has been a significant decrease in acquisition of HSV-1 infection in childhood and a substantial increase in the incidence of symptomatic HSV-2 infections in adults (2,51–55,58,59).

### Serologic Data

Serologic surveys indicate that HSV-1 infection is widespread. In Western countries until the 1950s, 80–90% of young adults had HSV-1 antibody (59). In recent decades, however, there has been a gradual decline in HSV-1 infection among middle and upper socioeconomic populations in Western developed countries. In studies performed in the United States and United Kingdom in the 1960s and 1970s, less than 50% of middle class young adults in their teens and 20s had HSV antibody (59,60).

Antibody to HSV-2 is rare in populations until puberty and then increases with age and sexual experience. In adults in the United States, HSV-2 antibody has been detected in 3% of nuns, 20–30% of adults in middle socioeconomic groups, 46–60% of persons in lower socioeconomic groups, and 80% of prostitutes (52,53). Seroprevalence tends to be higher in women as compared to men, perhaps reflecting increased efficiency of male-to-female transmission (51). In a recent study in Seattle, approximately one-half of homosexual men and one-quarter of heterosexual men had serologic evidence of past HSV-2 infection (8,55).

### Clinical Epidemiology

In a study in Yugoslavia, clinical evidence of primary herpes gingivostomatitis was found in 13% of children attending outpatient clinics. No cases were seen below 6 months of age, and 58% of cases were seen in children between 1 and 3 years of age (61). Estimates in the United States suggest there are approximately 500,000 cases of primary oral-labial herpes and approximately 100 million episodes of recurrent oral-labial herpes infections each year (62). More than half of persons with recurrent oral-labial herpes have two recurrences or fewer per year (63).

The number of first office visits for genital herpes in the United States increased ninefold between 1966 and 1984 (2,58), and the prevalence of genital HSV infections increased 12% per year between 1975 and 1982 in patients attending sexually transmitted disease clinics in the United Kingdom (64). Recent estimates by the Centers for Disease Control suggest there may be 500,000–700,000 or more symptomatic first episodes of genital herpes and more than 20 million episodes of recurrent genital herpes per year in the United States (2,58). The median number of genital herpes recurrences in adults with symptomatic genital herpes infection is approximately four per year (26,32,42).

Despite the higher seroprevalence of HSV-1 and HSV-2 infections in nonwhites and persons in lower socioeconomic groups (51), visits for symptomatic genital herpes are more common in whites versus nonwhites (2,58). Although these differences may relate in part to access to medical care, it is also likely that decreases in HSV-1 infections have contributed to an increased incidence of symptomatic first genital infections in middle class whites. Genital symptoms are more severe and prolonged when first-episode genital HSV-1 or HSV-2 infection occurs in the absence of prior HSV-1 antibody (26,42), and patients with severe symptoms may be more likely to seek medical care.

### Asymptomatic and Unrecognized HSV Infection

Overall, it is estimated that up to 90% of primary oral-labial HSV infections may be asymptomatic or unrecognized (52), and less than half of adults with HSV antibody in the Framingham Heart Study had a history of recent herpes labialis (65). Several recent studies employing type-specific HSV-

2 antibody have shown that of adults with HSV-2 antibody, two-thirds or more have no history of genital herpes or genital lesions (51,54,56). In a recent study at Stanford and Santa Clara Valley Hospitals, 76% of pregnant women with HSV-2 antibody had no history of genital herpes (57).

Asymptomatic viral shedding of HSV-1 in saliva has been reported in 1–5% of cultures in children and adults, and serial cultures have eventually yielded viral isolation in 30–50% of seropositive children and adults (66–71). Asymptomatic cervical and vulvar shedding has been most intensively studied in pregnant women. During pregnancy, up to 0.8% of cultures are positive (72). Prober et al. (57) recently reported that 14 (0.2%) of 6,904 genital cultures obtained at the time of delivery at Stanford and Santa Clara Valley Hospitals were positive for HSV-2, and only two (14%) of the 14 women had a history of genital herpes, sexual exposure to a partner with genital herpes, or serologic evidence of recent acquisition of HSV-2 infection.

### Transmission of HSV Infections

No epidemics of HSV-1 or HSV-2 have been described, although outbreaks of HSV-1 infection have been described in families, hospitals (e.g., in newborn nurseries, pediatric wards, and intensive care units), and in other closed populations such as orphanages or children's homes (61,71,73–76). Attack rates of 50–80% of susceptible children have been described, although attack rates as low as 10% over a 6-year period have also been reported (61,71,75). Finally, 37% of patients treated by a dental hygienist with primary herpetic whitlow developed symptomatic HSV pharyngitis (77). Although data documenting the state of HSV-1 infections in source contacts of persons with first episode oral-labial HSV-1 infection is limited, asymptomatic shedding of HSV-1 in saliva is felt to be an important source of transmission of HSV-1 infection.

In a recent study of 66 index patients with first-episode genital herpes and their 66 source contacts who had transmitted genital HSV infection, the mean ages were 29.5 years in source contacts and 28.2 years in index patients (56). HSV-1 was transmitted in five couples, and HSV-2 was transmitted in the remainder. The couples had had sexual contact for a median of 3 months prior to transmitting genital herpes, although the duration of the contact ranged from one sexual exposure to 14 years. Thirty-seven (56%) of the 66 source contacts denied a history of genital herpes or genital lesions at the time of transmission, and 23 of these 37 denied any history of genital herpes or lesions. Of interest, HSV-2 was isolated from the cervix of two source contacts who denied a history of genital herpes and who had no genital lesions by examination. Subsequent reports have provided additional support for the concept that transmission of genital herpes infections between sexual partners commonly results from contact during asymptomatic shedding (78), and other recent studies have found that the majority of women who transmit herpes at delivery have no history of genital herpes or symptoms suggestive of herpes at delivery (79–80).

This implies that exposure during periods of asymptomatic shedding is much more common than exposure to lesions, since the risk of transmission from a single exposure to active lesions is probably greater than the risk from a single exposure during asymptomatic shedding. The titer of HSV in active lesions is $10^2$–$10^3$ higher in active lesions versus during asymptomatic shedding (81), and the number of lesions, lesion area, and duration of viral shedding is far greater in first-episode versus recurrent genital herpes (26). Studies of transmission of neonatal herpes suggest that the risk of transmission at delivery from a mother with primary genital herpes may be as high as 50% as compared to less than 8% from mothers with recurrent genital herpes; the risk is probably much smaller during asymptomatic shedding (57,72,79,82).

The risk of transmission within couples with one partner with symptomatic recurrent genital herpes and one partner without a history of genital herpes has been estimated in three recent studies (10,83). In the first (10), 38 couples who had been sexual partners for a median of 10 months were followed prospectively for a median 6 months. Asymptomatic or unrecognized acquisition of HSV-2 had occurred in 10 couples prior to enrollment and in one exposed partner during prospective follow-up. The risk of transmission of HSV-2 was estimated to be approximately 12% per year in these couples, although the authors cautioned that there was incomplete information about source of infection in 6 of 11 couples. More recently, Bryson reported similar results in a prospective study in 29 couples (83). Subsequently, in a prospective, randomized, placebo-controlled vaccine study evaluating the risk of transmission in 162 couples with source partners with symptomatic genital HSV-2 infection and their seronegative exposed partners, we found a rate of transmission of approximately 10% per year and found that the risk of transmission was increased in couples with female exposed partners, exposed partners without HSV-1 antibody, and in couples who had sexual contact when the source partner had active lesions (G. J. Mertz, unpublished observations).

## CLINICAL MANIFESTATIONS

As indicated earlier, the immunological competence of the host and the presence or absence of past infection with virus of the same or heterologous type are the major determinants of the severity and duration of oral or genital HSV infections (26). Thus, primary or recurrent infections in severely immunocompromised patients may be severe and prolonged and may be complicated by visceral dissemination. In normal patients, first-episode infections tend to be more severe and prolonged than subsequent recurrent infections. Primary first episodes, those occurring in patients seronegative for both HSV-1 and HSV-2, tend to be more severe than those that occur in persons with past infection with HSV of the heterologous type (nonprimary first episodes) (26).

### Oral-Labial Facial Infections

Most primary oral infections are asymptomatic or unrecognized (52). Primary symptomatic infections are characterized by gingivostomatitis or pharyngitis and recurrent infections by herpes labialis (8,32,52,61, 84,85).

Symptoms of herpetic gingivostomatitis may include sore mouth or throat, fever, malaise, inability to eat, and irritability (8,52). Tender cervical lymphadenopathy is typically present, and lesions may involve the face, lip, hard and soft palate, tongue, gingiva, and buccal mucosa. Lesions progress through typical stages of erythema, vesicles, ulcers, and crusts before healing, although vesicles are less commonly seen on mucosal surfaces as compared to the outer lip and skin, and true crusted lesions are generally not seen on mucosal surfaces with either oral-labial or genital herpes. The mean duration of viral shedding may be as long as 23 days, and healing of lesions may take more than 3 weeks (84).

HSV pharyngitis, often accompanied by fever and cervical adenopathy, accounted for 11% of college students with pharyngitis in one study (67). When HSV pharyngitis is sexually transmitted, the onset or pharyngitis usually coincides with the onset of genital lesions; HSV of the same type and strain is isolated from both genital and pharyngeal lesions (26,32). Approximately one-third of persons with HSV pharyngitis will develop gingivostomatitis. In children, primary HSV infection is almost exclusively caused by HSV-1; in adults, primary infection can be caused by HSV-1 or HSV-2 (8,26,32).

Depending on the clinical presentation, HSV gingivostomatitis or pharyngitis must be differentiated from other causes of bacterial and viral pharyngitis, herpangina and hand-foot-mouth syndrome (both usually caused by coxsakie viruses), thrush, and noninfectious causes of oral and pharyngeal ulceration. Examples of the latter include mucousitis after high-dose chemotherapy or radiation therapy, and the Stevens-Johnson syndrome.

Recurrent herpes labialis in the normal host is preceded by a prodrome characterized by burning, itching, or pain for a few hours or days prior to development of lesions in more than half of patients (85). Lesions progress through typical stages of erythema, vesicles, ulcers, and crusts, and heal in a mean of approximately 8 days. Over 90% of lesions occur on the lip (usually the outer, vermillion border), with the remainder occurring on the skin of the chin, nose, or cheek, or within the mouth. Over 95% of patients have two lesions or fewer in a single location; approximately 25% have new lesion formation during the episode, usually in a contiguous site. Viral shedding is most likely from vesicular lesions in the first 24–48 hr of the outbreak, and positive cultures are uncommon after 5 or more days (85). Over 99% of recurrent herpes labialis infections are caused by HSV-1.

Differentiation of herpes labialis from other conditions such as apthous stomatitis is usually not difficult. The diagnosis of herpes labialis is usually clear if lesions begin as vesicles and occur on the outer lip or contiguous skin. Apthous ulcers are typically 3 mm or larger in size, are not vesicular, have an erythematous halo, and occur on mucous membranes in the anterior mouth. Recurrent herpes lesions of the mucous membranes are unusual, are generally 3 mm or less, and have an erythematous base. Most persons with recurrent herpes labialis do not have a history of herpetic gingivostomatitis or pharyngitis, so the absence of a history of the latter syndromes is usually not helpful in differentiating herpes labialis from apthous stomatitis.

### Genital Herpes Infections

As in the case of primary herpes gingivostomatitis and pharyngitis, most primary or nonprimary first-episode genital infections are probably asymptomatic or unrecognized. Among patients with symptomatic first episodes, episodes in persons without prior HSV-1 or-2 antibody (primary episodes) tend to be more severe and prolonged than first episodes in persons with antibody to HSV of the heterologous type (nonprimary episodes). In most series, 10–25% of primary genital HSV infections are caused by HSV-1, although rates of up to 50% have been noted in some series (26,86–88). HSV-2 is isolated from 75–90% of primary first episodes and 99% of nonprimary first episodes.

Symptomatic, primary first-episode genital herpes is characterized by a prolonged course, multiple bilateral lesions, local pain, sacral parethesias, and systemic complications (Table 1) (26). Systemic symptoms such as fever and malaise occur in over half of patients. Most patients have bilateral lesions, form crops of new lesions in the first or second week of illness, and heal in an average of approximately 3 weeks. The progression of lesion stages is similar to that described for oral-labial herpes infections. Systemic symptoms, meningitis, and dysuria are approximately twice as common in women as in men, and over 80% of women with primary genital herpes shed virus from the cervix.

HSV pharyngitis and extragenital lesions such as herpetic whitlow, usually acquired by autoinoculation, are seen in approximately 10% of patients with primary genital herpes.

Aseptic meningitis may complicate up to 25% of cases of primary genital herpes, but it is usually mild (8,26,86). Less than 1% of patients with primary genital herpes require hospitalization, usually for aseptic meningitis or urine retention (26,86). Urine retention may occur secondary to pain or from autonomic nervous system dysfunc-

**TABLE 1.** *Relation between viral type, presence of HSV antibody in acute phase sera, and severity of disease of first-episode genital herpes*[a]

| | Primary HSV-1 infection ($N = 20$) | Primary HSV-2 infection ($N = 189$) | Nonprimary HSV-2 infection ($N = 76$) |
|---|---|---|---|
| Patients with systemic symptoms (%) | 58 | 62 | 16 |
| Patients with meningitis symptoms (%) | 16 | 26 | 1 |
| Mean duration of local pain (days) | 12.5 | 11.8 | 8.7 |
| Mean number of lesions | 24.3 | 15.5 | 9.5 |
| Mean lesion area ($mm^2$) | 597 | 517 | 158 |
| Patients with bilateral lesions (%) | 100 | 82 | 45 |
| Patients forming new lesions during course of disease (%) | 68 | 75 | 45 |
| Mean duration viral shedding from genital lesions (days) | 11.1 | 11.4 | 6.8 |
| Mean duration lesions (days) | 22.7 | 18.6 | 15.5 |
| Patients developing extragenital lesions (%) | 10 | 18 | 8 |
| Patients shedding herpes simplex virus from cervix (%) | 80 | 88 | 65 |

[a]Only one patient with complement fixation and neutralizing antibody in acute phase sera had HSV-1 isolated from genital lesions. $p < 0.05$ for each comparison between nonprimary and primary HSV-2 infection ($\chi^2$ or Student's *t* test).

From Corey et al., ref. 26, with permission.

tion (26,86,89–94). When caused by pain, urine retention can usually be managed with pain medications and by having the patient urinate while sitting in warm water. When caused by autonomic nervous system dysfunction, intermittent catheterization may be required for days to weeks.

Nonprimary first-episode genital herpes tends to be intermediate in duration and severity between primary and recurrent genital herpes (26). Systemic symptoms such as fever and malaise are less common than in primary infection, and less than 1% of patients have symptoms suggesting aseptic meningitis. Viral shedding from the cervix is present in approximately two-thirds of women as compared to 80–90% in primary genital herpes and approximately 5% in recurrent genital herpes (Table 1).

The course of recurrent genital herpes outbreaks is similar to the course of herpes labialis (26,81). Like herpes labialis, lesions in recurrent genital herpes tend to be unilateral and well localized. Lesions typically involve the vulva in women or penis in men but may occur at a variety of sites including the buttocks in men and women and perianal areas, especially in women and homosexual men. The prodrome, which is similar to that described by patients with herpes labialis, occurs in approximately 50% of patients. The mean duration of viral shedding is 3–4 days, and healing occurs in a mean of 9–10 days. Tender inguinal adenopathy is present in approximately 25%, and mild systemic symptoms are noted in 5–13% of outbreaks. Complications such as recurrent aseptic meningitis have been reported but are exceedingly rare. HSV-2 is isolated from 98% of persons with recurrent genital herpes and in virtually 100% of episodes in normal adults with frequently recurring genital herpes (i.e., ≥6 episodes per year) (26,32,42).

For patients with typical first-episode or recurrent genital herpes, clinical diagnosis is usually not difficult, particularly when vesicles are observed by the clinician or when outbreaks are preceded by a typical prodrome accompanied by sacral paresthesias or other neurologic complications. However, atypical infections must be differentiated from syphilis, chancroid, lymphogranuloma veneveum (LGV), genital warts, scabies, molluscum contagiosum, fixed drug eruption, contact dermatitis, psoriasis, and trauma (86,95).

### Other HSV Infections

Ocular infections, neonatal herpes, and herpes encephalitis are covered in detail in other chapters. HSV is an uncommon cause of the urethral syndrome in women and of nongonococcal urethritis in men; salpingitis, endometritis, and prostatitis have been reported but are thought to be very rare (26,86,96,97).

HSV proctitis may be seen in men or women who have practiced receptive anal intercourse (26,86,90,91,98,99). Symptoms may include anorectal pain, tenesmus, constipation, discharge, and neurologic symptoms such as sacral parasthesias, impotence, and urine retention. Proctitis can generally be differentiated from proctitis-enteritis by the absence of diarrhea and crampy abdominal pain and by limitation of mucosal friability and discharge to the distal 10 cm of the rectum. HSV proctitis must be differentiated from proctitis caused by *Chlamydia trachomatis, Neisseria gonorrhea,* and *Treponema pallidum,* although infections with multiple pathogens are common. Neurologic symptoms and perianal vesicules or ulcers are present in approximately 50% of patients with herpes proctitis (99), although syphilis must be considered in the differential diagnosis of perianal or mucosal ulcers; none of the other causes of proctitis cause ulcers or neurologic symptoms. HSV proctitis and proctitis caused by the LGV serotypes of *Chlamydia trachomatis* tend to be associated with more severe symptoms as compared to gonococcal proctitis or *Chlamydia trachomatis* proctitis caused by other serotypes (98). In normal adults, proctitis results from primary or nonprimary infection. However, recurrent, persistent proctitis may occur in immunocompromised patients, especially men with AIDS (5,100,101).

Primary herpetic whitlow, an HSV infection of the finger, may be acquired from autoinoculation during primary gingivostomatitis or pharyngitis or primary genital herpes, or from direct contact with lesions in another person through sexual or nonsexual contact (8,26,102–109). Autoinoculation during recurrent episodes is uncommon. Health care workers appear to be at an increased risk of occupational acquisition of herpetic whitlow, but a recent study in Canada suggests that occupational acquisition is probably much less common than sexual acquisition of herpetic whitlow in adults (104). Primary infection may be associated with fever and painful epitroclear and axillary adenitis and may be difficult to differentiate from fungal or bacterial paronychia and cellulitis. Anecdotal experience suggests that the prodrome preceding recurrent herpetic whitlow tends to be more severe and prolonged as compared to prodromes preceding genital herpes or herpes labialis. Nosocomial transmission of HSV from health care workers with herpetic whitlow has been clearly documented, so health care workers should abstain from patient care or contact with materials touched by others until lesions heal (77). Similar advice would presumably be prudent in other, nonmedical, situations as well. Because of the potential loss of work associated with herpetic whitlow, early, aggressive episodic or suppressive therapy with oral acyclovir (ACV) may be appropriate (102,109–111).

### Complications in the Normal Host

In addition to the neurologic complications of primary genital herpes discussed previously, primary or recurrent oral or genital herpes may be complicated by erythema multiforme or by cutaneous or visceral dissemination in persons with eczema (eczema herpeticum) (112–117). Recurrent aseptic meningitis associated with recurrent genital herpes has been reported but is exceedingly rare (86,118,119).

### Infections in Immunocompromised Patients

Primary infection with HSV may cause severe disease with dissemination in immunocompromised hosts. However, since primary HSV infection precedes the onset of immunodeficiency in most patients, most HSV infections are recurrent infections resulting from reactivation of latent HSV infection (5–8,100,101,120–131). Primary infections in immunocompromised patients are most commonly seen in infants with malnutrition or severe combined immunodeficiency or in children with lymphoreticular malignancies (120,132–135).

Recurrent HSV infections in the immunocompromised host are characterized by severe, persistent mucocutaneous infection usually involving the mouth, face, genital, or perianal areas. In the absence of antiviral therapy, viral shedding may persist and lesions may progress until marrow function returns after marrow transplantation or induction chemotherapy (6–8,120–125), and viral shedding and lesions may persist indefinitely in patients with AIDS (5,100,101). Less commonly, visceral dissemination may occur. Any organ may be involved, but visceral dissemination most commonly involves the esophagus, lung, liver, adrenyl glands, and bone marrow (122,126–130). In most cases, visceral dissemination clearly occurs secondary to viremia, although local spread to the esophagus and lung may occur without viremia.

In some situations, the probability of developing severe recurrent mucocutaneous HSV infection is known to be high, and infections can be anticipated and treated or prevented with ACV therapy. For example, 85–90% of persons with HSV antibody who undergo bone marrow transplantation will develop mucocutaneous HSV infections, and many experts recommend suppressive oral ACV therapy in all HSV seropositive patients who undergo marrow transplantation (5,6,136).

## DIAGNOSIS

In the research setting, both viral cultures with typing and acute and convalescent antibody testing employing a type-specific antibody test are commonly employed to determine virus type and to differentiate primary first-episode, nonprimary first episodes and recurrent genital herpes (10,12–15,26,56,57). In the clinical setting, since the results of serologic tests will not be available in time to influence treatment, most clinicians make decisions based on their clinical impression and frequently do not employ serologic tests.

Although serologic testing is not widely performed outside the research setting, viral culture is strongly recommended if virologic confirmation has not been obtained in the past. Although some clinicians argue that virologic confirmation is often unnecessary when the clinical diagnosis is clear, there are several arguments in favor of obtaining virologic confirmation. First, typing of virus recovered from first episodes provides valuable prognostic information regarding the frequency and likelihood of subsequent recurrences (32,42). Second, a positive viral culture provides conclusive evidence of infection. In this case, the cost may be justified in light of counseling regarding the risk of transmission to sexual partners or at delivery and the potential cost of treatment or repeated clinical evaluations in persons who do not have a definitive diagnosis. Third, virologic confirmation, if positive, is extremely helpful in atypical HSV infections. Fourth, and finally, viral culture is clearly indicated in the immunocompromised host when HSV infection fails to respond to ACV therapy and ACV resistance is suspected (1,100,132–134,137). Viral culture is less clearly indicated in normal patients with recurrent herpes labialis or recurrent genital herpes who are comfortable accepting a clinical diagnosis, are not women of childbearing potential, and do not desire chronic suppressive ACV therapy.

In general, clinicians should be cautious about conclusions regarding the time and source of acquisition of HSV infections. Definitive determination of the time and source of genital HSV infection requires both comparison of viral DNA by restriction endonuclease analysis from viruses isolated from sexual partners and demonstration of seroconversion (10,13–15,27–29,56,57,109). In the case of nonprimary first episodes, demonstration of seroconversion requires utilization of type-specific assays (13–15). At present, both restriction endonuclease analysis and reliable serologic assays able to differentiate type-specific antibodies are confined to research laboratories. Recently, Bernstein et al. (15) reported that 75% of patients thought to have nonprimary first-episode genital herpes had an antibody to HSV-2 type-specific glycoproteins detected in acute serum specimens when tested by western blot analysis. Those with HSV-2 antibody thus had remote rather than recent acquisition of HSV-2 infection despite experiencing their first clinical episode. Thus, implication of a current sexual partner as the source of infection in these cases might be inappropriate, and determination of the time of acquisition would be impossible (10,15,56).

### Viral Diagnosis

Viral isolation in cell culture systems remains the gold standard for diagnosis; it is the most sensitive and specific laboratory method available. HSV grows well in a variety of cell types, and up to 90% of cultures will show characteristic cytopathic effects (CPE) within 72 hr of innoculation (138,139). Once CPE is present, typing can be performed with commercially available monoclonal antibodies to HSV-1 and HSV-2 (12). Rates of virus isolation of 80–90% or more can be expected from vesicles or ulcers in first-episode infections or infections, vesicles or ulcers in immunocompromised patients, and from vesicles in normal patients with recurrent disease. Isolation rates remain above 50% from ulcers in normal patients with recurrent disease but drop to 25% or less from crusted lesions (8,81,95,138,139).

Direct tests such as fluorescent antibody testing, indirect immunoperoxidase testing, or enzyme immunoassay (EIA) employing monoclonal antibodies have the advantages of lower cost, the potential for more rapid results, and do not require cell culture capability (8,12,138–140). None are as sensitive as tissue culture but most appear to have acceptable sensitivity (up to 80–90%) with typical, early lesions. None appear to have acceptable sensitivity for detection of cervical infection or asymptomatic shedding. Centrifugation of clinical specimens with susceptible cell lines followed by direct fluorescent antibody staining with monoclonal antibodies is a rapid, sensitive technique that combines the sensitivity of viral culture with the speed of direct techniques (141).

Tzank or Papanicolou smears can demonstrate herpes virus-induced changes in cells, but these techniques are less sensitive (50–60%) when compared with viral culture or the direct tests described and cannot differentiate between virus-induced changes caused by HSV-1, HSV-2, or VZV.

### Serologic Techniques

HSV antibody can be detected by a variety of techniques including complement fixation, microneutralization, or EIA (8,53,54,56,59,60,142). The techniques are highly sensitive and reliable in detecting past HSV infection, and, almost any technique can be used for screening for past infection prior to bone marrow transplant, organ transplant, or induction chemotherapy for leukemia to determine whether suppressive ACV therapy should be considered.

Complement fixation testing does not differentiate between HSV-1 and HSV-2 antibody, and antibody testing with microneutralization tests or currently available EIAs cannot reliably differentiate between infection with HSV-1 or HSV-2 and dual infection with both viruses (8,10,15). Several research laboratories have developed sensitive, specific serologic tests such as western blot assay, immunodot assay, and an EIA employing a type-specific monoclonal antibody that measure antibody to type-specific HSV-1 and HSV-2 glycoproteins (13–15,57). None of these assays is widely available.

## MANAGEMENT AND PREVENTION

Goals for the management and prevention of mucocutaneous herpes infection include safe and effective episodic treatment or suppression of mucocutaneous herpes episodes, eradication of established, latent infection, and prevention of transmission. Although there has been little progress in accomplishing the latter two goals, substantial progress has been made in the development of effective treatment for established infections. One antiviral agent, ACV, now enjoys wide clinical acceptance (1).

Fortunately, both *in vitro* screening techniques and animal models are available to guide the preclinical development of antiviral drugs, immune modulators, and vaccines. Although *in vitro* techniques and animal models each have limitations, both have proven valuable in the preclinical screening of antiviral agents.

### *In Vitro* Testing

Several *in vitro* screening tests are available for screening of antiviral drugs. The most commonly employed assays are plaque reduction assays or dye uptake assays that measure the degree of inhibition of infection of susceptible cell culture lines by HSV in the presence of antiviral agents (143,144); results are commonly expressed as an $ID_{50}$, the dose necessary to result in 50% inhibition of HSV infection.

### Animal Models

Animal models have proven useful for evaluation of HSV vaccines as well as topically and parenterally administered antiviral drugs. These models include (a) skin infections in shaved or depilitated rabbits, guinea pigs, or mice, or hairless mice (145–150), (b) infection of the lip, nasal mucosa, or pinna of the ear in mice (152–154), and (c) genital infections in female mice and guinea pigs (25,155–158). Most models are limited to evaluation of primary infections, but models of recurrent infection include ultraviolet radiation-induced infections in dorsal skin and the pinna of the ear in mice and external genital infections in guinea pigs (25,159–160). Efficacy parameters and end points vary with each model.

In animal models, ACV has been the most effective antiviral agent followed by phosphonoformate (foscarnet; PFA), phosphonoacetic acid (PAA), and systemic vidarabine (adenine arabinoside; ara-A) (146–158,161). Animal studies also indicate that systemic ACV treatment must be initiated before lesion onset to prevent establishment of latency in primary HSV infection and that systemic but not topical ACV therapy could suppress recurrent genital herpes in the giunea pig model. No antiviral agent has been shown to eradicate latent infection from sensory ganglia.

Among other agents tested, systemic vidarabine, and topical idoxuridine (IDU) in dimethylsulfoxide (DMSO), and exogenous dimethylsulfoxide (DMSO), and exogenous murine interferon and interferon inducers have shown some efficacy, whereas topical ara-A monophosphate (ara-AMP), topical IDU, topical ara-A, topical 2-deoxy-D-glucose have shown little or no efficacy (156,161–165).

genital herpes with Foscarnet (157,185; S. Sacks, unpublished observations). Future evaluation of antiviral agents may be aided by the recent development of experimental models where lip or buttock recurrences can be induced by measured doses of ultraviolet β irradiation (30).

**Clinical Trials of Antiviral Agents**

A series of placebo-controlled clinical trials in humans with topical, oral, and intravenous ACV have documented the efficacy of these preparations in a variety of mucocutaneous HSV infections and have led to licensure of all three preparations by the United States' Food and Drug Administration (FDA). These trials will be described in detail in subsequent sections.

In addition, a variety of agents have been evaluated in placebo-controlled trials and have failed to show any clinical benefit. These include bacille Calmette-Guérin (BCG) and smallpox vaccination, levamisole, topical ether or betadine, IDU, IDU in DMSO, vidarabine, and administration of γ-globulin (166–178). One study suggested that topical 2-deoxy-D-glucose accelerated healing in recurrent genital herpes, but concerns have been raised about the study design, and recent animal studies have shown no benefit from treatment with 2-deoxy-D-glucose (156,179). Although lysine treatment has been popular, clinical trials have shown conflicting results. In general, studies with adequate study design have shown no benefit from lysine treatment (180,181).

Several recent trials have suggested some clinical benefit from systematically administered interferons, but, to date, the virologic and clinical benefit demonstrated in these studies has been modest in comparison to that achieved with systemically administered ACV therapy (182–184). Topical therapy with Foscarnet (phosphonoformate) has produced conflicting results, but recent studies suggest there is little or no clinical benefit from topical treatment of recurrent

**Mechanism of Action of Acyclovir**

ACV, an acyclic analog of guanosine, must be phosphorylated to acyclovir triphosphate (ACV-TP) to exert its antiviral actions (1,186,187). Much of the specificity and safety of ACV as compared to other nucleoside analogs results from the relative inability of HSV-uninfected cells to phosphorylate ACV. In uninfected cells, cellular thymidine kinase (TK) is unable to phosphorylate ACV, whereas in HSV-infected cells, the TK specified by HSV readily phosphorylates acyclovir monophosphate (ACV-MP). ACV-MP is then phosphorylated to acyclovir diphosphate (ACV-DP) and ADV-TP by cellular enzymes.

ACV is a potent inhibitor of HSV DNA polymerase and is a competitive inhibitor of deoxyguanosine triphosphate. Enzyme inactivation appears to be the primary mechanism by which ACV inhibits HSV DNA polymerase. Secondly, once ACV-MP enters the DNA, chain-termination results. ACV-MP is incorporated into the DNA chain through formation of a 5′- to 3′-phosphodiester linkage between ACV-MP and the free 3′-hydroxyl group in the group chain. Chain termination results, because ACV is acyclic and has no 3′-hydroxyl group for subsequent 5′- to 3′-phosphodiester linkages, and ACV is not a substrate for the 3′-exonuclease activity of HSV DNA polymerase (Fig. 1).

The therapeutic index for ACV in HSV infections has been estimated to be 300–3,000. Levels of 70 μg/ml (300 μM) to 700 μg/ml (3,000 μM) are necessary to demonstrate toxicity in uninfected cells. The level of ACV required for $ID_{50}$ in HSV-infected

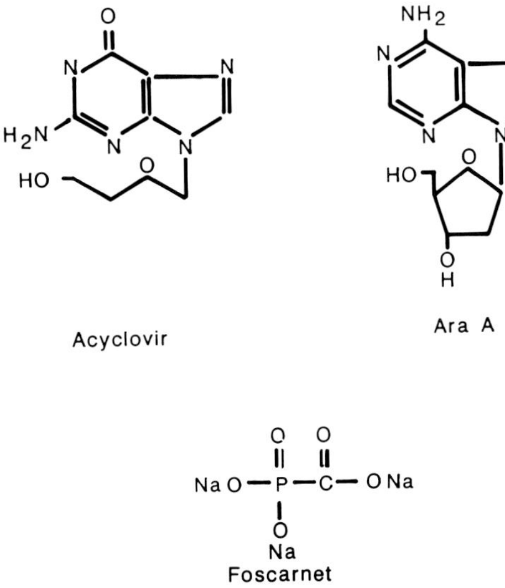

**FIG. 1.** Structure of antiviral drugs used in treatment of HSV infection.

cells is dependent on the assay and HSV strain, but strains with $ID_{50}$ less than 3.0 μg/ml (13 μM/L) are generally considered sensitive. Mean $ID_{50}$ values for clinical isolates of HSV-2 are generally less than 1.0 μg/ml, and $ID_{50}$ values for HSV-1 tend to be lower than those for HSV-2 (1,188).

### Mechanisms of Resistance to Acyclovir

ACV-resistant HSV strains can be selected *in vitro* that lack thymidine kinase (TK−), express thymidine kinase with altered substrate specificity, or express altered DNA polymerase (1,132–134,137). TK− mutants can be selected by growing HSV in subtherapeutic levels of ACV or by plaque purification of clinical isolates. These data suggest that TK− mutants occur at a low but predictable rate. TK− mutants are resistant to other nucleoside analogs such as ganciclovir (DHPG), which require phosphorylation by viral thymidine kinase, but TK− mutants remain sensitive to drugs such as ara-A and foscarnet, which do not require phosphorylation by viral TK (137). Sensitivity patterns are more variable with resistance from TK with altered substrate specificity or altered DNA polymerase.

### Treatment of First-Episode Genital Herpes

All three forms of ACV—the topical, oral, and intravenous preparations—have been shown to be effective in the treatment of first-episode genital herpes (189–194). In comparison to placebo groups, all three preparations significantly decrease the duration of viral shedding, time to healing of lesions, and duration of local symptoms of pain and itching (Table 2). As would be predicted from animal studies, the oral and intravenous preparations appear superior to topical treatment. The three preparations have not been compared with each other in placebo-controlled studies, but after controlling for differences in placebo groups, comparison of data collected from patients treated at the same clinic suggest that topical treatment is the least effective (195). The antiviral effect as measured by the duration of viral shedding was significantly greater with the oral and intravenous compared to the topical preparation (Fig. 2). Both the oral and intravenous preparation significantly decreased the duration of dysuria and suppressed the formation of new lesions, whereas, the topical preparation had no effect on these parameters (Table 2). Combined treatments with oral and topical ACV, and oral ACV and isoprinosine have been compared to treatment with oral ACV alone, and neither combined treatment regimen was more effective than oral ACV alone (196,197). Thus, there is no rationale for combination therapy.

Oral ACV, 200 mg orally five times daily for 10 days, has emerged as the treatment of choice for most patients with first-episode genital herpes. The clinical efficacy of the oral and intravenous preparations are probably about equal, but the oral preparation is far less expensive and more convenient to administer. With oral ACV treatment, the median duration of viral shedding

**TABLE 2.** *Signs and symptoms of first-episode primary genital herpes in acyclovir* (ACV) versus placebo-treated patients[a]

| Median number days after start of treatment | Topical ACV ($N = 28$) | Placebo ointment ($N = 23$) | Intravenous ACV ($N = 14$) | Placebo ($N = 13$) | Oral ACV ($N = 33$) | Placebo ($N = 27$) |
|---|---|---|---|---|---|---|
| Local itching | 4[b] | 8 | 2[c] | 8 | 4[b] | 6 |
| Local pain | 5[b] | 7 | 3[b] | 7 | 5[c] | 9 |
| Dysuria | 4 | 5 | 4[b] | 7 | 3[b] | 6 |
| Vaginal discharge | 6 | 7 | 4[c] | 11 | 6 | 8 |
| Percentages with systemic symptoms at 7 days of treatment (%) | 18 | 30 | 0[c] | 46 | 9 | 18 |
| Complete crusting of lesions | 8[b] | 13 | 6[c] | 13 | 7[c] | 13 |
| Complete healing of lesions | 11[b] | 15 | 9[c] | 21 | 13[c] | 20 |
| Percent forming new lesions after 48 hr of therapy (%) | 69 | 74 | 20[c] | 69 | 13[c] | 74 |

[a]All comparisons are between patients who had described symptoms at time of enrollment into the study.
[b]$p < 0.05$, Mantel-Cox Test.
[c]$p < 0.01$, Mantel-Cox Test.
From Corey et al., ref. 195, with permission.

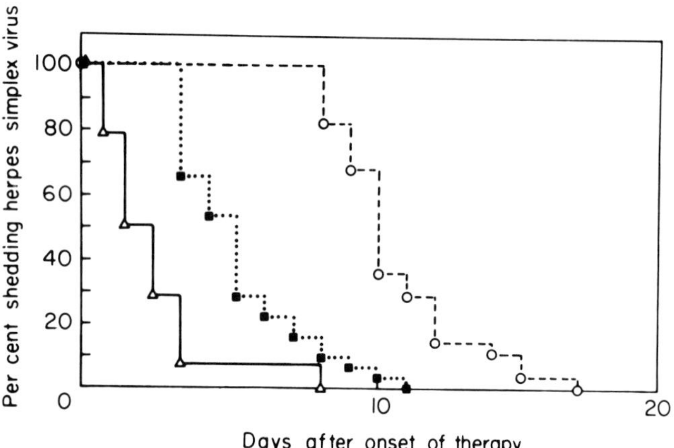


**FIG. 2.** Duration of viral shedding from genital lesions in patients with primary genital herpes after stratification for differences in viral shedding and healing times in placebo-treated patients. Comparison of virologic effects of intravenous, oral, and topical ACV. ($p < 0.001$ for comparison between intravenous and oral with topical ACV; Mantel-Cox test.) *Open circles,* topical ACV, $N = 25$; *open triangles,* intravenous ACV, $N = 15$; *solid squares,* oral ACV, $N = 26$. (From Corey et al., ref. 195, with permission.)

was reduced in one study from 9 to 2 days, and treatment led to a 4-day reduction in the duration of pain, a 7-day reduction in the time to healing, and a 60% reduction in the risk of forming crops of new lesions during therapy (Table 2) (195).

For patients ill enough to require hospitalization, therapy could be initiated with intravenous ACV (5 mg/kg/dose over 1 hr every 8 hr) followed by completion of a 10-day course of therapy with oral ACV once the patient begins to show clinical improvement. Aseptic meningitis is the most common complication of primary genital herpes leading to hospitalization, but fewer than 1% of patients with primary, first-episode genital herpes require hospitalization.

As would be predicted from animal models, initiation of ACV therapy after the onset of lesions does not prevent the establishment of latency nor does it appear to influence the frequency of subsequent episodes of recurrent genital herpes. When compared to placebo recipients, patients treated with topical, oral, or intravenous ACV during first-episode genital herpes are equally likely to experience recurrent episodes and have similar frequencies of episodes in the first year after treatment (191,192,194,198). Bryson et al. (199) reported a reduction in the frequency of episodes in the second year after oral ACV treatment, but Mertz et al. (200) found similar recurrence rates in the second year among patients who had been treated for primary genital herpes with oral ACV or placebo.

At present, there are no alternative forms of therapy for first-episode genital herpes. Although isoprinosine is licensed in some countries outside the United States, there is no data documenting efficacy in treatment of first-episode genital herpes. A recent placebo-controlled trial demonstrated accelerated healing and cessation of viral shedding in women treated with human leukocyte interferon, but the duration of pain was not influenced (183).

### Episodic Treatment of Recurrent Genital Herpes

Treatment of recurrent genital herpes episodes with oral ACV is effective in decreasing the duration of episodes, particularly when therapy is initiated at the first sign of a prodrome or lesion. However, the clinical benefit is not as clear as in treatment of first-episode genital herpes. Reichman et al. (201) reported the results of a placebo-controlled trial that compared the efficacy of ACV therapy (200 mg orally five times daily for 5 days) initiated by the physician within 48 hr of the onset of lesions with therapy initiated by the patient at the first sign of prodrome or lesions. Both physician- and patient-initiated therapy led to a significant reduction in the duration of viral shedding and time to healing, but both parameters were significantly shorter when treatment was patient-initiated (Fig. 3). Neither physician- nor patient-initiated therapy significantly decreased the duration of symptoms (Table 3).

Although these results are encouraging, it may be difficult to decide whether to recommend episodic oral ACV treatment to normal adults with recurrent genital herpes. Episodic treatment does not influence the frequency of recurrences, and the potential benefits of a mean reduction in time to healing of less than 2 days must be weighed against the cost of treatment of each episode, the potential for known adverse effects such as nausea, and the potential for unforseen toxicity. Episodic treatment has not been found to be associated with development of ACV resistance in the normal host, but a theoretical risk remains (202).

Episodic therapy should probably not be encouraged for patients who describe mild episodes that end in a week or less, but therapy should be considered in patients who describe multiple lesions, frequent new lesion formation, and healing in more than 7 days. Patients on episodic therapy should keep medication on hand and be in-

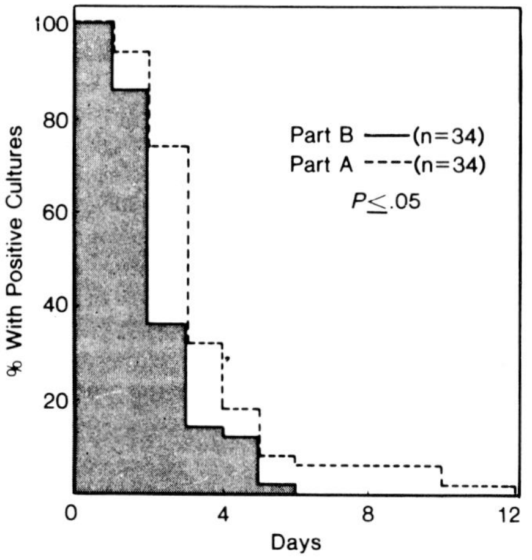


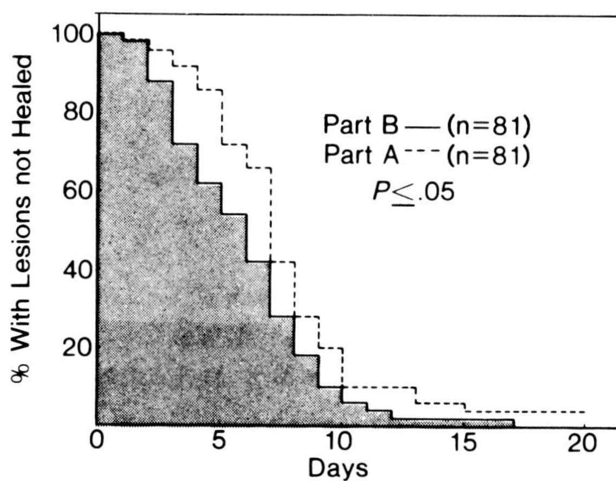


**FIG. 3.** Duration of virus snedding from all lesions (*left*) and time to healing of all lesions (*right*) of ACV recipients in parts A (physician-initiated therapy) and B (patient-initiated therapy). There is significant difference in duration of virus shedding and time to healing between two groups ($p < 0.05$; Gehan and Gilbert test). (From Reichman et al., ref. 201, with permission.)

structed to initiate treatment at the first sign or symptom suggesting a recurrence.

Episodic topical ACV therapy with the 5% ACV ointment available in the United States has not been shown to be effective in the normal host and is not generally recommended. Two trials, one where treatment was started within 48 hr of lesions and one started by the patient at the first sign or symptom, failed to demonstrate significant virologic or clinical benefit (191,203,204). A 5% cream is available in England and some other countries outside the United States. In one placebo-controlled study, patient ini-

**TABLE 3.** *Effect of orally administered ACV on the course of recurrent genital herpes*

| | Part A (physician-initiated therapy) | | Part B (patient-initiated therapy) | |
|---|---|---|---|---|
| | ACV | Placebo | ACV | Placebo |
| Lesions present at first clinic visit | | | | |
| Duration of virus shedding[a] | 2.0 ± 0.1[b] | 3.0 ± 0.3 | 2.1 ± 0.2[b] | 3.4 ± 0.3 |
| Time to crusting[a] | 2.1 ± 0.2 | 2.3 ± 0.2 | 2.4 ± 0.2[c] | 3.2 ± 0.3 |
| Time to healing[a] | 6.3 ± 0.3[d] | 7.0 ± 0.3 | 5.5 ± 0.3[e] | 6.5 ± 0.5 |
| All lesions | | | | |
| Duration of virus shedding[a] | 2.1 ± 0.2[b] | 3.1 ± 0.3 | 2.1 ± 0.2[b] | 3.9 ± 0.3 |
| Time to crusting[a] | 2.2 ± 0.2[e] | 2.7 ± 0.2 | 2.4 ± 0.2[b] | 3.9 ± 0.3 |
| Time to healing[a] | 6.3 ± 0.3[c] | 7.4 ± 0.3 | 5.7 ± 0.3[b] | 7.2 ± 0.5 |
| Duration of itching[a] | 2.5 ± 0.2 | 2.9 ± 0.3 | 2.8 ± 0.3[d] | 3.6 ± 0.3 |
| Duration of pain[a] | 2.8 ± 0.2 | 3.1 ± 0.3 | 3.0 ± 0.3[d] | 3.4 ± 0.3 |
| Development of new lesions during therapy (%) | 16.0 | 24.5 | 7.3 | 21.7 |

[a]Days (mean ± SEM), as measured from the first clinic visit.
[b]Duration significantly less than that observed in placebo group ($p \leq 0.001$), by logrank test.
[c]Duration significantly less than that observed in placebo group ($p \leq 0.01$), by logrank test.
[d]Duration not significantly less than that observed in the placebo group ($0.05 \leq p \leq 0.10$), by logrank test.
[e]Duration significantly less than that observed in placebo group ($p \leq 0.05$), by logrank test.
From Reichman et al., ref. 201, with permission.

tiated treatment with the 5% cream led to a significant reduction in the duration of viral shedding, duration of pain (from 5 to 2 days), and time to healing (from 6 to 4 days) (205). Thus, if the 5% cream is available, it might be considered as an alternative to episodic therapy with oral ACV.

### Suppressive ACV Therapy

To date, the most dramatic clinical benefit of oral ACV therapy in the normal adult has been from long-term suppression of frequently recurring genital herpes (202,206–217). Recently, Mertz et al. (202,206) reported the results of a multicenter, placebo-controlled trial comparing suppressive and episodic therapy for up to 2 years in patients with a history of a mean of 12.8 recurrences in the year prior to entry. Initially, almost 1,200 patients were randomized to receive ACV 400 mg twice daily or placebo; patients in either group with genital herpes episodes received standard episodic treatment with ACV. Only 2% of patients randomized to placebo were free of recurrences for 1 year, whereas 44% on suppressive therapy were recurrence-free for 1 year (Fig. 4). The mean frequency of recurrences was 11.4 per year in patients receiving episodic therapy versus 1.8 per year among those on suppressive therapy.

In the second year of the study, patients could choose the form of treatment, and 89% chose suppressive rather than episodic treatment. Among patients treated continuously for 2 years with suppressive treatment, 29% were free of recurrences for 2 years. Thus, patients with frequently recurring genital herpes experience substantial clinical benefit from suppressive treatment, and these patients clearly prefer suppressive to episodic treatment.

In published reports of trials continued for 3 months to 2 years and preliminary reports of trials continued for up to 4 years, suppressive therapy has been safe and well tolerated. Nausea was reported more often in patients on suppressive therapy in the first 3 months of the 2-year study. However, most patients described it as mild, and

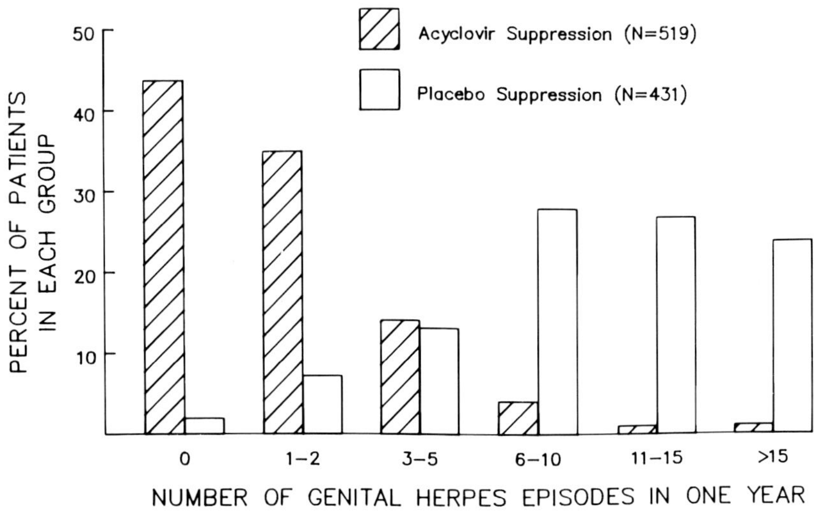


**FIG. 4.** Frequency of genital herpes episodes in one year among 519 patients receiving continuous suppression (*hatched bars*) with 400 mg of ACV orally twice daily for 1 year and among 431 patients (*open bars*) receiving placebo (episodic treatment) for 1 year. All patients received open-labeled ACV for 5 days during investigator-confirmed episodes of genital herpes. (From Mertz et al., ref. 202, with permission.)

**TABLE 4.** *ACV $ID_{50}$ concentrations in HSV*

| Treatment and temporal relation | Number of patients | Number of isolates | ACV $ID_{50}$ (μmol/L) Median | Range | Number of resistant isolates with $ID_{50} > 13$ μmol/L |
|---|---|---|---|---|---|
| Suppressive | | | | | |
| Before treatment | 53 | 54 | 3.6 | 0.5–17.8 | 2 |
| During treatment | 6 | 7 | 3.1 | 1.6–4.1 | 0 |
| After treatment | 48 | 55 | 3.8 | 0.5–10.9 | 0 |
| Episodic | | | | | |
| Before treatment | 54 | 59 | 3.5 | 0.4–13.7 | 1 |
| During treatment | 52 | 149 | 3.2 | 0.5–15.2 | 2 |
| After treatment | 32 | 34 | 4.5 | 1.2–13.8 | 1 |

$ID_{50}$, drug concentration producing a 50% reduction in CPE induced by HSV.
From Mertz et al., ref. 202, with permission.

only one discontinued therapy (202,206). No significant laboratory abnormalities have been associated with suppressive treatment, and routine laboratory monitoring does not appear to be necessary. In addition, no effect was noted on sperm motility or morphology in men using suppressive therapy for 6 months (218). Finally, although ACV-resistant HSV can occasionally be isolated before, during, or after suppressive or episodic therapy, there is little evidence that this is of clinical significance in the normal adult (202,215,217,219). Results in one study suggested an association with isolates recovered during suppressive therapy and ACV resistance, but subsequent isolates in these patients were sensitive to ACV (215). Subsequent studies have found no association with breakthrough episodes during suppressive therapy and ACV resistance (202,216,217,219) (Table 4).

As predicted by animal models, suppressive therapy does not appear to have any impact on the frequency of recurrences following discontinuation of therapy. Although two studies that did not include placebo group suggested a decrease in recurrence rates (209,217), two placebo-controlled studies have found no decrease in recurrence rates following discontinuation of suppressive therapy (207,214). However, in patients discontinuing suppressive therapy, Douglas et al. (207) noted that the time to the first recurrence was shorter than in placebo-treated patients and Mertz et al. (202) reported that the duration of the first recurrence was prolonged by a mean of 2 days in episodes occurring after discontinuation of suppressive therapy as compared to episodes in patients discontinuing episodic treatment.

### Recommendations for Suppressive Treatment

Suppressive therapy is generally reserved for patients who experience six or more episodes per year. Patients with frequent recurrences have been shown in one study to suffer greater psychological and social distress when compared to patients with infrequent episodes (G. J. Mertz, unpublished observations); thus, the former are presumably the most likely to benefit from suppressive therapy. However, clinicians tend to take multiple factors into consideration when making recommendations regarding suppressive therapy, and suppressive therapy may occasionally be appropriate in patients with relatively infrequent recurrences if accompanied by great psychological distress, if associated with serious complications such as erythema multiforme or eczema herpeticum, or if they lead to loss of work as in the case of herpetic whitlow in a health care worker.

Patients who wish to use suppressive

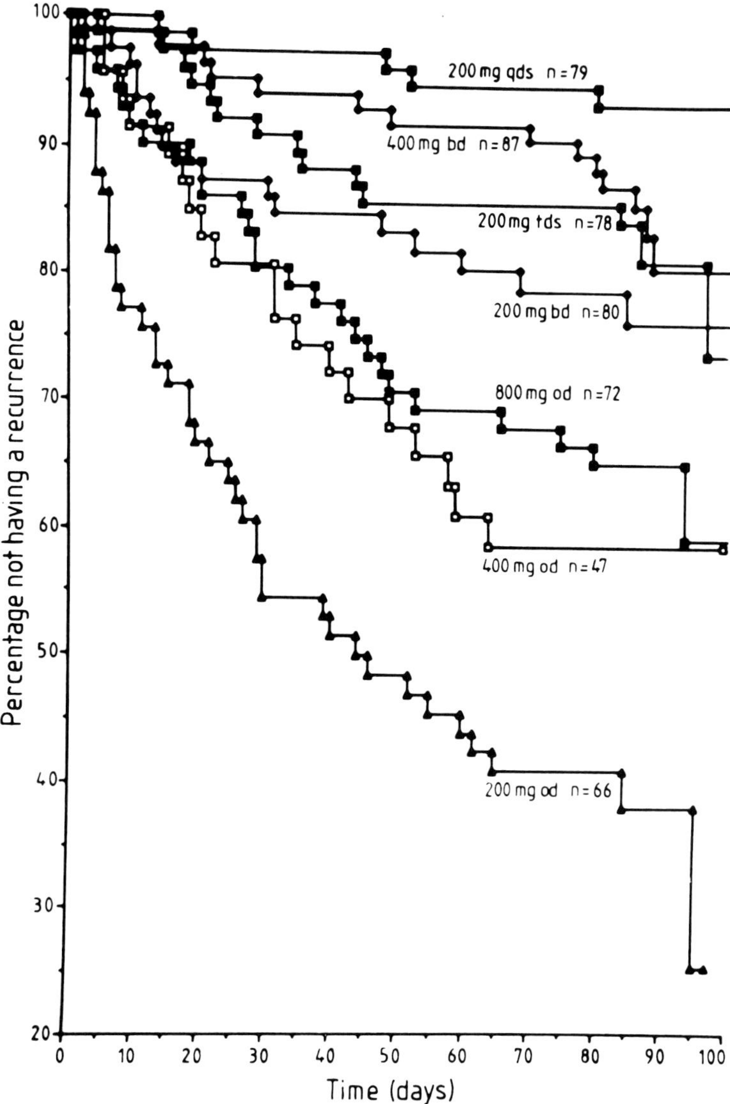


**FIG. 5.** Time to first recurrence with different doses of ACV. od, Once daily; bd, twice a day; tds, three times a day; qds, four times a day. (From Mindel et al., ref. 209, with permission.)

therapy to decrease the rates of transmission to a sexual partner should be warned that no studies have been performed to assess the risk of transmission during suppressive therapy. Viral shedding has been documented in episodes during suppressive therapy, and there are anecdotal and published reports of transmission during suppressive treatment (78,202,207,214). Sexual contact should be avoided during episodes regardless of the patient's treatment status, and couples may wish to use condoms between episodes to decrease the risk of transmission during asymptomatic shedding.

In the United States, suppressive therapy is currently approved at a dose of 200 mg three times daily for up to 6 months. When the FDA licensed oral ACV in 1985, only 3–6-month studies had been completed.

Now that safety and efficacy have been demonstrated for 2–4 years, recommendations for duration of treatment should probably be reevaluated (202,206,209,217). Regardless of the duration of suppressive therapy, most experts recommend periodically interrupting therapy to reassess the frequency of recurrences and the need for continued treatment (136,202,206,217). Although anecdotal experience suggests that most patients will again have frequent recurrences and will want to resume therapy, interruption of therapy may identify a subset of patients who do not require continued treatment (207,217).

In addition to the currently recommended dose of 200 mg three times daily; doses of 200 mg two, four, and five times daily; 400 mg twice daily; and 800 mg once daily have all been shown to be effective in suppressive therapy (202,206–217). Recently, Mindel et al. (209) reported the results of a 1-year, open, randomized trial comparing various regimens, each administered for up to 3 months. Although the open study design may have introduced bias, analysis of the time to first recurrence with each regimen suggests that the most effective regimens, in decreasing order, were 200 mg four times daily, 400 mg twice daily, 200 mg three times daily, and 200 mg twice daily (Fig. 5). At the least effective dose (200 mg once daily), the time to first recurrence was only approximately 40 days, as compared to 18 days in patients receiving placebo and 246 days in patients receiving ACV 400 mg twice daily in the study reported by Mertz et al. (202). Although 200 mg four times daily appeared very effective, the currently recommended dose of 200 mg three times daily and 400 mg twice daily also appeared highly effective and more convenient; 200 mg twice daily might be considered for patients concerned about cost who are willing to accept a slightly decreased level of efficacy. Treatment with 200 mg once daily should probably be discouraged, since it appears substantially less effective than 200 mg twice daily and may be only marginally more effective than placebo. Intermittent, weekend-only suppressive therapy has also been evaluated and found to be ineffective (220).

### Other Indications for Suppressive Acyclovir Therapy

As previously mentioned, therapy may be considered in patients with complications of recurrent genital or oral herpes such as recurrent erythema multiforme or eczema herpeticum or in persons with recurrent herpes whitlow, particularly if it interferes with work. Although large controlled trials have not been completed, anecdotal experience and small published series suggest that suppressive therapy may be effective (115,117).

### Treatment of Primary Herpes Gingivostomatitis or Pharyngitis

The majority of cases of primary gingivostomatitis occur in infants between 1 and 3 years of age, ages when oral administration of capsules is not practical. An oral suspension has been developed, but only limited studies have been performed with this, as yet, unlicensed formulation.

### Management of Herpes Labialis

In normal patients with recurrent herpes labialis, patient-initiated treatment with ACV 5% or 10% ointment at the first sign or symptom may decrease the duration of viral shedding, but it does not accelerate healing or decrease the duration of symptoms (221,222). Topical therapy of herpes labialis is, therefore, generally not recommended. Limited placebo-controlled trials evaluating both physician and patient-initiated treatment of herpes labialis with oral ACV have failed to demonstrate consistent benefit in time to healing or duration of symptoms, although the data suggest that patients who experience severe episodes complicated by second crops of lesions might benefit from therapy with oral ACV (223,224).

Short-term oral ACV suppression has been shown to decrease the incidence of sun-induced herpes labialis in skiers. In skiers with a history of herpes labialis following intense sun exposure, herpes labialis developed in 7% who were treated with 400 mg ACV orally twice daily compared to 26% who received placebo (30). Similarly, prophylactic oral ACV reduced the risk of herpes labialis following trigeminal surgery from 12 of 16 placebo recipients to three of 14 treated with 400 mg twice daily for 5 days (31).

### Management of Herpes Proctitis

Rompalo et al. (225) recently reported results of a placebo-controlled trial in which therapy with ACV 400 mg orally five times daily for 10 days decreased the duration of viral shedding and lesions but had limited effect on symptoms. Recurrent herpes proctitis occurs in patients who are immunocompromised from HIV infection, and anecdotal experience suggests that oral ACV therapy is also effective in this setting.

### Management of Herpetic Whitlow

Rather than employing chronic suppressive therapy in patients with herpetic whitlow, some investigations have advocated initiating episodic treatment at the first sign of prodrome. Clinical experience suggests that the prodrome is more prolonged in herpetic whitlow as compared to other infections, and a small, uncontrolled trial suggested that episodes could be aborted if episodic treatment was initiated during the prodrome (102). Results of an ongoing placebo-controlled trial are not yet available.

### Management of Mucocutaneous Herpes Infections in Immunocompromised Patients

Intravenous, oral, and topical ACV treatments have each been shown in placebo-controlled trials to provide substantial clinical benefit to immunocompromised patients with mucocutaneous oral-labial and genital herpes infections. For example, Wade et al. (226) reported that patients treated with intravenous ACV had a 4-day reduction in the median duration of pain and lesions and a 10-day reduction in the median duration of viral shedding; Shepp et al. (227) reported similar results in patients treated with oral ACV at a dose of 400 mg five times daily for 10 days.

Topical ACV treatment (applied to lesions six times daily) is effective for treatment of immunocompromised patients with outbreaks confined to the lip, face, or external genital area (121). However, I prefer to use oral ACV at a dose of 400 mg five times daily for treatment of most mild to moderate localized mucocutaneous herpes infections in the immunocompromised host. If lesions are extensive or if patients have severe symptoms, most clinicians prefer to initiate therapy with intravenous therapy (5 mg/kg/dose over 1 hr every 8 hr).

Few data are available regarding treatment of immunocompromised patients with visceral infections such as herpes esophagitis, hepatitis, or pneumonia, but treatment with intravenous ACV would be a reasonable choice for therapy. Intravenous vidarabine therapy could be considered, but to date vidarabine has generally appeared less effective than ACV for the treatment of serious HSV and VZV infections (1,228,229).

### Acyclovir-Resistant Infections in the Immunocompromised Host

Although uncommon, there are now a number of well-documented cases of ACV-resistant HSV infections in immunocompromised hosts (1,100,132–134,137,230). Although sporadic cases have been reported in a variety of immunocompromised patients, including patients undergoing bone marrow transplantation and a child with severe combined immunodeficiency, AIDS is now the most common form of immunodeficiency associated with ACV-resistant HSV infections (137). Researchers at the University of California at San Francisco have recently identified 12 ACV treatment failures associated with ACV-resistant TK− HSV infections in patients with AIDS (137). Research is needed to identify risk factors for the development of resistance, strategies to prevent development of resistance, and effective treatment for ACV-resistant HSV infections.

ACV resistant, TK− mutants have been shown to be less virulent in animal models (134,137). Although it is not known whether the diminished virulence found in animal models is of clinical importance, it is attractive to hypothesize that diminished virulence may in part explain the absence to date of recognized treatment failures in the normal host associated with ACV resistance.

Although ACV-resistant virus has been isolated from persons who have never been treated with ACV, most treatment failures in the immunocompromised host have occurred during episodic treatment in patients previously treated with ACV. AIDS patients who have failed treatment tend to have presented with large, chronic ulcers. Development of resistant infections during suppressive treatment in AIDS patients has not been described. It is not known whether it is because ACV-resistant mutants are more likely to be present in large lesions or simply because episodic treatment is employed more commonly than suppressive treatment. Similarly, although exposure to subtherapeutic levels of ACV *in vitro* encourages selection of ACV-resistant HSV (230), it is not known whether initial treatment of HSV infections in immunocompromised patients with intravenous ACV or higher doses of oral ACV would decrease the likelihood of selection of ACV-resistant HSV. Nonetheless, these theoretical concerns suggest a possible rationale for preferring suppressive to episodic therapy in immunocompromised patients and suggest that it may be appropriate to employ higher oral ACV doses (i.e., 400 mg rather than 200 mg).

ACV-resistant infections should be suspected when mucocutaneous infections remain culture positive, clinically worsen, or fail to show clinical improvement within a week of initiating systemic therapy. Isolates suspected of ACV resistance can be sent to a reference laboratory for *in vitro* sensitivity testing. To date, all clinical isolates showing resistance have been TK− or had TK with altered substrate specificity, and TK− isolates remain sensitive to vidarabine and foscarnet. If ACV-resistance is documented, a trial of systemic treatment with either vidarabine or Foscarnet could be considered. In the United States, the latter drug is available for investigative use only, but there are anecdotal reports of successful treatment of ACV-resistant HSV infections in AIDS patients with Foscarnet.

### ACV Prophylaxis in the Immunocompromised Host

In patients undergoing bone marrow or renal transplant or patients with leukemia undergoing induction chemotherapy, oral or intravenous ACV therapy has been shown to effectively suppress or modify the course of recurrent HSV episodes (6,120,231–238). Clinical experience suggests that prophylaxis is equally effective in patients with AIDS (100). Wade et al. (234) reported that prophylactic treatment with oral ACV for 1 week before and 4 weeks after bone marrow transplantation in HSV-seropositive patients reduced the number of patients with HSV episodes from 17 of 25 untreated patients to five of 24 ACV-treated patients.

Effective doses in patients with normal renal function include intravenous ACV, 250 mg/m$^2$ over 1 hr every 8 or 12 hr and oral ACV 200 or 400 mg two to five times daily (6,120,231,232,234,235,237,238). Treatment with intravenous ACV, 250 mg, once daily was not effective in patients with normal renal function (239). Oral and intravenous therapy appear almost equally effective in patients who can take oral medication, although some centers prefer prophylaxis with intravenous ACV (6). Doses of 200 mg two or three times daily have been successful in renal transplant patients (233,236). Treatment at these doses is safe and well tolerated. Routine laboratory monitoring for ACV toxicity is not generally necessary in patients receiving suppressive oral ACV therapy, but renal function should be monitored in those receiving intravenous ACV.

Although bone marrow suppression has been documented in patients treated with very high doses of ACV in attempts to treat CMV infection, marrow suppression has not been noted in patients with normal renal function treated with standard intravenous doses of 5 or 10 mg/kg/dose (the later dose being employed in serious infections such as HSV encephalitis or neonatal herpes) (1,6,226,232). In addition, oral ACV prophylaxis was associated in one study with more rapid marrow engraftment in patients undergoing bone marrow transplant with concurrent treatment with methotrexate (234).

In light of the clinical benefit and excellent safety record of ACV prophylaxis in the immunocompromised host, routine screening for HSV antibody is recommended for patients undergoing bone marrow or organ transplant or induction chemotherapy for leukemia, and prophylaxis is encouraged for seropositive patients (1,6,136). Although intravenous therapy can be employed perioperatively or when patients have mucositis, most patients can be treated with oral ACV. I generally use oral ACV at doses of 400 mg tid or qid in patients with normal renal function and 200 mg bid or tid in renal transplant patients. The optimal duration of prophylaxis is not clear. In general, following induction chemotherapy, prophylaxis can be stopped once the granulocyte count is > 500/mm$^3$, and prophylaxis can be discontinued 6–8 weeks after bone marrow and renal transplantation.

Patients with AIDS represent a special case because the immunodeficiency is chronic and progressive. In light of the morbidity of HSV infection in patients with AIDS, the limited life expectancy of most patients with AIDS, and the excellent safety profile of suppressive ACV therapy, an argument can be made for continuing suppressive treatment indefinitely in patients with AIDS.

### Pharmacokinetics and Dosing in Renal Failure

Peak serum concentrations after intravenous administration of 5 mg/kg body weight is approximately 9 μg/ml (40 μM/L) (240). Approximately 20% of an oral dose is absorbed, resulting in serum levels 2 hr after oral dosing with 200 mg, 400 mg, and 800 mg in normal adults of 0.2–0.7 μg/ml (0.9–3.2 μM/L), 0.7–1.4 μg/ml (3.2–6.4 μM/L), and 1.2–2.1 μg/ml (5.5–9.7 μM/L), respectively (241–243). Renal excretion is approximately 2.7 times creatinine clearance, and 85–90% is excreted unchanged in the urine (243,244).

Plasma half-life is approximately 3 hr in normal adults compared to 20 hr in anephric patients receiving hemodialysis (244). ACV is removed by hemodialysis, and 60–100% of loading dose should be administered after dialysis. Anephric patients can be treated intravenously with a loading dose of approximately 50% of the standard dosage followed by the same dose every 24 hr or 15% of a standard dose every 8 hr. Anephric patients can also be treated orally with 200 mg twice daily (1,136,244).

### Drug Interactions

Reports of drug interactions have been remarkably infrequent. Administration of probenecid with ACV prolongs the half-life of ACV by approximately 20% and increases serum ACV levels by approximately 50% (243). Preliminary results of studies evaluating combination therapy of ACV with zidovudine in HIV-infected patients suggest that the combination is well tolerated (246). The latter studies were stimulated by *in vitro* data showing synergy of ACV and zidovudine against HIV-1.

### Adverse Effects

Topical ACV 5% ointment may cause burning when applied, and it is not approved for application within the mouth or vagina (190). Oral ACV may cause nausea, but this is usually mild and generally resolves with continued use.

Intravenous ACV administration may cause local pain and phlebitis, but neither are common unless extravasation occurs. The most common serious adverse effect from intravenous ACV is reversible crystaline nephropathy, characterized by crystalization of ACV in renal tubules (247–251). Although uncommon in patients with normal renal function, elevations in renal function were seen in approximately half of elderly adults in one study who received intravenous ACV as outpatients for zoster (251). Crystaline nephropathy was commonly seen in early studies employing bolus infusion rather than the currently recommended 60-min infusion period. Rarely, use of intravenous ACV or other nucleoside analogs such as adenine arabinoside have resulted in neurotoxicity, including lethargy, tremor, delerium, and abnormal electroencephalograms (250,252).

## PREVENTION

In light of the important role of asymptomatic shedding in the transmission of HSV infection (10,15,51,54,56,78–80), strategies to increase recognition of HSV infection and prevention of exposure to lesions are unlikely to completely prevent transmission. Suppressive therapy with ACV has not been shown to prevent transmission of HSV infections, and, even if effective, widespread use to prevent transmission of infection would be prohibitively expensive. Animal studies suggest that short-term postexposure prophylactic treatment might effectively prevent transmission. However, no clinical trials of postexposure prophylaxis have been performed in man. Even effective postexposure prophylaxis would probably have only limited impact on transmission, since most transmission of HSV infection apparently occurs in the absence of recognized exposure to lesions (56).

Prevention of transmission of HSV infection will probably require development of an effective vaccine. Although a number of vaccines have been developed, significant problems remain in vaccine development for prevention of HSV infection. These problems include concerns about oncogenicity and potential pathogenicity of attenuated vaccines and oncogenicity of whole-virus, killed vaccines (253–259). Although a variety of attenuated live-virus, killed-virus, glycoprotein subunit and recombinant vaccines have been shown to be immunogenic, to decrease mortality and in some cases to prevent latency in animal models, none have provided 100% protection (260–270). Indeed, established infection with HSV in normal adults does not provide 100% protection from reinfection at a new site by the same strain or reinfection at the same site by a new strain of the same type (27,271). It appears likely from animal studies that a vaccine can be developed that will decrease the risk of acquisition of HSV infection and prevent severe primary episodes in those who acquire infection. However, it will be important to be sure that vaccines do not merely increase the number of persons acquiring and transmitting HSV infection asymptomatically.

The first vaccines developed were killed whole-virus vaccines (272–274). These were followed by a partially purified HSV-1 vaccine and glycoprotein HSV-1 and HSV-2 subunit vaccines (260–265). More recently, recombinant DNA technology has suggested a variety of approaches including insertion of HSV immunogens into other viruses, insertion of HSV-1– or HSV-2–specific immunogens into the heterologous type, deletion of areas in the genome responsible for establishment of latency, reactivation, or oncogenicity, or cloned glycoprotein vaccines employing single glycoproteins or a combination of antigens (266–269,274).

Only limited clinical trials have been performed in humans. Killed whole-virus HSV-1 and HSV-2 vaccines were licensed in Germany, but no clinical trials were performed to determine whether these vaccines decreased acquisition of HSV infection. Skinner et al. (262) administered their partially purified HSV-1 vaccine to sexual partners of persons with genital herpes, but the apparent efficacy of the vaccine has been questioned because of the use of a retrospective control group rather than a randomized, placebo-controlled design. More recently, a glycoprotein, subunit HSV-2 vaccine was administered to sexual partners of persons with genital herpes in a placebo-controlled trial after it was found to be immunogenic in humans (275–279). Preliminary analysis clearly indicates that the vaccine did not prevent transmission of genital herpes, but the vaccine lots employed in the efficacy study appear to have been less immunogenic than lots employed in the previous immunogenicity studies (G. J. Mertz, unpublished observations).

## REMAINING PROBLEMS AND NEEDS

Although a variety of rapid diagnostic tests have been developed, the role of these tests remains to be defined. Specifically, a sensitive rapid test for cervical shedding of HSV is needed as are rapid screening tests for *in vitro* ACV resistance. Sensitive, type-specific serologic tests currently available in the research laboratory have led to rapid advances in our understanding of the epidemiology and transmission of HSV infections, but these tests need to be adapted to the clinical laboratory.

Further studies are needed to evaluate the safety and efficacy of ACV treatment in primary gingivostomatitis, herpes pharyngitis, herpetic whitlow, erythema multiforme, and AIDS, and, in the latter, strategies are needed to prevent and treat ACV-resistant HSV infections. Additional antiviral agents should be developed. Further basic and clinical research is needed in vaccine development; licensing of a safe, effective vaccine is unlikely in the near future.

## REFERENCES


1. Dorsky DI, Crumpacker CS. Drugs five years later: acyclovir. *Ann Intern Med* 1987;107:859–74.
2. Genital herpes infection—United States, 1966–1984. *MMWR* 1986;35:402–4.
3. Winkelstein W Jr, Wiley JA, Padian NS, et al. The San Francisco men's health study: continued decline in HIV seroconversion rates among homosexual/bisexual men. *Am J Public Health* 1988;78:1472–4.
4. DeBuono BA, Zinner SH, McCormack WM. Comparative study of sexual behavior in college women, 1975 and 1986 [Abstract] In: *Program and Abstracts, International Society for STD Research, Atlanta, Georgia, August 2–5.* 1987;83.
5. Quinnan GV Jr, Masur H, Rook AH, et al. Herpesvirus infections in the acquired immune deficiency syndrome. *JAMA* 1984;252:72–7.
6. Saral R. Management of mucocutaneous herpes simplex virus infections in immunocompro-

mised patients. *Am J Med* 1988;85(suppl 2A):57–60.
7. Meyers JD, Flournoy N, Thomas ED. Infection with herpes simplex virus and cell-mediated immunity after marrow transplant. *J Infect Dis* 1980;142:338–46.
8. Corey L, Spear PG. Infections with herpes simplex viruses. Parts one and two. *N Engl J Med* 1986;314:686–91,749–57.
9. Buchman TG, Simpson T, Nosal C, Roizman B, Nahmias AJ. The structure of herpes simplex virus DNA and its application to molecular epidemiology. *Ann NY Acad Sci* 1980;354:279–90.
10. Mertz GJ, Coombs RW, Ashley R, et al. Transmission of genital herpes in couples with one symptomatic and one asymptomatic partner: a prospective study. *J Infect Dis* 1988;157:1169–77.
11. Spear PG. Glycoproteins specified by herpes simplex viruses. In: Roizman B, ed. *The herpesviruses. Vol 3.* New York: Plenum Press, 1985:315–56.
12. Goldstein LC, Corey L, McDougall JK, Tolentino E, Nowinski RC. Monoclonal antibodies to herpes simplex viruses: use in antigenic typing and rapid diagnosis. *J Infect Dis* 1983;147:829–37.
13. Bernstein DI, Bryson YJ, Lovett MA. Antibody response to type-common and type-unique epitopes of herpes simplex virus polypeptides. *J Med Virol* 1985;15:251–63.
14. Lee FK, Coleman RM, Pereira L, Bailey PD, Tatsuno M, Nahmias AJ. Detection of herpes simplex virus type 2-specific antibody with glycoprotein G. *J Clin Microbiol* 1985;22:641–4.
15. Bernstein DI, Lovett MA, Bryson YJ. Serologic analysis of first-episode nonprimary genital herpes simplex virus infection: presence of type 2 antibody in acute serum samples. *Am J Med* 1984;77:1055–60.
16. Vahlne A, Svennerholm B, Lycke E. Evidence for herpes simplex virus type-selective receptors on cellular plasma membranes. *J Gen Virol* 1979;44:217–25.
17. Vahlne A, Svennerholm B, Sandberg M, Hamberger A, Lycke E. Differences in attachment between herpes simplex type 1 and type 2 viruses to neurons and glial cells. *Infect Immun* 1980;28:675–80.
18. Stevens JG, Cook ML. Latent herpes simplex virus in spinal ganglia of mice. *Science* 1971; 173:843–5.
19. Baringer JR. Recovery of herpes simplex virus from human sacral ganglions. *N Engl J Med* 1974;291:828–30.
20. Warren KG, Brown SM, Wroblewska Z, Gilden D, Koprowski H, Subak-Sharpe J. Isolation of latent herpes simplex virus from the superior cervical and vagus ganglions of human beings. *N Engl J Med* 1978;298:1068–9.
21. Galloway DA, Fenoglio C, Shevchuk M, McDougall JK. Detection of herpes simplex RNA in human sensory ganglia. *Virology* 1979; 95:265–8.
22. Rock DL, Fraser NW. Detection of HSV-1 genome in central nervous system of latently infected mice. *Nature* 1983;302:523–5.
23. Puga A, Cantin EM, Wohlenberg C, Openshaw H, Notkins AL. Different sizes of restriction endonuclease fragments from the terminal repetitions of the herpes simplex virus type 1 genome latent in trigeminal ganglia of mice. *J Gen Virol* 1984;65:437–44.
24. Hill TJ. Herpes simplex virus latency. In: Roizman B, ed. *The herpesviruses. Vol. 3.* New York: Plenum Press, 1985:175–240.
25. Stanberry LR, Kern ER, Richards JT, Abbott TM, Overall JC Jr. Genital herpes in guinea pigs: pathogenesis of primary infection and description of recurrent disease. *J Infect Dis* 1982;146:397–404.
26. Corey L, Adams HG, Brown ZA, Holmes KK. Genital herpes simplex virus infections: clinical manifestations, course, and complications. *Ann Intern Med* 1983;98:958–72.
27. Buchman TG, Roizman B, Nahmias AJ. Demonstration of exogenous genital reinfection with herpes simplex virus type 2 by restriction endonuclease fingerprinting of viral DNA. *J Infect Dis* 1979;140:295–304.
28. Heller M, Dix RD, Baringer JR, Schachter J, Conte JE Jr. Herpetic proctitis and meningitis: recovery of two strains of herpes simplex virus type 1 from cerebrospinal fluid. *J Infect Dis* 1982;146:584–8.
29. Schmidt OW, Fife KH, Corey L. Reinfection is an uncommon occurrence in patients with symptomatic recurrent genital herpes. *J Infect Dis* 1984;149:645–6.
30. Spruance SL. Cutaneous herpes simplex virus lesions induced by ultraviolet radiation. A review of model systems and prophylactic therapy with oral acyclovir. *Am J Med* 1988;85(suppl 2A):43–5.
31. Schadelin J, Schilt HU, Rohner M. Preventive therapy of herpes labialis associated with trigeminal surgery. *Am J Med* 1988;85(suppl 2A):46–8.
32. Lafferty WE, Coombs RW, Benedetti J, Critchlow C, Corey L. Recurrences after oral and genital herpes simplex virus infection. Influence of site of infection and viral type. *N Engl J Med* 1987;316:1444–9.
33. Lopez C. Natural resistance mechanisms in herpes simplex virus infections. In: Roizman B, Lopez C, eds. *The herpesviruses: immunobiology and prophylaxis of human herpesvirus infections. Vol. 4.* New York: Plenum Press, 1985:37–68.
34. Oakes JE, Davis WB, Taylor JA, Weppner WA. Lymphocyte reactivity contributes to protection conferred by specific antibody passively transferred to herpes simplex virus-infected mice. *Infect Immun* 1980;29:642–9.
35. Rouse BT. Immunopathology of herpesvirus infections. In: Roizman B, Lopez C, eds. *The herpesviruses: immunobiology and prophylaxis of human herpesvirus infections. Vol. 4.* New York: Plenum Press, 1985:103–19.
36. Kapoor AK, Nash AA, Wildy P, Phelan J,

McLean CS, Field HJ. Pathogenesis of herpes simplex virus in congenitally athymic mice: the relative roles of cell-mediated and humoral immunity. *J Gen Virol* 1982;60:225–33.

37. Corey L, Reeves WC, Holmes KK. Cellular immune response in genital herpes simplex virus infection. *N Engl J Med* 1978;299:986–91.
38. Ashley RL, Corey L. Effect of acyclovir treatment of primary genital herpes on the antibody response to herpes simplex virus. *J Clin Invest* 1984;73:681–8.
39. Yasukawa M, Zarling JM. Human cytotoxic T cell clones directed against herpes simplex virus-infected cells. I. Lysis restricted by HLA class II MB and DR antigens. *J Immunol* 1984;133:422–7.
40. Cunningham AL, Merigan TC. Gamma interferon production appears to predict time of recurrence of herpes labialis. *J Immunol* 1983;130:2397–400.
41. Norrild B, Shore SL, Cromeans TL, Nahmias AJ. Participation of three major glycoprotein antigens of herpes simplex type 1 early in the infectious cycle as determined by antibody-dependent cell-mediated cytotoxicity. *Infect Immun* 1980;28:38–44.
42. Reeves WC, Corey L, Adams HG, Vontver LA, Holmes KK. Risk of recurrence after first episodes of genital herpes: relation to HSV type and antibody response. *N Engl J Med* 1981;305:315–9.
43. Rosenberg GL, Synderman R, Notkins AL. Production of chemotactic factor and lymphotoxin by human leukocytes stimulated with herpes simplex virus. *Infect Immun* 1974;10:111–5.
44. O'Reilly RJ, Chibbaro A, Anger E, Lopez C. Cell-mediated immune responses in patients with recurrent herpes simplex infections. II. Infection-associated deficiency of lymphokine production in patients with recurrent herpes labialis or herpes progenitalis. *J Immunol* 1977;118:1095–102.
45. Rasmussen LE, Jordan GW, Stevens DA, Merigan TC. Lymphocyte interferon production and transformation after herpes simplex infections in humans. *J Immunol* 1974;112:728–36.
46. Russell AS, Maini RA, Bailey M, Dumonde DC. Cell-mediated immunity to varicella-zoster antigen in acute herpes zoster (shingles). *Clin Exp Immunol* 1972;14:181–5.
47. Reichman RC, Dolin R, Vincent MM, Fauci AS. Cell-mediated cytotoxicity in recurrent herpes simplex virus infections in man. *Proc Soc Exp Biol Med* 1977;155:571–6.
48. Russell AS. Cell-mediated immunity to herpes simplex virus in man. *J Infect Dis* 1974;129:142–6.
49. Lopez C, O'Reilly RJ. Cell-mediated immune responses in recurrent herpesvirus infections. I. Lymphocyte proliferation assay. *J Immunol* 1977;118:895–902.
50. Corey L, Ashley R, Benedetti J, Selke S. The effect of prior HSV-1 infection on the subsequent natural history of genital HSV-2 [Abstract]. In: *Program and abstracts of the 28th Interscience Conference on Antimicrobial Agents and Chemotherapy, 23–26 October.* Washington, D.C.: American Society for Microbiology, 1988;257.
51. Nahmias A, Keyserling H, Bain R, et al. Prevalence of herpes simplex virus (HSV) type-specific antibodies in a U.S.A. prepaid group medical practice population [Abstract]. In: *Programme of the 6th International Meeting, International Society for STD Research, Brighton, England, 31 July–2 August.* 1985:40.
52. Nahmias AJ, Roizman B. Infection with herpes simplex virus 1 and 2. *N Engl J Med* 1973;289:667–74;719–25;781–9.
53. Nahmias AJ, Josey WE, Naib ZM, Luce CF, Duffey A. Antibodies to herpesvirus hominis types 1 and 2 in humans. I. Patients with genital herpetic infections. *Am J Epidemiol* 1970;91:539–46.
54. Stavraky KM, Rawls WE, Chiavetta J, Donner AP, Wanklin JM. Sexual and socioeconomic factors affecting the risk of past infections with herpes simplex virus type 2. *Am J Epidemiol* 1983;118:109–21.
55. Mann SL, Meyers JD, Holmes KL, Corey L. Prevalence and incidence of herpesvirus infections among homosexually active men. *J Infect Dis* 1984;149:1026–7.
56. Mertz GJ, Schmidt O, Jourden JL, et al. Frequency of acquisition of first-episode genital infection with herpes simplex virus from symptomatic and asymptomatic source contacts. *Sex Transm Dis* 1985;12:33–9.
57. Prober CG, Hensleigh PA, Boucher FD, Yasukawa LL, Au DS, Arvin AM. Use of routine viral cultures at delivery to identify neonates exposed to herpes simplex virus. *N Engl J Med* 1988;318:887–91.
58. Becker TM, Blount JH, Guinan ME. Genital herpes infections in private practice in the United States, 1966 to 1981. *JAMA* 1985;253:1601–3.
59. Smith IW, Peutherer JF, MacCallum FO. The incidence of herpesvirus hominis antibody in the population. *J Hyg (Camb)* 1967;65:395–408.
60. Wentworth BB, Alexander ER. Seroepidemiology of infections due to members of the herpesvirus group. *Am J Epidemiol* 1971;94:496–507.
61. Juretic M. Natural history of herpetic infections. *Helv Paediatr Acta* 1966;4:356–68.
62. Overall JC Jr. Antiviral chemotherapy of oral and genital herpes simplex virus infections. In: Nahmias AJ, Dowdle WR, Schinazi RF, eds. *The human herpesviruses: An interdisciplinary perspective.* New York: Elsevier North Holland, 1980:447–65.
63. Overall JC Jr, Kern ER, Schlitzer RL, Friedman SB, Glasgow LA. Genital herpesvirus hominis infection in mice. I. Development of an experimental model. *Infect Immun* 1975;11:476–80.
64. Sexually transmitted diseases. *Br J Vener Dis* 1983;59:134–7.
65. Blackwelder WC, Dolin R, Mittal KK, Mc-

Namara PM, Payne FJ. A population study of herpesvirus infections and HLA antigens. *Am J Epidemiol* 1982;115:569–76.
66. Kloene W, Bang FB, Chakraborty SM, Cooper MR, Kulemann H, Ota M, Shah KV. A two-year respiratory virus survey in four villages in West Bengal, India. *Am J Epidemiol* 1970; 92:307–20.
67. Glezen WP, Fernald GW, Lohr JA. Acute respiratory disease of university students with special reference to the etiologic role of herpesvirus hominis. *Am J Epidemiol* 1975;101:111–21.
68. Lindgren KM, Douglas RG Jr, Couch RB. Significance of herpesvirus hominis in respiratory secretions of man. *N Engl J Med* 1968;278:517–23.
69. Douglas RG Jr, Couch RB. A prospective study of chronic herpes simplex virus infection and recurrent herpes labialis in humans. *J Immunol* 1970;104:289–95.
70. Greenberg MS, Brightman VJ, Ship II. Clinical and laboratory differentiation of recurrent intraoral herpes simplex virus infections following fever. *J Dent Res* 1969;48:385–91.
71. Cesario TC, Poland JD, Wulff H, et al. Six years experience with herpes simplex virus in a children's home. *Am J Epidemiol* 1969; 90:416–22.
72. Arvin AM, Hensleigh PA, Prober CG, et al. Failure of antepartum maternal cultures to predict the infant's risk of exposure to herpes simplex virus at delivery. *N Engl J Med* 1986;315:796–800.
73. Scott TFM. Epidemiology of herpetic infections. *Am J Ophthalmol* 1957;43:134–47.
74. Linnemann CC Jr, Buchman TG, Light IJ, Ballard JL. Transmission of herpes-simplex virus type 1 in a nursery for the newborn: identification of viral isolates by DNA fingerprinting. *Lancet* 1978;1:964–6.
75. Hale BD, Rendtorff RC, Walker LC, Roberts AN. Epidemic herpetic stomatitis in an orphanage nursery. *JAMA* 1963;183:1068–72.
76. Anderson SG, Hamilton J. Epidemiology of primary herpes simplex infection. *Med J Aust* 1949;1:308–11.
77. Manzella JP, McConville JH, Valenti W, Menegus MA, Swierkosz EM, Arens M. An outbreak of herpes simplex virus type I gingivostomatitis in a dental hygiene practice. *JAMA* 1984;252:2019–22.
78. Rooney J, Felser JM, Ostrove JM, Straus SE. Acquisition of genital herpes from an asymptomatic sexual partner. *N Engl J Med* 1986;314:1561–4.
79. Whitley RJ, Nahmias AJ, Visintine AM, Fleming CL, Alford CA. The natural history of herpes simplex virus infection of mother and newborn. *Pediatrics* 1980;66:489–94.
80. Yeager AS, Arvin AM. Reasons for the absence of a history of recurrent genital infections in mothers of neonates infected with herpes simplex virus. *Pediatrics* 1984;73:188–93.
81. Guinan ME, MacCalman J, Kern ER, Overall JC Jr, Spruance SL. The course of untreated recurrent genital herpes simplex infection in 27 women. *N Engl J Med* 1981;304:759–63.
82. Prober CG, Sullender WM, Yasukawa LL, Au DS, Yeager AS, Arvin AM. Low risk of herpes simplex infections in neonates exposed to the virus at the time of vaginal delivery to mothers with recurrent genital herpes simplex virus infections. *N Engl J Med* 1987;316:240–4.
83. Bryson Y, Dillon M, Radolf J, Zakowski P, Bernstein D, Garratty E. Risk of acquisition of genital HSV-2 in sexual partners of patients with genital HSV: a prospective study [Abstract]. In: *Program and abstracts of the 28th Interscience Conference on Antimicrobiol Agents and Chemotherapy, 23–26 October.* Washington, D.C.: American Society for Microbiology, 1988;256.
84. Buddingh GJ, Schrum DI, Lanier JC, Guidry DJ. Studies of the natural history of herpes simplex infections. *Pediatrics* 1953;11:595–609.
85. Spruance SL, Overall JC Jr, Kern ER, Krueger GG, Pliam V, Miller W. The natural history of recurrent herpes simplex labialis: implications for antiviral therapy. *N Engl J Med* 1977; 297:69–75.
86. Mertz GJ, Corey L. Genital herpes simplex virus infections in adults. *Urol Clin North Am* 1984;11:103–19.
87. Ishiguro T, Ozaki Y, Matsunami M, Funakoshi S. Clinical and virological features of herpes genitalis in Japanese women. *Acta Obstet Gynecol Scand* 1982;61:173–6.
88. Kalinyak JE, Fleagle G, Docherty JJ. Incidence and distribution of herpes simplex virus types 1 and 2 from genital lesions in college women. *J Med Virol* 1977;1:175–81.
89. Caplan LR, Kleeman FJ, Berg S. Urinary retention probably secondary to herpes genitalis. *N Engl J Med* 1977;297:920–1.
90. Goldmeier D. Herpetic proctitis and sacral radiculomyelopathy in homosexual men [Letter]. *Br Med J* 1979;2:549.
91. Goldmeier D, Bateman JR, Rodin P. Urinary retention and intestinal obstruction associated with ano-rectal herpes simplex virus infection. *Br Med J* 1975;1:425.
92. Jacobs SC, Herbert LA, Piering WF, Lawson RK. Acute motor paralytic bladder in renal transplant patients with anogenital herpes infection. *J Urol* 1980;123:426–7.
93. Jacome DE, Yanez GF. Herpes genitalis and neurogenic bladder and bowel [Letter]. *J Urol* 1980;124:752.
94. Oates JK, Greenhouse PR. Retention of urine in anogenital herpetic infection. *Lancet* 1978; 1:691–2.
95. Corey L, Holmes KK. Genital herpes simplex virus infections: current concepts in diagnosis, therapy and prevention. *Ann Intern Med* 1983; 98:973–83.
96. Stamm WE, Wagner KF, Amsel R, Alexander ER, Turck M, Counts GW, Holmes KK. Causes of the acute urethral syndrome in women. *N Engl J Med* 1980;303:409–15.

97. Morrisseau PM, Phillips CA, Leadbetter GW Jr. Viral prostatitis. *J Urol* 1970;103:767–9.
98. Quinn TC, Corey L, Chaffee RG, Schuffler MD, Brancato FP, Holmes KK. The etiology of anorectal infections in homosexual men. *Am J Med* 1981;71:395–406.
99. Price RW, Walz MA, Wohlenberg C, et al. Latent infection of sensory ganglia with herpes simplex virus: efficacy of immunization. *Science* 1975;188:938–40.
100. Drew WL, Buhles W, Erlich KS. Herpesvirus infections (cytomegalovirus, herpes simplex virus, varicella-zoster virus). How to use ganciclovir (DHPG) and acyclovir. *Infect Dis Clin North Am* 1988;2:495–509.
101. Siegal FP, Lopez C, Hammer GS, et al. Severe acquired immunodeficiency in male homosexuals, manifested by chronic perianal ulcerative herpes simplex lesions. *N Engl J Med* 1981;305:1439–44.
102. Gill MJ, Arlette J, Tyrrell L, Buchan KA. Herpes simplex virus infection of the hand. *Am J Med* 1988;85(suppl 2A):53–6.
103. Glogau R, Hanna L, Jawetz E. Herpetic whitlow as part of genital virus infection. *J Infect Dis* 1977;136:689–92.
104. Gill MJ, Arlette J, Buchan K. Herpes simplex virus infection of the hand. A profile of 79 cases. *Am J Med* 1988;84:89–93.
105. Greaves WL, Kaiser AB, Alford RH, Schaffner W. The problem of herpetic whitlow among hospital personnel. *Infect Control* 1980; 1:381–5.
106. Kanaar P. Primary herpes simplex infection of fingers in nurses. *Dermatologica* 1967; 134:346–50.
107. Rowe HN, Heine CS, Kowalski CJ. Herpetic whitlow: an occupational disease of practising dentists. *J Am Dent Assoc* 1982;105:471–3.
108. Rosato FE, Rosato EF, Plotkin SA. Herpetic paronychia—an occupational hazard of medical personnel. *N Engl J Med* 1970;283:804–5.
109. Gill MJ, Den Hollander C. DNA restriction enzyme analysis of digital and genital isolates of herpes simplex virus from three patients [Letter]. *J Infect Dis* 1988;158:242.
110. Laskin OL. Acyclovir and suppression of frequently recurring herpetic whitlow. *Ann Intern Med* 1985;102:494–5.
111. Gill MJ, Arlette J, Buchan K, Tyrell DL. Therapy for recurrent herpetic whitlow [Letter]. *Ann Intern Med* 1986;105:631.
112. Wheeler CE Jr, Abele DC. Eczema herpeticum, primary and recurrent. *Arch Dermatol* 1966;93:162–73.
113. Bean SF, Quezada RK. Recurrent oral erythema multiforme. Clinical experience with 11 patients. *JAMA* 1983;249:2810–2.
114. Leigh IM, Mowbray JF, Levene GM, Sutherland S. Recurrent and continuous erythema multiforme—a clinical and immunological study. *Clin Exp Dermatol* 1985;10:58–67.
115. Leigh IM. Management of non-genital herpes simplex virus infections in immunocompetent patients. *Am J Med* 1988;85(suppl 2A):34–8.
116. David TJ, Longson M. Herpes simplex infections in atopic eczema. *Arch Dis Child* 1985;60:338–43.
117. Niimura M, Nishikawa T. Treatment of eczema herpeticum with oral acyclovir. *Am J Med* 1988;85(suppl 2A):49–52.
118. Craig CP, Nahmias AJ. Different patterns of neurologic involvement with herpes simplex virus types 1 and 2: isolation of herpes simplex virus type 2 from the buffy coat of two adults with meningitis. *J Infect Dis* 1973;127:365–72.
119. Steel JG, Dix RD, Baringer JR. Isolation of herpes simplex virus type 1 in recurrent (Mollaret) meningitis. *Ann Neurol* 1982;11:17–21.
120. Saral R, Burns WH, Prentice HG. Herpes virus infections: clinical manifestations and therapeutic strategies in immunocompromised patients. *Clin Haematol* 1984;13:645–60.
121. Whitley RJ, Levin M, Barton N, et al. Infections caused by herpes simplex virus in the immunocompromised host: natural history and topical acyclovir therapy. *J Infect Dis* 1984;150:323–9.
122. Ramsey PG, Fife KH, Hackman RC, Meyers JD, Corey L. Herpes simplex virus pneumonia: clinical, virologic, and pathologic features in 20 patients. *Ann Intern Med* 1982;97:813–20.
123. Pass RF, Whitely RJ, Whelchel JD, Diethelm AG, Reynolds DW, Alford CA. Identification of patients with increased risk of infection with herpes simplex virus after renal transplantation. *J Infect Dis* 1979;140:487–92.
124. Rand KH, Rasmussen LE, Pollard RB, Arvin A, Merigan TC. Cellular immunity and herpesvirus infections in cardiac-transplant patients. *N Engl J Med* 1977;296:1372–7.
125. Lam MT, Pazin GT, Armstrong JA, Ho M. Herpes simplex infection in acute myelogenous leukemia and other hematologic malignancies: a prospective study. *Cancer* 1981;48:2168–71.
126. Flewett TH, Parker RG, Philip WM. Acute hepatitis due to herpes simplex virus in an adult. *J Clin Pathol* 1969;22:60–6.
127. McDonald GB, Sharma P, Hackman RC, Meyers JD, Thomas ED. Esophageal infections in immunosuppressed patients after marrow transplantation. *Gastroenterology* 1985;88:1111–7.
128. Shortsleeve MJ, Gauvin GP, Gardner RC, Greenberg MS. Herpetic esophagitis. *Radiology* 1981;141:611–7.
129. Graham BS, Snell JD Jr. Herpes simplex virus infection of the adult lower respiratory tract. *Medicine (Baltimore)* 1983;62:384–93.
130. Tuxen DV, Cade JF, McDonald MI, Buchanan MR, Clark RJ, Pain MC. Herpes simplex virus from the lower respiratory tract in adult respiratory distress syndrome. *Am Rev Respir Dis* 1982;126:416–9.
131. Foley FD, Greenawald KA, Nash G, Pruitt BA Jr. Herpesvirus infection in burned patients. *N Engl J Med* 1970;282:652–6.
132. Crumpacker CS, Schnipper LE, Marlowe SI, Kowalsky PN, Hershey BJ, Levin MJ. Resistance to antiviral drugs of herpes simplex virus

isolated from a patient treated with acyclovir. *N Engl J Med* 1982;306:343–6.
133. Burns WH, Saral R, Santos GW, Laskin OL, Lietman PS, McLaren C, Barry DW. Isolation and characterization of resistant herpes simplex virus after acyclovir therapy. *Lancet* 1982;1:421–3.
134. Sibrack CD, Gutman LT, Wilfert CM, McLaren C, St. Clair MH, Keller PM, Barry DM. Pathogenicity of acyclovir-resistant herpes simplex virus type 1 from an immunodeficient child. *J Infect Dis* 1982;146:673–82.
135. Becker WB, Kipps A, McKenzie D. Disseminated herpes simplex virus infection. Its pathogenesis based on virologic and pathogenic studies in 33 cases. *Am J Dis Child* 1968;115:1–8.
136. Gold D, Corey L. Acyclovir prophylaxis for herpes simplex virus infection. *Antimicrob Agents Chemother* 1987;31:361–7.
137. Erlich KS, Mills J, Chatis P, et al. Acyclovir-resistant herpes simplex virus infections in patients with acquired immunodeficiency syndrome. *N Engl J Med* 1989;320:293–6.
138. Moseley RC, Corey L, Benjamin D, Winter C, Remington ML. Comparison of viral isolation, direct immunofluorescence, and indirect immunoperoxidase techniques for detection of genital herpes simplex virus infection. *J Clin Microbiol* 1981;13:913–8.
139. Mead PB. Proper methods of culturing herpes simplex virus. *J Reprod Med* 1986;31(suppl 5):390–4.
140. Richman DD, Cleveland PH, Redfield DC, Oxman MN, Wahl GM. Rapid viral diagnosis. *J Infect Dis* 1984;149:298–310.
141. Gleaves CA, Wilson DJ, Wold AD, Smith TF. Detection and serotyping of herpes simplex virus in MRC-5 cells by use of centrifugation and monoclonal antibodies 16 h postinoculation. *J Clin Microbiol* 1985;21:29–32.
142. Grauballe PC, Vestergaard BF. ELISA for herpes simplex virus type 2 antibodies [Letter]. *Lancet* 1977;2:1038–9.
143. Collins P, Appleyard GA, Oliver NM. Sensitivity of herpes virus isolates from acyclovir clinical trials. *Am J Med* 1982;73:380–2.
144. McLaren C, Ellis MN, Hunter GA. A colorimetric assay for the measurement of the sensitivity of herpes simplex viruses to antiviral agents. *Antiviral Res* 1983;3:223–34.
145. Force EE, Stewart RC, Haff RF. Herpes simplex skin infection in rabbits. I. Effect of 5-iodo-2′-deoxyruidine. *Virology* 1964;23:363–9.
146. Park NH, Pavan-Langston D, McLean SL, Lass JH. Acyclovir topical therapy of cutaneous herpes simplex virus infection in guinea pigs. *Arch Dermatol* 1980;116:672–5.
147. Tomlinson AH, MacCallum FO. The effect of 5-iodo-2′-deoxyuridine on herpes simplex virus infections in guinea-pig skin. *Br J Exp Pathol* 1968;49:277–82.
148. Shipkowitz NL, Bower RR, Appell RN, et al. Suppression of herpes simplex virus infection by phosphonoacetic acid. *Appl Microbiol* 1973; 26:264–7.
149. Klein RJ. Treatment of experimental latent herpes simplex virus infections with acyclovir and other antiviral compounds. *Am J Med* 1982;73:138–42.
150. Klein RJ, Friedman-Kien AE, DeStefano E. Latent herpes simplex virus infections in sensory ganglia of hairless mice prevented by acycloguanosine. *Antimicrob Agents Chemother* 1979;15:723–9.
151. Park NH, Pavan-Langston D, Hettinger ME, et al. Topical therapeutic efficacy of 9-(2-hydroxyethoxymethyl) guanine and 5-iodo-5′-amino-2′, 5′-dideoxy uridine on oral infection with herpes simplex virus in mice. *J Infect Dis* 1980;141:575–9.
152. Blyth WA, Harbour DA, Hill TJ. Effect of acyclovir on recurrence of herpes simplex skin lesions in mice. *J Gen Virol* 1980;48:417–9.
153. Field HJ, Bell SE, Elion GB, Nash AA, Wildy P. Effect of acycloguanosine treatment of acute and latent herpes simplex infections in mice. *Antimicrob Agents Chemother* 1979;15:554–61.
154. Hill TJ, Blyth WA, Harbour DA. Recurrent herpes simplex in mice: topical treatment with acyclovir cream. *Antiviral Res* 1982;2:135–46.
155. Kern ER. Acyclovir treatment of experimental genital herpes simplex virus infections. *Am J Med* 1982;73:100–8.
156. Kern ER, Glasgow LA, Klein RJ, Friedman-Kien AE. Failure of 2-deoxy-D-glucose in the treatment of experimental cutaneous and genital infections due to herpes simplex virus. *J Infect Dis* 1982;146:159–66.
157. Kern ER, Glasgow LA, Overall JC Jr, Reno JM, Boezi JA. Treatment of experimental herpesvirus infections with phosphonoformate and some comparisons with phosphonoacetate. *Antimicrob Agents Chemother* 1978;14:817–23.
158. Kern ER, Richards JT, Overall JC Jr, Glasgow LA. Genital herpesvirus hominis infection in mice. II. Treatment with phosphonoacetic acid, adenine arabinoside, and adenine arabinoside 5′-monophosphate. *J Infect Dis* 1977;135:557–67.
159. Blyth WA, Hill TJ, Field HJ, Harbour DA. Reactivation of herpes simplex virus infection by ultraviolet light and possible involvement of prostaglandins. *J Gen Virol* 1976;33:547–50.
160. Norval M, Howie SEM, Ross JA, Maingay JP. A murine model of herpes simplex virus recrudescence. *J Gen Virol* 1987;68:2693–8.
161. Harris SRB, Boyd MR. The activity of iododeoxyuridine, adenine arabinoside, cytosine arabinoside, ribavirin, and phosphonoacetic acid against herpes virus in the hairless mouse model. In: Oxford JS, Draser FA, Williams JD, eds. *Chemotherapy of herpes simplex virus infections*. London: Academic Press, 1977;91–8.
162. Richards JT, Kern ER, Overall JC Jr, Glasgow LA. Anti-herpes virus activity of adenine arabinoside analogues in tissue culture and a genital infection of mice and guinea pigs. *Antiviral Res* 1982;2:27–39.
163. Klein RJ, Friedman-Kien AE, Brady E. Herpes simplex virus skin infection in hairless

mice: treatment with antiviral compounds. *Antimicrob Agents Chemother* 1974;5:318–22.
164. Park NH, Pavan-Langston D, MacLean SL. Acyclovir in oral and ganglionic herpes simplex virus infections. *J Infect Dis* 1979;140:802–6.
165. Olsen GA, Kern ER, Overall JC Jr. Effect of treatment with exogenous interferon, polyriboinosinic polyribocytidylic acid, or polyriboinosinic polyribocytidylic acid poly-L-lysine complex on herpesvirus hominis infections in mice. *J Infect Dis* 1978;137:428–36.
166. Corey L, Reeves WC, Chiang WT, et al. Ineffectiveness of topical ether for the treatment of genital herpes simplex virus infection. *N Engl J Med* 1978;299:237–9.
167. Friedrich EG Jr, Masukawa T. Effect of povidone-iodine on herpes genitalis. *Obstet Gynecol* 1975;45:337–9.
168. Kern AB, Schiff BL. Smallpox vaccinations in the management of recurrent herpes simplex: a controlled evaluation. *J Invest Dermatol* 1959;33:99–102.
169. Bierman SM. BCG immunoprophylaxis of recurrent herpes progenitalis. *Arch Dermatol* 1976;112:1410–5.
170. Chang TW, Fiumara N. Treatment with levamisole of recurrent herpes genitalis. *Antimicrob Agents Chemother* 1978;13:809–12.
171. Guinan ME, MacCalman J, Kern ER, Overall JC Jr, Spruance SL. Topical ether and herpes simplex labialis. *JAMA* 1980;243:1059–61.
172. Jose DG, Minty CC. Levamisole in patients with recurrent herpes infection. *Med J Aust* 1980;2:390–4.
173. Russell AS, Brisson E, Grace M. A double-blind, controlled trial of levamisole in the treatment of recurrent herpes labialis. *J Infect Dis* 1978;137:597–600.
174. Adams HG, Benson EA, Alexander ER, et al. Genital herpetic infection in men and women: clinical course and effect of topical application of adenine arabinoside. *J Infect Dis* 1976;133:A151–9.
175. Burnett JW, Katz SL. A study of the use of 5-iodo-2′-deoxyuridine in cutaneous herpes simplex. *J Invest Dermatol* 1962;40:7–8.
176. Parker JD. A double-blind trial of idoxuridine in recurrent genital herpes. *J Antimicrob Chemother* 1977;3(suppl A):131–7.
177. MacCallum FO, Juel-Jenson BE. Herpes simplex virus skin infection in man treated with idoxuridine in dimethyl sulfoxide. Results of double-blind controlled trial. *Br Med J* 1966; 2:805–7.
178. Silvestri DL, Corey L, Holmes KK. Ineffectiveness of topical idoxuridine in dimethyl sulfoxide for therapy for genital herpes. *JAMA* 1982;248:953–9.
179. Blough HA, Giuntoli RL. Successful treatment of human genital herpes infections with 2-deoxy-D-glucose. *JAMA* 1979;241:2798–801.
180. Milman N, Scheibel J, Jessen O. Failure of lysine treatment in recurrent herpes simplex labialis [Letter]. *Lancet* 1978;2:942.
181. Milman N, Scheibel M, Jessen O. Lysine prophylaxis in recurrent herpes simplex labialis: a double-blind, controlled crossover study. *Acta Derm Venereol (Stockh)* 1980;60:85–7.
182. Pazin GJ, Armstrong JA, Lam MT, Tarr GC, Jannetta PJ, Ho M. Prevention of reactivated herpes simplex infection by human leukocyte interferon after operation on the trigeminal root. *N Engl J Med* 1979;301:225–30.
183. Pazin GJ, Harger JH, Armstrong JA, et al. Leukocyte interferon for treating first episodes of genital herpes in women. *J Infect Dis* 1987;156:891–8.
184. Kuhls TL, Sacher J, Pineda E, et al. Suppression of recurrent genital herpes simplex virus infection with recombinant alpha 2 interferon. *J Infect Dis* 1986;154:437–42.
185. Wallin J, Lernestedt JO, Lycke E. Therapeutic efficacy of trisodium phosphonoformate in treatment of recurrent herpes labialis [Abstract]. In: Nahmais AJ, Dowdle WR, Schinazi RF, eds. *The human herpesviruses: an interdisciplinary perspective*. New York: Elsevier North Holland, 1981:680–1.
186. Elion GB, Furman PA, Fyfe JA, de Miranda P, Beauchamp L, Schaeffer HJ. Selectivity of action of an antiherpetic agent, 9-(2-hydroxyethoxymethyl) guanine. *Proc Natl Acad Sci USA* 1977;74:5716–20.
187. Elion GB. History, mechanism of action, spectrum and selectivity of nucleoside analogues. In: Mills J, Corey L, eds. *Antiviral chemotherapy: new directions for clinical applications and research*. New York: Elsevier Science Publishing Co., 1986:118–37.
188. Crumpacker CS, Schnipper LE, Zaia JA, Levin MJ. Growth inhibition by acycloguanosine of herpesviruses isolated from human infections. *Antimicrob Agents Chemother* 1979;15:642–5.
189. Mindel A, Adler MW, Sutherland S, Fiddian AP. Intravenous acyclovir treatment for primary genital herpes. *Lancet* 1982;1:697–700.
190. Corey L, Fife KH, Benedetti JK, et al. Intravenous acyclovir for the treatment of primary genital herpes. *Ann Intern Med* 1983;98:914–21.
191. Corey L, Nahmias AJ, Guinan ME, Benedetti JK, Critchlow CW, Holmes KK. A trial of topical acyclovir in genital herpes simplex virus infections. *N Engl J Med* 1982;306:1313–9.
192. Mertz GJ, Critchlow CW, Benedetti J, et al. Double-blind placebo-controlled trial of oral acyclovir in first-episode genital herpes simplex virus infection. *JAMA* 1984;252:1147–51.
193. Nilsen AE, Aasen T, Halsos AM, et al. Efficacy of oral acyclovir in the treatment of initial and recurrent genital herpes. *Lancet* 1982;2:571–3.
194. Bryson YJ, Dillon M, Lovett M, et al. Treatment of first episodes of genital herpes simplex virus infection with oral acyclovir. A randomized double-blind controlled trial in normal subjects. *N Engl J Med* 1983;308:916–21.
195. Corey L, Benedetti J, Critchlow C, et al. Treatment of primary first-episode genital herpes simplex virus infections with acyclovir: results

of topical, intravenous and oral therapy. *J Antimicrob Chemother* 1983;12(suppl B):79–88.
196. Kinghorn GR, Abeywickreme I, Jeavons M, et al. Efficacy of combined treatment with oral and topical acyclovir in first episode genital herpes. *Genitourin Med* 1986;62:186–8.
197. Mindel A, Kinghorn G, Allason-Jones E, et al. Treatment of first-attack genital herpes—acyclovir versus inosine pranobex. *Lancet* 1987;1:1171–3.
198. Corey L, Mindel A, Fife KH, Sutherland S, Benedetti J, Adler MW. Risk of recurrence after treatment of first-episode genital herpes with intravenous acyclovir. *Sex Transm Dis* 1985; 12:215–8.
199. Bryson Y, Dillon M, Lovett M, Bernstein D, Garratty E, Sayre J. Treatment of first episode genital HSV with oral acyclovir: long-term follow-up of recurrences. A preliminary report. *Scand J Infect Dis [Suppl]* 1985;47:70–5.
200. Mertz GJ, Benedetti J, Critchlow C, Corey L. Long-term recurrence rates of genital herpes infections after treatment of first-episode genital herpes with oral acyclovir. In: Kano R, ed. *Herpes viruses and virus chemotherapy.* Amsterdam: Elsevier, 1985:141–4.
201. Reichman RC, Badger GJ, Mertz GJ, et al. Treatment of recurrent genital herpes simplex infections with oral acyclovir. A controlled trial. *JAMA* 1984;251:2103–7.
202. Mertz GJ, Jones CC, Mills J, et al. Long-term acyclovir suppression of frequently recurring genital herpes simplex virus infection. A multicenter double-blind trial. *JAMA* 1988; 260:201–6.
203. Luby JP, Gnann JW Jr, Alexander WJ, et al. A collaborative study of patient-initiated treatment of recurrent genital herpes with topical acyclovir or placebo. *J Infect Dis* 1984; 150:1–6.
204. Reichman RC, Badger GJ, Guinan ME, et al. Topically administered acyclovir in the treatment of recurrent herpes simplex genitalis: a controlled trial. *J Infect Dis* 1983;147:336–40.
205. Kinghorn GR. Topical acyclovir in the treatment of recurrent herpes simplex virus infections. *Scand J Infect Dis [Suppl]* 1985;47:58–62.
206. Mertz GJ, Eron L, Kaufman R, et al. Prolonged continuous versus intermittent oral acyclovir treatment in normal adults with frequently recurring genital herpes simplex virus infection. *Am J Med* 1988;85(suppl 2A):14–9.
207. Douglas JM, Critchlow C, Benedetti J, et al. A double-blind study of oral acyclovir for suppression of recurrences of genital herpes simplex virus infection. *N Engl J Med* 1984; 310:1551–6.
208. Halsos AM, Salo OP, Lassus A, et al. Oral acyclovir suppression of recurrent genital herpes. A double-blind, placebo-controlled crossover study. *Acta Derm Venereol [Stockh]* 1985; 65:59–63.
209. Mindel A, Faherty A, Carney O, Patou G, Freris M, Williams P. Dosage and safety of long-term suppressive acyclovir therapy for recurrent genital herpes. *Lancet* 1988;1:926–8.
210. Mindel A, Weller IV, Faherty A, et al. Prophylactic oral acyclovir in recurrent genital herpes. *Lancet* 1984;2:57–9.
211. Mostow SR, Mayfield JL, Marr JJ, Drucker JL. Suppression of recurrent genital herpes by single daily dosages of acyclovir. *Am J Med* 1988;85(suppl 2A):30–3.
212. Mattison HR, Reichman RC, Benedetti J, et al. Double-blind, placebo-controlled trial comparing long-term suppressive with short-term oral acyclovir therapy for management of recurrent genital herpes. *Am J Med* 1988;85(suppl 2A):20–5.
213. Portnoy J, Taussig A. A double-blind placebo-controlled six month trial of prophylactic oral acyclovir in recurrent genital herpes [Abstract]. Presented at the International Conjoint Sexually Transmitted Diseases Meeting, Montreal, 17–21 June, 1984:237.
214. Sacks SL, Fox R, Levendusky P, et al. Chronic suppression for six months compared with intermittent lesional therapy of recurrent genital herpes using oral acyclovir. Effect on lesions and nonlesional prodromes. *Sex Transm Dis* 1988;15:58–62.
215. Straus SE, Takiff HE, Seidlin M, et al. Suppression of frequently recurring genital herpes. A placebo-controlled double-blind trial of oral acyclovir. *N Engl J Med* 1984;310:1545–50.
216. Thin RN, Jeffries DJ, Taylor PK, et al. Recurrent genital herpes suppressed by oral acyclovir. A multicenter double-blind trial. *J Antimicrob Chemother* 1985;16:219–26.
217. Straus SE, Croen KD, Sawyer MH, et al. Acyclovir suppression of frequently recurring genital herpes. Efficacy and diminishing need during successive years of treatment. *JAMA* 1988;260:2227–30.
218. Douglas JM, Davis LG, Remington ML, et al. A double-blind placebo-controlled trial of the effect of chronically administered oral acyclovir on sperm production in men with frequently recurrent genital herpes. *J Infect Dis* 1988; 157:588–93.
219. Nusinoff Lehrman S, Douglas JM, Corey L, Barry DW. Recurrent genital herpes and suppressive oral acyclovir therapy: relationship between clinical outcome and in vitro drug sensitivity. *Ann Intern Med* 1986;104:786–90.
220. Straus SE, Seidlin M, Takiff HE, et al. Double-blind comparison of weekly and daily regimens of oral acyclovir for suppression of recurrent genital herpes. *Antiviral Res* 1986;6:151–9.
221. Spruance SL, Schnipper LE, Overall JC Jr, et al. Treatment of herpes simplex labialis with topical acyclovir in polyethylene glycol. *J Infect Dis* 1982;146:85–90.
222. Spruance SL, Crumpacker CS, Schnipper LE, et al. Early, patient-initiated treatment of herpes labialis with topical 10% acyclovir. *Antimicrob Agents Chemother* 1984;25:553–5.
223. Raborn GW, McGaw WT, Grace M, Tyrrell

LD, Samuels SM. Oral acyclovir and herpes labialis: a randomized, double-blind, placebo-controlled study. *J Am Dent Assoc* 1987; 115:38–42.
224. Raborn GW, McGaw WT, Grace M, Percy J. Treatment of herpes labialis with acyclovir: review of three clinical trials. *Am J Med* 1988;85(suppl 2A):39–42.
225. Rampalo AM, Mertz GJ, Davis LG, et al. Oral acyclovir for treatment of first-episode herpes simplex virus proctitis. *JAMA* 1988;259:2879–81.
226. Wade JC, Newton B, McLaren C, Flournoy N, Keeney RE, Meyers JD. Intravenous acyclovir to treat mucocutaneous herpes simplex virus infection after marrow transplantation: a double-blind trial. *Ann Intern Med* 1982;96:265–9.
227. Shepp DH, Newton BA, Dandliker PS, Flournoy N, Meyers JD. Oral acyclovir therapy for mucocutaneous herpes simplex virus infections in immunocompromised marrow transplant recipients. *Ann Intern Med* 1985;102:783–5.
228. Whitley RJ, Alford CA, Hirsch MS, et al. Vidarabine versus acyclovir therapy in herpes simplex encephalitis. *N Engl J Med* 1986; 314:144–9.
229. Shepp DH, Dandliker PS, Meyers JD. Treatment of varicella-zoster virus infection in severely immunocompromised patients. A randomized comparison of acyclovir and vidarabine. *N Engl J Med* 1986;314:208–12.
230. Field HJ, Darby G. Pathogenicity in mice of strains of herpes simplex virus which are resistant to acyclovir in vitro and in vivo. *Antimicrob Agents Chemother* 1980;17:209–16.
231. Gluckman E, Lotsberg J, Devergie A, et al. Oral acyclovir prophylactic treatment of herpes simplex infection after bone marrow transplantation. *J Antimicrob Chemother* 1983;12(suppl B):161–7.
232. Saral R, Burns WH, Laskin OL, Santos GW, Lietman PS. Acyclovir prophylaxis of herpes simplex virus infections. *N Engl J Med* 1981; 305:63–7.
233. Seale L, Jones CJ, Kathpalia S, et al. Prevention of herpesvirus infections in renal allograft recipients by low-dose oral acyclovir. *JAMA* 1985;254:3435–8.
234. Wade JC, Newton B, Flournoy N, Meyers JD. Oral acyclovir for prevention of herpes simplex virus reactivation after marrow transplantation. *Ann Intern Med* 1984;100:823–8.
235. Anderson H, Scarffe JH, Sutton RN, Hickmott E, Brigden D, Burke C. Oral acyclovir prophylaxis against herpes simplex virus in non-Hodgkin lymphoma and acute lymphoblastic leukemia patients receiving remission induction chemotherapy: a randomized double-blind, placebo-controlled trial. *Br J Cancer* 1984; 50:45–9.
236. Pettersson E, Hovi T, Ahonen J, et al. Prophylactic oral acyclovir after renal transplantation. *Transplantation* 1985;39:279–81.
237. Prentice HG. Use of acyclovir for prophylaxis of herpes infections in severely immunocompromised patients. *J Antimicrob Chemother* 1983;12(suppl B):153–9.
238. Straus SE, Seidlin M, Takiff H, Jacobs D, Bowen D, Smith HA. Oral acyclovir to suppress recurring herpes simplex virus infections in immunodeficient patients. *Ann Intern Med* 1984;100:522–4.
239. Shepp DH, Dandliker PS, Flournoy N, Meyers JD. Once-daily intravenous acyclovir for prophylaxis of herpes simplex virus reactivation after marrow transplantation. *J Antimicrob Chemother* 1985;16:389–95.
240. de Miranda P, Whitley RJ, Blum MR, et al. Acyclovir kinetics after intravenous infusion. *Clin Pharmacol Ther* 1979;26:718–28.
241. Van Dyke RB, Conner JD, Wyborny C, Hintz M, Keeney RE. Pharmacokinetics of orally administered acyclovir in patients with herpes progenitalis. *Am J Med* 1982;73:172–5.
242. McKendrick MW, Care C, Burke C, Hickmott E, McKendrick GD. Oral acyclovir in herpes zoster. *J Antimicrob Chemother* 1984;14: 661–5.
243. de Miranda P, Good SS, Krasny HC, Connor JD, Laskin OL, Lietman PS. Metabolic fate of radioactive acyclovir in humans. *Am J Med* 1982;73:215–20.
244. Laskin OL, Longstreth JA, Whelton A, et al. Effect of renal failure on the pharmacokinetics of acyclovir. *Am J Med* 1982;73:197–201.
245. Laskin OL, Longstreth JA, Saral R, de Miranda P, Keeney R, Lietman PS. Pharmacokinetics and tolerance of acyclovir, a new anti-herpesvirus agent, in humans. *Antimicrob Agents Chemother* 1982;21:393–8.
246. Fiddian AP, and European/Australian Collaborative Study Group. Zidovudine plus or minus acyclovir in patients with AIDS or ARC [Abstract]. In: *Program and abstracts of the 28th Interscience Conference on Antimicrobial Agents and Chemotherapy, 23–26 October.* Washington, D.C.: American Society for Microbiology, 1988;170.
247. Keeney RE, Kirk LE, Bridgen D. Acyclovir tolerance in humans. *Am J Med* 1982;73:176–181.
248. Bridgen D, Rosling AE, Woods NC. Renal function after acyclovir intravenous injection. *Am J Med* 1982;73:182–5.
249. Peterslund NA, Black FT, Tauris P. Impaired renal function after bolus injections of acyclovir [Letter]. *Lancet* 1983;1:243–4.
250. Speigal DM, Lau K. Acute renal failure and coma secondary to acyclovir therapy. *JAMA* 1986;255:1882–3.
251. Bean B, Aeppli D. Adverse effects of high-dose intravenous acyclovir in ambulatory patients with acute herpes zoster. *J Infect Dis* 1985;151:362–5.
252. Wade JC, Meyers JD. Neurologic symptoms associated with parenteral acyclovir treatment after marrow transplantation. *Ann Intern Med* 1983;98:921–5.
253. Galloway DA, McDougall JK. The oncogenic potential of herpes simplex viruses: evidence

for a "hit-and-run" mechanism. *Nature* 1983; 302:21–4.

254. Galloway DA, Nelson JA, McDougall JK. Small fragments of herpesvirus DNA with transforming activity contain insertion sequence-like structures. *Proc Natl Acad Sci USA* 1984;81:4736–40.
255. Jariwalla RJ, Aurelian L, Ts'o PO. Tumorigenic transformation induced by a specific fragment of DNA from herpes simplex virus type 2. *Proc Natl Acad Sci USA* 1980;77:2279–83.
256. Royston I, Aurelian L. The association of genital herpesvirus with cervical atypia and carcinoma *in situ*. *Am J Epidemiol* 1970;91:531–8.
257. Kaufman RH, Dreesman GR, Burek J, et al. Herpesvirus-induced antigens in squamous-cell carcinoma *in situ* of the vulva. *N Engl J Med* 1981;305:483–8.
258. Eglin RP, Sharp F, MacLean AB, Macnab JC, Clements JB, Wilkie NM. Detection of RNA complementary to herpes simplex virus DNA in human cervical squamous cell neoplasms. *Cancer Res* 1981;41:3597–603.
259. McDougall JK, Galloway DA, Fenoglio CM. Cervical carcinoma: detection of herpes simplex virus RNA in cells undergoing neoplastic change. *Int J Cancer* 1980;25:1–8.
260. Kitces EN, Morahan PS, Tew JG, Murray BK. Protection from oral herpes simplex virus infection by a nucleic acid-free virus vaccine. *Infect Immun* 1977;16:955–60.
261. Skinner GR, Williams DR, Moles AW, Sargent A. Prepubertal vaccination of mice against experimental infection of the genital tract with type 2 herpes simplex virus. *Arch Virol* 1980;64:329–38.
262. Skinner GR, Buchan A, Hartley CE, Turner SP, Williams DR. The preparation, efficacy, and safety of "antigenoid" vaccine NFU1 (S−L+) MRC toward prevention of herpes simplex virus infections in human subjects. *Med Microbiol Immunol (Berl)* 1980;169:39–51.
263. Cappel R, de Cuyper F, Rickaert F. Efficacy of a nucleic acid free herpetic subunit vaccine. *Arch Virol* 1980;65:15–23.
264. Price RW, Walz MA, Wohlenberg C, Notkins AL. Latent infection of sensory ganglia with herpes simplex virus: efficacy of immunization. *Science* 1975;188:938–40.
265. Hilleman MR, Larson VM, Lehman ED, Salerno RA, Conard PG, McLean AA. Subunit herpes simplex virus-2 vaccine. In: Nahmias AJ, Dowdle WR, Schinazi RF, eds. *The human herpesviruses: An Interdisciplinary Perspective.* New York: Elsevier North Holland, 1981: 503–6.
266. Berman PW, Gregory T, Crase D, Lasky LA. Protection from genital herpes simplex virus type 2 infection by vaccination with cloned type 1 glycoprotein D. *Science* 1985;227: 1490–2.
267. Lasky LA, Dowbenko DJ, Simonsen CC, Berman PW. Protection of mice from lethal herpes simplex virus infection by vaccination with a secreted form of cloned glycoprotein-D. *Bio-Technol* 1984;2:527–32.
268. Cremer KJ, Mackett M, Wohlenberg C, Notkins AL, Moss B. Vaccinia virus recombinant expressing herpes simplex virus type 1 glycoprotein D prevents latent herpes in mice. *Science* 1985;228:737–40.
269. Stanberry LR, Bernstein DI, Burke RL, Pachl C, Myers MG. Vaccination with recombinant herpes simplex virus glycoproteins: protection against initial and recurrent genital herpes. *J Infect Dis* 1987;155:914–20.
270. Scriba M. Protection of guinea pigs against primary and recurrent genital herpes infections by immunization with live heterologous or homologous Herpes simplex virus: implications for a herpes virus vaccine. *Med Microbiol Immunol (Berl)* 1978;166:63–9.
271. Blank H, Haines HG. Experimental human reinfection with herpes simplex virus. *J Invest Dermatol* 1973;61:223–5.
272. Allen WP, Rapp F. Concept review of genital herpes vaccines. *J Infect Dis* 1982;145:413–21.
273. Frank SB. Formolized herpes virus therapy and the neutralizing substance in herpes simplex. *J Invest Dermatol* 1938;1:267–82.
274. Nasemann T, Schaeg G. Herpes simplex-virus, type 2: Mikrobiologie und klinische erfahrungen mit einer abgetoteten vaccine. *Hautarzt* 1973;24:133–9.
275. Kitagawa K. Therapy of herpes simplex with heat inactivated herpes virus hominis type 1 and type 2. *Z Hautkr* 1973;48:533–5.
276. Roizman B, Warren J, Thuning CA, Fanshaw MS, Norrild B, Meignier B. Application of molecular genetics to the design of live herpes simplex virus vaccines. *Dev Biol Stand* 1982; 2:287–304.
277. Mertz GJ, Peterman G, Ashley R, et al. Herpes simplex virus type-2 glycoprotein-subunit vaccine: tolerance and humoral and cellular responses in humans. *J Infect Dis* 1984;150: 242–9.
278. Ashley R, Mertz G, Clark H, Schick M, Salter D, Corey L. Humoral immune response to herpes simplex virus type 2 glycoproteins in patients receiving a glycoprotein subunit vaccine. *J Virol* 1985;56:475–81.
279. Zarling JM, Moran PA, Brewer L, Ashley R, Corey L. Herpes simplex virus (HSV)-specific proliferative and cytotoxic T-cell responses in humans immunized with an HSV type 2 glycoprotein subunit vaccine. *J Virol* 1988;62: 4481–5.

*Antiviral Agents and Viral Diseases of Man, 3rd Edition,* edited by G. J. Galasso, R. J. Whitley, and T. C. Merigan, Raven Press, Ltd., New York © 1990.

# 9

# Human Papillomaviruses and Interferon Therapy

Richard C. Reichman

*Infectious Diseases Unit, Departments of Medicine, Microbiology, and Immunology, University of Rochester Medical Center, Rochester, New York 14642*



## HUMAN PAPILLOMAVIRUSES

Infection with human papillomaviruses (HPV) is widespread throughout the population. HPV produce epithelial tumors of the skin and mucous membranes, and have been associated closely with several genital tract malignancies, particularly carcinoma of the cervix. Papillomaviruses are highly species-specific, and cross-species infections occur rarely. Human warts were demonstrated to be caused by infectious agents in the late 19th century by investigators who inoculated subjects with wart extracts (1). Experiments conducted by Ciuffo (2) suggested that the infectious agent of warts was a virus when he transmitted this infection successfully using cell-free filtrates in 1907. Other early investigations examined the biologic behavior of the cottontail rabbit papillomavirus (CRPV) (3). These studies demonstrated that CRPV produces proliferative lesions containing large numbers of infectious virions in the epithelium of wild rabbits. On the other hand, CRPV infection of domestic rabbits produced proliferative lesions that contained few virus particles. In addition, lesions in domestic rabbits frequently underwent malignant degeneration, establishing CRPV as the earliest identified DNA tumor virus. Despite these interesting early observations, papillomaviruses have not been studied using standard virologic techniques, because they have not been propagated successfully in tissue culture or in common laboratory animals. This inability to propagate papillomaviruses in an experimental system has limited greatly our understanding of the biology of these viruses. For example, as recently as 15 years ago, it was generally believed that all human warts were caused by a single type of HPV.

Despite the lack of a suitable tissue culture system, recent advances in molecular biology have increased our ability to perform laboratory investigations of papillomaviruses. These advances have made it possible to clone viral DNA from tissue, identify multiple virus types, and have also led to an understanding of the genomic organization of HPV and the functions of different viral genes (4,5).

## Characteristics

### *Biophysical Properties*

HPVs are members of the A genus of the *Papovaviridae* family of viruses (6,7). HPV are nonenveloped viruses, approximately 55 nm in diameter, with icosahedral capsids consisting of 72 capsomers. The genome consists of circular, double-stranded DNA containing approximately 7,900 base pairs. Only one of the two strands is transcribed (8–10). Genomes of all papillomaviruses show a similar organization (Fig. 1) and are divided functionally into three separate regions (4). The early region contains five to seven open reading frames (ORFs) and codes for proteins that are involved in transformation and virus replication. The late region consists of ORFs *L1* and *L2,* which code for the virion capsid proteins. The third region is generally referred to as the "upstream regulatory region" or the "long control region" and appears to be important in the control of viral transcription and DNA replication (11).

HPV virions have a sedimentation coefficient of 300. The principal protein constituent of the virion particle is the major capsid protein, which has a molecular weight of approximately 56,000 and constitutes approximately 80% of the total weight. A larger, minor capsid protein, with a molecular weight of approximately 76,000, is also present, and histone-like proteins have been detected in some preparations of HPV.

Papillomaviruses have not been propagated successfully in tissue culture or in common animal models. In addition, significant quantities of virions are not present in most HPV lesions. For these reasons, well-characterized antigenic preparations of HPV are not available, and virus typing is dependent upon determination of nucleic acid homology (4). Using this criterion, DNA of a unique HPV type cross hybridizes, in liquid phase, to a maximum of 50% with the DNA of other classified viruses. At the present time, 57 different HPV types have been cloned (E.-M. de Villiers, unpublished observations). As indicated in Table 1, different types tend to be associated with specific diseases. HPV subtypes contain DNA which cross-hybridize more than 50% and have distinctive patterns when cut with restriction endonucleases.

Although a productive tissue culture system for papillomaviruses has not been established, some of these viruses can transform tissue culture cells. For example, bovine papillomavirus type 1 (BPV-1) can transform mouse C127 cells (12,13). Manipulation of this system has enabled investigators to determine certain functional characteristics of the papillomavirus genome (11). A novel experimental animal system has also been established in which HPV-11 virions are produced (14,15). Several laboratories have also recently employed DNA recombinant technology to generate HPV proteins (16,17). Further use of these recently developed techniques should make precise antigenic characterization of these viruses possible in the near future.

### *Transcription and Replication*

Current understanding of the transcription and replication of papillomavirus DNA has been derived from studies of the BPV-I transformation system in rodent cells (11). Manipulation of this system has produced a partial dissection of the function of different genomic elements. For example, the *E6* and *E5* ORFs have been demonstrated to

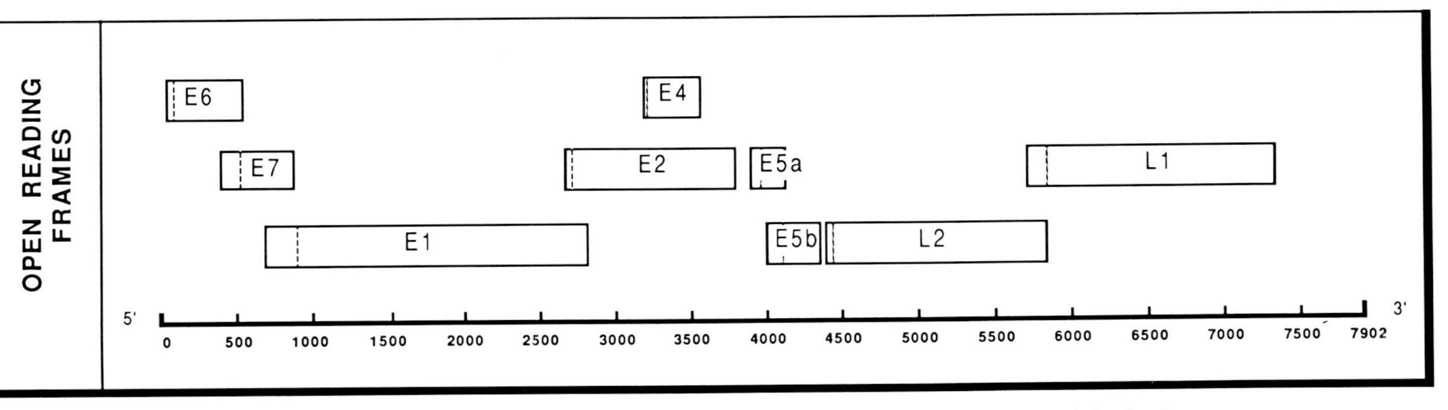


**FIG. 1.** Linearized genomic map of HPV-6B. ORFs are represented by *boxes,* and the *broken vertical line in each box* represents the position of the first potential start codon. ORFs of other sequenced papillomaviruses are positioned in similar locations. Adapted from Strike et al, ref. 17 and provided by W. Bonnez.

**TABLE 1.** *Association of HPV types with specific diseases*

| Disease | Virus type |
|---|---|
| Deep plantar warts | 1, 4 |
| Common warts | 1, 2, 4, 41 |
| Common warts of meat handlers | 7 |
| Flat warts | 3, 10, 27, 41 |
| Intermediate warts | 10, 26, 28 |
| Epidermodysplasia verruciformis | 5, 8, 9, 12, 14, 15, 17, 19–25, 36, 47 |
| Condyloma acuminatum | 6, 11, 10, 41, 42, 45, 51 |
| Intraepithelial neoplasias | 6, 11, 16, 18, 31, 33, 34, 35, 39, 42, 45, 51 |
| Laryngeal papillomas | 6, 11, 30 |
| Focal epithelial hyperplasia of Heck | 13, 32 |
| Conjunctival papillomas | 6, 11 |
| Other diseases | 37, 38 |

code for transforming proteins (18–21). These proteins alter phenotypic characteristics of cells, usually resulting in increased cellular growth potential. The *E7* ORF codes for a protein that appears to be important in maintaining episomal plasmids at a high copy number (22). The *E1* ORF codes for *trans*-acting factors that are necessary for stable plasmid replication (22–24). Two gene products are believed to be produced from the *E1* ORF, the *E1* modulator and the *E1* replicator (25). The *E2* ORF codes for two proteins that regulate an enhancer of the long control region (26). A recent study has established requirements of the *E2* products for plasmid replication, presumably indirectly through transcriptional regulatory mechanisms (27). The functions of the *E3* of BPV-1 and *E4* ORFs have not yet been established (28,29), although *E4* products have been demonstrated to constitute a major portion of extractable proteins in HPV-1–induced lesions (30) and are also present in lesions produced in the nude mouse model (15). In addition, a messenger RNA (mRNA) species containing the *E4* region appears to be the major message in condylomata acuminata produced by HPV-11 (31).

As discussed below, expression of *L1* and *L2* is limited to the more superficial keratinocytes of papillomavirus-induced lesions (32–34). These observations have been made by utilization of *in situ* hybridization and immunocytochemical techniques applied to virus-infected tissue. Expression of these late functions has not yet been observed in any tissue culture system. The *L1* ORF codes for the major capsid protein and contains the genus specific epitope (17). *L2* encodes a minor capsid protein that is not highly conserved among different HPV types (35).

## Manifestations of Infection

### *Cutaneous Warts*

Cutaneous warts include plantar warts, common warts, and flat warts (36,37). Plantar warts occur most commonly among adolescents and young adults. They appear as slightly elevated lesions that may be confused with calluses. However, shaving of plantar warts reveals punctate, bleeding, blood vessels, whereas similar manipulations of calluses do not. When located at pressure points, plantar warts are often quite painful. Similar lesions may appear on the palms of the hands.

Common warts are typically exophytic lesions that are sharply demarcated from surrounding normal skin. These hyperkeratotic papules have a rough surface and usually occur on the dorsum of the hand, between the fingers, or around the nails. Less commonly, lesions occur on the palms or soles, and may rarely be present on mucous membranes. Plain or flat warts are noted frequently among children. These slightly elevated papules have a smooth surface and an irregular contour. Most commonly, they are present on the face, neck, and hands. The natural history of all cutaneous warts is poorly understood. In one study, spontaneous resolution of common warts occurred in 50% of children within a 1-year period (38).

### *Epidermodysplasia Verruciformis*

Epidermodysplasia verruciformis (EV) is a poorly understood, rare condition that is characterized by extreme susceptibility to HPV infection and squamous cell carcinomas (39). Of interest, these patients do not appear to be unusually susceptible to other infections, and it is unclear whether or not they have an immune defect. A large number of HPV types have been detected among EV patients, as noted in Table 1. Most of these types have not been detected in other patient groups. HPV lesions in EV patients often resemble flat warts, may appear similar to pityriasis versicolor, and are most frequently located on the torso and upper extremities. When present on extensor surface, warts may coalesce and become hypertrophic. Squamous cell carcinomas occur in approximately one-third of patients and generally develop in sun-exposed areas.

### *Anogenital Warts*

Anogenital warts, or condylomata acuminata, are usually exophytic papules on normal appearing skin and/or mucous membranes. These lesions vary in appearance, ranging from smooth-surfaced papules to jagged, acuminate growths. Individual lesions may measure less than 1 mm in diameter or may merge into large plaques covering several square centimeters. In uncircumsized men, the preputial cavity is most commonly involved, whereas in circumsized men, the penile shaft is the most common site of infection (40–43). The urethral meatus may also be involved and can be associated with proximal extension into the urethra and, rarely, the bladder (40,43,44–46). Perianal lesions are commonly observed among homosexual men, although they may be present in heterosexual men as well (43,47,48). Adjacent areas including the scrotum, perineum, and groin are affected rarely. In women, most lesions are located in the posterior introitus, and less commonly on the labia majora and/or minora, and the clitoris. In addition, the vagina, anus, cervix, and urethra may also be involved (40,42).

Soaking of lesions and surrounding areas with dilute solutions of acetic acid, and use of colposcopy have led to an appreciation of more widespread disease in many patients. This procedure often produces areas of white patches with irregular borders containing capillary loops (49). External genital warts are often associated with cervical lesions including flat condylomas and cervical intraepithelial neoplasias (50). More recently, HPV vaginitis has also been described (51,52). This lesion often presents clinically with complaints of pruritis, and on physical examination appears as subtle abnormalities of normal skin and mucous membranes. Colposcopy and use of acetic acid has also led to an appreciation of more prevalent and extensive disease in men, particularly in recent studies of male sexual partners of women with HPV disease (53,54).

Most patients with condyloma acuminata are asymptomatic (42), although itching, burning, pain, and tenderness are encountered not uncommonly (42,51). The natural history of anogenital warts, particularly subclinical HPV disease, is poorly understood, although spontaneous remission has been observed in recently conducted, placebo-controlled trials (55–58).

Complications of anogenital warts include rare transformation into locally invasive carcinomas (59) and enlargement during pregnancy producing obstruction of the birth canal (60,61). A close association between HPV infection and genital tract malignancies has also been observed as described below. More recently, anorectal dysplasias and cancers have been observed among homosexual men with perianal HPV infection (62–64).

#### *Respiratory Papillomatosis*

Respiratory papillomatosis is associated with infection of the respiratory tract by HPV types commonly associated with condyloma acuminatum. Patients present with symptoms of obstruction of the respiratory tract including hoarseness, respiratory distress, and stridor. The disease may spread rarely to the trachea and lungs, leading to obstruction, infection, and respiratory failure. When present in young children, rapid growth of these lesions may lead to severe respiratory compromise and necessitate frequent surgical intervention. Patients who have received radiation may undergo malignant transformation (65–68).

#### *Other Warts*

Heck's disease, or focal epithelial hyperplasia, is associated primarily with HPV-13 infection and tends to regress spontaneously. HPV infections have also been observed in the oral cavity, conjunctiva, and nasal mucosa (69–71).

### Pathophysiology of Disease and Host Responses to Infection

#### *Pathogenesis*

Inoculation of human subjects with extracts of cutaneous warts led to initial estimates of the incubation period of HPV disease of 6 weeks to 2 years (1,2). Most commonly, warts developed in 3–4 months. A similar incubation period of anogenital warts was observed among wives of American soldiers returning from the Korean War (72). HPVs infect all types of squamous epithelium, but other tissues are rarely affected. Gross and histologic appearances of individual lesions tend to vary with the site of infection and virus type.

The pathogenesis of HPV infections is poorly understood. It is assumed that the virus life cycle begins with entry of particles into the basalar cells of the epithelium, and viral DNA has been detected in nuclei of these cells (33). HPV DNA replicates and transcribes as basal cells differentiate, and complete virions ultimately appear in the most superficial keratinocytes of the epithelium. HPV infection of epithelial tissues is generally associated with excessive proliferation of all epidermal layers excluding the basal cells (73). This process results in the histologic development of acanthosis, parakeratosis, and hyperkeratosis. In addition, deepening of the rete ridges occurs. These changes may develop in the absence of direct HPV infection, inasmuch as many cells in individual warts do not appear to contain HPV DNA (33). Some infected cells undergo koilocytotic changes producing large, squamous cells with shrunken nuclei lodged inside large cytoplasmic vacuoles. Of importance is the observation that grossly and histologically normal appearing epithelium may contain HPV DNA (74,75). Viral DNA is located extrachromosomally in the nuclei of infected cells in benign lesions associated with HPV infection. However, HPV DNA in severe dysplasias, cancers, and transformed cell lines is generally integrated (76). Integration occurs at specific sites within the HPV genome, although integration in host cell DNA appears to occur randomly.

#### *Host Responses*

Host defense responses to HPV infection are poorly understood. Lack of appropriate, uniform antigen preparations has severely hampered the elucidation of these mechanisms. Several clinical observations suggest that cell-mediated immune responses may be of importance in resolution of HPV disease. For example, these infections occur frequently and are often severe in patients with Wiscott-Aldrich syndrome, patients infected with immunodeficiency virus (HIV), and patients who have received allografts (77–80). However, most patients with HPV infections do not appear to have a discrete immune defect.

Immune responses to HPV infection have been summarized recently (77). Studies of both humoral and cell-mediated immunity to HPV antigens have been reported. However, most of these studies have been difficult to interpret because poorly characterized preparations were utilized as antigens and the clinical status of the patients from whom specimens were obtained have not been described clearly. Thus, although anti-HPV immune responses have been detected by several groups using a variety of techniques, the relative importance of these responses in protection from and resolution of HPV disease has not been determined. Recently conducted studies have employed HPV antigens produced using DNA recombinant techniques to detect antibodies in human sera. In one such study, β-galactosidase fusion proteins derived from the *L1* and *L2* ORFs of HPV-6b failed to detect antibodies in sera of HPV-6–infected patients (17). Other investigators found antibodies in sera from patients attending a sexually transmitted diseases clinic, which were directed against a TrpE fusion protein containing most of the major capsid protein of HPV-6b (16). Further investigations utilizing well-characterized proteins and/or HPV particles will be required to characterize adequately the immune responses to HPV antigens. In addition to characterizing humoral and peripheral blood mononuclear cell responses to HPV infection, future studies should also investigate the potential importance of local host defense mechanisms in the resolution of these diseases. Some studies have suggested that mononuclear cell infiltration of HPV lesions may be important in the resolution of these infections (81). Local defense mechanisms could be operative in the absence of detectable systemic immune responses.

## Epidemiology

### *Incidence and Prevalence*

Few systematically conducted studies of the epidemiology of most HPV infections have been performed. Such studies are difficult to conduct for several reasons. Laboratory techniques needed to make accurate diagnoses are not widely available. In addition, these techniques usually require biopsy specimens, and are expensive and labor intensive. Materials with which to conduct seroepidemiologic studies remain inadequate. Many, if not most HPV-induced diseases that come to medical attention are probably treated in some fashion, producing alterations in the natural history of disease. The magnitude of subclinical infection in the general population is at present impossible to estimate. Nevertheless, certain generalizations regarding the incidence and prevalence of these diseases can be made (82,83).

HPV infections are widespread throughout the general population. Three kinds of cutaneous warts are particularly common and appear to occur with equal frequency in members of both sexes. Common warts occur frequently among school-aged children and adolescents, and juvenile flat warts also occur commonly in somewhat younger age groups. Plantar warts are frequently observed among adolescents and young adults. Individuals whose occupations require them to handle fresh meat products frequently are also at high risk for the development of cutaneous warts (84–87). Patients with epidermodysplasia verruciformis generally develop widespread cutaneous HPV disease. Many individuals with this rare, probably autosomal recessive condition, also are at high risk for malignant transformation of their lesions (36,39).

Anogenital warts, or condyloma acuminatum, are sexually transmitted lesions that appear to be increasing rapidly in incidence (42,88–91). In the United States, data collected by the National Disease and Therapeutic Index indicate that the number of patient/physician interactions in a private practice setting increased almost sevenfold between 1966 and 1984. HPV infections of the cervix are the most common cause of squamous cell abnormalities on Papanicolau smears (92–100).

### Transmission

It is assumed that close personal contact is required for the transmission of most HPV infections, although strong epidemiologic evidence for this assumption does not exist. Minor trauma at the site of inoculation may also be of importance. Fomites may be responsible for the transmission of some types of HPV disease (101).

Considerable evidence exists to support the concept that anogenital warts are sexually transmitted. The age at which condyloma acuminatum is observed is similar to that of other sexually transmitted diseases, and approximately two-thirds of the sexual contacts of patients with anogenital warts go on to develop the disease (40,102). In addition, as outlined in Table 1, particular HPV types, most commonly HPV-6 and HPV-11, are associated with anogenital warts. These types are rarely found in lesions outside the genital tract.

Recurrent respiratory papillomatosis in children is probably acquired at birth. This hypothesis is based upon the observations that identical HPV types produce both respiratory papillomatosis and anogenital warts, and that a significant percentage of mothers of these children give a history of having had genital tract HPV disease. Nevertheless, cases of respiratory papillomatosis in children have been documented at birth, even after caesarean section (65–68). The mechanism of transmission of recurrent respiratory papillomatosis in adults is unknown. This disease may be acquired by oral-genital contact or may be a late complication of perinatally acquired infection.

### Association Between HPV and Malignancies

Several different types of information suggest a strong link between HPV infection and genital tract malignancies. Although thorough epidemiologic studies to demonstrate definitively a role for HPV in the development of genital tract cancers have not been performed (103), several epidemiologic observations support the association. For example, women with previous histories of genital warts are much more likely to develop cervical carcinoma *in situ* than are women without such a history (104). Women married to men who develop cancer of the penis are more likely to develop cervical cancer than are other women (105). Cohort studies indicate that patients with histories of genital warts are at increased risk for the development of cervical cancers (42). In addition, nuns rarely develop cervical cancer (106).

Certain HPVs have been intimately associated with genital tract neoplasias, particularly of the uterine cervix (107,108). As many as 90% of cervical cancers contain detectable HPV DNA, usually of types 16, 18, or 31. In addition, some longitudinal studies have indicated that dysplastic lesions that are associated with these same types are more likely to progress than are lesions associated with HPV types that are associated with condyloma acuminatum (types 6 and 11). When detected in tumors, HPV DNA is frequently integrated, whereas it is located extrachromosomally in benign lesions. In addition, HPV DNA of types 16 and 18 have been found in several "immortal" cell lines. In both malignant tissues and immortal cell lines, integrated HPV DNA is consistently interrupted in the same region of the viral genome. In certain *in vitro* systems, HPV-16 DNA has been shown to transform human cells (109,110).

## Clinical and Laboratory Diagnosis

Diagnosis of HPV infection is usually made accurately by gross physical examination. However, physical examination can be misleading, particularly in the evaluation of genital tract lesions, where approximately 10% of biopsy specimens yield different histopathologic diagnoses (W. Bonnez, R. C. Reichman, and M. H. Stoler, unpublished observations). Sensitivity of physical examination of anogenital lesions can be greatly increased by application of dilute solutions of acetic acid to areas surrounding typical warts in combination with colposcopy (54,111–113). So-called acetowhite lesions, which are produced by this procedure, frequently contain HPV DNA when biopsy specimens are examined using hybridization techniques to detect viral nucleic acids. Cytologic examination of cervical smears may detect characteristic changes of HPV infection, as well as dysplasias and cancer (114–116). Cytology may also be used to diagnose intra-anal HPV infection (62). When indicated, histologic examination of biopsy specimens should be performed. In addition to routine histologic techniques, confirmation of HPV infection can be made by use of antigen detection techniques that can be performed with commercially available antisera (117,118). The most sensitive and specific method of diagnosis currently available is demonstration of HPV nucleic acids in tissue specimens using either *in situ* or Southern hybridization techniques (119). Use of the recently developed polymerase chain reaction (120) will probably increase considerably the sensitivity of currently available techniques to detect HPV nucleic acids. Diagnosis of HPV infection cannot be made using culture or serologic techniques.

## Treatment

Design, execution, and interpretation of clinical trials of treatments for HPV infections are difficult to perform for several reasons (Table 2). The lack of adequate natural history data, as well as safe and effective treatment modalities, necessitates randomized, placebo-controlled designs. In addition, several clinical and virological parameters of potential importance must be taken into account. For example, virus type, which has been shown to be important in the study of antivirals for other diseases such as genital herpes infections, should be established prior to study enrollment. In addition, some recent studies have suggested that duration of disease prior to study entry may affect response to therapy (55), and appropriately conducted studies should take these observations into account. Potential effects of previous treatment should also be considered, and the immunologic status prior to study of patients should be established. Assessment of im-

**TABLE 2.** *Problems associated with the design, execution, and interpretation of clinical trials of treatment for HPV infections*

| |
|---|
| A lack of adequate natural history data |
| Potential importance of the following: |
| Immunologic status of patients |
| Virus type |
| Duration of disease prior to study entry |
| Effects of previous therapy |
| Sex |
| Sexual preference |
| Location of lesions |
| Paucity of objective measurements of disease |
| Size of lesions |
| Quantitative determinations of viral antigens and nucleic acids |
| Need for adequate follow-up |
| Need for histologic confirmation of clinical diagnoses |

munologic status should include determination of the presence of HIV infection, inasmuch as even asymptomatic HIV infection has been shown to affect response to treatment of anogenital warts (121). Studies of patients' immune status to papillomaviruses may also be important, although such studies are at the present time not possible to perform. Other factors that may be of potential importance include sex, sexual preference, and lesion location. Objective measurements of antiviral activity should be made in appropriately conducted clinical trials. However, although semiquantitative estimates of amounts of HPV antigens and nucleic acids can be determined using sequential biopsy specimens, serial biopsies are difficult to obtain and are subject to sampling error. Thus, at the present time, only size and numbers of lesions can be utilized as objective measurements of disease. Because HPV disease is known to recur frequently, adequate periods of follow-up should be included as a part of study design.

Some of the currently available modes of treatment for HPV diseases are listed in Table 3. Although most of these modes of therapy have been evaluated in reported investigations, they have not been, in general, studied in randomized, placebo-controlled trials. Such trials are needed because of the variability of the natural history of HPV infections and the lack of a suitable *in vitro* animal model system in which evaluations of different therapeutic modalities can be carried out. Most currently available therapies for HPV infections consist of physical or chemical destruction of grossly visible lesions and do not take into account the multifocal and subclinical characteristics of these diseases.

Cutaneous warts are benign, usually self-limited infections for which treatment is often not necessary. However, several different treatment approaches are commonly utilized (122–124). Application of salicylic and/or lactic acids is often used in treatment of common warts on the hand, producing cure rates of approximately 70%. Similar rates of disease resolution are obtained using cryotherapy. Deep plantar warts are also treated frequently with acid preparations and occasionally with podophyllin, glutaraldehyde, or 5-fluorouracil. Different surgical techniques, including curettage, electrosurgery, and electrocautery, may be utilized in the treatment of cutaneous warts.

There is general agreement that anogenital warts should be treated because they are sexually transmitted, and associated with genital tract dysplasias and malignancies. Optimal methods of treatment, however, have not been established, and the effects of currently available therapies on the rates of transmission or development of neoplasias are unknown. The Centers for Disease Control recommends cryotherapy and/or podophyllin for the treatment of external

**TABLE 3.** *Some modes of treatment for HPV-associated diseases*

| |
|---|
| Cutaneous warts |
| Salicylic, lactic acids |
| Cryotherapy |
| Podophyllin |
| Glutaraldehyde |
| 5-FU |
| Surgery |
| Anogenital warts |
| Cryotherapy |
| Podophyllin/podophyllotoxin |
| 5-FU |
| Trichoracetic and bichloracetic acids |
| Surgery |
| Electrosurgery |
| Laser |
| Infrared coagulation |
| Dinitrochlorobenzene |
| Interferons |
| Genital tract neoplasias |
| Cryotherapy |
| Laser |
| Surgery |
| Recurrent respiratory papillomatosis |
| Laser |
| Cryotherapy |
| Interferons |
| Epidermodysplasia verruciformis |
| 5-FU |
| Surgery |

genital warts (125). Cryotherapy is most often performed using liquid nitrogen (126–128). Podophyllin is a resin extract of the rhizome of *Podophyllum peltatum,* and has been a principal mode of therapy for condyloma acuminatum for many years (129). The active molecules are lignans, including podophyllotoxin. Podophyllin is a mitotic poison, but its mode of action in warts is unknown. Initial reports suggested high rates of complete resolution following application of podophyllin, although more recent studies have demonstrated cure rates of 20–40% (41,129,130). Both local and systemic side effects have been observed in association with application of podophyllin (129,131). Chemical burns are seen in as many as 50% of treated patients, and neurological, hematological, and febrile complications have been associated with topical administration. 5-Fluorouracil (5-FU) has also been used in treatment of anogenital warts. Topical administration has been recommended, particularly for intraurethral and vulvar warts (41,132–134). Application of 5-FU often produces local ulceration and pain. Trichloracetic and bichloracetic acids have also been used in the treatment of genital warts (135). Application of these acids is moderately painful, but is associated with efficacy rates similar to those of cryotherapy (126). A variety of surgical techniques have been employed for the treatment of anogenital warts. Conventional surgery provides immediate eradication of visible lesions, but has been associated with recurrent disease in approximately one-third of patients and is commonly complicated by scarring (136,137). Electrosurgical techniques have produced results similar to those of cryotherapy (138). Rates of cure as high as 80–90% have been reported using $CO_2$ laser, although laser therapy may not be superior to conventional surgery (139–142). Infrared coagulation has also been utilized (143).

Recent studies have employed interferons administered topically, intralesionally, and parenterally for the treatment of anogenital warts. These studies are reviewed in detail in the section on interferons.

Internal genital warts are frequently associated with dysplasias and malignancies. Because of the special skills and techniques required for optimal diagnosis and management of these lesions, patients with internal lesions should be managed by an experienced surgical specialist. Several different forms of therapy for anal, rectal, urethral, vaginal, and cervical warts and/or dysplasias are available and include podophyllin, 5-FU, laser, cryotherapy, and conventional surgery (41,43,144–152).

### Prevention

No effective methods of preventing transmission of HPV infection are currently available, other than avoiding contact with infectious lesions. Limited studies have given contradictory results regarding the effectiveness of barrier methods of contraception in preventing sexual transmission of HPV infection (153,154). The sexual partners of patients with anogenital warts should be examined and treated as indicated (125). A number of obstacles to development of effective vaccines exist, and such preparations are not currently available (155).

## INTERFERON THERAPY

### Pharmacology and Toxicology

The pharmacokinetics of exogenously administered interferons are determined by the interferon type and the route of administration (156). In the absence of active infection, endogenously produced interferons are rarely present in detectable amounts in serum. Viral infections induce large amounts of endogenous interferon, which has a short half-life in the circulation, probably due to binding to cellular receptors throughout the body and metabolism by the kidney and liver.

Intravenously administered interferon-α disappears rapidly from plasma, and less than 0.1% of large doses remains in the circulation 24 hr after administration. These interferons are filtered by the renal glomeruli and reabsorbed by the tubular cells where they are destroyed by proteolysis (157,158). In contrast to intravenous administration, intramuscular or subcutaneous administration of interferon-α results in more prolonged plasma levels. Following administration by these routes, peak plasma levels of interferon occur in 1–6 hr, remain stable for 6–12 hr, and slowly reach undetectable levels after 18–36 hr (158).

The pharmacokinetics of interferon-β and interferon-γ differ markedly from those of interferon-α. Interferon-γ and interferon-β do not appear in significant concentrations in plasma after intramuscular injection, and they are metabolized primarily by the liver rather than by the kidney (159–165). Despite low serum levels, intramuscular or subcutaneous injection of these interferons produces systemic effects. For example, natural killer (NK) cells are activated as readily by intramuscularly administered interferon-β and interferon-γ as by intramuscularly administered interferon-α (166). Alterations in cellular enzyme systems are also readily detectable following intramuscular injection with these preparations, despite low or undetectable plasma levels.

Characteristic side effects are produced by administration of significant quantities of exogenously administered interferons. These side effects have been reported after administration of interferons from each of the major classes, although doses that produce these effects may differ according to interferon class. Subcutaneous or intramuscular administration of 3–5 million units or more of interferon-α preparations produces side effects in the majority of patients. The principal clinical side effect produced by interferon administration is the development of an influenza-like syndrome consisting of fever, headache, chills, myalgia, malaise, and fatigue. Fever usually develops within 3–4 hr after initial injection, and spontaneously resolves within 12–24 hr. When interferon is administered daily, tachyphylaxis to fever usually develops after one or two doses. Occasionally, fever may occur after daily injections for several days. Development and disappearance of the other symptoms listed above tends to correlate with fever. Administration of antipyretics tends to alleviate these symptoms. After several weeks of continuous administration of significant amounts of interferon, many patients develop chronic fatigue.

In addition to the clinical symptoms and signs mentioned above, characteristic abnormalities in routine laboratory tests commonly occur after administration of interferon. Neutropenia usually develops within 24 hr after the initial dose. Neutropenia may persist, and occasionally necessitates dosage reduction, or termination of interferon therapy. Thrombocytopenia also occurs commonly and tends to coincide with the development of neutropenia. Anemia develops occasionally, usually when interferons are administered for prolonged periods of time. Elevations of serum transaminases are observed not uncommonly among patients treated with moderate doses of exogenously administered interferons, and abnormalities of renal function tests are occasionally observed also.

Less commonly observed adverse effects of interferon have been reported. These effects have been observed generally in patients with severe underlying diseases who have been given large doses of parenterally administered interferons. These side effects include central nervous system (CNS) toxicity, consisting of lethargy, confusion, coma, psychomotor slowing, visual disorientation, and seizures. Also reported rarely are cardiac arrhythmias, hypotension, and renal failure.

### Clinical Uses

In recent years, improvements in tissue culture techniques, broad application of

DNA recombinant technology, and the subsequent development of highly purified products have led to the availability of large quantities of interferons for performance of clinical trials. Clinical trials of interferons have been performed for a variety of cancers, as well as infectious diseases. Because of their antiproliferative and broad spectrum antiviral activity, there was initially great optimism that interferons would produce beneficial effects in a wide variety of these disease processes. Although many well-conducted trials have subsequently failed to confirm this initial optimism, such studies have begun to delineate roles for the clinical use of these agents. The use of interferons for several different viral infections, including respiratory diseases, herpes virus infections, and hepatitis is discussed in other chapters in this book. Use of interferons for the treatment of papillomavirus infections and some malignancies is discussed below.

## HPV Infections

### Anogenital Warts

Different interferons, administered by different routes, have been evaluated in the treatment of some HPV infections, particularly anogenital warts. Initial studies suggested that interferon-α and interferon-β may be effective when administered topically (167–170). However, in a recently conducted, placebo-controlled evaluation of topically administered natural interferon-α in women, no beneficial effects of interferon, with or without nonoxynol-9, were demonstrated as compared to placebo (171). Discrepancies in results of reported studies of topically administered interferons for treatment of condyloma acuminatum may be a result of differences in study design or patient populations that have been evaluated. Alternatively, these preparations may not deliver adequate quantities of interferon to relevant cells in infected tissues.

In contrast to topical administration, administration of interferons intralesionally has been demonstrated definitively to be efficacious in the treatment of condyloma acuminatum. The four completed, placebo-controlled trials that have established the efficacy of intralesionally administered interferon in this setting are summarized in Table 4 (55–58,172). In two of the trials, a single wart was injected, whereas in the other investigations, multiple warts were injected with interferon or placebo. Multiple doses per week were administered in these studies, for periods of up to 8 weeks. Rates of complete resolution of interferon-injected warts were similar among the four studies, ranging from 36% to 62%. In all four trials, approximately 20% of placebo-injected lesions completely regressed. Side effects associated with administration of interferon were observed primarily in those studies in which multiple lesions were injected and correspondingly larger amounts of interferon were administered. Side effects consisted of an influenza-like syndrome, as well as decreases in white cell counts and slight elevations of liver enzymes. Pain on injection was frequently noted in these studies, but was brief and rarely severe.

All four of these studies employed interferon-α preparations as well as placebo. In one study, interferon-β was also utilized, as well as interferon-$\alpha_{n1}$ and interferon-$\alpha_{2b}$ (58). In this study, no differences in rates of complete lesion resolution were noted among the three interferon groups, and recipients of each interferon were significantly more likely to experience complete resolution of the injected lesion than were recipients of placebo. Also of interest in this study was the observation that among lesions that ultimately did not resolve, warts that were injected with interferon were significantly smaller than were placebo-injected lesions at weeks 4, 6, and 8 of study. This difference disappeared at week 10, suggesting that more prolonged therapy with interferon may produce higher rates of complete lesion regression. In most of the

**TABLE 4.** *Randomized, placebo-controlled trials of intralesionally administered interferons for the treatment of condyloma acuminatum*

| Author (reference) | Number of warts injected/patient | Treatment schedule and duration | Treatment arm | Interferon dose | Number of patients available for efficacy analysis | Complete response rates (%) | Dropouts due to adverse reactions interferon/placebo |
|---|---|---|---|---|---|---|---|
| Vance et al. (57) | 1 | 3×/week × 3 weeks | Interferon-$\alpha_{2b}$ | $10^6$ IU/wart | 30 | 53[a] | 1/1 |
| | | | Interferon-$\alpha_{2b}$ | $10^5$ IU/wart | 32 | 19 | |
| | | | Placebo | | 29 | 14 | |
| Eron et al. (55) | Up to 3 | 3×/week × 3 weeks | Interferon-$\alpha_{2b}$ | $10^6$ IU/wart | 125 | 36[b] | 11/2 |
| | | | Placebo | | 132 | 17 | |
| Friedman-Kien et al. (56) | All | 2×/week × 8 weeks | Interferon-α, natural | 2.5–5.0 × $10^5$ IU/25 $mm^2$ wart | 66 | 62[b] | 9/0 |
| | | | Placebo | | 66 | 21 | |
| Reichman et al. (58) | 1 | 3×/week × 4 weeks | Interferon-$\alpha_{2b}$ | $10^6$ IU/wart | 23 | | 0/1 |
| | | | Interferon-$\alpha_{n1}$ | $10^6$ IU/wart | 15 | 47[c] | |
| | | | Interferon-β | $10^6$ IU/wart | 20 | | |
| | | | Placebo | | 18 | 22 | |

[a]Significantly more recipients in the $10^6$ IU/wart group experienced complete resolution of the injected wart than did subjects in either the $10^5$ IU/wart group or the placebo group ($p < 0.01$ for each comparison).

[b]Significantly more interferon recipients experienced complete resolution of injected lesions than did placebo recipients ($p < 0.001$).

[c]Significantly more interferon recipients than placebo recipients experienced complete resolution of injected lesions ($p < 0.05$). Differences in rates of lesion resolution among the three interferon groups were not significant.

reported studies, insufficient follow-up was obtained to determine rates of recurrence in different treatment groups. However, in one study, nine of 26 interferon recipients experienced recurrence of disease compared to zero of four placebo recipients (58). In another, approximately 25% of patients who initially cleared their lesions subsequently developed recurrent disease regardless of initial form of treatment (56).

In a subset of 43 patients enrolled in one of these studies (58), patients were subdivided into two different categories according to histologic and virologic criteria (173). One category consisted of patients with "documented HPV infected" lesions, as determined by characteristic histopathology including koilocytosis and/or detection of papillomavirus antigens and/or nucleic acids in pretherapy biopsies. The other category consisted of patients whose biopsies were consistent with HPV infection, but which did not contain these characteristic features. Using this subclassification, patients with "HPV-infected lesions" were significantly more likely to respond to interferon than were patients whose biopsies did not meet these criteria.

In most studies, beneficial effects of interferon on noninjected lesions have not been observed. However, there was a suggestion of beneficial effects of interferon on noninjected lesions in one investigation (58). In this study, when the three interferon groups were combined and compared to placebo, survival analysis indicated a trend towards a greater rate of complete lesion resolution in the interferon group as compared to the placebo group. These effects could be mediated directly by circulating interferon or perhaps by triggering of host defense mechanisms.

Parenteral administration of interferons has also been evaluated for the treatment of condyloma acuminatum. Most of these investigations have utilized interferon-α preparations and have employed open, uncontrolled designs. An exception was one study that employed interferon-β compared to placebo (174). In this study, nine of 11 interferon recipients experienced complete resolution of all lesions compared to two of 11 patients in the placebo group. All patients were women with disease of relatively short duration. Diagnoses were not confirmed by histologic examination in all cases, and a cross-over design was used, prohibiting accurate determination of recurrence rates. The results of this study need to be confirmed in additional investigations.

Studies of parenterally administered interferon-α in the treatment of condyloma acuminatum have focused on patient populations with disease of long duration that has been refractory to conventional modes of treatment (175–178). Most of these studies have employed substantial doses of interferon and have been associated with significant toxicity. These side effects have included influenza-like syndromes, depression of white cell and platelet counts, and, less commonly, abnormalities of liver and kidney function. These adverse reactions, although reversible, have frequently necessitated dosage reductions. One of these investigations compared low and moderate dose regimens of interferon-$\alpha_{n1}$ (176). In this study, 30 women received 1 million units/$m^2$ daily for 2 weeks, followed by the same dose given three times per week for 4 more weeks. Twenty-seven additional women received 3 million units/$m^2$ in the same fashion. Although the moderate dose group experienced significantly greater rates of side effects and laboratory abnormalities than did the low dose group, efficacy rates between the two groups were similar. Thus, tolerable doses of interferon may produce beneficial effects comparable to those achieved with regimens that are poorly tolerated by patients with a nonmalignant disease.

Although most studies of parenterally administered interferons for the treatment of condyloma acuminatum have not been placebo-controlled, one recently conducted investigation compared interferon-$\alpha_{2a}$, interferon-$\alpha_{2b}$, and interferon-$\alpha_{n1}$ with placebo in the therapy of this common sexually transmitted disease (179). When the three interferon groups were combined and compared with the placebo group, no significant differences between the two were observed in rates of complete lesion resolution. However, statistically significant differences between interferon and placebo recipients were observed when smaller reductions in rates of decreases in lesion area were compared. In this study, women were more likely than men to experience complete resolution of lesions, regardless of therapy. No significant differences in rates of lesion resolution were observed among the three interferon groups. Interferon recipients in this study had more influenza-like symptoms and developed more decreases in white blood cell and platelet counts than did placebo recipients. However, rates of dropout did not differ between interferon and placebo groups, and decreases in interferon dosage were not required.

In a recently reported study, parenteral administration of interferon-$\gamma$ with and without cryotherapy was investigated (180). Twenty-eight patients with anogenital warts that were refractory to conventional therapy were enrolled in this study. Results suggested that regimens employing interferon with conventional modes of therapy should be evaluated in subsequent studies.

In summary, intralesionally administered interferons have been demonstrated to be more effective than intralesionally administered placebo in the treatment of anogenital warts. Approximately 50% of interferon-injected lesions resolve completely, compared to approximately 20% of placebo-injected lesions. Further studies will need to be conducted to determine the relapse rates associated with intralesionally administered interferon. Potential effects of intralesional administration on uninjected lesions also need to be clarified. Intralesionally administered recombinant-derived interferon-$\alpha_{2b}$ has been licensed recently by the Food and Drug Administration (FDA) for treatment of anogenital warts (181). In addition to the beneficial effects produced by intralesionally administered interferon-$\alpha$, parenteral administration of these preparations has been demonstrated to be at least partially effective in the treatment of condyloma acuminatum. Additional studies will need to be performed to determine optimal interferon preparations, routes of administration, and treatment regimens in the treatment of this disease.

### *Recurrent Respiratory Papillomatosis*

Several open, uncontrolled studies have suggested that interferons may be effective in the treatment of recurrent respiratory papillomatosis (182–184). One recently reported study evaluated the efficacy and toxicity of interferon-$\alpha$ plus surgery compared to surgery alone (185). One hundred and twenty-three patients were enrolled in this randomized, multicentered study. In the first 6 months of this 2-year investigation, patients who received interferon experienced significantly lower rates of papilloma growth than did placebo recipients. However, this beneficial effect was not sustained, and the authors concluded that interferon was neither curative nor of substantial value in the management of patients with this disease.

The mechanism of action of interferons in the treatment of HPV diseases is unclear. In one *in vitro* system, interferon was demonstrated to eradicate papillomavirus genomes from transformed tissue culture cells (186). However, attempts to detect an antiviral effect *in vivo* have produced contradictory results (187,188). Lesions associated with different HPV types may or may not respond differently to administration of exogenous interferons (188,189).

## **Malignancies**

Different interferon preparations have been evaluated in many studies designed to determine the efficacy and toxicity of these molecules in the treatment of several malignant diseases. Reviews of these studies have been published recently (190,191). These investigations have evaluated the use of interferons in the treatment of both hematologic and solid tumors.

### *Hematologic Malignancies*

Hairy cell leukemia is a malignant disease of B cells that is characterized clinically by pancytopenia, splenomegaly, the presence of characteristic cells in peripheral blood, and increased susceptibility to both bacterial and fungal infections. Splenectomy appears to produce an increased rate of survival, but the disease tends to progress and has been associated with a median survival of approximately 4 years (192). Several studies have indicated that administration of interferon-α is effective in the treatment of this disease, and these preparations have been licensed by the FDA for this indication (193–198). Development of antibodies to recombinant-derived products appears to be associated with the development of recurrent disease (199). Evaluation of interferon-β and interferon-γ preparations for the treatment of hairy cell leukemia is underway currently.

Chronic myelogenous leukemia (CML) is a hematopoetic cancer that affects stem cells as well as myeloid, monocytic, megakaryocytic, and erythroid cells (200). CML is characterized usually by an initial indolent course of approximately 3 years' duration, followed by a rapid acceleration that results in death in 3–6 months (201). Reductions in total white cell counts, as well as decreases in platelet counts, have been observed in patients treated with interferon-α preparations (202–205).

Several clinical trials have suggested strongly that interferons produce beneficial effects in the treatment of multiple myeloma (206–210). Other hematologic malignancies that may be affected favorably by interferon treatment include cutaneous T-cell lymphomas (211), non-Hodgkin's lymphomas (212,213), and chronic lymphocytic leukemia.

### *Solid Tumors*

Several studies have suggested that different interferon preparations may be effective in the treatment of malignant melanoma (214–218). Results that have been observed are similar to results associated with administration of traditional chemotherapeutic agents.

The poor results associated with endocrine and chemotherapy of metastatic renal cell carcinoma have made this disease a candidate for treatment with alternative forms of therapy (219). Promising results, although usually associated with response rates of less than 50%, have been obtained with interferon therapy (220–225).

Other solid tumors in which administration of interferon preparations has been associated with beneficial effects include breast carcinoma (226–229), Kaposi's sarcoma in the setting of acquired immunodeficiency syndromes (AIDS) produced by HIV infection (230,231), ovarian carcinoma (232–236), carcinoid (237,238), bladder cancer (239), nasopharyngeal carcinoma (240), and cervical carcinoma (241).

## REFERENCES

1. Goldschmidt H, Klingman AM. Experimental inoculation of humans with ectodermotropic viruses. *J Invest Dermatol* 1958;31:175–82.
2. Ciuffo G. Imnesto positivo con filtrato di verruca volgare. *Giorn ital Mal Venereol* 1907;48:12–7.
3. Shope RE. Immunization of rabbits to infectious papillomatosis. *J Exp Med* 1937;68: 219–31.
4. Broker TR. Structure and genetic expression of papillomaviruses. *Obstet Gynecol Clin North Am* 1987;14:329–48.
5. Syrjanen K, Gissmann L, Koss LG. *Papillomaviruses and human disease*. Berlin: Springer Verlag, 1987.
6. Melnick JL, Allison AC, Butel JS, et al. Papoviridae. *Intervirology* 1974;3:106–20.

7. Shah KV. Papoviruses. In: Fields BN, Knipe DM, Chanock RM, Melnick JL, Roizman B, Shope RE, eds. *Virology*. New York: Raven Press, 1985:371–91.
8. Amtmann E, Sauer G. Bovine papilloma virus transcription: polyadenylated RNA species and assessment of the direction of transcription. *J Virol* 1982;43:59–66.
9. Engel LW, Heilman CA, Howley PM. Transcriptional organization of the bovine papillomavirus type 1. *J Virol* 1983;47:516–28.
10. Heilman CA, Engel L, Lowy DR, et al. Virus-specific transcription in bovine papillomavirus-transformed mouse cells. *Virology* 1982; 119:22–34.
11. Lambert PF, Baker CC, Howley PM. The genetics of bovine papillomavirus type 1. *Annu Rev Genetics* 1988;22:235–58.
12. Meischke HRC. *In vitro* transformation by bovine papilloma virus. *J Gen Virol* 1979;43: 473–87.
13. Dvoretzky I, Shober R, Chattopadhyay SK, et al. A quantitative *in vitro* focus assay for bovine papilloma virus. *Virology* 1980;103:369–75.
14. Kreider JW, Howett MK, Leure-Dupree AE, et al. Laboratory production *in vivo* of infectious human papillomavirus type 11. *J Virol* 1987; 61:590–3.
15. Brown DR, Chin MT, Strike DG. Identification of human papillomavirus type 11 E4 gene products in human tissue implants from athymic mice. *Virol* 1988;165:262–7.
16. Jenison SA, Firzlaff JM, Langenberg A, et al. Identification of immunoreactive antigens of human papillomavirus type 6b by using *Escherichia coli*-expressed fusion proteins. *J Virol* 1988;62:2115–23.
17. Strike DG, Bonnez W, Rose R, et al. Expression in *Escherichia coli* of seven DNA segments comprising the complete L1 and L2 open reading frames of human papillomavirus type 6b and localization of the "common antigen" region. *J Gen Virol* 1989;70:543–55.
18. Schiller JT, Vass WC, Lowy DR. Identification of a second transforming region in bovine papillomavirus DNA. *Proc Natl Acad Sci USA* 1984;81:7880–4.
19. Schiller JT, Vass WC, Vousdan KH, et al. The E5 open reading frame of bovine papillomavirus type 1 encodes a transforming gene. *J Virol* 1986;57:1–6.
20. Yang Y-C, Okayama H, Howley PM. Bovine papillomavirus contains multiple transforming genes. *Proc Natl Acad Sci USA* 1985;82: 1030–4.
21. Yang Y-C, Spalholz BA, Rabson MS, et al. Dissociation of transforming and transactivating functions for bovine papillomavirus type 1. *Nature* 1985;318:575–7.
22. Lusky M, Botchan MR. Genetic analysis of bovine papillomavirus type 1 transacting replication factors. *J Virol* 1985;53:955–65.
23. Sarver N, Rabson MS, Yang YC, et al. Localization and analysis of bovine papillomavirus type 1 transforming functions. *J Virol* 1984; 52:377–88.
24. Rabson MS, Yee C, Yang Y-C, et al. Bovine papillomavirus type 1 3′ early region transformation and plasmid maintenance functions. *J Virol* 1986;60:626–34.
25. Lusky M, Botchan MR. A bovine papillomavirus type 1-encoded modulator function is dispensable for transient viral replication but is required for establishment of the stable plasmid state. *J Virol* 1986;60:729–42.
26. Spalholz BA, Yang Y-C, Howley PM. Transactivation of a bovine papillomavirus transcriptional regulatory element by the E2 gene product. *Cell* 1985;42:183–91.
27. DiMaio D, Settleman J. Bovine papillomavirus mutant temperature sensitive for transformation, replication and transactivation. *EMBO J,* 1988;7:1197–204.
28. Hermonat PL, Howley PM. Mutational analysis of the 3′ open reading frames and the splice junction at nucleotide 3225 of bovine papillomavirus type 1. *J Virol* 1987;61:3889–95.
29. Neary K, Horwitz BH, DiMaio D. Mutational analysis of open reading frame E4 of bovine papillomavirus type 1. *J Virol* 1987;61:1248–52.
30. Doorbar J, Campbell D, Grand RJA, et al. Identification of the human papilloma virus-1a E4 gene products. *EMBO J* 1986;5:355–62.
31. Chow LT, Hirochika H, Nasseri M, et al. Human papillomavirus gene expression. In: Steinberg BM, Brandsma JL, Taichman LB, eds. *Cancer cells. 5. Papillomaviruses*. Cold Spring Harbor, New York: Cold Spring Harbor Press, 1987:57–71.
32. Orth G, Breitburd F, Favre M. Papillomavirus: possible role in human cancer. In: Hiatt HH, Watson JD, Winsten JA, eds. *Origins of human cancer*. Cold Spring Harbor, New York: Cold Spring Harbor Press, 1977:1043–68.
33. Stoler MH, Broker TR. *In situ* hybridization detection of human papilloma virus DNA and messenger RNA in genital condylomas and a cervical carcinoma. *Human Pathol* 1986; 17:1250–8.
34. Howley PM. The molecular biology of papillomavirus transformation: Warner-Lambert Parke-Davis award lecture. *Am J Pathol* 1983; 113:413–21.
35. Komly CA, Breitburd F, Croissant O, et al. The L2 open reading frame of human papillomavirus type 1a encodes a minor structural protein carrying type-specific antigens. *J Virol* 1986;60:13.
36. Grussendorf-Conen E-I. Papillomavirus-induced tumors of the skin: Cutaneous warts and epidermodysplasia verruciformis. In: Syrjanen K, Gissmann L, Koss LG, eds. *Papillomaviruses and human disease*. Berlin: Springer Verlag, 1987:158–81.
37. Jablonska S, Orth G, Obalek S, et al. Cutaneous warts. Clinical, histologic, and virologic correlations. *Clin Dermatol* 1985;3:71–82.
38. Massing AM, Epstein WL. Natural history of

warts. A two year study. *Arch Dermatol* 1963;87:306–10.

39. Lutzner MA, Blanchet-Bardon C. Epidermodysplasia verruciformis. *Curr Probl Dermatol* 1985;13:164–85.
40. Oriel JD. Natural history of genital warts. *Br J Vener Dis* 1971;47:1–13.
41. von Krogh G. Podophyllotoxin for condylomata acuminata eradication. Clinical and experimental comparative studies on Podophyllum lignans, colchicine and 5-fluorouracil. *Acta Derm Venereol (Stockh)* 1981;suppl 98:1–48.
42. Chuang T-Y, Perry HO, Kurland LT, et al. Condyloma acuminatum in Rochester, Minn., 1950–1978 (parts I and II). *Arch Dermatol* 1984;120:469–83.
43. Rosemberg SK, Jacobs H, Fuller T. Some guidelines in the treatment of urethral condylomata with carbon dioxide laser. *J Urol* 1982;127:906–8.
44. Sand PK, Bowen LW, Blischke SO, et al. Evaluation of male consorts of women with genital human papilloma virus infection. *Obstet Gynecol* 1986;68:679–81.
45. de Benedictis JT, Marmar JL, Praiss DE. Intraurethral condylomata acuminata: management and a review of the literature. *J Urol* 1977;118:767–9.
46. Masse S, Tosi-Kruse A, Carmel M, et al. Condyloma acuminatum of the bladder. *Urology* 1981;17:381–2.
47. Goorney BP, Waugh MA, Clarke J. Anal warts in heterosexual men. *Genitourin Med* 1987; 63:216.
48. Oriel JD. Anal warts and anal coitus. *Br J Vener Dis* 1971;47:373–6.
49. Reid R, Laverty CR, Coppleson M, et al. Noncondylomatous cervical wart virus infection. *Obstet Gynecol* 1980;55:476–83.
50. Walker PG, Colley NV, Grubb C, et al. Abnormalities of the uterine cervix in women with vulvar warts. *Br J Vener Dis* 1983;59:120–3.
51. Growdon WA, Fu YS, Lebherz TB, et al. Pruritic vulvar squamous papillomatosis. Evidence for human papillomavirus etiology. *Obstet Gynecol* 1985;66:564–8.
52. Manoharan V, Sommerville JM. Benign squamous papillomatosis: case report. *Genitourin Med* 1987;63:393–5.
53. McCance DJ, Singer A. The importance of HPV infections in the male and female genital tract and their relationship to cervical neoplasia. In: Peto R, zur Hausen H, eds. *Viral etiology of cervical cancer. Banbury report 21.* New York: Cold Spring Harbor Laboratory, 1986:311–9.
54. Barrasso R, de Brux J, Croissant O, et al. High prevalence of papillomavirus-associated penile intraepithelial neoplasia in sexual partners of women with cervical intraepithelial neoplasia. *N Engl J Med* 1987;317:916–23.
55. Eron LJ, Judson F, Tucker S, et al. Interferon therapy for condylomata acuminata. *N Engl J Med* 1986;315:1059–64.
56. Friedman-Kien A, Eron LJ, Conant M, et al. Natural interferon alpha for the treatment of condylomata acuminata. *JAMA* 1988;259: 533–8.
57. Vance JC, Bart BJ, Hansen RC, et al. Intralesional recombinant alpha-2 interferon for the treatment of patients with condyloma acuminatum or verruca plantaris. *Arch Dermatol* 1986;122:272–7.
58. Reichman RC, Oakes D, Bonnez W, et al. Treatment of condyloma acuminatum with three different interferons administered intralesionally. A double-blind, placebo-controlled trial. *Ann Intern Med* 1988;108:675–9.
59. Shafeek MA, Osman MI, Hussein MA. Carcinoma of the vulva arising in condylomata acuminata. *Obstet Gynecol* 1979;54:120–3.
60. Gorthey RL, Krembs MA. Vulvar condylomata acuminata complicating labor. *Obstet Gynecol* 1954;4:67–74.
61. Young RL, Acosta AA, Kaufman RH. The treatment of large condylomata acuminata complicating pregnancy. *Obstet Gynecol* 1973; 41:65–73.
62. Frazer IH, Crapper RM, Meddley G, et al. Association between anorectal dysplasia, human papillomavirus, and human immunodeficiency virus infection in homosexual men. *Lancet* 1986;2:657–60.
63. Gal AA, Meyer PR, Taylor CR. Papillomavirus antigens in anorectal condyloma and carcinoma in homosexual men. *JAMA* 1987;257:337–40.
64. Nash G, Allen W, Nash S. Atypical lesions of the anal mucosa in homosexual men. *JAMA* 1986;256:873–6.
65. Mounts P, Shah KV. Respiratory papillomatosis: etiological relation to genital tract papillomaviruses. *Prog Med Virol* 1984;29:90–114.
66. Kashima HK, Shah K. Recurrent respiratory papillomatosis. Clinical overview and management principles. *Obstet Gynecol Clin North Am* 1987;14:581–8.
67. Steinberg BM, Abramson AL. Laryngeal papillomas. *Clin Dermatol* 1985;3:130–8.
68. Kashima H, Mounts P. Tumors of the head and neck, larynx, lung and esophagus and their possible relation to HPV. In: Syrjanen K, Gissman L, Koss LG, eds. *Papillomaviruses and human disease.* Berlin: Springer Verlag, 1987:138–57.
69. Syrjanen SM. Human papillomavirus infections in the oral cavity. In: Syrjanen K, Gissmann L, Koss LG, eds. *Papillomaviruses and human disease.* Berlin: Springer Verlag, 1987:104–37.
70. Lass JH, Grove AS, Papale JJ, et al. Detection of human papillomavirus DNA sequences in conjunctival papilloma. *Am J Ophthalmol* 1983;96:670–4.
71. Schuster DS. Snorter's warts. *Arch Dermatol* 1987;123:571.
72. Barrett TJ, Silbar JD, McGinley JP. Genital warts—a venereal disease. *JAMA* 1954; 154:333–4.
73. Jenson AB, Kurman RJ, Lancaster WD. Tissue effects of and host response to human papillomavirus infection. In: Reid R, ed. *Obstetrics*

*and gynecology clinics of North America, vol. 14.* Philadelphia: WB Saunders Company, 1987:397–406.
74. Ferenczy A, Mitao M, Nagai N, et al. Latent papillomavirus and recurring genital warts. *N Engl J Med* 1985;313:784–8.
75. Steinberg BM, Gallagher T, Stoler M, et al. Persistence and expression of human papillomavirus during interferon therapy. *Arch Otolaryngol Head Neck Surg* 1988;114:27–32.
76. Howley PM. The role of papillomaviruses in human cancer. In: de Vita V, Hellman S, Rosenberg SA, eds. *Important advances in oncology, 1987.* Philadelphia: J. B. Lippincott Co., 1987:55–73.
77. Kirchner H. Immunobiology of human papillomavirus infection. *Prog Med Virol* 1986;33: 1–41.
78. Matis WL, Triana A, Shapiro R, et al. Dermatologic findings associated with human immunodeficiency virus infection. *J Am Acad Dermatol* 1987;17:746–51.
79. Boyle J, Briggs JD, Mackie RM, et al. Cancer, warts, and sunshine in renal transplant patients. A case-control study. *Lancet* 1986;1:702–5.
80. Rudlinger RM, Smith IW, Bunney MH, et al. Human papillomavirus infections in a group of renal transplant recipients. *Br J Dermatol* 1986;115:681–92.
81. Oguchi M, Komura J, Tagami H, et al. Ultrastructural studies of spontaneously regressing plane warts. Macrophages attack verruca-epidermal cells. *Arch Dermatol Res* 1981;270: 403–11.
82. Koutsky LA, Galloway DA, Holmes KK. Epidemiology of genital human papillomavirus infection. *Epidemiol Rev* 1988;10:122–63.
83. Reichman RC, Bonnez W. Papillomaviruses. In: Mandell GL, Douglas RG Jr, Bennett JE, eds. *Principles and practice of infectious diseases.* 3rd ed. New York: John Wiley & Sons, 1990;1191–200.
84. DePeuter M, DeClercq B, Minette A, et al. An epidemiological survey of virus warts of the hands among butchers. *Br J Dermatol* 1977;96:427–31.
85. Jennings LC, Ross AD, Faoagali JL. The prevalance of warts on the hands of workers in a New Zealand slaughterhouse. *N Z Med J* 1984;97:473–6.
86. Rudlinger R, Bunney MH, Grob R, et al. Warts in fishhandlers. *Br J Dermatol* 1989;120:375–81.
87. Taylor SWC. A prevalence of warts on the hands in a poultry processing and packing station. *J Soc Occup Med* 1980;30:20–3.
88. Becker TM, Blount JF, Guinan ME. Trends in genital herpes infections among private practitioners in the United States, 1966–1981. *JAMA* 1985;253:1601–3.
89. Becker TM. Genital human papillomavirus infection: an epidemiological perspective. In: Norrby SR, ed. *New Antiviral Strategies.* London: Churchill Livingstone, 1988;44–9.
90. U.S. Department of Health and Human Services. *Sexually transmitted disease statistics, 1985. Issue no. 135.* Atlanta, Georgia: Public Health Service, 1987.
91. Chief Medical Officer of the Department of Health and Social Security for the year 1983. Extract from the annual report. Sexually transmitted diseases. *Genitourin Med* 1985;61: 204–7.
92. deVilliers E-M, Schneider A, Miklaw H, et al. Human papillomavirus infections in women with and without abnormal cytology. *Lancet* 1987;2:703–6.
93. Ludwig ME, Lowell DM, LiVolsi VA. Cervical condylomatous atypia and its relationship to cervical neoplasia. *Am J Clin Pathol* 1981;76:255–62.
94. Meisels A, Fortin R, Roy M. Condylomatous lesions of the cervix. II. Cytologic, colposcopic, and histopathologic study. *Acta Cytol* 1977;21:379–90.
95. Garrido JL. Pathological incidence study of human papilloma virus (HPV) carried out on 1,439 patients between 1982–1985 in Panama. *Eur J Gynaecol Oncol* 1988;9:144–148.
96. Venereal Disease Control Division, Bureau of State Services, CDC. Current trends: nonreported sexually transmissible diseases-United States. *MMWR* 1979;28:61–3.
97. Lacey CJN, Mulcahy FM, Sutton J. Koilocyte frequency and prevalence of cervical human papillomavirus infection. *Lancet* 1986;1:557–8.
98. Armstrong BK, Allen OV, Brennan BA, et al. Time trends in prevalence of cervical cytological abnormality in women attending a sexually transmitted diseases clinic and their relationship to trends in sexual activity and specific infections. *Br J Cancer* 1986;54:669–75.
99. Meisels A, Morin C. Human papillomavirus and cancer of the uterine cervix. *Gynecol Oncol* 1981;12:S111–23.
100. Drake M, Mitchell H, Medley G. Human papillomavirus infection of the cervix in Victoria, 1982–1985. *Med J Aust* 1987;147:57–9.
101. Rowson KEK, Mahy BWJ. Human papova (wart) virus. *Bacteriol Rev* 1967;31:110–31.
102. Campion MJ, Singer A, Clarkson PK, et al. Increased risk of cervical neoplasia in consorts of men with penile condylomata acuminata. *Lancet* 1985;1:943–6.
103. Munoz N, Bosch X, Kaldor JM. Does human papillomavirus cause cervical cancer? The state of the epidemiological evidence. *Br J Cancer* 1988;57:1–5.
104. Franchesci S, Doll R, Gallwey J, et al. Genital warts and cervical neoplasm: an epidemiological study. *Br J Cancer* 1983;48:621–8.
105. Graham S, Priore R, Graham M, et al. Genital cancer in wives of penile cancer patients. *Cancer* 1979;44:1870–4.
106. Fraumeni JF, Lloyd JM, Smith EM, et al. Cancer mortality among nuns: role of the marital status in etiology of neoplastic disease in women. *JNCI* 1969;42:455–68.

107. zur Hausen H. Genital papillomavirus infections. *Prog Med Virol* 1985;32:15–21.
108. Gissmann L, Durst M, Oltersdorf T, et al. Human papillomaviruses and cervical cancer. In: Steinberg BM, Brandsma JL, Taichman LB, eds. *Cancer cells, vol. 5*. Cold Spring Harbor, New York: Cold Spring Harbor Laboratory, 1987:275–80.
109. Pirisi L, Yasumoto S, Feller M, et al. Transformation of human fibroblasts and keratinocytes with human papillomavirus type 16 DNA. *J Virology* 1987;61:1061–6.
110. McCance DJ, Kopan R, Fuchs E, et al. Human papillomavirus type 16 alters human epithelial cell differentiation *in vitro*. *Proc Natl Acad Sci USA* 1988;85:7169–73.
111. Sedlacek TV, Cunnane M, Carpiniello V. Colposcopy in the diagnosis of penile condyloma. *Am J Obstet Gynecol* 1986;154:494–6.
112. Krebs H-B, Schneider V. Human papillomavirus-associated lesions of the penis: colposcopy, cytology, and histology. *Obstet Gynecol* 1987;70:299–304.
113. Singer A, Campion MJ, Clarkson PK, et al. Recognition of subclinical human papillomavirus infection of the vulva. *J Reprod Med* 1986;31:985–6.
114. Saigo PE. Cytology of the uterine cervix. *Semin Diagn Pathol* 1986;3:204–10.
115. Purola E, Savia E. Cytology of gynecologic condyloma acuminatum. *Acta Cytol* 1977; 21:26–31.
116. Syrjanen KJ, Heinonen U-M, Kauraniemi T. Cytologic evidence of the association of condylomatous lesions with dysplastic and neoplastic changes in the uterine cervix. *Acta Cytol* 1981;25:17–22.
117. Jenson AB, Kurman RJ, Lancaster WD. Detection of papillomavirus common antigens in lesions of skin and mucosa. *Clin Dermatol* 1985;3:56–63.
118. Wilbur DC, Reichman RC, Stoler MH. Detection of infection by human papillomavirus in genital condylomata. A comparison study using immunocytochemistry and *in situ* nucleic acid hybridization. *Am J Clin Path* 1988;89:505–10.
119. Schneider A. Methods of identification of human papillomaviruses. In: Syrjanen K, Gissmann L, Koss LG, eds. *Papillomaviruses and human disease*. Berlin: Springer Verlag, 1987:19–39.
120. Shibata DK, Arnheim N, Martin WJ. Detection of human papilloma virus in paraffin-embedded tissue using the polymerase chain reaction. *J Exp Med* 1988;167:225–30.
121. Douglas JM Jr, Rogers M, Judson FN. The effect of asymptomatic infection with HTLV-III on the response of anogenital warts to intralesional treatment with recombinant alpha-2 interferon. *J Infect Dis* 1986;154:331–4.
122. Bunney MH, Nolan MW, William DA. An assessment of methods of treating viral warts by comparative treatment trials based on a standard design. *Br J Dermatol* 1976;94:667–9.
123. Bunney MH. *Viral warts: their biology and treatment*. Oxford: Oxford University Press, 1982.
124. Rees RB. The treatment of warts. *Clin Dermatol* 1985;3:179–84.
125. 1985 STD treatment guidelines. *Morbid Mortal Week Rep* 1985;34(suppl 4S):335–605.
126. Godley MJ, Bradbeer CS, Gellan M, et al. Cryotherapy compared with trichloracetic acid in treating genital warts. *Genitourin Med* 1987;63:390–2.
127. Bashi SA. Cryotherapy versus podophyllin in the treatment of genital warts. *Int J Dermatol* 1985;24:535–6.
128. Matsunaga J, Bergman A, Bhatia NN. Genital condylomata acuminata in pregnancy: effectiveness, safety and pregnancy outcome following cryotherapy. *Br J Obstet Gynaecol* 1987;94:168–72.
129. Miller RA. Podophyllin. *Int J Dermatol* 1985; 24:491–8.
130. Simmons PD. Podophyllin 10% and 25% in the treatment of ano-genital warts. A comparative double-blind study. *Br J Venereol Dis* 1981;57:208–9.
131. Beutner KR. Podophyllotoxin in the treatment of genital human papillomavirus infection: a review. *Semin Dermatol* 1987;6:10–8.
132. Dretler SP, Klein LA. The eradication of intraurethral condyloma acuminata with 5 per cent 5-fluorouracil cream. *J Urol* 1975;113: 195–8.
133. Wallin J. 5-Fluorouracil in the treatment of penile and urethral condylomata acuminata. *Br J Venereol Dis* 1977;53:240–3.
134. Krebs H-B. Prophylactic topical 5-fluorouracil following treatment of human papillomavirus-associated lesions of the vulva and vagina. *Obstet Gynecol* 1986;68:837–41.
135. Richart RM, Kaufman RM, Woodruff JD. Advances in managing condylomas. *Contemp OB/GYN* 1982;20:1641–93.
136. Jensen SL. Comparison of podophyllin application with simple surgical excision in clearance and recurrence of perianal condylomata acuminata. *Lancet* 1985;2:1146–8.
137. McMillan A, Scott GR. Outpatient treatment of perianal warts by scissor excision. *Genitourin Med* 1987;63:114–5.
138. Simmons PD, Langlet F, Thin RNT. Cryotherapy versus electrocautery in the treatment of genital warts. *Br J Vener Dis* 1981;57:273–4.
139. Baggish MS. Improved laser techniques for the elimination of genital and extragenital warts. *Am J Obstet Gynecol* 1985;153:545–50.
140. Fuselier HA, McBurney EI, Brannan W, et al. Treatment of condylomata acuminata with carbon dioxide laser. *Urology* 1980;15:265–6.
141. Reid R. Physical and surgical principles governing expertise with the carbon dioxide laser. *Obstet Gynecol Clin North Am* 1987;14:513–35.
142. Duus BR, Philipsen T, Christensen JD, et al. Refractory condylomata acuminata: a controlled clinical trial of carbon dioxide laser versus conventional surgical treatment. *Genitourin Med* 1985;61:59–61.

143. Bekassy Z, Westrom L. Infrared coagulation in the treatment of condyloma acuminata in the female genital tract. *Sex Transm Dis* 1987; 14:209–12.
144. Ng N, Vuignier BI, Hart LL. Fluorouracil in condyloma acuminatum. *Drug Intell Clin Pharm* 1987;21:175–6.
145. Sand PK, Shen W, Bowen LW, et al. Cryotherapy for the treatment of proximal urethral condyloma acuminatum. *J Urol* 1987;137: 874–6.
146. Halverstadt DB, Parry WL. Thiotepa in the management of intraurethral condylomata acuminata. *J Urol* 1969;101:729–31.
147. Gigax JH, Robison JR. The successful treatment of intraurethral condyloma acuminata with colchicine. *J Urol* 1971;105:809–11.
148. Dodi G, Infantino A, Moretti R, et al. Cryotherapy of anorectal warts and condylomata. *Cryosurgery* 1982;19:287–8.
149. Billingham RP, Lewis RG. Laser versus electrical cautery in the treatment of condylomata acuminata of the anus. *Surg Gynecol Obstet* 1982;155:865–7.
150. Krebs HB. Treatment of vaginal condylomata acuminata by weekly topical application of 5-fluorouracil. *Obstet Gynecol* 1987;70:68–71.
151. Ferenczy A. Treating genital condyloma during pregnancy with the carbon dioxide laser. *Am J Obstet Gynecol* 1984;148:9–12.
152. Wertheimer A. Indirect colposcopy and laser vaporization in the management of vaginal condylomata. *J Reprod Med* 1986;31:39–42.
153. Syrjanen K, Vayrynen M, Castren O, et al. Sexual behaviour of women with human papillomavirus (HPV) lesions of the uterine cervix. *Br J Venereol Dis* 1984;60:243–8.
154. Richardson AC, Lyon JB. The effect of condom use on squamous cell cervical intraepithelial neoplasia. *Am J Obstet Gynecol* 1981;140: 909–13.
155. Schreier AA, Allen WP, Laughlin C, et al. Prospects for human papillomavirus vaccines and immunotherapies. *JNCI* 1988;80:896–9.
156. Mannering GJ, Deloria LB. The pharmacology and toxicology of the interferons: an overview. *Annu Rev Pharmacol Toxicol* 1986;26:455–515.
157. Bino T, Edery H, Gertler A, et al. Involvement of the kidney in catabolism of human leukocyte interferon. *J Gen Virol* 1982;59:39–45.
158. Bocci V. Evaluation of routes of administration of interferon in cancer: a review and a proposal. *Cancer Drug Delivery* 1984;1:337–51.
159. Billiau A, Heremans H, Ververken D, et al. Tissue distribution of human interferons after exogenous administration in rabbits, monkeys, and mice. *Arch Virol* 1981;68:19–25.
160. Bocci V, Pacini A, Bandienelli L, et al. The role of the liver in the catabolism of human alpha and beta interferon. *J Gen Virol* 1982;60:397–400.
161. Abreau SL. Pharmacokinetics of rat fibroblast interferon. *J Pharmacol Exp Ther* 1983; 226:197–200.
162. Cantell K, Fiers W, Hirvonen S, et al. Circulating interferon in rabbits after simultaneous intramuscular administration of human alpha and gamma interferons. *J Interferon Res* 1984;4:291–3.
163. Gutterman JU, Rosenblum MG, Rios A, et al. Pharmacokinetic study of partially pure gamma interferon in cancer patients. *Cancer Res* 1984;44:4164–71.
164. Satoh YL, Kasama K, Kajita A, et al. Different pharmacokinetics between natural and recombinant human interferon beta in rabbits. *J Interferon Res* 1984;4:411–22.
165. Bocci V, Pacini A, Pessina GP, et al. Catabolic sites of human interferon gamma. *J Gen Virol* 1985;66:887–91.
166. Lucero MA, Magdelenat H, Fridman WH, et al. Comparison of effects of leukocyte and fibroblast interferon on immunological parameters in cancer patients. *Eur J Cancer Clin Oncol* 1982;18:243–51.
167. Ikic D, Bosnie N, Smerdel S, et al. Double-blind clinical study with human leukocyte interferon in the therapy of condyloma acuminata. In: *Proceedings of the Symposium on Clinical Use of Interferon*. Zagreb, Yugoslavia: Yugoslav Academy of Sciences and Arts, 1975:229–33.
168. Ikic D, Brnobic A, Jurkovic-Vukelicv V, et al. Therapeutic effect of human leukocyte interferon incorporated into ointment and cream on condyloma acuminata. In: *Proceedings of the Symposium on Clinical Use of Interferon*. Zagreb, Yugoslavia: Yugoslav Academy of Sciences and Arts, 1975:235–238.
169. Vesterinen E, Meyer B, Purola E, et al. Treatment of vaginal flat condyloma with interferon cream. *Lancet* 1984;1:157.
170. Vesterinen E, Meyer B, Cantell K, et al. Topical treatment of flat vaginal condyloma with human leukocyte interferon. *Obstet Gynecol* 1984;64:535–8.
171. Keay S, Teng N, Eisenberg M, et al. Topical interferon for treating condyloma acuminata in women. *J Infect Dis* 1988;158:934–9.
172. Reichman RC, Bonnez W. Intralesional interferons in the treatment of condyloma acuminatum. In: Mills J, Corey L, eds. *Antiviral chemotherapy*. 2nd ed. New York: Elsevier, 1989;143–9.
173. Reichman RC, Stoler MH, Oakes D. Human papillomaviruses and treatment of condyloma acuminatum with intralesionally administered interferon. In: Norrby SR, ed. *New antiviral strategies*. London: Churchill Livingston, 1988: 36–43.
174. Schonfeld A, Nitke S, Schattner A, et al. Intramuscular human interferon-beta injections in treatment of condylomata acuminata. *Lancet* 1984;1:1038–42.
175. Alawattegama AB, Kinghorn GR. Human lymphoblastoid interferon in genital warts. *Lancet* 1984;1:1468.
176. Reichman RC, Micha JP, Weck PK, et al. In-

terferon alpha-n1 for refractory genital warts: efficacy and tolerance of low dose systemic therapy. *Antiviral Res* 1988;10:41–57.

177. Gall SA, Hughes CE, Mounts P, et al. The efficacy of human lymphoblastoid interferon (Wellferon) in the therapy of resistant condyloma acuminata. *Obstet Gynecol* 1986;67:643–51.
178. Trofatter KF, Olsen EA, Kucera PK, et al. Combination of non-steroidal anti-inflammatory drug and Wellferon: a controlled clinical trial in genital warts. In: Scheliekens H, Stewart WA, eds. *The biology of the interferon system*. Amsterdam: Elsevier, 1985.
179. Reichman RC, Farchione A, Whitley R, et al. A placebo-controlled trial of three different interferon preparations administered parenterally for condyloma acuminatum [Abstract]. In: *Program and abstracts, 28th Interscience Conference on Antimicrobial Agents and Chemotherapy*. Washington, D.C.: American Society for Microbiology, 1988:365.
180. Kirby PK, Kiviat N, Beckman A, et al. Tolerance and efficacy of recombinant human interferon gamma in the treatment of refractory genital warts. *Am J Med* 1988;85:183–8.
181. Interferon for treatment of genital warts. *The Medical Letter*. 1988;30:70–2.
182. Lusk RP, McCabe BR, Clark KF. Interferon and laryngeal papillomatosis: a follow-up of the Iowa experience. In: Zoon KC, Noguchi PD, Liu T-Y, eds. *Interferon: research, clinical application and regulatory considerations*. New York: Elsevier, 1984:169–79.
183. Goepfert H, Sessions RB, Gutterman J, et al. Leukocyte interferon in patients with juvenile laryngeal papillomatosis. *Ann Otol Rhinol Laryngol* 1982;91:431–6.
184. McCabe BF, Clark KF. Interferon and laryngeal papillomatosis: the Iowa experience. *Ann Otol Rhinol Laryngol* 1983;92:2–7.
185. Healy G, Gelber RD, Trowbridge AL, et al. Treatment of recurrent respiratory papillomatosis with human leukocyte interferon. *N Engl J Med* 1988;319:401–7.
186. Turek LP, Byrne JC, Lowy DR, et al. Interferon induces morphologic reversion with elimination of extrachromosomal viral genomes in bovine papillomavirus-transformed mouse cells. *Proc Natl Acad Sci USA* 1982;79:7914–8.
187. Androphy EJ, Dvoretzky I, Maluish AE, et al. Response of warts in epidermodysplasia verruciformis to treatment with systemic and intralesional alpha interferon. *J Am Acad Dermatol* 1984;11:197–202.
188. Steinberg BM, Gallagher T, Stoler MJH, et al. Relationship between human papillomavirus types in laryngeal papillomatosis and response to interferon-alpha. In: Steinberg BM, Brandsma JL, Taichman LB, eds. *Papillomaviruses*. Cold Spring Harbor, New York: Cold Spring Harbor Laboratory Press, 1987:403–9.
189. Schneider A, Papendick U, Gissmann L, et al. Interferon treatment of human genital papillomavirus infection: importance of viral type. *Int J Cancer* 1987;40:610–4.
190. Borden EC. Effects of interferons on neoplastic diseases of man. *Pharmacol Ther* 1988;37:213–29.
191. Ozer H, Golomb HM. Introduction. *Semin Oncol* 1988;15(suppl 5):1.
192. Golde DW. Therapy of hairy cell leukemia. *N Engl J Med* 1982;307:495–6.
193. Ouesada JR, Reuben J, Manning JT, et al. Alpha interferon for induction of remission in hairy-cell leukemia. *N Engl J Med* 1984; 310:15–8.
194. Ratain MJ, Golomb HM, Vardiman JW, et al. Treatment of hairy cell leukemia with recombinant alpha-2 interferon. *Blood* 1985;65:644–8.
195. Flandrin H, Sigaux F, Castaigne S, et al. Quantitative analysis by bone marrow changes during treatment of hairy cell leukemia with interferon alpha. *Cancer Treat Rep* 1985;12B:17–22.
196. Naeim F, Jacobs AD. Bone marrow changes in patients with hairy cell leukemia treated by recombinant alpha-2 interferon. *Human Pathol* 1985;16:1200–5.
197. Hofmann V, Fehr J, Sauter C, et al. Hairy cell leukemia: an interferon deficient disease? *Cancer Treat Rev* 1985;12B:33–7.
198. Golomb HM, Fefer A, Golde DW, et al. Report of a multi-institutional study of 193 patients with hairy cell leukemia treated with interferon-alpha2b. *Semin Oncol* 1988;15(suppl 5): 7–9.
199. Steis RG, Smith JW, Urba WJ, et al. Resistance to recombinant interferon alpha-2a in hairy-cell leukemia associated with neutralizing anti-interferon antibodies. *N Engl J Med* 1988; 318:1409–13.
200. Fialkow PJ, Denman AM, Jacobson RJ, et al. Chronic myelocytic leukemia: origin of some lymphocytes from leukemia stem cells. *J Clin Invest* 1978;62:815–23.
201. Canellos G. Chronic granulocytic leukemia. *Med Clin North Am* 1976;60:1001–18.
202. Talpaz M, McCredie KB, Mavligit GM, et al. Leukocyte interferon-induced myeloid cytoreduction in chronic myelogenous leukemia. *Blood* 1983;62:689–92.
203. Talpaz M, Mavligit GM, Keating MJ, et al. Human leukocyte interferon to control thrombocytosis in chronic myelogenous leukemia. *Ann Intern Med* 1983;99:789–92.
204. Talpaz M, Kantarjian HM, McCredie K, et al. Hematologic remission and cytogenic improvement induced by recombinant human interferon alpha (A) in chronic myelogenous leukemia. *N Engl J Med* 1986;314:1065–9.
205. Alimena G, Morra E, Lazzarino M, et al. Interferon alpha-2b as therapy for Ph'-positive chronic myelogenous leukemia: a study of 82 patients treated with intermittent or daily administration. *Blood* 1988;72:642–7.
206. Gutterman JU, Blumenschein GR, Alexanian R. Leukocyte interferon-induced tumor regression in human metastatic breast cancer, multi-

ple myeloma, and malignant melanoma. *Ann Intern Med* 1980;93:399–406.
207. Mellstedt H, Ahre A, Bjorkholm M, et al. Interferon therapy in myelomatosis. *Lancet* 1979;1:245–7.
208. Osserman EF, Sherman WH, Alexanian R, et al. Human leukocyte interferon in multiple myeloma: The American Cancer Society sponsored trial. In: DeMaeyer E, Galasso G, Schellekens H, eds. *The biology of the interferon system*. Amsterdam: Elsevier/North Holland Biomedical Press, 1981;409–13.
209. Alexanian R, Gutterman J, Levy H. Interferon treatment for multiple myeloma. *Clin Haematol* 1982;11:211–20.
210. Cooper MR. Interferons in the management of multiple myeloma. *Semin Oncol* 988;15(suppl 5):21–5.
211. Bunn PA, Foon KA, Ihde DC, et al. Recombinant leukocyte A interferon: an active agent in advanced cutaneous T-cell lymphomas. *Ann Intern Med* 1984;101:484–7.
212. Wagstaff J, Scarffe JH, Crowther D. Interferon in the treatment of multiple myeloma and the non-Hodgkin's lymphomas. *Cancer Treat Rep* 1985;12B:39–44.
213. O'Connell MJ, Colgan JP, Oken MM, et al. Clinical trial of recombinant leukocyte A interferon as initial therapy for favorable histology non-Hodgkin's lymphomas and chronic lymphocytic leukemia. An ECOG pilot study. *J Clin Oncol* 1986;4:128–36.
214. Krown SE, Burk MW, Kirkwood JM, et al. Human leukocyte (alpha) interferon in metastatic malignant melanoma: The American Cancer Society Phase II trial. *Cancer Treat Rep* 1984;68:723–6.
215. Creagan ET, Ahmann DL, Green SJ. Phase II study of recombinant leukocyte A interferon (rINF-alpha-A) in disseminated malignant melanoma. *Cancer* 1984;54:2844–9.
216. Creagan ET, Ahmann DL, Green SJ. Phase II study of low dose recombinant leukocyte A interferon in disseminated malignant melanoma. *J Clin Oncol* 1984;2:1002–5.
217. Goldberg RM, Ayoob M, Silgals R, et al. Phase II trial of lymphoblastoid interferon in metastatic malignant melanoma. *Cancer Treat Rep* 1985;69:813–6.
218. Kirkwood JM, Ernstoff MS. Melanoma: therapeutic options with recombinant interferons. *Semin Oncol* 1985;12(suppl 5):7–12.
219. Muss HB. The role of biological response modifiers in metastatic renal cell carcinoma. *Semin Oncol* 1988;15(suppl 5):30–4.
220. Quesada JR, Swanson DA, Trindale A, et al. Renal cell carcinoma: antitumor effects of leukocyte interferon. *Cancer Res* 1983;43:940–7.
221. Kirkwood J, Harris J, Vera R, et al. A randomized study of low and high doses of leukocyte alpha-interferon in metastatic renal cell carcinoma: The American Cancer Society collaborative trial. *Cancer Res* 1985;45:863–71.
222. Krown SE. Therapeutic options in renal cell carcinoma. *Semin Oncol* 1985;12:13–7.
223. Trump DL, Elson PR, Borden EC, et al. High-dose lymphoblastoid interferon in advanced renal cell carcinoma. *Cancer Treat Rep* 1987; 71:165–9.
224. Abdi EA, Kamitomo BI, McPherson TA, et al. Extended phase I study of human beta-interferon in human cancers. *Clin Invest Med* 1986;9:33–40.
225. Rinehart J, Malspeis L, Young D, et al. Phase I/II trial of human recombinant beta-interferon in patients with renal cell carcinoma. *Cancer Res* 1986;46:5364–7.
226. Borden EC, Gutterman JU, Holland JF, et al. Interferons in breast carcinoma: a combined analysis of the M.D. Anderson Hospital and American Cancer Society trials. In: Sikora K, ed. *Interferon and cancer*. London: Plenum Publishing, 1983:103–12.
227. Horning S, Levine JF, Miller RA, et al. Clinical and immunologic effects of recombinant leukocyte A interferon in eight patients with advanced cancer. *JAMA* 1982;247:1718–22.
228. Sherwin SA, Mayer D, Ochs JJ, et al. Recombinant leukocyte A interferon in advanced breast cancer: results of a Phase II efficacy trial. *Ann Intern Med* 1983;98:598–602.
229. Nethersell A, Smedley H, Katrak M, et al. Recombinant interferon in advanced breast cancer. *Br J Cancer* 1984;49:615–20.
230. Real FX, Oettgen HF, Krown SE. Kaposi's sarcoma and the acquired immunodeficiency syndrome: treatment with high and low doses of recombinant leukocyte A interferon. *J Clin Oncol* 1986;4:544–51.
231. Groopman JE, Gottlieb MS, Goodman J, et al. Recombinant alpha-2 interferon therapy for Kaposi's sarcoma associated with the acquired immunodeficiency syndrome. *Ann Intern Med* 1984;100:671–6.
232. Willson JKV, Bittner G, Borden EC. Antiproliferative activity of human interferons against ovarian cancer cells grown in human tumor stem cell assay. *Interferon Res* 1984;4:441–7.
233. Willson JKV, Yordan E, Sielaff KM, et al. High-dose human lymphoblastoid interferon (HLBI) administered as a ten-day continuous infusion in ovarian cancer. *Clin Res* 1984; 32:424A.
234. Niloff JM, Knapp RC, Jones G, et al. Recombinant leukocyte alpha interferon in advanced ovarian carcinoma. *Cancer Treat Rep* 1985; 69:895–6.
235. Burek JS, Hacker NF, Lichtenstein A, et al. Intraperitoneal recombinant alpha-interferon for salvage immunotherapy in Stage III epithelial ovarian cancer: a gynecologic oncologic group study. *Cancer Res* 1985;45:4447–53.
236. Welander CE. Interferon in the treatment of ovarian cancer. *Semin Oncol* 1988;15(suppl 5):26–9.
237. Oberg K, Funa K, Alm G. Effects of leukocyte interferon on clinical symptoms and hormone levels in patients with mid-gut carcinoid tumors and carcinoid syndrome. *N Engl J Med* 1983;309:129–32.

238. Spiegel RJ. Additional indications for interferon therapy: basal cell carcinoma, carcinoid, and chronic active hepatitis. *Semin Oncol* 1988;15(suppl 5):41–5.
239. Williams RD. Intravesical interferon alpha in the treatment of superficial bladder cancer. *Semin Oncol* 1988;15(suppl 5):10–3.
240. Connors JM, Andiman WA, Howarth CB, et al. Treatment of nasopharyngeal carcinoma with human leukocyte interferon. *J Clin Oncol* 1985;3:813–7.
241. Krusic J, Kirhmajer V, Knezeric M, et al. Influence of human leukocyte interferon on squamous cell carcinoma of uterine cervix: clinical, histological, and histochemical observations. *Cancer Res* 1981;101:309–15.

*Antiviral Agents and Viral Diseases of Man, 3rd Edition,* edited by G. J. Galasso, R. J. Whitley, and T. C. Merigan, Raven Press, Ltd., New York © 1990.

# 10

# Respiratory Diseases

Robert B. Couch

*Departments of Microbiology, Immunology, and Medicine, Baylor College of Medicine, Houston, Texas 77030*



The viruses that induce the various acute respiratory diseases are known collectively as the "respiratory viruses." These viruses are quite diverse in their properties and replication strategies. Similarly, the illnesses they induce are diverse; they involve the upper and lower respiratory tract and include mild, almost inconsequential illness, as well as severe illness leading to death. Included among the various syndromes are the most common human illness—the common cold—and the last of the pandemic diseases of history—influenza. All ages, all seasons, all populations, and all geographic locations experience illnesses caused by respiratory viruses; an extraordinary amount of time is lost from school and work because of the acute respiratory illnesses. The impact of these illnesses on human health is difficult to overestimate.

Considerable attention has been devoted to study of the viruses that cause acute respiratory illness and to the development of vaccines for their prevention. This effort has produced only two vaccines currently in use: inactivated influenza virus vaccine, and types 4 and 7 adenovirus given in enteric-coated capsules. The former vaccine is principally used to prevent severe influenza and death among those at high risk for complications, and the latter is used to prevent epidemics of acute respiratory disease among military recruits. New approaches are now being utilized to develop other vaccines for the acute respiratory diseases, and it is probable that this effort will succeed for some of the viruses.

The identification of the major viruses causing acute respiratory illness led to an effort to develop antivirals effective for prevention and treatment of these illnesses. This effort has produced only two antivirals currently in use: amantadine for prevention and treatment of influenza caused by the type A viruses, and ribavirin for treatment of severe respiratory illnesses caused by respiratory syncytial virus (RSV). Pertinent to the development of the latter treatment was the development of methods for administration of the drug by aerosol.

Despite the paucity of available antivirals for treatment of the acute respiratory viral illnesses, there are a number of active developmental programs underway for identifying new antivirals and new approaches to their use. In this regard, the precise understanding of viral structure and replication emanating from recent basic virologic research is providing a rational basis for design of these new antivirals and for understanding of their mechanism of action. It seems likely that some of the approaches will lead to identification of new and useful compounds.

## RESPIRATORY VIRAL DISEASES

Estimates of the incidence of acute conditions in the United States are obtained annually by a health interview survey, and a recurring pattern of these conditions is seen. The incidence of acute conditions that were medically attended or restricted activity for the year 1985 is shown in Fig. 1; the incidence of acute respiratory conditions far exceeds those of other acute conditions (1). Females experience a few more illnesses than males, but infants and children experience many more illnesses than adults; the incidence of these moderate and severe respiratory illnesses is two to four times greater among children than among adults. The most common illness syndromes reported are the common cold and influenza; together, they account for over 80% of illnesses and respectively represent over 71 and 94 million significant illnesses annually. Among the notable age-related differences are the high incidence of common colds and pneumonia among very young children and the greater frequency of influenza among school-aged children. Approximately half of the illnesses are medically attended, and each illness leads to an average of 3.2 days of restricted activity and 1.6 days in bed. Other studies in families include milder illnesses; these report frequencies of two to 12 illnesses per person per year (2). Thus, the acute respiratory illnesses constitute an impressive burden of illness that could benefit from effective means for prevention and therapy.

The incidence of acute respiratory illnesses is about the same in different geographic areas of the United States, and in cities and rural/suburban areas. The incidence varies, however, by season. During

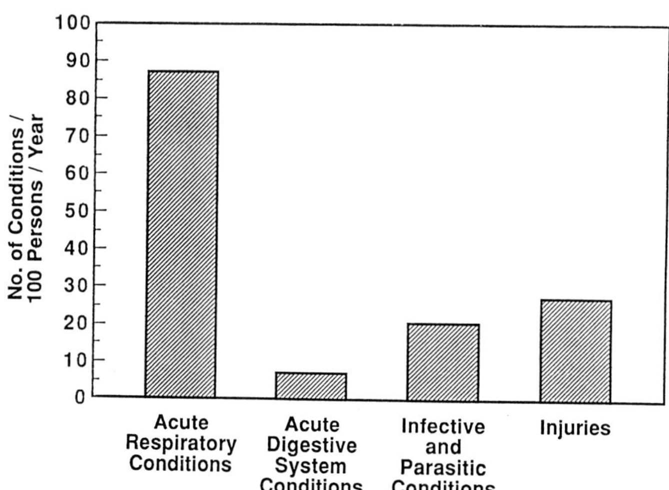


**FIG. 1.** Incidence of acute conditions that caused persons in the United States to visit a physician or lose 2 days of work or school, 1985. From National Health Survey.

**TABLE 1.** *Viruses causing respiratory disease in humans*

| Virus group | Serotypes: Number | Serotypes: Number causing respiratory illness | Serotypes commonly producing respiratory disease in: Infants, <2 years | Children, 2–18 years | Adults, > 18 years |
|---|---|---|---|---|---|
| *Adenoviridae* | 41 | 9 | 1, 2, 3, 5, 7 | 1, 2, 3, 5, 7 | 3, 4, 7, 14, 21 |
| *Coronaviridae* | 3 | 3 | | 229E, OC43, B814 | 229E, OC43, B814 |
| *Herpesviridae* | | | | | |
| HSV | 2 | 1 | 1 | 1 | 1 |
| EBV | 1 | 1 | | EBV | EBV |
| *Orthomyxoviridae* | | | | | |
| Influenza viruses | 3 | 3 | A, B | A, B | A, B |
| *Paramyxoviridae* | | | | | |
| Parainfluenza viruses | 4 | 4 | 1, 3 | 1, 3 | |
| RSV | 1 | 1 | 1 | 1 | |
| *Picornaviridae* | | | | | |
| Enteroviruses | 72 | 19 | | Cox A2, 4, 5, 6, 8, 10 | Cox A21 |
| Rhinoviruses | >100 | >100 | | All | All |

winter months in the United States, the incidence is about twice that in summer; the incidence is intermediate in spring and fall (1). In tropical climates, acute respiratory illnesses are reported to be increased during the rainy season, a finding supportive of the prevalent belief that crowding, with an increased opportunity for transmission, is the primary reason for the increase in incidence in temperate climates during winter months (3).

### Viruses

Over 200 distinct viruses are capable of infecting the human respiratory tract, and most can produce an acute respiratory illness. The major virus families, and the number of different serotypes and those commonly producing respiratory disease at different ages are shown in Table 1. Six virus families contain the viruses most commonly causing acute respiratory illness. Approximately 20 different serotypes in addition to the rhinoviruses account for nearly all illnesses; represented are viruses that contain DNA and RNA, that are cubic (icosahedral) and helical, and that are enveloped and nonenveloped (Table 2). A number of other viruses (not listed) may cause respiratory symptoms but are better known for other disease syndromes. These include measles (rubeola), mumps, rubella, chicken pox (varicella), and cytomegalovirus (CMV). These viruses and the diseases they cause are described elsewhere.

The variability in virion characteristics of the respiratory viruses is also reflected in the variability in patterns of replication

**TABLE 2.** *Major virion characteristics of the respiratory viruses*

| Virus family | Nucleic acid | RNA polarity | Nucleocapsid symmetry | Enveloped |
|---|---|---|---|---|
| *Herpesviridae* | DSDNA | | Icosahedral | Yes |
| *Adenoviridae* | DSDNA | | Icosahedral | No |
| *Coronaviridae* | SSRNA | + | Helical | Yes |
| *Orthomyxoviridae* | SSRNA (segmented) | − | Helical | Yes |
| *Paramyxoviridae* | SSRNA | − | Helical | Yes |
| *Picornaviridae* | SSRNA | + | Icosahedral | No |

DSDNA, double-stranded deoxyribonucleic acid; SSRNA, single-stranded ribonucleic acid.

**TABLE 3.** *Cellular site for the major steps in virus replication*

| Virus family | Genome replication | Nucleocapsid assembly | Virion assembly | Virus release |
|---|---|---|---|---|
| *Herpesviridae* | Nucleus | Nucleus | Nucleus | Budding at nuclear membrane; release by lysis or reverse phagocytosis |
| *Adenoviridae* | Nucleus | Nucleus | Nucleus | Cell lysis |
| *Coronaviridae* | Cytoplasm | Cytoplasm | Cytoplasm | Budding at cell membrane |
| *Orthomyxoviridae* | Nucleus | Nucleus | Cytoplasma | Budding at cell membrane |
| *Paramyxoviridae* | Cytoplasm | Cytoplasm | Cytoplasm | Budding at cell membrane |
| *Picornaviridae* | Cytoplasm | Cytoplasm | Cytoplasm | Cell lysis |

(4,5). Except for the orthomyxoviruses, the patterns conform to those generally applicable to DNA and RNA viruses; i.e., DNA viruses replicate their genome and assemble the nucleocapsid in the nucleus, whereas RNA viruses replicate their genome and assemble the nucleocapsid in the cytoplasm (Table 3). The orthomyxoviridae are RNA viruses that undergo these events in the nucleus (6). Assembly of DNA-containing virions occurs in the nucleus, whereas assembly of RNA-containing virion occurs in the cytoplasm. Enveloped viruses acquire their envelope by a process of budding through the cell or nuclear membrane. Virion release of enveloped RNA viruses occurs by budding through the cell membrane, whereas herpesviruses are released by reverse phagocytosis and cell lysis after budding through the nuclear membrane. Nonenveloped virions are released by cell lysis.

Since an understanding of the action of existing antivirals and the development of new antivirals is, to a considerable extent, dependent upon understanding the cycle of virus replication, a summary of present knowledge of the replication cycle and major features of each of the respiratory virus families is presented.

### *Adenoviridae*

The adenoviridae are nonenveloped, icosahedral, double-stranded DNA viruses (7,8). The capsid is made up of 240 capsomers called "hexons" (surrounded by six neighbors) and 12 capsomers called "pentons" (surrounded by five neighbors), which are at the vertices. Each penton consists of a base and a fiber of varying length that extends from the base. Type-specific antigens that define adenovirus serotypes are present on the fiber and the hexon.

The vertex fiber is the physical unit attaching to cell-surface receptors. Following attachment, penetration is by pinocytosis and partial uncoating is initiated immediately in the endosome. A subviral particle is released into the cytoplasm; it traverses microtubules to the nucleus where early messenger RNAs (mRNAs) are transcribed. As with other double-stranded DNA viruses, an early and late phase characterize the replication cycle. Approximately 40% of the genome is transcribed during the early phase. Prominent in the early phase are synthesis of proteins required for DNA replication; these include a terminal protein, a DNA-binding protein, and polymerase. Viral DNA synthesis and transcription of late mRNAs begins approximately 6 hr after infection. By 12–14 hr, synthesis of host cell proteins ceases and viral structural protein synthesis predominates. The structural proteins are synthesized on polyribosomes and transported to the nucleus where assembly takes place. Only approximately 10–15% of new viral DNA and protein is incorporated into virions. Assembled virus tends to remain cell-associated; replication ceases 24–36 hr after initiation and virus is eventually released by cell lysis.

### *Orthomyxoviridae*

The influenza viruses make up the orthomyxoviridae. They are enveloped, helical, single-stranded RNA viruses (4,6). The genome is segmented and of opposite polarity (−) to mRNA; as a result, the genome can only serve as a template for transcription and the virion must contain the polymerase required for initial transcription. Two surface glycoproteins extend from the envelope, the hemagglutinin (HA), and the neuraminidase. Both the HA and the neuraminidase exhibit antigenic variation, the basis for recurring epidemics of influenza in human populations.

Attachment of influenza viruses to cell surfaces is mediated by the HA subunit. The cell receptor is *N*-acetylneuraminic acid (NANA). Penetration is by pinocytosis into endosomes, and uncoating results from fusion between the lipid bilayer and the plasma membrane. Fusion is triggered by the acid pH within the endosome; this alters the conformation of the HA, and an exposed hydrophobic amino acid sequence then inserts into the plasma membrane, thereby promoting fusion and subsequent uncoating. By an unknown mechanism, the viral genome is transported into the nucleus where RNA replication occurs. Unlike other RNA viruses, replication requires synthesis of host cell mRNA as a source of primer for viral mRNA. The nucleocapsid is assembled in the nucleus; virion assembly takes place at the plasma membrane, and mature virus is released by budding. The lipid bilayer is acquired from the host cell during the latter process. During assembly and budding, proteolytic cleavage of the HA by host cell enzymes or enzymes in secretions takes place; this is required for released particles to be infectious.

Newly synthesized virions possess surface glycoproteins containing NANA as part of their carbohydrate structure. A major function of the neuraminidase is the enzymatic removal of these NANA residues to disrupt or prevent the occurrence of aggregates and thereby increase the number of free infectious particles. The entire replicative process requires only approximately 6 hr, and cell death results from the infection.

### *Paramyxoviridae*

Like the influenza viruses, the paramyxoviruses are enveloped, helical, single-stranded RNA viruses with a genome of opposite polarity to mRNA (4,5,9). They share many properties with the influenza viruses, but their genome is not segmented. Two surface glycoproteins extend from the surface; one represents the attachment protein, and the other is the fusion protein. For RSV, attachment and fusion are the only described activities; the attachment protein of the parainfluenza viruses also exhibits HA and neuraminidase activity.

The replication cycle for the paramyxoviruses is generally similar to that for the influenza viruses. The receptor for the parainfluenza viruses is NANA, whereas that for RSV is not yet defined. Uncoating is not pH-dependent and takes place at the plasma membrane. Replication occurs in the cytoplasm and, unlike orthomyxoviruses, does not utilize host cell mRNA. The nucleocapsid is assembled in the cytoplasm. Virion assembly takes place at the plasma membrane, and virus is released by budding. A characteristic feature of infection with the paramyxoviridae is the formation of syncytia; and F protein mediates this event (10).

### *Picornaviridae*

The picornaviruses are nonenveloped, icosahedral, single-stranded RNA viruses

(4,5,11). The genome of picornaviruses can serve as mRNA and initiate the replication process.

The picornaviruses utilize a number of different but undefined receptors as attachment sites. Penetration is by pinocytosis; uncoating involves pH-induced surface alterations. The parental virus RNA strands bind to ribosomes and are translated into a polyprotein. The polymerase derived from the polyprotein then transcribes the parental RNA into strands of minus polarity. Progeny plus-strands are transcribed repeatedly from the minus-strand templates by a peeling-off type of mechanism. These progeny plus-strands are either translated or encapsidated into new virions. Multiplication occurs in the cytoplasm, and functional proteins are mainly or entirely produced by posttranslational cleavage of precursor. Host cell protein synthesis is inhibited as viral synthesis increases.

After synthesis, viral coat proteins are assembled with RNA into complete virions and virus is released by cell lysis. The replication cycle requires 5–10 hr, and 25,000–100,000 viral particles may be produced by each cell.

### *Coronaviridae*

The coronaviruses are enveloped, helical, single-stranded RNA viruses (4,5,12). A distinctive feature of the coronaviruses is the very large club-shaped surface projections that represent the attachment subunit; they contain epitopes for neutralizing antibody. Like picornaviruses, the genome can serve as mRNA and initiate the replication process. Replication takes place in the cytoplasm and follows a sequence similar to picornaviruses. However, coronavirus mRNA is synthesized in a unique manner; a single leader sequence apparently serves as a primer for transcription of all mRNAs. Virus is released by budding into cytoplasmic vacuoles. Replication is optimal at 33°C and is relatively slow.

## Syndromes

The major respiratory illness syndromes seen in children and adults and the major viruses causing each syndrome are shown in Tables 4 and 5. The listed syndromes indicate the anatomic site of major symptoms; however, symptoms referable to other respiratory sites are usually present but less prominent. In addition, some patients are best designated as diffuse acute respiratory disease (ARD), as no clear site of anatomic localization is noted. Each of the major syndromes listed may be caused by a number of different viruses, and each virus may cause several syndromes. Nevertheless, when age, time of year, and other information is considered, the number of possible viruses causing a given syndrome in an individual patient is narrowed considerably.

### *Common Cold*

The most common ARD syndrome is the common cold. It is an acute, self-limited illness characterized by prominence of nasal obstruction, discharge, and sneezing.

It is well established that viruses cause most and possibly all infectious colds (13). The viruses causing colds in infants and children (Table 4) reflect the virus infections prevalent in these age groups at a particular time. Thus, during the annual RSV epidemic, this virus will be the predominant cause of colds among infants while it is also causing severe disease of the lower respiratory tract requiring hospitalization. A similar circumstance is true during periods of prevalence of influenza and parainfluenza viruses. Rhinoviruses, adenoviruses, and coronaviruses are also prominent causes of upper respiratory illnesses in children, including the common cold.

Rhinoviruses are the predominant cause of colds among adults; they have been isolated from throat swabs of up to 30% of adults experiencing colds (14). A consider-

**TABLE 4.** *Relative importance of the respiratory viruses in disease syndromes in children*

| Virus | Common cold | Pharyngitis | Tracheobronchitis | Laryngotracheobronchitis (croup) | Bronchiolitis | Pneumonia |
|---|---|---|---|---|---|---|
| RSV | + + | + + | + + + | + | + + + | + + + |
| Parainfluenza type 3 | + + | + + | + + + | + + | + + | + + + |
| Parainfluenza type 1 | + + | + + | + + | + + + | + + | + |
| Influenza type A | + + | + + | + + + | + + | + + | + + |
| Influenza type B | + + | + + | + + | + | + | + |
| Rhinovirus, >100 types | + + + | + + | + | + | + | + |
| Parainfluenza type 2 | + | + | + | + + | + | + |
| Adenovirus types 1, 2, 3, and 5 | + | + + | + | + + | + | + |
| Coronaviruses | + + | + | + | + | − | − |
| Coxsackie A viruses | + | + + | + | + | − | + |
| HSV-1 | − | + + | − | − | − | − |
| Coxsackie B, echo, and polioviruses | + | + | + | − | − | − |

Relative frequency as cause of syndrome: −, rare or not a cause; +, causes some cases; + +, common cause; + + +, major cause of cases.

**TABLE 5.** *Relative importance of the respiratory viruses in disease syndromes in adults*

| Virus | Common cold | Pharyngitis | Tracheobronchitis | Pneumonia |
|---|---|---|---|---|
| Rhinovirus, >100 types | + + + | + + | + | − |
| Influenza type A | + + | + + | + + + | + + + |
| Influenza type B | + + | + + | + + | + |
| Coronaviruses | + + | + | + | − |
| HSV | − | + + | − | − |
| EBV | − | + | − | − |
| Adenoviruses | + | + + | + | + |
| RSV | + | + | − | − |
| Parainfluenza viruses | + | + | − | − |
| Coxsackie A and B, echo, and polioviruses | + | + + | + | + |

Relative frequency as causes of syndrome: −, rare or not a cause; +, causes some cases; + +, common cause of syndrome; + + +, major cause of syndrome.

ation of the low sensitivity of throat swabs suggests that rhinoviruses cause 40–60% of colds among adults (15). Coronaviruses cause approximately 20% of colds in adults, and the other viruses listed account for the remainder of cases associated with a known virus (16,17). Altogether, the viruses listed in Tables 4 and 5 cause approximately 70% of colds. The remaining colds are of unknown cause and may be attributable to undiscovered agents.

### *Acute Pharyngitis*

Acute pharyngitis is usually a more severe disease than the common cold. Fever is common, may reach levels of 104°F, and may persist for several days. Although the major respiratory complaints are referable to the throat, patients with acute pharyngitis also exhibit other respiratory symptoms.

In both children and adults, no virus or virus group predominates as a cause of acute pharyngitis. The syndrome is one of those seen during epidemics caused by a number of the viruses listed in Tables 4 and 5. Viruses that exhibit a predilection for causing pharyngitis are the coxsackie A viruses that produce herpangina, a syndrome of febrile pharyngitis usually seen in children, and adenoviruses, herpes simplex virus type 1 (HSV-1), and the Epstein-Barr herpes virus (EBV). During the latter infection, which is prominent in teenagers and young adults, pharyngitis is prominent and sometimes severe, although other findings of this infection lead to a diagnosis of infectious mononucleosis. Adenoviruses, particularly types 4 and 7, were extremely common in the past among military recruits, where they caused a pattern of annual epidemics in some military groups and near continuous presence in others (18). Pharyngitis as well as other respiratory illness syndromes, including diffuse respiratory disease and pneumonia, were seen during these outbreaks. The routine immunization of all incoming recruits by means of ingestion of an enteric-coated capsule containing live types 4 and 7 adenovirus that produces an asymptomatic intestinal infection has been highly successful in preventing this respiratory infection (19).

### *Acute Tracheobronchitis and Laryngotracheobronchitis*

Acute tracheobronchitis is the appropriate designation for an illness with symptoms referable primarily to the trachea and larger bronchial passages. The characteristic feature of this illness is the prominence of nonproductive cough, which frequently occurs in paroxysms.

The syndrome of acute tracheobronchitis may be caused by any of the respiratory viruses, but is particularly prominent among infants and small children with RSV and parainfluenza virus infection and in both older children and adults during infection with an influenza virus (20). Indeed, among adults, the influenza viruses are the viruses most commonly causing tracheobronchitis.

Acute laryngotracheobronchitis is the anatomic designation for a childhood illness better known as "croup." The characteristic feature of croup is a barking, metallic cough followed by inspiratory stridor. Parainfluenza viruses are primarily responsible for croup, particularly type 1, although RSV, the other parainfluenza viruses and the influenza viruses are also common causes of the syndrome (21).

### *Bronchiolitis and Pneumonia*

Bronchiolitis is a syndrome seen almost exclusively in infants. Only 10–30% of ill infants exhibit fever, but all exhibit expiratory wheezing on auscultation of the lungs, the characteristic feature of bronchiolitis. On many occasions, a child may appear clinically to have bronchiolitis but a chest x-ray is interpreted as exhibiting pneumonia.

This syndrome in infants is primarily caused by RSV, and an increase in frequency of cases in a community may be used as an indicator of onset of the annual RSV epidemic (22). Other viruses may produce bronchiolitis in infants, particularly parainfluenza types 1 and 3 and type A influenza virus (23). When an acute, wheezing, asthma-like syndrome is seen in adults with acute respiratory virus infection, the cause is usually infection with an influenza virus.

Pneumonia is a syndrome characterized by fine rales on auscultation of the lungs and presence of an infiltrate on chest x-ray. It is common in infants and leads to high frequencies of hospitalization (1,24,25). Viruses causing this syndrome in infants are numerous, but RSV, type 3 parainfluenza virus, and type A influenza virus are most prominent (25,26). Virus pneumonia in older children and adults is most commonly produced by type A influenza viruses but is not uncommon with adenovirus or coxsackie A virus infection in some populations (18,27–29).

On occasion, influenza viruses and adenoviruses may produce an extensive bilateral pneumonia among adults. This occurrence is well documented for type A influenza virus, and its occurrence is prominent among persons with underlying heart and lung disease. Extreme respiratory difficulty, cyanosis, and extremis characterize this syndrome; it leads to death in almost 50% of subjects (30).

## Pathogenesis

The acute respiratory viral infections are transmitted from person to person by transfer of virus-containing respiratory secretions from an infected person to a susceptible recipient. The ability of a respiratory virus to spread to some extent in all human populations where circumstances of exposure must vary greatly suggests that the respiratory viruses can spread by more than a single means. Influenza is generally considered to be transmitted primarily by the airborne route, and available data suggests that the adenovirus types 4 and 7 epidemics in the military were similarly transmitted (31,32).

Rhinovirus infections were thought to be transmitted primarily by contact but a recent series of controlled room exposure experiments showed that airborne transmission can occur (33). Conditions shown to enhance rhinovirus spread are presence of high titers of virus in secretions, presence of virus on the hands of an ill person, presence of moderate to severe illness in transmittors, and spending of many hours together (34). These latter findings conform to a principle of transmission of respiratory viruses that appears valid; i.e., persons with the most severe infections contain the most virus in secretions, are most symptomatic, shed the most virus into the environment, and are the major source of virus that induces infection in susceptible persons.

Less is known about spread of RSV and parainfluenza virus infections, but comparison of various preventive measures for nosocomial spread in hospitals indicated that spread included a contact route (35).

The incubation period to onset of illness varies between 1 and 14 days among the various respiratory viruses. Virus shedding into secretions can be detected before or at the time of onset of illness. Quantities of virus are initially low but concentrations increase with time to levels of $10^3$–$10^7$ median tissue culture infective doses ($TCID_{50}$) per ml of secretions (36–38). Persons with higher concentrations of virus are more ill; with influenzal pneumonia, concentrations of $10^9$ $TCID_{50}$ per ml have been detected in secretions (39). Although viremia has been detected on rare occasions in severely ill patients, illness is accounted for entirely by infection of the respiratory mucosa.

Because of the benign nature of most acute respiratory illnesses, histology among ill patients is not generally available. Tissues obtained from severely ill influenza patients have shown an extensive mucosal infection, with cellular sloughing into the lumen of the lower respiratory passages (40). In contrast, histologic studies of biopsies obtained from persons experiencing rhinovirus common colds generally reveal little or no apparent histologic alteration (41). This latter finding has caused Gwaltney to postulate physiologic abnormalities induced by kinin secretion as causing the symptoms and signs of colds (42).

A common feature of the acute reaction to injury is the appearance of edema, transudation of serous fluids, and infiltration of polymorphonuclear cells. Nevertheless, lymphocytes and macrophages soon become the predominant cell type in the submucosal area. When the edema accompanying inflammation is sufficient to narrow respiratory passages, obstruction to airflow may occur and lead to wheezing. This is most notable in infants and small children, where caliber of bronchi and bronchioles is small; it may lead to the air trapping and atelectasis seen in bronchiolitis caused by RSV infection. Peribronchial lymphocytic infiltrates occur in persons with lower respiratory diseases and on occasion may be so extensive as to produce appearance of a bronchopneumonia on chest x-ray. In some cases of pneumonia, extensive interstitial infiltrates, alveolar edema, and hyaline membrane formation may occur; in others, a predominance of a cellular infiltrate and fibrosis may be seen. The reparative process for the mucosal surfaces and lung may be prolonged when pathology is extensive.

### Immune Responses and Immunity

Infection with a respiratory virus elicits both a humoral and a cell-mediated immune response. Recovery mechanisms from infection are complex and incompletely understood. Nevertheless, current concepts attribute recovery from a primary infection to a combination of interferon and nonspecific cytotoxic and phagocytic mechanisms that limit growth and spread of virus (43).

Immunity to reinfection is mediated by antibody (43). A degree of immunity is manifested in all normal persons following recovery from infection. It may, however, be incomplete and variable among the various viruses. Reinfection with RSV is frequent during the first few years of life, but recent information indicates that passively acquired antibody can mediate protection and that there is an inverse relationship between level of antibody and occurrence of reinfection, indicating that antibody can mediate immunity to RSV infection (44). On the other hand, recent data suggests that homotypic immunity to influenza may last for more than 20 years (45). Antibody persists for decades in serum but appears less persistent in nasal secretions.

### Diagnosis

The decision to prescribe an antiviral for prevention or treatment of a viral respiratory infection must be based on proof or a strong presumption that the patient will be exposed to or is experiencing a specific viral infection. The information used by the physician for these decisions involves knowledge of infections occurring at the community level as well as that occurring in a specific patient. The epidemiologic patterns of the major respiratory viruses are well described; when presence of an epidemic is confirmed at the community level, then administration of an antiviral for prophylaxis can begin. For some infections, herald illnesses may be used to indicate the beginning of an epidemic; these illnesses include bronchiolitis in infants as an indicator for RSV, croup for the parainfluenza viruses, and influenza in school children for influenza. Most indicator illnesses occur in children, but infections in adults may eventually be extensive.

Although illness information is useful, a community virologic surveillance program is a better way to identify the epidemic period of a respiratory virus (Fig. 2). Surveillance has been provided in the past only through research programs and some community health departments; however, viral diagnostic laboratories are becoming so prevalent that an organized reporting of virus identifications could provide a measure of community surveillance.

A presumptive clinical diagnosis of a specific virus infection can be made with a reasonable degree of accuracy in most serious viral respiratory illnesses. The information used for such a diagnosis includes categorizing the syndrome exhibited by the patient, and taking into consideration the patient's age, the time of year, and the population group from which the patient arises; this provides a differential of possible etiologic agents. If a characteristic pattern of illnesses is occurring in the community, then a presumptive diagnosis can be made in most cases; knowledge that a specific virus is epidemic in the community increases the certainty of the diagnosis.

A definitive diagnosis of a viral respiratory infection requires demonstration of presence of a specific virus in the patient, rise in titer of a specific antibody, or detection of a significant titer of an immunoglobulin M (IgM) antibody. Exceptions to the requirement for one of these criteria are rare. The laboratory methods that may be used for diagnosis of viral infections are described in Chapter 5.

### Approaches to Chemoprophylaxis and Chemotherapy

#### *Chemoprophylaxis*

The options for chemoprophylaxis of viral respiratory infections are seasonal prophylaxis, prophylaxis for the duration of an epidemic, or prophylaxis for a short period before or just after exposure. Seasonal prophylaxis would encompass a 6 to 9-month period; for this purpose, a broad spectrum of activity would be needed. The hope that interferon would fulfill this role has now been abandoned because of the side effects induced by chronic administration (46). Alternatives to interferon for safe, long-term use and broad spectrum effectiveness have not been described.

Chemoprophylaxis for the epidemic period is a feasible concept and has been successful with use of amantadine or rimantadine for type A influenza virus infection and illness (see below). Viruses for which epidemic prophylaxis can be considered, the epidemic pattern, and the primary tar-

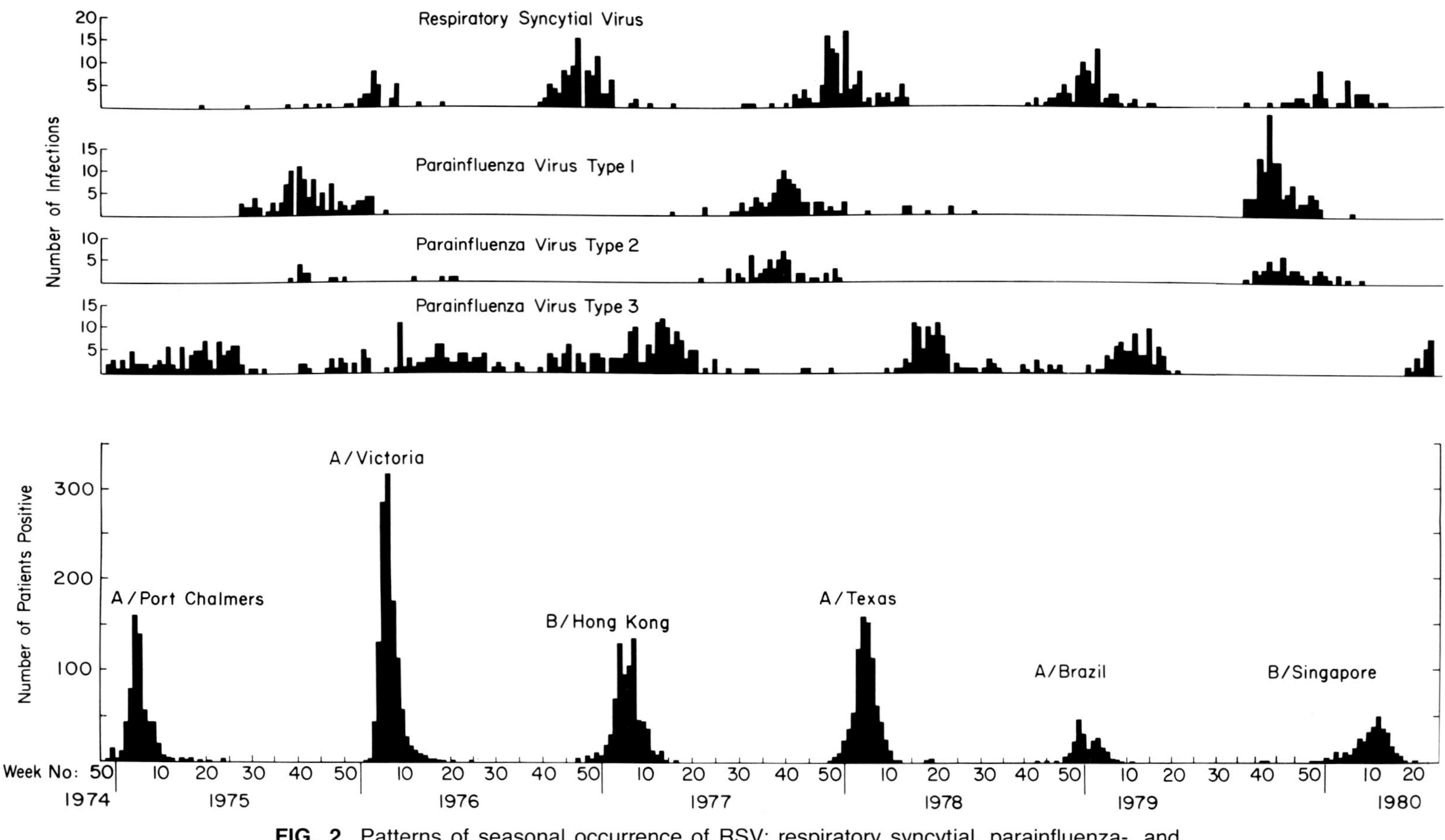


**FIG. 2.** Patterns of seasonal occurrence of RSV: respiratory syncytial, parainfluenza-, and influenza-virus–associated respiratory illnesses, in Houston, Texas, 1974–80.

**TABLE 6.** *Potential targets for chemoprophylaxis during epidemic period*

| Virus | Epidemic pattern | Target populations |
|---|---|---|
| Type A influenza virus | Winter, 6–8 weeks duration, most years, affects all ages | School children, high-risk persons[a] |
| Type B influenza virus | Winter, 6–8 weeks duration, approximately 1 in 3 years, affects all ages | School children, high-risk persons[a] |
| RSV | Winter or spring, 8–12 weeks duration, annual | Infants |
| Type 1 parainfluenza virus | Fall, 8–12 weeks duration, biennial | Small children |
| Rhinoviruses | Fall and/or spring, 8–12 weeks, annual | Chronic lung disease/asthma |

[a]As defined by recommendations for use of influenza virus vaccine.

get populations are shown in Table 6; the target populations designated for prophylaxis are those experiencing either the highest attack rates or the most serious illnesses. Short-term chemoprophylaxis for persons entering an outbreak situation or because of exposure in a circumstance with high secondary attack rates has a potential for widespread application and a high degree of effectiveness.

The requirements for optimal utilization of chemoprophylaxis are an antiviral suitable for prolonged administration and a means for identifying the beginning and end of an outbreak. The properties desired in an antiviral for prophylaxis are an extreme degree of safety, moderate to high degree of effectiveness, ease of administration, and low cost. Any compromise in these properties will impair utilization of the antiviral.

### *Chemotherapy*

Effective specific antiviral therapy is desirable for all viral respiratory illnesses because of their high frequency and common severity. However, the major targets for chemotherapy are RSV and type 3 parainfluenza viruses when they are causing serious disease in infants, type 1 and sometimes type 2 parainfluenza viruses and type A influenza viruses when they are causing croup, and type A and B influenza viruses when they are causing a serious illness regardless of age. Despite their tendency to cause mild illness, therapy for rhinoviruses and coronaviruses is desirable because of their high frequency and tendency to lead to serious illness in some unhealthy populations.

### *Aerosol Therapy*

Knight et al. (47) recently have developed a method for aerosol therapy of respiratory viral infections and demonstrated its clinical utility. The method used is based on a number of studies of amantadine and ribavirin therapy of experimental influenza virus infection in mice (48,49). A Collison aerosol generator was adapted so as to make it easily portable; a diagram of the unit is shown in Fig. 3. The Collison generator produces an aerosol at ambient temperature and humidity that is heterogenous in size over a range of $<1$–$6\ \mu m$ in diameter but with a mass median diameter of approximately $1.3\ \mu m$ (47). The site of deposition in the respiratory tract is a function of particle size. Aerosols used for treatment (aqueous solutions of drug) are hygroscopic and change in size when relative humidity increases or decreases. Equilibration of particles to the high humidity of the respiratory tract ($>95\%$) during nose breathing will provide an estimated deposition of approximately 40% of the aerosol in the nose; another 40% will be approximately equal-

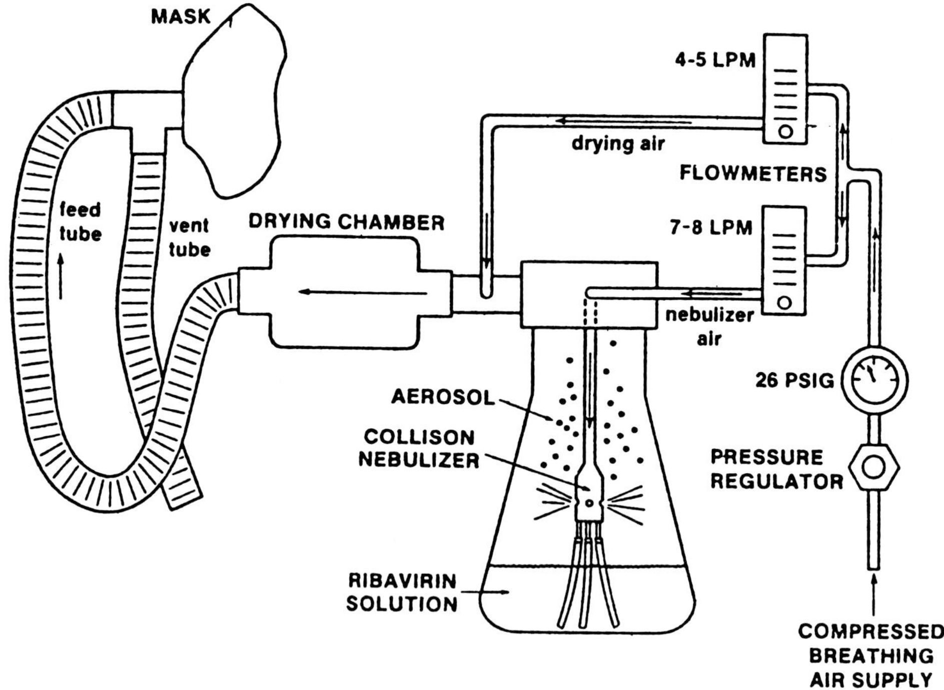


**FIG. 3.** Collison generator for human treatment with ribavirin aerosol. (From Knight et al., ref. 47, with permission.)

ly divided between tertiary bronchi/bronchioles and alveolar ducts, whereas approximately 15–20% of the aerosol will be exhaled (47). Actual alveolar surface deposition is low because air mixing at this site is by diffusion; deposition is also low in primary and secondary bronchi because of rapid air flow. Deposition in the lower respiratory tract will increase with mouth breathing, a circumstance that is common among persons experiencing viral respiratory illness and is the circumstance when aerosol is administered to intubated patients. However, with mouth breathing, overall drug deposition would decrease.

Dosage can be calculated from variables that control deposition. These are the minute volume (tidal volume times number of respirations per minute) the fractional deposition, the aerosol concentration of drug, and the duration of treatment (50). Since tidal volume is related to body weight, the dosage can be estimated from readily available values.

## ANTIVIRALS FOR RESPIRATORY VIRAL INFECTIONS

### Clinically Useful Antivirals

#### *Amantadine and Rimantadine*

Amantadine (L-adamantanamine hydrochloride) is a primary amine with a 10-carbon alicyclic ring structure (Fig. 4). Rimantadine (α-methyl-L-adamantane methylamine hydrochloride) is a closely related analog (Fig. 4). Both drugs are very stable, water-soluble, crystalline powders that are acid salts of weak bases.

Amantadine was first reported as effective for type A influenza over two decades ago and it was approved for use in the

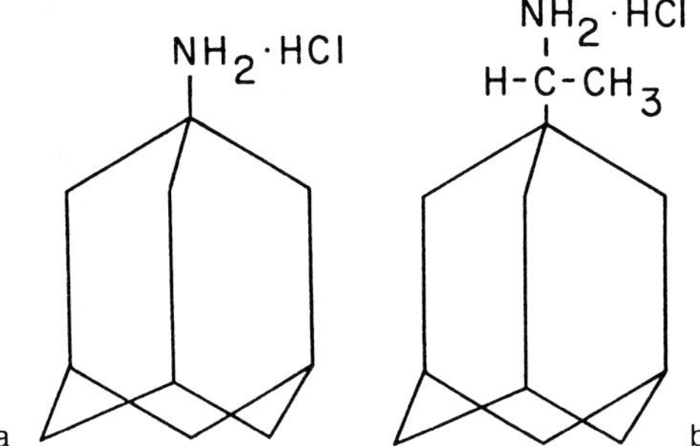


**FIG. 4.** Chemical structures of amantadine hydrochloride **(A)** and rimantadine hydrochloride **(B)**.

United States in 1966 (51). Despite being the only effective drug for this important and common infection, it has taken almost 20 years for the drug to achieve a measure of acceptance by physicians. The reasons are multiple and include an inappropriate emphasis on adverse effects by some, a failure of the Food and Drug Administration (FDA) to provide approval for all type A viruses and of public health agencies to recommend its use, its availability only by prescription, and lingering questions regarding its clinical value. Despite being approved for all type A virus infections in 1976, the increase in use of the drug has been slow, largely because of difficulty in overcoming past problems. There is little doubt that the amantadine experience acted as a disincentive for a commitment to antiviral development by the pharmaceutical industry. Fortunately, the drug is now experiencing acceptance by the medical profession, and rimantadine, a drug commonly used in the Soviet Union, is said to be nearing market availability in the United States.

### *Antiviral Effects*

Amantadine was identified in an antiviral screening system as effective against type A influenza viruses and was soon shown to be effective against all type A variants (51–53). It is effective at low concentrations (<1 μg/ml) that are achievable in humans with recommended doses and schedules. At these concentrations, it is ineffective against type B influenza viruses. The spectrum of activity of amantadine at higher concentrations (10–50 μg/ml) is broadened considerably and includes a variety of viruses and virus families (Table 7); these concentrations, however, are not achievable by oral therapy (53–55). Although not systematically evaluated, the level of drug required to inhibit susceptible strains does not appear to be host-cell–related.

Amantadine has been shown as effective for type A influenza in a number of animal systems, including mice, ferrets, and chickens (52,54). Davies showed effectiveness in mice against challenge with a type A (H2N2) influenza virus at doses of 0.6–40 mg/kg when given by the oral, subcutaneous, or peritoneal route; a dose response was noted, and effectiveness was detected for up to 72 hr postinoculation (51). Grunert et al. (56) later showed that amantadine was effective when given by the nasal or aerosol route to mice; when given prophylactically, a single dose was effective, but multiple doses were required for treatment. Walker et al. (48) extended the work with aerosol treatment of influenza using a collison atomizer system later refined by Knight et al. (47) for aerosol therapy of humans (see above). He showed that therapy with aero-

**TABLE 7.** *Reported antiviral spectrum of amantadine-sensitive viruses according to drug concentration*

| Low and high concentration | High concentration only (>10 μg/ml) |
|---|---|
| Influenza A[a] | Influenza B and C<br>Parainfluenza 1, 2, 3[a]<br>RSV[a]<br>Rubella[a]<br>Avian and murine retroviruses[a]<br>Dengue 1–4[a]<br>Semliki Forest[a]<br>LCM-Tacaribe[b] viruses |

[a]Same result obtained for rimantadine.
[b]LCM is lymphocytic choriomeningitis.

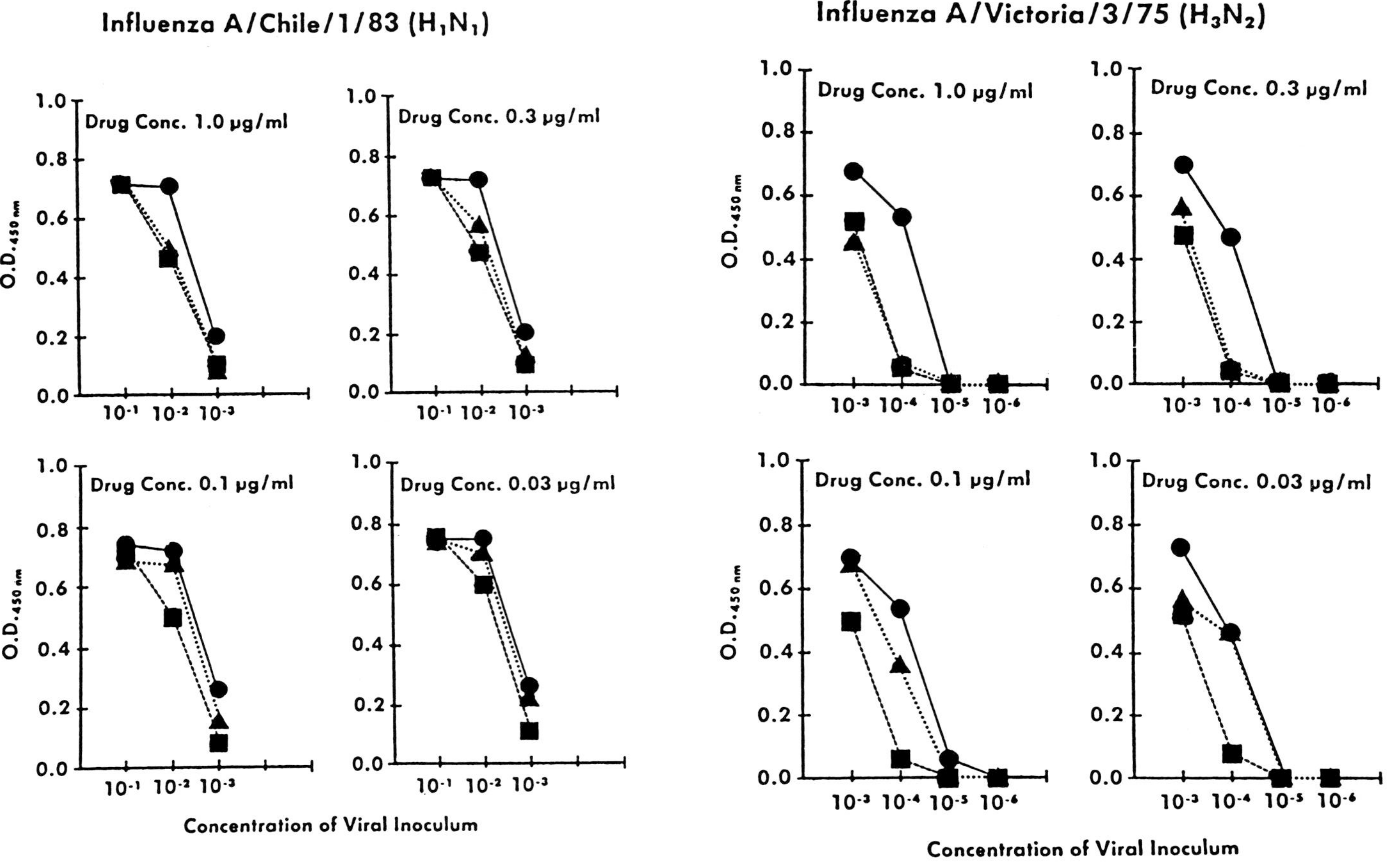


**FIG. 5.** Comparisons of amantadine (*solid triangles*) and rimantadine (*solid squares*) to control (*solid circles*) in *in vitro* tests of drug sensitivity. Virus growth is measured by optical density at different drug and virus input concentrations (From Belshe et al., ref. 57, with permission.)

solized drug at 4 mg/kg/day was superior to 40 mg/kg/day given by the peritoneal route (48). This work was confirmed and extended by Wilson et al. (49) to include comparisons to ribavirin and to a combination of amantadine and ribavirin by aerosol. In the mouse system, there is little doubt that amantadine is more effective for treatment by aerosol than by the intraperitoneal route.

Rimantadine is also effective against type A influenza viruses at low concentrations (≤1 μg/ml). Where tested, its antiviral spectrum is the same as that for amantadine (Table 7). Both amantadine and rimantadine exhibit 50% plaque reduction inhibitory concentrations for clinical strains of 0.1–0.4 μg/ml. In simultaneous comparisons of both H1N1 and H3N2 strains, rimantadine is somewhat more effective at the same concentration (57) (Fig. 5). In ferret tracheal ring cultures, rimantadine is also more effective at similar concentrations (58). Finally, in influenza challenges of mice, Shulman (59) showed that rimantadine given intraperitoneally reduced mortality, pulmonary virus titers, and the ability of mice to transmit infection to uninfected cage mates; comparable doses of amantadine were slightly less effective. There seems little doubt that rimantadine is somewhat more effective against type A influenza viruses at equal concentrations.

### *Mechanism of Action*

Initial studies on the mechanism of action of rimantadine indicated inhibition of an early event in the replication cycle (52–54). The drug has no viricidal properties and does not inhibit attachment of viruses to host cell receptors. Using resistant and susceptible viruses for preparation of a number of reassortant viruses containing genes from both parents indicated that both the matrix (M) and HA proteins may be involved in resistance and susceptibility (60). Resistance to high concentrations (>50 μg/ml) was resolved following definition of the uncoating process for enveloped viruses. Most enveloped viruses enter the cell by endocytosis through clathrin-coated pits (61). The pH of virus is then lowered through an ATP-driven proton pump. For influenza A viruses, the low pH induces a conformational change in the HA protein, exposing the amino terminus region of the $HA_2$ polypeptide (62). This region has a hydrophobic character, and its exposure triggers a fusion event between the endosomal membrane and the virus envelope. The pH optima for fusion of influenza viruses is 5.0–5.5, and high concentrations of amantadine are capable of buffering the endosome so that these acidic conditions do not occur. Viruses resistant to high concentrations were shown to exhibit a pH optima for fusion of greater than 5.5 and to have mutations in the gene coding for the HA protein (62). It seems likely that this endosomal buffering effect of amantadine also accounts for the broad spectrum of viruses inhibited by amantadine at high concentrations.

More recent data has indicated clearly that viruses resistant only to low concentrations of virus (≤1 μg/ml) exhibit mutations in the gene coding for the M protein (63,64). This concentration of amantadine does not alter the pH of endosomes. Hay and Zambon (65) have suggested different mechanisms of action of amantadine via the M protein. They demonstrated the usual inhibition of replication of a sensitive human strain only when drug was added to cultures before the addition of virus; however, an avian influenza A strain was inhibited by amantadine when added 60 min after virus. Further analysis of the avian strain indicated that synthesis of RNA and viral proteins was unaffected, whereas the amount of HA protein incorporated into progeny virus particles were markedly reduced. These data suggest that amantadine had impaired assembly of viral particles for the avian strain. Progeny of both the human and avian strains selected for resistance to amantadine exhibited mutations that were clustered near the middle of the gene coding for a second M protein, the $M_2$ protein. This segment of the gene codes for a string of hydrophobic amino acids that span the viral membrane. Recent studies have suggested that rimantadine interferes with hydrogen ion penetration of the matrix protein. Dissociation of the protein at low pH appears necessary for release of RNA; without release replication is not initiated (Belshe, *personal communication*).

Rimantadine has been less extensively studied than amantadine, but its mechanism for action appears identical to that of amantadine. Viruses resistant or susceptible to amantadine exhibit an identical spectrum for rimantadine (63,66). There is no increase in antiviral effects of mixtures of the two drugs, and strains selected for resistance to rimantadine also exhibit amino acid substitutions in the hydrophobic region of the $M_2$ protein similar to those of strains selected for resistance to amantadine (66).

### *Pharmacokinetics*

Amantadine is available in 100-mg capsules and as a syrup containing 50 mg/5 ml; rimantadine has been used as 100-mg tablets and in a syrup of similar concentration. Neither drug is available in injectable form.

Despite their structural similarity, amantadine and rimantadine differ significantly in their pharmacokinetics. Plasma concentrations in young and elderly adults after a single 200-mg dose of each drug are shown in Fig. 6 (55). Amantadine is rapidly and completely absorbed with a time to peak plasma level of approximately 2 hr. The peak plasma concentrations after a 100-mg dose in young adults are 0.2–0.3 μg/ml and 0.5–0.7 μg/ml after a 200-mg dose. Peak concentrations in elderly persons are more than 50% higher, a finding attributable to a delay in renal clearance.

Amantadine is entirely eliminated through urinary excretion. The half-life for amantadine in healthy young adults is variable, but averages approximately 15 hr, whereas the half-life among elderly persons is approximately 30 hr (55,67,68). Amantadine is excreted by both glomerular filtration and tubular secretion. Nevertheless, creatinine clearance appears to be a useful guide for adjusting dosage, as there is a significant inverse correlation between creatinine clearance and plasma half-life. These findings clearly indicate a need for dosage reduction among elderly persons so as to reduce the likelihood of undesirable side effects. For healthy adults, a dosage of 100 mg twice daily is used, whereas a dosage of only 100 mg/day is recommended for elderly persons. Because of a nonlinear increase in plasma concentration with continual dosing, Aoki and Sitar (67) have recommended selecting a dose that produces a trough concentration at steady state of 0.3 μg/ml. For healthy young and elderly adults, this is 3 and 1.5 mg/kg/day, respectively, doses that will be near the recommended 200 and 100 mg per day for an average sized person.

The volume of distribution of amantadine is large, and this accounts for the minimal removal of drug during hemodialysis (55,67). In humans, nasal mucous concentrations are approximately the same as those in plasma, and the drug is known to be excreted in breast milk (55,69).

Rimantadine is also completely absorbed after an oral dose, but absorption is considerably delayed when compared to amantadine (55,68). The time to peak plasma concentration in young adults after a 100- or 200-mg dose orally is approximately twice that of amantadine (mean of approximately 5 hr), and concentrations are approximately one-half of those for amantadine (0.1 μg/ml for a 100-mg dose and 0.2–0.3 μg/ml for a 200-mg dose). In contrast to amantadine, the time to peak plasma concentration after a 100-mg and 200-mg dose orally are approximately the same among elderly persons as among young adults. Rimantadine plasma levels increase after continual dosing; steady state concentrations after a pe-

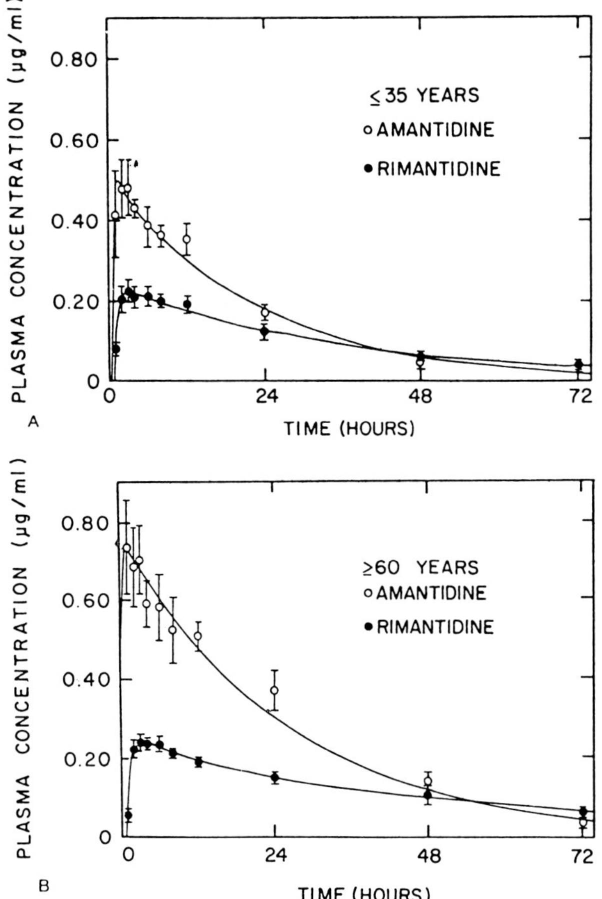


**FIG. 6.** Plasma concentrations of amantadine (*open circles*) and rimantadine (*solid circles*) observed after the administration of a single 200-mg dose in young **(A)** or elderly **(B)** adults. (From Hayden et al., ref. 55, with permission.)

riod of multiple doses of 100 mg once daily or twice daily are 0.2 µg and 0.4 µg/ml, respectively. At steady state in elderly nursing home patients, however, a dosage of 100 mg twice daily produced an average plasma concentration of 1.2 µg/ml (70). Although the condition of these patients was not reported, these data suggest that dosages may need modification in some elderly patients.

Rimantadine is metabolized and eliminated through urinary excretion. The half-life for rimantadine in healthy young adults averages approximately 30 hr, and it is similar among patients over age 65 (55,71). Only a small percentage of rimantadine is recoverable in urine, as most of the drug is metabolized to the inactive hydroxyl or glucuronidate derivative. Single-dose pharmacokinetics in patients with cirrhosis were similar to those in healthy patients. Patients with chronic renal disease exhibit an increase in the half-life of rimantadine, indicating need for a reduced dose among such persons (72).

The volume of distribution of rimantadine is large and, as for amantadine, accounts for minimal removal of drug during hemodialysis. In humans, nasal mucous concentrations are greater than those in serum, suggesting a concentration of drug in this body fluid (55).

### *Adverse Reactions*

Amantadine exhibits central nervous system (CNS) stimulatory activity, presumably through its demonstrated effect on catecholamine release (73). This presumably accounts for the CNS side effects and for its beneficial effect in therapy of Parkinson's disease. Rimantadine does not exhibit an effect on catecholamine metabolism; it is ineffective for Parkinson's disease, and yet it has been reported to exhibit CNS side effects when plasma concentrations are comparable to those of amantadine (74). Both amantadine and rimantadine exhibit gastrointestinal side effects and both produce local stinging when given by aerosol (75,76). These findings suggest a local cellular toxic effect, and a depression of ciliary activity was noted in ferret tracheal ring cells exposed to the concentrations that might be present at surface sites (77).

Amantadine is generally well tolerated when given by the oral route at recommended dosages. The most commonly reported adverse effects are minor CNS and gastrointestinal symptoms (52,55,78–82). CNS symptoms include nervousness, insomnia, dizziness, and difficulty concentrating; on occasion, drowsiness, somnolence, and listlessness may develop. Gastrointestinal symptoms include nausea, vomiting, and dyspepsia. These adverse reactions reportedly occur in approximately 10% of normal adults given 200 mg/day for prophylaxis. Complaints typically develop during the first 2–3 days of drug use. On continued dosing, the percentage of persons complaining will fall to approximately 5%; side effects promptly disappear on cessation of the drug. During trials for prophylaxis, an excess of persons taking amantadine in a double-blind fashion will withdraw from study because of side effects. In a comparative trial among college students that showed effectiveness for amantadine, 16% of subjects withdrew before completion because of side effects, whereas only 5% in the placebo group withdrew (82).

Side effects from amantadine are related to drug dosage and correlate with plasma concentration (55). Dosages of 300 mg/day have been tried and are poorly tolerated because of side effects; side effects reported by persons given 100 mg/day do not appear to be different from those in placebo. Patients with impaired renal function may develop high plasma drug concentrations (>1 μg per ml); such patients have exhibited confusion, hallucinations, seizures, and other findings of CNS toxicity. Long-term usage of amantadine in patients with Parkinson's disease has been associated with an increase in livedo reticularis and peripheral edema (83).

Rimantadine at dosages similar to amantadine has been accompanied by fewer side effects. In an extensive report of side effects, including unreported studies, Reale (84) reported that rimantadine was well tolerated by persons of all ages, but a slight increase in gastrointestinal and CNS-related adverse reactions was seen in geriatric patients when compared to children and young adults. CNS and gastrointestinal complaints were similar to those described for amantadine. At a dosage of 200 mg/day in adults and 5 mg/kg/day in children, reports of side effects were no different than seen among persons given placebo. Large-scale trials in the Soviet Union also indicate the infrequency of side effects from use of rimantadine (85).

Higher dosages of rimantadine can, however, induce side effects. Dosages of 300 mg/day have produced an increase in CNS and gastrointestinal complaints in comparison to placebo. Hayden et al. (55) and Tominak and Hayden (68) have suggested that toxicity is similar for rimantadine and amantadine among persons with similar plasma concentrations and that the lower frequency of complaints among rimantadine recipients at the 200 mg/day dosage is because of the difference in pharmacokinetics. Among residents of nursing homes, a dosage of 200 mg/day was associated with occurrence of nausea and anxiety (70). As with amantadine, side effects promptly disappear on discontinuation of the drug.

### *Clinical Effectiveness: Prophylaxis*

Both amantadine and rimantadine are effective for prevention of type A influenza virus infection and illness. The initial demonstration of clinical effectiveness of amantadine was provided by Jackson et al. (86) in a controlled study employing volunteers challenged with an H2N2 virus. This demonstration of effectiveness was followed by a series of trials involving artificial challenge that demonstrated effectiveness for prevention of infection and illness caused by an H2N2 or an H3N2 influenza A virus (52,87,88). Most of these studies employed amantadine at a dose of 200 mg/day in a young adult population. Amantadine at a dose of 100 mg/day was recently shown to be effective for preventing illness among volunteers following challenge with an influenza A virus of the H1N1 subtype (89). These studies employing artificial challenge clearly indicate effectiveness of amantadine for prevention of type A influenza virus infection and illness caused by all 3 subtypes of type A and absence of effectiveness for type B influenza virus infection and illness. A study employing rimantadine at a dose of 400 mg/day indicated effectiveness for prevention of illness following challenge with a type A (H2N2) influenza virus (90).

A number of studies have also demonstrated the effectiveness of amantadine and rimantadine for prevention of naturally occurring infection and illness caused by type A influenza viruses. A summary of 34 separate studies is shown in Table 8 (52,80–82,85,88,91–98). Approximately 30,000 persons have been involved in studies that included children, healthy adults, and elderly persons. Amantadine has been tested against all three virus subtypes of influenza A, and rimantadine has been tested against the H1N1 and H3N2 subtypes. The majority of studies demonstrated significant protection against both infection and illness. The reasons for lack of uniformity in demonstrating protection is not always clear, but insufficient numbers of subjects was responsible in some studies. Studies in families where members exposed to an index case were given prophylaxis demonstrated effectiveness against a type A Asian (H2N2) virus and not against type A Hong Kong (H3N2) virus 1 year later (99). The author suggested that the absence of any prior immunity among exposed persons in the latter study caused less protection. In immunized elderly nursing home residents, administration of 200 mg/day of rimantadine to vaccinated persons during an epidemic significantly improved protection over vaccine alone (95).

A summary of four recent studies in

**TABLE 8.** *Summary of studies of amantadine and rimantadine for prophylaxis of naturally occurring influenza A virus infection and illness*

| Virus | Drug[a] | Number of studies[b] | Approximate number of subjects (Range per study)[c] | Number of studies with significant decreases in drug group (%) | |
|---|---|---|---|---|---|
| | | | | Illness | Infection |
| Type A H2N2 | Amantadine | 6 | 5,500 (96–3,990) | 5 (83) | 5 (83) |
| Type A H3N2 | Amantadine | 9 | 20,000 (110–8,170) | 7 (78) | 4/6 (67) |
| | Rimantadine | 11 | 13,000 (57–6,000) | 10 (91) | 5/5 (100) |
| Type A H1N1 | Amantadine | 3 | 700 (214–275) | 3 (100) | 3 (100) |
| | Rimantadine | 5 | 500 (76–202) | 3 (60) | 4 (80) |

[a]Includes studies employing 100 and 200 mg/day of amantadine and 50–200 mg/day of rimantadine in adults.
[b]Two studies employed both amantadine and rimantadine.
[c]Includes placebo controls.

**TABLE 9.** *Recent trials of amantadine and rimantadine for prevention of type A influenza*

| Age group and viral subtype | Drug group | Infected | Infected and ill | CNS side effects |
|---|---|---|---|---|
| Young adults, A/H1N1 and A/H3N2 | Placebo | 32/132 (24%) | 27/132 (21%) | 6/148 (4%) |
| | Amantadine | 7/113 (6%) | 2/113 (2%) | 19/145 (13%) |
| | Rimantadine | 11/133 (8%) | 4/133 (3%) | 9/147 (6%) |
| Young adults, A/H1N1 | Placebo | 42/139 (30%) | 28/139 (20%) | 2%, 6%[a] |
| | Amantadine | 26/142 (18%) | 8/136 (6%) | 8%, 13%[a] |
| Children | | | | |
| A/H1N1 | Placebo | 13/41 (32%) | 7/41 (17%) | 2/41 (5%) |
| | Rimantadine | 1/35 (3%) | 0/35 (0%) | 0/35 (0%) |
| A/H3N2 | Placebo | 9/29 (31%) | 7/29 (24%) | 1/27 (4%) |
| | Rimantadine | 2/27 (7%) | 0/27 (0%) | 2/27 (7%) |

[a]Percent with mental depression and nervousness, respectively. Other CNS symptoms same in both groups.

healthy persons is shown in Table 9 (80, 82,97,98). Both amantadine and rimantadine were given daily for 5–7 weeks at a dosage of 200 mg/day in adults, and rimantadine was given as 5 mg/kg/day to children. Protection against infection varied between 39% and 91%, whereas protection against illness varied between 71% and 100%. Generally speaking, amantadine and rimantadine usually prevent approximately two-thirds of infections and approximately three-fourths of infection-related illnesses. Of interest is the higher frequency of reports of adverse reactions among those taking amantadine; reactions among those taking rimantadine were not different than placebo. The lowest effective dose for prophylaxis has not been clearly determined, but some studies have suggested that 100 mg/day of amantadine and 50 mg/day of rimantadine are effective for prevention of type A infection and illness among adults (85).

### *Therapy*

Both amantadine and rimantadine are effective for treatment of type A influenza virus infections. A summary of 25 treatment studies is shown in Table 10 (52,85,88,100–108). All studies were conducted in healthy children or adults, and both rimantadine and amantadine were evaluated against

**TABLE 10.** *Summary of studies of amantadine and rimantadine for treatment of naturally occurring influenza A virus infection and illness*

| Virus | Drug[a] | Number of studies[b] | N[c] | Number of studies with significant reduction in drug group (%): Illness | Virus shedding[d] |
|---|---|---|---|---|---|
| Type A H2N2 | Amantadine | 4 | 554 | 4 (100) | NT |
| | Rimantadine | 2 | 80 | 2 (100) | 0/1 (0) |
| Type A H3N2 | Amantadine | 5 | 740 | 5 (100) | 2 (40) |
| | Rimantadine | 8 | 1125 | 8 (100) | 2/2 (100) |
| Type A H1N1 | Amantadine | 2 | 50 | 2 (100) | 2 (100) |
| | Rimantadine | 4 | 186 | 3 (75) | 3/3 (100) |

[a]Includes studies employing 200 mg/day of amantadine and 150–300 mg/day of rimantadine in adults.
[b]Two studies employed both amantadine and rimantadine.
[c]Includes placebo controls.
[d]Evaluations were virus isolation only or virus isolation and quantitation.
NT, not tested.

each of the subtypes of type A influenza virus. All but one study (108) report statistically significant beneficial effects on signs and symptoms of acute influenza. Early studies employing virus isolation frequency as the only variable for assessing effects on virus shedding did not identify an antiviral effect. Later studies have sometimes shown a reduction in frequency of isolations, but a significant reduction in quantity of virus in respiratory secretions at some time during the course of infection was uniformly detected when this variable was evaluated. Thus, the significant clinical benefit was associated with a significant antiviral effect. In studies where aspirin or acetaminophen were used as controls, a superior effect of amantadine or rimantadine was usually noted either on fever or symptoms or both (105,107).

A comparison of the effect of amantadine and rimantadine in clinical influenza among college students treated during an A/USSR/77 (H1N1) epidemic is shown in Fig. 7. Students with influenza for less than 48 hr were given drug at a dose of 100 mg twice daily for 5 days. At 48 hr after commencing treatment, significantly more students given drug were afebrile and symptomatically improved; in addition, they shed less virus and returned to class sooner. Amantadine patients tended to improve somewhat more rapidly than the rimantadine-treated patients, a finding that has been attributed to the differences in pharmacokinetics of the two drugs since beneficial effects were equal at 48 hr. Because of the short duration of clinical influenza in healthy persons, it is not possible to show beneficial effects of treatment in those ill for more than 2 days before initiation of therapy.

Studies of peripheral airways function among students experiencing naturally occurring type A influenza indicated abnormalities during the acute and early convalescence period (109,110). In a study employing amantadine therapy, a more rapid return to normal function was seen among these given drugs compared to placebo. This suggests a beneficial effect

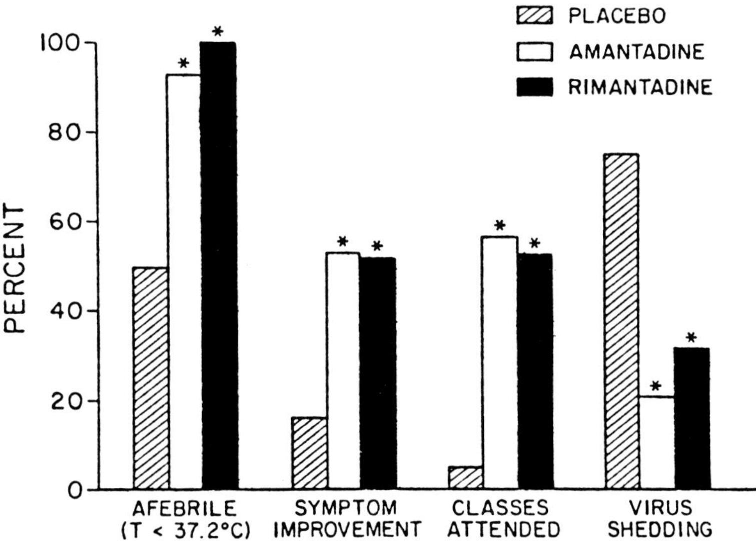


**FIG. 7.** Comparative therapeutic effectiveness of amantadine, rimantadine, and placebo in uncomplicated influenza A/USSR/77 (H1N1) infection of students. At 48 hr after initiating therapy, the percent of subjects with temperature less than 37.2°C, the percent symptom improvement from enrollment, the percent of subjects shedding virus, and the drug-treated group differed significantly (*$p < 0.05$) from the placebo group. (From Vann Voris et al., ref. 104, with permission.)

might be seen in persons with chronic peripheral airways dysfunction when experiencing influenza; a test of this possibility has not been reported. Treatment of 11 persons apparently experiencing primary influenzal pneumonia with 400–500 mg/day was followed by death in five, a finding not clearly different from that for untreated persons (88). Whether early treatment of persons in high-risk groups will reduce the frequency of complications has not been tested.

Treatment of persons with acute influenza with aerosols containing amantadine or rimantadine has also been reported. A modest benefit was seen among persons given intermittent amantadine in this way (111). Wilson et al. (75) reported on tolerance and clinical use of the Collision atomizer for prolonged therapy with amantadine. Some minor nasal stinging was noted in normals with aerosol administration, but patients treated with amantadine by small-particle aerosol tolerated drug well and experienced a prompt recovery. More recently, Atmar et al. (76) have used a small-particle aerosol generator to treat patients with acute influenza with rimantadine. Patients experienced nasal stinging, sometimes unpleasant, with inhalations of concentrations designed to deliver approximately 150 mg/day to a normal adult, but they tolerated 75 mg/day without difficulty.

Recent studies of virus isolates from children treated for 5 days with rimantadine revealed the appearance of rimantadine-resistant strains during and following therapy (107). The M protein of these strains has been examined, and an amino acid change in the hydrophobic region of the M2 protein was detected (66). More recently, it has been noted that rimantadine-resistant strains can transmit to other persons and produce clinical influenza (57). Although it seems unlikely that rimantadine resistance will become a characteristic of influenza strains in general, the possibility that high-risk persons on rimantadine prophylaxis would be exposed to rimantadine-resistant virus during epidemic periods is somewhat disconcerting. Findings such as these have been reported earlier by Webster et al. (112) among chickens experiencing epidemic avian influenza. They suggested that a widespread use of vaccine would be desirable to reduce the risk of disease from drug-resistant strains.

### *Recommendations for Clinical Use of Amantadine and Rimantadine*

It should be emphasized that immunization is the primary means for control of influenza. A variety of persons and circumstances can, however, benefit from use of amantadine or rimantadine for prophylaxis or therapy of type A influenza. Although rimantadine is not yet approved for clinical use in the United States, it is recommended as an alternative to amantadine, and dosages are given for both drugs. Because of lower toxicity at effective doses, rimantadine will probably replace amantadine when approved for clinical use. Amantadine is not approved for use in infants under 1 year of age or in pregnant women, because of lack of safety data. It is not recommended for nursing mothers because drug is excreted in breast milk. A similar restriction on the use of rimantadine is recommended at present, although available data on rimantadine in infants under 1 year of age indicate safety (113).

#### *Prophylaxis*

As indicated in Table 11, amantadine or rimantadine should be given throughout the epidemic season to persons at risk of serious complications of influenza if they have not been immunized with influenza virus vaccine or the vaccine used is known to be a poor antigenic match for epidemic virus. Persons in the high-risk group are adults and children with chronic disease of the heart or lungs requiring regular medical care, children with asthma, residents of

**TABLE 11.** *Recommendations for clinical use of amantadine and rimantadine*

| |
|---|
| Prophylaxis |
| Unimmunized high-risk persons |
| Unimmunized persons caring for and/or in home with high-risk persons |
| Immunized high-risk persons when vaccine and epidemic virus are a poor antigenic match |
| All residents and personnel in institutions containing high-risk persons during an institutional outbreak |
| Persons with immunodeficiency |
| As an adjunct to late immunization among high-risk persons (2-week period) |
| Consider as routine adjunct to immunization among high-risk persons |
| Consider for persons exposed in the household (2 weeks) |
| Treatment |
| All high-risk persons with type A influenza |
| Persons with severe type A influenza including pneumonia |

nursing homes and other chronic-care facilities housing patients of any age with chronic diseases, persons over age 65, adults and children requiring regular medical care for chronic metabolic disorders, renal disease, a hemoglobinopathy, or immunosuppression, and children receiving long-term aspirin therapy that may put them at risk for Reyes' syndrome after an influenza virus infection (114). Prophylaxis with amantadine or rimantadine should be given to unimmunized persons in close contact with high-risk persons in the home and those who care for them in medical institutions. This recommendation is aimed at reducing the exposure of high-risk persons to type A influenza virus.

Experience with use of amantadine during institutional outbreaks of influenza has led to a recommendation for short-term prophylaxis (2–3 weeks) of all residents and personnel of institutions containing high-risk persons as soon as an outbreak is recognized at the institution (114). In this circumstance, all persons should be given drug regardless of vaccination status. In order to be effective, such programs should be organized before the influenza season.

Amantadine or rimantadine should also be given to persons with an immunodeficiency throughout the epidemic period, even though they were vaccinated, because of their suboptimal responses to influenza virus vaccine. A similar use of drug as an adjunct to vaccine among high-risk persons should be considered, as this would constitute optimal prophylaxis currently. Amantadine and remantadine can also be used for a period of 2 weeks to provide protection during an immediate postvaccination period when immunization is given early in the outbreak period. Finally, the drug can be effective for prevention of influenza in persons exposed in households.

### *Treatment*

Amantadine and rimantadine can shorten the duration of fever, symptoms, pulmonary function abnormalities, and virus shedding when used for treatment early in the course of acute influenza (see above). In this circumstance, a 32% reduction in secondary infection frequencies was seen in families where acute illnesses were treated in comparison to families where persons with acute illness were given placebo (115). Efficacy for amantadine or rimantadine requires commencing therapy early, preferably within 24 hr of onset, but at least within 48 hr. Whether therapy of severe influenza such as in children with croup, persons with pneumonia, and persons requiring hospitalization can be initiated later and still provide benefit has not been determined. Nevertheless, because of the gravity of these illnesses, late initiation of therapy is recommended in hopes that it will be of some benefit.

Therapy of acute influenza A illness is recommended for all persons in the high-risk group regardless of whether they received vaccine. In addition, to clinical benefit, it is hoped that early treatment of such persons will reduce the frequency of complications; a study to evaluate this possibility is underway. Finally, therapy is recommended for healthy persons ill enough to seek health care at a medical facility, particularly for persons providing essential community services. A return to work 1–2 days earlier as a consequence of treatment is worthwhile.

### *Dosage*

Dosage recommendations for both amantadine and rimantadine are shown in Table 12, although the latter is not yet approved for use. Doses for prophylaxis are similar for both drugs among healthy adults and children and persons over age 65. Although it is less clear that rimantadine needs to be reduced to 100 mg/day among those over age 65, this is recommended because of the reported delay in elimination and accumulation of high blood levels among elderly persons (55,67,68). A dosage adjustment for renal insufficiency is recommended for both amantadine and rimantadine.

Therapy with amantadine or rimantadine has been recommended for a period of 5 days. In view of the demonstration of development of resistance in children treated for 5 days, the recommendation is for treatment only as long as incapacitating symptoms such as fever, myalgias, and severe cough are present. In most cases, a 3-day course of therapy will be adequate.

**TABLE 12.** *Dosage recommendations for amantadine*[a]

| | |
|---|---|
| Ages 1–9 years | 5 mg/kg/day<br>Not to exceed 150 mg/day |
| Ages 10–64 years | 200 mg daily |
| Age 65 years and older | 100 mg daily |
| Renal insufficiency | Initial dose as above for day 1, then reduce dose so *average* daily dose thereafter is approximately equivalent to (creatinine clearance/100) × 200 mg. |

[a]Daily dosage can be given once daily or in divided doses (every 12 hr).

## *Ribavirin*

Ribavirin (1-β-ribofuranosyl-1H-1,2,4-triazole-3-carboxamide) is a colorless, water-soluble compound with a molecular weight of 244.2 (Fig. 8). It was synthesized in 1972 by Witkowski and Robins and shown shortly thereafter to exert antiviral effects against a variety of RNA- and DNA-containing viruses (116,117).

### *Antiviral Effects*

Ribavirin is effective *in vitro* against the influenza viruses, parainfluenza viruses, and RSV (118). It is less effective against adenoviruses, coxsackie A viruses, rhinoviruses, and coronaviruses (118).

Ribavirin has also been efficacious in animal model systems against a variety of the respiratory viruses; included are influenza A and B virus and parainfluenza virus (Sendai) in mice, respiratory syncytial virus in cotton rat, and influenza in monkeys (49,119–121). Although effective when given by a parenteral route, ribavirin was more effective for treatment of influenza A and B virus infection in mice and for RSV in cotton rats when given by small particle aerosol (119–121). The most effective therapy for influenza A virus pneumonia in mice was administration of a combination of ribavirin and amantadine by small-particle aerosol; aerosol treatment of infected mice could be delayed for up to 120 hr postinoculation and still be effective.

### *Mechanism of Action*

Ribavirin closely resembles guanosine and is converted to the mono-, di-, and triphosphate derivatives by cellular enzymes (122). This similarity led to a proposal that ribavirin might be utilized competitively in place of guanosine. Guanosine has been shown in many systems to reverse the inhibitory effects of ribavirin; however, the inhibition of influenza virus and RSV *in vi-*

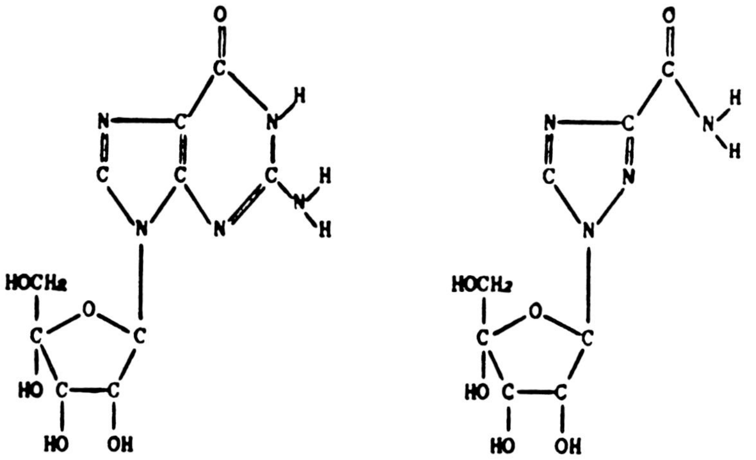

**FIG. 8.** Formula for ribavirin and guanosine. Note the similarity of the two formulas.

*tro* is not completely reversed by the addition of guanosine to the system (122,123). This indicates that, at least for these two viruses, the potent inhibition of inosine monophosphate (IMP) dehydrogenase exhibited by ribavirin monophosphate with the resulting decrease in pool size of guanosine triphosphate (GTP) is not the sole action that inhibits their replication.

The mechanism of action of ribavirin has been studied in detail for the influenza viruses. Three possible mechanisms for an inhibitory effect have been proposed: a decrease in the intracellular concentration of GTP due to the competitive inhibition of IMP dehydrogenase, inhibition of 5′ cap formation of mRNA, and inhibition of the virus-coded RNA polymerase complex. Wray et al. (123), showed a reduction in GTP pool size, with increasing concentrations of ribavirin, but a continued increase in concentration beyond 25 μM did not result in a further reduction, and, yet, antiviral effects progressively increased. Moreover, the 1,4,5-triazole derivative is a potent inhibitor of IMP dehydrogenase and has no antiviral activity (124). Ribavirin triphosphate inhibits the GTP-dependent capping of the 5′ end of viral mRNA (122). Since influenza requires the simultaneous synthesis of host mRNA as a source of capped primer for viral mRNA, inhibition of host-capping enzymes may contribute to inhibition of influenza virus.

Ribavirin triphosphate has been shown to inhibit the influenza virus polymerase complex (125,126). Synthesis of the mRNA of influenza virus involves priming and initiation of synthesis, probably via the PB1 and PB2 polymerase proteins. Initiation is mediated by the incorporation of a guanosine residue onto the 3′ end of the capped primer fragment; elongation of the mRNA is then most probably mediated by the PB1 enzyme. Ribavirin triphosphate inhibits both initiation and elongation but is more active on the latter process. This possible action of ribavirin on different steps of the replication process may explain the inability to detect viral isolates resistant to ribavirin. Support for inhibition of mRNA synthesis as the major mechanism for inhibition of RSV is provided by the observation that ribavirin inhibits viral but not cellular polypeptide synthesis in RSV-infected cells (127).

### *Pharmacokinetics*

Ribavirin is approved for treatment of RSV by small-particle aerosol only. The available data on pharmacokinetics of ribavirin given by the oral route, however, provides a basis for interpreting some of the pharmacokinetics of small-particle aerosol therapy. When administered orally, approximately 50% of ribavirin is absorbed from the gastrointestinal tract (128). Approximately 50% of ribavirin is excreted as undegraded or deribosylated ribavirin in 72 hr. The half-life of ribavirin in plasma in 10–12 hr, whereas that in red blood cells is 40 days; the latter is explained by inefficient dephosphorylation (128).

Less than 1% of ribavirin given to monkeys by the oral route is present in the lung at 8 hr, whereas the small-particle aerosol route will provide approximately 70% of inhaled drug to the lung (129,130). Concentrations of ribavirin in secretions of infants during administration by small-particle aerosol are very high, whereas they fall by 24 hr after cessation of treatment (130). The half-life in secretions was estimated to be approximately 2 hr, whereas that in plasma of aerosol-treated infants was approximately 9 hr. Infants given aerosol therapy with a reservoir containing 20 mg/ml of ribavirin for 2.5 hr/day for 3 days had a plasma level of 0.76 μM, whereas those given aerosol for 20 hr for 5 days had levels ranging from 1.5 to 14.3 M, with a mean of 6.8 μM (130).

### *Adverse Effects*

A variety of adverse effects were described in preclinical toxicology evaluations of ribavirin, but use of ribavirin in humans has been remarkably free of toxicity. Transient elevations of serum bilirubin and occurrence of mild anemia have been noted in persons given ribavirin orally or intravenously (131,132). Studies in monkeys showed rapid extravascular clearing of erythrocytes and, at high doses, the suppression of the release of late erythroid elements from the bone marrow (133). The bilirubin elevations probably represent the more rapid elimination of red cells containing ribavirin triphosphate. No adverse effect has clearly been attributable to aerosol therapy with ribavirin, although reports of adverse effects during or following aerosol therapy of infants with RSV-induced illness have included bronchospasm, pulmonary function changes, pneumothorax (in ventilated patients), apnea, cardiac arrest, hypotension, and digitalis toxicity (134).

Concern has been expressed by many about the safety of administering ribavirin by small-particle aerosol to infants receiving assisted ventilation. Cases cared for in pediatric intensive care units by persons knowledgable about respiratory function and attentive to respirator function have not encountered difficulty, although therapy using a respirator is not yet an approved method for aerosol therapy.

Some concern has been expressed for the safety of persons in the room with infants being treated with ribavirin by aerosol, particularly women in the child-bearing age group since the drug is teratogenic for rodents; it was not, however, teratogenic in baboons (135). Rodriguez et al. (136) reported on the study of 19 nurses exposed to 20–35 hr of ribavirin therapy over a 3-day period given via a ventilator, oxygen tent, or oxygen hood (136). Urine and blood were collected before, 1 hr after completion of therapy, and 3–5 days later. No ribavirin was detected in urine, plasma, or red blood cells using an assay with a sensitivity of 0.01 μM of drug. Another recent test of eight workers exposed in rooms where therapy was being conducted evaluated air concentrations of ribavirin in the vicinity of personnel and cases as well as in body fluids (137). Air concentrations around ventilators were lowest (<1 to 6 μg/M$^3$), whereas those around oxygen tents were highest (69–316 μg/M$^3$). Thirty samples of blood and urine of the eight employees were tested for ribavirin; plasma and urine samples were all negative, but one red cell sample reportedly contained 0.44 μg/ml of ribavirin. This nurse had cared for an infant being treated via oxygen tent. These findings indicate that awareness and caution on the part of personnel would effectively prevent significant environmental exposure; a portable aerosol-removal device for the tent and hood area has recently been developed, and its use should increase environmental safety.

### *Clinical Effectiveness: Prophylaxis*

Limited studies of prophylaxis have been conducted in volunteers artificially infected with influenza virus. Results were varied, although one study where 1,000 mg/day was given orally starting 6 hr after inoculation demonstrated a beneficial effect on illness and infection (131). All other trials have been therapeutic; ribavirin is not now proposed as a drug for prophylaxis of respiratory viral infection and illness.

### *Treatment of Influenza*

Although initial reports suggested a therapeutic effect of oral ribavirin therapy for acute influenza, subsequent studies have shown minimal to no effect of this therapy. Smith et al. (132), in a double-blind multicenter trial during a naturally-occurring outbreak with A/Brazil/11/78 (H1N1)–like virus in young adults, failed to find a therapeutic or antiviral effect of ribavirin begun within 48 hr of disease onset and given orally at a dose of 1,000 mg/day (132). A recent trial using a loading dose of 3,600 mg orally and then 1,200 mg at 12-hr intervals for 48 hr showed a minimal therapeutic effect and no effect on virus shedding (138).

Treatment of acute influenza with ribavirin by small-particle aerosol has, however, been effective. Over a period of 4 years, Knight et al. (47,139,142) and others (140,141) conducted placebo-controlled clinical trials of ribavirin aerosol treatment of college students experiencing acute influenza. Students were admitted to the study if they had an oral temperature of over 101°F and had been ill for less than 24 hr. A summary of ribavirin aerosol treatment of type A and B influenza virus infections in college students is shown in Table 13. A total of 64 treated and 72 control patients were studied. Ribavirin aerosol therapy was associated with a significant shortening of the duration of fever in four studies, borderline in one, and not significant in one. The absence of an effect in 1 year was thought to be related to the mildness of illness. Estimated dosage in the first 36–40 hr varied between 1.15 gm and 3.12 gm (mean dosage of 2.0 ± 0.8 gm), but dosage did not correlate with therapeutic effect. Each trial that showed a beneficial effect on fever also revealed a beneficial effect on virus shedding. Thus, it appears clear that ribavirin aerosol therapy is effective for treatment of acute influenza caused by either type A or type B influenza virus.

Experience with treatment of hospital-

**TABLE 13.** *Mean hours from start of treatment to afebrile (<100°F)*

| Virus | Year | Patients: Control | Patients: Treated | *p* Value |
|---|---|---|---|---|
| H3N2 | 1983 | 55.5 (3) | 25.1 (2) | 0.017 |
| B | 1982 | 55.0 (7) | 36.1 (9) | 0.047 |
| H1N1 | 1984 | 48.6 (20) | 29.9 (18) | 0.004 |
| | 1983 | 33.5 (14) | 30.3 (13) | 0.300 |
| | 1982 | 42.7 (11) | 31.4 (8) | 0.066 |
| | 1981 | 35.5 (17) | 21.1 (14) | 0.015 |

Values for fever represent time in hours. Value in parentheses are number of patients studied. *p* Values were obtained from analysis of data by Students *t* test, two-tailed.

ized cases of acute influenza has, thus far, been limited. Six cases of influenza pneumonia were treated with ribavirin aerosol therapy, and all recovered (143).

### *Treatment of RSV Infections*

Initial reports of treatment of infants with aerosol ribavirin indicated a beneficial effect of therapy. Taber et al. (144) used a 12-hr daily course of therapy among infants with a clinical diagnosis of bronchiolitis and showed a significant benefit on symptom score at day 3 of therapy but no effect on virus shedding. Hall et al. (145) used a 20-hr daily course for 3–6 days and showed a significant improvement in severity score (Fig. 9) and improvement in arterial oxygen among treated cases at the end of therapy (Fig. 10). Similarly, at the end of the treatment period, ribavirin-treated infants were shedding significantly less virus. No adverse effects were noted from aerosol therapy in these studies.

A summary of six reported studies of ribavirin aerosol therapy is shown in Table 14 (144–149). Each showed a significant beneficial effect of treatment on signs, symptoms, and/or severity of illness. This beneficial effect in controlled studies is supported by a perception among pediatricians that this therapy is beneficial, particularly for the infant with underlying bronchopulmonary or cardiac disease. A significant antiviral effect was detected only in the trials reported by Hall et al. (145,146). The reductions in virus shed were not noted until the end of therapy (days 4–6) and related to virus quantity only. Only the study by Taber et al. (144) performed similar evaluations of virus shedding, and they treated for a 12-hr period only. It seems clear that ribavirin in aerosol therapy is beneficial for serious disease in infants caused by RSV.

An additional potentially beneficial effect of ribavirin aerosol therapy was reported by Rosner et al. (150). They noted a lower frequency of development of RSV-specific IgE and IgA antibody in respiratory secretions. It is postulated that the IgE antibody may have a role in producing the recurrent bronchospasm and wheezing that may occur on reinfection with RSV; the suppression of an IgE antibody response may prevent the subsequent bronchospastic disease. On the other hand, the reduction in

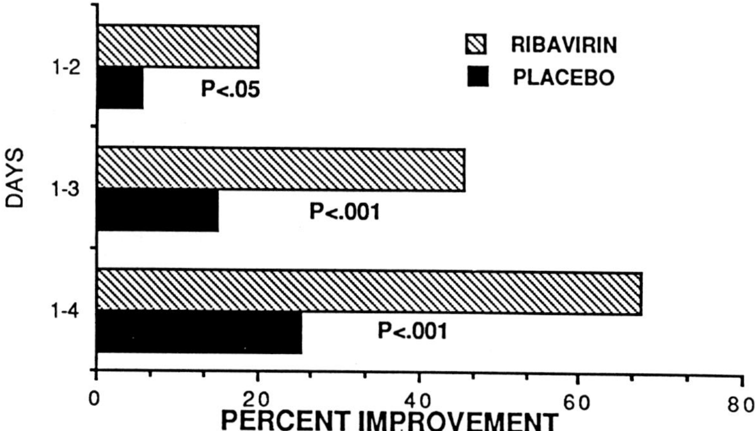


**FIG. 9.** Percent improvement in illness severity scores from day one to days two, three, and four of aerosol ribavirin therapy among infants with RSV illness. (Modified by Hall from data in ref. 145, used with permission.)

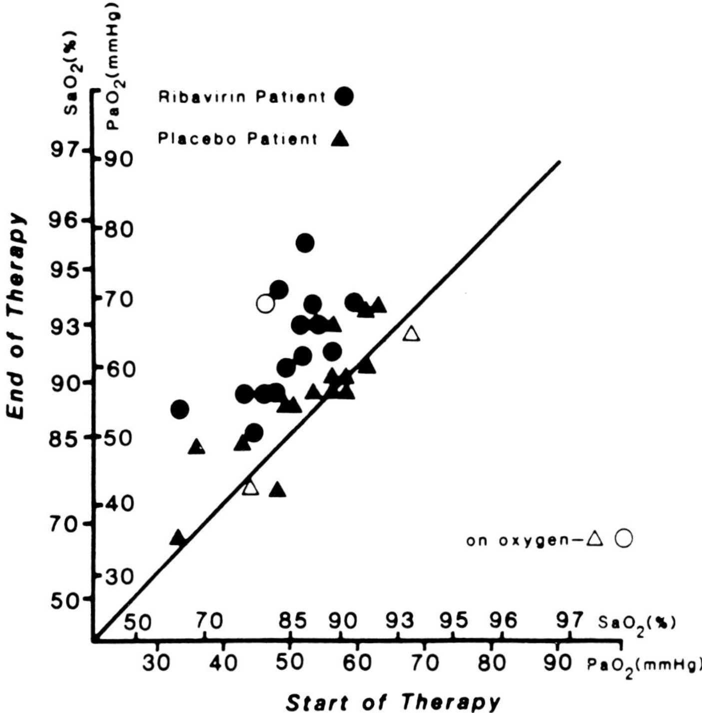


**FIG. 10.** Arterial blood-gas levels at the beginning and end of therapy with ribavirin (*solid circles*) or placebo (*solid triangles*). The diagonal represents the line of identity—i.e., no change in values over the course of the therapy. $SaO_2$, arterial oxygen saturation; $PaO_2$, arterial oxygen tension. All infants were breathing room air, except those three indicated by *open symbols*. (From Hall et al., ref. 145, with permission.)

**TABLE 14.** *Treatment of severe lower respiratory disease in infants with ribavirin aerosol*[a]

| Ref. | *N*, infants | | Treatment schedule | Significant beneficial effect on | | Side effects |
|---|---|---|---|---|---|---|
| | Treated | Control | | Illness | Virus shedding | |
| 145 | 16 | 17 | 20 hr × 3–6 days | + | + | 0 |
| 146 | 14 | 12 | 20 hr × 5 days | + | + | 0 |
| 144 | 12 | 14 | 12 hr × 5 days | + | 0 | 0 |
| 147 | 20 | 10 | 20–22 hr × 3 days | + | 0[2] | 0 |
| 148 | 14 | 12 | 18 hr × 3+ days | + | 0[2] | 0 |
| 149 | 33 | 97 | 12–20 hr × 3–8 days | + | NT | 0 |

[a]Included croup, bronchiolitis, pneumonia, cases with underlying disease, and cases where respirators were used.
[b]One study evaluated shedding for 3 days only, and the other only evaluated isolation frequency.
NT, not tested.

IgA antibody responses in this study and the reduction in serum neutralizing antibody responses in another study among infants given ribavirin therapy may impair resistance to reinfection (144,150).

*Parainfluenza Virus Infections*

Three infants with severe combined immune deficiency virus pneumonia were treated with ribavirin aerosol, and results were reported (151). One infant had RSV, one had RSV and parainfluenza 3 virus infection, and one had parainfluenza 3 virus only. Each child was treated with several courses of ribavirin aerosol over a period of weeks and experienced clinical and virologic benefit from each course (Fig. 11). These data support a benefit for treatment of parainfluenza virus infections.

*Recommendations for Clinical Use of Ribavirin Aerosol*

Infants hospitalized with lower respiratory disease caused by RSV are candidates for ribavirin aerosol therapy (Table 15). Treatment should be given to infants at high risk for severe and complicated RSV illness; these include infants with a variety of reasons for severe illness and complications. Infants at risk of progressing to severe illness (<6 weeks of age with underlying illness) and infants who are severely ill also should be treated. The latter may be defined by a low arterial $O_2$ or rising $CO_2$.

Treatment is also recommended for infants with immunodeficiency who develop parainfluenza virus lower respiratory disease. This has been beneficial in controlling infection until bone marrow transplantation can be given (151). Infants and adults hospitalized with severe influenza virus pneu-

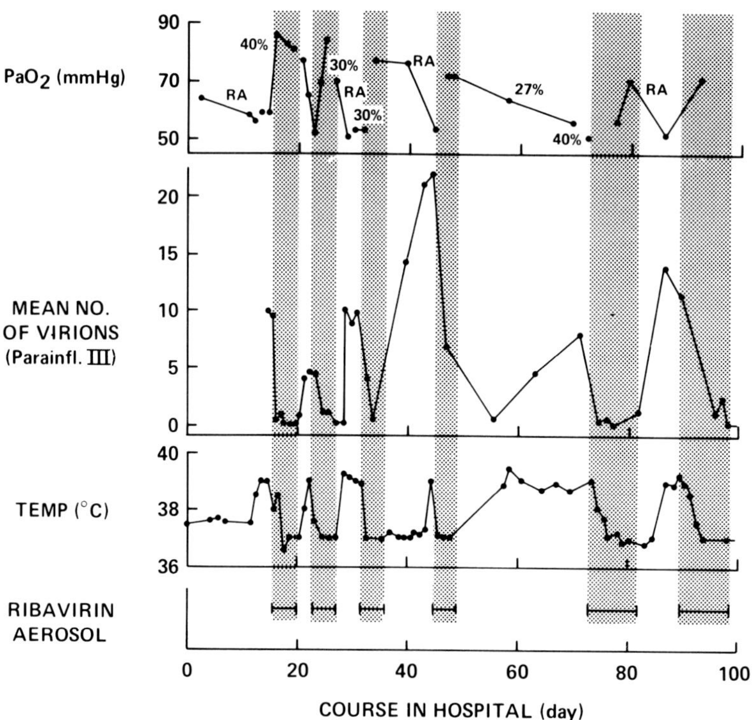


**FIG. 11.** Ribavirin aerosol treatment of parainfluenza virus, type 3, infection in an infant with severe combined immune deficiency disease. Inspired oxygen concentrations shown in *upper panel.* (From Gelfand et al., ref. 151, with permission.)

**TABLE 15.** *Recommendations for clinical use of ribavirin aerosol therapy*

| |
|---|
| RSV |
| Hospitalized infants at high risk for severe or complicated illness |
| Congenital heart disease |
| Bronchopulmonary dysplasia |
| Premature infants |
| Immunodeficiency |
| Transplant recipients |
| Cancer chemotherapy |
| Hospitalized infants <6 weeks of age with underlying chronic illness |
| Hospitalized infants who are severely ill |
| Parainfluenza virus |
| Hospitalized infants with severe illness and immunodeficiency |
| Influenza virus |
| Hospitalized infants, children, and adults with pneumonia |

monia should be treated, although proof of beneficial effect is not available at this time.

### *Dosage*

Dosage estimates for infants and adults may be calculated using variables noted earlier. Recent determinations by Knight et al. (50) indicate that a greater air exchange per kg per unit time occurs in infants, so dosage for a given reservoir concentration will be greater for this age group. It is generally agreed that near-continuous therapy for 3–5 days is desirable for infants with severe lower respiratory disease; this will mean daily therapy should be for approximately 20 hr of each 24-hr period.

College students with acute influenza have recovered rapidly with an initial 16-hr duration of therapy followed by an additional 2 days of therapy of 12-hr duration. Treatment of influenza penumonia has been for periods of 16–20 hr daily for 3–5 days.

## Antivirals with Potential for Clinical Use

### *Interferons*

The observation that prior inoculation of chick embryos with irradiated influenza virus inhibited subsequent growth of infectious virus led to the discovery by Isaacs and Lindemann (152) that a protein mediated this effect. Because it mediated interference, they called it "interferon." Since the initial reports, study of the interferons has occupied the attention of many investigators and the subject area has expanded in complexity. We now know that three families of interferons exist and that a great variety of effects on cellular function may be mediated by the interferons; their antiviral effects constitute only one potential clinical use for these chemicals.

The recent availability of interferon produced in *Escherichia coli* by recombinant DNA has permitted a reevaluation of all early basic and clinical studies. One of the original hopes for interferon was that this natural body substance would be nontoxic and effective for all virus infections, including the respiratory viral infections. Yet when given by the parenteral route in effective doses, the interferons were found to produce fever, myalgias, malaise, and other adverse effects (153). For this reason, trials for acute respiratory illness have been limited to topical administration. The status of development of topical administration of interferon for prevention and treatment of respiratory viral infections will be briefly summarized.

#### *Description*

The interferons are proteins or glycoproteins with a molecular weight of approximately 17,000 (Table 16). Virus infection stimulates production of interferon-α and interferon-β presumably via nucleic acid replication; double-stranded RNA is a potent inducer of interferon. Interferon-γ is released by T cells activated by antigen or mitogens; it is weak as an inducer of the antiviral state in comparison with interferon-α and interferon-β. A number of different species of interferon are known to exist, as about 18 different genes for interferon-α have been identified and two for interferon-

**TABLE 16.** *Properties of the three families of interferons*

| Property | Alpha (leukocyte) | Beta (fibroblast) | Gamma (immune) |
|---|---|---|---|
| Cell source | Macrophages, lymphocytes | Fibroblasts, epithelial cells | T lymphocytes |
| Inducer | Nucleic acid, virus infection | Nucleic acid, virus infection | Antigens, mitogens |
| Number of genes | 18 | 2 | 1 |
| Chemical structure | Protein | Glycoprotein | Glycoprotein |
| Molecular weight | 17,000 | 17,000 | 17,000 |
| Acid stability (pH2) | Stable | Stable | Labile |
| Relative antiviral effect | + + + | + + + | + |

β. Only a small number have been used in clinical trials (see also Chapter 2).

Interferon is quantitated by reference to a standard and expressed as international units (IU). Initial leukocyte (α) interferon preparations contained up to $1 \times 10^6$ IU/mg of protein, whereas recombinant DNA (rDNA) produced interferon preparations containing up to $1 \times 10^8$ IU/mg.

### *Mechanism of Action*

The mechanism for induction of interferon remains to be determined; however, considerable information is available on how it induces the antiviral state. Interferon-α and interferon-β attach to a receptor on the cell surface encoded by chromosome 21 (154). Internalization of interferon triggers a series of events that influence the metabolic processes required for viral replication. A protein kinase is induced that modifies the function of initiation factor. In addition, 2′, 5′-oligoadenosine is synthesized by an induced synthetase, and the oligoadenosine activates an RNAase that digests the mRNA of the virus (155). Other enzymes appear to be induced and may also affect virus replication.

### *Pharmacokinetics*

Topically applied interferon has been shown to clear rapidly from the nasal mucosa. An almost immediate 10-fold reduction in concentration was noted in clearance studies of interferon-α; this was followed by a slower clearance over the next 24 hr, but overall clearance appears rapid (156). This rapid clearance may partially explain the large dose requirements for obtaining an antiviral effect.

Initial trials with administration of interferon by intranasal instillations or by aerosol were short term, and no toxicity was detected. However, when rDNA-produced interferon became available, longer durations of use were evaluated and local adverse effects were encountered. A dose- and duration-dependent toxicity has been clearly noted for interferon-α (157,158). Side effects are primarily nasal stuffiness, blood-tinged mucus, and occurrence of mucosal erosions. Nasal biopsies from persons experiencing these effects revealed submucosal infiltrations with lymphocytes and other mononuclear cells, and the degree of infiltration correlated with the severity of nasal symptoms (159). Symptoms and cellular infiltrates resolved with cessation of interferon use. The side effects begin to appear approximately 5 days after initiating interferon use, so only short-term use of effective doses can be considered.

Interferon-β has been less completely studied, and interferon-γ has not been used intranasally, so comparative toxicity is not yet available.

### *Clinical Effectiveness*

Soviet investigators reported effectiveness of topical interferon for prevention of influenza in controlled studies (160). In a subsequent controlled trial in volunteers, Merigan et al. (161) were unable to show a beneficial effect for influenza with a higher dose. They did, however, show a beneficial effect for prevention of a rhinovirus illness. This focused attention on the possibility that interferon could prevent common colds; rhinovirus infections then received the most attention as targets for interferon use. A summary of clinical trials of topical interferon for rhinovirus infections, the most commonly studied infection, is shown in Table 17 (157,161–177).

### *Prophylaxis*

The study by Merigan et al. (161) used what was then considered to be a very large dose (14 × $10^6$ IU); this suggested the dose requirement might be large. In a series of physiologic studies, Greenberg et al. (178) showed that a 10-fold lower dose could be made effective, but only when used in a cotton pledget and when antihistamines were added. His studies suggested the major reason for the high-dose requirement was the lack of cellular contact with interferon.

The availability of rDNA-produced interferon removed the interferon availability restrictions. Initial trials with rDNA produced interferon, and artificial challenge with a rhinovirus indicated a potent preventive effect of intranasal interferon; 60–100% of colds were prevented with doses of 10 × $10^6$ IU/day, and infection was prevented or reduced as well (Table 17). Dose-response

**TABLE 17.** *Summary of controlled studies of interferon-α for rhinovirus infections*

| Type of study (reference) | Interferon dose and schedule | Significant reduction in: Illness | Virus shedding |
|---|---|---|---|
| Leukocyte interferon | | | |
| Experimental challenge | | | |
| prophylaxis | | | |
| Merigan (161) | 3.5 × $10^6$ × 6 days | + | + |
| Greenberg (163) | 1–3× $10^6$ × 1–2 days | 0 | 0 |
| Scott (162) | 22.5 × $10^6$ × 4 days | + | + |
| Natural infection | | | |
| Prophylaxis | | | |
| Scott (164) | 0.4, 1.5, 4.4 × $10^6$ × 28 days | T | NT |
| rDNA interferon, | | | |
| Experimental challenge | | | |
| Prophylaxis | | | |
| Phillpotts (166) | 11 × $10^6$ × 4 days | + | + |
| Scott (165) | 22.5 × $10^6$ × 4 days | + | + |
| Hayden (167) | 45.6 × $10^6$ × 4 days | + | + |
| Samo (157,158) | 2.4–10 × $10^6$ × 4 days | + | 0 |
| Therapy | | | |
| Hayden (168) | 27 × $10^6$ × 5 days | ± | ± |
| Natural infection | | | |
| Preexposure prophylaxis | | | |
| Farr (169) | 10 × $10^6$ × 22 days | T | + |
| Douglas (170) | 2 × $10^6$ × 28 days | T | + |
| Monto (171) | 3 × $10^6$ × 28 days | T | + |
| Betts (172) | 5 × $10^6$ × 28 days | T | + |
| Postexposure prophylaxis | | | |
| Douglas (173) | 5 × $10^6$ × 7 days | + | + |
| Hayden (174) | 5 × $10^6$ × 7 days | + | + |
| Foy (175) | 5 × $10^6$ × 7 days | 0 | 0 |
| Herzog (176) | 1.5 × $10^6$ × 5 days | + | 0 |
| Therapy | | | |
| Hayden (177) | 40–80 × $10^6$ × 5 days | 0 | + |

+, Significant; ±, borderline; 0, not significant; T, toxicity so assessment not possible; NT, no test.

studies indicated the minimal effective dose was approximately $3 \times 10^6$ IU/day (158). Clinical trials then moved to a seasonal (preexposure) prophylaxis approach to prevention of respiratory viral infection and illness, but the nasal toxicity described earlier was encountered so that such an approach did not appear feasible (157). Lower doses and alternative interferon preparations have not overcome this problem.

The seasonal prophylaxis studies did, however, provide a clear indication of effectiveness of interferon for preventing naturally occurring rhinovirus infections (169–172). In order to exploit this effect in an approach to prophylaxis designed to minimize the side effects, trials were organized to give interferon to family members for 7 days when an index case of respiratory illness appeared in a family member (173–176). In two studies, this approach reduced the overall frequency of colds in exposed family members by approximately 40%, but approximately 85% of rhinovirus colds were prevented (173–174). Side effects of treatment occurred, but they appeared minimal. Two other studies, however, did not show such a significant beneficial effect (175,176). Disappointing, however, was the finding of little to no effectiveness of this approach for prevention of influenza or parainfluenza virus infections occurring during the study period.

The use of intranasal interferon for short periods in the family exposure circumstance remains as a potential clinical use. It would, however, have greater potential for use if a means for rapid identification of rhinovirus infection in index cases were available. Alternatively, it has been suggested that persons with chronic underlying disease such as chronic bronchitis and emphysema might have an acceptable risk-benefit from seasonal prophylaxis because rhinovirus infection has been shown to provoke serious decompensation (179).

Other studies with lymphoblastoid and interferon-β have reported equal effectiveness for prevention of rhinovirus infections induced by artificial challenge, but they are insufficiently evaluated to discern whether side effects will be limiting at effective doses (180,181). Other trials evaluated rDNA-produced interferon against artificial challenge with influenza virus or coronavirus (182,183). In these trials, topical interferon has appeared relatively ineffective for prevention of illness and infection caused by influenza viruses, whereas limited data suggests an effectiveness for coronaviruses comparable to rhinoviruses.

#### *Treatment*

Large doses of rDNA-produced interferon have been used for treatment of rhinovirus infection and illness. Some minimal beneficial effects have been noted, but the investigators concluded that the effect was not sufficient to support further studies on this application (168,177).

### *Antirhinovirus Antivirals*

Considerable effort has been devoted toward developing antivirals for rhinovirus infections because of the large market a safe and effective compound would command. This effort has involved a large number of clinical trials; it has yielded a number of interesting compounds, and clinical benefit has been demonstrated for some. None are, however, nearing approval at the present time.

#### *Enviroxime*

Enviroxime (Fig. 12) is a benzimidazole derivative with a high degree of activity *in vitro* against 83 of 83 rhinovirus serotypes (184). The 50% inhibition dose ($ID_{50}$) varies from <0.01 to 0.12 μg/ml; concentrations required for *in vitro* toxicity are considerably higher (>20 μg/ml), suggesting a high degree of selectivity for the compound.

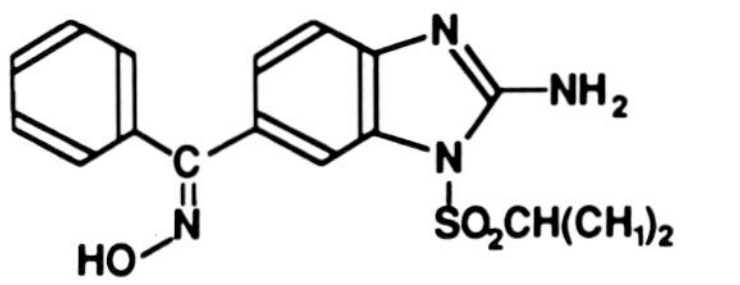

**Enviroxime**

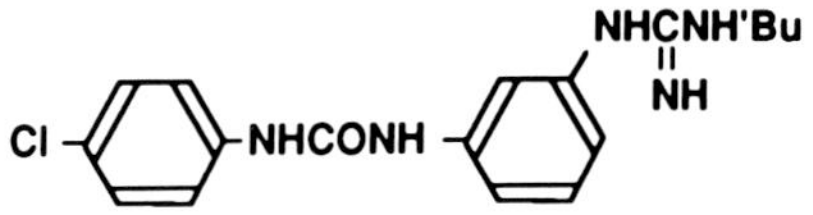

**ICI 73602**
**1 - (p-chlorophenyl) - 3 - (m - 3 - isobutylguanidinophenyl) urea hydrochloride**

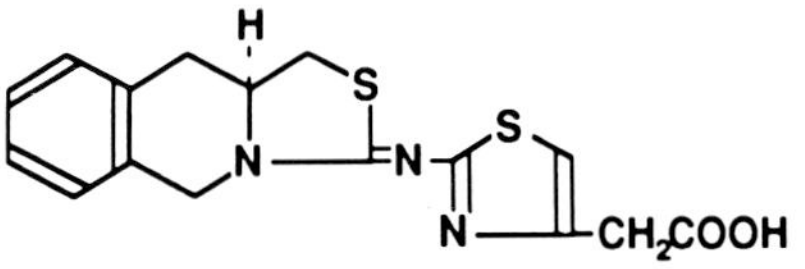

**44081**
**2 - [(1, 5, 10, 10a - tetrahydro - 3H - thiazolo (3, 4b] - isoquinolin - 3 - ylidine) amino] - 4 - thiazole acetic acid**

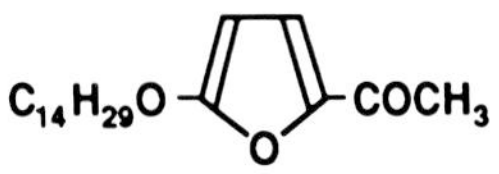

**RMI 15731**
**1 - (5 - Tetracecyloxy - 2 - furanyl) ethanone**

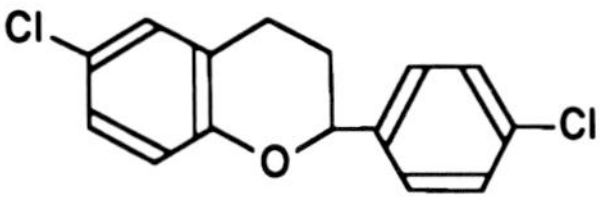

**4'6' Dicloroflavan**

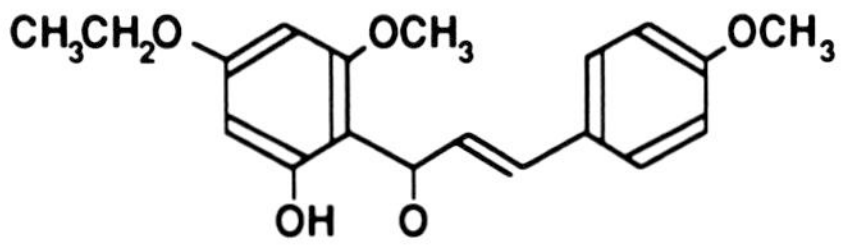

**RO 09-0410**
**4' - Ethoxy - 2' - hydroxy - 4, 6' - dimethoxychalcone**

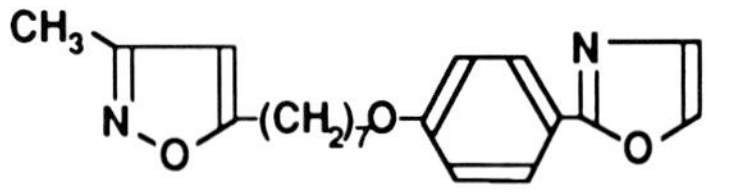

**WIN 151711**
**(5 - [7 - [4 - (4, 5 - dihydro - 2 - oxazolyl] phenoxy] heptyl] - 3 - methylisoxazole)**

**FIG. 12.** Formulas of antiviral compounds with effectiveness *in vitro* against rhinoviruses.

The mechanism of action of enviroxime is not known, but it acts on a process after uncoating such that formation of the RNA polymerase complex is inhibited (185).

Preclinical trials with oral enviroxime revealed nausea in volunteers at doses that were not considered adequate for clinical use, so an intranasal spray was developed to permit topical administration. Because of its low solubility in water, an alcohol carrier was used and the final product produced some nasal irritation. The initial clinical trial used oral and intranasal administration in a prophylactic design that employed artificial challenge of normal volunteers with a rhinovirus (186). Each intranasal dose was 24 μg, and each oral dose was 25 mg; both were given four times daily starting before and continuing after inoculation. Nausea and vomiting was a problem among treated persons, but the reduction in symptoms and virus titer in nasal wash specimens caused the authors to believe the drug had clinical potential.

Subsequent trials involved several locations and several different rhinoviruses; topical administration only was used. Some trials showed a beneficial effect, and others did not; those with beneficial effects had reductions in colds ranging form 25% to 60% of colds (184,186,187). Simultaneous therapeutic trials among artificially infected volunteers also showed some effect, although a trial of early treatment against naturally occurring colds indicated only a minimal therapeutic benefit (188). Because of these minimal and inconsistent results, the manufacturer chose not to further study this compound.

### *ICI 73602 and 44081 R.P.*

ICI 73602 inhibits action of the viral RNA polymerase. It was shown to be effective *in vitro* against a number of serotypes of rhinovirus and appeared to have selectivity, as the cellular toxicity concentration was 20- to 100-fold higher than the effective antiviral concentrations (0.2–1.6 μg/ml) (189). Nevertheless, in trials in volunteers, little activity was detected (190). Compound 44081 R.P. was shown to inhibit uncoating and to be effective in cells pretreated before challenge; it also had a high degree of selectivity (191). In volunteer trials, it exerted no significant benefit against rhinovirus challenge when given as a self-administered spray; concentrations of compound 44081 R.P. in nasal secretions were, however, variable and frequently below the minimal inhibitory concentration (MIC) for the virus (192). The authors suggested that a very high intranasal dose to MIC ratio was required for effectiveness; the ratio was approximately $10^6$ for effective doses of interferon, which was effective for prevention, whereas the value for compound 44081 R.P. was $10^3$.

### *Inhibitors of Uncoating*

A number of compounds have been developed recently that bind to viral capsid protein and inhibit uncoating of rhinovirus after adsorption and penetration. This is the mechanism of action for compounds RMI 15731, 4′,6′-dichloroflavan, RO 09-0410, WIN 51711, and possibly compound 44081 described above (193–198). More is known about the action of WIN 51711 than the others; it is an isoxazole derivative of arildone, a compound shown many years ago to possess activity against a number of enteroviruses (196). WIN 51711 had high activity against poliovirus type 2 and rhinovirus type 2; further studies indicated activity against many enteroviruses and rhinoviruses including rhinovirus type 14 (199). Rhinovirus type 14 has been crystallized, and the three-dimensional structure described (200). Viral proteins (VP) 1, 2, and 3 form the exterior of the particle, with folding that creates a canyon on the viral surface surrounding each of the 12 vertices of the virus particle. The WIN compound was added to rhinovirus type 14 crystals, and diffraction analysis was performed. The compound was detected within the VP1 structure, which makes up the majority of the canyon floor (Fig. 13). This configuration apparently does not interfere with adsorption and penetration, but uncoating is impaired. The molecular mechanism for interference is not yet certain, but it is proposed that the compound might compete with a molecule that appears in the canyon and promotes membrane interactions after receptor binding (200).

Studies by Ishitsuka et al. (198) have shown a similar mechanism of action for RM 15731, 4′,6′-dichloroflavan, and RO 09-0410. In addition, they have shown that mutant viruses selected for resistance to each of the compounds exhibit cross-resistance to the other compounds. These compounds inhibit rhinovirus replication *in vitro* at very low concentrations in some cases (0.002 μg/ml), although a range of sensitivities is seen. Again, a high degree of selectivity is exhibited by these compounds.

4′,6′-Dichloroflavan is well absorbed after oral administration; however, when volunteers were given 1 mg/kg three times daily starting before and continuing after rhinovirus challenge, no beneficial effect was seen (201). The chalcone RO 09-0410 is not well absorbed after oral administration, but a phosphorylated precursor to the ac-

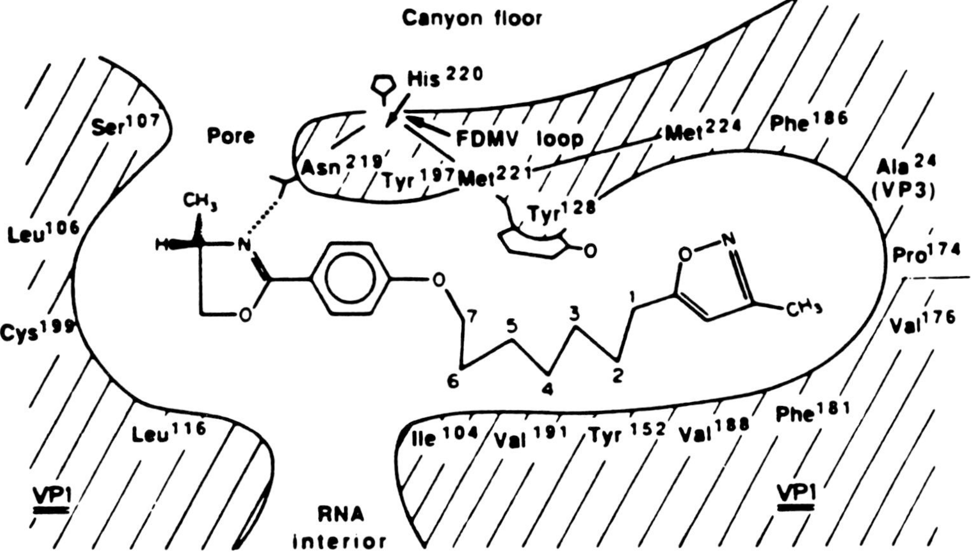


**FIG. 13.** Diagram of WIN 15711 binding site within capsid protein ($VP_1$) of human rhinovirus type-14, showing amino acid residues within 3.6A of the bound drug. (From Smith et al., ref. 200, with permission.)

tive compound is well absorbed. The precursor was administered at a dose of 1,200 mg twice daily for 7 days starting before challenge with rhinovirus type 9 (202). As with the flavan, plasma concentration in excess of those required to inhibit virus *in vitro* were obtained; nevertheless, no beneficial effect was seen. In order to evaluate topical therapy, a suspension of the flavan was prepared and given repeatedly before and after inoculation with rhinovirus; this approach was also clinically ineffective (203). Since the 4′,6′-Dichloroflavan is hydrophobic, topical therapy may present a problem of access to mucosal cells similar to that seen with enviroxime.

These clinical trials with antivirals for rhinovirus infection have been almost uniformly discouraging. Little to no clinical benefit was realized, despite availability of compounds with a high degree of effectiveness *in vitro* and a wide margin of safety. The reason suggested for failure of orally administered drug was that it did not reach mucosal cells and surrounding fluids in concentrations sufficient for a significant antiviral effect. Similarly, it was proposed that topically administered drug was cleared so rapidly or penetrated mucus so poorly that pericellular fluids never contained sufficient drug for an antiviral effect. Thus, the problem no longer appears to be identifying potent and safe antivirals for rhinovirus infections, but, rather, it appears to be developing methods for optimal administration to the nasal mucosa so as to obtain full benefit from the antiviral.

## FINAL COMMENTS

The identification of the individual viruses causing most of the acute respiratory viral illnesses during the 1950s and 1960s provided a basis for hope that effective vaccines and antivirals would soon be available. However, development of safe and effective vaccines and antivirals for these infections proved to be a significant scientific problem. Only now does it appear that new and useful antivirals will soon be available. This optimism can be attributed to the elucidation of the details of viral replication. The technology of molecular biology is permitting search for antiviral compounds with a specific action. Obstacles remain, however, to implementation of any effective compound identified.

The acute respiratory viral illnesses are localized, mostly mild illnesses that are of short duration. These features indicate that a useful antiviral must obtain rapid access to the respiratory system and exhibit a high degree of safety. In order to initiate the required prompt use, an antiviral must be immediately available to the ill person; a requirement for physician contact or parenteral administration will permit use for severe and prolonged illnesses only. Knowledge of the specific virus causing the infection is needed in order to know when a particular antiviral is appropriate. The diverse nature of viruses causing the acute respiratory illnesses indicates the probable need for a diverse set of antivirals; this is both a problem for development and a problem for implementation. Increased community surveillance for prevalent viruses and methods for rapid viral diagnosis are needed for directing the proper use of antivirals.

A resolution of the difficulties facing development and recommendations for use of antivirals for respiratory illnesses may not be sufficient to ensure their widespread use. Many believe that the mild nature of most acute respiratory illnesses will lead to a low incentive for their use. That this is unlikely (unless cost becomes a disincentive to use) is suggested by the extensive use of symptomatic medications for these illnesses. A more likely problem in usage is the fact that the medical care system in developed societies is oriented toward therapeutic medicine and not preventive medicine. Antivirals are likely to be most effective when used to prevent infection and illness. For this application, a redirection of the practice of medicine is needed; such a redirection of emphasis would also have benefits in other areas of medicine. Thus, the future of antivirals for the acute respiratory viral infections holds problems as well as promise, but there is ample reason for optimism that a resolution of problems will be realized.

### Addendum

R61837 is a recently described pyridazinamine that inhibits uncoating of rhinoviruses by binding to capsid protein. When combined with a cyclodextrin (a cyclic carbohydrate) that is water soluble, the relatively insoluble R61837 given topically resulted in a beneficial effect on infection and illness. The cyclodextrin is presumed to have provided improved access to the nasal mucosa permitting *in vivo* activity for this compound which was highly active *in vitro* (Al-Nakib, W, Higgins PG, Barrow BI, et al. Suppression of colds in human volunteers challenged with rhinovirus by a new synthetic drug (R61837) Antimicrob Agents Chemother, 1989, 33:522–525.

## REFERENCES


1. *Vital and health statistics. Current estimates from the National Health Interview Survey, United States, 1985*. DHHS publication no. (PHS) 86-1588. Hyattsville, Maryland: National Center for Health Statistics, September 1986.
2. Fox JP, Hall CE. *Viruses in families*. Littleton: PSG Publishing Co., Inc., 1980.
3. Tyrrell DAJ. *Common colds and related diseases*. Baltimore: The Williams & Wilkins Co., 1965.
4. Joklik WK. Basic virology. In : *Zinsser Microbiology*. Norwalk: Appleton and Lange, 1988:624–756.
5. Fields BN. *Virology*. New York: Raven Press, 1985.
6. Lamb RA, Choppin PW. The gene structure and replication of influenza viruses. *Annu Rev Biochem* 1983;52:467.
7. Doerfler W. The molecular biology of adenoviruses. *Curr Top Microbiol Immunol* 1983; 109:1—232.
8. Doerfler W. The molecular biology of adenoviruses. *Curr Top Microbiol Immunol* 1984; 110:1–265.
9. Bishop DHL, Compans RW. *Nonsegmented negative strand viruses: paramyxoviruses and rhabdoviruses*. New York: Academic Press, 1984.
10. Choppin PW, Richardson CD, Merz DC, et al. The functions and inhibition of the membrane glycoproteins of paramyxoviruses and myxoviruses and the role of the measles virus M pro-

tein in subacute sclerosing panencephalitis. *J Infect Dis* 1981;143:352–63.
11. Strauss EG, Strauss JH. Replication strategies of the single-stranded RNA viruses of eukaryotes. *Curr Top Microbiol Immunol* 1983; 105:1–184.
12. Sturman LS, Holmes KV. The molecular biology of coronaviruses. *Adv Virus Res* 1986; 28:36.
13. Gwaltney JM Jr. The common cold. In: Mandell GL, Douglas RG, Jr, Bennett JE, eds. *Principles and practice of infectious diseases*. New York: John Wiley & Sons, 1985:351–5.
14. Gwaltney JM Jr. Rhinoviruses. *Yale J Biol Med* 1975;48:17–45.
15. Cate TR, Couch RB, Johnson KM. Studies with rhinovirus in volunteers: production of illness, effect of naturally acquired antibody, and demonstration of a protective effect not associated with serum antibody. *J Clin Invest* 1964;43:56–67.
16. McIntosh K, Kapikian AZ, Turner HC, et al. Seroepidemiologic studies of coronavirus infection in adults and children. *Am J Epidemiol* 1970;91:585–92.
17. Monto AS, Lim SK. The Tecumseh study of respiratory illness. VI. Frequency of and relationship between outbreaks of coronavirus infection. *J Infect Dis* 1974;129:271–6.
18. Dingle J, Langmuir AD. Epidemiology of acute respiratory disease in military recruits. *Am Rev Respir Dis* 1968;97:1–65.
19. Top FH Jr. Control of adenovirus acute respiratory disease in US army trainees. *Yale J Biol Med* 1975;48:185–95.
20. Gwaltney JM Jr. Acute bronchitis. In: Mandell GL, Douglas RG Jr, Bennett JE, eds. *Principles and practice of infectious diseases*. New York: John Wiley & Sons, 1985:385–7.
21. Hall CB. Acute laryngotracheobronchitis, croup. In: Mandell GL, Douglas RG Jr, Bennett JE, eds. *Principles and practice of infectious diseases*. New York: John Wiley & Sons, 1985:385–7.
22. Hall CB, Douglas RG Jr. Respiratory syncytial virus and influenza: practical community surveillance. *Am J Dis Child* 1976;130:615–20.
23. Henderson FW, Clyde WA Jr., Collier AM, et al. The etiologic and epidemiologic spectrum of bronchiolitis in pediatric practice. *J Pediatr* 1979;95:183–90.
24. Foy HM, Cooney MK, Maletzky AJ, et al. Incidence and etiology of pneumonia croup and bronchiolitis in preschool children belonging to a prepaid medical care group over a four year period. *Am J Epidemiol* 1973;97:80.
25. Glezen WP. Viral pneumonia as a cause and result of hospitalization. *J Infect Dis* 1983; 147:765–70.
26. Glezen WP, Paredes A, Taber LH. Influenza in children: relationship to other respiratory agents. *JAMA* 1980;243:1345–9.
27. Fry J. Lung involvement in influenza. *Br Med J* 1951;2:1374–7.
28. Mufson MA, Chang V, Gill V, et al. The roles of viruses, mycoplasmas and bacteria in acute pneumonia in civilian adults. *Am J Epidemiol* 1967;86:526–44.
29. Couch RB, Cate TR, Gerone PJ, et al. Production of illness with a small particle aerosol of coxsackie A-21. *J Clin Invest* 1965;44:535–42.
30. Burk RF, Schaffner W, Koenig MG. Severe influenza virus pneumonia in the pandemic of 1968–1969. *Arch Intern Med* 1971;127:1122–8.
31. Couch RB Cate TR, Douglas RG Jr, et al. Effect of route of inoculation on experimental respiratory viral disease in volunteers and evidence for airborne transmission. *Bacteriol Rev* 1966;30:517–29.
32. Moser MR, Bender JR, Margolis HS, et al. An outbreak of influenza aboard a commercial airliner. *Am J Epidemiol* 1979;110:1–6.
33. Dick EC, Jennings LC, Mink KA, et al. Aerosol transmission of rhinovirus colds. *J Infect Dis* 1987;156:442–8.
34. D'Alessio DJ, Peterson JA, Dick CR, et al. Transmission of experimental rhinovirus colds in volunteer married couples. *J Infect Dis* 1976;133:28–36.
35. Hall CB, Douglas RG Jr. Modes of transmission of respiratory syncytial virus. *J Pediatr* 1981;99:100–3.
36. Couch RB, Cate TR, Fleet WR, et al. Aerosol-induced adenovirus illness resembling the naturally-occurring illness in military recruits. *Am Rev Resp Dis* 1966;93:529–35.
37. Douglas RG Jr, Couch RB, Cate TR, et al. Quantitative rhinovirus shedding patterns in volunteers. *Am Rev Resp Dis* 1966;94:159–67.
38. Couch RB, Douglas RG Jr, Fedson DS, et al. Correlated studies of a recombinant influenza virus vaccine. III. Protection against experimental influenza in man. *J Infect Dis* 1971;124:473–80.
39. LeFrak EA, Stevens PA, Pitha J, et al. Extracorporeal membrane oxygenation for fulminant influenza pneumonia. *Chest* 1974;66:385–8.
40. Mulder J, Hers JF. *Influenza*. Groningen: Wolters-Noordhoff Publishing, 1972.
41. Douglas RG Jr, Alford BR, Couch RB. Atraumatic nasal biopsy for studies of respiratory virus infection in volunteers. *Antimicrob Agents Chemother* 1986:340–3.
42. Naclerio RM, Proud D, Lichtenstein LM, et al. Kinins are generated during experimental rhinovirus colds. *J Infect Dis* 1988;157:133–42.
43. Mims CA, White DO. *Viral pathogenesis and immunology*. Oxford: Blackwell Scientific Publications, 1984.
44. Glezen WP, Taber LH, Frank AL, et al. Risk of primary infection and reinfection with respiratory syncytial virus. *Am J Dis Child* 1986;140:543–6.
45. Couch RB, Kasel JA. Immunity to influenza in man. *Annu Rev Microbiol* 1983;37:529–49.
46. Tyrrell DAJ. Interferons and their clinical value. *Rev Infect Dis* 1987;9:243–9.
47. Knight LV, Gilbert BE, Wilson SZ. Ribavirin small particle aerosol treatment of influenza and respiratory syncytial virus infections. In: Stapleton T, ed. *Studies with a broad spectrum*

*antiviral agent*. London: Royal Society of Medicine, 1986:37–56.
48. Walker JS, Stephen EL, Spertzel RO. Small-particle aerosols of antiviral compounds in treatment of type A influenza pneumonia in mice. *J Infect Dis* 1976;133S:A140–4.
49. Wilson SZ, Knight V, Wyde PR, et al. Amantadine and ribavirin aerosol treatment of influenza A and B infection in mice. *Antimicrob Agents Chemother* 1980;17:642–8.
50. Knight V, Yu CD, Gilbert BE, et al. Ribavirin aerosol dosage according to age of patient and other variables. *J Infect Dis* 1988;158:443–8.
51. Davies WL, Grunert RR, Haff RF, et al. Antiviral activity of 1-adamantanamine (amantadine). *Science* 1964;144:862–3.
52. Hoffman CE. Amantadine HCI and related compounds. In: Carter WA, ed. *Selective inhibitors of viral functions*. Cleveland: CRC Press, 1973:199–211.
53. Couch RB, Six HR. The antiviral spectrum and mechanism of action of amantadine and rimantadine. In: Mills J, Corey L, eds. *New directions in antiviral chemotherapy*. Amsterdam: Elsevier Science Publishing Co., 1985:50–7.
54. Oxford JS, Galbraith A. Antiviral activity of amantadine: a review of laboratory and clinical data. *Pharmol Ther* 1980;11:181–262.
55. Hayden FG, Minocha A, Spyken DA, et al. Comparative single-dose pharmacokinetics of amantadine hydrochloride and rimantadine hydrochloride in young and elderly adults. *Antimicrob Agents Chemother* 1985;28:216–21.
56. Grunert RR, McGahern JW, Davies WL. The *in vivo* antiviral activity of 1-adamantanamine (amantadine). I. Prophylactic and therapeutic activity against influenza viruses. *Virology* 1965;26:262–9.
57. Belshe RB, Burk B, Newman F, et al. Resistance of influenza A virus to amantadine and rimantadine: results of one decade of surveillance. *J Infect Dis* 1989;159:430–75.
58. Burlington DB, Meiklejohn G, Mostow SR. Anti-influenza A virus activity of amantadine hydrochloride and rimantadine hydrochloride in ferret tracheal ciliated epithelium. *Antimicrob Agents Chemother* 1982;21:794–9.
59. Schulman JL. Effect of 1-amantanamine hydrochloride (amantadine Hcl) and methyl-1-adamantanethylamine hydrochloride (rimantadine HCl) on transmission of influenza virus infection in mice. *Proc Soc Exp Biol Med* 1968;128:1173–8.
60. Scholtissek C, Faulkner GP. Amantadine-resistant and sensitive influenza A strains and recombinants. *J Gen Virol* 1979;38:807–15.
61. White J, Kielian M, Helenius A. Membrane fusion proteins of enveloped animal viruses. *Q Rev Biophys* 1983;16:151–95.
62. Daniels RS, Downie JC, Hay AJ, et al. Fusion mutants of the influenza virus hemagglutinin glycoprotein. *Cell* 1985;40:431–9.
63. Lubeck MD, Schulman J, Palese P. Susceptibility of influenza A viruses to amantadine is influenced by the gene coding for M protein. *J Virol* 1978;12:710–16.
64. Hay AS, Walstenholme AJ, Skehel JJ, et al. The molecular basis of the specific anti-influenza action of amantadine. *EMBO J* 1985;4:3021–4.
65. Hay AJ, Zambon MC. In: Becker Y, ed. *Antiviral drugs and interferon. The molecular basis of their activity*. Boston: Martinus-Nijhoff Pub., 1983;301–15.
66. Belshe RB, Smith MH, Hall CB, et al. Genetic basis of resistance to rimantadine emerging during treatment of influenza virus infection. *J Virol* 1988;62:1508–12.
67. Aoki FY, Sitar DS. Amantadine kinetics in healthy elderly men: implications for influenza prevention. *Clin Pharmacol Ther* 1985;37:137–44.
68. Tominack RL, Hayden FG. Rimantadine hydrochloride and amantadine hydrochloride use in influenza A virus infections. In: Knight V, Gilbert BE, eds. *Antiviral chemotherapy. Infectious disease clinics of North America, vol. 1*. 1987:459–78.
69. Bleidner WE, Harmon JB, Hewes WE, et al. Absorption, distribution and excretion of amantadine hydrochloride. *J Pharmacol Exp Ther* 1965;150:1–7.
70. Patriarca PA, Kater NA, Kendal AP, et al. Safety of prolonged administration of rimantadine hydrochloride in the prophylaxis of influenza A virus infections in nursing homes. *Antimicrob Agents Chemother* 1984;26:101–3.
71. Wills RJ, Farolino DA, Choma N, et al. Rimantadine pharmacokinetics after single and multiple doses. *Antimicrob Agents Chemother* 1987;31:826–8.
72. Wills RJ. The clinical pharmacokinetics of rimantadine. *J Respir Dis* 1987;8:S39–50.
73. Vernier VG, Harmon JB, Stump JM, et al. The toxicologic and pharmacologic properties of amantadine hydrochloride. *Toxicol Appl Pharmacol* 1969;15:642–65.
74. Hayden FG, Gwaltney JM, Van de Castle RL, et al. Comparative toxicity of amantadine hydrochloride and rimantadine hydrochloride in healthy adults. *Antimicrob Agents Chemother* 1981;19:226–33.
75. Wilson SZ, Knight V, Moore R, et al. Amantadine small-particle aerosol: generation and delivery to man. *Proc Soc Exp Biol Med* 1979;161:350–4.
76. Atmar R, Greenberg SB, Quarles J, et al. Tolerance of aerosolized rimantadine in normal volunteers and during influenza-like illnesses [Abstract]. In: *Abstracts of 28th Interscience Conference on Antimicrobial Agents and Chemotherapy*. Los Angeles: American Society for Microbiology, 1988.
77. Burlington DB, Meiklejohn G, Mostow SR. Toxicity of amantadine and rimantadine for the ciliated epithelium of ferret tracheal rings. *J Infect Dis* 1981;144:77.
78. Bryson YJ, Monahan C, Pollack M, et al. A prospective double-blind study of side effects associated with the administration of amantadine for influenza A virus prophylaxis. *J Infect Dis* 1980;141:543–7.

79. Miller VM, Dreisbach M, Bryson YJ. Double-blind controlled study of central nervous system side effects of amantadine, rimantadine, and chlorpheniramine. *Antimicrob Agents Chemother* 1982;21:1–4.
80. Monto AS, Gunn RA, Bandyk MG, et al. Prevention of Russian influenza by amantadine. *JAMA* 1979;241:1003–7.
81. Quarles JM, Couch RB, Cate TR, et al. Comparison of amantadine and rimantadine for prevention of type A (Russian) influenza. *Antiviral Res* 1981;1:149–55.
82. Dolin R, Reichman RC, Madone HP, et al. A controlled trial of amantadine and rimantadine in the prophylaxis of influenza A infection. *N Engl J Med* 307:580–4.
83. Schwab RS, Poskanzer DC, England AC, et al. Amantadine in Parkinson's disease. *JAMA* 1972;222:792–3.
84. Reele SB. Adverse drug experiences during rimantadine trials. *J Respir Dis* 1987;8:S81–96.
85. Zlydnikov DM, Kubar OI, Kovaleva TP, et al. Study of rimantadine in the USSR: a review of the literature. *Rev Infect Dis* 1981;3:408–21.
86. Jackson GG, Muldoon RL, Akers LW. Serological evidence for prevention of influenzal infection in volunteers by an anti-influenza drug, adamantanamine hydrochloride. *Antimicrob Agents Chemother* 1964:703–7.
87. Togo Y, Hornick RB, Dawkins AT Jr. Studies on induced influenza in man. 1. Double-blind studies designed to assess prophylactic efficacy of amantadine hydrochloride against A2/Rockville/1/65 strain. *JAMA* 1968;203:1089–94.
88. Couch RB, Jackson GG. Antiviral agents in influenza: summary of influenza workshop VIII. *J Infect Dis* 1976;134:516–27.
89. Sears SD, Clements ML. Protective efficacy of low-dose amantadine in adults challenged with wild-type influenza A virus. *Antimicrob Agents Chemother* 1987;31:1470–3.
90. Dawkins AT, Jr, Gallager LR, Togo Y, et al. Studies on induced influenza in man. II. Double-blind study designed to assess the prophylactic efficacy of an analogue of amantadine hydrochloride. *JAMA* 1968;203:1095–9.
91. Finklea JF, Hennessy AV, Davenport FM. A field trial of amantadine prophylaxis in naturally-occurring acute respiratory illness. *Am J Epidemiol* 1967;85:403–12.
92. Oker-Blom N, Hovi T, Leinikki P, et al. Protection of man from natural infection with influenza A2 Hong Kong virus by amantadine: a controlled field trial. *Br Med J* 1970;3:676–8.
93. Smorodintsev AA, Karpuchin GI, Zlydinkov DM, et al. The prospect for amantadine for prevention of influenza A2 in humans (effectiveness of amantadine during influenza A2/Hong Kong epidemics in January–February, 1969 in Leningrad). *Ann NY Acad Sci* 1970;173:44–61.
94. O'Donoghue JM, Ray CG, Terry DW, et al. Prevention of nosocomial influenza infection with amantadine. *Am J Epidemiol* 1973;97:276–82.
95. Dolin R, Betts RF, Treanor JJ, et al. Rimantadine prophylaxis in the elderly [abstract] In: *Abstracts of the 23rd Interscience Conference on Antimicrobial Agents and Chemotherapy*. Washington D.C.: American Society of Microbiology, 1983.
96. Payler DK, Purdham PA. Influenza A prophylaxis with amantadine in a boarding school. *Lancet* 1984;1:502–4.
97. Clover RD, Crawford SA, Abell TD, et al. Effectiveness of rimantadine prophylaxis of children within families. *Am J Dis Child* 1986;140:706–9.
98. Crawford SA, Clover KRD, Abell TD, et al. Rimantadine prophylaxis in children: a follow-up study. *Pediatr Infect Dis J* 1988;7:379–83.
99. Galbraith AW, Oxford JS, Schild GC, et al. Protective effect of 1-adamantanamine hydrochloride on influenza A2 infections in the family environment. A controlled double-blind study. *Lancet* 1969;2:1026–8.
100. Wingfield WL, Pollack D, Grunert RR. Therapeutic efficacy of amantadine HCI and rimantadine HCI in naturally occurring influenza A2 respiratory illness in man. *N Engl J Med* 1969;281:579–84.
101. Knight V, Fedson D, Baldini J, et al. Amantadine therapy of epidemic influenza A2 (Hong Kong). *Infect Immun* 1970;1:200–4.
102. Togo Y, Hornick RB, Felitti VJ, et al. Evaluation of therapeutic efficacy of amantadine in patients with naturally occurring A2 influenza. *JAMA* 1970;211:1149–56.
103. Rabinovich S, Baldini JT, Bannister R. Treatment of influenza. The therapeutic efficacy of rimantadine HCI in a naturally occurring influenza A2 outbreak. *Am J Med Sci* 1969;257:328–35.
104. Van Voris LP, Betts RF, Hayden FG, et al. Successful treatment of naturally occurring influenza A/USSR/77 H1N1. *JAMA* 1981;245:1128–31.
105. Younkin SW, Betts RF, Roth FK, et al. Reduction in fever and symptoms in young adults with influenza A/Brazil/78 H1N1 infection after treatment with aspirin or amantadine. *Antimicrob Agents Chemother* 1983;23:577–82.
106. Hayden FG, Monto AS. Oral rimantadine hydrochloride therapy of influenza A virus H3N2 subtype infection in adults. *Antimicrob Agents Chemother* 1986;29:339–41.
107. Hall CB, Dolin R, Gala CL, et al. Children with influenza A infection: treatment with rimantadine. *Pediatrics* 1987;80:275–82.
108. Thompson J, Fleet W, Lawrence E, et al. A comparison of acetaminophen and rimantadine in the treatment of influenza A infection in children. *J Med Virol* 1987;21:249–55.
109. Little JW, Hall WJ, Douglas RG Jr, et al. Amantadine effect on peripheral airways abnormalities in influenza. *Ann Intern Med* 1976;85:177–82.
110. Little JW, Hall WJ, Douglas RG, Jr et al. Attenuation of airway hyperreactivity by amantadine in natural influenza A infection. *Am Rev Respir Dis* 1987;118:295–303.
111. Hayden FG, Hall WJ, Douglas RG Jr. Thera-

peutic effects of aerosolized amantadine in naturally acquired infection due to influenza A virus. *J Infect Dis* 1980;141:535–42.

112. Webster LRG, Kawaoka Y, Bean WJ. Vaccination as a strategy to reduce the emergence of amantadine- and rimantadine-resistant strains of A/Chick/Pennsylvania/83 (H5N2) influenza virus. *J Antimicrob Chemother* 1986;18:157–64.
113. Nahata MC, Brady MT. Serum concentrations and safety of rimantadine in paediatric patients. *Eur J Clin Pharm* 1986;30:719–22.
114. CDC. Prevention and control of influenza: recommendations of the Immunization Practices Advisory Committee. *MMWR* 1988;37:361–73.
115. Couch RB, Kasel JA, Glenzen WP, et al. Influenza: its control in persons and populations. *J Infect Dis* 1986;153:431–40.
116. Sidwell RW, Huffman JH, Khare GP, et al. Broad-spectrum antiviral activity of Virazole: 1-B-D-ribofuranosyl-1, 2,4-triazole-3-carboxamide. *Science* 1972;177:705–6.
117. Huffman JH, Sidwell RW, Khare GP, et al. *In vitro* effect of 1-b-D-ribofuranosyl-1,2,4-triazole-3-carboxamide (virazole, ICN 1229) on deoxyribonucleic acid and ribonucleic acid viruses. *Antimicrob Agents Chemother* 1973; 3:235–41.
118. Sidwell RW. Ribavirin: in vitro antiviral activity. In: Smith RA, Kirkpatrick W, eds. *Ribavirin: a broad spectrum antiviral agent.* New York: Academic Press, 1980:23–42.
119. Allen LB. Review of in vivo efficacy of ribavirin. In: Smith RA, Kirkpatrick W, eds. *Ribavirin: a broad spectrum antiviral agent.* New York: Academic Press, 1980:43–58.
120. Stephen EL, Dominik JW, Moe JB, et al. Therapeutic effects of ribavirin given by the intraperitoneal or aerosol route against influenza virus infections in mice. *Antimicrob Agents Chemother* 1976;10:549–54.
121. Hruska JF, Bernstein JM, Douglas RG Jr, et al. Effects of ribavirin on respiratory syncytial virus in vitro. *Antimicrob Agents Chemother* 1980;17:770–5.
122. Gilbert BE, Knight V. Biochemistry and clinical applications of ribavirin. *Antimicrob Agents Chemother* 1986;30:201–5.
123. Wray SK, Gilbert BE, Noall MW, et al. Mode of action of ribavirin: effect of nucleotide pool alterations on influenza virus ribonucleoprotein synthesis. *Antiviral Res* 1985;5:29–37.
124. Smith RA. Background and mechanisms of action of ribavirin. In: Smith RA, Knight V, Smith JAD, eds. *Clinical applications of ribavirin.* New York: Academic Press, 1984:1–18.
125. Eriksson BE, Helgstrand NG, Johnsson A, et al. Inhibition of influenza virus ribonucleic acid polymerase by ribavirin triphosphate. *Antimicrob Agents Chemother* 1977;11:946–51.
126. Wray SK, Gilbert BE, Knight V. Effect of ribavirin triphosphate on primer generation and elongation during influenza virus transcription *in vitro*. *Antiviral Res* 1985;5:29–37.
127. Smith RA, Wade MJ. Ribavirin: a broad spectrum antiviral agent. In: Stapleton T, ed. *Studies with a broad spectrum antiviral agent. International congress and symposia series.* London: Royal Society of Medicine, 1986:3–23.
128. Catlin DH, Smith RA, Samuels AI. $^{14}$C-ribavirin: distribution and pharmacokinetics studies in rats, baboons and man. In: Smith RA, Kirkpatrick W, eds. *Ribavirin: a broad spectrum antiviral agent.* New York: Academic Press, 1980:83–98.
129. Ferrara EA, Oishi JS, Wannemacher RW Jr, et al. Plasma disappearance, urine excretion, and tissue distribution of ribavirin in rats and Rhesus monkeys. *Antimicrob Agents Chemother* 1981;19:1042–9.
130. Connor JD, Hintz M, Van Dyke R, et al. *Clinical applications of ribavirin.* New York: Academic Press, 1984:107–23.
131. Magnussen CR, Douglas RG Jr, Betts RF, et al. Double-blind evaluation of oral ribavirin (Virazole) in experimental influenza A virus infection in volunteers. *Antimicrob Agents Chemother* 1977;12:498–502.
132. Smith CB, Charette RP, Fox JP, et al. Lack of effect of oral ribavirin in naturally occurring influenza A virus (H1N1) infection. *J Infect Dis* 1980;141:548–54.
133. Canonico PG, Kastello MD, Cosgriff TM, et al. Hematological and bone marrow effects of ribavirin in Rhesus monkeys. *Toxicol Appl Pharmacol* 1984;74:163–72.
134. Rodriguez WJ, Parrott RH. Ribavirin aerosol treatment of serious respiratory syncytial virus infection in infants. In: Knight V, Gilbert BE, eds. *Infectious disease clinics of North America.* Philadelphia: WB Saunders Co., 1987; 1:425–39.
135. Hillyard IW. The preclinical toxicology and safety of ribavirin. In: *Ribavirin: a broad spectrum antiviral agent.* New York: Academic Press, 1980:59–71.
136. Rodriguez WJ, Dang Bui RHD, Conner JD, et al. Environmental exposure of primary care personnel to ribavirin aerosol when supervising treatment of infants with respiratory syncytial virus infections. *Antimicrob Agents Chemother* 1987;31:1143–6.
137. CDC. Assessing exposures of health-care personnel to aerosols of ribavirin. *MMWR* 1988;37:560–3.
138. Stein DS, Creticos CM, Jackson, GG, et al. Oral ribavirin treatment of influenza A and B. *Antimicrob Agents Chemother* 1987;31:1285–7.
139. Knight V, McClung H, Wilson SZ, et al. Ribavirin small-particle aerosol treatment of influenza. *Lancet* 1981;2:945–9.
140. McClung HW, Knight V, Gilbert BE, et al. Ribavirin aerosol treatment of influenza B virus infection. *JAMA* 1983:249:2671–4.
141. Gilbert BE, Wilson SZ, Knight V, et al. Ribavirin small-particle aerosol treatment of infections caused by influenza virus strains

A/Victoria/7/83 (H1N1) and B/Texas/1/84. *Antimicrob Agents Chemother* 1985;27:309–13.
142. Knight V, Gilbert BE. Ribavirin aerosol treatment of influenza. *Antivir Chemother* 1987; 1:441–57.
143. Knight V, Gilbert B. Antiviral therapy with small particle aerosols. *Eur J Clin Microb Infect Dis* 1988;7:721–31.
144. Taber LH, Knight V, Gilbert BE, et al. Ribavirin aerosol treatment of bronchiolitis associated with respiratory syncytial virus infection in infants. *Pediatrics* 1983;72:613–8.
145. Hall CB, McBride J, Watch E, et al. Aerosolized ribavirin treatment of infants with respiratory syncytial virus infection. *N Engl J Med* 1983;308:1443–7.
146. Hall CB, McBride JT, Gala CL, et al. Ribavirin treatment of syncytial viral infection in infants with underlying cardiopulmonary disease. *JAMA* 1985;254:3047–51.
147. Rodriquez WJ, Kim HW, Brandt CD, et al. Aerosolized ribavirin in the treatment of patients with respiratory syncytial virus disease. *Pediatr Infect Dis J* 1987;6:159–63.
148. Barry W, Cockburn F, Cornall R, et al. Ribavirin aerosol for acute bronchiolitis. *Arch Dis Child* 1986;61:593–7.
149. Conrad DA, Christenson JC, Waner JL, et al. Aerosolized ribavirin treatment of respiratory syncytial virus infection in infants hospitalized during an epidemic. *Pediatr Infect Dis J* 1987;6:152–8.
150. Rosner IK, Welliver RC, Edelson PJ, et al. Effect of ribavirin therapy on respiratory syncytial virus-specific IgE and IgA responses after infection. *J Infect Dis* 1987;155:1043–7.
151. Gelfand EW, McCurdy D, Rao DP, et al. Ribavirin treatment of viral pneumonitis in severe combined immunodeficiency disease. *Lancet* 1983;2:732–3.
152. Isaacs A, Lindenmann J. Virus interference. I. The interferon. *Proc R Soc Lond [Biol]* 1957;147:258–67.
153. Ingimarsson S, Cantell K, Strander H. Side effects of long-term treatment with human leukocyte interferon. *J Infect Dis* 1979;140:560–3.
154. Trent JM, Olson S, Lawn RM. Chromosomal localization of human leukocyte, fibroblast, and immune interferon genes by means of *in situ* hybridization. *Proc Natl Acad Sci USA* 182;79:7809–13.
155. Greenberg SB. Human interferon in viral diseases. In: Knight V, Gilbert BE, eds. *Infectious disease clinics of North America, vol. 1*. Philadelphia: WB Saunders Co., 1987:383–423.
156. Johnson PE, Greenberg SB, Harmon MW, et al. Recovery of applied human leukocyte interferon from the nasal mucosa of chimpanzees and humans. *J Clin Microbiol* 1976;4:106–7.
157. Samo TC, Greenberg SB, Couch RB, et al. Efficacy and tolerance of intranasally applied recombinant leukocyte A interferon in normal volunteers. *J Infect Dis* 1983;148:535–42.
158. Samo TC, Greenberg SB, Palmer JM, et al. Intranasally applied recombinant leukocyte A interferon in normal volunteers. II. Determination of minimal effective and tolerable dose. *J Infect Dis* 1984;150:181–8.
159. Hayden FG, Mills SE, Johns ME. Human tolerance and histopathologic effects of long-term administration of intranasal interferon-A2. *J Infect Dis* 1983;148:914–21.
160. Solov'ev VD. The results of controlled observations on the prophylaxis of influenza with interferon. *Bull WHO* 1969;41:683–8.
161. Merigan TC, Hall TS, Reed SE, et al. Inhibition of respiratory virus infection by locally applied interferon. *Lancet* 1973;1:563–7.
162. Scott GM, Phillpotts RJ, Wallace J, et al. Purified interferon as protection against rhinovirus infection. *Br Med J* 1982;284:1822–5.
163. Greenberg SB, Harmon MW, Couch RB, et al. Prophylactic effect of low doses of human leukocyte interferon against infection with rhinovirus. *J Infect Dis* 1982;145:542–6.
164. Scott GM, Onwubalili JK, Robinson JA, et al. Tolerance of one-month intranasal interferon. *J Med Virol* 1985;17:99–106.
165. Scott GM, Wallace J, Greiner J, et al. Prevention of rhinovirus colds by human interferon alpha-2 from *Escherichia coli*. *Lancet* 1982; 2:186–8.
166. Phillpotts RJ, Scott GM, Higgins PG, et al. An effective dosage regimen for prophylaxis against rhinovirus infection by intranasal administration of HuIFN-$\alpha_2$. *Antiviral Res* 1983;3:121–36.
167. Hayden FG, Gwaltney JM Jr. Intranasal interferon-$\alpha_2$ for prevention of rhinovirus infection and illness. *J Infect Dis* 1983;148:543–50.
168. Hayden FG, Gwaltney JM Jr. Intranasal interferon-$\alpha_2$ treatment of experimental rhinoviral colds. *J Infect Dis* 1984;150:174–80.
169. Farr BM, Gwaltney JM Jr, Adams KF, et al. Intranasal interferon-$\alpha_2$ for prevention of natural rhinovirus colds. *Antimicrob Agents Chemother* 1984;26:31–4.
170. Douglas RM, Albrecht JK, Miles HB, et al. Intranasal interferon-$\alpha_2$ prophylaxis of natural respiratory virus infection. *J Infect Dis* 1985;151:731–6.
171. Monto AS, Schope TC, Swartz SA, et al. Intranasal interferon-$\alpha_{2b}$ for seasonal prophylaxis of respiratory infection. *J Infect Dis* 1986;154:128–33.
172. Betts RF, Erb S, Roth F, et al. A field trial of intranasal interferon [Abstract]. In: *Proceedings of 13th International Congress Chemotherapy*. Vienna, 1983.
173. Douglas RM, Moore BW, Miles HB, et al. Prophylactic efficacy of intranasal alpha interferon against rhinovirus infections in a family setting. *N Engl J Med* 1986;314:65–70.
174. Hayden FG, Albrecht JK, Kaiser DL, et al. Prevention of natural colds by contact prophylaxis with intranasal alpha$_2$-interferon. *N Engl J Med* 1986;314:71–5.
175. Foy HM, Fox JP, Cooney MK, et al. Efficacy of alpha$_2$-interferon against the common cold (Letter). *N Engl J Med* 1986;315:513.

176. Herzog C, Berger R, Fernex M, et al. Intranasal interferon (rIFN-aA, Ro 22-8181) for contact prophylaxis against common cold: a randomized, double-blind and placebo-controlled field study. *Antiviral Res* 1986;6:171–6.
177. Hayden FG, Kaiser DL, Albrecht JK. Intranasal recombinant alpha-2b interferon treatment of naturally occurring common colds. Antimicrob Agents Chemother 1988;32:224–30.
178. Greenberg SB, Harmon MW, Johnson PE, et al. Antiviral activity of intranasally applied human leukocyte interferon. *Antimicrob Agents Chemother* 1978;14:596–600.
179. Smith CB, Golden CA, Kanner RE, et al. Association of viral and *Mycoplasma pneumoniae* infections with acute respiratory illness in patients with chronic obstructive pulmonary diseases. *Am Rev Respir Dis* 1980;121:225–32.
180. Phillpotts RJ, Higgins PG, Willman JS, et al. Intranasal lymphoblastoid interferon ("Wellferon") prophylaxis against rhinovirus and influenza virus in volunteers. *J Interferon Res* 1984;4:535–41.
181. Higgins PG, Al-Nakib W, Willman J, et al. Interferon-$B_{ser}$ as prophylaxis against experimental rhinovirus infection in volunteers. *J Interferon Res* 1986;6:153–9.
182. Dolin R, Betts R, Treanor J, et al. Intranasally administered rIFN-α as prophylaxis against experimentally induced influenza in man [Abstract]. In: *Proceedings of the 13th International Congress of Chemotherapy.* Vienna, 1983.
183. Turner RB, Felton A, Kosak K, et al. Prevention of experiment coronavirus colds with intranasal α-2b interferon. *J Infect Dis* 1986; 154:443–7.
184. DeLong DC. Effect of enviroxime on rhinovirus infections in humans. In: Leive L, Schlessinger D, eds. *Microbiology.* Washington D.C. ASM, 1984:431–4.
185. Wu CYE, Nelson JD, Warren BR, et al. Virus inhibition studies with AR-336 II: mode of action studies [Abstract]. In: *Abstracts of annual meeting of American Society for Microbiology.* 1978:234.
186. Phillpotts RJ, DeLong DC, Wallace J, et al. The activity of enviroxime against rhinovirus infection in man. *Lancet* 1981;1:1342–4.
187. Hayden FG, Gwaltney JM Jr. Prophylactic activity of intranasal enviroxime against experimentally induced rhinovirus type 39 infection. *Antimicrob Agents Chemother* 1982;21:892–7.
188. Miller FD, Monto AS, DeLong DC, et al. Controlled trial of enviroxime against natural rhinovirus infections in a community. *Antimicrob Agents Chemother* 1985;27:102–6.
189. Swallow DL, Bucknall RA, Stanier WE, et al. A new antirhinovirus compound. ICI 73602: structure, properties and spectrum of activity. *Ann NY Acad Sci* 1977;284:305–309.
190. Swallow DL, Kampfner GL. The laboratory selection of antiviral agents. *Br Med Bull* 1985;41:322–32.
191. Alarcon B, Zerial A, Dupiol C, et al. Antirhinovirus compound 44 081 RP inhibits virus uncoating. *Antimicrob Agents Chemother* 1986;30:31–4.
192. Zerial A, Werner GH, Phillpotts JS, et al. Studies on 44 081 RP, a new antirhinovirus compound in cell cultures and in volunteers. *Antimicrob Agents Chemother* 1985;27:846–50.
193. Ishitsuka H, Ninomiya YT, Ohsawa C, et al. Direct and specific inactivation of rhinovirus by chalcone Ro 09-0410. *Antimicrob Agents Chemother* 1982;22:617–21.
194. Ninomiya Y, Ohsawa C, Aoyama M, et al. Antivirus agent, Ro 09-0410, binds to rhinovirus specifically and stabilizes the virus conformation. *Virology* 1984;134:269–76.
195. Ninomiya Y, Aoyama M, Umeda I, et al. Comparative studies on the modes of action of the antirhinovirus agents Ro 09-0410, Ro 09-0179, RMI-15,731, 4′,6′-dichloroflavan, and enviroxime. *Antimicrob Agents Chemother* 1985;27: 595–9.
196. Diana GD, Otto MJ, McKinlay MA. Inhibitors of picornavirus uncoating as antiviral agents. *Pharmacol Ther* 1985;29:287–97.
197. Fox MP, Otto MJ, McKinlay MA. Prevention of rhinovirus and poliovirus uncoating by WIN 51711, a new antiviral drug. *Antimicrob Agents Chemother* 1986;30:110–6.
198. Ishitsuka H, Ninomiya Y, Suhara Y. Molecular basis of drug resistance to new antirhinovirus agents. *J Antimicrob Chemother* 1986;18:11–8.
199. Otto MJ, Fox MP, Fancher MJ, et al. *In vitro* activity of WIN 51711, a new broad spectrum antipicornavirus drug. *Antimicrob Agents Chemother* 1985;27:883–6.
200. Smith TJ, Kremer MJ, Luo M, et al. The site of attachment in human rhinovirus 14 for antiviral agents that inhibit uncoating. *Science* 1986;233:1286–93.
201. Tisdale M, Selway JWT. Effect of dichloroflavan (BW683C) on the stability and uncoating of rhinovirus type 1B. *J Antimicrob Chemother* 1984;14:97–105.
202. Phillpotts RJ, Higgins PG, Willman JS, et al. Evaluation of the antirhinovirus chalcone Ro 09-0415 given orally to volunteers. *J Antimicrob Chemother* 1984;14:403–9.
203. Tyrrell DAJ, Al-Nakib W. Prophylaxis and treatment of rhinovirus infections. In: DeClercq E, ed. *Clinical use of antiviral drugs.* Boston: Martinus Nijhoff Publishing, 1988: 241–76.

*Antiviral Agents and Viral Diseases of Man, 3rd Edition*, edited by G. J. Galasso, R. J. Whitley, and T. C. Merigan, Raven Press, Ltd., New York © 1990.

# 11

# Viral Infections of the Gastrointestinal Tract

John Treanor and Raphael Dolin

*Infectious Diseases Unit, University of Rochester School of Medicine and Dentistry, Rochester, New York 14642*



Viruses that infect the gastrointestinal tract can be conveniently divided into two general groups: those that induce disease primarily within the gastrointestinal tract, i.e., gastroenteritis, and those that initially replicate in the gastrointestinal tract, but induce disease in other organ systems, e.g., in the myocardium or central nervous system (CNS). The first group of viral infections result in "acute viral gastroenteritis," which is an exceedingly widespread and common illness, second in frequency only to the common cold as a disease experience among families in the United States (1). Based on figures compiled by the National Health Interview Survey, the incidence of acute gastrointestinal disease in the United States is 11.2% per year, with an estimated 23.7–26.0 days lost from work or school per 100 individuals per year as a result of illness (2). Worldwide, it is estimated that more than 700 million episodes of acute diarrheal disease occur in children below the age of 5 years alone, with as many as 5 million deaths associated with such illnesses, primarily in developing countries (3). On rare occasions, gastroenteritis has been reported as a cause of death in neonates in developed countries as well (4). In addition, several other population groups have been noted to be at high risk for acute gastrointestinal disease, including the elderly in institutional settings (5) and certain immunosuppressed patients (6). Because the etiology of much of acute gastrointestinal disease remains unknown, the proportion of such illnesses caused by viral agents has not been established. However, studies employing recently developed methods for detection of newly described agents (Norwalk-like agents and rotaviruses) indicate that viral agents are major causes of acute gastroenteritis, as will be discussed below. Thus, acute viral gastroenteritis is a significant public health problem for which there are no adequate control measures. The relevance of antiviral chemotherapy and/or prophylaxis as potential control measures for these infections will be the focus of this chapter.

The second group of viral infections of the gastrointestinal tract, i.e., those caused by enteroviruses, have gastrointestinal illness as a minor or occasional feature of infection, but the major clinical manifestations occur outside of the gastrointestinal tract. These viral infections are considered elsewhere in this text, and the potential application of antivirals will be discussed only briefly here.

## NORWALK-LIKE AGENTS OF ACUTE GASTROENTERITIS

### Biophysical Properties of Agents

The term "Norwalk-like agents" refers to several agents obtained from outbreaks of acute gastroenteritis that share certain properties in common. The name of each agent was derived from the location of the outbreak, e.g. Norwalk, Ohio; Snow Mountain, Colorado (7). These agents have been detected in the stools of acutely ill patients during outbreaks of gastrointestinal illness and, in some cases, have induced acute gastroenteritis after oral administration to normal volunteers (8–10). As will be discussed below, the Norwalk-like agents have not been successfully propagated *in vitro*. Information regarding their characteristics have been derived from direct visualization of particles in stool by electron microscopy (EM) (10–12), indirectly from physicochemical manipulation of infectious inocula (13), and recently by partial purification and analysis by radioimmunoassay (14,15). These agents are similar in size and morphology and, therefore, have been grouped together under the heading of "Norwalk-like agents" (16). Nucleic acid has not been extracted from these agents, and since relatively limited information is available concerning their biochemical properties and antigenic characteristics, definitive classification of this "group" awaits further characterization.

A summary of the Norwalk-like agents and their associated properties is presented in Table 1. The agents are 27–34 nm in diameter, have cubic symmetry, and are nonenveloped. Buoyant density of these agents in cesium chloride has been variously reported to be 1.33–1.41 gr/cc (10,12,17). Among those agents that have been tested,

**TABLE 1.** *Norwalk-like agents*

| Agent | Size (nm) | Density in cesium chloride (g/cc) |
|---|---|---|
| Norwalk | 27–32 | 1.38–1.41 |
| Hawaii | 26–29 | 1.37–1.39 |
| Snow Mountain | 27–32 | 1.33–1.34 |
| Taunton | 32–34 | 1.36–1.41 |

relative heat stability and resistance to acid and lipid solvents have been noted (13,18). The prototype and best studied of these agents is the Norwalk agent, which was derived from a large outbreak in an elementary school (7). The Hawaii agent was derived from a family outbreak in that state (12), the Taunton agent was associated with a hospital outbreak in the United Kingdom (19), and the Snow Mountain agent (SMA) (20) was associated with a water-borne outbreak of gastroenteritis at a camp in Colorado.

Biochemical characterization of these agents has not been achieved, although some information concerning the polypeptides associated with the Norwalk agent and SMA is available. Immunoprecipitation and subsequent polyacrylamide gel electrophoresis (PAGE) of partially purified stool preparations that contain the Norwalk agent or SMA have been carried out, and a single virion-associated protein of a molecular mass of 59,000–62,000 daltons and a soluble protein of a molecular mass of 29,000–30,000 daltons have been detected (14,15). This pattern and size of polypeptides most closely resembles those associated with caliciviruses, and it has been suggested that the Norwalk-like agents may be related to the calicivirus family.

Because of the inability to grow these agents *in vitro* and the lack of conventional detection tests (see below), only limited analyses of the antigenic relatedness among these agents have been carried out. The antigenic topology of these agents does not appear to be complex, since a single monoclonal antibody to the SNA was able to block the binding of polyclonal serum to this agent (21). It appears that at least three, and perhaps more, antigenic types exist. Norwalk and Hawaii agents have been compared directly in cross-challenge studies in human volunteers (22) and by immuno electron microscopy (IEM) (10,12). These studies indicate that Norwalk and Hawaii agents are antigenically distinct. SMA appears to be antigenically distinct from Norwalk and Hawaii agents by IEM (10), radioimmunoassay (RIA) (23), and enzyme-linked immunosorbent assay (ELISA) (24), although serologic cross reactions occur among all three of these agents, particularly between SMA and Hawaii agents (25). Recently, serologic cross-reactions between Norwalk and human calicivirus infections have been reported, further supporting the suggestion that these two groups of viruses may be related (26). The antigenic relationships between Taunton and the other Norwalk-like agents are unknown at present.

### Epidemiology

As has been discussed earlier, the type of gastrointestinal illness from which the Norwalk-like agents have been derived appears to be extremely common, and these agents have been detected in widespread geographic locations. Disease has been described in all age groups, in both open and closed populations. Explosive outbreaks as well as sporadic cases have been noted. However, it has been only recently that methods have been developed with which to perform large-scale population surveys for infection with several of these agents, in particular, the Norwalk and Hawaii agents, and SMA. Studies employing RIA have demonstrated that antibody to the Norwalk agent is present in 50–80% of individuals above the age of 10 years in developed countries and is present with even higher frequencies in developing countries (27). The acquisition of serum antibody to the Norwalk agent occurs largely after 3 years of age in the United States, in contrast to the earlier acquisition of antibody in developing countries. Preliminary studies with the SMA show that similar serum antibody patterns of prevalence exist (23).

RIA has also been used to examine the role of the Norwalk agent in outbreaks of acute gastroenteritis of unknown etiology. In serum specimens from 70 outbreaks that were examined by RIA, 20 (34%) of the outbreaks were associated with the Norwalk agent (28). In an overlapping study conducted by the Centers for Disease Control (CDC), the Norwalk agent was implicated in 42% of outbreaks that were studied (29). Thus, the Norwalk agent appears to be an important cause of outbreaks of acute gastroenteritis in the United States. SMA has been implicated in six outbreaks of gastroenteritis in various parts of the United States (30), although systematic seroepidemiologic studies with this agent or with the Hawaii agent have not yet been carried out.

### *In Vitro* Detection Methods

Conventional methods to detect viral agents, e.g., tissue culture, have not been successful in identification of the Norwalk-like agents, and these agents were first detected *in vitro* by the use of IEM (10–12). Because of the small size and unremarkable morphology of these viral agen , and because of the presence of particulate matter with similar morphology in stool preparations, identification of virus in negatively stained stool preparations by standard EM techniques has only rarely been possible. However, the reaction of stool preparations with antibody to the agent results in the aggregation of viral particles in a characteristic cluster shown in Fig. 1. Conversely, if a source of known antigen (particle) is employed, the amount of antibody in a serum sample can be estimated by the appearance of the aggregate, in which the antibody content is rated on a semiquantitative basis against known standards. Thus, IEM can be employed to detect either antigen or antibody to individual agents.

Because of the laborious and cumber-

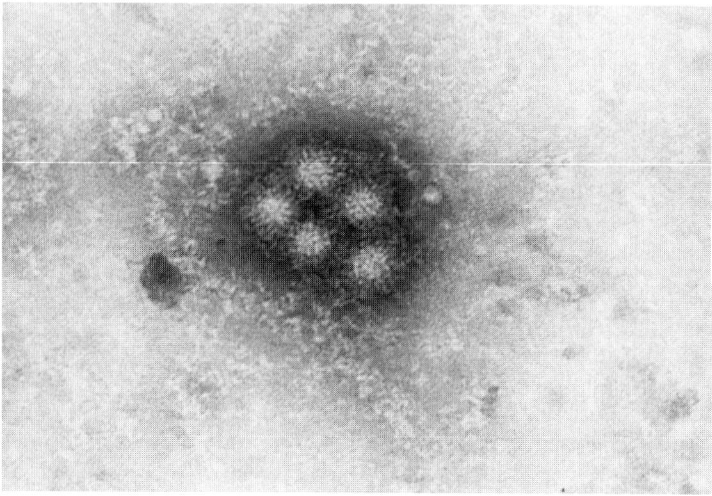

**FIG. 1.** SMA in stool filtrate from volunteer with experimentally induced disease as visualized by immune electron microscopy. Particles are 27–32 nm in diameter and are stained with 2% phosphotungsstic acid.

some nature of IEM, only limited numbers of samples can be examined by this technique. Recently, highly efficient and sensitive RIAs and ELISAs for the Norwalk agent (31–33), the SMA (23,24), and the Hawaii agent (34) have been developed, which represent significant advances in the field. These assays can detect either antigen or antibody, and they provide the basis for ongoing seroepidemiologic and laboratory studies of these agents.

## Clinical Characteristics of Illness

The clinical characteristics of illness induced by oral administration of the Norwalk agent to normal volunteers are presented in Fig. 2. The incubation period for illness is 24–48 hr, and disease manifestations generally last 48–72 hr. Volunteer A manifested vomiting without diarrhea, whereas volunteer B experienced diarrhea but no vomiting. Often, both vomiting and diarrhea occur, along with myalgia, malaise, and low-grade fever. Illness induced by each of the Norwalk-like agents listed in Table 1 appears to be clinically indistinguishable.

Virus shedding in stools as detected by IEM or RIA is maximal over the first 24–48 hr after illness (10,35). In volunteer studies, virus has been rarely detected beyond 72 hr after the onset of vomiting or diarrhea (10,35).

## Pathophysiology

Acute illness induced by Norwalk (36,37) and Hawaii (38,39) agents is associated with a reversible histopathologic lesion in the jejunum, with apparent sparing of the stomach and rectum (Fig. 3). The mucosa remains intact, but the villi are blunted, and there is round cell and polymorphonuclear leukocytic infiltration of the lamina propria. On EM examination, the epithelial cells also appear to be intact, but the microvilli are shortened, and there are widened intercellular spaces (36,38). These pathologic changes appear as early as 24 hr after chal-

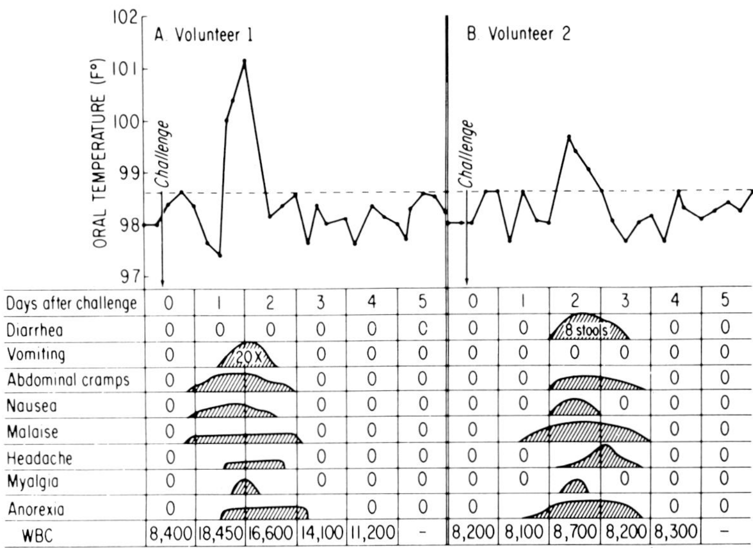


**FIG. 2.** Clinical response of two normal volunteers after oral administration of Norwalk agent. Height of shaded curve is proportional to severity of sign or symptom. (From Dolin et al., ref. 91, with permission.)

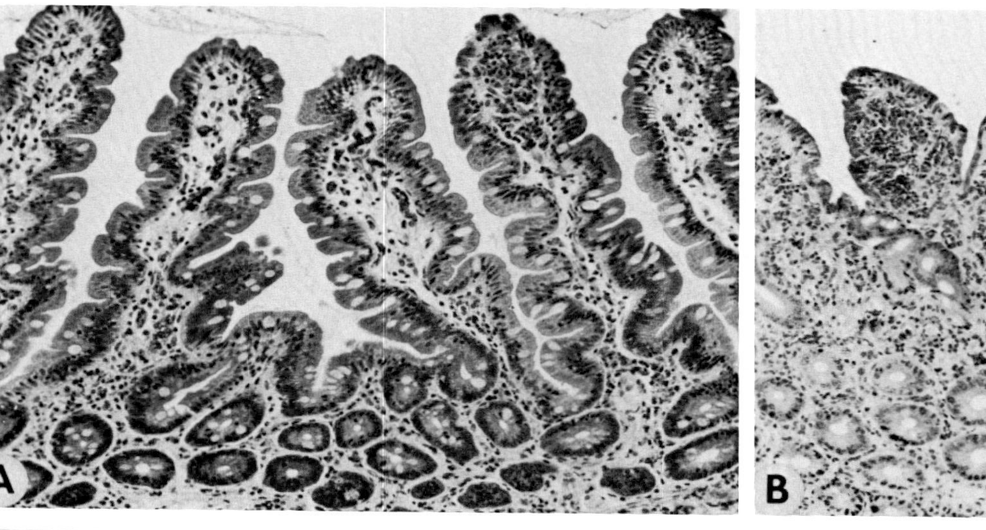


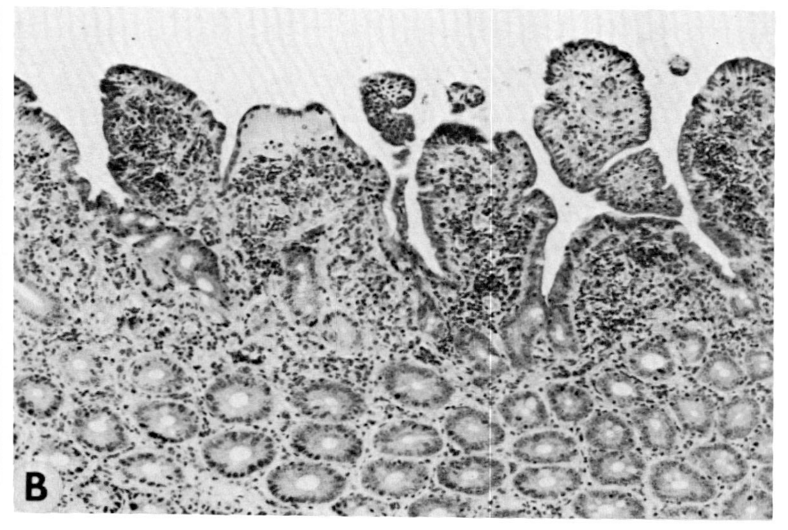


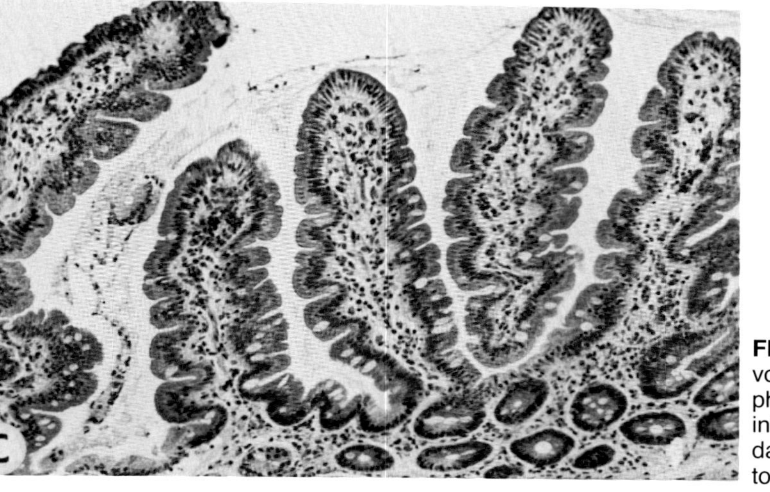


**FIG. 3.** Light micrographs of sections of jejunal mucosal biopsies from a volunteer with Hawaii-agent–induced disease. **A:** Prior to challenge, morphology is normal. **B:** Forty-eight hours after challenge. Blunted villi and inflammatory cell infiltrate in the lamina propria are present. **C:** Fourteen days after challenge, morphology has returned to normal. ×140, hematoxylin and eosin. (From Dolin et al., ref. 94, with permission.)

lenge, persist for a variable period after acute illness, and resolve within 10 days to 6 weeks after challenge. Similar histopathology may also be seen in individuals who experience subclinical infections with these agents (37). The lack of destruction of intestinal mucosa is also reflected in the absence of fecal leukocytes in diarrheal stools (40).

Acute illness with the Norwalk agent is associated with a transient malabsorption of D-xylose and fat, as well as with decreased activity of the brush border enzymes, alkaline phosphatase, sucrase, and trehalase (8). Absorption activity and brush border enzyme levels return to normal by 2 weeks after challenge.

The specific mechanism by which viral infection with these agents results in diarrhea and/or vomiting is unclear at present. Production of intestinal fluid, although highly variable in experimentally induced illness, may be markedly increased on occasion. However, infection with Norwalk and Hawaii agents has not been associated with increased jejunal mucosal levels of cyclic AMP (41). Assays for enterotoxins produced during infection have been similarly negative (R. Dolin, H. P. Madore, and J. Treanor J., unpublished observations, 1988). The precise pathogenesis of viral diarrhea and/or vomiting remains a major, unresolved question in this area.

### Humoral and Local Immunity

Immunity to the Norwalk-like agents is not well understood. Resistance to rechallenge with the homologous agent persists for 6–14 weeks after challenge (22,42) but apparently wanes within 24–42 months (42). Some individuals manifest a poorly characterized long-term resistance to infection. The above studies of immunity to the Norwalk-like agents have been hampered by difficulties measuring specific antibody responses. Serum antibody has been measured primarily by IEM, or by RIA or ELISA, which can detect antibody rises 2 weeks after illness (23,24,34). However, in volunteer studies, illness has been induced over a wide range of prechallenge serum antibody titers, which therefore correlate poorly with protection from infection. It has been suggested that local antibody in the gut may play an important role in protection, similar to that played by intestinal secretory immunoglobulin A (IgA) in poliovirus infections. However, direct measurements of intestinal antibody to the Norwalk agent by IEM and RIA (28) have failed to demonstrate a correlation with protection from infection. Studies of local immunity with the other Norwalk-like agents have not yet been carried out.

### Cell-Mediated Immunity and Interferon Production

Acute infections with Norwalk and Hawaii agents are associated with a transient lymphopenia that involves thymus-derived, bone-marrow–derived, and null cell subpopulations (Figs. 4 and 5) (43). The response of circulating lymphocytes to mitogenic stimulation with phytohemagglutin and concanavalin A remains intact or even supranormal. It has been suggested that the kinetics of the lymphopenia may represent an acute redistribution of circulating lymphocytes to the site of viral infection in the gut (43).

Despite the accumulation of lymphocytes in the lamina propria and histopathologic involvement of the mucosa, examinations of jejunal biopsies have not detected interferon activity in the mucosa or in intestinal aspirates from acute Norwalk or Hawaii-induced disease (44). It is not clear whether the failure to detect interferon in intestinal samples represents a rapid degradation of interferon by intestinal enzymes, whether the Norwalk-like agents are weak inducers of interferon, or even whether the intestine is a poor producer of interferon. Attempts to induce interferon in human fetal organ

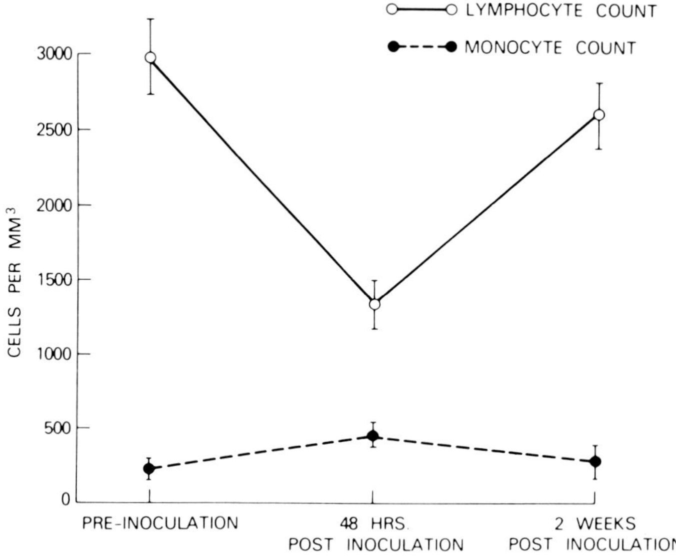


**FIG. 4.** Circulating lymphocyte and monocyte counts in volunteers with Hawaii-agent–induced gastroenteritis. Values represent means ± SEM at various time points after inoculation. (From Dolin et al., ref. 96, with permission.)

culture with a variety of inducers have also been unsuccessful (45).

### *In Vitro* Systems for Study

The Norwalk-like agents have not been successfully cultivated *in vitro*. Considerable efforts have been expended in attempts to grow the Norwalk-like agents in both tissue culture and in human fetal intestinal organ culture (HFIOC) (46). These latter cultures are full-thickness explants of human fetal gut, which can be maintained for approximately 3 weeks. Two blind passage experiments wherein organ culture harvests inoculated with the Norwalk agent

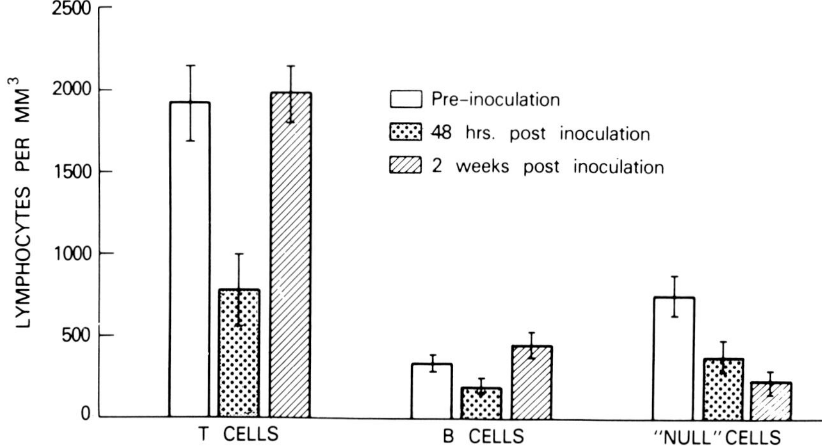


**FIG. 5.** Circulating lymphocyte subpopulations in Hawaii-agent–induced gastroenteritis. Height of bar represents mean ± SEM cell counts. (From Dolin et al., ref. 96, with permission.)

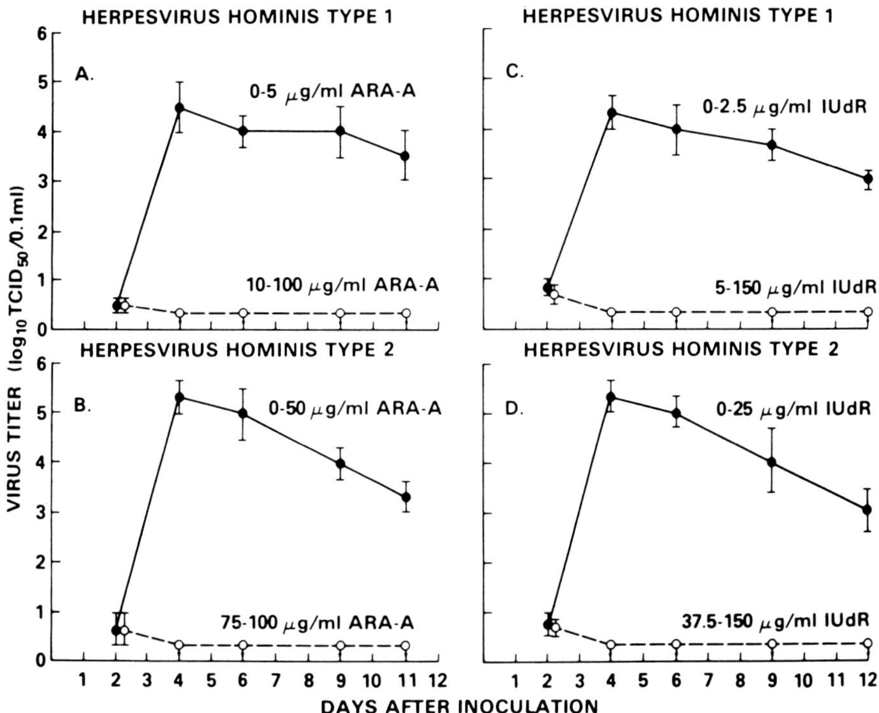


**FIG. 6.** Growth of herpesvirus hominis, types 1 and 2, in HFIOC in the presence of high (*closed circles*) and low (*open circles*) concentrations of adenine arabinoside (ARA-A) and idoxuridine (IUdR). Fluid was harvested every 2–3 days and assayed in tissue cultures. Values represent mean titers ± SD for a single strain. (From Dolin and Smith, ref. 99, with permission.)

were administered to normal volunteers yielded inconclusive results (8), and the Norwalk agent has not been detected in the cultures by immunofluorescence (IF), IEM, or RIA. Such organ cultures support the growth of a wide variety of other viruses to high titers and have proved to be suitable *in vitro* systems in which to detect antiviral activity (47) (Fig. 6).

### Animal Models

Although a wide variety of animals have been inoculated with the Norwalk-like agents, experimental infection has been achieved only in chimpanzees, which shed small amounts of Norwalk antigen and manifested seroresponses (48). However, gastrointestinal illness was not associated with these infections, and, thus, the absence of an experimental model for illness remains a major limitation in the field.

## CALICIVIRUSES

### Biophysical Properties and Replication

Caliciviruses are nonenveloped icosahedral viruses that are 31–35 nm in diameter. They were formerly classified as a genus within the family of picornaviruses, but are now recognized as a separate family and have been isolated from a variety of animal species (49). The name "calicivirus" is derived from the appearance of the viral particles under EM, in which "cup-like" indentations and a scalloped border can be noted, from which the Latin name *chalice* or *calyx* is derived (Fig. 7). Caliciviruses contain a single, plus stranded RNA genome with a 3′ poly (A) tail (49). The virion has a single major structural protein of approximately 60,000 daltons in mass, and a smaller soluble protein of approximately 30,000 daltons has been variably reported (49–51). A small protein of approximately 10,000 daltons in mass, covalently linked to calicivirus RNA, has also been described (50). Human caliciviruses have been difficult to cultivate *in vitro,* although adaptation of one strain to growth in tissue culture has been reported (52), and, thus, relatively little biochemical information is available regarding their replication. Some animal caliciviruses, however, readily replicate in tissue culture, among which feline calicivirus has been studied most extensively (50). In this latter system, calicivirus replication and maturation appear to occur entirely within the cytoplasm of infected cells. Syn-

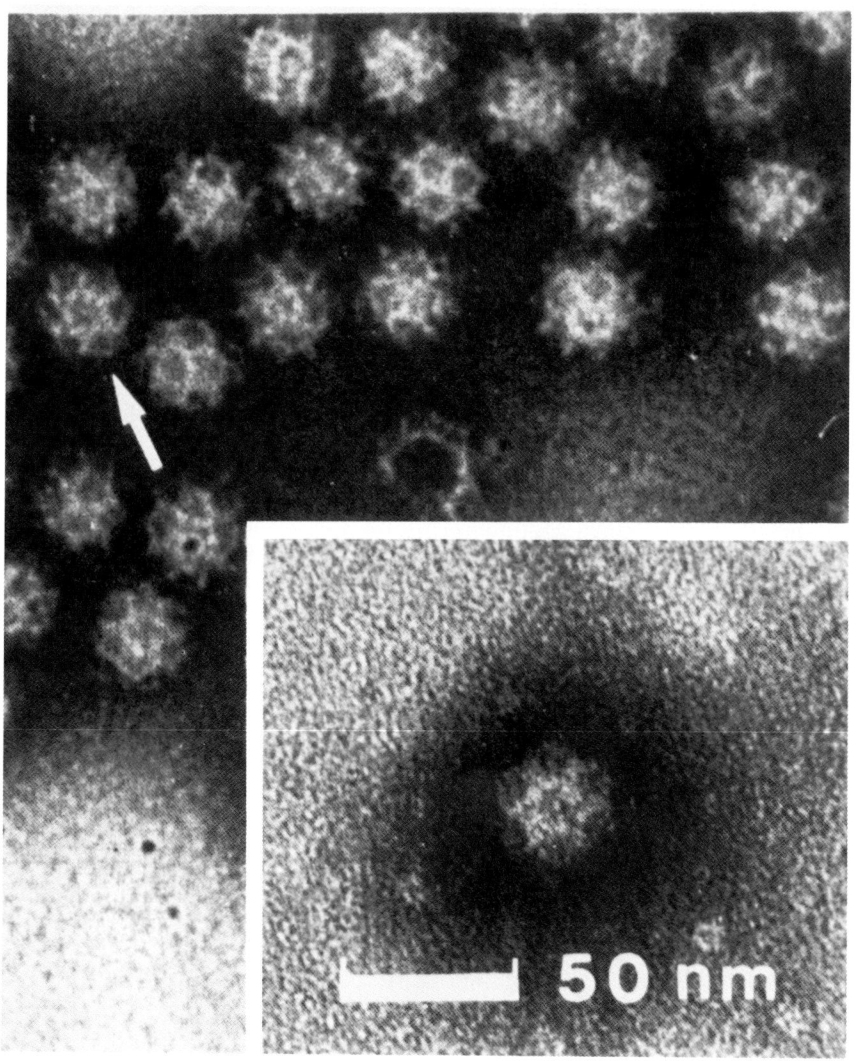


**FIG. 7.** Calicivirus particles in fecal extract from a child with gastroenteritis. (From Chiba, ref. 59 with permission.)

thesis of viral RNA can be detected within 3 hr after infection and continues for up to 7 hr. Virions can be detected by EM in the cytoplasm within 4 hr after infection. Subsequently, virions accumulate in clusters and crystalline arrays. Two or three species of single-stranded RNA in infected cells have been described, ranging from 18S to 36S. Details of calicivirus RNA replication have not been reported, although it has been suggested that it may resemble that of Alphaviruses (50).

At present, four or five serologic types of human caliciviruses have been described that apparently do not cross-react with known animal caliciviruses (26,30). As noted earlier, serologic cross-reactions have been noted between infections with human caliciviruses and the Norwalk agent, suggesting a potential relatedness between these two groups of viruses (26).

### Epidemiology

Human infections with caliciviruses were first noted in 1976 when virus particles were detected in the stools of children with gastroenteritis (53) and have subsequently been reported primarily from children in community-wide and nosocomial outbreaks, as well from sporadic cases of gastroenteritis in various parts of the world (54–59). Seroepidemiological studies carried out in Japan and the United Kingdom indicate that antibody is acquired early in childhood and is present in up to 90% of older children and adults (60,61). Infection with human caliciviruses also appears to be widely prevalent in Southeast Asia (62).

### *In Vitro* Detection

Caliciviruses have been primarily detected in stool specimens by EM. RIA has been recently developed for caliciviruses but is not widely available (63).

### Clinical Illness

The majority of reports of gastrointestinal illness associated with human caliciviruses have involved young children. Disease has consisted of vomiting and/or diarrhea, abdominal cramps, and low-grade fever, all of which have been generally mild and self-limited. The estimated incubation period for illness has been 24–72 hr, and disease manifestations have generally lasted from 1–3 days (48,53–56,59,64).

### Pathogenesis and Immune Response

Little is known regarding the pathogenesis of calicivirus-induced illness in humans. In animals, calicivirus infections have been associated with atrophy of the small intestinal mucosa and mild infiltration of lamina propria with inflammatory cells (65,66).

The parameters of immunity of calicivirus infections in humans are also not well understood. The presence of preexisting serum antibody was associated with lower rates of illness during an outbreak of calicivirus infection in an orphanage in Japan (67).

## ASTROVIRUSES

### Biophysical Properties and Replication

Astroviruses are nonenveloped viruses that are 28–30 nm in diameter and have a characteristic morphology that consists of a round, smooth edge, with multiple triangular electron lucent areas, and an electron dense center (68,69). This results in the appearance of a five- or six-pointed star from which the virus derives its name (Fig. 8) (70). Astroviruses have been difficult to cultivate *in vitro*, although some human astrovirus strains have been serially passaged in tissue culture (71). Astroviruses contain a positive single-stranded 35S RNA genome with a poly (A) tail (72). The virion

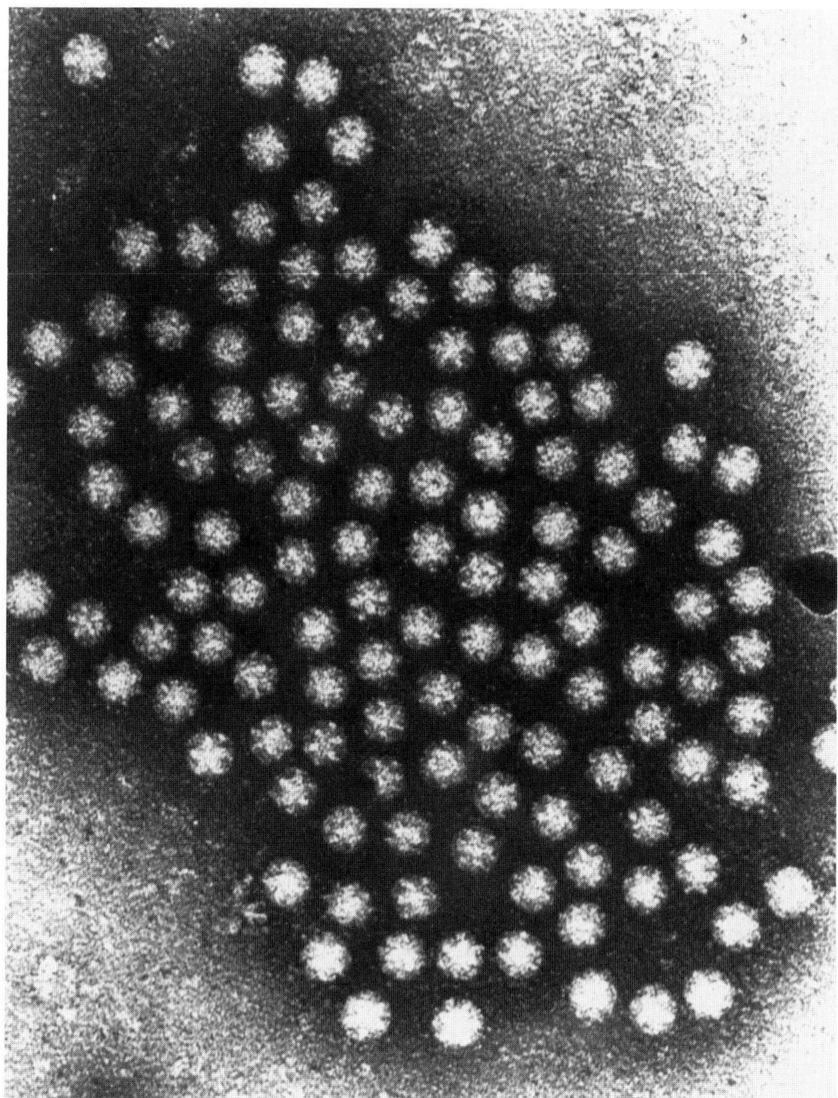

**FIG. 8.** Astrovirus in intestinal contents of gnotobiotic lambs. Particles are 30 nm in diameters. (From Snodgrass and Gray, ref. 376, with permission.)

has a density of 1.35–1.37 gr/cc in cesium chloride. Sodium dodecylsulfate (SDS)/PAGE analysis of human astrovirus has revealed four polypeptides ranging in molecular mass from 36,500 to 32,000 daltons (73). At least five serotypes of human astroviruses have been recognized in the United Kingdom, and these appear to be serologically unrelated to Norwalk-like viruses, to which they have been compared (74).

### Epidemiology

Astroviruses have been detected in diarrheal stools from outbreaks in young children, in both schools and hospitals, and from outbreaks among elderly nursing home residents (68,69,75–77). Systematic studies of the epidemiology of astrovirus infections in humans have not been carried out, although seroprevalence studies in the United Kingdom have shown that detectable serum antibody is present in 75% of children between 3 and 4 years of age (78).

### *In Vitro* Detection

Because astroviruses have not been able to be cultivated efficiently *in vitro*, virus is detected most frequently by EM. In contrast to Norwalk-like agents and caliciviruses, astroviruses are often shed in large amounts in stool and can be detected by EM, even without immune aggregation. If infection in tissue culture can be established, astroviruses can be identified by IF or by IEM (73), and an ELISA has also been recently reported (79).

### Clinical Illness

Illness attributed to astroviruses has consisted primarily of diarrhea, headache, malaise, and nausea, whereas vomiting appears to be less common. Low-grade fever is also frequently present. The incubation period of illness has been estimated to be approximately 3–4 days, and disease manifestations generally last only 2–3 days, but occasionally have been reported to be longer.

### Pathogenesis and Immune Response

The pathogenesis of astrovirus-induced illness is poorly understood. The histopathology of astrovirus infection in animals consists of small intestinal villus shortening and mild inflammatory infiltration of the lamina propria (66,80). Oral administration of stool filtrates that contained astroviruses to normal volunteers resulted in infection but induced illness very infrequently, suggesting that astroviruses may be "less pathogenic" in adults than Norwalk-like agents (81).

Information regarding immunity to human astrovirus infection is currently not available.

## STUDIES OF ANTIVIRALS AND INFECTIONS WITH NORWALK-LIKE AGENTS, CALICIVIRUSES, AND ASTROVIRUSES

### *In Vitro* and *In Vivo* Studies

Because of the absence of both animal models and *in vitro* systems in which to evaluate the activity of antiviral substances against the Norwalk-like agents, few studies have been carried out to examine antivirals in infections with those agents. The effect of therapy with bismuth subsalicylate (BSS) was examined in experimental infection in volunteers who developed illness after challenge with the Norwalk agent in one study (82). Volunteers received either 30 cc of BSS or placebo preparations orally every half hour, for a total of eight doses. This regimen was begun when illness was first noted and was repeated 24 hr after the onset of illness. BSS recipients had a modest but statistically significant reduction in the severity and duration of abdominal cramps, and in the median duration of total gastrointestinal symptoms. No difference was noted in number, weight, or content of stools, nor in the rates of virus shedding when compared to placebo recipients. The precise mechanism of action of BSS in this setting is unknown, although it has been suggested that it may act through antiinflammatory or antisecretory effects rather than through antiviral effects (82).

Ribavirin has also been reported to be active against feline calicivirus in tissue culture (83) and has also been studied *in vivo* in the feline model. One day after aerosol challenge of cats with $10^8$ median tissue culture infective dose ($TCID_{50}$), ribavirin was administered at a dose of 75 mg/kg/day in three doses for 10 days (84). However, no beneficial effect on clinical illness or virus shedding was noted. The author described areas of hemorrhage in ribavirin-treated animals, apparently as a result of thrombocytopenia, as well as decreases in both red cell and white cell counts. The author suggested that aerosol administration of ribavirin in this system might be more effective (84). Calicivirus replication *in vitro* was not inhibited by actinomycin D (85), halogenated uridine deoxiribosides (86), guanidine, or hydroxybenzyl benzimidizole (87). Recombinant human interferon (Hu-$\alpha_A$), the hybrid interferon (Hu-$\alpha_{A/D}$), and feline interferon have been reported to reduce the yield of feline calicivirus by 1.5 to 4.3 $\log_{10}$ PFU (plaque forming unit/ml) when added to feline lung cells 18–24 hr before viral challenge (88). This effect was observed over interferon concentrations of $10^3$–$10^4$ U/ml and over $10^2$–$10^3$ PFU of challenge virus. The authors concluded that feline calicivirus was sensitive to the actions of interferon *in vitro,* although somewhat less sensitive than VSV in the same system.

Information regarding the effects of antivirals on astrovirus infections is not currently available.

### Potential Application of Antivirals

Currently available information indicates that multiple antigenic types exist among the Norwalk-like agents, caliciviruses, and astroviruses. The critical parameters of immunity, and the epidemiologic significance of infection with the various serotypes are not well defined currently. However, if immunity is of short duration, as appears to be the case in some individuals who experience infection with the Norwalk-like agents, or if different serotypes within each group of agents are of similar epidemiologic importance and do not confer cross-protection, then it would appear unlikely that effective immunoprophylaxis (vaccines) can be developed to control the bulk of disease caused by infection with such agents. Successful prevention may depend, instead, on the application of measures that have broadly protective effects or that do not depend on the stimulation of specific immune responses. Therefore, infections with these gastrointestinal viruses are logical targets for antiviral prophylaxis and/or therapy. *In vitro* culture and animal model systems are available for certain caliciviruses and to some extent with astroviruses, as well, which can be used to approach the development of antivirals. However, *in vitro* systems and animal models with which to study the Norwalk-like agents are not available, and, thus, the potential utility of antiviral compounds for those infections is difficult to assess.

The development of effective antiviral prophylaxis and/or therapy for gastrointestinal infections may also depend on the availability of an appropriate delivery system for antiviral substances. Enteritis induced by the above viral agents appears to be a superficial infection that involves the jejunal mucosa, and, to be effective, antivirals will likely have to manifest activity at this mucosal site. Topical application of antiviral compounds that are active on intestinal mucosal surfaces and that are not absorbed systemically appear to be particularly promising approaches for investigation.

The relatively short incubation period and short duration of disease induced by these viruses, in which peak viral shedding occurs in the first 24–48 hr of illness, suggests that antiviral compounds must be administered early after exposure or onset of illness to be useful. Administration of antivirals could be undertaken if outbreaks were recognized early in community or institutional settings, or if index cases were detected in family groups. Early recognition of cases will require the development of rapid, accurate diagnostic methods, which would be applicable for use in clinical or public health settings.

## ROTAVIRUSES

### Classification

The rotaviruses are 67–70-nm viruses with a distinct inner and outer capsid (89)

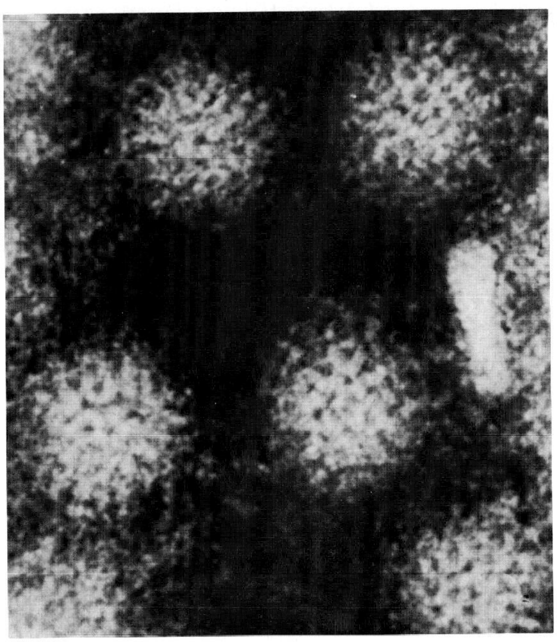

**FIG. 9.** Rotavirus particles in stool of a child with gastroenteritis as visualized by electron microscopy. Particles are 66–77 nm in diameter and are stained with 2% phosphotungstic acid. (Courtesy of R. G. Wyatt, National Institutes of Health, Bethesda, Maryland.)

(Fig. 9). The double-shelled particle has a smooth appearance by EM, whereas the inner capsid is an icosahedron with T = 13 (90,91). The genome consists of 11 segments of double-stranded RNA, with a total molecular weight of 11–12 × $10^6$ daltons. The buoyant density of intact double-shelled particles in cesium chloride is 1.36 g/cc (92) (Table 2). The rotaviruses are thus currently classified as members of the reovirus family, which include three animal genera, the orthoreoviruses, orbiviruses, and rotaviruses, and three genera of plant viruses (93). Rotavirus infections are ubiquitous in nature, and a large number of human and animal rotaviruses have been described (94–100).

**TABLE 2.** *Biophysical properties of rotavirus*

| | |
|---|---|
| Size: | 66–70 nm |
| Capsid structure: | double |
| Outer capsid: | distinct |
| Nucleic acid: | RNA, double-stranded, 11 segments, 11–12 × $10^6$ daltons |
| Structural polypeptides: | 7 |
| Nonstructural polypeptides: | 4 |
| Buoyant density: | 1.36 g/cc in cesium chloride |

The rotaviruses are further subdivided into groups, subgroups, and serotypes. Serotypes are defined as viruses with 20-fold or greater differences in neutralization titer using hyperimmune sera (101). At least seven rotavirus serotypes, including four occurring in humans, are currently recognized (102–107). Several additional human (108,109) and animal (110) rotavirus serotypes have been proposed. The major determinant of rotavirus serotype is the outer capsid protein VP7 encoded by rotavirus gene segment 7, 8, or 9 (111). However, it has recently been recognized that antibody directed against the outer capsid protein VP4, encoded by gene segment 4, may also neutralize infectivity, and that these two gene segments may segregate independently during mixed infection (112,113). Thus, it is possible that a more complex system of serotype designation that takes into account both of these proteins will eventually be needed (113).

Subgroups are defined on the basis of reactivity with hyperimmune sera, as measured by enzyme immunoassay (EIA) or complement fixation (CF) (114). At least two subgroups, denoted subgroup I and II, are recognized (115). Subgroup specificity is primarily determined by the major inner capsid protein VP6 (116–120). Thus, subgroup and serotype specificity may also segregate independently during mixed infection (121).

Finally, rotaviruses that do not react in standard detection tests have been described (122–124). It has recently been proposed that such viruses be classified by the presence of a group specific antigen on VP6 into groups A, B, and C, with group A denoting the more commonly recognized rotavirus group (125). The epidemiologic significance of the group B and C rotaviruses is currently under investigation; however, it is clear that viruses belonging to both groups also cause disease in humans (126–129).

## Genetics

A variety of methods have been used to determine the specific coding assignments of the segmented rotavirus genome. The coding assignments of the gene segments of the simian rotavirus SA-11 are summarized in Table 3 (130–132). The specific gene order may differ for other rotaviruses due to naturally occurring variations in the electrophoretic mobility of the gene segments. Important features of the rotavirus structural polypeptides are outlined below.

The inner capsid is composed primarily of the virus protein VP6, with smaller amounts of VP1, VP2, and VP3 (130,131). It should be noted that the product of RNA segment 3 has only recently been identified as an 88,000-dalton protein, which has been denoted VP3 (130). The outer capsid protein formerly referred to as VP3 is therefore now denoted VP4. VP6 contains the major group antigen of group A rotaviruses (117,120) as well as bearing antigenic determinants responsible for division of group A rotaviruses into subgroups (10,117,120,133). VP6 is also necessary for *in vitro* transcription catalyzed by purified virus cores (134). Purified VP6 can self assemble *in vitro* into spherical particles resembling single-shelled virions (135), indicating that this protein also plays a role in virus assembly. The role of the minor inner capsid proteins VP1, VP2, and VP3 in virus replication is not clear, but it is likely that at least one of them has a polymerase function, based on the synthesis of double-stranded RNA by virus cores (136,137).

**TABLE 3.** *Polypeptides encoded by gene segments of rotavirus SA-11*

| Gene segments | Molecular weight of primary gene product (designation) | Location |
|---|---|---|
| 1 | 125,000 (VP1) | Inner capsid |
| 2 | 94,000 (VP2) | Inner capsid |
| 3 | 88,000 (VP3) | Inner capsid |
| 4 | 88,000 (VP4) | Outer capsid |
| 5 | 53,000 (NS) | Nonstructural |
| 6 | 41,000 (VP6) | Outer capsid |
| 7 | 34,000 (NS) | Nonstructural |
| 8 | 35,000 (NS) | Nonstructural |
| 9 | 37,000 (VP7) | Outer capsid |
| 10 | 20,000 (NS) | Nonstructural |
| 11 | 29,000 (VP9) | ? Outer |

After Middleton et al., ref. 194.

The outer capsid is composed of the major proteins VP4 and VP7, and possibly a minor polypeptide VP9 (132). The most abundant virus protein on the outer capsid is VP7, a 37,000-dalton glycoprotein product of gene segment 7, 8, or 9, depending on virus. Monoclonal antibody to VP7 inhibits adsorption of virus to cells, suggesting that VP7 is the attachment protein (138,139). Analysis of reassortants and of the reactivity of VP7 with monoclonal antibodies has also identified VP7 as the major determinant of rotavirus serotype (111,140). Therefore, definition of the antigenic topology and extent of antigenic variation of VP7 is of considerable interest. Neutralizing monoclonal antibodies directed at VP7 have defined a single large neutralization site on this protein containing multiple overlapping epitopes (141–145). Escape mutants generated in the presence of these antibodies have amino acid changes in two distinct regions of VP7 denoted A and C (145,146). Although these two regions are separated on the linear sequence of the molecule, the ability of the corresponding monoclonal antibodies to compete with each other for binding suggests that they are juxtaposed on the folded protein (145–147). The three-dimensional structure of this protein thus appears to be important for its immunogenicity, as also suggested by the failure of many monoclonal antibodies against VP7 to react with reduced forms of this protein (139,141).

Naturally occurring human and animal rotaviruses display marked sequence conservation of VP7 within serotype, to the extent that serotype can be predicted from sequence analysis (148,149). However, some antigenic variation within serotypes can be detected in VP7 with monoclonal antibodies (143). In addition, an escape mutant generated in the presence of a monoclonal antibody to VP7 also had a slightly decreased neutralization titer with polyclonal sera (141). Further studies of the reactivity of human rotavirus isolates with neutralizing monoclonal antibodies should help to determine the extent of antigenic drift in human rotaviruses.

The second most abundant outer capsid protein is VP4, the product of gene segment 4. VP4 is synthesized as an approximately 88,000-dalton protein, which is subsequently cleaved by trypsin into the two outer capsid proteins VP5 (55,000 molecular weight) and VP8 (27,000 molecular weight). Several important functions have been identified for VP4, including determination of growth in tissue culture, entry into cells, and virulence.

The restricted ability of human rotaviruses to grow in tissue culture was originally associated with gene segment 4 by studies of reassortants between human rotaviruses and a temperature-sensitive bovine rotavirus that grew well in tissue culture (116,150,151). Subsequently, it was found that treatment of rotaviruses with trypsin greatly enhanced growth in tissue culture (152,153) and that this effect was associated with the cleavage of VP4 into VP5 and VP8 (154–156). Recent studies have suggested that trypsin-mediated cleavage of VP4 is necessary for entry of infectious virus cores into the cell (157).

Sequence data for gene segment 4 of several animal and human rotaviruses are now available. A potential trypsin cleavage site has been identified in the VP4 of several rotaviruses (158–162), and a putative fusion peptide has also been identified in the VP4 of rhesus rotavirus (163). The sequence of the cleavage site and regions flanking it are conserved in most human rotaviruses associated with diarrhea (160,162), but analysis of gene segment 4 from human rotaviruses isolated from asymptomatic neonates has revealed a sequence dimorphism of this gene that appears to correlate with virulence (158,159). Three of six amino acids in the connecting peptide differed between rotaviruses associated with diarrhea and those associated with asymptomatic shedding, and all together 45 amino acids could be identified in VP4 that differed between such viruses (159). The role of VP4 in specifying virulence is further indicated by studies with reassortants in which the dose of virus necessary to induce diarrhea in suckling mice was correlated with the parental origin of gene 4 (164). The role of a protease-sensitive protein in specifying virulence has parallels in both reoviruses and influenza A viruses.

VP4 also plays an important role in virus neutralization and protection from disease. Monoclonal antibodies to VP4 neutralize infectivity *in vitro* (140,165), and passive oral immunization with such monoclonal antibodies protects animals from disease (158,159,165). Monoclonal antibodies to

VP4 apparently do not inhibit attachment of virus to the host cell, but prevent the trypsin-mediated internalization of virus necessary for productive infection (138). Both serotype-specific and serotype cross-reactive monoclonal antibodies to VP4 have been described (141,166,167). At least three operationally distinct heterotypic neutralization epitopes have been defined for VP4 (168), and sequence analysis of escape mutants to these heterotypically neutralizing monoclonal antibodies has localized amino acid changes in the larger cleavage product of VP4, VP5 (168,169). Serotype-specific monoclonal antibodies, on the other hand, select mutations in five different regions in the smaller cleavage product VP8 (163). Of note, antigenic variants of VP4 selected by monoclonal antibodies did not have altered virulence when tested in neonatal mice (122). The extent of naturally occurring antigenic variation in VP4 is currently under study. The reported isolation of two otherwise identical rotaviruses from a nursery 2 months apart that differed in their reactivity with VP4 monoclonal antibodies suggests that antigenic drift in this protein may occur (141).

### Replication

Attachment of rotavirus to intestinal epithelial cells probably occurs by interaction of virus with specific receptors, mediated by VP7. Sialic acid may be a component of this receptor (170,171). After attachment, the virus may enter the cell through one of two mechanisms, either by endocytosis (172,173) or by direct penetration (157,174). Recent evidence suggests that virus that enters the cell by endocytosis is not infectious and that direct penetration leads to productive infection (138,157,174). Trypsin-mediated cleavage of VP4 is necessary for utilization of the direct penetration pathway (138). EM studies have suggested that rotavirus RNA may be injected directly into the cell in a manner analogous to that of bacteriophage (174).

Loss of the outer capsid proteins triggers activation of the virus transcriptase (175,176). Transcription of viral RNA then proceeds in an asymmetrical fashion similar to that of reovirus in which positive strand RNAs are copied from the genomic negative strand (177) and then used as templates for production of double-stranded RNA (178–180). Both positive and negative strand synthesis proceed throughout infection, but at different relative rates (181). Eventually, completed daughter segments are packaged together into complete copies of the viral genome. The mechanism ensuring a complete copy of the genome in each virus is unknown.

The role of specific viral proteins in these processes is currently under investigation. Subviral particles with associated replicase activity are enriched for VP1 and VP2, suggesting these proteins are involved in replicase activity (136,182). The nonstructural proteins NS 34 and NS 35 are also observed in these particles (137). VP6 has an important role in transcription, since removal of VP6 from viral cores abolishes transcriptase activity, which can be restored by addition of VP6 (134).

New protein synthesis is detected as early as 1–2 hr postinfection (183). Inner capsid proteins are synthesized throughout the cytoplasm, whereas outer capsid proteins are synthesized in the rough endoplasmic reticulum (184,185). Addition of the outer capsid is associated with budding into the endoplasmic reticulum (ER) and acquisition of a transient viral envelope (173,186,187). Inhibition of glycosylation of VP7 and NS 28 results in accumulation of enveloped forms in the ER (188,189). Release of virus is by cell lysis. A single cycle of virus replication in a permissive cell takes approximately 8–24 hr (183,186,190).

### Detection

A variety of methods are currently available for the detection of rotaviruses in stool samples (191–199). The most widely utilized are immunoassays that in general detect the rotavirus group antigen present on VP6 (200–203). Such assays frequently involve binding of rotavirus antigen to a solid phase with a capturing antibody, followed by detection with a second, labeled antibody or antibody-coated particle (204,205). Recently tests based on monoclonal antibodies have been developed that are able to determine the serotype of rotavirus directly in stool samples (206,207).

Other methods of detection of rotavirus in stool samples have included hybridization of radiolabeled nucleic acid probes to viral RNA (208,209), or PAGE analysis of viral RNA from stool either with (210,211) or without (192,212) prior deproteinization. Finally, EM remains a useful technique for detection of rotavirus. Because of the distinctive morphology and high titer of rotavirus particles in stool, immunoaggregation of virus has generally not been required, although it may prove helpful (213,214). EM is especially useful for detection of group B and C rotaviruses, which are not detected by commonly available rotavirus immunoassays.

A major advance in the study of these viruses has been the development of techniques for the direct isolation of human rotaviruses from stool samples (153,215). Rotavirus inocula are pretreated with trypsin, which is maintained in the media throughout the culture, and the virus is grown on a continuous primate kidney cell line such as MA-104 cells with continuous rolling. Primary monkey kidney cells may be even more efficient for initial isolation. Cytopathic effect (CPE) is clearly seen especially at later passages, and many viruses can be adapted to form plaques in cell culture (153,216–218). The combination of initial isolation in cell culture followed by detection of antigen in first passage material by immunoassay may be a particularly sensitive technique for rotavirus detection (219). The development of efficient systems for propagation of human rotavirus has generated considerable new information on the epidemiology and biology of these viruses.

### Epidemiology

Rotaviruses have emerged over the past several years as major causes of diarrheal diseases world wide. Rotaviruses have accounted for 42–55% of cases of gastroenteritis in children hospitalized in different parts of the world (Table 4) (220–224). Prospective studies have suggested that 2.9 million episodes of rotavirus-induced diarrhea in children less than 5 years old occur per year in the United States, accounting for 22,000 hospitalizations (225). In developing countries, diarrheal diseases, of which rotaviruses are a major cause, account for as many as 5–10 million deaths per year (226).

The incidence of symptomatic rotavirus infections varies with age. The group primarily at risk appears to be those between 6 months and 2 years of age (149,227–233). Infections in neonates, i.e., those younger

**TABLE 4.** *Proportion of children hospitalized with acute gastroenteritis associated with rotavirus infection*

| Geographic location | Reference | Number of cases | Percentage with rotavirus infection |
|---|---|---|---|
| Washington, D.C. | Kapikian et al. (246) | 143 | 42 |
| Atlanta, Georgia | Gomez-Barreto et al. (451) | 29 | 55 |
| Birmingham, U.K. | Flewett et al. (452) | 73 | 54 |
| Oslo, Norway | Orstavik et al. (453) | 35 | 54 |
| Melbourne, Australia | Davidson et al. (280) | 378 | 52 |

Adapted from Gomez-Barreto et al., ref. 451.

than 6 months, tend to be asymptomatic (234–238), but symptomatic infections have also been reported in this age group (234,239,240). Rotaviruses have also been associated with symptomatic infections in adults (241), in sporadic cases (242–244), in parents of affected children (225,236,245–247), and in cases of traveler's diarrhea (248–251). Rotaviruses have been implicated as important pathogens in several institutional settings. These include hospitals (252–255), day care centers (256–258), and nursing homes (259–261) with high attack rates and severe illness in the latter group.

The major route of transmission of rotavirus is likely to be fecal-oral since virus is shed in large quantity in the stool of infected individuals and is highly infectious when administered orally. Under appropriate circumstances, as few as one to 10 infectious particles are sufficient to cause disease (262,263). Since virus may be shed by both symptomatic and asymptomatic individuals (19,253,258), ample opportunities for virus transmission exist. A respiratory route of transmission has also been proposed based on the high frequency of respiratory symptoms in affected children, but direct evidence of this route is lacking.

A consistent feature of rotavirus epidemiology has been seasonal variation of disease incidence. Rotavirus-induced gastroenteritis occurs primarily during the cooler months, reaching peaks in December and January in the northern hemisphere (228,231,233,264–268) and in June and July in the southern (269–271). In tropical countries, rotavirus gastroenteritis occurs throughout the year (227,230,237,272).

The ability to cultivate rotaviruses and development of typing systems based on monoclonal antibodies has allowed preliminary determinants of the relative frequency of rotavirus serotypes. Serotype 1 has emerged in most studies as the currently most frequent serotype (206,207,273–275), but additional serotypes frequently cocirculate (274–277).

### Pathogenesis

Descriptions of the histopathology of rotavirus-induced gastroenteritis have been obtained from peroral small intestinal biopsies performed 24–129 hr after onset of illness (278). The jejunal and duodenal mucosa appear to have patchy irregularities, which consist of shortening and blunting of villi, and increased infiltration of the lamina propria with mononuclear cells. EM reveals numerous rotavirus particles in the epithelial cells. Biopsies obtained 4–8 weeks after onset of illness demonstrate apparently normal histology (279). IF studies have demonstrated rotaviral antigen in the cytoplasm of terminal villous epithelial cells in the duodenum and jejunal mucosa (280), whereas the stomach and large intestine are relatively spared (279,280).

The pattern of virus shedding in symptomatic cases closely parallels the temporal development of illness. Virus can be detected coincident with or slightly before the onset of illness (258,281), and in 94% of specimens 1–4 days and 76% 4–8 days after onset. Occasionally, virus can be found in stool 2 weeks or longer after illness (231,258).

Acute illness is associated with decreased levels of intestinal brush border enzymes such as maltase, sucrase, and lactase (278). The diminished activity of these enzymes is reflected in the findings of lactose and D-xylose malabsorption in acutely infected children (282–284) and the presence of reducing substances in diarrheal stool (284). Similar findings have been demonstrated in experimentally infected piglets. In these studies, virus antigen is found by IF in villous tip cells, associated with villous atrophy, decreased levels of mucosal lactase, sucrase, and Na/K ATPase, and lactose malabsorption (285,286). A hypothetical sequence of events to explain rotavirus-induced diarrhea has been proposed, in which infection and destruction of differentiated villous epithelial cells leads to brush border enzyme deficiency, complex sugar malabsorption, and osmotic diarrhea (285,286). The success of oral rehydration under these circumstances may reflect the patchy nature of the mucosal abnormality (284). The mechanisms by which rotavirus infection results in nausea and vomiting are unknown.

### Clinical Characteristics of Illness

Studies of both hospitalized individuals and outpatients with rotavirus infection have demonstrated a spectrum of disease ranging from asymptomatic shedding (287,288) to severe dehydration and even death (289,290). Typical symptoms are nonspecific and include vomiting, diarrhea, and fever (108,231,236, 291,292). Studies of hospitalized children have indicated that cases of gastroenteritis associated with rotavirus have tended to be more severe than cases in which rotavirus was not detected, with more severe dehydration and higher incidences of vomiting and fever (105,294–295). Disease manifestations in hospitalized children have lasted an average of 8 days (291), although protracted episodes have been noted on occasion. Clinical manifestations in adults appear similar, with frequent vomiting, but are somewhat less severe (225,244). Respiratory symptoms may be seen in 30–50% of children with rotavirus gastroenteritis (225,293,294,296,297), and, in one study, rotavirus antigen was detected by immunoassay in the nasopharyngeal secretions of four children with pneumonia (298). However, ill children are frequently simultaneously infected with both respiratory and gastrointestinal viruses, making interpretation of these findings more difficult (299). A variety of additional syndromes have also been associated with rotavirus infection (300–304), including an association with necrotizing enterocolitis in neonates (239,305) and chronic infection in immunodeficiency (6,306).

Laboratory studies in symptomatic children are generally unremarkable. Dehydration with elevations in the blood urea nitrogen and hyperchloremic metabolic acidosis is a common finding (105,307). Peripheral blood leukocyte counts are usually normal in uncomplicated cases. Mild elevations in the serum aspartase aminotransferase (AST) have been reported during acute illness without other evidence of hepatic injury (308), and these elevations may reflect damage to intestinal epithelial cells. Diarrheal stools are described as watery or yellow without mucus or blood. Minimal to moderate numbers of fecal leukocytes are seen in approximately one-third of samples (244,292,294).

Current therapy consists of rehydration and correction of metabolic abnormalities in severe cases. Oral rehydration with solutions containing glucose and electrolytes similar to those used in cholera have been very successful (227,309,310).

### Immune Responses

The humoral immune response of children to rotavirus infection is highly complex, with stimulation of antibody of multiple classes and specificities in both local and systemic compartments. Several techniques can be used to measure antibody to rotavirus, including CF and EIA (213,311), which can determine antibody class specific responses. Most studies have shown rotavirus specific IgM in sera taken shortly after illness, followed by an IgG and IgA response in convalescent sera (312–316). Rotavirus-specific antibody can also be detected in stool (coproantibody) following acute illness and appears to be an accurate reflection of the response in duodenal secretions (316). The coproantibody response includes IgM, IgA, and IgG (314,315,317, 318). When measured directly by aspiration, the level of IgG in duodenal secretions is low and may represent a transudate from the systemic compartment rather than local production (313,314). Antirotaviral IgA has also been detected in nasopharnygeal secretions, saliva (314,318), and breast milk (107,319). The antibody response after infection is directed against both structural and nonstructural proteins by radioimmunoprecipitation analysis (320).

Neutralizing antibody is seen in both serum and duodenal secretions following challenge (321). Both serotype specific and heterotypic neutralizing antibody responses may be seen (322–324). The frequency of heterotypic responses appears to increase with increasing age, suggesting that priming may boost the heterotypic response (322–324), but heterotypic responses can also occur after apparently primary infection (322). Heterotypic neutralization may reflect antibody to cross-reactive neutralizing epitopes on VP7 or to the more broadly cross-reactive VP4, or both. In adults, the majority of the neutralizing antibody response appears to be directed at VP4 (325).

Relatively less is known about the cellular immune response to rotavirus infection. In mice, both serotype-specific and cross-reactive HLA restricted cytotoxic T cells develop after infection (326). Delayed-type hypersensitivity, as measured by foot pad injection, apparently does not develop after infection of neonatal mice (327). The relative importance of cellular immunity in recovery from rotavirus is unknown, since T-cell deficient mice recover normally from infection (328), but mice with combined immunodeficiency become chronically infected (329).

The decreasing incidence of symptomatic rotavirus infection with age and the efficacy of rotavirus vaccines (see below) suggest that the immune response to infection provides some protection against symptomatic reinfection. The specific components of the response outlined above most responsible for this protection are currently under study. Some human challenge studies (321) and epidemiologic studies (330) have shown a correlation between the presence of serum antibody and protection, whereas others (263,291) have not. These studies may be difficult to compare because the antibody that was measured has not always had neutralizing activity. Nonhumoral mechanisms have also been postulated to play a role, since infected neonates are protected from subsequent disease without a measurable antibody response (331).

### Immunoprophylaxis

Both active and passive forms of immunoprophylaxis against rotavirus infections have been investigated. In mice, oral administration of neutralizing monoclonal antibodies against VP4 or VP7, or of breast milk from dams immunized with VP4 or VP7, protects neonatal mice from subsequent challenge (332,333). Similarly, oral administration of antirotavirus antibody to calves also protects against rotavirus (334). In humans, oral administration of $\gamma$-globulin protects low-birth-weight infants from diarrhea caused by rotavirus (335). Recently, bovine milk immunoglobulin concentrates containing high levels of rotavirus neutralizing activity have been prepared from the milk and colostrum of cows hyperimmunized against rotavirus (336). In a preliminary study, administration of such concentrates to infants with naturally acquired rotavirus gastroenteritis shortened the duration of virus shedding but had no other clinical effect (339). Further studies on the use of oral immunoglobulins in the prophylaxis or therapy of rotavirus are currently under way.

A variety of approaches to the development of a rotavirus vaccine have also been undertaken. To date, live, attenuated rotavirus vaccines have received the greatest attention. The most promising vaccine candidates currently being evaluated are rotaviruses isolated from animals that manifest attenuated virulence for humans (337). These include the rhesus monkey rotavirus RRV MMU 18006 (338,340–342) and the bo-

viruses, echoviruses, and enteroviruses 69–71 grow well in tissue culture. Coxsackie A viruses grow variably in tissue culture, particularly on initial isolation, and certain serotypes have not been cultivated *in vitro* and must be inoculated into suckling mice for detection (366).

The majority of infections and illnesses with enteroviruses occur in children, although severe illnesses such as meningitis and myocarditis have been recognized in adults (366). Infection and illness with these agents is most frequent during the summer months and in early autumn (368). Enteroviruses have been associated with diarrheal disease in immunosuppressed patients (6) and with persistent CNS infections in patients with agammaglobulinemia (369). Echoviruses have been cultured from the cerebrospinal fluid (CSF) of such patients over a period varying from 2 months to 3 years. Patients with agammaglobulinemia also have a higher incidence of paralytic disease following oral administration of live poliovirus vaccine (370,371).

**TABLE 5.** *Diseases associated with enteroviruses*

| |
|---|
| Echoviruses |
| Acute undifferentiated illness (summer grippe) |
| Aseptic meningitis[a] |
| Gastroenteritis |
| Group A Coxsackieviruses |
| Acute undifferentiated illness |
| Aseptic meningitis[a] |
| Herpangina |
| Hand-foot-and-mouth disease |
| Exanthems |
| Acute lymphonodular pharyngitis |
| Acute hemorrhagic conjunctivitis |
| Group B Coxsackieviruses |
| Acute undifferentiated illness |
| Aseptic meningitis[a] |
| Myocarditis (newborn and older) |
| Pleurodynia |
| Orchitis |
| Poliovirus |
| Acute undifferentiated illness |
| Aseptic meningitis |
| Paralytic poliomyelitis |
| Enteroviruses (types 69–71) |
| Acute hemorrhagic conjunctivitis (pandemic) |
| Meningoencephalitis |
| Acute respiratory disease |

[a]Uncommonly associated with paresis.

## Clinical Characteristics of Illness

Enteroviruses cause a wide variety of illnesses, as depicted in Table 5. The most common manifestations of infection with coxsackie and echoviruses are "acute undifferentiated illnesses," which are often referred to as "summer grippe" (365,366). These short-lived, self-limited illnesses may have respiratory components, and fever is variably present as well. Although vomiting or diarrhea may occasionally be present in enterovirus infection, large-scale studies have not implicated enteroviruses as major causes of acute gastroenteritis. Isolation of several echovirus serotypes have been reported in cases of acute gastroenteritis, and echovirus 18 has been implicated in a newborn nursery outbreak (372). The newly described enteroviruses have been associated with outbreaks of conjunctivitis and, occasionally, paralytic disease (366,367). The potential role of antivirals in the therapy of enterovirus associated conjunctivitis is described elsewhere (Chapter 6).

Incubation periods of illness induced by enteroviruses vary markedly with enteroviral syndromes, but are generally within the range of 1 to 15 days (366,367). Most of the common illnesses appear to have incubation periods of 2–5 days. Although the duration of illness is also highly variable, enteroviruses can be cultured from throat and stool in high titer early in the illness, and for variable periods after illness. Shedding of virus in stools for weeks after illness is not uncommon.

## Pathogenesis

The pathogenesis of enterovirus infections is based primarily on studies with polioviruses (373,374). Initial viral replication occurs in the pharynx and in the gut, where it may or may not be associated with a minor illness. Viremia can follow initial replication of virus in the gut, and end organ replication of virus after hematogenous spread accounts for distant or disseminated manifestations. Invasion of the CNS could occur either by neural spread from the original site of virus implantation or by bloodborne routes. Certain enteroviruses have been demonstrated to require the presence of virus-specific receptors on cell surfaces to initiate infection (268,375). It has been suggested that the specificity of such receptors may account for tissue tropisms of certain enteroviruses, e.g., for the central CNS or for the myocardium (268,375).

### Studies with Antivirals

Antiviral substances have received relatively little attention with respect to enteroviral infections in humans. However, a large number of compounds have been shown to have *in vitro* activity against enteroviruses (376,377), and many of these compounds also are active *in vivo*. In these latter studies, the mouse model has been most frequently employed, although subhuman primates have also occasionally been used. These drugs could potentially inhibit enterovirus replication at a number of steps and are reviewed below.

Virus uncoating is the target of several antienterovirus drugs. 4-(6-(2-Chloro-4-methoxyphenoxy)-hexyl)-3, 5-heptane dione (arildone) is an acyclic diketone with *in vitro* activity against both DNA and RNA viruses, including rhinovirus, poliovirus, and coxsackie virus A9 (378). Both orally and intraperitoneally administered arildone prevented paralysis and death in neonatal mice infected intracerebrally with a lethal dose of poliovirus, with protection seen even when medication was delayed until 48 hr after infection (379). However, the drug appears to be less effective when administered to older mice, possibly due to more rapid elimination (380). Arildone exerts its greatest antiviral effect *in vitro* when added within 4 hr of infection, but does not directly inactivate virus and does not inhibit adsorption of virus to cells (381–384). Instead, arildone appears to bind directly to the virus capsid (381), thereby inhibiting virus uncoating (384). VP1 has been identified as potentially important in the action of arildone, since resistant mutants have an altered VP1 protein by peptide mapping (385). 5-(7-(4-(4,5-Dihydro-2-oxazoyl) phenoxy)heptyl)-3-methylisoxazol (WIN 51711) also has broad-spectrum antiviral activity against both rhinovirus and enteroviruses (386). Both oral and parenteral therapy are effective in suckling mice in preventing paralysis induced by poliovirus (387) and echovirus 9 (388), even when administered 48 hr after infection. WIN 51711 also binds to the virus capsid, stabilizing it (389) and thereby preventing pH dependent uncoating in endosomes (390). X-ray crystallographic studies of WIN 51711 complexed with rhinovirus 14 indicate that WIN 51711 interacts with the B barrel structure of the VP1 protein (391). (2-Thio-4-oxothiazolidine (rhodanine) is a selective inhibitor of the multiplication of echovirus 12 in tissue culture (392–394). This agent exhibits an unexplained selectivity for echovirus type 12 but not other enteroviruses (392). Rhodanine also appears to act to prevent virus uncoating through direct interaction with the virus capsid (395).

The requirement for proteolytic cleavage of a protein precursor by a viral protease in the replication of picornaviruses makes such enzymes a logical target for antiviral drugs. Relatively few studies have been done along these lines; however, the cysteine proteinase inhibitor, chicken cystatin, has been reported to inhibit the growth of poliovirus *in vitro* (396). Further studies of the interactions between virus proteases and their inhibitors may allow additional antiviral agents to be developed.

A large number of inhibitors of enteroviral replication have been described that inhibit the replication of viral RNA. Flavenoids are a class of plant extracts that have been investigated for their activity against enteroviruses (397). Quercetin, 3-methyl-quercetin, and 4′,5′-dihydroxy-3,3′,7-trimethoxyflavone (Ro 90-0179) have *in vitro* activity against a broad spectrum of enteroviruses (398). All of these agents have *in vivo* activity as well in murine models of enterovirus infection (399–402). The antiviral activity of Ro 09-0179 appears to be related to a block in the formation of the viral RNA polymerase complex, and not due to inhibition of the function of the intact polymerase (395). 3-Methylquercetin is a selective inhibitor of poliovirus RNA and protein synthesis in infected cell and cell free systems (403,404). The mechanism of the antiviral activity of quercetin is unknown. Interestingly, silica treatment abolishes the *in vivo* activity of quercetin in mengo-virus–infected mice, suggesting that macrophages may be necessary for this effect (401).

Guanidine is a natural constituent of animal serum that is a selective inhibitor of several picornaviruses *in vitro* (406) and is considered here with the benzimidazoles, 2-(α-hydroxybenzyl) benzimidazole (HBB) (407) and enviroxime, because of a possible synergistic effect of these agents *in vivo*. Guanidine inhibits viruses from all enterovirus groups (408), whereas HBB inhibits polioviruses, group B coxsackieviruses, echoviruses, and coxsackie A9 (409,410). Enviroxime has been evaluated primarily as an antirhinovirus compound (239,411), but also inhibits other picornaviruses *in vitro,* including coxsackie, polio, and echoviruses (412). HBB appeared to be effective in treatment of coxsackie A9 and variably effective in echovirus 9 infection in mice (413), whereas guanidine has minimal to no effect on these infections when used alone (410). Both guanidine and HBB were ineffective in chemotherapy of poliovirus infection in cynomologous monkeys, with drug-resistant mutants developing rapidly with each compound (414,415). However, simultaneous administration of HBB and guanidine has a synergistic effect on echovirus 9 and coxsackie A9 infections in newborn mice, without the development of resistant virus (410,413). Enviroxime protected infant mice from these infections, but was not synergistic with either HBB or guanidine (410).

These agents also appear to act at the level of viral RNA synthesis. Guanidine and HBB both inhibit viral RNA synthesis *in vitro* (409,416), and viral RNA and protein synthesis are reduced in infected, enviroxime-treated cells (322,412). Guanidine exerts its greatest effect early in infection, at the initiation of RNA synthesis (406,417). Mutants of poliovirus that have become resistant to the action of guanidine are easily isolated in culture and have changes in the nonstructural protein pX, which has been postulated to play a role in RNA synthesis (406).

Antiviral agents that act by modulating the susceptibility of the host to viral infection are also effective to a certain extent against enteroviruses. Interferon has been demonstrated to inhibit the growth of several enteroviruses *in vitro,* including echovirus types 9 and 11, and poliovirus (47,417,418). Interferon has conferred protection when administered prophylactically in encephalomyocarditis (EMC) virus infections of mice (419–422), and human interferon produced by recombinant DNA techniques also has been shown to protect squirrel monkeys from EMC infection (423). Administration of interferon inducers, such as poly I:C and tilorone, is also effective in the prophylaxis of picornavirus infections in mice (420,421,424,425). Single-stranded RNAs have also been shown to protect mice against EMC infection independently of interferon production (426–429). The mechanism of *in vivo* activity of these agents is unclear; however, silica treatment abolishes the effect, suggesting that macrophages play a role (430). Finally, isoprinosine has been reported to have *in vitro* activity against poliovirus (431) and demonstrates synergistic activity with interferon in EMC infections of mice (432).

Conflicting data have been generated concerning the antiviral activity of isoprinosine, but both suppression of viral RNA synthesis and immunomodulation of the host have been described (94,432,433).

A number of other compounds have shown some activity against human and animal enteroviruses *in vitro*. These include the substituted thiosemicarbazones, such as methisazone (434,435), dipyridamole and its derivatives (396,436,437,438), derivatives of phenylthiourea (439,440) and derivatives of 2-aminooxazole (441,442), and nitrobenzene (443,444). In addition, a variety of products from plants and animals have been investigated for antiviral properties. Products with activity against enteroviruses include B penicillamine (445), phleomycin (446), gliotoxin (447,448), and the didemnins, a class of depsipeptides from a Carribean tunicate (449,450). Relatively little is known concerning the *in vivo* efficacy and toxicity of these agents.

In summary, a large number of agents with some antiviral activity against enteroviruses have been investigated. Many of these compounds have been useful in elucidating the steps of picornavirus replication. To date, agents useful in the prophylaxis or treatment of enterovirus infections in human are not available. However, studies of the most promising of these compounds in animal models and continued development of new compounds should provide information with which to assess the potential utility of these substances in human enterovirus infections.

## SUMMARY

Acute viral gastroenteritis is a major public health problem of worldwide importance, for which there are as yet no adequate control measures. Recent advances in the study of viral infections of the gastrointestinal tract have led to the emergence of new groups of etiologic agents. Although understanding of the basis of immunity against those viruses is at an early stage, it appears that the development of vaccines against many of these viruses presents formidable problems. With the description of yet additional viral "groups" as likely causes of gastroenteritis, the development of control measures for viral gastrointestinal infections confront obstacles that are similar to those encountered in the control of viral respiratory tract infections. The inability to cultivate the Norwalk-like agents *in vitro* and the lack of animal models remain major obstacles to the investigation of potentially efficacious antiviral substances against those agents. Studies of human caliciviruses and astroviruses are at an early stage, but progress in adaptation of certain strains to *in vitro* cultivation has been achieved, and information on the effect of antivirals on those viruses should be forthcoming. Human rotaviruses can now be cultivated efficiently in tissue culture, and animal models are available as well. Thus, an increasing number of studies on the effect of antivirals in rotavirus infections can be expected. The successful application of antiviral chemoprophylaxis and/or therapy in acute viral gastroenteritis will also depend on the availability of rapid diagnostic methods for these infections. Such methods are currently widely available for rotaviruses and are being developed for the other viral agents of gastroenteritis as well. A large number of compounds have been demonstrated to have *in vitro* activity against enteroviruses, but relatively limited studies *in vivo* have been carried out. Although the need for antiviral therapy of enterovirus infections is less well defined at this time, such therapy may be useful in severe or widespread disease, or in certain immunocompromised patients.

## REFERENCES

1. Dingle JH, Badger GF, Feller AE, et al. A study of illness in a group of Cleveland families. I. Plan of study and certain general observations. *Am J Hyg* 1953;58:16–30.

2. National Center for Health Statistics, U.S. Department of Health, Education and Welfare. Current estimates from the Health Interview Survey, United States—1972. *Vital and health statistics publication no. (HRA)74-1512*. Series 10, no. 85. 1973.
3. Snyder JD, Merson MH. The magnitude of the global problem of acute diarrheal disease: a review of active surveillance data. *Bull WHO* 1982;60:605–13.
4. Middleton JA, Szymanski MT, Abbott GD, et al. Orbivirus acute gastroenteritis of infancy. *Lancet* 1974;1:1241–7.
5. Halvorsund J, Orstavik I. An epidemic of rotavirus associated gastroenteritis in a nursing home for the elderly. *Scand J Infect Dis* 1980;12:161–4.
6. Yoken RH, Bishop CA, Townsend TR, et al. Infectious gastroenteritis in bone marrow transplant recipients. *N Engl J Med* 1982;306:1009–12.
7. Adler JL, Zickl R. Winter vomiting disease. *J Infect Dis* 1969;119:668–93.
8. Blacklow NR, Dolin R, Fedson DS, et al. Acute infectious non-bacterial gastroenteritis: etiology and pathogenesis. *Ann Intern Med* 1972;76:993–1008.
9. Dolin R, Blacklow NR, Dupont H, et al. Transmission of acute infectious nonbacterial gastroenteritis to volunteers by administration of stool filtrates. *J Infect Dis* 1971;123:307–12.
10. Dolin R, Reichman RC, Roessner KD, et al. Detection by immune electron microscopy of the Snow Mountain agent of acute viral gastroenteritis. *J Infect Dis* 1982;146:184–9.
11. Kapikian AZ, Wyatt RG, Dolin R, et al. Visualization of a 27 nm particle associated with acute infectious non-bacterial gastroenteritis. *J Virol* 1972;10:1075–81.
12. Thornhill TS, Wyatt RG, Kalica AR, et al. Detection by immune electron microscopy of 26–27 nm virus-like particles associated with two family outbreaks of gastroenteritis. *Infect Dis* 1977;138:20–6.
13. Dolin R, Blacklow NR, Dupont H, et al. Biological properties of Norwalk agent of acute infectious nonbacterial gastroenteritis. *Proc Soc Exp Biol Med* 1972;140:578–83.
14. Greenberg HB, Valdesuso J, Kalica AR. Proteins of Norwalk virus. *J Virol* 1981;37:994–9.
15. Madore HP, Treanor JJ, Dolin R. Characterization of the Snow Mountain agent of viral gastroenteritis. *J Virol* 1986;58:487–92.
16. Kapikian AZ, Greenberg HB, Wyatt RG, et al. Norwalk group of viruses-agents associated with epidemic viral gastroenteritis. In: Tyrrell DAJ, Kapikian AZ, eds, *Virus infections of the gastrointestinal tract*. New York: Marcel Dekker, 1982:147–77.
17. Kapikian AZ, Gerin JL, Wyatt RG, et al. Density in cesium chloride of the 27 mm "8FIIa" particle associated with acute infectious nonbacterial gastroenteritis: determination by ultracentrifugation and immune electron microscopy. *Proc Soc Exp Biol Med* 1973;140:578–83.
18. Clark SKR, Cook GT, Egglestone SI, et al. A virus from epidemic vomiting disease. *Br Med J* 1972;3:86–9.
19. Caul EO, Ashley C, Pether JVS. "Norwalk-like" particles in epidemic gastroenteritis in the U.K. *Lancet* 1979;2:1292.
20. Morens DM, Sweighaft RM, Vernon TM, et al. A waterborne outbreak of gastroenteritis with secondary person-to-person spread. Association with a viral agent. *Lancet* 1979;1:964–66.
21. Treanor JJ, Dolin R, Madore HP. Production of a monoclonal antibody against the Snow Mountain agent of gastroenteritis by *in vitro* immunization of murine spleen cells. *Proc Natl Acad Sci USA* 1988;85:3613–7.
22. Wyatt RG, Dolin R, Blacklow NR, et al. Comparison of three agents of acute infectious nonbacterial gastroenteritis by virus challenge in volunteers. *J Infect Dis* 1974;129:709–14.
23. Dolin R, Roessner KD, Treanor JJ, et al. Radioimmunoassay for detection of the Snow Mountain agent of a viral gastroenteritis. *J Med Virol* 1986;19:11–8.
24. Madore HP, Treanor JJ, Pray KA, et al. Enzyme-linked immunosorbent assays for Snow Mountain and Norwalk agents of viral gastroenteritis. *J Clin Microbiol* 1986;24:456–9.
25. Madore HP, Treanor JJ, Buja R, et al. Antigenic relatedness among the Norwalk-like agents by serum antibody rises [Abstract]. Presented at the 28th Interscience Congress on Antimicrobial Agents of Chemotherapy, Los Angeles, California. 1988.
26. Cubitt WD, Blacklow NR, Herrmann JE, et al. Antigenic relationships between human caliciviruses and Norwalk virus. *J Inf Dis* 1987;156:806–14.
27. Greenberg HB, Valdesuso J, Kapikian AZ, et al. Prevalence of antibody to the Norwalk virus in various countries. *Infect Immun* 1979;26:270–3.
28. Greenberg HB, Wyatt RG, Kalica AR, et al. New insights in viral gastroenteritis. *Perspectives in Virology* 1981;11:163–87.
29. Kaplan JE, Feldman R, Compbell DS, et al. The frequency of a Norwalk-like pattern of illness in outbreaks of acute gastroenteritis. *Am J Public Health* 1982;72:1329–32.
30. Dolin R, Treanor JJ, Madore HP. Novel agents of viral enteritis in humans. *J Infect Dis* 1987;155:365–76.
31. Gary GW Jr, Kaplan JE, Stine SE, et al. Detection of Norwalk virus antibodies and antigen with a biotinavidin immunoassay. *J Clin Microbiol* 1985;22:274–8.
32. Greenberg HB, Wyatt RG, Valdesuso J, et al. Solid phase microtiter radioimmunoassay for detection of Norwalk strain of acute nonbacterial epidemic gastroenteritis and antibodies *J Med Virol* 1978;2:97–108.
33. Hermann JE, Nowak NA, Blacklow NR. Detection of Norwalk virus in stools by enzyme immunoassay. *J Med Virol* 1985;17:127–33.
34. Treanor JJ, Madore HP, Dolin R. Enzyme-linked immunoassay for detection of Hawaii

agent of viral gastroenteritis. *J Virol Methods* 1988 (in press).
35. Thornhill TS, Kalica AR, Wyatt RG, et al. Pattern of shedding of the Norwalk particle in stools during experimentally induced gastroenteritis in volunteers as determined by immune electron microscopy. *J Infect Dis* 1975;132:28–34.
36. Agus SG, Dolin R, Wyatt RG, et al. Acute infectious nonbacterial gastroenteritis: Intestinal histopathology. *Ann Intern Med* 1973;79:18–25.
37. Schreiber DS, Blacklow NR, Trier JS. The mucosal lesion of the proximal small intestine in acute infectious nonbacterial gastroenteritis. *N Engl J Med* 1973;288:1318–23.
38. Dolin R, Levy AG, Wyatt RG, et al. Viral gastroenteritis induced by the Hawaii agent: jejunal histopathology and serologic response. *Am J Med* 1975;59:761–8.
39. Schreiber DS, Blacklow NR, Trier JS. The small intestinal lesion induced by Hawaii agent acute infectious nonbacterial gastroenteritis. *J Infect Dis* 1974;129:705–8.
40. Harris JC, Dupont HL, Hornick RB. Fecal leukocytes in diarrheal illness. *Ann Intern Med* 1972;76:697–703.
41. Levy AG, Widerlite L, Schwartz CJ, et al. Jejunal adenylate cyclase activity in human subjects during viral gastroenteritis. *Gastroenterology* 1976;70:321–6.
42. Parrino TA, Schreiber DS, Trier JS, et al. Clinical immunity in acute gastroenteritis caused by Norwalk agent. *N Engl J Med* 1977;297:86–9.
43. Dolin R, Reichman RC, Fauci AS. Lymphocyte populations in acute viral gastroenteritis. *Infect Immun* 1976;14:422–8.
44. Dolin R, Baron S. Absence of detectable interferon in jejunal biopsies, jejunal aspirates and sera in experimentally induced viral gastroenteritis in man. *Proc Soc Exp Biol Med* 1975;140:337–9.
45. Albright DJ, Whalen RAS, Blacklow NR. Sensitivity of human fetal intestine to interferon. *Nature* 1974;247:218–20.
46. Dolin R, Blacklow NR, Malmgrem RA, et al. Establishment of human fetal intestinal organ cultures for growth of viruses. *J Infect Dis* 1970;122:227–31.
47. Dolin R, Smith HA. Antiviral activity of adenine arabinoside and iododeoxyuridine in human fetal intestinal and tracheal organ cultures. *J Infect Dis* 1975;132:287–95.
48. Wyatt RG, Greenberg HB, Dalgard DN, et al. Experimental infection of chimpanzees with the Norwalk agent of epidemic viral gastroenteritis. *J Med Virol* 1978;2:89–96.
49. Schaffer FL, Bachrach HL, Brown F, et al. Caliciviridae. *Intervirol* 1980;14:1–6.
50. Schaffer FL. Caliciviruses. In: Frankel-Conmrat H, Wagner RR, eds. *Newly characterized vertebrate virus. Comprehensive virology, vol. 14.* New York: Plenum Press, 1979:249–94.
51. Terashima H, Chiba S, Sakuma Y, et al. The polypeptide of a human calicivirus. *Arch Virol* 1983;78:1–7.
52. Cubitt WD, Barrett ADT. Propagation of human candidate calicivirus in cell culture. *J Gen Virol* 1984;65:1123–6.
53. Madeley CR, Cosgrove BP. Caliciviruses in man [Letter]. *Lancet* 1976;1:199–200.
54. Chiba S, Sakuma Y, Kogasaka R, et al. An outbreak of gastroenteritis associated with calicivirus in an infant home. *J Med Virol* 1979;4:249–54.
55. Flewett TH, Davies H. Caliciviruses in man [Letter]. *Lancet* 1976;1:311.
56. Kjeldsberg E. Small spherical viruses in faeces from gastroenteritis patients. *Acta Pathol Microbiol Immunol Scand* 1977;85:351–4.
57. McSwiggan DA, Cubitt D, Moore W. Calicivirus associated with winter vomiting disease. *Lancet* 1978;1:1215.
58. Oishi I, Maeda A, Yamazaki K, et al. Calicivirus detected in outbreaks of acute gastroenteritis in school children. *Biken J* 1980;23:163–8.
59. Spratt HC, Marks MI, Gomersall M, et al. Nosocomial infantile gastroenteritis associated with minirotavirus and calicivirus. *J Pediatr* 1978;93:922–6.
60. Cubitt D, McSwiggan D. A seroepidemiologic survey of the prevalence of antibodies to a strain of human calicivirus. *J Infect Dis* (in press).
61. Sakuma Y, Chiba S, Kogasaka R, et al. Prevalence of antibody to human calicivirus in the general population of Northern Japan. *J Med Virol* 1981;7:221–5.
62. Nakata S, Chiba S, Terashima H, et al. Prevalence of antibody to human calicivirus in Japan and Southeast Asia determined by radioimmunoassay. *J Clin Microbiol* 1985;22:519–21.
63. Nakata S, Chiba S, Terashima H, et al. Microtiter solid-phase radioimmunoassay for detection of human calicivirus in stools. *J Clin Microbiol* 1983;17:198–201.
64. Chiba S, Sakuma Y, Kogasaka R, et al. Fecal shedding of virus in relation to the days of illness in infantile gastroenteritis due to calicivirus. *J Infect Dis* 1980;142:247–9.
65. Saif LJ, Bohl EHJ, Theil KW, et al. Rotavirus-like, calicivirus-like, and 23-nm virus-like particles associated with diarrhea in young pigs. *J Clin Microbiol* 1980;12:105–11.
66. Woode GN, Bridgers JC. Isolation of small viruses resembling astroviruses and caliciviruses from acute enteritis of calves. *J Med Microbiol* 1978;11:441–52.
67. Nakata S, Chiba S, Terashima H, et al. Humoral immunity in infants with gastroenteritis caused by human calicivirus. *J Infect Dis* 1985;152:274–9.
68. Ashley CR, Caul EO, Paver WK. Astrovirus-associated gastroenteritis in children. *J Clin Pathol* 1978;31:939–43.
69. Madeley CR, Cosgrove BP. 28nm particles in faeces in infantile gastroenteritis [Letter]. *Lancet* 1975;2:451.
70. Snodgrass DR, Gray EW. Detection and transmission of 30 nm virus particles (astroviruses)

in the faeces of lambs with diarrhoea. *Arch Virol* 1977;55:287–91.
71. Lee TW, Kurtz JB. Serial propagation of astrovirus in tissue culture with the aid of trypsin. *J Gen Virol* 1981;57:421–4.
72. Herring AJ, Gray EW, Snodgrass DR. Purification and characterization of ovine astrovirus. *J Gen Virol* 1981;53:47–55.
73. Kurtz JB, Lee TW. Astroviruses: human and animal. In: Bock G, Whelan J, eds., *Novel diarrhoea viruses*. Chichester, England: John Wiley and Sons, 1987:92–107.
74. Kurtz JB, Lee TW. Human astrovirus serotypes [Letter]. *Lancet* 1984;2:1405.
75. Konno T, Suzuki H, Ishida N, et al. Astrovirus-associated epidemic gastroenteritis in Japan. *J Med Virol* 1982;9:11–7.
76. Kurtz JB, Lee TW, Pickering D, et al. Astrovirus associated gastroenteritis in a children's ward. *J Clin Pathol* 1987;30:948–52.
77. Oshiro LS, Haley CE, Roberto RR, et al. A 27 nm virus isolated during an outbreak of acute infectious nonbacterial gastroenteritis in a nursing home. *J Infect Dis* 1981;143:791.
78. Kurtz L, Lee T. Astrovirus gastroenteritis age distribution of antibody. *Med Microbiol Immunol (Berl)* 1978;166:227–30.
79. Herrmann JE, Hudson RW, Perron-Henry DM. Antigenic characterization of cell cultivated serotypes and development of astrovirus-specific monoclonal antibodies. *J Infect Dis* 1988;158:182–5.
80. Snodgrass DR, Angus KW, Gray EW, et al. Pathogenesis of diarrhoea caused by astrovirus infections in lambs. *Arch Virol* 1979;60:217–26.
81. Kurtz JB, Lee TW, Craig JW, et al. Astrovirus infection in volunteers. *J Med Virol* 1979;3:221–30.
82. Steinhoff MC, Douglas RG, Greenberg HB, et al. Bismuth subsalycylate therapy of viral gastroenteritis. *Gastroenterology* 1980;78:1495–9.
83. Povey RC. In vitro antiviral efficacy of ribavirin against feline calicivirus, feline viral rhinotracheitis virus, and canine parainfluenza virus. *Am J Vet Res* 1978;39:175–8.
84. Povey RC. Effect of orally administered ribavirin in experimental feline calicivirus infection in cats. *Am J Vet Res* 1978;39:1337–41.
85. Oglesby AS, Schaffer FL, Madin SH. Biochemical and biophysical properties of vesicular exanthema of swine virus. *Virology* 1971;44:329–35.
86. Smith AW, Prato CM, Skilling DE. Characterization of two new serotypes of San Miguel sea lion virus. *Intervirology* 1977;8:30–7.
87. Burki F, Pichler L. Further biochemical testing of feline picornavirus. *Arch Gesamte Virusforsch* 1971;33:126–31.
88. Fulton RW, Burge LT. Susceptibility of feline herpesvirus 1 and a feline calicivirus to feline interferon and recombinant human leukocyte interferons. *Antimicrob Agents and Chemother* 1985;28:698–9.
89. Madeley CR, Cosgrove BP. Viruses in infantile gastroenteritis. *Lancet* 1975b;1:124.
90. Roseto A, Esedig J, Delain E. et al. Structure of rotaviruses as studied by the freezing-drying technique. *Virology* 1979;98:471–5.
91. Venkataram Prasad BV, Wang GJ, Clerx JPM, et al. Three-dimensional structure of rotavirus. *J Mol Biol* 1988;199:269–75.
92. Bridger JC, Woode GN. Characterization of two particle types of calf rotavirus. *J Gen Virol* 1976;31:245–50.
93. Ohnishi H, Kosuzume H, Inaba H, et al. Mechanism of host defense suppression induced by viral infection: mode of action of inosiplex as an antiviral agent. *Infect Immun* 1982;38:243–50.
94. Adams WR, Kraft LM. Epizootic diarrhea of infant mice: identification of the etiologic agent. *Science* 1963;141:359–60.
95. Bryden AS, Thouless ME, Flewett TH. Letter: rotavirus and rabbits. *Vet Rec* 1976;99:323.
96. Flewett TH, Bryden AS, Davies H. Letter: virus diarrhea in foals and other animals. *Vet Rec* 1975;96:477.
97. Hoshino Y, Baldwin CA, Scott FW. Isolation and characterization of feline rotavirus. *J Gen Virol* 1981;54:313–23.
98. Lecce JG, King MW, Mock R. Reovirus-like agent associated with fatal diarrhea in neonatal pigs. *Infect Immun* 1976;14:816–25.
99. Malherbe HH, Strickland-Cholmley M. Simian virus SA 11 and the related O agent. *Arch Ges Virusforsch* 1968;22:235–45.
100. Snodgrass DR, Smith W, Gray EW, et al. A rotavirus in lambs with diarrhea. *Res Vet Sci* 1976;20:113–4.
101. Wyatt RG, Greenberg HB, James WD, et al. Definition of human rotavirus serotypes by plaque reduction assay. *Infect Immun* 1982;37:110–5.
102. Beards GM, Pilford JN, Thouless ME, et al. Rotavirus serotypes by serum neutralization. *J Med Virol* 1980;5:231–7.
103. Flewett TH, Thouless ME, Pilford JN, et al. More serotypes of human rotavirus. *Lancet* 1978;11:632.
104. Hoshino Y, Wyatt RG, Greenberg HB, et al. Serotypic similarity and diversity of rotavirus of mammalian and avian origin as studied by plaque-reduction neutralization. *J infect Dis* 1984;149:694–702.
105. Kovacs A, Chan L, Hotrakitya C, et al. Rotavirus gastroenteritis. Clinical and laboratory features and use of the rotazyme test. *Am J Dis Child* 1987;141:161–6.
106. Shepherd RW, Truslow S, Walker-Smith JA, et al. Infantile gastroenteritis: a clinical study of reovirus-like agent infections. *Lancet* 1975;2:1082–4.
107. Totterdell RM, Chrystie IL, Banatvala JE. Cord blood and breast milk antibodies in neonatal rotavirus infection. *Br Med J* 1980;280:828–30.
108. Clark HF, Hoshino Y, Bell LM, et al. Rotavirus isolate WI16 representing a presumptive new human serotype. *J Clin Microbiol* 1987;25:1757–62.

109. Matsuno S, Hazegawa A, Mukoyama A, et al. A candidate for a new serotype of human rotavirus. *J Virol* 1985;54:623–4.
110. Ruiz AW, Lopez IV, Lopes S, et al. Molecular and antigenic characterization of porcin rotavirus YM, a possible new rotavirus serotype. *J Virol* 1985;62:4331–6.
111. Kantharidis P, Dyall-Smith ML, Holmes IH. Completion of the gene coding assignments of SA11 rotavirus: Gene products of segments 7, 8, and 9. *J Virol* 1983;48:330–4.
112. Greenberg HB, Valdesuso J, van Wyke K, et al. Production and preliminary characterization of monoclonal antibodies directed at two surface proteins of rhesus rotavirus. *J Virol* 1983;47:267–75.
113. Hoshino Y, Sereno MM, Midthun K, et al. Independent segregation of two antigenic specificities (VP3 and VP7) involved in neutralization of rotavirus infectivity. *Proc Natl Acad Sci USA* 1985;82:8701–4.
114. Bastardo JW, McKimm-Breschkin JL, Sonza S, et al. Preparation and characterization of antisera to electrophoretically purified SA-11 virus polypeptides. *Infect Immun* 1981;34:641–7.
115. Zissis G, Lambert JP. Serotypes of human rotavirus. *Lancet* 1978;1:38.
116. Greenberg HB, Flores J, Kalica AR, et al. Gene coding assignments for growth restriction, neutralization, and subgroup specificities of the W and DS-1 strains of human rotavirus. *J Gen Virol* 1983;64:313–20.
117. Greenberg HB, McAuliffe V, Valdesuso J, et al. Serological analysis of the subgroup protein of rotavirus, using monoclonal antibodies. *Infect Immun* 1983;39:91–9.
118. Kalica AR, Greenmberg HB, Espejo RT, et al. Distinctive ribonucleic acid patterns of human rotavirus subgroups 1 and 2. *Infect Immun* 1981;33:958–61.
119. Kalica AR, Greenberg HB, Wyatt RG, et al. Genes of human (strain Wa) and bovine (strain OK) rotaviruses that code for neutralization and subgroup antigens. *Virology* 1981;112:385–90.
120. Taniguchi K, Urasawa T, Urasawa S, et al. Production of subgroup-specific monoclonal antibodies against human rotaviruses and their application to an enzyme-linked immunosorbent assay for subgroup determination. *J Med Virol* 1984;14:115–25.
121. Kapikian AZ, Cline WL, Greenberg HG, et al. Antigenic characterization of human and animal rotaviruses by immune adherence hemagglutination assay (IAHA): evidence for distinctness of IAHA and neutralization antigens. *Infect Immun* 1981;33:415–25.
122. McNulty MS, Allan GM, Todd D, et al. Isolation from chickens of a rotavirus lacking the rotavirus group antigen. *J Gen Virol* 1983;55:405–13.
123. Nicolas JC, Cohen J, Fortier B, et al. Isolation of a human pararotavirus. *Virology* 1983;124:181–4.
124. Snodgrass DR, Harring AJ, Campbell I, et al. Comparison of atypical rotaviruses from calves, piglets, lambs and man. *J Gen Virol* 1984;65:909–14.
125. Pedley S, Bridger JC, Brown JF, et al. Molecular characterization of rotavirus with distinct group antigens. *J Gen Virol* 1983;64:2093–101.
126. Bridger JC, Pedley S, McCrae MA. Group C rotaviruses in humans. *J Clin Microbiol* 1986;23:760–3.
127. Eiden J, Vonderfecht S, Yolken RH. Evidence that a novel rotavirus-like agent of rats can cause gastroenteritis in man. *Lancet* 1985;2:8–10.
128. Nakata S, Estes MK, Graham DY, et al. Antigenic characterization and ELISA detection of adult diarrhea rotaviruses. *J Infect Dis* 1986;154:448–54.
129. Nakata S, Estes MK, Graham DY, et al. Detection of antibody to group B adult diarrhea rotaviruses in humans. *J Clin Microbiol* 1987;25:812–8.
130. Liu M, Offit PA, Estes MK. Identification of the simian rotavirus SA 11 genome segment 3 product. *Virology* 1988;163:26–32.
131. Mason BB, Graham DY, Estes MK. *In vitro* transcription and translation of simian rotavirus SA 11 gene products. *J Virol* 1980;33:1111–21.
132. Mason BB, Graham DY, Estes MK. Biochemical mapping of the simian rotavirus SA 11 genome. *J Virol* 1983;46:413–424.
133. Singh N, Sereno MM, Flores J, et al. Monoclonal antibodies to subgroup 1 rotavirus. *Infect Immun* 1983;42:835–7.
134. Sandino AM, Jashes M, Faundez G, et al. Role of the inner protein capsid on *in vitro* human rotavirus transcription. *J Virol* 1986;60:797–802.
135. Ready KF, Sabara M. *In vitro* assembly of bovine rotavirus nucleocapsid protein. *Virology* 1987;157:189–98.
136. Patton JT. Synthesis of simian rotavirus SA 11 double-stranded RNA in a cell-free system. *Virus Res* 1986/87;6:217–33.
137. Patton JT, Gallegos CO. Structure and protein composition of the rotavirus replicase particle. *Virology* 1988;166:358–65.
138. Fukuhara N, Yoshie O, Kitaoka S, et al. Role of VP3 in human rotavirus internalization after target cell attachment via VP7. *J Virol* 1988;62:2209–18.
139. Sabara M, Gilchrist JE, Hudson GR, et al. Preliminary characterization of an epitope involved in neutralization and cell attachment that is located on the major bovine rotavirus clycoprotein. *J Virol* 1985;53:58–66.
140. Offit PA, Blavat G. Identification of the two rotavirus genes determining neutralization specificities. *J Virol* 1986;57:376–8.
141. Coulson BS, Fowler KJ, Bishop RF, et al. Neutralizing monoclonal antibodies to human rotavirus and indications of antigenic drift among strains from neonates. *J Virol* 1985;54:14–20.
142. Gerna G, Sarasini A, DiMatteo A, et al. The

outer capsid glycoprotein VP7 of simian rotavirus SA 11 contains two distinct neutralization epitopes. *J Gen Virol* 1988;69:937–44.
143. Morita Y, Taniguch K, Urasawa T, et al. Analysis of serotype-specific neutralization epitopes on VP7 of human rotavirus by the use of neutralizing monoclonal antibodies and antigenic variants. *J Gen Virol* 1988;69:451–8.
144. Shaw RD, Vo PT, Offit PA, et al. Antigenic mapping of the surface proteins of Rhesus rotavirus. *Virology* 1986;155:434–51.
145. Taniguchi K, Hoshino Y, Nishikawa K, et al. Cross-reactive and serotype specific neutralization epitopes on VP7 of human rotavirus: nucleotide sequence analysis of antigenic mutants selected with monoclonal antibodies. *J Virol* 1988;62:1870–4.
146. Dyall-Smith ML, Lazdins I, Tregear GW, et al. Identification of the major antigenic sites involved in rotavirus serotype-specific neutralization. *Proc Natl Acad Sci USA* 1986;3465–8.
147. Mackow ER, Shaw RD, Matsui SM, et al. Characterization of homotypic and heterotypic VP7 neutralization sites of Rhesus rotavirus. *Virology* 1988;165:511–7.
148. Green KY, Sears JF, Taniguchi K, et al. Prediction of human rotavirus serotype by nucleotide sequence analysis of the VP7 protein gene. *J Virol* 1988;62:1819–23.
149. Gunn PR, Sato F, Powell KFH, et al. Rotavirus neutralizing protein VP7: antigenic determinants investigated by sequence analysis and peptide synthesis. *J Virol* 1985;54:791–7.
150. Greenberg HB, Wyatt RG, Kapikian AZ. Rescue and serotype characterization of non-cultivatable human rotavirus by gene reassortment. *Infect Immun* 1982;37:104–9.
151. Kalica AR, Flores J, Greenberg HB. Identification of the rotaviral gene that codes for hemagglutination and protease-enhanced plaque formation. *Virology* 1983;125:194–205.
152. Ramia S, Sattar SA. Simian rotavirus SA11 plaque formation in the present of trypsin. *J Clin Microbiol* 1979;10:609–14.
153. Sato K, Inaba Y, Shinozaki T, et al. Isolation of human rotavirus in cell cultures. *Arch Virol* 1981;69:155–60.
154. Clark SM, Roth JR, Clark ML, et al. Trypsin enhancement of rotavirus infectivity: mechanisms of enhancement. *J Virol* 1981;39:816–22.
155. Espejo RT, Lopez S, Arias C. Structural polypeptides of simian rotavirus SA11 and the effect of trypsin. *J Virol* 1981;37:156–60.
156. Estes MK, Graham DY, Mason BB. Proteolytic enhancement of rotavirus infectivity: molecular mechanisms. *J Virol* 1981;39:879–88.
157. Kaljot KT, Shaw RD, Rubin DH, et al. Infectious rotavirus enters cells by direct cell membrane penetration, not by endocytosis. *J Virol* 1988;62:1136–44.
158. Flores J, Midthun K, Hoshino Y, et al. Conservation of the fourth gene among rotaviruses recovered from asymptomatic newborn infants and its possible role in attenuation. *J Virol* 1986;60:972–9.
159. Gorziglia M, Hoshino Y, Buckler-White A, et al. Conservation of amino acid sequence of VP8 and cleavage region of 4-kDa outer capsid protein among rotaviruses recovered from symptomatic neonatal infection. *Proc Natl Acad Sci* 1986;83:7039–43.
160. Kantharidis P, Dyall-Smith ML, Holmes IH. Marked sequence variation between segment 4 genes of human RV-5 and simian SA11 rotaviruses. *Arch Virol* 1987;93:111–21.
161. Lopez S, Arias CF, Bell JR, et al. Primary structure of the cleavage site associated with trypsin enhancement of rotavirus SA11 infectivity. *Virology* 1985;144:11–9.
162. Lopez S, Arias CF, Mendez E, et al. Conservation in rotaviruses of the protein region containing the two sites associated with trypsin enhancement of infectivity. *Virology* 1986;154:224–7.
163. Mackow ER, Shaw RD, Matsui SM, et al. The rhesus rotavirus gene encoding protein VP3: Location of amino acids involved in homologous and heterologous rotavirus neutralization and identification of a putative fusion region. *Proc Natl Acad Sci USA* 1988;85:645–9.
164. Offit PA, Blavat G, Greenberg HB, et al. Molecular basis of rotavirus virulence: role of gene segment 4. *J Virol* 1986;57:46–9.
165. Streckert HJ, Brussow H, Werchau H. A synthetic peptide corresponding to the cleavage region of VP3 from rotavirus SA11 includes neutralizing antibodies. *J Virol* 1988;62:4265–9.
166. Coulson BS, Tursi JM, McAdam WJ, et al. Derivation of neutralizing monoclonal antibodies to human rotaviruses and evidence that an immunodominant neutralization site is shared between serotypes 1 and 3. *Virology* 1986;154:302–12.
167. Taniguchi K, Urasawa S, Urasawa T. Preparation and characterization of neutralizing monoclonal antibodies with different reactivity patterns to human rotaviruses. *J Gen Virol* 1985;66:1045–53.
168. Taniguchi K, Morita Yu, Urasawa T, et al. Cross-reactive neutralization epitopes on VP3 of human rotavirus: analysis with monoclonal antibodies and antigenic variants. *J Virol* 1987;61:1726–30.
169. Taniguchi K, Maloy WL, Nishikawa K, et al. Identification of cross-reactive and serotype 2-specific neutralization epitopes on VP3 of human rotavirus. *J Virol* 1988;62:2421–6.
170. Keljo DJ, Smith AK. Characterization of binding of simian rotavirus SA-11 to cultured epithelial cells. *J Pediatr Gastroenter Nutr* 1988;7:249–56.
171. Yolken RH, Willoughby R, Wee S-B, et al. Sialic acid glycoproteins inhibit *in vitro* and *in vivo* replication of rotaviruses. *J Clin Invest* 1987;79:148–54.
172. Ludert JE, Michelangeli F, Gil F, et al. Penetration and uncoating of rotaviruses in cultured cells. *Intervirology* 1987;27:95–101.
173. Quan CM, Doane FW. Ultrastructural evidence for the cellular uptake of rotavirus by endocytosis. *Intervirology* 1983;20:223–231.

174. Suzuki H, Kitaoka S, Sato T, et al. Further investigation of the mode of entry of human rotavirus into cells. *Arch Virol* 1986;91:135–44.
175. Flores J, Myslinski J, Kalica AR, et al. *In vitro* transcription of two human rotaviruses. *J Virol* 1982;43:1032–7.
176. Spencer E, Arias ML. *In vitro* transcription catalyzed by heat-treated human rotavirus. *J Virol* 1981;40:1–10.
177. Ward CW, Elleman TC, Azad AA, et al. Nucleotide sequence of gene segment 9 encoding a nonstructural protein of UK bovine rotavirus. *Virology* 1984;134:249–53.
178. Bernstein J, Hruska JF. Characterization of RNA polymerase products of calf diarrhea virus and SA11 rotavirus. *J Virol* 1981;37:1071-4.
179. Estes MK, Palmer EL, Obijeski JF. Rotaviruses: a review. *Curr Top Microbiol Immunol* 1983;105:123–84.
180. Holmes IH. Rotaviruses. In: Joklik WK, eds. *The reoviridae*. New York: Plenum Press, 1983:359–423.
181. Stacy-Phipps S, Patton JT. Synthesis of plus- and minus-strand RNA in rotavirus-infected cells. *J Virol* 1987;61:3479–84.
182. Helmberger-Jones M, Patton JT. Characterization of subviral particles in cells infection with simian rotavirus SA11. *Virology* 1986;155:655–65.
183. Carpio MM, Babiak LA, Misra V, et al. Bovine rotavirus-cell interactions: effect of virus infection on cellular integrity and macromolecular synthesis. *Virology* 1981;114:86–97.
184. Petrie BL, Graham DY, Hanssin H, et al. Localization of rotavirus antigens in infected cells by ultrastructural immunocytochemistry. *J Gen Virol* 1982;63:457–67.
185. Richardson SC, Mercher LE, Sonza S, et al. Intracellular localization of rotaviral proteins. *Arch Virol* 1986;88:251–64.
186. Altenberg BC, Graham DY, Estes MK. Ultrastructural study of rotavirus replication in cultured cells. *J Gen Virol* 1980;46:75–85.
187. Petrie BL, Graham DY, Estes MK. Identification of rotavirus particle types. *Intervirology* 1981;16:20–8.
188. Petrie BL, Estes MK, Graham DY. Effects of tunicamycin on rotavirus morphogenesis and infectivity. *J Virol* 1983;46:270–4.
189. Suzuki H, Sato H, Konno T, et al. Effect of tunicamycin of human rotavirus morphogenesis and infectivity. *Arch Virol* 1984;81:363–9.
190. McCrae MA, Faulkner-Valle GP. Molecular biology of rotavirus. *J Virol* 1981;39:490–6.
191. Birch CJ, Lehrmann NI, Hawker AJ, et al. Comparison of EM, Elisa, solid phase RIA and indirect IF for detection of human rotavirus antigen in feces. *J Clin Pathol* 1979;32:700–5.
192. Dolan KT, Twist EM, Horton-Slight P, et al. Epidemiology of rotavirus electropherotypes determined by a simplified diagnostic technique with RNA analysis. *J Clin Microbiol* 1985;21:753–8.
193. Kalica AR, Purcell RH, Sereno MM, et al. A microtiter solid phase radioimmunoassay for detection of the human reovirus-like agent in stools. *J Immunol* 1977;118:1275–9.
194. Middleton PJ, Holdaway MD, Patrick M, et al. Solid-phase radioimmunoassay for the detection of rotavirus. *Infect Immun* 1977;16:439–44.
195. Middleton PJ, Petric M, Hewitt CM, et al. Counter-immunoelectro-osmophoresis for the detection of infantile gastroenteritis virus (orbi-group) antigen and antibody. *J Clin Pathol* 1976;21:191–7.
196. Rubenstein D, Milne RG, Buckland R, et al. The growth of the virus of epidemic diarrhea of infant mice (EDIM) in organ cultures of intestinal epithelium. *Br J Exp Pathol* 1971;52:442–5.
197. Sarkkinen HR, Halonen PE, Aristila PP. Comparison of 4-layer RIA and EM for detection of human rotavirus. *J Med Virol* 1979;4:255–60.
198. Spence L, Fauvel M, Bouchard S, et al. Letter: test for reovirus-like agent. *Lancet* 1975;2:322.
199. Wall RA, Mulars BJ, Luton P, et al. Comparison of ELISA, Space and EM for the routine diagnosis of rotavirus infection. *J Clin Pathol* 1982;35:104–6.
200. Cromien JL, Himmelreich CA, Class RI, et al. Evaluation of new commercial enzyme immunoassay for rotavirus detection. *J Clin Microbiol* 1987;25:2359–62.
201. Hornsleth A, Aaen K, Gundestrup M. Detection of respiratory syncytial virus and rotavirus by enhances chemiluminescence enzyme-linked immunosorbent assay. *J Clin Microbiol* 1988;26:630–5.
202. Inouye S, Matsuno S, Yamaguchi H. Efficient coating of the solid phase with rotavirus antigens for enzyme-linked immunosorbent assay of immunoglobulin A antibody in feces. *J Clin Microbiol* 1984;19:259–63.
203. Thomas EE, Puterman ML, Kawano E, et al. Evaluation of seven immunoassays for detection of rotavirus in pediatric stool samples. *J Clin Microbiol* 1988;26:1189–93.
204. Brandt CD, Arndt CW, Evans GL, et al. Evaluation of a latex test for rotavirus detection. *J Clin Microbiol* 1987;25:1800–2.
205. Sanekata T, Okada H. Human rotavirus detection by agglutination of antibody-coated erythrocytes. *J Clin Microbiol* 1983;17:1141–7.
206. Birch CJ, Heath RL, Gust ID. Use of serotype-specific monoclonal antibodies to study the epidemiology of rotavirus infection. *J Med Virol* 1988;24:45–53.
207. Taniguchi K, Urasawa T, Morita Y, et al. Direct serotyping of human rotavirus stools by an enzyme-linked immunosorbent assay using serotype 1-, 2-, 3- and 4-specific monoclonal antibodies to VP7. *J Infect Dis* 1987;155:1159–66.
208. Dimitrov DH, Graham DY, Estes MK. Detection of rotaviruses by nucleic acid hybridization with cloned DNA of simian rotavirus SA11 genes. *J Infect Dis* 1985;152:293–300.
209. Flores J, Purchell RH, Perez I, et al. A dot hybridization assay for detection of rotavirus. *Lancet* 1983;555–9.
210. Kasempimolporn S, Louisirirotchanul S, Sin-

arachatanant P, et al. Polyacrylamide gel electrophoresis and silver staining for detection of rotavirus in stools from diarrheic patients in Thailand. *J Clin Microbiol* 1988;26:158–60.

211. Pacini DL, Brady MT, Budde CT, et al. Polyacylamide gel electrophoresis of RNA compared with polyclonal-and monoclonal-antibody-based enzyme immunoassays for rotavirus. *J Clin Microbiol* 1988;26:194–7.
212. Estes MK. Letter to editor. Simplified method of rotavirus RNA analysis. A word of caution. *J Clin Microbiol* 1986;2:806.
213. Kapkian AZ, Yolken RH, Greenberg HB, et al. In: Lennette EH, Schmidt NJ, eds. *Diagnostic procedures for viral, rickettsial and chlamydial infections*. 5th ed. Washington, D.C.: American Public Health Association, 1979:927–96.
214. Nicolaieff A, Omert G, Ryan-Martel MHV. Detection of rotavirus by serological trapping on antibody coated EM grids. *J Clin Microbiol* 1980;12:101–4.
215. Wyatt RG, James HD Jr, Pittman AL, et al. Direct isolation in cell culture of human rotaviruses and their characterization into four serotypes. *J Clin Microbiol* 1983;18:310–7.
216. Taniguchi K, Urasawa S, Urasawa T. Electrophoretic analysis of RNA segments of human rotavirus cultivated in cell culture. *J Gen Virol* 1982;60:171–5.
217. Urasawa T, Urasawa S, Taniguchi K. Sequential passages of human rotaviruses in MA-104 cells. *Microbiol Immunol* 1981;25:1025–35.
218. Urasawa S, Urasawa T, Taniguchi K. Three human rotavirus serotypes demonstrated by plaque neutralization of isolated strains. *Infect Immun* 1982;38:781–4.
219. Christy C, Madore HP, Pichichero ME, et al. Field trial of rhesus rotavirus vaccine in infants. *Pediatr Infect Dis J* 1988;7:645–50.
220. Oishi F, Maeda A, Kirimera T, et al. Epidemiological and virological studies on outbreaks of acute gastroenteritis associated with rotavirus in primary schools on Osaka. *Biken J* 1979;22:61–9.
221. Paul MO, Erinle EA. Influence of humidity on rotavirus prevalence among Nigerian infants and young children with gastroenteritis. *J Clin Microbiol* 1981;15:212–5.
222. Sack DA, Gilman RH, Kapikian AZ, et al. Seroepidemiology of rotavirus infection in rural Bangladesh. *J Clin Microbiol* 1980;11:530–2.
223. Taraska SP, Rhodes KH, Smith TF, et al. Etiology of pediatric gastroenteritis in Rochester, Minnesota. *Mayo Clin Proc* 1979;54:151–6.
224. Taylor B, Golding J, Wadsworth J, et al. Breastfeeding, bronchitis and admissions for lower respiratory illness and gastroenteritis during the first 5 years. *Lancet* 1982;1:1227–9.
225. Rodriguez WJ, Kim HW, Brandt CD, et al. Longitudinal study of rotavirus infection and gastroenteritis in families served by a pediatric medical practice: clinical and epidemiologic observations. *Pediatr Infect Dis* 1987;6:170–6.
226. Kapikian AZ, Chanock RM. Rotaviruses. In: Fields BN, Knipe DM, Chanock RM, Melnick J, Roizman B, Shope R, eds. *Virology*. 1st ed. New York: Raven Press, 1985:863–906.
227. Black RE, Merson MH, Rahman ASMM, et al. A two year study of bacterial viral and parasitic agents associated with diarrhea in rural Bangladesh. *J Infect Dis* 1980;142:606–64.
228. Brandt CD, Kim HW, Yolken RH, et al. Comparative epidemiology of two rotavirus serotypes and other viral agents associated with pediatric gastroenteritis. *Am J Epidemiol* 1979;110:243–54.
229. Engleberg NC, Holbart EN, Barrett TJ, et al. Epidemiology of diarrhea due to rotavirus on an indian reservation: risk factors in the home environment. *J Infect Dis* 1982;145:894–8.
230. Hull BP, Spence L, Basset D, et al. The relative importance of rotavirus and other pathogens in the etiology of gastroenteritis in Trinidadian children. *Am J Trop Med Hyg* 1982;31:142–8.
231. Konno T, Suzuki H, Imai A, et al. A long term survey of rotavirus infection in Japanese children with acute gastroenteritis. *J Infect Dis* 1978;138:569–76.
232. Paul MO, Erinle EA. Rotavirus infection in Nigerian infants and young children. *Am J Trop Med Hyg* 1982;31:374–5.
233. Rodriguez WJ, Kim HW, Brandt CD, et al. Rotavirus gastroenteritis in the Washington, D.C. area. *Am J Dis Child* 1980;134:777–9.
234. Murphy A, Albery M, Hay P. Rotavirus infections in neonates. *Lancet* 1975;i:297.
235. Renterghem LV, Borre P, Tilleman J. Rotavirus and other viruses in the stool of premature babies. *J Med Virol* 1980;5:137–42.
236. Rodriguez WJ, Kim HW, Brandt CD, et al. Common exposure outbreak of gastroenteritis due to type 2 rotavirus with high secondary attack rate within families. *J Infect Dis* 1979;140:353–7.
237. Soenarto Y, Sebodo T, Ridho R, et al. Acute diarrhea and rotavirus infection in newborn babies and children in Yogaharta, Indonesia from June, 1978 to June, 1979. *J Clin Microbiol* 1981;14:123–9.
238. Totterdell RM, Chrystie IL, Banatvala JE. Rotavirus infection in a maternity unit. *Arch Dis Child* 1976;51:924–8.
239. Dearlove J, Latham P, Dearlove J, et al. Clinical range of neonatal rotavirus gastroenteritis. *Br Med J* 1983;286:1473–5.
240. Rodriguez WJ, Kim HW, Brandt CD, et al. Rotavirus: a cause of nosocomial infection in the nursery. *J Pediatr* 1982;101:274–7.
241. Von Bonsdorff CH, Jovi T, Makela P, et al. Rotavirus associated with acute gastroenteritis in adults. *Lancet* 1976;2:423.
242. Jewkes J, Larson HE, Price AB, et al. Aetiology of acute diarrhoea in adults. *Gut* 1981;22:388–92.
243. Loosli J, Gyr K, Stalder H, et al. Etiology of acute infectious diarrhea in a highly industrialized area of Switzerland. *Gastroenterology* 1985;88:75–9.
244. Pryor WM, Bye WA, Curran DH, et al. Acute

diarrhoea in adults: a prospective study. *Med J Aust* 1987;147:490–2.
245. Haug KW, Orstavik I, Kvelstad G. Rotavirus infections in families: a clinical and virological study. *Scand J Infect Dis* 1978;10:265–9.
246. Kapikian AZ, Kim HW, Wyatt RG, et al. Human reovirus-like agent as the major pathogen associated with "winter" gastroenteritis in hospitalized infants and young children. *N Engl J Med* 1976;294:965–72.
247. Monto AS, Koopman JS, Longini IM, et al. The Tecumseh study. XII. Enteric agents in the community, 1976–1981. *J Infect Dis* 1983;148:284–91.
248. Echeverria P, Ramirez G, Blacklow NR, et al. Traveler's diarrhea among U.S. Army troups in South Korea. *J Infect Dis* 1979;139:215–9.
249. Keswick GH, Blacklow NR, Cukor GC, et al. Norwalk virus and rotavirus in travellers' diarrhea in Mexico. *Lancet* 1982;1:109–10.
250. Sheridan JF, Aurelian L, Barbour G, et al. Travelers diarrhea associated with rotavirus infection: Analysis of virus specific immunoglobulin classes. *Infect Immun* 1981;31:419–29.
251. Vollet JJ, Ericsson CD, Gibson G, et al. Human rotavirus in an adult population with travelers diarrhea and its relationship to the location of food consumption. *J Med Virol* 1979;4:81–7.
252. Chrystie IL, Totterdell B, Baker MJ. Rotavirus infection in a maternity unit. *Lancet* 1975; 2:79.
253. Eiden JJ, Verleur DG, Vonderfecht SL, et al. Duration and pattern of asymptomatic rotavirus shedding by hospitalized children. *Pediatr Infect Dis J* 1988;7:564–9.
254. Hjelt K, Krasilnikoff A, Graubella PC, et al. Nosocomial acute gastroenteritis in a paediatric department, with special reference to rotavirus infections. *Acta Paediatr Scand* 1985;74:89–95.
255. Rodriguez WJ, Kim HW, Brandt CD, et al. Use of electrophoresis of RNA from human rotavirus to establish the identity of strains involved in outbreaks in a tertiary care nursery. *J Infect Dis* 1983;148:34–40.
256. Barron-Romero BL, Barreda-Gonzalez J, Doval-Ugalde R, et al. Asymptomatic rotavirus infections in day care centers. *J Clin Microbiol* 1985;22:116–8.
257. Bartlett AV, Reves RR, Pickering LK. Rotavirus in infant-toddler day care centers: epidemiology relevant to disease control strategies. *J Pediatr* 1988;113:435–41.
258. Pickering LK, Bartlett AV, Reves RR, et al. Asymptomatic excretion of rotavirus before and after rotavirus diarrhea in children in day care center. *J Pediatr* 1988;112:361–5.
259. Cubitt WD, Hozel H. An outbreak of rotavirus infection in a long stay ward of a general hospital. *J Clin Pathol* 1980;33:306–8.
260. Halvorsund J, Orstavik I. An epidemic of rotavirus associated gastroenteritis in a nursing home for the elderly. *Scand J Infect Dis* 1980;12:161–4.
261. Marrie TJ, Lee HS, Faulkner RS, et al. Rotavirus infection in a geriatric population. *Arch Intern Med* 1982;142:313–6.
262. Graham DY, Dufour GR, Estes MK. Minimal infective dose of rotavirus. *Arch Virol* 1987;92:261–71.
263. Ward RL, Bernstein DI, Young EC, et al. Human rotavirus studies in volunteers: determination of infectious dose and serological response to infection. *J Infect Dis* 1986;154:871–80.
264. Brandt CD, Kim HW, Rodriquez WJ, et al. Rotavirus gastroenteritis and weather. *J Clin Microbiol* 1982;16:478–82.
265. Kibrick S. Current status of coxsackie and echo viruses in human disease. *Prog Med Virol* 1964;6:27–70.
266. Konno T, Suzuki H, Katsushima N, et al. Influence of temperature and relative humidity on human rotavirus infection in Japan. *J Infect Dis* 1983;147:125–8.
267. Lonberg-Holm K, Phillipson L. Early interaction between animal viruses and cells. *Monogr Virol* 1974;9:1–148.
268. Suzuki H, Amaro Y, Kinebuehi H. Rotavirus infection in children with acute gastroenteritis in Ecuador. *Am J Trop Med Hyg* 1981;30;293–4.
269. Davidson GP, Bishop RF, Townley RRW, et al. Importance of a new virus in acute sporadic enteritis in children. *Lancet* 1975;1:242–6.
270. Muchinik GR, Grinstein S. Rotavirus in Buenos Aires, Argentina. *Intervirology* 1980;13:253–6.
271. Williamson HG, Bowden DK, Birch CJ, et al. Human rotavirus infections in Efate, Vanuatu. *Am J Trop Med Hyg* 1982;31:136–41.
272. Black RE, Greinberg HB, Kapikian AZ, et al. Acquisition of serum antibody to Norwalk virus and rotavirus and relation to diarrheas in a longitudinal study of young children in rural Bangladesh. *J Infect Dis* 1983;145:483–9.
273. Coulson BS. Variation in neutralization epitopes of human rotaviruses in relation to genomic RNA polymorphism. *Virology* 1987;159:209–16.
274. Georges-Courbot MC, Beraud AM, Beards GM, et al. Subgroups, serotypes, and electrophoretypes of rotavirus isolated from children in Bangui, Central Africa Republic. *J Clin Microbiol* 1988;26:668–71.
275. Urasawa T, Urasawa S, Chiba Y, et al. Antigen characterization of rotavirus isolated in Kenya from 1982 to 1983. *J Clin Microbiol* 1987;25:1891–986.
276. Flores J, Taniguchi K, Green K, et al. Relative frequencies of rotavirus serotypes 1, 2, 3, and 4 in Venezuelan infants with gastroenteritis. *J Clin Microbiol* 1988;26:2092–5.
277. Follett EAC, Desselberger V. Circulation of different rotavirus strains in a local outbreak of infantile gastroenteritis: monitoring by rapid and sensitive nucleic acid analysis. *J Med Virol* 1983;11:39–52.
278. Bishop RF, Davidson GP, Holmes IH, et al. Virus particles in epithelial cells of duodenal mucosa from children with acute non-bacterial gastroenteritis. *Lancet* 1973 :1281–3.

279. Barnes GL, Townley RRW. Duodenal mucosal damage in 31 infants with gastroenteritis. *Arch Dis Child* 1973;43:343–9.
280. Davidson GP, Goller I, Bishop RF, et al. Immunofluorescence in duodenal mucosa of children with acute enteritis due to a new virus. *J Clin Pathol* 1975;28:263–6.
281. Konno T, Suzuki H, Aki I, et al. Reovirus-like agent in acute epidemic gastroenteritis in Japanese infants: fecal shedding and serologic response. *J Infect Dis* 1977;135:259–66.
282. Hyams JS, Krause PJ, Gleason PA. Lactose malabsorption following rotavirus infection in young children. *J Pediatr* 1981;99:916–8.
283. Mavronrehalis J, Evans N, McNeish AS, et al. Intestinal damage in rotavirus and adenovirus gastroenteritis assessed by D. xylose malabsorption. *Arch Dis Child* 1977;52:589–91.
284. Sack DA, Rhoads M, Molla A, et al. Carbohydrate malabsorption in infants with rotavirus diarrhea. *Am J Clin Nutr* 1982;36:1112–8.
285. Davidson GP, Gall DG, Petric M. Human rotavirus enteritis induced in conventional piglets. *J Clin Invest* 1977;60:1402–9.
286. Graham DY, Sackman JW, Estes MK. Pathogenesis of rotavirus-induced diarrhea. *Dig Dis Sci* 1984;29:1028–35.
287. Champsaur H, Henry-Amar N, Goldsmith D, et al. Rotavirus carriage, asymptomatic infection, and disease in the first two years of life. II. Serological response. *J Infect Dis* 1984;149:675–82.
288. Champsaur H, Questiauz E, Prevot J, et al. Rotavirus carriage, asymptomatic infection, and disease in the first two years of life. I. Virus shedding. *J Infect Dis* 1984;149:667–74.
289. Carlson JAK, Middleton PJ, Szymanski MT. Fatal rotavirus gastroenteritis. *Am J Dis Child* 1978;132:477–9.
290. Shukry S, Zaki AM, DuPont HL, et al. Detection of enteropathogens in fatal and potentially fatal diarrhea in Cairo, Egypt. *J Clin Microbiol* 1986;24:959–62.
291. Gurwith M, Wenman W, Hinde D, et al. A prospective study of rotavirus in infants and young children. *J Infect Dis* 1981;144:218–44.
292. Rodriguez WJ, Kim HW, Arrobio JO, et al. Clinical features of acute gastroenteritis associated with human neovirus-like agent in infants and young children. *J Pediatr* 1977; 1:188–93.
293. Bhan MK, Bhandari N, Svensson L, et al. Role of enteric adenoviruses and rotaviruses in mild and severe acute enteritis. *Pediatr Infect Dis J* 1988;7:320–3.
294. Hieber JP, Shelton S, Nelson JD. Comparison of human rotavirus disease in tropical and temperate settings. *Am J Dis Child* 1978; 132:853–8.
295. Hjelt K, Krasilnikoff A, Graubella PC, et al. Clinical features in hospitalized children with acute gastroenteritis. *Acta Paediatr Scand* 1985;74:96–101.
296. Goldwater PN, Chrystie IL, Banatvala JE. Rotavirus and the respiratory tract. *Br Med J* 1979;2:1551.
297. Lewis HM, Parry JV, Davies HA. A year's experience of the rotavirus syndrome and its association with respiratory illness. *Arch Dis Child* 1979;54:339–46.
298. Santosham M, Yolken RH, Quiroz E, et al. Detection of rotavirus in respiratory secretions of children with pneumonia. *J Pediatr* 1983;103:583–5.
299. Brandt CD, Kim HW, Rodriquez WJ, et al. Simultaneous infections with different enteric and respiratory tract viruses. *J Clin Microbiol* 1986;23:177–9.
300. Kitaoka S. Human rotavirus and intersusception. *N Engl J Med* 1977;297:945.
301. Konno T, Suzuki H, Kutsuzawa T, et al. Human rotavirus infection in infants and young children with intersusception. *J Med Virol* 1978;2:265–9.
302. Matsuno S, Utagawa E, Sugiura A. Association of rotavirus infection with Kawasaki syndrome. *J Infect Dis* 1983;148:177.
303. Mulcahy DZ, Kanath KR, DeSilva LM, et al. A 2 part study of the aetiological role of rotavirus in intersusception. *J Med Virol* 1982;9:51–5.
304. Nichols JC, Ingrand D, Fortier B, et al. A one year virologic survey of acute intersusception in children. *J Med Virol* 1982;9:267–71.
305. Rotbart HA, Nelson WL, Glode MP, et al. Neonatal rotavirus-associated necrotising enterocolitis: case control study and prospective surveillance during an outbreak. *J Pediatr* 1988;112:87–93.
306. Saulsbury FT, Winkelstein JA, Yolken RJ. Chronic rotavirus infection in immunodeficiency. *J Pediatr* 1980;97:61–5.
307. Tallett S, MacKenzie C, Middleton P, et al. Clinical, laboratory, and epidemiologic features of viral gastroenteritis in infants and children. *Pediatrics* 1977;60:217–22.
308. Grimwood K, Coakley JC, Hudson IL, et al. Serum asparate aminotransferase levels after rotavirus gastroenteritis. *J Pediatr* 1987;112:597–600.
309. Flores J, Nakagomi O, Nakogomi T, et al. The role of rotaviruses in pediatric diarrhea. *Pediatr Infect Dis* 1986;5:S53–62.
310. Taylor PR, Mason MH, Black RE. Oral rehydration therapy for treatment of rotavirus diarrhea in a rural treatment center in Bangladesh. *Arch Dis Child* 1980;55:376–9.
311. McLean B, Sonza S, Holmes IH. Measurement of immunoglobulins A, G and M class rotavirus antibodies in serum and mucosal secretions. *J Clin Microbiol* 1980;12:314–9.
312. Angeretti A, Magi MT, Merlino C, et al. Specific serum IgA rotavirus gastroenteritis. *J Med Virol* 1987;23:345–9.
313. Davidson GP, Hogg RJ, Kirubakaran GP. Serum and intestinal immune response to rotavirus enteritis in children. *Infect Immun* 1983;40:447–52.

314. Grimwood K, Lund JCS, Coulson BS, et al. Comparison of serum and mucosal antibody responses following severe acute rotavirus gastroenteritis in young children. *J Clin Microbiol* 1988;26:732–8.
315. Riepenhoff-Talty M, Bogger-Goren S, Li P, et al. Development of serum and intestinal antibody response to rotavirus after naturally acquired rotavirus infection in man. *J Med Virol* 1981;8:215–22.
316. Yolken RH, Wyatt RG, Kim HW, et al. Immunological response to infection with human reovirus-like agent: measurement of anti-human reovirus-like agent immunoglobulin G and M levels by the method of enzyme-linked immunosorbent assay. *Infect Immun* 1978;19:540–6.
317. Sonza S, Holmes IH. Corproantibody response to rotavirus infection. *Med J Aust* 1980;2:496–9.
318. Stals F, Walther FJ, Bruggeman CA. Faecal and pharyngeal shedding of rotavirus and rotavirus IgA in children with diarrhoea. *J Med Virol* 1984;14:333–9.
319. Mclean B, Holmes IH. Transfer of antirotavirus antibodies from mothers to their infants. *J Clin Microbiol* 1980;12:320–5.
320. Svensson L, Sheshberadaran H, Vene S, et al. Serum antibody responses to individual viral polypeptides in human rotavirus infections. *J Gen Virol* 1987;68:643–51.
321. Kapikian AZ, Wyatt RG, Levine MM, et al. Oral administration of human rotavirus to volunteers: Induction of illness and correlates of resistance. *J Infect Dis* 1983;147:95–106.
322. Brussow H, Werchau H, Lerner L, et al. Seroconversion patterns of four human rotavirus serotypes of hospitalized infants with acute rotavirus gastroenteritis. *J Infect Dis* 1988;158:588–92.
323. Brussow H, Werchau H, Leidtke W, et al. Prevalence of antibodies to rotavirus in different age-groups of infants in Bochum, West Germany. *J Infect Dis* 1988;157:1014–22.
324. Urasawa S, Urasawa T, Taniguchi K, et al. Serotype determination of human rotavirus isolates and antibody prevalence in pediatric population in Hokkaido, Japan. *Arch Virol* 1984;84:1–12.
325. Ward RL, Knowlton DR, Schiff GM, et al. Relative concentrations of serum neutralizing antibody to VP3 and VP7 protein in adults infected with a human rotavirus. *J Virol* 1988;62:1543–9.
326. Offit PA, Dudzik KI. Rotavirus-specific cytotoxic T lymphocytes cross-react with target cells infected with different rotavirus serotypes. *J Virol* 1988;62:127–31.
327. Sheridan JF, Eyedelloth RS, Vonderfecht SL, et al. Virus-specific immunity in neonatal and adult mouse rotavirus infection. *Infect Immun* 1983;39:917–27.
328. Eiden J, Lederman HM, Vonderfecht S, et al. T-cell-deficient mice display normal recovery from experimental rotavirus infection. *J Virol* 1986;57:706–8.
329. Riepenhoff-Talty M, Dharakul T, Kowalski E, et al. Persistent rotavirus infection in mice with severe combined immunodeficiency. *J Virol* 1987;61:3345–8.
330. Ryder RW, Singh N, Reeves WC, et al. Evidence of immunity induced by naturally acquired rotavirus and Norwalk virus infection on two remote Panamanian islands. *J Infect Dis* 1985;151:99–105.
331. Bishop RF, Barnes GL, Cipriani E, et al. Clinical immunity after neonatal rotavirus infection. A prospective study in young children. *N Engl J Med* 1983;1988:72–6.
332. Offit PA, Clark HF, Blavat G, et al. Reassortant rotaviruses containing structural proteins vp3 and vp7 from different parents induce antibodies protective against each parental serotype. *J Virol* 1986;60:491–6.
333. Offit PA, Shaw RD, Greenberg HB. Passive protection against rotavirus-induced diarrhea by monoclonal antibodies to surface proteins vp3 and vp7. *J Virol* 1986;58:700–3.
334. Besser TE, Gay CC, McGuire TC, et al. Passive immunity to bovine rotavirus infection associated with transfer of serum antibody into the intestinal lumen. *J Virol* 1988;62:2238–42.
335. Barnes GL, Hewson PH, McLellan JA, et al. A randomized trial of oral gammaglobulin in low-birth weight infants infected with rotavirus. *Lancet* 1982;1:1371–3.
336. Brussow H, Hilpert H, Walther I, et al. Bovine milk immunoglobulins for passive immunity in infantile rotavirus gastroenteritis. *J Clin Microbiol* 1987;25:982–6.
337. Kapikian AZ, Flores J, Hoshino Y, et al. Rotavirus: the major etiologic agent of severe infantile diarrhea may be controllable by a "Jennerian" approach to vaccination. *J Infect Dis* 1986;153:815–20.
338. Anderson EL, Belshe RB, Bartram J, et al. Evaluation of rhesus rotavirus vaccine (MMU 18006) in infants and young children. *J Infect Dis* 1986;153:823.
339. Hilpert H, Brussow H, Mietens C, et al. Use of bovine milk concentrate containing antibody to rotavirus to treat rotavirus gastroenteritis in infants. *J Infect Dis* 1987;156:158–66.
340. Losonsky GA, Rennels MB, Kapikian AZ, et al. Safety, infectivity, transmissibility and immunogenicity of rhesus rotavirus vaccine (MMU 18006) in infants *Pediatr Infect Dis J* 1986;5:25–9.
341. Clark HF, Furukawa T, Bell LM, et al. Immune response of infants and children to low-passage bovine rotavirus (strain WC3). *Am J Dis Child* 1986;140:350–6.
342. Vesikari T, Isolauri E, D'Hondt E, et al. Protection of infants against rotavirus diarrhoea by RIT 4237 attenuated bovine rotavirus strain vaccine. *Lancet* 1984;1:977–81.
343. Vesikari T, Ruuska T, Delem A, et al. Neonatal rotavirus vaccination with RIT 4237 bovine rotavirus vaccine: a preliminary report. *Pediatr Infect Dis J* 1987;6:164–9.
344. Clark HF, Offit PA, Dolan KT, et al. Response

of adult human volunteers to oral administration of bovine and bovine-human reassortant rotaviruses. *Vaccine* 1986;4:25–31.

345. Midthun K, Greenberg HB, Hoshino Y, et al. Reassortant rotaviruses as potential live rotavirus vaccine candidates. *J Virol* 1985;53:949–54.
346. Midthun K, Hoshino Y, Kapikian AZ, et al. Single gene substitution rotavirus reassortants containing the major neutralization protein (VP7) of human rotavirus serotype 4. *J Clin Microbiol* 1986;24:822–6.
347. Kapikian AZ, Wyatt RG, Greenberg HS, et al. Approaches to immunization of infants and young children against gastroenteritis due to rotavirus. *Rev Infect Dis* 1980;2:459–69.
348. Sabara M, Barrington A, Babiuk LA. Immunogenicity of a bovine rotavirus glycoprotein fragment. *J Virol* 1985;56:1037–40.
349. Estes MK, Crawford SE, Penaranda ME, et al. Synthesis and immunogenicity of the rotavirus major capsid antigen using a baculovirus expression system. *J Virol* 1987;61:1488–94.
350. Andrew ME, Boyle DB, Coupar BEH, et al. Vaccinia virus recombinants expressing the SA11 rotavirus VP7 glycoprotein gene induce serotype-specific neutralizing antibodies. *J Virol* 1987;61:1054–60.
351. Dagenais L, Pastoret PP, Van den Broecke C, et al. Susceptibility of bovine rotavirus to interferon. *Arch Virol* 1981;70:377–9.
352. McKimm-Breschkin JL, Holmes IH. Conditions required for induction of interferon by rotaviruses and for their sensitivity to its action. *Infect Immun* 1982;36:857–63.
353. LaBonnardiere C, deVaureix C, L'Haridon R, et al. Weak susceptibility of rotavirus to bovine interferon in calf kidney cells. *Arch Virol* 1980;64:167–70.
354. Huffman JH, Sidwell RW, Khare G, et al. *In vitro* effect of 1-B-D-ribofuranosyl-1,2,4-triazole-3-cenboxamide (Virazole, 1 CN 1229) on deoxyribonucleic acid and ribonucleic acid viruses. *Antimicrob Agents Chemother* 1973;3:235–41.
355. Smee DF, Sidwell RW, Clark SM, et al. Inhibition of reoviruses *in vitro* by selected antiviral substances. *Antiviral Res* 1981;1:315–23.
356. Schoub BD, Prozesky DN. Antiviral activity of ribavirin in rotavirus gastroenteritis of mice. *Antimicrob Agents Chemother* 1977;12:543–4.
357. Smee DF, Sidwell RW, Clark SM, et al. Inhibition of rotaviruses by selected antiviral substances: mechanisms of viral inhibition and *in vivo* activity. *Antimicrob Agents Chemother* 1982;21:66–73.
358. Kitaoka S, Konno T, DeClercq E. Comparative efficacy of broad-spectrum antiviral agents as inhibitors of rotavirus replication *in vitro*. *Antiviral Res* 1986;6:57–65.
359. Caul ED, Egglestone SI. Coronaviruses in humans. In: Tyrrell DAS, Kapikian AZ, eds. *Virus infections of the gastrointestinal tract*. New York: Marcell Dekker, 1982:179–93.
360. Appleton HS, Pereira MS. A possible etiology in outbreaks of food poisoning from cockles. *Lancet* 1977;1:780–1.
361. Appleton HZ, Buckley M, Thom BT, et al. Virus-like particles in winter vomiting disease. *Lancet* 1977;1:409–11.
362. Christopher PJ, Grohmann GS, Millson RH, et al. Parvovirus gastroenteritis-A new entity for Australia. *Med J Aust* 1978;1:121.
363. Pauer WK, Caul EO, Ashley CR, et al. A small virus in human faeces. *Lancet* 1973;1:237–40.
364. Richmond SJ, Dunn SM, Caul ED, et al. An outbreak of gastroenteritis in young children caused by adenoviruses. *Lancet* 1979;1:1178–80.
365. Artenstein MS, Cadigan FC, Buescher EL. Clinical and epidemiological features of coxsackie group B virus infections. *Ann Intern Med* 1965;63:597–603.
366. Dolin R. Enteroviral diseases. In: Wyngaarden JB, Smith LH, eds. *Cecil's textbook of medicine*. Philadelphia, Pennsylvania: W.B. Saunders, 1982:1663–70.
367. Melnick JL. Enteroviruses. In: Evans AS, eds. *Viral infections of humans*. New York: Plenum, 1982:187–251.
368. Gelfand HM, Holgiun AH, Marchetti GE, et al. A continuing surveillance of enterovirus infections in healthy children in six United States cities. *Am J Hyg* 1963;78:358–75.
369. Wilfert CM, Buckley RH, Mohanakumarz T, et al. Persistent and fatal central-nervous-system echovirus infections in patients with agammaglobulinemia. *N Engl J Med* 1977;26:1485–9.
370. Chang T-W, Weinstein L, MacMahon HE. Paralytic poliomyelitis in a child with hypogammaglobulinemia: probable implication of type 1 vaccine strain. *Pediatrics* 1961;37:630–6.
371. Wyatt H. Poliomyelitis in hypogammaglobulinemics. *J Infect Dis* 1973;128:802–6.
372. Eichenwald HF, Arabio A, Arky AM, et al. Epidemic diarrhea in premature and older infants caused by ECHO virus type 18. *JAMA* 1958;166:1563–6.
373. Horstmann DM, McCollum RW. Poliomyelitis virus in human blood during the "minor illness" and the asymptomatic infection. *Proc Soc Exp Biol Med* 1953;82:434–7.
374. Sabin AB. Pathogenesis of poliomyelitis. *Science* 1956;123:1151–7.
375. Miller PA, Miller J, Dev GV, et al. Human chromosome 19 carries a poliovirus receptor gene. *Cell* 1974;1:167–9.
376. Deschamps J, DeClercq E. Broad spectrum antiviral activity of pyrazofurin (Pyrazomycin). In: *Current chemotherapy: proceedings of the 10th International Congress of Chemotherapy*. Washington, D.C.: American Society for Microbiology, 1978:354–7.
377. Halperen S. Inhibition of echovirus-12 multiplication by *N*-carbobenzoxy-D-glucosamine. *J Gen Virol* 1976;33:389–401.
378. Kim KS, Sapienza VJ, Carp RI. Antiviral activity of arildone on deoxyribonucleic acid and ribonucleic acid viruses. *Antimicrob Agents Chemother* 1980;18:276–80.
379. McKinlay MA, Miralles JV, Brisson CJ, et al. Prevention of human poliovirus-induced paralysis and death in mice by the novel antiviral

agent, arildone. *Antimicrob Agents Chemother* 1982;22:1022–5.
380. Eggers HJ. Antiviral agents against picornaviruses. *Antiviral Res* 1985; suppl 1:57–65.
381. Caliguiri LA, McSharry JJ, Lawrence GW. Effect of arildone on modifications of poliovirus *in vitro*. *Virology* 1980;105:86–93.
382. Diana GD, Salvador VJ, Zalay ES, et al. Antiviral activity of some B diketones. 2. Aryloxy alkyldiketones. *In vitro* activity against both RNA and DNA viruses. *J Med Chem* 1977;20:757–61.
383. Diana GD, Salvador VJ, Zalay ES, et al. Antiviral activity of some B diketones. 1. Aryl alkyl diketones. *In vitro* activity against both RNA and DNA viruses. *J Med Chem* 1977; 20:750–6.
384. McSharry JJ, Caliguiri LA, Eggers HJ. Inhibition of uncoating of poliovirus by arildone, a new antiviral drug. *Virology* 1979;97:307–15.
385. Eggers HJ, Rosenwirt, B. Isolation and characterization of an arildone-resistant poliovirus 2 mutant with an altered capsid protein VP1. *Antiviral Res* 1988;9:23–36.
386. Otto MJ, Fox MP, Fanmcher MJ, et al. *In vitro* activity of WIN 51711, a new broad-spectrum antipicornavirus drug. *Antimicrob Agents Chemother* 1985;27:883–6.
387. McKinlay MA, Steinberg BA. Oral efficacy of WIN 51711 in mice infected with human poliovirus. *Antimicrob Agents Chemother* 1986;29:30–2.
388. McKinlay MA, Frank JA, Benziger DP, et al. Use of WIN 51711 to prevent echovirus type 9-induced paralysis in suckling mice. *J Infect Dis* 1986;154:676.
389. Fox MP, Otto MJ, McKinlay MA. Prevention of rhinovirus and poliovirus uncoating by WIN 51711, a new antiviral drug. *Antimicrob Agents Chemother* 1986;30;110–6.
390. Zeichhardt H, Otto MJ, McKinlay MA, et al. Inhibition of poliovirus uncoating by disoxaril (WIN 51711). *Virology* 1987;160:281–5.
391. Smith TJ, Kremer MJ, Luo M, et al. The site of attachment in human rhinovirus 14 for antiviral agents that inhibit uncoating. *Science* 1986;233:1286–93.
392. Eggers HF, Koch MA, Furst A, et al. Rhodanine: A selective inhibitor of the multiplication of echovirus 12. *Science* 1970;167:294–7.
393. Rosenwirth B, Eggers HJ. Echovirus 12-induced host cell shutoff is prevented by rhodanine. *Nature* 1977;267:370–1.
394. Rosenwirth B, Eggers HJ. Early processes of echovirus 12-infection: elution, penetration, and uncoating under the influence of rhodanine. *Virology* 1979;97:241–55.
395. Eggers HF, Bode B, Brown DT. Cytoplasmic localization of the uncoating of picornaviruses. *Virology* 1979;92:211–8.
396. Korant BD, Towatari T, Ivanoff L, et al. Viral therapy: prospects for protease inhibitors. *J Cell Biochem* 1986;3:91–5.
397. Beladi I, Pusztai R, Mucsi I, et al. Activity of some flavonoids against viruses. *Ann NY Acad Sci* 1977;284:358–64.
398. Vrijsen R, Everaert L, Boeye A. Antiviral activity of flavones and potentiation by ascorbate. *J Gen Virol* 1988;69:1749–51.
399. Guttner J, Veckenstedt A, Heinecke H, et al. Effect of quercetin on the course of mengovirus infection in immunodeficient and normal mice: a histological study. *Acta Virol* 1982;26: 148–55.
400. Ishitsuka H, Ohsawa C, Ohiwa T, et al. Antipicornavirus flavone Ro 09-0179. *Antimicrob Agents Chemother* 1983;22:611–6.
401. Veckenstedt A, Beladi I, Mucsi I. Effect of treatment with certain flavonoids on mengovirus-induced encephalitis in mice. *Arch Virol* 1978;57:255–60.
402. Veckenstedt A, Pusztai R. Mechanism of antiviral action of quercetin against cardiovirus infection in mice. *Antiviral Res* 1981;1:249–61.
403. Castrillo JL, Carrasco L, et al. Action of 3-methylquercetin on poliovirus RNA replication. *J Virol* 1987;61:3319–21.
404. Vrijsen R, Everaert L, Van Hoff LM, et al. The poliovirus-induced shut-off of cellular protein synthesis persists in the presence of 3-methylquercetin, a flavonoid which blocks viral protein and RNA synthesis. *Antiviral Res* 1987;7:35–42.
405. Linnemann CC Jr, May DB, Shubert WK. Fatal viral encephalitis in children with X-linked hypogammaglobulinemia. *Am J Dis Child* 1973;126:100–3.
406. Anderson-Sillman K, Bartal S, Tershak DR. Guanidine-resistant poliovirus mutants produce modified 37-kilodalton proteins. *J Virol* 1984:50:922–8.
407. Sehgal PB, Tamm I. Benzimidazoles and their nucleosides. *Antibiot Chemother* 1979;27: 93–138.
408. Tershak DR. Inhibition of poliovirus polymerase by guanidine *in vitro*. *J Virol* 1982;41:313–8.
409. Caliguiri LA, Tamm I. Guanidine and 2-(α-hydroxybenzyl)-benzimidazole (HBB): Selective inhibitors of picornavirus multiplication. In: Carter WA, eds. *Selective Inhibitors of viral functions*. Cleveland: CRC Press, 1973:257–94.
410. Herrmann EC, Herrmann JA, Delong DC. Comparison of the antiviral effects of substituted benzimidazoles and guanidine *in vitro* and *in vivo*. *Antiviral Res* 1981;1:301–14.
411. Phillpotts RJ, Delong DC, Wallace J, et al. The activity of enviroxime against rhinovirus infection in man. *Lancet* 1981;1:1342–4.
412. *Enviroxime clinical investigation manual*. Indianapolis: Lilly Research Laboratories, 1980.
413. Eggers HJ. Successful treatment of enterovirus-infected mice by 2-(α-hydroxybenzyl)-benzimidazole and guanidine. *J Exp Med* 1976;143: 1367–81.
414. Barrera-Oro JG, Melnick JL. The effect of guanidine: (1) On experimental poliomyelitis induced by oral administration of virus to cynomolgus monkeys; (2) On naturally occurring

enteroviruses of cynomolgus monkeys. *Tex Rep Biol Med* 1961;19:529–836.
415. Fara GM, Cockran KW. Antiviral activity of selected benzimidazoles. *Boll Ist Sieroter Milan* 1963;42:630–5.
416. Caliguiri LA, Tamm I. Action of guanidine on the replication of poliovirus RNA. *Virology* 1968;35:408–17.
417. Buckley CE, Wong KT, Baron S. Induction of the interferon system by various interferon inducers. *Proc Soc Exp Biol Med* 1968;127:1258–62.
418. Ho M, Enders JF. Further studies on an inhibitor of viral activity appearing in infected cell cultures and its role in chronic viral infections. *Virology* 1959;9:446–77.
419. Baron R, Buckler CD, Friedman RM, et al. Role of interferon during viremia. II. Protective action of circulating interferon. *J Immunol* 1966;96:12–6.
420. Gresser I, Bourali C, Thomas MT, et al. Effect of repeated inoculation of interferon preparations on infection of mice with encephalomyocarditis virus. *Proc Soc Exp Biol Med* 1968;127:491–6.
421. Olsen GA, Kern ER, Glasgow LA, et al. Effect of treatment with exogenous interferon, polyinosinic acid-polycytidylic acid, or polyinosinic acid, polycytidylic acid-poly-L-lysine complex on encephalomyocarditis virus infections in mice. *Antimicrob Agents Chemother* 1974; 10:668–78.
422. Weck PK, Rindleknecht E, Estell DA, et al. Antiviral activity of bacteria derived human alpha interferons against encephalomyocarditis virus infections of mice. *Infect Immun* 1982;35:660–5.
423. Weck PK, Harkins RN, Stebbing N. Antiviral effects of human fibroblast interferon from E. coli against encephalomyocarditis virus infection of squirrel monkeys. *J Gen Virol* 1983;64:415–9.
424. Stebbing N, Lindley IJD, Dawson KM. Variations in the combination of induced interferon and adjuvanticity to the antiviral effect of different polyinosinic acid, polycytiacylic acid formations in mice infected with encephalomyocarditis virus. *Infect Immun* 1980;29: 960–5.
425. Veckenstedt A, Witkowski W, Hoffmann S. Comparison of antiviral properties in mice of bis-pyrrolidine acetamido-fluorenone (MLU-B75), bis-dipropyl-aminoaceta-mido-flourenone (MLU-B76) and tilorone hydrochloride. *Acta Virol* 1979;23:153–8.
426. Stebbing N. Protection of mice against infection with wild type mingovirus and an interferon sensitive mutant (1S-1) by polynucleotides and interferons. *J Gen Virol* 1979;44:255–60.
427. Stebbing N, Grantham CA, Carey NH. Antiviral activity of single-stranded homopolynucleotides against EMC virus and semliki forest virus in adult mice without interferon induction. *J Gen Virol* 1976;30:21–39.
428. Stebbing N, Lindley JD, Grantham CA. Protection of mice against encephalomyocarditis virus infection by chemically modified transfer RNAs. *J Gen Virol* 1977;36:351–5.
429. Stewart AG, Grantham CA, Dawson KM, et al. The antiviral activity of ribosomal polynucleotides against encephalomyocarditis virus infection of mice. *Arch Virol* 1980;66:283–91.
430. Stebbing N, Grantham CA, Kaminski F, et al. Protection of mice against encephalomyocarditis virus infection by preparations of transfer RNA. *J Gen Virol* 1977;34:73–85.
431. Gordon P, Brown ER. The antiviral activity of isoprinosine. *Can J Microbiol* 1972;18:1463–70.
432. Chany C, Cerutti I. Enhancement of antiviral protection against encephalomyocarditis virus by a combination of isoprinosine and interferon. *Arch Virol* 1977;55:255–31.
433. Simon LN, Settineri R, Coats H, et al. Isoprinosine: integration of the antiviral and immunoproliferative effects. In: *Current chemotherapy. Proceedings of the 10th International Congress of Chemotherapy*. Washington, D.C.: American Society for Microbiology, 1978:366–8.
434. Tonew E, Lober G, Tonew M. The influence of antiviral isatinisothio semicarbazones on RNA dependent RNA polymerase in mengovirus-infected FL cells. *Acta Virol* 1974;18:185–92.
435. Tonew M, Tonew E, Heinisch L. Antiviral thiosemicarbazones and related compounds. II. Antiviral action of substituted isatinisothiosemicarbazones. *Acta Virol* 1974;18:17–24.
436. Galabov AS, Mastikova M. Dipyridamole is an interferon inducer. *Acta Virol* 1982;26: 137–47.
437. Tonew M, Laass W, Tonew E, et al. Antiviral activity of dipyridamole derivatives. *Acta Virol* 1978;22:287–95.
438. Tonew M, Tonew E, Mentel R. The antiviral activity of dipyridamole. *Acta Virol* 1977;21:146–50.
439. Galabov AS. Thiourea derivatives as specific inhibitors of picornaviruses. *Arzneimittelforschung* 1979;29:1863–68.
440. Galabov AS, Galabov BS, Neykova NA. Structure activity relationship of diphenylthiomes antivirals. *J Med Chem* 1981;23:1048–51.
441. Bonina L, Orzalesi G, Merendino R, et al. Structure activity relationships of new antiviral compounds. *Antimicrob Agents Chemother* 1982;22:1067–9.
442. Tonew M, Tonew E. Inhibitory activity of 2-amino-oxazole derivatives against coxsackie B1 virus in FL cells. *Acta Virol* 1980;24:207–14.
443. Powers RD, Gwaltney JM, Hayden FG. Activity of 2-(3,4-Dichlorophenoxy)-5-Nitrobenzonitrite (MDL-860) against picornaviruses *in vitro*. *Antimicrob Agents Chemother* 1982;22:639–42.
444. Torey HL, Dulworth JK, Steward DL. Antiviral activity and mechanism of action of 2-(3,4-dichlorophenoxy)-5-nitrobenzonitrite (MDL-860). *Antimicrob Agents Chemother* 1982;22:635–8.
445. Merryman P, Jaffe IA, Ehrenfeld E. Effect of D-penicillamine in poliovirus replication in HeLa cells. *J Virol* 1974;13:881–7.

446. Hecht TT, Summers DF. The effect of phleomycin on poliovirus RNA replication. *Virology* 1970;40:441–7.
447. Miller PA, Milstrey KP, Trown PW. Specific inhibition of viral ribonucleic acid replication by gliotoxin. *Science* 1968;159:431–2.
448. Richtsel WA, Schneider HG, Sloan BJ, et al. Antiviral activity of gliotoxin and gliotoxin acetate. *Nature* 1966;204:1333–4.
449. Rinehart KL, Gloer JB, Hughes RG, et al. Didemnins: antiviral and antitumor depsipeptides from a Caribbean tunicate. *Science* 1981;212:933–5.
450. Rinehart KL, Gloer JB, Cook JC. Structures of the didemnins, antiviral and cytotoxic depsipeptides from a Caribbean tunicate. *J Am Chem Soc* 1981;103:1857–9.

*Antiviral Agents and Viral Diseases of Man, 3rd Edition,*
edited by G. J. Galasso, R. J. Whitley, and
T. C. Merigan, Raven Press, Ltd., New York © 1990.

# 12

# Antiviral Therapy of Viral Hepatitis

Jay H. Hoofnagle and *Adrian M. Di Bisceglie

*Division of Digestive Diseases and Nutrition and *Liver Diseases Section, National Institute of Diabetes and Digestive and Kidney Diseases, National Institutes of Health, Bethesda, Maryland 20892*



Viral hepatitis encompasses at least five different diseases caused by five separate agents: hepatitis A or infectious hepatitis caused by hepatitis A virus (HAV) (1), hepatitis B or classical serum hepatitis due to hepatitis B virus (HBV) (2); delta or type D hepatitis due to hepatitis D virus (HDV) (3); classically, parenterally transmitted non-A, non-B (NANB) hepatitis due to a recently described, medium-sized RNA virus, which has been tentatively called "hepatitis C virus" (HCV) (4–7); and, finally, epidemic or enterically transmitted NANB hepatitis due to a small RNA virus tentatively called "hepatitis E virus" (HEV) (8). The major features of these five agents are given in Table 1.

All five forms of viral hepatitis can lead to an acute hepatitis; only type B, delta, and classical NANB hepatitis can also lead to a chronic hepatitis. The clinical features of the five forms of viral hepatitis are similar, and the five diseases cannot be distinguished on the basis of symptoms or signs of disease or biochemical laboratory tests. Fortunately, sensitive and specific sero-

**TABLE 1.** *Comparison of the five types of viral hepatitis*

| Feature | Hepatitis A | Hepatitis B | Hepatitis D | Classical NANB | Epidemic NANB |
|---|---|---|---|---|---|
| Virus | HAV | HBV | HDV | HCV | HEV |
| Virus class | Picornavirus | Hepadnavirus | Satellite virus | ?Flavivirus | ?Calici virus |
| Virus size | 27 nm | 42 nm | 40 nm | 30–60 nm | 27–34 nm |
| Genome | ssRNA(+) | dsDNA | ssRNA(−) | ssRNA(+) | ?RNA |
| | 7.8kb | 3.2kb | 1.7kb | 10.5kb | ? |
| Antigens | HA Ag (VP1-4) | $HB_sAg$ | HDV Ag | HCV Ag | HEV Ag |
| | | $HB_cAg$ | | | |
| | | $HB_eAg$ | | | |
| Spread | Enteric | Parenteral and sexual | Parenteral largely | Parenteral largely | Enteric |
| Incubation period (range) | 25 days (15–45 days) | 75 days (40–120 days) | 50 days (25–75 days) | 50 days (15–90 days) | 40 days (20–80 days) |
| Chronicity | None | 3–10% | 2–70%[a] | 40–70% | None |
| Fulminant | 0.2% | 0.2% | 2–20% | 0.2% | 0.2–10%[b] |

[a]High rate of chronicity when delta occurs as a superinfection.
[b]High rate of mortality in pregnant women.

logic assays are available for diagnosis of hepatitis A, B, and delta hepatitis. Non-A, non-B hepatitis is currently a diagnosis of exclusion (6), although research assays for antibody to HCV have been described that may soon make a positive serologic identification of this disease possible (5). Assays for antibody to HEV (anti-HEV) are difficult and cumbersome [immune electron microscopy (IEM)] and available in only a few research institutions. However, epidemic NANB hepatitis is extremely rare in the United States and Western Europe; the disease has been described only in underdeveloped areas of the world.

Acute viral hepatitis is a common and serious illness. For the past several years, the reported incidence of acute hepatitis in the United States has been rising. In 1986, there were approximately 60,000 cases reported to the Center for Diseases Control (9). This reported incidence is undoubtedly lower than the true incidence; previous studies have suggested that the actual rate of disease is three- to eight-fold higher than the reported rate. These findings suggest that the true incidence of acute, symptomatic viral hepatitis in the United States is one per thousand population per year.

Serologic investigation of reported cases of acute viral hepatitis in four "sentinel" counties in the United States have shown that approximately 25% of cases are hepatitis A, 40% hepatitis B, and 35% NANB hepatitis (9,10). The incidence of delta hepatitis has not been adequately assessed in these studies, but it probably represents only 5–20% of cases reported as hepatitis B. Epidemic NANB hepatitis has been evaluated in a small number of sporadic cases of acute NANB hepatitis, and as yet no case of this disease has been identified as occurring sporadically in the United States (11).

Discussion of antiviral therapy of viral hepatitis has to begin with an understanding of the natural history and course of this disease as well as the actual viral agents that can cause acute and chronic hepatitis.

## TYPICAL ACUTE VIRAL HEPATITIS

The typical course of acute viral hepatitis is shown in Fig. 1. The course is divided into incubation period, preicteric phase, icteric phase, and convalescence.

### Incubation Period

The incubation period of viral hepatitis ranges from 2 weeks to 6 months. Incubation period is short for hepatitis A (mean, 25 days) and epidemic non-A, non-B hepatitis (mean, 30 days), longer for delta hepatitis (30–50 days) and classical NANB hepatitis (mean, 50 days), and longest for hepatitis B (mean, 75 days). During the incubation period, viral replication in the liver begins. The level of viral replication as assessed by excretion of virus in stool (hepatitis A and epidemic NANB) or in serum (hepatitis B and delta hepatitis) typically reaches its peak during the incubation period while the patient is still asymptomatic and usually unaware of having been infected.

### Preicteric Phase

The symptomatic onset of acute viral hepatitis can be sudden or insidious. The initial symptoms are typically fatigue and lassitude followed by anorexia, nausea, and right upper quadrant or diffuse abdominal pain. These nonspecific symptoms precede the onset of jaundice and dark urine by 3–14 days. Symptoms during this preicteric phase can also include fever, headache, influenza-like symptoms, or diarrhea. In 5–15% of cases and especially in cases of hepatitis B, the preicteric phase is marked by an immune-complex-like syndrome of fever, arthralgias, and rash (usually hives). During the preicteric phase, levels of virus are usually high, and serum aminotransferases [alanine aminotransferase (ALT) and aspartate aminotransferase (AST)] begin to rise. In most forms of acute hepatitis, virus-

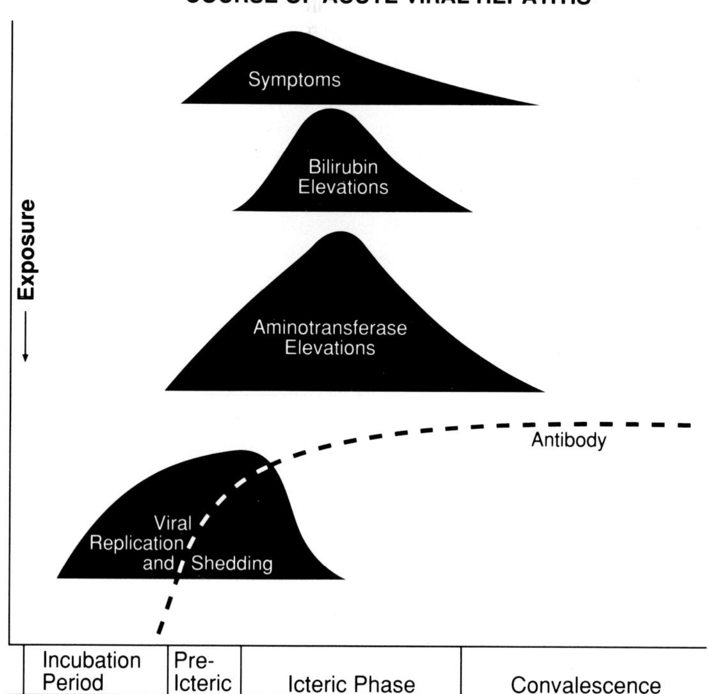


**FIG. 1.** The course of acute viral hepatitis.

specific antibody is first detectable during this early phase.

### Icteric Phase

The icteric phase of acute viral hepatitis is marked by the onset of jaundice or dark urine. With onset of jaundice, other symptoms tend to worsen. The exception to this is fever, arthralgias, and hives, which typically resolve when jaundice appears. Prolonged jaundice is also accompanied by lightening of the color of stools and pruritus. Weight loss usually occurs, averaging 5–15 pounds. The duration of clinical symptoms varies greatly, but averages 2–8 weeks. A return of appetite is often the first symptom to improve; fatigue is usually the last. Some patients have easy fatiguability for months into convalescence.

By the onset of the icteric phase, serum ALT and AST are at least 10-fold elevated and serum bilirubin levels are above 3 mg/dl (51 μmol/L). The peak in symptoms and biochemical evidence of hepatic injury usually corresponds to the time of clearance of virus and rising levels of antibody.

### Convalescence Phase

The convalescence phase begins with the disappearance of jaundice and amelioration of symptoms. Virus is usually no longer detectable in serum or stool, and specific antibody is present. Serum ALT and AST levels are either normal or are decreasing towards the normal range.

Acute viral hepatitis is usually self-limiting, and recovery is complete. In view of the typically benign outcome, antiviral therapy of typical acute viral hepatitis has not been a major focus of basic or clinical research studies. There are also several reasons why antiviral treatments should not be used in acute viral hepatitis. Most antiviral agents are not completely innocuous. The hepatic injury that accompanies acute hepatitis predisposes to defective or abnormal drug metabolism, activation, and clearance. In this setting, drug toxicity can worsen symptoms and may even contribute to further hepatic injury. Care has to be taken in administering any medication to a patient with acute icteric hepatitis.

The major focus of antiviral therapy in viral hepatitis has been the complications of acute disease. These complications include fulminant hepatitis, prolonged or relapsing hepatitis, and chronic hepatitis.

## FULMINANT HEPATITIS

Fulminant hepatitis represents the extreme end of the clinical spectrum of severity of acute viral hepatitis. It comprises 0.2–2% of clinically apparent cases of acute disease (12). The incidence of fulminant disease relates partly to the form of hepatitis, being highest in delta hepatitis and lowest in hepatitis A. Its incidence also relates to host factors; thus, acute hepatitis is usually more severe in the elderly, and some forms (especially epidemic NANB) are more severe during pregnancy. The onset is marked by the appearance of signs of hepatic encephalopathy with abnormal behavior, drowsiness, confusion, somnolence, and, finally, coma. Deep jaundice and coagulation abnormalities are usually present. Once coma is present, the mortality rate is high. There are no specific therapies for fulminant hepatitis. Currently, a major approach to this dire syndrome is emergency hepatic transplantation (13).

The high mortality rate of fulminant hepatitis makes it a particularly attractive target for antiviral therapy. However, the features that make therapy of acute hepatitis difficult make treatment of fulminant disease even more troublesome. Patients with fulminant hepatitis have severely compromised hepatic function and cannot be expected to metabolize or activate medications normally. The marginal nature of their hepatic reserve makes the addition of medications potentially dangerous. In addition, once hepatic failure appears, viral replication has usually ceased (14,15). Thus, antiviral therapy is likely to be too late and possibly too risky in patients with fulminant hepatic failure.

## PROLONGED OR RELAPSING HEPATITIS

In up to 10% of patients with acute viral hepatitis, the disease is prolonged (for longer than 8 weeks) or is marked by repeated relapses. A relapsing or polyphasic course is particularly common in acute hepatitis A (16,17). A biphasic course is common in acute delta hepatitis (3,18).

Antiviral therapy for prolonged or relapsing viral hepatitis seems indicated. The disease can be extremely debilitating, associated with loss of time from work, severe weight loss, depression, and weakness. However, use of antiviral therapy in the individual case is difficult. This course of the disease is quite variable. Acute relapses are likely to be followed by spontaneous remissions. Furthermore, ultimate recovery is typical. The addition of an antiviral agent during this unpredictable period has to be weighed carefully. Nevertheless, the possibility that relapses in viral hepatitis are due to recurrence of viral replication during convalescence (17) makes antiviral therapy an attractive approach to ameliorating or shortening the course of prolonged or relapsing disease. Although there have been case reports of therapy of patients with prolonged or relapsing disease, there have been no adequate, prospective trials of treatment of this form of acute hepatitis.

## CHRONIC VIRAL HEPATITIS

Acute infections with HBV, HDV, and the agent of classical NANB hepatitis (HCV) can lead to persistent infection and chronic viral hepatitis. Actually, chronic hepatitis is more likely to eventuate from a mild, subclinical acute illness than from a severe, icteric acute hepatitis. Therefore, the evolution of acute to chronic disease often goes undetected. Indeed, the majority of patients with chronic hepatitis do not recall a history of acute disease or jaundice, and many patients are asymptomatic of the liver disease (19). These features make determination of the incidence or prevalence of chronic viral hepatitis difficult. It is estimated that 0.5–1% of the population of the United States have chronic hepatitis B and 1–2% have chronic NANB hepatitis (19). Chronic delta hepatitis is rare, affecting only 5–10% of patients with chronic hepatitis B (i.e., less than 0.05% of the population of the United States) (3).

Symptoms of chronic viral hepatitis are exceedingly variable. At least half of patients have no symptoms of liver disease (19). The most common symptom in the remainder is mild, intermittent fatigue. Patients with more severe disease may also have poor appetite, nausea, right upper quadrant abdominal pain, myalgias, and arthralgias. In any case, symptoms are often mild and intermittent.

The characteristic serum biochemical abnormalities of chronic viral hepatitis are mild elevations of serum aminotransferases (between two and ten times the upper limit of the normal range). Elevations in serum bilirubin and alkaline phosphatase, or decreases in serum albumin or clotting factor concentrations rarely occur unless the chronic hepatitis is particularly severe or cirrhosis is present.

Serologic testing indicates that chronic viral hepatitis is accompanied by persistence of viral replication. This has been best shown in chronic hepatitis B in which persistent disease activity has been found to be invariably accompanied by persistence of HBV DNA in serum or hepatitis B core antigen with replicative intermediates of HBV DNA in liver (19). Similarly, chronic delta hepatitis HDV RNA or antigen can be demonstrated in serum and/or liver in almost all patients (3,20). The state of viral replication in chronic NANB hepatitis remains unclear, but may be resolved once molecular probes for this agent are available (4).

Once complications of chronic viral hepatitis develop, the signs and symptoms as well as laboratory and serologic test results can change. The major complication of chronic viral hepatitis is the development of cirrhosis of the liver with its attendant problems of portal hypertension and loss of hepatocyte function. Worldwide, chronic viral hepatitis and, specifically, chronic HBV infection are the most common causes of cirrhosis. In the United States, chronic viral hepatitis probably accounts for only 20–30% of cases of cirrhosis, the majority of the remainder being due to alcoholism. Once cirrhosis is present, patients are more likely to have symptoms of liver disease, the most common being chronic fatigue, poor appetite, wasting, and weakness. Complications of portal hypertension include fluid retention, edema, and ascites as well as variceal and gastrointestinal hemorrhage. Mortality from hemorrhage or hepatic failure is common.

Immune complex or extrahepatic phenomena occur with some forms of chronic viral hepatitis. Arthralgias and even frank arthritis occur in a proportion of patients, particularly women with chronic hepatitis B. Both polyarteritis nodosa and membranous glomerulonephritis have been found to occur in chronic hepatitis B (21,22); whether they also develop in some cases of chronic NANB hepatitis remains unclear. Minor arthralgias, a nondeforming polyarthritis, cryoglobulinemia, and skin rashes also can accompany chronic hepatitis B. A rare but usually fatal complication of acute or chronic hepatitis (especially NANB hepatitis) is aplastic anemia (23).

A final complication of chronic viral hepatitis is primary hepatocellular carcinoma (HCC) (24–26). Both epidemiological and molecular biological evidence has firmly linked HCC with chronic HBV infection. Worldwide, HCC is one of the major causes of cancer mortality in humans, and chronic HBV infection appears to be the single major etiologic factor in the development of this tumor. Recent studies also indicate that chronic NANB hepatitis can lead to HCC (27). The majority of patients with HCC, regardless of etiology, are found to have cirrhosis.

Therapy in chronic viral hepatitis can be directed at ameliorating the disease itself or at prevention of its complications. Some patients with chronic viral hepatitis have troublesome or even incapacitating symptoms to disease, particularly fatigue. These symptoms can be severe despite the absence of cirrhosis or severe disease activity as assessed by serum biochemical tests or liver histology. Other patients with chronic viral hepatitis request treatment because of concerns regarding infectivity. This is particularly a concern to medical care workers and sexually active persons with chronic hepatitis B.

The major focus of therapy in chronic viral hepatitis, however, has been prevention of progressive hepatic injury and cirrhosis. Cirrhosis generally develops after several years of chronic hepatitis disease activity, the period preceding the establishment of cirrhosis ranging from as short as 1 year to as long as 30–40 years (19). Beneficial therapy or induction of a remission in disease at an early stage might prevent cirrhosis from occurring or at least delay its appearance. Even treatment of patients with established cirrhosis may be beneficial in halting the disease at an early "compensated" stage before intractable portal hypertension or hepatic failure supervenes.

Therapy of chronic viral hepatitis can also be directed at the extrahepatic manifestations of disease. Thus, resolution of the chronic hepatitis is usually accompanied by resolution of the extrahepatic manifestations (21,22).

Finally, therapy of chronic viral hepatitis can be directed at prevention of HCC. This desirable outcome may, however, not be responsive even to beneficial therapy. HCC seems to be a long-term complication of chronic viral hepatitis, developing after 10–50 years of disease. The role of the chronic viral replication and hepatitis disease activity in the development of HCC is controversial. Control of HCC would be better accomplished by prevention of hepatitis infection in general.

## HEPATITIS A

### HAV

Hepatitis A is caused by a 27-nm picornavirus that has been tentatively designated as an enterovirus (1). HAV has a single molecule of a single-stranded RNA that is 7,478 bases in length and demonstrates positive (plus) polarity (28,29). Hepatitis A is very contagious; it is spread by the fecal oral route, often by close personal exposure or by contamination of food or drink (1,30). The virus is highly resistant to environmental stresses surviving for long periods in water as well as in the acid pH of the human stomach. The virus passes through the gastrointestinal mucosa by an unknown mechanism (perhaps by an initial phase of replication in the intestinal wall) and spreads to the liver. Once inside the hepatocyte, the RNA genome is released and serves both as a template for translation of viral proteins as well as for transcription of replicative intermediates of negative RNA strands, which then serve as templates for the virion, genomic RNA strands (29). HAV RNA in liver exists as both single-stranded and partially double-stranded molecules. The translation product of HAV RNA is a polyprotein, which is then cleaved into structural, proteolytic, and replicative enzymic proteins. The structural polypeptides of HAV (VP1-4) assemble to form the nucleocapsid particle and are secreted in vesicles into bile and, to a lesser extent, into serum.

### Clinical Course

The typical course of hepatitis A is shown in Fig. 2. The incubation period averages 25 days (range, 15–45 days). During the incubation period, HAV and HAV-related antigen are detectable in stool. With the onset of disease, antibody to HAV (anti-HAV) appears in the serum. The initial antibody response is largely immunoglobulin M (IgM) class. IgM anti-HAV is, however, relatively short-lived and is no longer detectable after 6–12 months of onset. IgG anti-HAV, in contrast, slowly rises and is sustained for life. Serodiagnosis rests usually upon the finding of IgM anti-HAV in the serum of a patient with acute hepatitis. Specific and sensitive assays for IgM anti-HAV are commercially available.

### Experimental Models of Hepatitis A

HAV has been grown in cell culture and thus can be evaluated for its susceptibility to antiviral agents *in vitro*. Interestingly, in cell culture, HAV often leads to a persistent and noncytopathic infection (31). Vallbracht and co-workers (31) demonstrated that interferon-α inhibits replication of HAV in cell culture and can terminate persistent infections. Siegel and Eggers (32) demonstrated that several antiviral compounds that were effective against other picornaviruses had little effect on HAV rep-

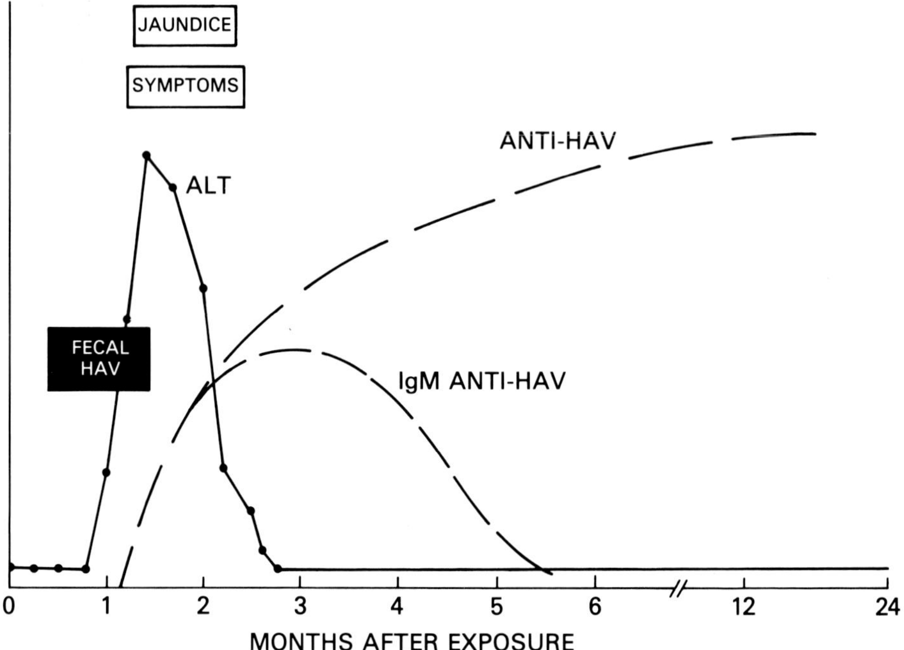


**FIG. 2.** The clinical, serum biochemical and serologic course of a typical case of acute hepatitis A. HAV, hepatitis A virus; anti-HAV, antibody to hepatitis A virus; ALT, alanine aminotransferase activity.

lication except at doses that were toxic to cells. Passagot and co-workers (33) screened 16 antiviral agents for efficacy in inhibiting HAV replication and found significant reductions in titer of virus with minimal evidence of cellular toxicity with seven substances: ribavirin, 2-deoxy D-glucose, protamine, amantadine, glucosamine, toxifolin, and atropine. Widell et al. (34) screened 20 antiviral substances and found maximal inhibition of HAV replication with amantadine and ribavirin, but at doses at which mild cellular toxicity was noted. Despite these promising *in vitro* studies, no antiviral agent has been evaluated in a controlled, prospective manner in experimental animals or humans.

### Therapy of Acute Hepatitis A

In humans, HAV infection causes an acute hepatitis only, not leading to chronic hepatitis or a carrier state (1). In view of the usually benign ultimate outcome of hepatitis A, the need for antiviral therapy must be questioned. Two situations, however, might require treatment: when the disease is particularly severe or fulminant, and when there is prolonged or relapsing illness.

Fulminant hepatitis A is rare, making it difficult to study a suitable number of cases of this disease to draw conclusions regarding the benefit of antiviral therapy. Levin and Hahn (35) treated seven patients with sporadic fulminant hepatitis using human interferon-α. Five of the 7 patients, including the single patient with fulminant hepatitis A, survived. These findings led the authors to suggest that interferon-α therapy might attenuate the course of fulminant viral hepatitis. Obviously, these results require further verification.

Hepatitis A can also result in a prolonged or relapsing course (16). Relapses can be severe and debilitating. At least one report has suggested that relapses are accompanied by reappearance of HAV excretion as measured by virus and viral RNA detected in stool (17). There have been no reports of therapy of relapsing hepatitis with antiviral agents.

### Summary

Thus, hepatitis A is usually a benign, self-limiting illness. However, the disease can be severe, prolonged, relapsing, and even fatal. Further studies in cell culture and in animal models to evaluate antiviral agents of potential use in hepatitis A are needed. Preliminary information suggests that trials of interferon-α or antiviral agents such as ribavirin for severe or relapsing acute hepatitis A are in order.

## HEPATITIS B

### HBV

Hepatitis B is caused by a 42-nm double-shelled DNA virus that is the prototype member of the family of viruses known as "hepadnaviruses" (hepatotropic DNA viruses) (2). The virus has an outer, envelope component of hepatitis B surface antigen ($HB_sAg$) and an inner, nucleocapsid component of hepatitis B core antigen ($HB_cAg$). Inside of the nucleocapsid core is an endogenous DNA polymerase activity with a single molecule of partially double-stranded, circular DNA (Fig. 3).

During acute and chronic infection with HBV, $HB_sAg$ is present in serum and liver in high concentrations, which makes detection of this antigen in serum a reliable marker for this infection (19). $HB_cAg$ is usually not detectable in serum unless special techniques are used to extract virions and remove $HB_sAg$, but $HB_cAg$ can be readily detected in liver, especially in chronic infections. Interestingly, a third antigen, $HB_eAg$, is detectable in serum and closely correlates with the presence of $HB_cAg$ in liver. Molecular biologic studies reveal that $HB_eAg$ is synthesized from the core gene but is not incorporated into the

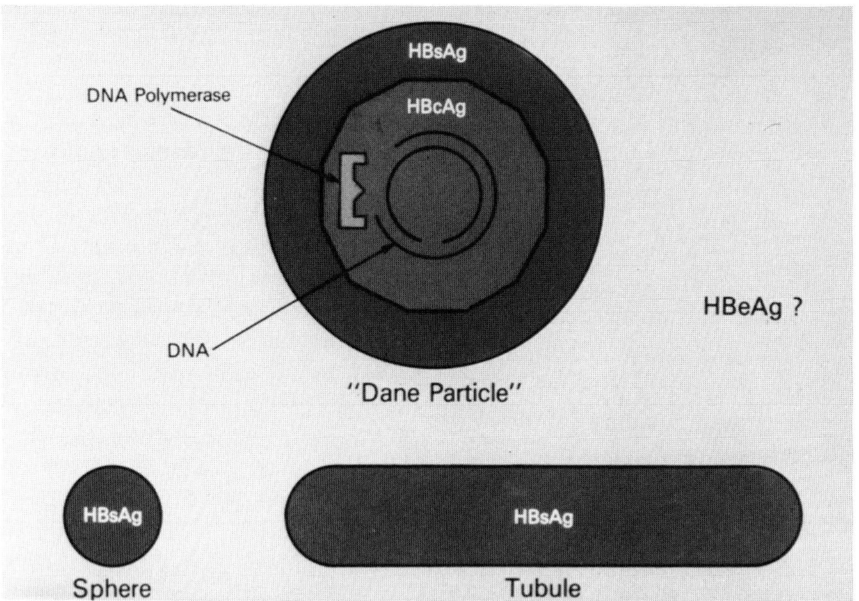


**FIG. 3.** The structure of the hepatitis B virus (HBV). $HB_sAg$, hepatitis B surface antigen; $HB_cAg$, hepatitis B core antigen; $HB_eAg$, hepatitis B e antigen.

nucleocapsid because of a leader, signal peptide that directs it to be secreted rather than to be associated with the endoplasmic reticulum (36). DNA polymerase activity and HBV DNA can be detected in serum during the early "replicative" phases of infection. These two markers are reliable means of assessing the activity of the infection and level of viral replication. Not all patients who have $HB_sAg$ in serum, however, have detectable HBV DNA and DNA polymerase activity. Such patients may be recovering from acute hepatitis B or may be carriers of $HB_sAg$, who produce $HB_sAg$ in serum but who do not appear to have active viral replication. These healthy carriers of $HB_sAg$ also do not have $HB_cAg$ detectable in liver or $HB_eAg$ in serum, and usually have inactive liver disease.

### HBV Genome

The HBV DNA genome is complex. One of the DNA strands (plus) is incomplete and the other strand (minus) is nicked (2). The 5′ end of the incomplete, plus strand is fixed in location (bp 1230) and is capped with a small protein (VPg). The 3′ end of the plus strand is variable in location so that the HBV DNA molecule has a single-stranded region that can vary from 10% to 60% of the genome. The negative strand of the HBV DNA genome is full-length, but its 5′ and 3′ ends are not covalently attached. This nick in the negative strand is fixed in location; the molecule is held in a circular conformation because of overlapping base pairs on either side of the nick. The reason for the peculiar structure of the HBV genome is not clear.

All of the genomic information is contained on the long, negative strand of HBV DNA. This strand has four open reading frames, *S* ($HB_sAg$), *C* ($HB_cAg$), *P* (polymerase), and *X*. The *S* gene has three potential initiation codons that divide the gene into pre-*S1*, pre-*S2*, and *S* regions (2,37). The gene also encodes for at least two glycosylation sites. As a result, there are multiple polypeptide forms of $HB_sAg$. The major S protein is 226 amino acids in length and exists in glycosylated (GP27) and nonglycosylated forms (P24). Medium S protein consists of the S protein with the 55 amino acid pre-*S2* region; it can exist in two glycosylated forms (GP32 and GP36). Large S protein consists of the S and pre-S2 proteins, with an initial 123 amino acid pre-S1 region; it exists in two forms (GP39 and GP42). The majority of $HB_sAg$ produced is in the small S forms. The pre-S antigens are relatively enriched on virions. The function of the pre-S antigens are unknown, but they may serve as receptors for the virion. The pre-S antigens may also be more immunologic than the major S antigen (37).

The *C* gene is also complex and has two initiation sites that divide it into a pre-*C* and *C* region. Synthesis of protein starting with the pre-*C* region results in the production of small molecular weight $HB_eAg$, which is secreted from the cell (36). Synthesis of protein starting with the *C* region results in the production of $HB_cAg$ (p26), which self-assembles in the cytoplasm into core particles.

The *P* gene is a large region that overlaps both the *C* and *S* region. The gene product is a polymerase that probably directs synthesis of DNA from both a DNA as well as an RNA template.

The *X* gene is a small protein of uncertain significance. Transfection assays suggest that the X protein is a transactivating factor that may be important in regulation of viral replication (38).

### HBV Replication

HBV replicates largely in the liver (Fig. 4). How the virus enters the hepatocyte is unclear; no specific receptors for HBV on hepatocytes have been identified. Once in the cell, the genome is released and the incomplete (plus) strand is completed by the DNA polymerase reaction. In addition, the long (minus) strand is ligated, covalently closing the nick and converting the genome to a covalently closed, circular "supercoiled" form (39). This form of HBV DNA is found in the nucleus of infected cells and probably serves as the progenome from which HBV RNA is synthesized. HBV is unique, in that the DNA is replicated asymmetrically through an RNA intermediate. Thus, the HBV RNA serves not only as a template for protein synthesis but also as a template for reverse transcription of HBV DNA. The HBV RNA "pre-genome" is taken up into $HB_cAg$ particles and reverse transcribed into DNA (minus strand). The single-stranded DNA is then used as a template to produce the plus strand. The virion is encapsidated with $HB_sAg$ and secreted before the plus strand is complete, yielding the typical HBV particle with its partially double-stranded molecule of DNA. This complex replicative cycle is typical of all the hepadnaviruses.

Review of the replicative cycle of HBV suggests several sites at which antiviral agents might interrupt viral replication (Fig. 4, steps 1–8). Most emphasis has been placed on inhibition of reverse transcription (step 6) or DNA synthesis (step 7), which would result in block in virion production. However, unless the pregenomic, supercoiled DNA is degraded, virion synthesis will start again as soon as the inhibition of DNA synthesis has ceased. To date, most antiviral agents that inhibit HBV replication have largely a temporary effect on virion synthesis, and virus production rises to pretreatment levels as soon as the antiviral agent is stopped.

The ability to degrade the more stable pregenomic forms of HBV DNA or to delete cells that contain this key form in viral replication is central to developing a successful therapy for acute or chronic HBV infection. Several possibilities exist. First, there may be natural host enzymes that gradually degrade virion DNA, even in a stable, supercoiled double-stranded form. Therefore, with prolonged inhibition of DNA synthesis, and thus blockage of formation of new HBV DNA molecules, permanent clearance of infectious virus may

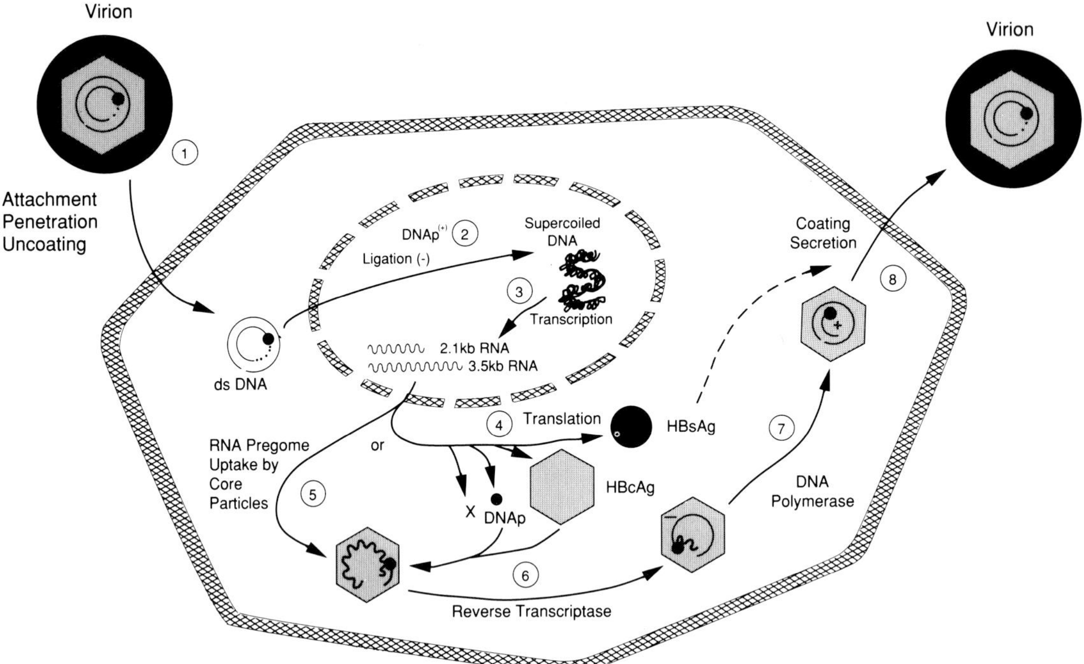


**FIG. 4.** The replicative cycle of the HBV. From *left* to *right,* the HBV enters the hepatocyte, the double-stranded (ds) DNA is completed by DNA polymerase activity ($DNA_p$) and a ligase to form supercoiled DNA. The supercoiled DNA is transcribed into two major RNA forms (2.1 kb and 3.5 kb), the larger of which (the RNA pregenome) can either be transcribed into viral proteins ($HB_sAg$, $HB_cAg$, DNAp or $HB_xAg$) or can be packaged into core particles and reverse transcribed into minus-strand DNA, which serves as a template for plus-strand DNA. The core particles with the HBV DNA are then coated and excreted (2).

be possible as levels of the supercoiled DNA decreased with time. Alternately, cells with the pregenomic DNA may gradually be deleted by immune clearance of HBV-containing hepatocytes. If there is not further production of infectious virions, infection will not spread further and viral replication may cease as new hepatocytes that do not contain infectious DNA are regenerated. These remain theoretical possibilities to explain successful outcomes of antiviral therapy.

## Clinical Course

The course and outcome of acute hepatitis B are variable (37). The serologic and biochemical events that accompany a "typical" case of acute hepatitis B are shown in Fig. 5. HBV markers appear in the serum during the incubation period of the disease. Initially, $HB_sAg$ is detected, followed shortly by $HB_eAg$, HBV DNA, and DNA polymerase activity. During this early, replicative phase, serum levels of HBV are highest.

After an incubation period of 1–4 months, clinical symptoms and biochemical evidence of liver injury appear. The disease typically lasts 2–8 weeks. Serum titers of HBV and HBV antigens begin to decrease with the course of the illness. The peak of serum aminotransferase activities usually coincides with the disappearance of HBV DNA and $HB_eAg$ from the serum. $HB_sAg$, in contrast, may persist throughout the illness and into convalescence, but is prob-

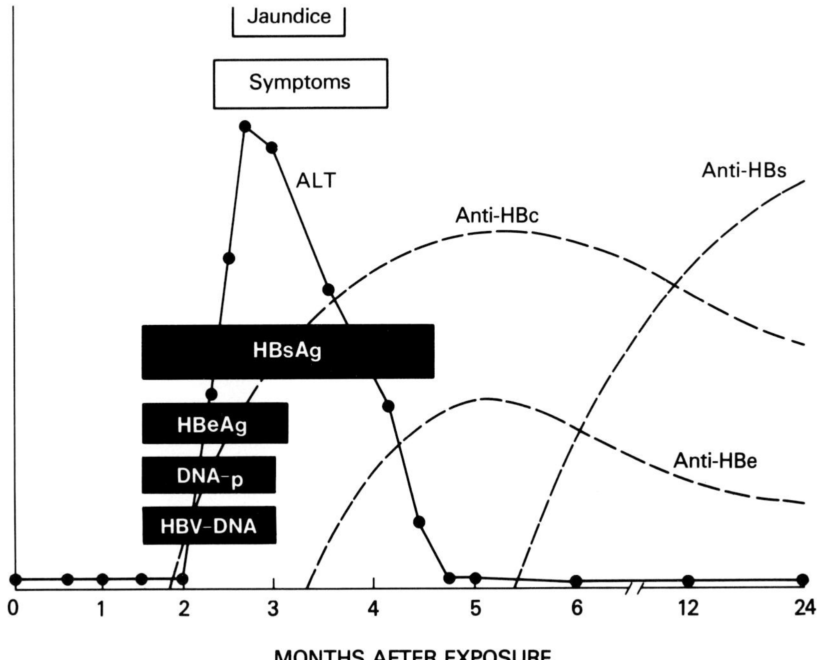


**FIG. 5.** The clinical, serum biochemical, and serologic course of a typical case of acute hepatitis B. $HB_sAg$, hepatitis B surface antigen; $HB_eAg$, hepatitis B e antigen; DNA-p, DNA polymerase activity; HBV, hepatitis B virus; ALT, alanine aminotransferase; Anti-$HB_s$, antibody to $HB_sAg$; Anti-$HB_c$, antibody to hepatitis B core antigen; Anti-$HB_e$, antibody to $HB_eAg$.

ably no longer being produced by the liver: the continued presence of this antigen being caused by the slow rate of clearance of $HB_sAg$. Patients who clear $HB_sAg$, however, recover from the hepatitis and are left with no residual liver injury or viral persistence.

Antibodies of HBV antigens appear sequentially during acute hepatitis B. Antibody to $HB_cAg$ (anti-$HB_c$) arises at the onset of illness and is a reliable serologic marker for ongoing or previous HBV infection. The initial anti-$HB_c$ response is largely IgM antibody, and specific tests for IgM anti-$HB_c$ can be used to make the diagnosis of acute hepatitis B. This diagnosis usually rests on the finding of $HB_sAg$ in serum of a patient with acute hepatitis. However, $HB_sAg$ can be present as the result of chronic infection, and $HB_sAg$ occasionally is short-lived and is no longer detectable at the onset of illness. In both of these situations, the correct diagnosis can be made by tests for IgM anti-$HB_c$.

Antibody to $HB_sAg$ (anti-$HB_s$) rarely develops during the acute disease but arises during convalescence, well after the loss of $HB_sAg$ from serum. This antibody is a reliable marker of immunity and recovery from hepatitis B. Patients with acute hepatitis often make only low levels of anti-$HB_s$; indeed, 10–15% of patients never make this antibody despite clearing HBV infection.

Antibody to $HB_eAg$ (anti-$HB_e$) appears in most patients with acute hepatitis B, shortly after loss of $HB_eAg$ from serum. This antibody can be short-lived and is usually not present in very high titer as a result of acute infection.

Not all patients with acute hepatitis B recover completely. A proportion develop chronic hepatitis B. The frequency of development of the hepatitis B carrier state varies based upon age, sex, and immuno-

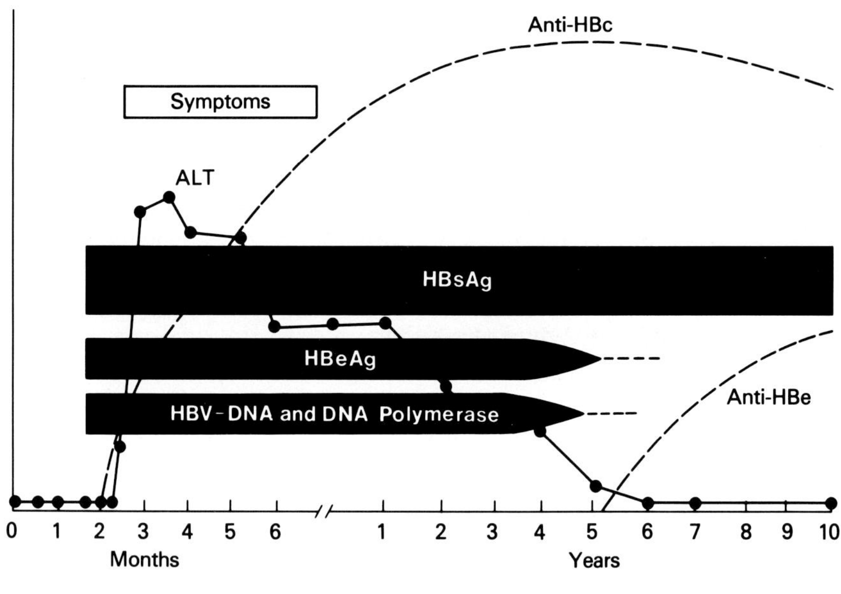


**FIG. 6.** The clinical, serum biochemical, and serologic course of a typical case of chronic hepatitis B. After a 5-year period of chronic hepatitis, there is a spontaneous improvement in disease, with fall of serum aminotransferase activities into the normal range and loss of serum markers of HBV replication despite continued presence of $HB_sAg$. $HB_sAg$, hepatitis B surface antigen; $HB_eAg$, hepatitis B e antigen; DNA-p, DNA polymerase activity; HBV, hepatitis B virus; ALT, alanine aminotransferase; Anti-$HB_c$, antibody to hepatitis B core antigen; Anti-$HB_e$, antibody to $HB_eAg$.

logic status (37). Newborn infants almost always develop chronic infection as a result of HBV exposure. In contrast, 20–30% of children and only 2–7% of adults develop chronic hepatitis B as a result of acute infection.

The course of a "typical" case of chronic hepatitis B is shown in Fig. 6. These individuals develop $HB_sAg$, $HB_eAg$, and HBV DNA in the serum during the incubation period of the disease. The subsequent clinical illness that accompanies the onset of chronic HBV infection is often subclinical and anicteric. Fewer than half of patients with chronic hepatitis B remember an episode of illness that might have occurred at the onset of infection (19). In addition, the rise in the serum aminotransferase activities is not accompanied by a fall in serum HBV DNA or antigens. Indeed, patients who develop chronic hepatitis B develop the highest levels of HBV markers in the serum. In these patients, $HB_sAg$, $HB_eAg$, and serum HBV DNA persist for years, if not for life. The antibody response is usually restricted to anti-$HB_c$ that arises at the onset of illness and usually reaches high levels. Anti-$HB_s$ is not detectable or is present in low titers only.

The clinical course of chronic hepatitis B is variable, and the activity and severity of the disease can change markedly with time. In some patients, the disease is rapidly progressive, the virus remains detectable, and the patient develops cirrhosis and disability from liver disease within a few years of onset of infection. In other patients, the disease waxes and wanes in severity, periods of mild disease activity are followed by exacerbations of disease, and the patient may develop cirrhosis after many years of infection. In other patients, the disease is mild or moderate, but ultimately the patient enters a spontaneous remission.

The example of chronic hepatitis B shown in Fig. 6 demonstrates an important feature of this disease: the presence of disease activity correlates with the presence of serological evidence of viral replication. Thus, the patient shown undergoes a spontaneous remission in disease activity after 5 years of having chronic hepatitis. Serum aminotransferase activities fall into the normal range, clinical symptoms resolve, and liver histology improves. This type of remission in disease is almost always preceded by loss of HBV DNA, DNA polymerase activity, and $HB_eAg$ from serum, and is often followed by the development of anti-$HB_e$. Thus, the termination of viral replication marks onset of remission in chronic hepatitis B. The continued presence of $HB_sAg$ despite the lack of serologic evidence of persistent viral replication is probably due to production of $HB_sAg$ by molecules of integrated HBV DNA that are capable of producing viral antigen but are not capable of reliably producing intact virions (2,25).

The seroconversion from $HB_eAg$ to anti-$HB_e$ is an important serologic event in the course of chronic hepatitis B that has both virologic and clinical implications. The loss of $HB_eAg$ from serum is the most sensitive and reliable serologic marker for eradication of viral replication, and patients who lose $HB_eAg$ from serum usually manifest a marked clinical and serum biochemical improvement in disease activity despite the continued presence of $HB_sAg$. For these reasons, the seroconversion from $HB_eAg$ to anti-$HB_e$ is usually used as the end point of successful antiviral therapy.

### Experimental Models of Hepatitis B

A major advance in the ability to assess new approaches to therapy of hepatitis B has been the identification of animal models of this infection. Four animal viruses similar to HBV have been identified and characterized: the woodchuck hepatitis virus (WHV) (40), the ground squirrel hepatitis virus (GSHV) (41), the duck hepatitis B virus (DHBV) (39,42), and the heron hepatitis virus (43). These agents share a similar morphology, genomic structure, and replicative cycle with human HBV and have been used with great success in analyzing the replication (39), natural history, and carcinogenic potential of hepadnaviruses (44).

Several of the animal hepadnavirus infections are appropriate models for evaluating antiviral agents for potential efficacy in hepatitis B. The Pekin duck chronically infected with DHBV and, to a lesser extent, the woodchuck infected with WHV have been used to analyze the antiviral effects of agents such as phosphonoformate, suramin, acyclovir (ACV), adenine arabinoside (vidarabine), dideoxynucleosides and Phyllanthus amarus (45–50). It must be stressed, however, that these animals are good models of the infection, but are poor models of the disease in humans. Most of the models are marked by a lack of active underlying liver disease and by very high levels of viral replication, two features that correlate well with a lack of a long-term beneficial response to antiviral medications in human chronic hepatitis B.

Also of potential importance in evaluating antiviral substances have been the recently reported tissue culture systems that support HBV replication. Continuous HCC cell lines have been transfected with cloned HBV DNA and made to produce virus in a pattern of replication similar to the human infection (51,52). In addition, infection of primary liver cell cultures with DHBV and WHV has been accomplished, which may ultimately lead to a tissue culture system that can be used to evaluate accurately agents of potential efficacy in inhibiting human HBV replication (53–55).

### Therapy of Acute Hepatitis B

Few reports on therapy of acute hepatitis B have been published. Indeed, patients with uncomplicated, acute icteric hepatitis B almost invariably recover without sequelae, and those patients who develop chronic hepatitis B usually have a mild, anicteric onset of disease (19). This was confirmed recently in a study from Greece using up-to-date serologic tests for acute hepatitis B that allowed for exclusion of cases of superimposed acute hepatitis (i.e., hepatitis A; delta, or non-A, non-B) in which all of 176 cases of acute, icteric hepatitis B recovered with clearance of $HB_sAg$ from serum and without residual liver disease (56). In view of these features of acute hepatitis B, antiviral therapy has been focused upon treatment of protracted or fulminant disease.

Levin and Hahn (35) treated seven patients with fulminant hepatitis using interferon-α, and five recovered, which suggested to them that interferon therapy was beneficial in fulminant viral hepatitis. No data were presented regarding the serologic markers of disease or effects of therapy on viral levels. Iwarson et al. (57) from Sweden treated a single case of protracted hepatitis B with human leukocyte interferon. The patient improved after 10 days of treatment with clearance of $HB_sAg$ and resolution of abnormal liver biochemical tests. These promising results must be viewed with caution as the usual outcome of protracted hepatitis B is recovery and clearance of virus.

Sanchez-Tapias et al. (58) from Barcelona, Spain treated 12 patients with fulminant hepatitis using recombinant human interferon-α. Nine patients had delta hepatitis (seven coinfection and two superinfection), two had hepatitis B alone, and one had hepatitis A. All except two patients with delta hepatitis died. Most patients no longer had detectable serum levels of HBV DNA when therapy was begun. These findings suggested that interferon-α therapy had no beneficial effects on the course of fulminant hepatitis B or delta.

In actuality, there is inadequate information on the effects of interferon-α or any antiviral agents as therapy of acute hepatitis B. No controlled observations of therapy have been published. Most patients that have been treated had advanced disease, and inhibition of viral replication probably would no longer be of benefit. Several multicenter trials of interferon-α therapy of acute hepatitis B are now underway. Antiviral therapy in acute hepatitis should be focused on amelioration of symptoms and shortening of the illness in patients with severe or protracted hepatitis, and not necessarily on improving mortality in fulminant cases alone.

### Therapy of Chronic Hepatitis B

#### *Early Studies*

The majority of efforts in antiviral therapy of hepatitis B and of viral hepatitis in general has been in treatment of chronic hepatitis B. This field was initiated after Merigan and co-workers from Stanford University reported on the successful therapy of a small number of patients with chronic hepatitis B using human leukocyte interferon and vidarabine (59–62). They demonstrated that both agents inhibited HBV replication as assessed by serial levels of serum HBV DNA and DNA polymerase. In many patients, this inhibition of viral replication was transient, and HBV DNA returned to pretreatment levels within a few weeks of stopping therapy. However, some patients had a sustained response, as indicated by a disappearance of HBV DNA and DNA polymerase from serum followed by a clearance of $HB_eAg$ and improvement in serum biochemical evidence of disease. Indeed, occasional patients not only lost $HB_eAg$ from serum, but also became $HB_sAg$-negative and developed anti-$HB_s$.

### *Three Responses*

The early studies of Merigan and co-workers generated great interest in antiviral therapy of chronic hepatitis B. These studies also laid the groundwork for understanding the mechanism of action of antiviral therapies in this disease by defining three types of response or outcome of treatment.

#### *Transient Response*

A transient response is defined by a lowering of HBV levels that is not sustained once therapy is stopped. Most patients treated with either interferon-α or vidarabine demonstrate an immediate decrease in serum HBV levels as monitored by either HBV DNA or DNA polymerase activity. Yet, the transient inhibition of virus does not appear to be particularly helpful, as there is no accompanying improvement in liver disease or long-term remission in hepatitis. An example of a transient response to interferon-α therapy in a patient with chronic hepatitis B is shown in Fig. 7. In this example, there was a decrease in serum aminotransferases after 3 months of therapy, although serum HBV DNA and $HB_eAg$ persisted. Once therapy was discontinued, serum aminotransferase activities returned to pretreatment levels, the patient remained symptomatic of liver disease, and follow-up liver biopsy showed no change in disease activity.

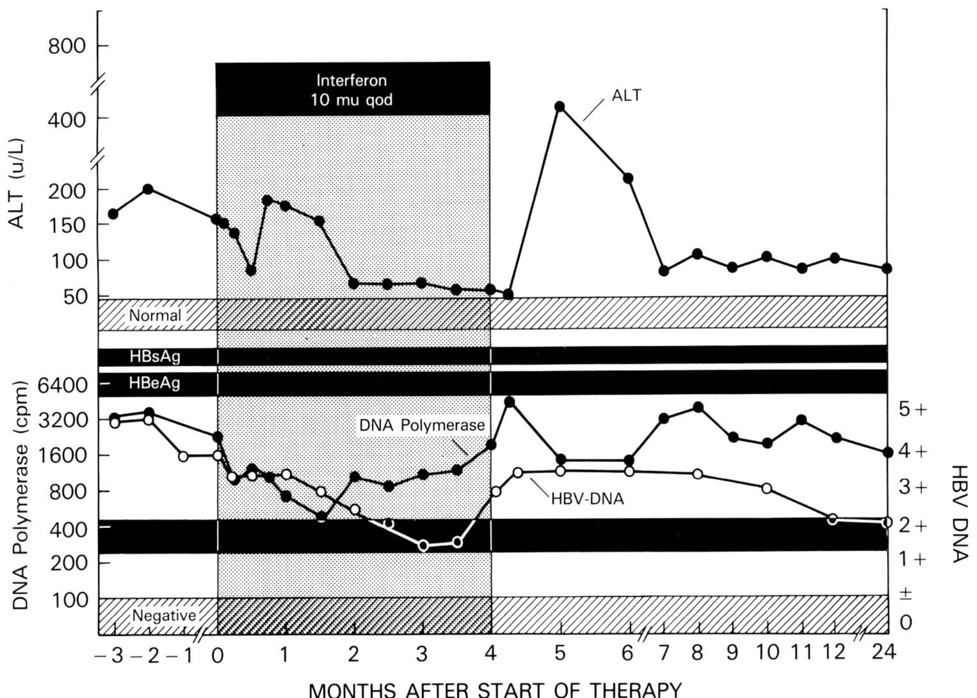


**FIG. 7.** The clinical, serum biochemical, and serologic course of a patient with chronic hepatitis B who had only a transient response to treatment with recombinant human interferon-α. During therapy, serum hepatitis B virus (HBV) DNA and DNA polymerase decreased, but hepatitis B e antigen ($HB_eAg$) and hepatitis B surface antigen ($HB_sAg$) persisted in the serum. Serum alanine aminotransferase (ALT) levels improved mildly during interferon therapy but later returned to pretreatment values (82).

*Partial Response*

A partial response to antiviral therapy is indicated by a disappearance of detectable serum HBV, as assessed by serum HBV DNA and DNA polymerase, along with clearance of $HB_eAg$ and improvement in the accompanying liver disease, but persistence of serum $HB_sAg$. An example of a partial response is shown in Fig. 8. These patients often have an exacerbation of the hepatitis with increases in serum aminotransferase activities while on therapy. The flare in disease activity usually occurs after 1–3 months of therapy and coincides with the disappearance of HBV DNA and $HB_eAg$ from serum. Once HBV is cleared, the accompanying liver disease improves despite the fact that $HB_sAg$ remains detectable in serum. Symptoms generally resolve, and follow-up liver biopsy reveals an improvement in the hepatocyte necrosis and inflammation. The remission in disease is usually sustained and represents a transition from chronic hepatitis B to the "healthy" $HB_sAg$ carrier state (19,63,64). Underlying the transition is the disappearance of active viral replication. HBV DNA is no longer detected in serum, and $HB_cAg$ is no longer detected in liver. Most revealing, however, is that replicative intermediates of HBV DNA, including supercoiled, single-stranded, and partially double-stranded molecules of HBV DNA, can no longer be detected in the liver (63). The continued presence of $HB_sAg$ in serum appears to be

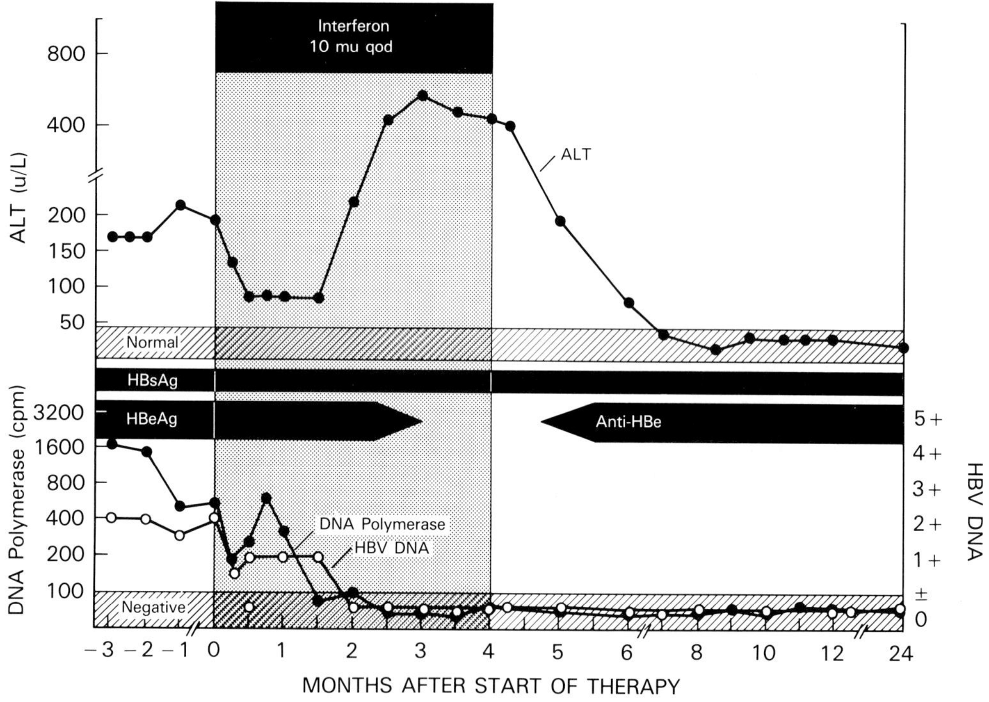


**FIG. 8.** The clinical, serum biochemical, and serologic course of a patient with chronic hepatitis B who had a partial response to treatment with recombinant human interferon-α. During therapy, HBV DNA and DNA polymerase fell to undetectable levels and $HB_eAg$ disappeared and was followed by the development of antibody (anti-$HB_e$). This patient remained positive for $HB_sAg$ but had a clinical remission in disease with serum ALT levels falling to normal. Four years later, this patient is still an $HB_sAg$ carrier but has no symptoms of liver disease and has normal serum aminotransferase levels (82).

produced by integrated molecules of HBV DNA, which retain an intact *S* gene but do not produce intact virions.

### *Complete Response*

A complete response to antiviral therapy is indicated not only by a loss of HBV DNA, DNA polymerase activity, and $HB_eAg$ but also $HB_sAg$ from serum (Fig. 9). The loss of $HB_eAg$ and $HB_sAg$ is followed by improvement in the liver disease, with a fall of serum aminotransferase activities into the normal range. This is the most optimal response to treatment but is uncommon. Many patients with this response ultimately develop anti-$HB_s$ and, therefore, have the serologic pattern of a resolved hepatitis B infection. These patients also have no $HB_cAg$ in liver and no replicative intermediates of HBV DNA in liver biopsies. However, some do have continued presence of low levels of integrated HBV DNA in liver. Although these patients have no evidence of progressive liver disease after having become $HB_sAg$ negative, some are left with an inactive cirrhosis as a result of the chronic hepatitis B and may yet suffer the consequences of portal hypertension or hepatocellular carcinoma. In this regard, it should be pointed out that 10–30% of patients with HCC that is suspected to have resulted from chronic HBV infection are no longer $HB_sAg$ positive when they present with liver cancer (63–65). These in-

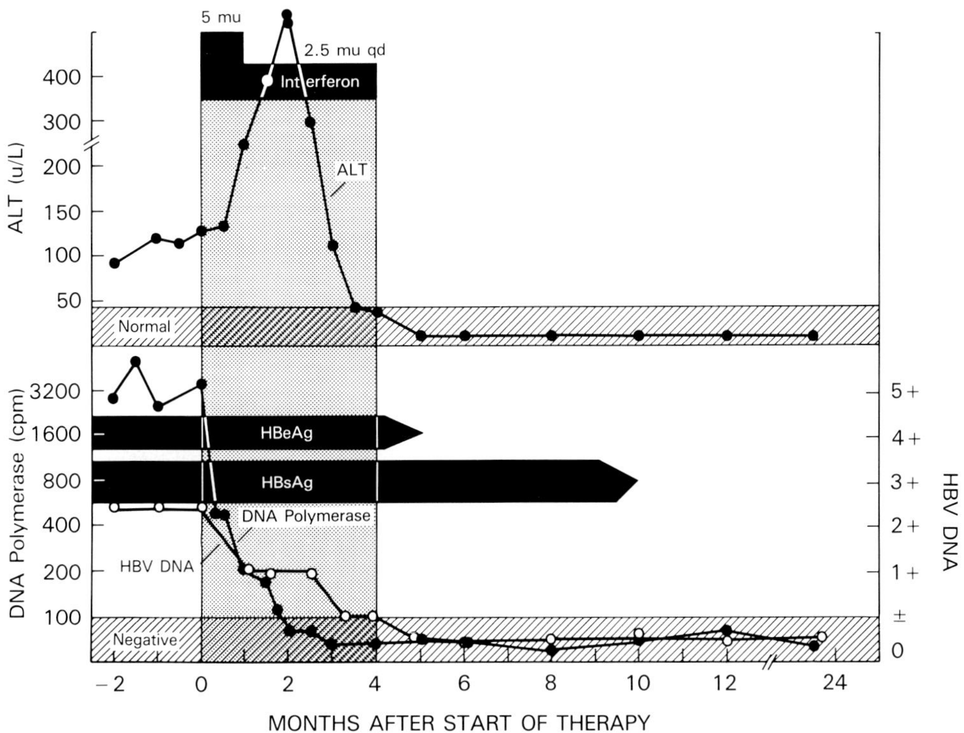


**FIG. 9.** The clinical, serum biochemical, and serologic course of a patient with chronic hepatitis B who had a complete response to treatment with recombinant human interferon-$\alpha$. During therapy, serum HBV DNA and DNA polymerase activity fell to undetectable levels. The patient later became $HB_eAg$ and $HB_sAg$ negative, but never developed antibodies. Three years later, the patient has no symptoms of liver disease and has normal serum aminotransferase activities (82).

dividuals, like the patients with a complete response to antiviral treatment, have anti-$HB_s$ in serum but may have cirrhosis along with integrated HBV DNA in liver tissue (25,65).

### *Adenine Arabinoside*

Initial studies on antiviral therapy of chronic hepatitis B focused largely on adenine arabinoside (ara-A; vidarabine) and its water-soluble derivative, adenine arabinoside monophosphate (ara-AMP) (62). Ara-AMP rapidly replaced vidarabine as the major drug of interest because it could be given by intramuscular injections whereas vidarabine had to be given by slow intravenous infusions. Table 2 summarizes six major, prospectively randomized, controlled trials of ara-AMP in chronic hepatitis B. Interestingly, three studies from the United States all failed to show any benefit of ara-AMP therapy: the rate of loss of $HB_eAg$ and HBV DNA from serum with therapy was no higher than what occurred without treatment (66,67) or with placebo injections (68). In contrast, three studies from Europe all demonstrated a statistically more frequent remission in disease after ara-AMP therapy than occurred in untreated controls (69–71).

Initial reviews of ara-AMP claimed that the low response rates to ara-AMP could be accounted for by the fact that most patients treated in United States studies were male homosexuals who were likely to have abnormalities of the immune system and not respond to antiviral treatment (72). However, in studies in the United States, the response rates were no lower among male homosexuals than among male heterosexuals (66–68,73). Furthermore, response rates in French male homosexuals were similar to the response rates in male heterosexuals (71). Other differences in these trials may relate to ethnic variations in response rates to antiviral therapy. Indeed, most trials of antiviral agents conducted on Mediterranean populations have yielded much higher response rates than trials on Northern European and especially Oriental populations (72,74). The reasons for these differences are unclear.

Thus, ara-AMP has not consistently been shown to be effective in eradicating chronic HBV replication. Another difficulty is the high incidence of neuromuscular toxicity that occurs with ara-AMP (73). These toxicities led to the withdrawal of this agent from clinical trials in the United States. The partial efficacy of ara-AMP should serve as encouragement for trials of other, less toxic antiviral agents.

**TABLE 2.** *Controlled trials of ara-AMP in chronic hepatitis B*

| First author (ref.) | *N* | Percent responding[a] | |
|---|---|---|---|
| | | Ara-AMP | Controls |
| Hoofnagle (66) | 20 | 20 | 20 |
| Perrillo (67) | 35 | 6 | 6 |
| Garcia (68) | 64 | 8 | 15 |
| Weller (69) | 29 | 40 | 0[b] |
| Ouzan (70) | 52 | 52 | 22[b] |
| Marcellin (71) | 43 | 33 | 0[b] |

[a]Response = loss of $HB_eAg$ within 1 year of starting therapy.
[b]$p < 0.05$.

### *Interferon*

The interferons are a group of host proteins that have antiviral effects on cells (75,76). Interferons are usually separated into three forms: $\alpha$, $\beta$, and $\gamma$ based upon cell of origin and antigenicity. A thorough discussion of interferon is given in Chapter 2.

Several forms of human interferon-$\alpha$ have been developed for use in humans, the most well known being lymphoblastoid interferon (Wellferon; Burroughs Wellcome, Research Triangle Park, NC), recombinant human interferon-$\alpha$A (Roferon; Hoffmann-La Roche, Nutley, NJ), and recombinant human interferon-$\alpha_{2b}$ (Intron-A; Schering Corporation, Kenilworth, NJ).

All three commercial forms of interferon-α seem to have the same spectrum of activity and toxicities, and studies using these three agents will be discussed together.

Interferon-α was first used in chronic hepatitis B by investigators from Stanford University (59–61). They reported the results of treating four patients using a buffy coat-derived interferon provided by the Finnish Red Cross (76). In three patients, serum levels of HBV DNA and DNA polymerase activity fell with treatment, and in two these viral markers as well as $HB_eAg$ eventually disappeared. In follow-up studies, one patient became $HB_sAg$-negative.

Further studies using leukocyte-derived interferon-α, carried out at Stanford University and in Europe, failed to yield as high a response rate to interferon-α as was originally reported (77). After an experience of treating 32 patients, the Stanford investigators concluded that interferon-α alone was usually not adequate to induce a long-term remission in disease (60,61). They went on to study a combination of interferon-α with ara-AMP, which in early studies was associated with a 40–50% response rate. However, in a prospective randomized trial, this combination was found to be less effective and led to a neuromuscular pain syndrome in over 90% of patients (68).

In a randomized, placebo-controlled trial of buffy coat-derived interferon from the Netherlands, interferon-α was found to decrease serum levels of HBV, but therapy for 1 month was not associated with a higher remission rate than that which occurred in controls (77). This study was faulted for using relatively low doses of interferon-α for 1 month only. Moreover, at the time of these studies, the only interferon-α available for use was expensive to produce and in short supply (76). These features dampened enthusiasm for interferon-α, at least until the middle 1980s when large amounts of highly purified recombinant and lymphoblastoid interferons-α became available.

When modern interferons-α became commercially available, several small pilot studies from the United States, Europe, Africa, and Asia suggested that 3–6-month courses of interferon-α would induce remissions in disease in 25–50% of patients and that a proportion of responders not only lost $HB_eAg$, but also lost $HB_sAg$ and developed anti-$HB_s$ (78–81). These pilot studies led to a large number of randomized, controlled trials conducted on six continents involving hundreds of patients. To date, only three of these randomized, prospective controlled trials have been published in complete form (81–83). Several other trials have been reported in abstracts and at scientific meetings. The results of these trials have been remarkably consistent: between 25% and 50% of interferon-α–treated patients have responded to therapy with loss of HBV DNA and $HB_eAg$ from serum, and subsequent clinical and serum biochemical remission. In contrast, only 0–15% of untreated controls had a spontaneous remission in disease during a comparable follow-up period. The results of three controlled trials conducted in Western countries are given in Table 3.

### *Interferon Dose and Schedule*

In all trials of interferon-α to date, the response rate to treatment has been higher than the spontaneous remission rate of concurrently followed, control subjects. The various trials have used different doses, schedules of administration, formulations,

**TABLE 3.** *Controlled trials of interferon-α therapy of chronic hepatitis B*[a]

| First author (ref.) | N | Percent responding[b] Interferon | Controls |
|---|---|---|---|
| McDonald (79) | 37[c] | 43% (18%) | 0% (0%) |
| Hoofnagle (82) | 45 | 32% (7%) | 7% (0%) |
| Alexander (83) | 46 | 26% (14%) | 0% (0%) |

[a]Two controlled trials from the Orient (85,86) are not included in this analysis.

[b]Response = rate of loss of $HB_eAg$ (in parenthesis is rate of loss of $HB_sAg$) from serum.

[c]Anti-HIV negative patients only.

and durations of therapy. Most schedules have not been adequately compared, but several general guidelines have become evident.

The duration of therapy with interferon in different studies has varied from 2 weeks to 6 months (78–83). Trials using only a few weeks of treatment have yielded poor results. Indeed, the serologic response to interferon therapy usually does not occur until after 8–12 weeks of therapy. These features have led to the recommendation that interferon therapy be given for at least 3 months. Longer periods of therapy have not been adequately evaluated, but in small numbers of patients, it appears that continuation of interferon-α for longer than 3–4 months does not increase the response rate to therapy (81). Most trials in the United States have used a 4-month course.

The dose of interferon-α used in most studies has been 1–18 million units (mu) given daily, every other day or three times weekly. The higher doses are associated with more side effects, but also with higher degrees of viral inhibition and higher ultimate response rates. Direct comparison of daily versus every other day interferon treatment has shown no difference in degree of viral inhibition (82). Furthermore, comparison of different trials suggests that high doses and intermittent therapy are optimal. A compilation of results from three studies conducted at the National Institutes of Health are given in Table 4 (82; and unpublished observations). The various schedules used were not compared in a concurrent, randomized fashion but were used in three sequential trials of interferon-α that employed identical designs and entry criteria. These and other studies suggest that three-times-weekly therapy with high doses of interferon-α yields the highest rates of response in chronic hepatitis B. Three-times-weekly therapy is also associated with better tolerance and compliance than daily treatment.

Thus, a 3- to 6-month course of interferon-α given in doses of 5–10 mu three

**TABLE 4.** *Interferon-α therapy of chronic hepatitis B response rates with different regimens*[a]

| Interferon-α dose regimen | | *N* | Number (percent) responding | |
|---|---|---|---|---|
| | | | $HB_eAg$ - | $HB_sAg$ - |
| 1 mu | qd | 10 | 1 (10%) | 0 (0%) |
| 3 mu | qd | 10 | 3 (30%) | 2 (20%) |
| 5 mu | qd | 16 | 4 (25%) | 1 (6%) |
| 10 mu | qod | 15 | 6 (40%) | 3 (20%) |
| 10 mu | tiw | 13 | 5 (38%) | 2 (15%) |

[a]All patients were treated for four months.

mu, million units; qd, daily; qod, every other day; tiw, three times weekly.

From ref. 82, and Dr. Adrian Di Bisceglie unpublished data.

times weekly to patients with chronic hepatitis B with well-compensated liver disease and $HB_eAg$ in serum can be expected to result in a remission in disease (partial response: loss of $HB_eAg$ and improvement in liver histology) in 30–45% of patients and an apparent cure of the chronic infection (complete response: loss of $HB_eAg$ and $HB_sAg$) in 5–25% of patients.

The early results of interferon-α therapy in chronic hepatitis B have been promising and important. However, many difficult issues remain unresolved: How can one identify patients who are most likely to respond to treatment? How can the response rate be improved? What can be done for nonresponders? What is the most appropriate therapy for patients with decompensated liver disease, extrahepatic manifestations, complicating diseases, or immunosuppression? How should one treat patients who do not have $HB_eAg$ or HBV DNA in serum but who have active liver disease apparently due to hepatitis B?

### *Determinants of Response*

Most large studies on therapy of chronic hepatitis B have attempted to analyze what features correlate with a successful outcome of treatment (82–84). The major features that have been found to predict a response to interferon-α therapy in published studies are summarized in Table 5.

In almost all studies, the features that correlated best with a response to treatment have been the initial activity of the liver disease as assessed by serum aminotransferase and the level of viral replication as assessed by serum levels of HBV DNA or DNA polymerase activity. In view of the typical pattern of these markers during a response to therapy (Figs. 8 and 9), it seems appropriate that the higher the aminotransferases and lower the HBV DNA levels at the start, the more likely that treatment will be successful.

Several trials of antiviral therapy have suggested that women with chronic hepatitis B are more likely to respond to therapy than men (61,82). However, this disease is rare in women: in studies from the United States and Western Europe, men have comprised 80–90% of patients with this disease. Thus, women are not only less likely to develop chronic hepatitis B, but are more likely to resolve it with treatment. A confounding feature in analyzing gender as a predictor of response to therapy has been the ethnic background of patients. Comparison of studies from Asia with studies from Europe and the United States has shown a remarkably lower response rate to antiviral therapy among Oriental patients (72,81,85,86). Ethnic variations in response to interferon-α have also been sited as the reasons for very high rates of response to interferon-α among Mediterranean patients and in blacks. The reasons for the ethnic differences in responses to antiviral therapy have been unclear. Human leukocyte antigen (HLA) differences do not seem to correlate with responses to treatment (82).

**TABLE 5.** *Features that predict a response to interferon-α therapy of chronic hepatitis B*

| |
|---|
| Disease activity (high serum aminotransferases) |
| Level of HBV (low levels of HBV DNA in serum) |
| Ethnic background (non-oriental patients) |
| Female sex |
| Absence of other disease (HIV positivity, renal disease diabetes, immunosuppression) |
| ?Age (adults) |
| ?Lack of homosexual exposures |

Data from references 80–86.

Ethnic differences in responses to interferon-α therapy may also account for the apparent low rate of response among children (86). Trials of antiviral therapy in chronic hepatitis B in children may be largely limited to Asian countries where low response rates have been reported. The other confounding feature in analyzing results among children is the fact that chronic hepatitis B is often mild in children who typically have low serum aminotransferase activities and high serum levels of HBV DNA. Thus, further studies in children with chronic hepatitis B are still needed.

Early studies suggested that male homosexual patients and patients with or without antibody to human immunodeficiency virus (anti-HIV) were less likely to respond to antiviral therapy than heterosexual patients (72). However, large prospective studies have failed to show a correlation between lack of response to treatment and sexual preference or even anti-HIV status (82). In addition, male homosexuals, and particularly those who are anti-HIV positive, are likely to have relatively low serum aminotransferase activities and high serum levels of HBV DNA (87). Thus, the confounding factors of disease activity and level of viral replication may be responsible for the relatively low rate of response in these patients. On the other hand, long-term follow-up studies indicate that anti-HIV positive patients are prone to have a relapse or "reactivation" of chronic hepatitis B, redeveloping HBV DNA and $HB_eAg$ in serum along with a recurrence of the chronic hepatitis (73). Reactivation of chronic hepatitis B can be transient or persistent and is often severe. Patients who have had a reactivation of disease after successful antiviral therapy have been retreated with interferon-α, sometimes with success. Thus, male homosexual patients should not be excluded from studies of antiviral therapy for chronic hepatitis B. However, the presence of HIV infection may adversely alter outcome.

Perhaps the major negative predictor of a response to antiviral therapy is the presence of a complicating illness or immunosuppression. These features have not been adequately evaluated prospectively because patients with other illnesses or who are on immunosuppressive agents are usually excluded from therapeutic trials. Small numbers of patients with renal failure, immunologic abnormalities, severe diabetes, and/or concurrent immunosuppressive therapy have been treated with interferon-α or ara-AMP. Results have been poor. The role of interferon in treating these patients deserves more thorough evaluation, especially in the situation of patients on chronic renal dialysis or patients who have received kidney, heart, or liver transplants, in whom chronic hepatitis B can be a major problem.

### *Increasing the Response Rate*

The major approach to increasing the response rate to interferon-α in chronic hepatitis B has been the use of combination therapy (60). Several combinations have been used, and many antiviral agents are currently being evaluated as possible single or combined agents for therapy of this disease. Table 6 lists some of the antiviral agents that are currently being evaluated as therapy for hepadnavirus infection in humans or experimental animals (45–50, 88–98).

Recombinant human interferon-β has recently been shown to have potent effects in inhibiting HBV and is promising as an alternative therapy for chronic hepatitis B (88). The effects of interferon-β in this disease, however, are not surprising in that interferon-β shares at least 70% homology with interferon-α and both interact with a common cell surface receptor (75). Interferon-α and interferon-β probably have

**TABLE 6.** *Antiviral agents of potential use in chronic hepatitis B*

| |
|---|
| Interferon-α (59–61,77–86) |
| Interferon-α (88) |
| Interferon-α (88–91) |
| Interleukin 2 (94) |
| Granulocyte-macrophage colony-stimulating factor |
| Thymosin (95) |
| Phyllantus amarus (47,96) |
| Levamisole (97) |
| Vidarabine (60–62,66–74) |
| Acyclovir (50,92,93) |
| Foscarnet (49) |
| Suramin (45) |
| Azidothymidine (46) |
| Dideoxynucleosides (48) |
| Ribavirin (98) |

similar actions and toxicities (88). The relative advantages of interferon-β over interferon-α are not clear, and it is likely that their toxicities are additive.

Interferon-γ has no homology with interferon-α and interferon-β, and acts on different cell surface receptors. Interferon-γ has been evaluated as therapy for chronic hepatitis B in several prospective studies (88–91). Unfortunately, interferon-γ has less antiviral activity against HBV but far more troublesome side effects than interferon-α. The combination of interferon-γ and interferon-α does not seem to provide any advantage over interferon-α alone (91).

ACV is a potent antiviral agent that has been used to treat herpes virus infections. It has mild inhibitory effects on HBV replication as well and has been studied in several therapeutic trials in chronic hepatitis B (92,93). Results of prolonged treatment have been disappointing. ACV is currently being evaluated in combination with interferon-α in this disease.

None of the other agents listed in Table 7 have been subjected to adequate clinical evaluation to assess their potential role as a single agent or combination agent in the therapy of chronic hepatitis B. Some are promising, whereas others are of doubtful efficacy or are impractical for use in humans, either because of difficulty of administration or toxicity.

### *Prednisone and Interferon*

Perhaps the most promising approach to increasing the response rate to interferon-α has been the use of a short course (pulse) of corticosteroids before starting interferon. The rationale for this approach arose out of the original observations by the Stanford investigators that concurrent corticosteroid therapy seemed to block the effects of interferon, but that withdrawal of corticosteroids immediately before starting interferon was associated with a high rate of partial or complete responses to interferon-α (60,99). Retrospective and prospective studies showed that corticosteroid therapy in chronic hepatitis B led to transient decreases in serum aminotransferase activities but marked increases in serum levels of HBV (99–102). These features suggested that immunosuppression caused an enhancement of HBV replication, a hypothesis supported by the finding of high levels of HBV DNA and $HB_eAg$ in immunosuppressed patients such as renal dialysis patients, patients on chemotherapy, and patients with acquired immunodeficiency syndromes (AIDS) (87). As a correlate to these findings, withdrawal of immunosuppression was often associated with a transient exacerbation of chronic hepatitis B and a decrease in serum HBV DNA and $HB_eAg$ levels that occurred 4–8 weeks afterwards (99–102).

A short course of prednisone by itself has been evaluated in small controlled trials (101,102). The results have been controversial. A pulse of prednisone may be harmful: it is rarely followed by clearance of HBV DNA, $HB_eAg$, or $HB_sAg$ from serum, and it may be followed by a severe and prolonged exacerbation of disease (100). This flare of hepatitis can be particularly severe in a patient with preexisting cirrhosis in whom variceal hemorrhage, hepatic encephalopathy, or marked ascites can develop during the exacerbation (101).

A short course of prednisone in combination with a subsequent course of ara-AMP or interferon has been evaluated in uncontrolled trials by several groups of investigators (103–105). Most studies have reported a high rate of remission in disease. Unfortunately, none of these studies have sufficiently controlled both for the spontaneous rate of remission in this disease and the rate of improvement with interferon-α alone. Prospective, concurrently randomized, controlled trials comparing interferon alone to prednisone followed by interferon are now underway (105). Until the role of prednisone pretreatment is clarified by controlled trials, it is prudent to reserve this approach for patients who have already failed treatment with interferon-α alone or patients who have mild disease.

In trials of short course of prednisone for chronic hepatitis B, the usual regimen employed has been a 4–6-week course of prednisone (or prednisolone) starting at doses of 40–60 mg/day and decreasing every 1–2 weeks. This approach should not be used in patients with cirrhosis, as such treatment can result in a severe, life-threatening flare of disease (102).

### *Atypical Patients*

Most prospective trials of therapy in chronic hepatitis B have studied patients with well-compensated liver disease, no complicating illnesses, and the typical serologic pattern of having HBV DNA and $HB_eAg$ in serum. Extrapolating results in this homogeneous group of patients to those with unusual features is not always possible. Three special groups of patients deserve comment: those with extrahepatic manifestations of HBV infection, those with decompensated liver disease, and those who lack detectable levels of $HB_eAg$ or HBV DNA in serum.

#### *Extrahepatic Manifestations*

Extrahepatic manifestations of chronic hepatitis B are uncommon; they include glomerulonephritis, polyarteritis nodosa, Raynaud's phenomenon, childhood papular acrodermatitis, mucocutaneous vasculitis, and arthritis (19,21,22). Two studies of patients with glomerulonephritis have demonstrated that a high percentage of patients with this complication of HBV infection respond to interferon-α therapy with a loss of HBV markers as well as with improvement in the renal disease (five of seven patients reported) (106,107). The temporal correlation between the amelioration of the glomerulonephritis and the loss of $HB_eAg$ supports the hypothesis that immune complexes of $HB_eAg$ and immunoglobulin account for the renal lesion. These results indicate that interferon-α rather than corticosteroids should be the treatment of HBV-related glomerulonephritis.

There have been no reported cases of polyarteritis nodosa due to HBV infection that have been treated with interferon. However, the poor prognosis of this condition when it is untreated compared to its good prognosis with prednisone treatment indicates that antiviral therapy should be withheld until immunosuppressive treatment has been evaluated (21). The good results of prednisone in HBV-related polyarteritis nodosa stand in contradistinction to the poor effects of corticosteroid therapy in uncomplicated chronic hepatitis B (100,108,109).

The other, less severe, extrahepatic complications of chronic hepatitis B are not common and should not be an impediment to the use of antiviral agents for the underlying condition. Indeed, correlations of the symptoms and signs of these manifestations with the outcome of therapy may help define the pathogenesis of these unusual features of this liver disease.

### *Decompensated Chronic Hepatitis B*

Patients with decompensated chronic hepatitis B represent a difficult group to evaluate in experimental trials of antiviral agents. The extremely poor prognosis of advanced cirrhosis due to chronic hepatitis B makes this group of patients prime candidates for some form of therapy (110). Currently, all that can be recommended is liver transplantation, which itself has a poor relative outcome in this disease as compared to other forms of cirrhosis (111). Small numbers of patients with advanced chronic hepatitis B have been studied in uncontrolled trials of interferon-α therapy (112). In several cases, therapy appeared to be dramatically beneficial. However, interferon therapy was almost always complicated in these patients by severe side effects. Most patients experienced an immediate and clinically apparent exacerbation of the underlying chronic hepatitis B with onset of antiviral therapy. The exacerbation, however, was accompanied by a decrease in serum levels of HBV DNA and was sometimes followed by a long-lasting remission in disease activity and gradual improvement in the clinical and serum biochemical features of disease. Patients with clinically apparent cirrhosis usually tolerated interferon poorly, and the dose had to be decreased rapidly to one-half to one-tenth of the starting dose.

Guidelines for therapy of patients with advanced disease are different from those for patients with mild to moderately severe chronic hepatitis B. Of course, patients who are moribund or who have extremely poor hepatic function (spontaneous hepatic encephalopathy or deep jaundice) have too little hepatic reserve to tolerate therapy and, even if therapy were successful in halting disease activity, are unlikely to survive with the little hepatic reserve that is left. On the other hand, patients with mild hepatic decompensation may tolerate therapy and an accompanying exacerbation of disease sufficiently to be treated with an adequate dose for a long enough period of time (2–4 months). Therapy of these patients should be undertaken only by physicians with experience with interferon-α therapy and availability of sensitive serologic markers for HBV levels. Deciding how to alter dose and how long to continue therapy requires information on the week-to-week changes in clinical status, disease activity, and serum biochemical and serologic findings, which include HBV DNA levels.

### $HB_eAg$ Negative

A final group of atypical patients with chronic hepatitis B that deserve comment are those who have active liver disease apparently due to HBV but who are $HB_eAg$-negative. The serologic pattern of HBV DNA without $HB_eAg$ in serum is uncommon in the United States and England but is frequent in other areas of the world, especially in the Mediterranean countries. Patients with antibody to $HB_eAg$ (anti-$HB_e$) and chronic hepatitis B may have severe liver disease and warrant some form of intervention (112–114). Results of antiviral therapy in a few patients in this category have yielded promising results; indeed, the response rate among anti-$HB_e$–positive patients may be higher than among $HB_eAg$-positive patients. An important factor, however, has been a high rate of relapse or reactivation among such patients. Studies from Italy suggest that these patients benefit from therapy but may require multiple courses (114).

### *Side Effects of Interferon*

The characteristics of the interferons, biologic activities, pharmacologic features, and side effects are presented in detail in Chapter 2. Several of the side effects of interferon-α need to be stressed in any discussion of therapy of chronic hepatitis B. Side effects are usually separated into two patterns: the early side effects that occur during the first days of therapy and the late side effects that appear thereafter.

At doses of interferon-α of 1 mu or greater, the first day of therapy is marked by the sudden appearance of fever, chills, fatigue, muscle aches, headaches, and nausea 4–8 hr after the first injection. The peak of fever may be 39°C and accompanied by shaking chills. Some patients report abdominal cramps and diarrhea. Because of these symptoms, patients should be kept in the hospital or at home for the first few days of therapy. This influenza-like syndrome usually lasts 4–12 hr, and its severity is clearly dose-related. In doses of 20 mu or greater, these early side effects can be severe and associated with confusion, delirium, seizures, hypotension, and cyanosis (78–80,115–117). There have been isolated reports of deaths from myocardial infarction in patients with preexisting heart disease given high single doses of interferon.

The early side effects with the first few injections of interferon can be ameliorated by acetaminophen given a few hours before the expected onset of symptoms. The side effects decrease with subsequent injections, so that by the second week of therapy there is usually minimal amounts of muscle aches and low-grade, if any, fever appearing a few hours after each injection. At this time, the late or chronic side effects of interferon-α begin to appear.

The most troublesome side effects of prolonged interferon-α therapy are fatigue and muscle aches, which can be dose-limiting. Many patients also report a difficulty in concentrating, and intellectual or academic performance can deteriorate. In 5–10% of patients, psychological side effects are severe enough that therapy must be altered or discontinued (115,117). The most typical psychologic side effects are irritability and depression. Some patients develop marked emotional lability. All of these symptoms resolve within 3–5 days of discontinuation of treatment.

Severe side effects from interferon-α are rare. The interferons are myelosuppressive, and therapy with 1–10 mu three times weekly leads to a 25–50% decrease in peripheral white blood cells (predominantly neutrophils) and platelet counts (82). Bone marrow suppression is most marked in patients with cirrhosis who may have preexisting decreases in peripheral blood cell counts because of hypersplenism (112). Patients with preexisting anemia can develop marked decreases in red blood cell counts. The myelosuppressive effects of interferon-α are reversed within a few weeks of stopping therapy.

Bacterial infections are the most important complication of interferon-α therapy. Perhaps as a result of the decrease in neutrophil count, patients on interferon-α demonstrate an increased susceptibility to bacterial infections, particularly urinary tract infections, sinusitis, and bronchitis. Cases of septicemia, lung abscess, brain abscess, and bacterial peritonitis during interferon-α therapy have been reported (80,82,112,115). Infections are particularly common in patients with preexisting cirrhosis. Any fever that appears after the first week of therapy should be quickly and carefully evaluated.

Acute psychosis, extreme agitation, and severe depression can occur with interferon-α therapy and all respond to discontinuation of treatment (115). These extreme examples of psychiatric side effects of interferon-α usually occur in patients with preexisting neurologic damage (hepatic encephalopathy, history of seizures or head trauma).

A further side effect of interferon-α therapy has been the development of autoantibodies with or without autoimmune disease. Autoantibodies develop frequently in patients treated with interferon-α (118), and these are sometimes accompanied by the appearance of autoimmune conditions, the most common being autoimmune thyroid disease, either hypo- or hyperthyroidism (119,120). Although more than 50% of patients develop autoantibodies, only rare individuals develop clinical symptoms or signs of autoimmune diseases. This complication of prolonged interferon-α therapy is still under intense evaluation, and the appearance of signs of autoimmunity during therapy may relate to an underlying autoimmune diathesis.

### *Summary*

Thus, antiviral therapy for chronic hepatitis B is still experimental. Recent studies suggest that a 3–6-month course of interferon-α in doses of 5–10 mu three times weekly will result in a clinical, biochemical, and serologic remission in 30–40% of patients with well-compensated liver disease and HBV DNA and $HB_eAg$ in serum. Features that predict a response to treatment include high initial serum aminotransferase activities and low levels of circulating HBV DNA. Oriental patients and children may be less likely to respond to treatment than Caucasian adults. Pretreatment of patients with a 4–6-week course of high doses of prednisone may help to increase the response rate to interferon-α alone, but this approach should be limited to patients with mild disease and perhaps to patients who have previously failed to respond to interferon-α alone. The best approach to treatment of patients with complications of chronic hepatitis B and atypical serologic patterns is still uncertain. The limited efficacy and the side effects of interferon-α therapy should be carefully weighed in the decision to treat patients with chronic hepatitis B. Future studies should focus upon the use of newer antiviral agents with or without interferon-α.

## δ (TYPE D) HEPATITIS

### HDV

Delta hepatitis is caused by a 37–40-nm RNA virus, HDV, which was initially described as a new and unique antigen found in the liver of patients with hepatitis B (121). Subsequent investigations showed that delta antigen was associated with a novel RNA virus, resembling a plant satellite virus or viroid, and that delta was a defective virus and could replicate only in the presence of HBV infection (3,122). Delta hepatitis occurs only in patients who have

$HB_sAg$ in serum and adds to the morbidity and mortality of acute and chronic hepatitis B.

The delta hepatitis virus is detectable in serum as a hybrid 37–40-nm particle that has an envelop protein of $HB_sAg$ and a nucleocapsid protein of hepatitis delta antigen (Fig. 10) (123). The HDV antigen exists as two related forms: 24 and 27 kd in size (124). Associated with HDV antigen is a small, 1.7-kb, circular molecule of single-stranded RNA with negative polarity (125–127). In the serum of patients with delta hepatitis, one finds $HB_sAg$, but in addition, one usually can detect HDV antigen (by Western blotting) and the genomic strand of HDV RNA (by Northern blotting). Titers of virus in serum can be as high as $10^{12}$ virions/ml (3).

In the liver, HDV antigen is found in the nuclei of infected hepatocytes, often in large amounts (3,121). Small amounts of HDV antigen can be detected in cytoplasm. The virus appears to replicate only in the liver and only in the presence of $HB_sAg$. In hepatocytes, HDV RNA exists in both genomic (minus) and antigenomic (plus) strands, some of which are greater than genomic length (126). These features have led to the suggestion that HDV employs the rolling circle model of replication, similar to that of viroids and plant satellite viruses (Fig. 11) (127). In addition, HDV has a "viroid" like region in its genome that has two autocatalytic sites that can self-cleave and ligate with small changes in cationic concentration (127), so that the replicative cycle does not require an endogenous endonuclease or ligase activity to cleave and reanneal the circular molecule of RNA.

HDV RNA has been cloned and sequenced. The genome is 1,689 bases in length, which makes it the smallest known animal virus genome (125,126). The genome has six open reading frames, but only one appears to encode a protein: the 24–27-kd delta antigen. Although the RNA molecule is circular in conformation, it also has many areas of homology and probably exists as a rod-like structure due to internal base pairing.

Several unusual features of the HDV replicative cycle and its association with HBV infection are relevant to a discussion of therapy. HDV requires $HB_sAg$ for replication, but the function of $HB_sAg$ appears to allow for HDV to enter and exit the hepatocyte as the replicative cycle itself can occur independent of HBV replication and antigens. Nevertheless, eradication of $HB_sAg$ would appear to ensure eradication of HDV infection. Unfortunately, clearance of

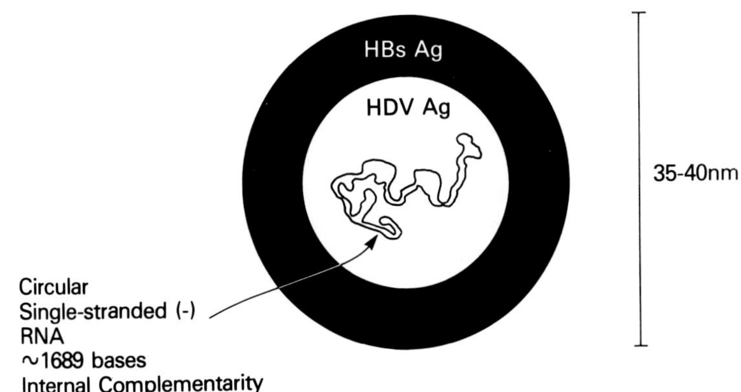


**FIG. 10.** The structure of the hepatitis delta virus (HDV). The outer envelope is hepatitis B surface antigen ($HB_sAg$), and the nucleocapsid is HDV antigen in association with which is a small, single-stranded circular molecule of HDV RNA (3).

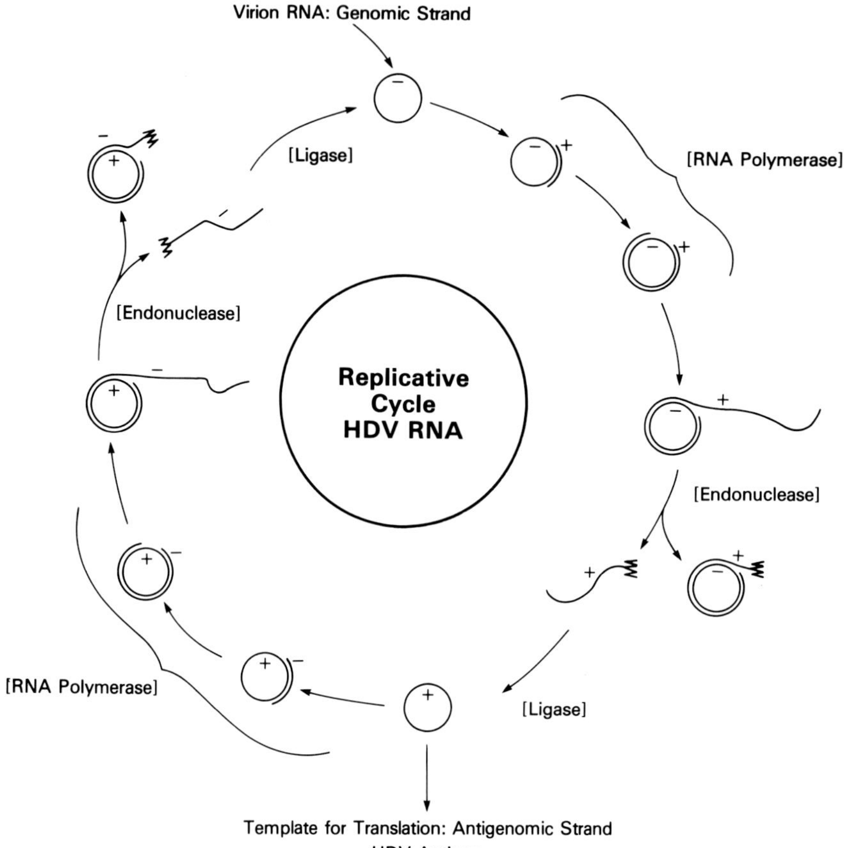


**FIG. 11.** The rolling circle model of replication of circular RNA genomes. In the case of HDV, the endonuclease and ligase activities are nonenzymatic and are performed at an autocatalytic site on the HDV genome (124–126).

$HB_sAg$ with antiviral therapy is rarely accomplished and may be even more difficult to achieve if there is concurrent delta infection (70–83).

The cycle of HDV RNA replication includes several points at which double-stranded RNA is present, which suggests a possible role for interferon-α in interrupting or inhibiting replication (75). Moreover, the similarity of HDV and plant viruses may allow for *in vitro* assessments of antiviral drugs. Finally, the availability of woodchucks infected with WHBV as well as HDV may provide a means of rapidly screening antiviral drugs of potential use (128).

## Clinical Course

Delta hepatitis can occur as either an acute or chronic hepatitis (3). Both forms tend to be severe; indeed, delta hepatitis stands out as the most severe form of viral hepatitis and as an important cause of fulminant hepatitis.

Acute delta hepatitis occurs in two forms: coinfection and superinfection. The term "coinfection" is used to describe simultaneous infection with both HBV and HDV, whereas "superinfection" refers to HDV infection occurring in a chronic $HB_sAg$ carrier. Both forms of acute delta hepatitis tend to be severe, and they cannot be distinguished from each other by clinical or serum biochemical findings alone. However, they can be separated on the basis of serologic markers as well as usual clinical outcome (122). Acute delta coinfection is, by definition, associated with acute hepatitis B, which is readily recognized by the presence in serum of IgM antibody to hepatitis B core antigen (IgM anti-$HB_c$) (Fig. 12). Acute delta superinfection is associated with the chronic $HB_sAg$ carrier state and often presents as a sudden deterioration or worsening of chronic hepatitis B (Fig. 13). Patients with delta superinfection test negative for IgM anti-$HB_c$. Both coinfection and superinfection can result in a severe or fulminant acute hepatitis. Coinfection usually resolves and rarely results in chronic infection. In contrast, most patients with delta superinfection develop chronic delta hepatitis.

Chronic delta hepatitis is usually the result of HDV superinfection of an $HB_sAg$ carrier. Chronic HDV infection often is severe and leads to cirrhosis of the liver in 60–70% of patients (129). The progression to cirrhosis can be quite rapid, and chronic delta hepatitis has a poor prognosis regardless of age or underlying health of the patient. Indeed, the severity of chronic delta hepatitis led to early attempts to treat this disease.

The diagnosis of acute delta hepatitis can be difficult. Acute infection is associated with a brief period of HDV antigen and RNA in serum followed by the appearance of anti-HDV (both IgG and IgM) (18,122). Titers of anti-HDV, however, are often low, and the antibody response can be transient. Thus, patients may not be correctly identified as having delta hepatitis if testing is restricted to serum antibodies. Unfortunately, tests for HDV antigen (124) and RNA (123) remain difficult research assays, which are not available to most physicians.

The diagnosis of chronic delta hepatitis is easier than that of acute disease. Patients will have $HB_sAg$ and high titers of anti-HDV in serum. The diagnosis can be confirmed by finding HDV antigen or RNA in

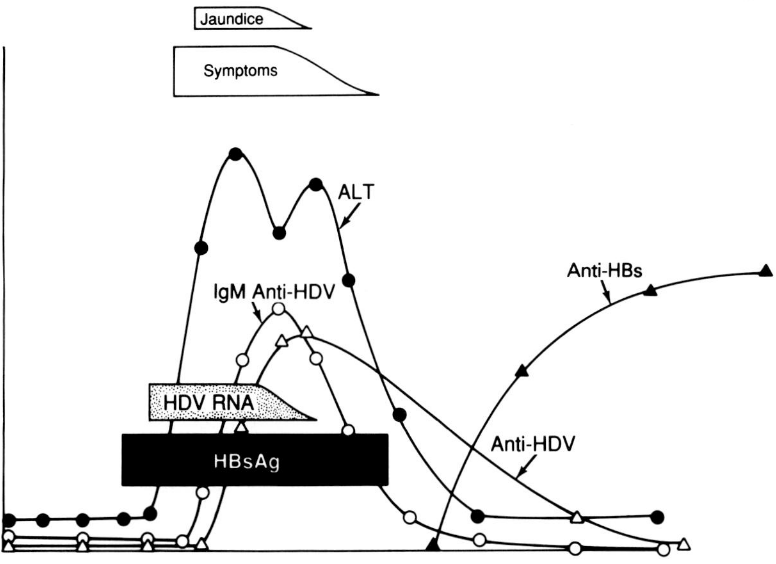


**FIG. 12.** The clinical, serum biochemical, and serologic course of a patient with acute delta coinfection. HDV, hepatitis delta virus; anti-HDV, antibody to HDV; $HB_sAg$, hepatitis B surface antigen; Anti-$HB_s$, antibody to $HB_sAg$; ALT, alanine aminotransferase.

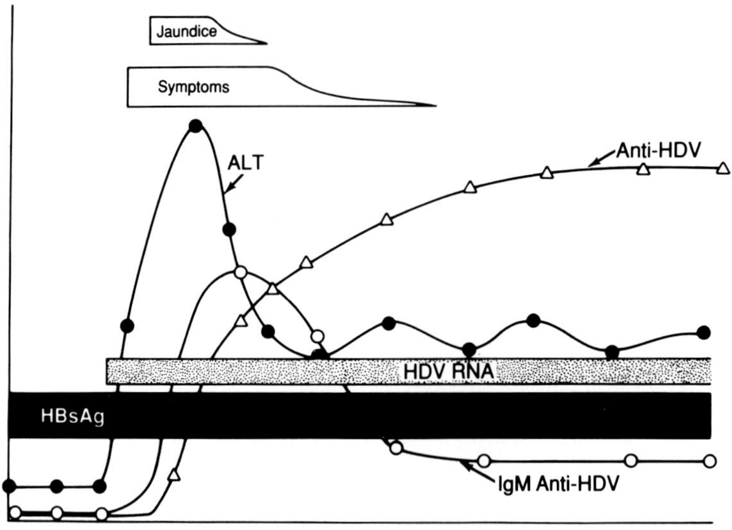


TIME AFTER EXPOSURE

**FIG. 13.** The clinical, serum biochemical, and serologic course of a patient with acute delta superinfection who develops chronic delta hepatitis. HDV, hepatitis delta virus; anti-HDV, antibody to HDV; $HB_sAg$, hepatitis B surface antigen; Anti-$HB_s$, antibody to $HB_sAg$; ALT, alanine aminotransferase.

serum or liver. Sensitive immunoperoxidase tests for HDV antigen in liver are available (130). In assessing effects of antiviral therapy, however, tests for HDV antigen and RNA in serum are important: indeed, the rapid decrease in these serum markers with antiviral therapy is the best evidence for efficacy of interferon-α treatment in this disease.

### Antiviral Therapy

There is currently no established therapy for either acute or chronic delta hepatitis. Interferon-α has shown most promise but is still experimental.

Investigators from Barcelona treated nine patients with acute, fulminant delta hepatitis with recombinant human interferon-α (58). Only two patients survived, one of whom developed chronic delta hepatitis and cirrhosis. These results suggested that interferon had little effect in this disease. Further studies are needed, especially in patients with severe acute or subacute disease. Currently, antiviral therapy of fulminant delta hepatitis should only be used in a situation where liver transplantation is available if the disease progresses. Survival after liver transplantation for fulminant delta hepatitis has ranged from 50% to 70% (111,131).

Investigators from Sweden have recently reported the use of foscarnet (phosphonoformate) in three patients with fulminant delta hepatitis, all of whom survived and recovered fully (132). Subsequently, another case of apparently successful therapy of severe delta hepatitis with foscarnet has been published (133). These preliminary results are encouraging, but foscarnet is still experimental and not commercially available for use in humans in the United States.

Most studies on antiviral therapy of delta hepatitis have focused on chronic disease. Retrospective analyses of large series of cases of chronic delta hepatitis demonstrated that corticosteroids are probably not effective in altering the severity or outcome of this disease (129). The lack of response to immunosuppressive agents and the severity of acute and chronic delta hepatitis led to trials of antiviral agents in this disease. The use of interferon-α has been most extensively evaluated.

Pilot studies from the United Kingdom (134) and the National Institutes of Health (135) suggested that interferon-α therapy decreased serum levels of HDV RNA and antigen and resulted in amelioration of disease in approximately 50% of patients. With therapy, serum levels of virus and serum aminotransferase activities decreased rapidly (Fig. 14). Follow-up liver biopsies revealed improvement in the necroinflammatory disease and disappearance of HDV antigen from the liver. However, discontinuation of treatment, even after 1 year of therapy, was invariably followed by relapse of disease and reappearance of serum and liver markers of HDV replication. Several patients in these series have now been treated continuously for several years with sustained benefit. Although the patients remain negative for HDV RNA and antigen in serum, liver biopsy has revealed a low level of HDV antigen (by Western blotting) and mild disease activity.

Investigators from Turin, Italy have conducted a randomized controlled trial of a 3-month course of interferon-α in chronic delta hepatitis (136). Twelve patients were treated with recombinant interferon-α, and 12 acted as untreated controls. Serum aminotransferase activities decreased in eight of 12 treated patients and became normal in four. Improvement in liver disease was invariably associated with a decrease in the amount of HDV RNA detectable in serum. In the control group, no significant change was noted in serum aminotransferase levels, although HDV RNA became undetectable in one case. Unfortunately, the effects of interferon-α were not sustained when treatment was stopped. Twelve months later, only one of the 12 treated patients maintained the biochemical and virologic improvement.

#### Summary

Interferon-α therapy results in a significant improvement in biochemical and histologic features of chronic delta hepatitis in at least 50% of patients. This improvement in disease is associated with decreases in serum and liver HDV RNA and antigen. Unfortunately, this improvement is not sustained, and relapses with return of disease activity and HDV RNA after treatment have occurred even with prolonged therapy. Therapy of chronic delta hepatitis should only be undertaken by investigators with availability of serologic markers for HDV replication and experience in using interferon-α. Therapy should begin with a dose of 5 mu daily and continued for at least 2 months. If a beneficial effect on HDV levels and serum aminotransferase activities is found, therapy should be continued indefinitely. The dose of interferon-α should only be decreased if side effects are intolerable. The decision to discontinue interferon-α should only be made if $HB_sAg$ becomes undetectable or if liver biopsy shows no evidence of continued disease activity or either HDV antigen or RNA by sensitive techniques.

It is obvious that other approaches to therapy of delta hepatitis are needed. Other agents such as ACV, ribavirin, and dideoxynucleosides deserve evaluation as therapy of this severe disease. Animal models of chronic delta hepatitis have recently been developed and hold promise as tools to screen antiviral agents for possible use in delta hepatitis in humans.

## CLASSICAL NANB HEPATITIS (HEPATITIS C)

### HCV

The genome of the viral agent that causes the majority of cases of NANB hepatitis in the United States and Western Europe has recently been isolated and characterized.

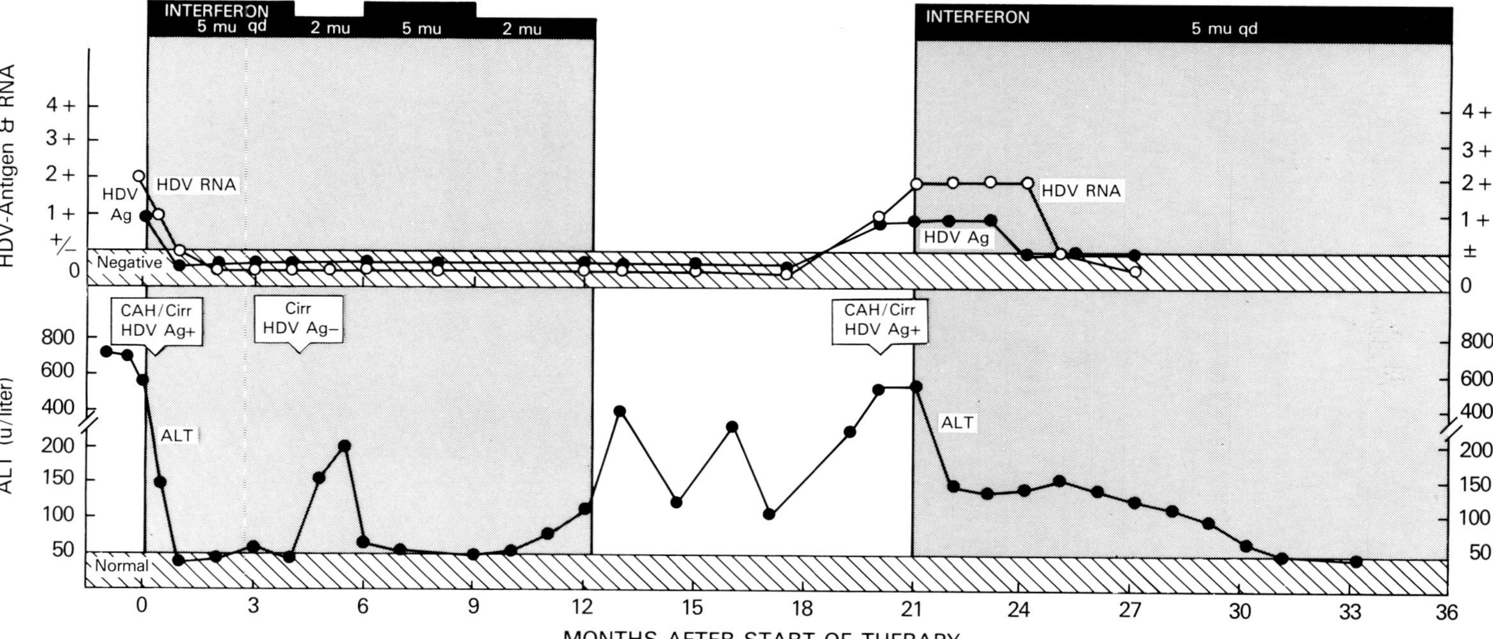


**FIG. 14.** The clinical, serum biochemical, and serologic course of a patient with chronic delta hepatitis treated with interferon-α for several years. Serum alanine aminotransferase (ALT) activity decreased with treatment, and serum levels of heptatitis delta virus (HDV) RNA and antigen (Ag) became undetectable with treatment. However, decreasing the dose of interferon or discontinuing therapy led to a relapse in disease. mu, million units; qd, daily; CAH, chronic active hepatitis; Cirr, cirrhosis.

Houghton et al. (4) from the Chiron, Corporation in California cloned an RNA from the serum of a chimpanzee that had been shown to be highly infectious in serial transmission studies in experimental animals. The RNA was single-stranded, approximately 10 kb in length, and demonstrated positive polarity and a single open reading frame. The nucleotide sequence has yet to be published, but characteristics of the genome and the size of the viral agent (30–60-nm by filtration studies) indicate that it is probably a flavivirus similar to yellow fever virus and other arboviruses. These findings allow for this agent to be called "HCV" and the disease it causes "hepatitis C."

Hepatitis C accounts for over 90% of cases of posttransfusion in the United States and for 20–35% of sporadic viral hepatitis (5–7). This disease is transmitted by exposure to blood and blood products, but the frequency of this infection in the general population suggests that other modes of spread are common. Whether these other modes are sexual exposure, fecal-oral exposure, or insect vectors (as is typical for other flaviviruses) is still unknown.

Using the cloned RNA of HCV, Kuo et al. (5) developed immunoassays for detection of anti-HCV. These assays allowed for the screening of blood samples for serologic evidence of HCV infection. Population surveys suggested that 0.7% to 1.4% of normal blood donors have anti-HCV. The antibody was detected in 50–90% of cases of posttransfusion hepatitis, in 50–60% of cases of sporadic NANB hepatitis, and in 60–90% of cases of suspected chronic NANB hepatitis. Furthermore, the majority of blood donors implicated in transmitting NANB hepatitis have tested positive for anti-HCV. These results suggested that testing for anti-HCV was a reliable means of detecting NANB hepatitis and would provide a valuable means of screening blood for this virus.

Unfortunately anti-HCV appears late during the course of acute NANB hepatitis, so that many patients test negative for this antibody when they first present to the physician (5). Thus, the assay may be less reliable as a serologic marker of acute NANB hepatitis. Serologic assays for anti-HCV may soon become commercially available and will permit screening of blood for this agent as well be a means of diagnosis of this disease. Questions still remain concerning the sensitivity and specificity of this serologic test and whether all cases of NANB hepatitis can be attributed to this virus. At present, it appears that the majority of cases of both transfusion acquired and sporadic NANB hepatitis in the United States can be attributed to HCV.

### Clinical Course

Classical, parenterally transmitted NANB hepatitis resembles other forms of viral hepatitis clinically (6,7,19,137). At least 75% of cases are anicteric. A fluctuating course of aminotransferase activities (ranging from normal to 10-fold elevated) is typical of hepatitis C. Most characteristic of this disease, however, is its propensity to progress to chronic hepatitis. In prospective studies after blood transfusion, over 50% of cases of acute NANB hepatitis have been left with chronic aminotransferase elevations, and liver histology in these cases usually shows some form of chronic hepatitis (137–139). Recent studies indicate that sporadic cases of NANB hepatitis are also likely to result in chronic hepatitis (140). The frequency of chronicity after hepatitis C (50–70%) is at least 10-fold higher than the frequency of chronicity after acute hepatitis B (1–7%).

Chronic hepatitis C is often mild and asymptomatic. However, 10–25% of cases eventually progress to cirrhosis, and a proportion of these patients will die of hepatic failure or the complications of portal hypertension (137–139). An example of the course of a patient with chronic, posttransfusion hepatitis C who developed cirrhosis within 2 years and who later died of hepatic failure is shown in Fig. 15. The course of chronic hepatitis C can also be prolonged and insidious, and patients may not develop symptoms for many years after onset of the chronic infection. Instances of hepatocellular carcinoma related to chronic NANB hepatitis have recently been reported (27). Most patients who develop liver cancer have had disease for more than a decade and have an underlying cirrhosis as a result.

### Antiviral Therapy

Conventional treatments are not effective for acute or chronic NANB hepatitis. The role of corticosteroids is not clear, but anecdotal evidence suggests that they are not helpful and may be detrimental (141).

There have been no reports of therapy of acute NANB hepatitis with antiviral agents. As in other forms of hepatitis, liver transplantation is currently offered as the best approach to improving the survival rate of fulminant hepatitis (17).

The knowledge that NANB hepatitis was caused by a transmissible agent led to attempts to treat this disease with antiviral agents. A pilot study of ACV carried out in five patients with chronic NANB hepatitis showed that a 10-day course of intravenous treatment had no apparent short- or long-term beneficial effects on levels of serum aminotransferase activities or liver biopsy histology (142). More prolonged courses of oral ACV appeared to be similarly ineffective.

Because of the marked effects of interferon-α therapy in chronic hepatitis B, pilot studies were started using this agent in chronic NANB hepatitis (143). Without markers for the viral agent, the only means of assessing the effects of therapy were liver biopsy and frequent determinations of the serum aminotransferase activities. Furthermore, diagnosis of NANB hepatitis rested on clinical and epidemiologic features (a history of exposure to blood or blood products before the onset of hepatitis). Using these criteria, a pilot study was begun at the National Institutes of Health

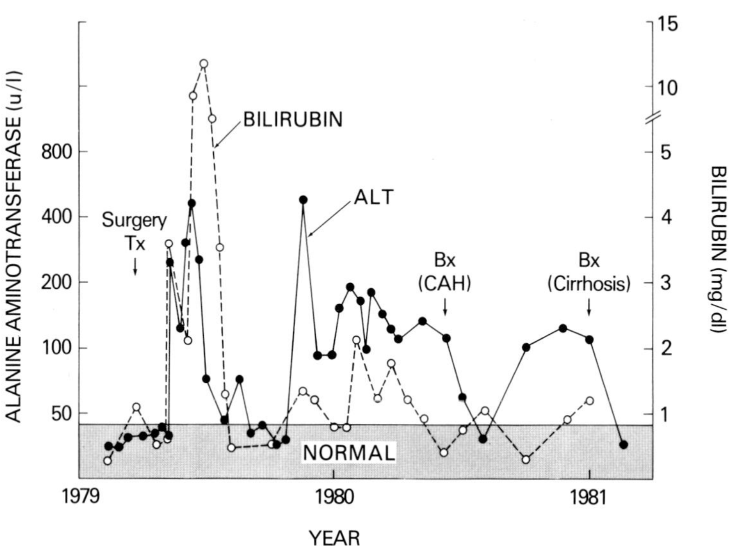


**FIG. 15.** The clinical and serum biochemical course of a patient who developed posttransfusion non-A, non-B hepatitis that progressed to chronic liver disease and cirrhosis within 2 years of onset. This patient later died of hepatic failure (137). ALT, alanine aminotransferase; Tx, transfusion; Bx, liver biopsy; CAH, chronic active hepatitis.

in 10 patients with well-documented NANB hepatitis (143,144). Eight of the 10 patients had a marked response to therapy, with decreases in serum aminotransferases within 1–2 months of starting treatment (Fig. 16). By the end of 4 months of therapy, serum aminotransferase activities were normal in six patients and minimally elevated in two more. Attempts to stop interferon after 4 months of treatment were followed by rises in serum aminotransferase activities to pretreatment values. However, subsequent retreatment was followed by improvement in serum aminotransferases, and sustained therapy was accompanied by sustained improvements in serum biochemical tests. After 1 year of therapy, all eight patients who had responded to treatment underwent a second liver biopsy, which revealed marked improvement in the degree of lobular inflammation, hepatocyte necrosis, and portal infiltration.

In this pilot study, interferon-α therapy was continued for 1 year in the eight patients who responded to treatment initially. Stopping treatment was followed by relapse in disease activity in two patients, but the remaining six patients have continued to be asymptomatic and five have continued to have normal (Fig. 17) and one minimally elevated serum aminotransferase activities 1–3 years after stopping treatment. These results suggested that a majority of patients with chronic NANB hepatitis respond to interferon therapy with an improvement in serum aminotransferase activities and histologic evidence of disease activity. Furthermore, the improvement in biochemical tests could be sustained in most patients with rather low doses of interferon-α (1–5 mu three times weekly). Therapy for 1 year resulted in sustained improvements in disease in over 50% of patients.

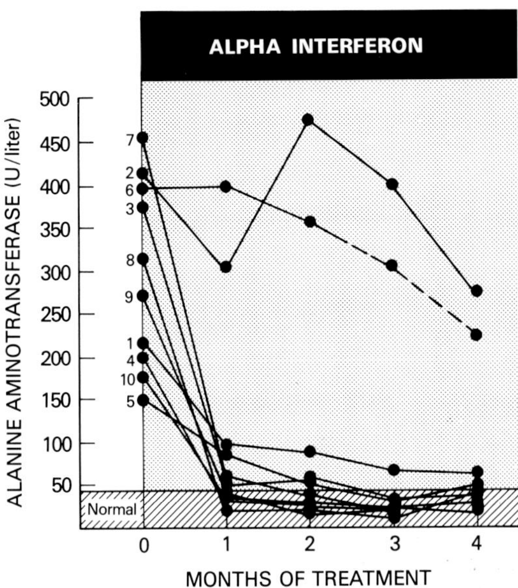


**FIG. 16.** Serial serum alanine aminotransferase activities in 10 patients with chronic non-A, non-B hepatitis who were treated in a pilot study of recombinant human interferon-α (143). Serum aminotransferases fell rapidly in eight patients and were within the normal range in six patients at the end of 4 months of treatment.

The results from this pilot study were encouraging and were supported by studies of leukocyte interferon from the United Kingdom (145) as well as by studies of interferon-β from Japan (146,147). These preliminary results led to a series of large-scale randomized, controlled trials of varying doses of interferon-α in patients with chronic NANB hepatitis (148–150). The results of these trials have not been fully reported. However, preliminary results support the findings of the pilot studies and suggest that 70–80% of patients with this disease will have improvements in serum aminotransferase activities with therapy, and in 40–50% of patients these biochemical tests of hepatitis disease activity will become normal. Therapy for prolonged periods is necessary to induce a permanent improvement in disease activity, and current findings suggest that a 12-month course of treatment is usually necessary.

Retrospective testing of serum specimens from patients participating in these studies of interferon-α therapy has shown that 80–90% of patients had anti-HCV (149,150). However, the absence of anti-HCV did not predict lack of response to interferon-α, and the presence of the anti-

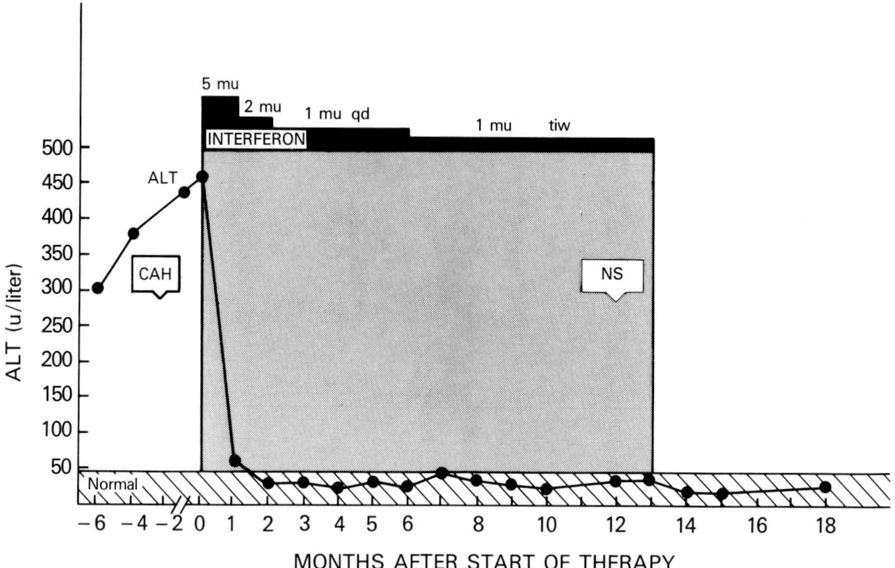


**FIG. 17.** The clinical, serum biochemical, and serologic course of a patient with chronic post-transfusion non-A, non-B hepatitis who was treated with interferon-α for 1 year and had a sustained clinical and serum biochemical remission in disease activity. Serum alanine aminotransferase (ALT) levels fell to normal within 2 months of starting therapy. Despite decreasing the dose of interferon, the liver disease remained in remission and liver biopsy, which revealed chronic active hepatitis (CAH) before therapy, showed nonspecific reactive changes at the end of therapy. This patient still has normal ALT levels and no symptoms of liver diseases 2 years after stopping therapy.

body did not predict a beneficial response to treatment. Obviously, molecular hybridization studies for the presence and level of virus in serum and liver are needed to fully assess the effects of interferon-α on chronic hepatitis C.

The availability of serologic assays for hepatitis C should allow many advances in the understanding of this viral infection and its prevention and treatment. Obviously, animal models are needed for this infection, and means of assessing antiviral agents *in vitro* would be helpful. The flaviviruses are RNA viruses that are quite sensitive to inhibition by interferon-α and several other antiviral agents including ribavirin.

## Summary

Interferon-α (and possibly interferon-β) shows great promise as beneficial therapeutic agents in chronic NANB hepatitis. Definitive studies that are at present underway should establish the role of interferon-α therapy for this condition with certainty. Future studies need to be directed at establishing the correct dose of interferon-α and the correct duration of therapy. Alternative therapies should be sought for those patients who either do not respond to interferon-α therapy at all or who have only a partial response with recurrence of hepatitis when interferon therapy is discontinued.

At the present time, antiviral therapy of chronic NANB hepatitis should be reserved for patients in controlled clinical trials. However, interferon-α is commercially available and may soon be listed as an indicated therapy for chronic NANB hepatitis. Because of the presence of severe disease that is rapidly progressive, some patients may warrant interferon-α therapy before it is approved as routine treatment for chronic NANB hepatitis. The recommendations given below are provisional and cautious.

Patients to be treated with interferon-α should first receive a full explanation of the state of knowledge about this disease and its treatment. The diagnosis of NANB hepatitis should be carefully made to exclude other forms of liver disease and confirm the diagnosis, if possible, by anti-HCV testing. The correct dose of interferon-α is still not known. We recommend starting treatment at a dose of 5 mu three times weekly. If there is no response in serum aminotransferase activities within 2 months, therapy should be stopped. If interferon-α therapy appears to be having a beneficial effect, therapy should be continued for at least 6–12 months. An increase in the dose of interferon-α may be appropriate in patients who seem to have a partial response only; i.e., serum aminotransferase levels have decreased by more than 50% but have not yet returned to normal after 2 months of treatment. If side effects are troublesome, the dose can be gradually decreased to as low as 1 mu three times weekly. However, lower doses of interferon-α appear to be less effective, and "breakthrough" with rises in serum aminotransferases to pretreatment levels is common when low doses are used. When treatment is stopped, frequent monitoring of serum aminotransferase activities is warranted. However, retreatment should not be commenced until serum aminotransferase activities have been elevated for at least 3–6 months.

## EPIDEMIC NANB HEPATITIS (HEPATITIS E)

### HEV

Epidemic NANB hepatitis was first described in 1978, when investigations of several large, water-borne outbreaks of hepatitis from India and Pakistan revealed that these epidemics were not due to either hepatitis A or B (151). Subsequently, Balayan and co-workers from Moscow identified a 27–34-nm nonenveloped, virus-like particle in the stools of patients during the incubation period of this disease (152). Convalescent serum from patients involved in outbreaks of this disease was able to agglutinate these stool-derived particles. Furthermore, inoculation of experimental animals with stool preparations harboring these virus-like particles was followed by the development of hepatitis and excretion of similar particles in the stools (152). These findings were confirmed and extended by several groups of investigators (8,11,153). The viral agent has not been fully characterized, but molecular hybridization studies suggest that this is a small RNA virus that may belong to the family of viruses called "caliciviruses." This disease has been called "epidemic" or "enterically-transmitted" NANB hepatitis, but with the identification of a viral agent it probably deserves to be called "hepatitis E" and the virus "HEV."

### Clinical Course

Outbreaks of hepatitis E have been described largely from underdeveloped areas of the world including India, Pakistan, Nepal, Burma, Russia, Central Africa, Algeria, Peru, and Mexico (8). These outbreaks have provided the basis for clinical descriptions of this disease. Imported, but no endemic cases, have been described from the United States.

Clinically, epidemic NANB hepatitis is a self-limited hepatitis that is often cholestatic (8,154). Hepatitis E does not lead to chronic hepatitis or cirrhosis, and no carrier state of the infection has been identified. The most striking clinical characteristic of this disease has been a high mortality rate in pregnant women: the fatality rate in pregnant women in epidemics of hepatitis E has been approximately 10% as compared to a rate of less than 1% among nonpregnant women and men. The reason for the high fatality rate in pregnancy is unknown.

Antibody to HEV (anti-HEV) can be detected by IEM in the serum of most patients with hepatitis during epidemics of this disease (152,153). Recently, a HEV-associated antigen has been detected in the hepatocytes of experimental animals (tamarins) infected with HEV (11). This fluorescence test can be modified to assay for anti-HEV. Anti-HEV was detected in all large outbreaks of epidemic NANB hepatitis. Interestingly, none of more than 30 cases of sporadic NANB hepatitis from the United States and Europe were found to be associated with anti-HEV. In contrast, several sporadic cases of NANB hepatitis from India and Pakistan have demonstrated anti-HEV reactivity. These results suggest that epidemic NANB hepatitis is a major cause of acute hepatitis in the underdeveloped world but is a rare cause of hepatitis in the United States. Obviously, this form of NANB hepatitis (hepatitis E) differs greatly from classical, blood-borne NANB hepatitis (hepatitis C).

### Antiviral Therapy

Enterically-transmitted NANB hepatitis is usually a self-limited illness requiring no therapy. Secondary spread from case to case is also rare, and the disease can be controlled by preventing contamination by sewage of sources of drinking water (8). However, the severity of this illness among pregnant women argues for search for a therapy of this disease. Full characterization of the agent of epidemic NANB hepatitis would help to guide investigators to appropriate antiviral agents. At present, interferon-α would seem to be the most promising agent to investigate in this disease.

### Summary

Thus, epidemic NANB hepatitis or hepatitis E is an acute, self-limited disease that has a high fatality rate in pregnant women. Hepatitis E occurs largely in underdeveloped areas of the world and is usually associated with a contaminated water supply. Antiviral agents have not been used in this disease and are probably not warranted in most cases. Identification and characterization of the hepatitis E virus may help to direct future investigations into therapy for severe cases or hepatitis occurring during pregnancy.

## REFERENCES


1. Lemon SM. Type A viral hepatitis. New developments in an old disease. *N Engl J Med* 1985;313:1059–67.
2. Tiollais P, Pourcel C, Dejean A. The hepatitis B virus. *Nature* 1985;317:489–95.
3. Rizzetto M. The delta agent. *Hepatology* 1983;3:729–37.
4. Choo Q-L, Kuo G, Weiner AM, Overby LR, Bradley DW, Houghton M. Isolation of a cDNA clone derived from a blood-borne non-A, non-B viral hepatitis genome. *Science* 1989;244:359–62.
5. Kuo G, Choo Q-L, Alter HJ, et al. An assay for circulating antibodies to a major etiologic virus of human non-A, non-B hepatitis. *Science* 1989;244:362–4.
6. Dienstag JL. Non-A, non-B hepatitis. I. Recognition, epidemiology, and clinical features. *Gastroenterology* 1983;85:439–62.
7. Dienstag JL. Non-A, non-B hepatitis. II. Experimental transmission, putative virus agents and markers, and prevention. *Gastroenterology* 1983;85:743–68.
8. Gust ID, Purcell RH. Report of a workshop: waterborne non-A, non-B hepatitis. *J Infect Dis* 1987;156:630–5.
9. Centers for Disease Control. *Hepatitis surveillance report. No. 51.* May 1987.
10. Francis DP, Hadler SC, Prendergast TJ, et al. Occurrence of hepatitis A, B, and non-A, non-B hepatitis in the United States: CDC Sentinel County Hepatitis Study I. *Am J Med* 1984;76:69–75.
11. Kraczynski K, Bradley DW, Kane MA. Virus associated antigen of epidemic non-A, non-B hepatitis and specific antibodies in outbreaks and in sporadic cases of NANB hepatitis. *Hepatology* 1988;8:1223.
12. Bernuau J, Rueff B, Benhamou J-P. Fulminant and subfulminant liver failure: definition and causes. *Semin Liver Dis* 1986;6:97–106.
13. Peleman RR, Gavaler JS, Van Thiel DH, Starzl TE. Orthotopic liver transplantation for acute and subacute hepatic failure. *Hepatology* 1987;7:484–9.
14. Krogsgaard K, Kryger P, Aldershvile J, Andersson P, Brechot C, Copenhagen Hepatitis

Acuta Programme. Hepatitis B virus DNA in serum from patients with acute hepatitis B. *Hepatology* 1985;5:10–3.

15. Brechot C, Bernuau J, Thiers V, et al. Multiplication of hepatitis B virus in fulminant hepatitis B. *Br Med J* 1984;288:270–1.
16. Gordon SC, Reddy KR, Schiff L, et al. Prolonged intrahepatic cholestasis secondary to acute hepatitis A. *Ann Intern Med* 1984;101:635–7.
17. Sjogren MH, Tanno H, Fay O, et al. Hepatitis A virus in stool during clinical relapse. *Ann Intern Med* 1987;106:221–6.
18. Aragona M, Macagno S, Caredda F, et al. IgM anti-HD in acute hepatitis D: diagnostic and prognostic significance. In: Rizzetto M, Gerin JL, Purcell RH, eds. *Hepatitis delta virus and its infection*. New York: Alan R. Liss, 1987:243–8.
19. Hoofnagle JH, Alter HJ. Chronic viral hepatitis. In: Vyas GN, Dienstag JL, Hoofnagle JH, eds. *Viral hepatitis and liver disease*. New York: Grune & Stratton, 1984:97–113.
20. Smedile A, Baroudy BM, Bergmann KF, et al: Clinical significance of HBV RNA in HDV disease. In: Rizzetto M, Gerin JL, Purcell RH, eds. *Hepatitis delta virus and its infection*. New York: Alan R. Liss, 1987:231–4.
21. McMahon BJ, Heyward WL, Templin DW, Clement D, Lanier AP. Hepatitis B-associated polyarteritis nodosa in Alaskan Eskimos: clinical and epidemiologic features and long-term follow-up. *Hepatology* 1989;9:97–101.
22. Takekoshi Y, Tanaka M, Shida N, Satake Y, Saheki Y, Matsumoto S. Strong association between membranous nephropathy and hepatitis B surface antigen in Japanese children. *Lancet* 1979;2:1065–8.
23. Zeldis JB, Dienstag JL, Gale RP. Aplastic anemia and non-A, non-B hepatitis. *Am J Med* 1983;74:64–7.
24. Beasley RP, Hwang LY, Lin CC, et al. Hepatocellular carcinoma and hepatitis B virus: a prospective study of 22,707 men in Taiwan. *Lancet* 1981;2:1129–33.
25. Shafritz DA, Kew MC. Identification of integrated hepatitis B virus DNA sequences in human hepatocellular carcinomas. *Hepatology* 1981;1:1–8.
26. Popper H, Shafritz DA, Hoofnagle JH. Relation of the hepatitis B virus carrier state to hepatocellular carcinoma. *Hepatology* 1987;7:764–72.
27. Okuda H, Obata H, Motoike Y, Hisamitsu T. Clinicopathological features of hepatocellular carcinoma: comparison of seropositive and seronegative patients. *Hepatogastroenterology* 1984;31:64–8.
28. Ticehurst JR. Hepatitis A virus: clones, cultures, and vaccines. *Semin Liver Dis* 1986;6:46–55.
29. Cohen JI, Ticehurst JR, Purcell RH, Buckler-White A, Baroudy BM. Complete nucleotide sequence of wild-type hepatitis A virus: comparison with different strains of hepatitis A virus and other picornaviruses. *J Virol* 1987;61:50–9.
30. Mijch AM, Gust ID. Clinical, serologic, and epidemiologic aspects of hepatitis A virus infection. *Semin Liver Dis* 1986;6:42–5.
31. Vallbracht A, Hofmann L, Wurster KG, Flehmig B. Persistent infection of human fibroblasts by hepatitis A virus. *J Gen Virol* 1984;65:609–15.
32. Siegl G, Eggers HJ. Failure of guanidine and 2(alpha-hydroxybenzyl)-benzimidazole to inhibit replication of hepatitis A virus *in vitro*. *J Gen Virol* 1982;61:111–4.
33. Passagot J, Biziagos E, Crance JM, Deloince R. Effect of antiviral substances on hepatitis A virus replication. In: Zuckerman A, ed. *Viral hepatitis and liver disease*. New York: Alan R. Liss, 1988:953–5.
34. Widell A, Hansson BG, Oberg B, Nordenfelt E. Influence of twenty potentially antiviral substances on *in vitro* multiplication of hepatitis A virus. *Antiviral Res* 1986;6:103–12.
35. Levin S, Hahn T. Interferon system in acute viral hepatitis. *Lancet* 1982;1:592–4.
36. Ou J, Laub O, Rutter W. Hepatitis B virus gene function: the precore region targets the core antigen to cellular membranes and causes the secretion of the e antigen. *Proc Natl Acad Sci USA* 1986;83:1578–82.
37. Hoofnagle JH, Schafer DF. Serologic markers of hepatitis B virus infection. *Semin Liver Dis* 1986;6:1–10.
38. Siddiqui A, Jameel S, Mapoles J. Transcriptional control elements of hepatitis B surface antigen gene. *Proc Natl Acad Sci USA* 1986;83:566–70.
39. Summers J, Mason WS. Replication of the genome of a hepatitis B-like virus by reverse transcription of an RNA intermediate. *Cell* 1982;29:403–15.
40. Summers J, Smolec J, Snyder R. A virus similar to human hepatitis B virus associated with hepatitis and hepatoma in woodchucks. *Proc Natl Acad Sci USA* 1978;75:4533–7.
41. Marion PL, Oshiro LS, Regnery DS, et al. A virus in Beechey ground squirrels which is related to hepatitis B virus of man. *Proc Natl Acad Sci USA* 1980;77:2941–5.
42. Mason WS, Seal S, Summers J. Virus of Pekin ducks with structural and biological relatedness to human hepatitis B virus. *J Virol* 1980;36:829–36.
43. Sprengel R, Kaleta EF, Will H. Isolation and characterization of a hepatitis B virus endemic in herons. *J Virol* 1988;62:3832–9.
44. Popper H, Roth L, Purcell RH, et al. Hepatocarcinogenicity of the woodchuck hepatitis virus. *Proc Natl Acad Sci USA* 1986;83:4543–6.
45. Tsiquaye K, Zuckerman A. Suramin inhibits duck hepatitis B virus DNA polymerase activity. *J Hepatol* 1985;1:663–9.
46. Tsiquaye KN, Collins P, Zuckerman AJ. Screening of antiviral drugs for treatment of hepatitis B. *J Hepatol* 1986;3:S45–8.
47. Venkateswaran PS, Millman I, Blumberg BS. Effects of an extract from *Phyllanthus niruir* on hepatitis B and woodchuck hepatitis viruses. *In vitro* and *in vivo* studies. *Proc Natl Acad Sci USA* 1987;84:274–8.

48. Kassianides C, Hoofnagle JH, Miller RH, et at. Effects of 2′,3′-dideoxycytidine on duck hepatitis B virus. *Gastroenterology* 1988; 94:A552.
49. Sherker Ah, Hirota K, Omata M, Okuda K. Foscarnet decreases serum and liver duck hepatitis B virus DNA in chronically infected ducks. *Gastroenterology* 1986;91:818–24.
50. Hantz O, Allaudeen HS, Ooka T, De Clerq, Trepo C. Inhibition of human and woodchuck hepatitis virus DNA polymerase by the triphosphates of acyclovir, 1-(2′deoxy-2′-fluoro-B-D-arabinofuranosyl)-5-iodocytosine and E-5-(2-bromovinyl)-2′-deoxyuridine. *Antiviral Res* 1984;4:187–99.
51. Sells MA, Chen M-L, Acs G. Production of hepatitis B virus in Hep G2 cells transfected with cloned hepatitis B virus DNA. *Proc Natl Acad Sci USA* 1987;84:1005–9.
52. Sureau C, Romet-Lemonne J-L, Mullins JI, et al. Production of hepatitis B virus by a differentiated human hepatoma cell line after transfection with cloned circular HBV DNA. *Cell* 1986;47:37–47.
53. Tuttleman JS, Pugh JC, Summers JW. *In vitro* experimental infection of primary duck hepatocyte cultures with duck hepatitis B virus. *J Virol* 1986;58:17–25.
54. Taylor J, Mason W, Summers J, et al. Replication of human hepatitis delta virus in primary cultures of woodchuck hepatocytes. *J Virol* 1987;61:2891–5.
55. Fourel I, Gripon P, Hantz O, et al. Prolonged duck hepatitis B virus replication in epithelial cells: a useful system for antiviral testing. *Hepatology* 1989;10:186–91.
56. Roumeliotou-Karayannis A, Tassopoulos N, Richardson SC, Kalafatas P, Papaevangelou G. How often does chronic liver disease follow acute hepatitis B in adults? *Infection* 1985; 13:174–6.
57. Iwarson S, Norkrans G, Nodenfelt E, Hagberg R. Interferon treatment in acute hepatitis B infection with prolonged course. *Scand J Infect Dis* 1980;12:233–4.
58. Sanchez-Tapias JM, Mas A, Bruguera M, et al. Recombinant alpha-2c-interferon therapy in fulminant viral hepatitis. *J Hepatology* 1987;5:205–10.
59. Greenberg HB, Pollard RB, Lutwick LI, et al. Effect of human leukocyte interferon on hepatitis B virus infection in patients with chronic active hepatitis. *N Engl J Med* 1976;295:517–22.
60. Scullard GH, Pollard RB, Smith JL, et al. Antiviral treatment of chronic hepatitis B virus infection. I. Changes in viral markers with interferon combined with adenine arabinoside. *J Infect Dis* 1981;143:722–83.
61. Scullard GH, Andres L, Greenberg HB, et al. Antiviral treatment of chronic hepatitis B virus infection: improvement in liver disease with interferon and adenine arabinoside. *Hepatology* 1981;1:228–32.
62. Pollard RB, Smith JL, Neal A, Gregory PB, Merigan TC, Robinson WS. Effect of vidarabine on chronic hepatitis B virus infection. *JAMA* 1978;239:1648–50.
63. Di Bisceglie AM, Waggoner JG, Hoofnagle JH. Hepatitis B virus deoxyribonucleic acid in liver of chronic carriers. *Gastroenterology* 1987;93:1236–41.
64. Hoofnagle JH, Shafritz DA, Popper H. Chronic type B hepatitis and the "healthy" $HB_sAg$ carrier state. *Hepatology* 1987;7:758–63.
65. Shafritz DA, Kew MC. Identification of integrated hepatitis B virus DNA sequences in human hepatocellular carcinomas. *Hepatology* 1:1:1–8.
66. Hoofnagle JH, Hanson RG, Minuk GY, et al. Randomized controlled trial of adenine arabinoside monophosphate for chronic type B hepatitis. *Gastroenterology* 1984;86:150–7.
67. Perillo RP, Regenstein FG, Bodicky CJ, Campbell CR, Sanders GE, Sunwoo YT. Comparative efficacy of adenine arabinoside 5′ monophosphate and prednisone withdrawal followed by adenine arabinoside 5′ monophosphate in the treatment of chronic active hepatitis B. *Gastroenterology* 1985;88:780–6.
68. Garcia G, Smith CI, Weissberg JI, et al. Adenine arabinoside monophosphate in combination with human leukocyte interferon in the treatment of chronic hepatitis B. A randomized, double-blind, placebo-controlled trial. *Ann Intern Med* 1987;107:278–85.
69. Weller IVD, Lok ASF, Mindel A, et al. Randomized controlled trial of adenine arabinoside 5′-monophosphate (ara-AMP) in chronic hepatitis B virus infection. *Gut* 1985;26:745–51.
70. Ouzan D, Chevallier M, Laffranchi B, et al. Therapeutic efficacy of ara-AMP in symptomatic $HB_eAg$ positive CAH. A randomized placebo control study in heterosexuals. *Hepatology* 1986;6:1151.
71. Marcellin P, Ouzan D, Degos F, et al. Randomized controlled trial of adenine arabinoside 5′ monophosphate (ara-AMP) in chronic active hepatitis B: comparison of the efficacy in heterosexual and homosexual patients. *Hepatology* 1989;10:328–31.
72. Novick DM, Lok ASF, Thomas HC. Diminished responsiveness of homosexual men to antiviral therapy for $HB_sAg$-positive chronic liver disease. *J Hepatol* 1984;1:29–35.
73. Hoofnagle JH. Therapy of chronic type B hepatitis with adenine arabinoside and adenine arabinoside monophosphate. *J Hepatology* 1986; 3:S73–80.
74. Guardia J, Esteban R, Buti M, Jardi R, Allende H, Esteban JI. Prolonged inhibition of hepatitis B virus replication with vidarabine monophosphate in chronic active type B hepatitis. *Liver* 1986;6:118–22.
75. Peters MG, Davis GL, Dooley JG, Hoofnagle JH. The interferon system in acute and chronic viral hepatitis. In: Popper H, Schaffner F, eds. *Progress in liver diseases, vol. 8.* New York: Grune & Stratton, 1986:453–67.
76. Cantell K, Hirvonen S, Mogensen KE, et al. Human leukocyte interferons. Production, pu-

rification, stability and animal experiments. The production and use of interferon for treatment of human virus infection. *In Vitro* 1974;3:35–8.

77. Weimar W, Heijtink RA, Ten Kate FJP, Schalm SW, Masurel N, Schellekens H. Double-blind study of leukocyte interferon administration in chronic $HB_sAg$-positive hepatitis. *Lancet* 1980;1:336–8.
78. Dooley JS, Davis GL, Peters M, Waggoner JG, Goodman Z, Hoofnagle JH. Pilot study of recombinant human interferon-α for chronic type B hepatitis. *Gastroenterology* 1986;90:150–7.
79. McDonald JA, Caruso L, Thomas HC. A randomised controlled trial of recombinant interferon-α in treatment of HBV infection. *Gut* 1989;31:1116–22.
80. Dusheiko G, Di Bisceglie A, Boyer A, et al. Recombinant leukocyte interferon treatment of chronic hepatitis B. *Hepatology* 1985;5:556–60.
81. Thomas HC. Treatment of hepatitis B viral infection. In: Zuckerman AJ, ed. *Viral hepatitis and liver disease*. New York: Alan R. Liss, 1988:817–22.
82. Hoofnagle JH, Peters MG, Mullen KD, et al. Randomized controlled trial of a four-month course of recombinant human alpha interferon in chronic type B hepatitis. *Gastroenterology* 1988;95:1318–25.
83. Alexander GJM, Brahm J, Fagan EA, et al. Loss of $HB_sAg$ with interferon therapy in chronic hepatitis B virus infection. *Lancet* 1987;1:66–8.
84. Brook MG, Karayiannis P, Thomas HC. Which patients with chronic hepatitis B virus infection will respond to alpha interferon therapy? A statistical analysis of predictive factors. *Hepatology* 1989; (in press).
85. Lok ASF, Lai CL, Wu PC, Leung EKY. Long-term follow-up in a randomised controlled trial of recombinant interferon-$\alpha_2$ in Chinese patients with chronic hepatitis B infection. *Lancet* 1988;2:298–302.
86. Lai CL, Lok ASF, Lin HJ, et al. Placebo-controlled trial of recombinant interferon-$\alpha_2$ in Chinese $HB_sAg$-carrier children. *Lancet* 1987; 2:877–80.
87. Perrillo RP, Regenstein FG, Roodman ST. Chronic hepatitis B in asymptomatic homosexual men with antibody to the human immunodeficiency virus. *Ann Intern Med* 1986;105:382–3.
88. Bissett J, Eisenberg M, Gregory P, et al. Recombinant fibroblast interferon and immune interferon for treating chronic hepatitis B virus infection. Patient's tolerance and the effect on viral markers. *J Infect Dis* 1988;157:1076–80.
89. Porres JC, Mora I, Gutlez J, et al. Antiviral effect of recombinant gamma interferon in chronic hepatitis B virus infection. A pilot study. *Hepatogastroenterology* 1988;35:5–9.
90. Caselmann WH, Eisenburg J, Hofschneider PH, Koshy R. Beta and gamma interferon in chronic active hepatitis B. A pilot trial of short-term combination therapy. *Gastroenterology* 1989;96:449–55.
91. Di Bisceglie AM, Kassianides C, Lisker-Melman M, et al. Treatment of chronic type B hepatitis with recombinant human alpha and gamma interferon in combination. A dose-finding study. *Hepatology* 1987;7:1116.
92. Alexander GJM, Fagan E, Hegarty JE, et al. Controlled clinical trial of acyclovir in chronic hepatitis B virus infection. *J Med Virol* 1987;21:81–7.
93. Schalm SW, Heijtink RA, Van Buren HR, de Man H. Acyclovir enhances the antiviral effect of interferon in chronic hepatitis B. *Lancet* 1985;2:358–60.
94. Nishioka M, Kagawa H, Shirai M, Terada S, Watanabe S. Effects of human recombinant interleukin 2 in patients with chronic hepatitis B. A preliminary report. *Am J Gastroenterol* 1987;82:438–42.
95. Mutchnick MG, Lee HH, Haynes GD, Hoofnagle JH, Appelman HO. Thymosin treatment of chronic active hepatitis B. A preliminary report on a controlled, double-blind study. *Hepatology* 1988;8:1270.
96. Thyagarajan SP, Subramantian S, Thirunalasundari T, Venkateswaran PS, Blumberg BS. Effect of *Phyllanthus amarus* on chronic carriers of hepatitis B virus. *Lancet* 1988;2:764–6.
97. Fattovich G, Brollo L, Pontisso P, et al. Levamisole therapy in chronic type B hepatitis: results of a double-blind randomized trial. *Gastroenterology* 1986;91:692–6.
98. Jain S, Thomas HC, Oxford JS, Sherlock S. Trial of ribavirin for the treatment of $HB_sAg$ positive chronic liver disease. *J Antimicro Chemo* 1978;4:367–73.
99. Scullard GH, Gregory PB, Robinson WS, Merigan TC. The effect of immunosuppressive therapy on hepatitis B viral infection in patients with chronic hepatitis B. *Gastroenterology* 1981;81:987–91.
100. Hoofnagle JH, Davis GL, Pappas SC, et al. A short course of prednisolone in chronic type B hepatitis. Report of a randomized double-blind, placebo controlled trial. *Ann Intern Med* 1986;104:12–7.
101. Rakela J, Redeker AG, Weliky B. Effect of short-term prednisone therapy on aminotransferase levels and hepatitis B virus markers in chronic type B hepatitis. *Gastroenterology* 1983;84:956–60.
102. Nair PV, Tong MJ, Stevenson D, et al. Effects of short-term, high-dose prednisone treatment of patients with $HB_sAg$-positive chronic active hepatitis. *Liver* 1985;5:8–12.
103. Yokosuka O, Omata M, Imazeki F, et al. Combination of short-term prednisone and adenine arabinoside in the treatment of chronic hepatitis B. A controlled study. *Gastroenterology* 1985;89:246–51.
104. Perrillo R, Regenstein F, Peters M, et al. Prednisone withdrawal followed by recombinant interferon-α in the treatment of chronic type B hepatitis. A randomized controlled trial. *Ann Intern Med* 1988;109:95–100.
105. Perillo R, Davis G, Bodenheimer H, et al. A

randomized, controlled multicenter trial of recombinant interferon-$\alpha_{2b}$, alone and following prednisone withdrawal, in chronic type B hepatitis. *Hepatology* 1987;7:1148.

106. Garcia G, Scullard G, Smith C, et al. Preliminary observations of hepatitis B–associated membranous glomerulonephritis after treatment with interferon. *Hepatology* 1985;5:317–20.
107. Lisker-Melman M, Webb D, Di Bisceglie AM, et al. Successful treatment of hepatitis B virus–associated glomerulonephritis with recombinant human alpha interferon. *Hepatology* 1988;8:1269.
108. Lam KC, Lai CL, Ng RP, et al. Deleterious effect of prednisolone in $HB_sAg$-positive chronic active hepatitis. *N Engl J Med* 1981;304:380–6.
109. A Trial Group of the European Association for the Study of the Liver. Steroids in chronic B-hepatitis. A randomized, double-blind, multinational trial on the effect of low-dose, long-term treatment on survival. *Liver* 1986;6:227–32.
110. Weissberg J, Andres LL, Smith CI, et al. Survival in chronic hepatitis B. An analysis of 379 patients. *Ann Intern Med* 1984;101:613–6.
111. Maddrey WC, Van Thiel DH. Liver transplantation. An overview. *Hepatology* 1988;8:948–59.
112. Kassianides C, Di Bisceglie AM, Hoofnagle JH, et al. Alpha interferon therapy in patients with decompensated chronic type B hepatitis. In: Zuckerman AJ, ed. *Viral hepatitis and liver disease*. New York: Alan R. Liss, 1988:840–3.
113. Fattovich G, Brollo L, Stenico D, Boscaro S, Alberti A, Realdi G. Long term follow-up of anti-$HB_e$ positive chronic active hepatitis. *Hepatology* 1988;1651–4.
114. Brunetto MR, Oliveri F, Bonino F, et al. Natural course and response to interferon of chronic hepatitis B accompanied by antibody to hepatitis B e antigen. *Hepatology* 1989;10: 198–202.
115. Renault PF, Hoofnagle JH, Park Y, et al. Psychiatric complications of long-term interferon alpha therapy. *Arch Intern Med* 1987;147:1577–80.
116. Gutterman JJ, Fine S, Quesada J, et al. Recombinant leukocyte A interferon. Pharmacokinetics, single dose tolerance and biologic effects in cancer patients. *Ann Intern Med* 1982;26:549–56.
117. McDonald EM, Mann AH, Thomas HC. Interferons as mediators of psychiatric morbidity. An investigation in a trial of recombinant alpha-interferon in hepatitis B carriers. *Lancet* 1987;2:1175–7.
118. Burman P, Totterman TH, Oberg K, Karlsson FA. Thyroid autoimmunity in patients on long-term therapy with leukocyte-derived interferon. *J Clin Endocrinol Metab* 1986;63:1086–90.
119. Mayet W-J, Hess G, Gerken G, et al. Treatment of chronic type B hepatitis with recombinant alpha-interferon induces autoantibodies not specific for autoimmune chronic hepatitis. *Hepatology* 1989; (in press).
120. Lisker-Melman M, Di Bisceglie AM, Usala SJ, Weintraub B, Murray LM, Hoofnagle JH. Autoimmune thyroid disease associated with recombinant human alpha interferon therapy in patients with chronic hepatitis B. Submitted.
121. Rizzetto M, Canese MG, Arico S, et al. Immunofluorescence detection of new antigen-antibody system (δ/anti-δ) associated to hepatitis B virus in liver and serum of $HB_sAg$ carriers. *Gut* 1977;18:997–1003.
122. Hoofnagle JH. Type D (delta) hepatitis. *JAMA* 1989;261:1321–5.
123. Bonino F, Hoyer B, Ford E, Shih J, Purcell RH, Gerin JL. The δ agent: $HB_sAg$ particles with δ antigen in the serum of an HBV carrier. *Hepatology* 1981;127:127–31.
124. Bergmann KF, Gerin JL. Antigens of hepatitis delta virus in the liver and serum of humans and animals. *J Infect Dis* 1986;154:702–6.
125. Chen P-J, Kalpana G, Goldberg J, et al. Structure and replication of the hepatitis D virus. *Proc Natl Acad Sci USA* 1986;83:8774–8.
126. Wang K-S, Choo W, Weiner AJ, et al. Structure sequence and expression of the hepatitis delta viral genome. *Nature* 1986;323:508–11.
127. Branch AD, Benenfeld BJ, Baroudy BM, Wells FV, Gerin JL, Robertson HD. An ultraviolet-sensitive RNA structural element in a viroid-like domain of the hepatitis delta virus. *Science* 1989;243:649–52.
128. Ponzetto A, Forzani B, Smedile A, et al. Acute and chronic delta infection in the woodchuck. In: Rizzetto M, Gerin JL, Purcell RH, eds. *Delta hepatitis virus and its infection. Vol. 234.* New York: Alan R. Liss, 1987:37–45.
129. Rizzetto M, Verme G, Recchia S, et al. Chronic $HB_sAg$ hepatitis with intrahepatic expression of delta antigen. An active and progressive disease unresponsive to immunosuppressive treatment. *Ann Intern Med* 1983;98:437–41.
130. Recchia S, Rizzi R, Acquaviva F, et al. Immunoperoxidase staining of the HBV-associated delta antigen in paraffinated liver specimens. *Pathologica* 1981;73:773–7.
131. Marinucci G, Valeri L, Alfani D, Rossi M, Di Giacomo C, Cortesini R. Delta infection and liver disease recurrence in hepatic allografts. *Transplant Proc* 1986;18:1401–4.
132. Hedin G, Weiland O, Ljunggren K, et al. Treatment with foscarnet of fulminant hepatitis B and fulminant hepatitis B and D coinfection. In: Zuckerman AJ, ed. *Viral hepatitis and liver disease*. New York: Alan R. Liss, 1988:947–52.
133. Price JS, France AJ, Moaven LD, Welsby PD. Foscarnet in fulminant hepatitis B. *Lancet* 1986;2:1273.
134. Thomas HC, Lever AML, Scully LJ, Pignatelli M. Approaches to the treatment of hepatitis B virus and delta-related liver disease. *Seminar Liver Disease* 1986;6:34–41.
135. Hoofnagle JH, Di Bisceglie AM. Therapy of chronic viral hepatitis: chronic hepatitis D and non-A, non-B hepatitis. In: Zuckerman AJ, ed.

*Viral hepatitis and liver disease*. New York: Alan R. Liss, 1988:823–30.

136. Rosina F, Saracco G, Actis GC, et al. Treatment of chronic delta hepatitis with $\alpha_2$ recombinant interferon (IFN). *Gastroenterology* 1986;90:1762.
137. Alter HJ, Hoofnagle JH. Non-A, non-B. Observations on the first decade. In: Vyas GN, Dienstag JL, Hoofnagle JH, eds. *Viral hepatitis and liver disease*. Orlando: Grune & Stratton, 1984:345–55.
138. Realdi G, Alberti A, Rugge M, et al. Long-term follow-up of acute and chronic non-A, non-B post-transfusion hepatitis: evidence of progression to liver cirrhosis. *Gut* 1982;23:270–5.
139. Koretz RL, Stone O, Gitnick GL. The long-term course of non-A, non-B post-transfusion hepatitis. *Gastroenterology* 1980;79:893–8.
140. Alter MJ, Gerety RJ, Smallwood LA, et al. Sporadic non-A, non-B hepatitis: frequency and epidemiology in an urban US population. *J Infect Dis* 1982;145:886–93.
141. Hoofnagle JH. Chronic hepatitis: the role of corticosteroids. In: Szmuness W, Maynard JE, Alter HJ, eds. *Viral hepatitis: The 1981 International Symposium*. Philadelphia: Franklin Institute Press, 1981:573–83.
142. Pappas SC, Hoofnagle JH, Young N, et al. Treatment of chronic non-A, non-B hepatitis with acyclovir: pilot study. *J Med Virol* 1985;15:1–9.
143. Hoofnagle JH, Mullen KM, Jones DB, et al. Pilot study of recombinant human alpha interferon in chronic non-A, non-B hepatitis. *N Engl J Med* 1986;315:1575–8.
144. Hoofnagle JH. Management of post-transfusion hepatitis. *Transfusion Medicine Reviews* 1989;2:215–20.
145. Thomson BJ, Doran M, Lever AMI, Webster ADB. Alpha-interferon therapy for non-A, non-B hepatitis transmitted by gammaglobulin replacement therapy. *Lancet* 1987;i:539–41.
146. Kiyosawa K, Sodeyama T, Yoda H, et al. Treatment of chronic non-A, non-B hepatitis with beta-interferon. In: Zuckerman AJ (ed). *Viral hepatitis and liver disease*. New York: Alan R. Liss, 1988:895–7.
147. Arima T, Nagashima H, Shimomura H, et al. Treatment of chronic non-A, non-B hepatitis with human beta-interferon. In: Zuckerman AJ, ed. *Viral hepatitis and liver disease*. New York: Alan R. Liss, 1988:898–901.
148. Jacyna MR, Brooks MG, Loke RHT, Main J, Murray-Lyon IM, Thomas HC. Randomised controlled trial of interferon-α (lymphoblastoid interferon) in chronic non-A, non-B hepatitis. *Br Med J* 1989;298:80–2.
149. Di Bisceglie AM, Kassianides C, Lisker-Melman M, et al. Randomized, double-blind, placebo-controlled trial of alpha interferon therapy for chronic non-A, non-B hepatitis. *Hepatology* 1988;8:1222.
150. Davis GL, Balart L, Schiff E, et al. Multicenter randomized controlled trial of alpha interferon treatment for chronic non-A, non-B hepatitis. *Gastroenterology* 1989;96:A591.
151. Wong DC, Purcell RH, Sreenivasan MA, Prasad Sr, Pavri KM. Epidemic and endemic hepatitis in India. Evidence for non-A/non-B hepatitis virus etiology. *Lancet* 1980;2:876–78.
152. Balayan MS, Andzhaparidze AG, Savinskaya SS, et al. Evidence for a virus in non-A, non-B hepatitis transmitted via the fecal oral route. *Intervirology* 1983;20:23–31.
153. Kane MA, Bradley DW, Shrestha SM, et al. Epidemic non-A, non-B hepatitis in Nepal. Recovery of a possible etiologic agent and transmission studies in marmosets. *JAMA* 1984;252:3140–5.
154. Khuroo MS, Teli MR, Skidmore S, Lofo MA, Khuroo MI. Incidence and severity of viral hepatitis in pregnancy. *Am J Med* 1981;70:252–5.

*Antiviral Agents and Viral Diseases of Man, 3rd Edition,*
edited by G. J. Galasso, R. J. Whitley, and
T. C. Merigan, Raven Press, Ltd., New York © 1990.

# 13

# Viral Infections of the Central Nervous System

Diane E. Griffin

*Departments of Medicine and Neurology, Johns Hopkins University School of Medicine, Baltimore, Maryland 21205*



Viral infections of the central nervous system (CNS) occur uncommonly and usually represent complications of systemic viral infection. Spread from a peripheral site of virus replication to the nervous system can occur by several routes, but hematogenous spread is most frequent. Nervous system infection may result in clinical syndromes recognized as meningitis, encephalitis, or myelitis, which suggest primary involvement of the leptomeninges, brain parenchyma, or spinal cord, respectively. Compound terms such as "encephalomyelitis" or "meningoencephalitis" are often more appropriate descriptions of the disease manifestations. Proper diagnosis and therapy of viral infections of the CNS depend on an understanding of the epidemiology, pathogenesis, and clinical features of the potential causes of CNS infection and on an understanding of the special circumstances that govern entry of infectious and potential therapeutic agents into the CNS.

## BLOOD-BRAIN BARRIER

Ehrlich (1) first recognized the presence of the blood-brain barrier after observing that the intravenous injection of certain dyes, now known to bind to albumin, stained essentially all organs of the body except the brain and spinal cord. The anatomic basis of this barrier is the cerebral capillary endothelial cell tight junction (2,3). These endothelial cell tight junctions greatly restrict access of blood constituents, both soluble and cellular, to the parenchyma of the CNS. The extent of the exclusion is determined for soluble substances primarily by their lipid solubility and the presence of carrier systems (4,5), for cells by the presence of surface adhesion molecules (6), and for viruses by surface charge (7) and cellular attachment proteins. When CNS infection occurs, the blood-brain barrier is often disrupted, as manifested by an increase in serum proteins in the cerebrospinal fluid (CSF).

A complete understanding of the interchange of substances between blood and brain also involves an analysis of the barriers between the blood and CSF and between the CSF and brain parenchyma (5,8). CSF is produced primarily by the choroid plexus, which has "leaky" capillary endothelial cell connections but relatively tight junctions between choroidal epithelial cells. Substances enter the interstitial spaces of the choroid plexus relatively easily, but may or may not pass through the choroidal epithelial cells into the CSF (9,10). Protein entry is determined by size (11) and charge (12). Once in the CSF, there is little restriction to movement across the ependyma into the brain parenchyma (13). Therefore, substances (viruses, drugs, antibodies, etc.) that enter the CSF can usually enter the brain parenchyma by diffusion with little restriction and vice versa. For this reason, blood-brain barrier penetration of a substance is usually assessed by comparing the level in blood to that in the CSF. Since diffusion is a relatively slow process compared to bulk flow of CSF, this may not always be an accurate assessment (14).

Entry of pharmacologic agents into the CNS is a major consideration for treatment of CNS infections. Inability to deliver sufficient concentrations of antiviral drugs for therapeutic efficacy is a problem potentially limiting the application of a number of drugs to viral infections of the CNS. Ability to achieve therapeutic levels in the CNS is determined both by the penetration of the agent and by the therapeutic index for the drug under consideration. If higher blood levels than necessary for treatment of systemic infection can be achieved without toxicity, then therapeutic CNS levels may be achievable even though penetration of the drug is relatively poor. Penetration is determined by the size, relative hydrophobicity, and charge of the drug. In general, the smaller, more hydrophobic, and more positively charged the agent, the more readily it will enter the CNS. The absolute level of drug will also be influenced by the presence in the CNS of mechanisms for active or passive transport or removal of the compound (15). Fortunately for some antiviral agents, entry of nucleosides other than thymidine is aided by an active transport system (16,17). In the individual patient, the integrity of the blood-brain barrier, which often changes during the course of infection, may influence drug levels. Knowledge of the CNS penetration of currently available antiviral agents is summarized in Table 1.

## PATHOGENESIS

Most viral infections of the CNS represent uncommon complications of common viral infections. The virus enters and repli-

**TABLE 1.** *CNS penetration of currently available antiviral drugs*

| Therapeutic agent | Brain | CSF/serum | References |
|---|---|---|---|
| ACV | | 50% | (18,19) |
| Amantadine | 26% | 50–60% | (20,21) |
| AZT | <1% | 25–75% | (22–24) |
| DHPG | | 25–50% | (25) |
| Interferon | | <1% | (26) |
| Ribavirin | 4% | 65–90% | (27–29) |
| Rimantadine | 88% | — | (20) |
| Vidarabine | | 50–100% | (30,31) |

cates at a peripheral site, then spreads to the CNS. The likelihood of symptomatic CNS disease in an infected individual varies with the virus, the host, and often with the route and dose of virus inoculation. There are two primary routes of entry into the CNS: from the blood by crossing the blood-brain barrier and from the periphery by direct transport up nerve axons to the CNS. Entry from the blood is by far the most common route of entry, and a viremia occurs during many viral infections. Thus, the potential to infect the nervous system exists frequently, but the normal barriers to infection are usually effective and CNS infection is infrequent. Virus from the blood may enter the brain parenchyma by infecting cerebral capillary endothelial cells or epithelial cells of the choroid plexus or by crossing the cerebral capillary blood-brain barrier to reach susceptible cells within the substance of brain or spinal cord (32,33). The rapidity with which virus is cleared from the blood directly affects the opportunity for CNS infection. Factors affecting clearance such as the size of the virus and the presence of antiviral factors (e.g., antibody, complement, etc.) in the blood will help to determine the likelihood of CNS infection (32,34,35).

A second mechanism for entry into the CNS is by retrograde axonal transport from the periphery. Neurons with cell bodies within the CNS have axonal processes that extend to skin and muscle and continuously transport substances to and from the CNS (36). The axonal route is the only route by which rabies virus enters the CNS (37), and axonal transport contributes significantly to the clinical features of reactivated herpes simplex virus (HSV) and varicella-zoster virus (VZV) infections, though their mechanism for entry into brain parenchyma is less clear (38). A variation on this theme is viral entry into the CNS by way of the olfactory mucosa. The endings of olfactory neurons are in direct contact with the surface of the olfactory mucosa and potentially exposed to infectious agents that replicate in the upper respiratory tract or are present in the air and could be transported directly to the CNS. This route is of established importance in experimental infections (39) but is of unproven importance in natural infections, although aerosol-associated CNS infections with rabies virus probably involved entry by the olfactory route (40).

Once a viral infection is established within the brain or spinal cord, only certain cells may be susceptible to infection. The type of cell infected will determine the clinical manifestations. Infection of neurons may produce electrical irritability and seizures, of motor neurons focal paralysis, and of sensory neurons dysesthesias. Selective infection and destruction of oligodendroglia can lead to demyelination. Infection of the ependyma may result in hydrocephalus due to closure of the aqueduct. Infection of immature cells may cause congenital malformations dependent on the time in gestation when infection occurred. Once within the CNS, the viral infection may remain localized or spread extensively through the nervous system. The mode of spread is determined in part by the tropism of the virus for particular cells (32). Viruses that replicate in the choroid plexus, the leptomeninges, or the ependyma will be shed into the CSF, allowing rapid spread of the infection throughout the CNS. Viruses that replicate solely in parenchymal cells may spread only cell to cell, causing focal disease. If neurons are infected, spread from one area to another may occur by axonal transport, potentially resulting in infection at distinctive anatomic sites determined by the projections of the neurons originally infected.

## IMMUNE RESPONSE

The immune response within the CNS is similar to that in other organs, but is complicated by the presence of the blood-brain barrier. Infections in the immunocompetent host elicit a cellular and a humoral immune response to the infecting agent. The cellular response to most viral infections is manifest by a mononuclear cell infiltrate that includes CD4- and CD8-positive T cells, B cells, and monocyte/macrophages. In addition, natural killer (NK) cells are likely participants early in the infectious process. Some of these cells (particularly T lymphocytes) also appear in the CSF, especially if the leptomeninges are involved in infection (41).

B cells in the parenchyma differentiate and produce antibody locally. Intrathecally produced antibody appears in the interstitial fluid of the brain and moves from there into the CSF (41,42). Antibody found in the CSF in the absence of infection comes from the blood (43). In the presence of an intact blood-brain barrier, antibody is present in CSF at approximately 0.5–1% of the concentration in blood. If the blood-brain barrier is not intact (usually evidenced by increased total protein in the CSF), then the CSF to serum antibody ratio must be corrected for this fact. Correction is based on the concentration of albumin relative to immunoglobulin G (IgG) in both the CSF and the serum (the IgG index) (44,45). Increased amounts of antibody in the CSF are evidence of local antibody synthesis and suggest parenchymal infection with the agent against which the antibody is directed (46–52). Depending on the extent of systemic infection and on the stimulation of antibody synthesis in peripheral tissue versus CNS tissue amounts of antibody in the CSF during CNS viral infection may equal or exceed that found in the serum.

## SPECIFIC CAUSES OF CNS VIRAL INFECTIONS

### Enteroviruses

The enteroviruses belong to the picornavirus family of small, nonenveloped, positive-stranded RNA viruses and are among the most common causes of CNS infection. The enterovirus group includes the polioviruses (three types), Coxsackie viruses (29 types), echoviruses (31 types) and five miscellaneous enteroviruses, which include hepatitis A virus (HAV) (enterovirus 72). Almost all enteroviruses are spread primarily by the fecal-oral route and replicate initially in the gastrointestinal tract and the gut-associated lymphatic tissue. Enteroviruses spread to the CNS primarily through the blood (53–55). A secondary role for entry by the neural route has been suggested by some, particularly for polio (53,54), and spread of poliovirus within the parenchyma of the nervous system is primarily neural (54). Infections are most common in the late summer and early fall, but also occur sporadically throughout the year (53). Many enteroviruses can cause meningitis, encephalitis, paralysis, or cerebellar ataxia, but the frequency of particular neurologic syndromes varies with the virus (46). Overall, the enteroviruses account for 70–80% of all cases of aseptic meningitis and 11–22% of viral encephalitis (55).

#### *Clinical Features*

Current knowledge of the pathogenesis of enterovirus infection is due largely to the intensive study given to poliovirus in the effort to combat the epidemics of "infantile paralysis" occurring in the developed world during the 1940s and 1950s. During this period, *in vitro* cell culture of the virus was accomplished (56), and it was observed that there are three distinct serotypes (57) and that primary viral replication is in the gastrointestinal rather than in the respiratory tract (58,59), with subsequent spread to the CNS through the blood (60,61). Most poliovirus infections are asymptomatic or associated only with fever and malaise, without localizing signs or symptoms (62). When

CNS infection occurs, it may result in meningitis, encephalitis (principally in infants), or the more classic picture of "poliomyelitis" with predominant infection of the motor neurons of the spinal cord (spinal polio) or brain stem (bulbar polio) (54). Frank paralysis occurs in approximately 1 in 1,000 poliovirus infections. A prodromal illness of fever, headache, anorexia, and myalgia is often present prior to the onset of paralysis and muscle pain. The paralysis is typically flaccid and asymmetric and may progress over 2–3 days while the patient remains febrile. The best estimates of the incubation period of poliomyelitis are 9–12 days from infection to the onset of the prodrome and 11–17 days to the onset of paralysis (44). Wild-type poliovirus is endemic in much of the world, but has been essentially eliminated from the United States. Therefore, cases of polio seen in the United States are rare and are usually imported or vaccine-induced (62,63).

### *Coxsackie Viruses and Echoviruses*

Most Coxsackie virus infections are asymptomatic or associated with nonneurologic diseases such as rash, pleurodynia, myocarditis, and pericarditis (55,64). Echoviruses are disproportionately isolated from cases of meningitis and encephalitis and infrequently from cases of paralysis (64). Meningitis due either to Coxsackie or echovirus is usually benign; symptoms last only a few days; recovery is uneventful. Disease is more serious when echovirus (particularly type 11) (65) and Coxsackie virus (66) infections are acquired perinatally. Approximately 25% of infants infected with an echovirus *in utero* near term or shortly after birth have evidence of CNS infection, and 19% of these infants die (65). There is a similarly high mortality in newborns with disseminated Coxsackie B virus infections (66). For both viruses, mortality is much lower when infection is acquired even a few days after birth, although the question of significant neurological sequelae resulting from infantile enterovirus meningoencephalitis remains unanswered (66).

### *Miscellaneous Enteroviruses*

Cases of meningoencephalitis due to HAV have recently been reported (67,68). The neurologic symptoms may appear prior to frank jaundice although evidence of abnormal hepatic function is usually present at the time of neurologic disease. Outbreaks of paralysis resembling poliomyelitis, and cases of encephalitis and meningitis, have been associated with enterovirus 71 infection (69).

### ***Immunocompromised Individuals***

Children with defects in antibody synthesis are particularly susceptible to chronic enteroviral infection (55,62,70) (Table 2). CNS infection is usually manifested by chronic meningitis, encephalitis, and slowly progressive neurologic deterioration associated with seizures and loss of developmental milestones. Other features may include weakness, lethargy, headaches, hearing loss, ataxia, and paresthesias. The most common pathogens isolated are echoviruses, particularly type 11 (70). Virus can be recovered from the CSF for prolonged periods of time.

**TABLE 2.** *Viruses causing slowly progressive neurologic disease in the immunocompromised host*

| | References |
|---|---|
| Immunoglobulin deficiency | |
| Enteroviruses | |
| Polio | (70) |
| Coxsackie | (70) |
| Echo | (70) |
| T-cell deficiency | |
| Paramyxoviruses; measles | (152) |
| Retroviruses; HIV | (185–189) |
| Papovaviruses; JC (PML) | (285) |
| Herpesviruses; CMV | (277–280) |

Other organ systems may also be involved, producing hepatitis, rashes, edema, and a dermatomyositis-like syndrome (70). Children with deficiencies in B cell function appear uniquely susceptible to enterovirus infections, suggesting that the ability to develop antibody to these agents is essential for recovery.

### *Diagnosis*

Enteroviral CNS infection is often suspected based on the community epidemiology. The echoviruses, polioviruses, and Coxsackie B viruses are relatively easily grown in tissue culture cells in the viral diagnostic laboratory permitting isolation of the pathogen (53). Isolation attempts should be made from throat, stool, and urine as well as CSF. Several Coxsackie A viruses can be recovered only by inoculation of suckling mice (53). The importance of an isolate from a peripheral source should be confirmed with acute and convalescent phase serology since virus present in stool may or may not be significant for the CNS disease. Hepatitis A is diagnosed by the presence of IgM antibody in acute phase serum. Intrathecal synthesis of enterovirus-specific antibody may also be useful for retrospective diagnosis (47).

### *Prevention*

Two forms of vaccine each containing all three poliovirus serotypes are available: an inactivated vaccine that is given intramuscularly and an attenuated live virus vaccine given orally. Both vaccines are effective in preventing the CNS complications of poliovirus infection (71). Inactivated poliovirus vaccine (IPV) induces circulating serum antibodies that prevent spread of virus from the gastrointestinal tract to the CNS (72). Booster injections every few years are desirable (54). Three injections of the enhanced-potency IPV are required for protective immunity (73). Orally administered attenuated live poliovirus vaccine (OPV) induces local gut immunity and inhibits the initial replication of wild-type virus in the intestinal tract in addition to inducing serum antibody (72). Three oral doses are given during the first 6 months of life, with a booster at 18 months (54). OPV also spreads to unvaccinated individuals, increasing the level of immunity in the community. The type 3 strain has shown a tendency to revert to virulence (74) and has been the primary serotype isolated from cases of vaccine-associated poliomyelitis (75). Unimmunized adults and immunocompromised individuals of all ages are at increased risk for CNS infection by the vaccine virus and should receive IPV (73). The relative merits of IPV and OPV for routine immunization of children in different parts of the world remains an area of active discussion (71).

Currently, there is no available vaccine for Coxsackie, echo, or hepatitis A viruses, but mortality and long-term morbidity after infection with these viruses are comparatively infrequent. Immune globulin is effective in preventing clinical disease due to hepatitis A infection and is given in a dose of 0.2 ml/kg for short-term exposure and 0.6 ml/kg every 5 months for long-term exposure (76).

### *Therapy*

Therapy in the immunocompetent individual is primarily supportive. Hypogammaglobulinemic children with chronic enteroviral meningoencephalitis have improved with the intravenous administration of $\gamma$-globulin preparations containing antibody to the infecting serotype (70,77). For CNS infection, this has been most effective when given intrathecally, and a few children have apparently been cured with such treatment (70,78).

### Arthropod-Borne Viruses

The arthropod-borne viruses (arboviruses) are important causes of encephalitis in many areas of the world and are also discussed in Chapter 18. Arboviruses replicate in both their invertebrate and vertebrate hosts and include members of the alphavirus, flavivirus, and bunyavirus families. Over 20 arboviruses cause encephalitis but are restricted geographically and seasonally by their specific vectors so that in any one part of the world only a few of these viruses are found (Table 3). Many are named for the geographical site of the original virus isolation (79).

Arboviruses are inoculated subcutaneously or intravenously by injection of infected saliva from the insect vector and replicate locally in muscle or subcutaneous tissue to produce a viremia. Spread to the CNS is usually through the blood (79), although in experimental infection entry by the olfactory route has been demonstrated (39). Initial CNS infection in experimental models is of capillary endothelial or choroid epithelial cells, and spread within the CNS can be cell to cell or through the CSF (80).

**TABLE 3.** *Arboviruses causing encephalitis*

| Virus | Vector | Geographic location |
|---|---|---|
| *Togaviridae* | | |
| Alphavirus | | |
| Eastern equine | Mosquitoes (Culiseta, Aedes) | Eastern and Gulf coasts of United States, Caribbean & South America |
| Western equine | Mosquitoes (Culiseta, Culex) | Western United States and Canada |
| Venezuelan equine | Mosquitoes (Aedes, Culex, etc.) | South and Central America<br>Florida and Southwest United States |
| *Flaviviridae* | | |
| West Nile complex | | |
| St. Louis | Mosquitoes (Culex) | Widespread in United States |
| Japanese | Mosquitoes (Culex) | Japan, China, Southeast Asia, and India |
| Murray Valley | Mosquitoes (Culex) | Australia and New Guinea |
| West Nile | Mosquitoes (Culex) | Africa and Mideast |
| Ilheus | Mosquitoes (Psorophora) | South and Central America |
| Rocio | Mosquitoes (?) | Brazil |
| Tick-borne-complex | | |
| Far Eastern | Ticks (Ixodes) | Eastern USSR |
| Central European | Ticks (Ixodes) | Central Europe |
| Kyasanur Forest | Ticks (Haemophysalis) | India |
| Louping-ill | Ticks (Ixodes) | England, Scotland, and Northern Ireland |
| Powassan | Ticks (Ixodes) | Canada and Northern United States |
| Negishi | Ticks (?) | Japan |
| *Bunyaviridae* | | |
| Bunyavirus | | |
| California | Mosquitoes (Aedes) | Western United States |
| La Crosse | Mosquitoes (Aedes) | Mid and Eastern United States |
| Jamestown Canyon | Mosquitoes (Culiseta) | United States and Alaska |
| Snowshoe Hare | Mosquitoes (Culiseta) | Canada, Alaska, and Northern United States |
| Tahyna | Mosquitoes (Aedes, Culiseta) | Czechoslovakia and Yugoslavia, Italy and Southern France |
| Inkoo | Mosquitoes (?) | Finland |
| Phlebovirus | | |
| Rift Valley | Mosquitoes (Culex, Aedes) | East Africa |
| *Reoviridae* | | |
| Orbivirus | | |
| Colorado tick fever | Ticks (Dermacentor) | Rocky Mountains of United States |

Adapted from Johnson, ref. 79.

The incubation period for arboviral encephalitis has been estimated between 4 days and 3 weeks. Typically, there is a prodromal illness of a few days with fever, headache, and malaise. Symptoms then intensify, with confusion followed by obtundation and frequently coma. Seizures are common, particularly in children. CSF shows a pleocytosis with mononuclear predominance. Protein is usually modestly elevated and the glucose normal (79).

### *Clinical Features*

#### *Alphaviruses*

The alphaviruses belong to the togavirus family of small, enveloped, positive-stranded RNA viruses. In North and South America, the alphaviruses, Eastern equine, Western equine and Venezuelan equine encephalitis viruses, are important causes of arthropod-borne encephalitis. All are transmitted by mosquitoes and have birds as their primary hosts (80,81).

Eastern equine encephalitis virus is endemic along the eastern and Gulf coasts of the United States, in the Caribbean, and in South America and causes small localized outbreaks of equine and human encephalitis in the summer (81). Eastern equine encephalitis is associated with a high case fatality rate (50–75%) in all ages. The encephalitis tends to be fulminant and associated with fever, headache, altered consciousness, and seizures. Sequelae are common, with more than 80% of survivors having significant neurological residua (80–82).

Western equine encephalitis virus produces epidemics of equine and human encephalitis, primarily in the western and midwestern United States (81). Western equine encephalitis has signs and symptoms similar to those of Eastern encephalitis, but a lower case fatility rate (10%). There is an increased risk with advanced age (83). Severe disease, fatal encephalitis, and significant sequelae are more likely to occur in infants and young children than in older children and adults (80,81,84).

Venezuelan equine encephalitis virus occurs in the northern parts of South America, Central America, and the Southern United States (81). Infection can occur by the respiratory route, as well as by mosquito inoculation, as evidenced by a number of laboratory-acquired infections (85). Venezuelan equine encephalitis virus usually causes a mild illness in adults (mortality < 1%) associated with fever, headache, myalgia, and pharyngitis. Encephalitis occurs infrequently. More severe disease, including fulminant reticuloendothelial system infection and encephalitis, may occur in young children (80,81,85,86).

#### *Flaviviruses*

The flaviviruses are small, enveloped, positive-stranded RNA viruses that are morphologically similar to the togaviruses, but have a distinctive genomic organization and replication cycle (87). Flavivirus encephalitis has been reported from all continents except Antarctica. Encephalitic strains are transmitted either by mosquitoes or by ixodid ticks.

#### *Mosquito-Borne Flaviviruses*

The mosquito-borne flaviviruses that cause encephalitis are all members of the West Nile antigenic complex and are found worldwide. The largest number of cases of encephalitis occur in Asia, where Japanese encephalitis is endemic and epidemic. Sporadic outbreaks also occur in the Americas (St. Louis, Rocio), Australia (Murray Valley), and Africa (West Nile) (88).

Japanese encephalitis is widely distributed in Asia including Japan, China, the Soviet Union, the Philippines, and all of Southeast Asia and India. Japanese encephalitis is the most important of the arbovirus-induced encephalitides in terms of worldwide morbidity and mortality, with tens of thousands of cases occurring annually (88). In endemic areas such as southern Thailand, children are most often affected; older age groups have preexisting immunity. Cases occur throughout the year (89). In epidemic areas such as China, all ages are susceptible and equally affected, and cases occur in outbreaks usually beginning in late summer (89). Infection may be asymptomatic, or manifested by fever alone, aseptic meningitis, or encephalitis. The onset of encephalitis is rapid, beginning with a 2–3-day prodrome of headache, fever, chills, malaise, and nausea. In children, abdominal symptoms may be prominent. The acute stage lasts 2–4 days and is marked by sustained fever (usually > 104°F), meningismus, photophobia, confusion, and delirium. Characteristic neurological signs include a Parkinsonian-like picture of mask-like facies, rigidity and involuntary movements, altered consciousness, and generalized or localized paralysis. Seizures are frequent in children, but occur in < 10% of adults. Tremor is present in 90% of patients (90,91).

St. Louis encephalitis is the most common flavivirus-induced encephalitis in the United States and is widely distributed. Numerous outbreaks have been documented usually in August, September, and October—somewhat later than the spring and early summer outbreaks for most arboviruses (88). The virus can have both urban (epidemic) and rural (endemic) cycles (92). The risk of illness increases sharply with age (93,94). After a prodrome of several days, there is the abrupt onset of severe generalized headache, nausea, and vomiting, followed by disorientation, irritability, and stupor. Low serum sodium due to inappropriate secretion of antidiuretic hormone and pyuria with elevated blood urea nitrogen are relatively common laboratory findings (93–95). Mortality is low in the young but over 20% in the elderly (94). Convalescence may be prolonged, and significant neurologic residua are present in 20% of survivors (88).

Rocio virus is endemic in Brazil and has caused numerous outbreaks of encephalitis in that country (88). Murray Valley encephalitis virus causes infrequent outbreaks of encephalitis in Australia and New Guinea during the summer after high rainfall for 2 consecutive years (88). West Nile virus is widely distributed throughout Africa, the Middle East, Europe, the Soviet Union, India, and Indonesia. Infection is common, but meningitis and encephalitis are rare complications occurring primarily in the elderly (88).

### *Tick-Borne Flaviviruses*

The tick-borne flaviviruses form a separate antigenic group and are most prominent in Europe and Asia. Transmission by ingestion of infected goat milk in addition to tick transmission has been documented (88). The tick-borne encephalitis complex includes six closely-related viruses that cause encephalitis in humans: Kyasanur Forest, louping-ill, Powassan, Negishi, and two strains of tick-borne encephalitis, Far Eastern (Russian spring-summer) and Central European encephalitis viruses.

The Far Eastern and Central European strains of tick-borne encephalitis virus are endemic over a wide area of Europe and the Soviet Union and cause thousands of cases of encephalitis each year, primarily in adults working or vacationing in wooded areas (88). The onset of Far Eastern encephalitis is gradual, progressing from fever and headache to meningismus, paralysis, and seizures over many days. Evidence of lower motor neuron disease with loss of tone and reflexes, and localized muscle weakness, usually limited to the upper extremities, reflect selective involvement of the motor neurons of the cervical spinal cord. The case fatality rate is approximately 20%. Neurologic sequelae occur in 30–60% of survivors. Especially characteristic is a residual flaccid paralysis of the shoulder girdle and arms (88,96,97). In addition, chronic CNS infection may account for some cases of epilepsy partialis continua in the Soviet Union (98).

Central European encephalitis is milder than Far Eastern and exhibits a typical diphasic course in half of the cases. The first phase is a nonspecific flu-like illness lasting approximately 1 week, followed by a 1–3-day remission. The neurologic phase may manifest as aseptic meningitis or encephalitis with tremor, diplopia, altered mental status, and paresis. The case fatality rate is 1–5%, and approximately 20% of survivors have mild neurologic residua (88,96,99,100).

Other members of the tick-borne complex are associated with fewer cases of encephalitis. Louping ill is endemic in the British Isles and causes encephalitis in sheep. Most human infections have followed laboratory exposure, but transmission by ticks and by direct contact with sick sheep also occurs (88). Like Central European encephalitis, louping ill is a biphasic disease in both sheep and in humans. No human deaths have been reported. Powassan virus has a widespread distribution in the United States and Canada but has been associated with only 20 reported cases of encephalitis. Negishi virus is a rare cause of encephalitis in Japan. Kyasanur Forest virus causes 50–200 virologically documented cases of a hemorrhagic fever syndrome occasionally complicated by encephalitis in the Mysore State of India each year (88).

### *Bunyaviruses*

The bunyaviruses are a large group of enveloped, negative-stranded RNA viruses. The bunyavirus family has more than 200 members, but the most important causes of encephalitis belong to the California serogroup (101). This serogroup includes La Crosse virus [the most frequent arbovirus cause of encephalitis in the United States (Fig. 1)]; Jamestown Canyon, snowshoe hare, and California encephalitis viruses, which are found in North America; and Inkoo and Tahyna viruses, found in Europe. All of these viruses are endemic in their particular locations and cause encephalitis primarily in children (102,103). Both urban and rural cases occur since one vector *Aedes triseriatus* can breed in containers such as old tires (101). The recent introduction and spread in the United States of another container-breeding mosquito *Aedes albopictus*, an efficient vector

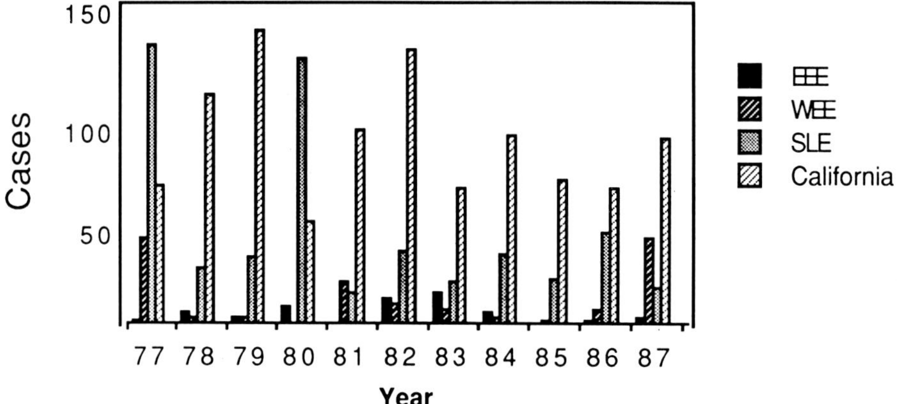


**FIG. 1.** Annual incidence of specific types of arbovirus encephalitis in the United States. EEE, Eastern equine encephalitis; WEE, Western equine encephalitis; SLE, St. Louis encephalitis; California, California serogroup mainly La Crosse encephalitis. (Data from Centers for Disease Control, refs. 83, 104, and 305.)

for the California serogroup viruses, as well as for yellow fever and dengue viruses, has led to concern about the potential for a significant increase in these infections (104,105).

Encephalitis due to La Crosse virus occurs nearly exclusively among children (103,106). The case fatality rate is less than 1%. During the acute illness, seizures occur in 50% and focal weakness, paralysis, or other neurologic signs occur in 25%. Some neurological residua (usually seizure disorders) are noted in approximately 10% (106).

Rift Valley fever is caused by a mosquito-transmitted bunyavirus of the phlebovirus group. Rift Valley fever virus has been associated with large epizootics of hepatic necrosis and abortion in sheep and cattle in sub-Saharan Africa. Humans are infected by contact with infected animals or the mosquito vector. Most patients infected with Rift Valley fever virus have the acute onset of a severe, but self-limited febrile illness. In 5% of cases, infection is complicated acutely by hepatitis or in later stages by encephalitis or retinitis. Encephalitis is associated with vertigo, disorientation, hallucinations, decerebrate rigidity, choreiform movements, and hemiparesis. The case fatality rate is estimated at 10%. Most patients recover slowly and without sequelae (101,107).

### *Diagnosis*

Although most arboviruses enter the CNS by virtue of a viremia, virus is usually cleared from the blood by the time of the onset of encephalitis, and isolations of virus from blood are rare. Occasionally, isolation from CSF is succesful but requires inoculation of suckling mice. Therefore, diagnosis is usually dependent on detection of specific antibodies in the serum or CSF of the patient by complement fixation (CF), hemagglutination inhibition (HI), immunofluorescence (IF), or enzyme immunoassay (EIA). IgM-specific EIAs have been developed for Japanese and tick-borne encephalitides that provide rapid, reliable diagnostic information, particularly when applied to CSF (108,109).

### *Prevention*

The primary approach used for the prevention of most arthropod-borne diseases is to decrease contact with the vector by use of screens, insect repellents, and protective clothing. In addition, attempts at vector control may include campaigns to eliminate breeding habitats, aerial spraying of insecticides, and the introduction of biological larvicides (79,81,88,102).

Vaccines for Eastern, Western, and Venezuelan equine encephalitis are available for horses and, on an experimental basis, for investigators working with these agents in the laboratory (81). Several vaccines are available for prevention of Japanese encephalitis in humans and horses, and to prevent abortion in swine. Vaccines consisting of inactivated virus or attenuated virus grown in primary baby hamster kidney cells are used in India and China. The greatest experience with the human vaccines has been with an inactivated suckling mouse brain vaccine produced in Japan. This vaccine is efficacious (89,110), and individuals from nonendemic areas spending time in rural areas of Asia during the rainy season should be immunized. Pasteurization of milk prevents oral transmission of tick-borne encephalitis, and vaccines consisting of inactivated tissue culture or egg-grown virus are available in Russia and Eastern Europe (88,111) for persons at high risk of exposure. Prevention of Rift Valley fever has concentrated on control of infection in domestic animals, which amplify the disease, by immunizing sheep and cattle. An experimental inactivated vaccine has been used for laboratory personnel and other persons at high risk (101,112).

### *Therapy*

Therapy of arboviral encephalitis is not well established. There is some experience using antiserum or ribonuclease for tick-borne encephalitis in the Soviet Union (113), but no trials with other agents have been reported and animal studies have not been encouraging (Chapter 18). Survival and the quality of recovery depend in part on supportive care. Remarkable recoveries can occur even after prolonged coma. Therefore, vigorous supportive therapy and avoidance and treatment of complications are essential. Respiratory support may be necessary. Fluids and electrolytes should be carefully monitored since water, glucose, and salt control may be compromised during encephalitis. Seizures must be treated and increased intracranial pressure should be controlled with osmotic agents or steroids, if necessary, but routine use of steroids has not proven beneficial (79).

## Rubella Virus

Acute rubella is not associated with neurologic disease except for the occasional case of postinfectious encephalomyelitis (114). Congenital infection with rubella produces persistent infection of multiple organs including the nervous system. Virus is excreted for months postnatally, but is eventually cleared (115). A small proportion of children with congenital rubella syndrome develop a late progressive, neurologic disease—progressive rubella panencephalitis—in the second or third decade of life (116,117) (Table 4). The disease is manifest by a progressive decline in cognitive function, spasticity, ataxia, and seizures. Virus has been recovered from CNS tissue in one case (117), and the pathology suggests a chronic generalized encephalitis. Immunoglobulin is increased in CSF, and antibody to rubella virus is greatly increased in serum and CSF. Treatment with isoprinosine has been attempted (118), but no effective therapy has been identified.

## Rabies Virus

Rabies virus is a member of the rhabdovirus family of enveloped negative-stranded RNA viruses. Rabies is an important cause of human disease, primarily in countries of Asia and Africa where endemic canine rabies in a continuing problem. Rabies has been completely eliminated only from a few island countries such as England, Australia, and Japan. In many other places in the world, such as Europe and the United States, rabies has been controlled in domestic animals by immunization and licensing requirements but remains endemic in wild animals, primarily skunks, raccoons, bats, and foxes. In countries with rabies in wildlife, rabies virus continues to cause sporadic human disease and remains a major concern because of the essentially 100% mortality in infected persons (119).

### *Clinical Features*

Rabies virus replicates almost exclusively in neural tissue. After limited local replication at the site of inoculation, the virus is taken up by nerve endings in the area and transported to the CNS (37,120).

**TABLE 4.** *Viruses causing slowly progressive neurologic disease in the immunocompetent host*

| Virus | Disease | References |
|---|---|---|
| Togavirus; rubella | Progressive rubella panencephalitis | (116,117) |
| Paramyxovirus; measles | Subacute sclerosing panencephalitis | (155–157) |
| Retrovirus; HTLV-I | Tropical spastic paraparesis | (173,174) |
| Spongiform agents; kuru, | Kuru | (292) |
| Creutzfeldt Jacob | Creutzfeldt-Jacob disease | (294–297) |

Within the CNS, rabies virus is spread transynaptically (121). The incubation period is widely variable from a minimum of 9 days up to 19 years, although the usual is between 20 and 60 days (122). The length of incubation is determined partly by the proximity of the injury to the CNS and by the amount of virus initially introduced. Not all persons bitten by a known rabid animal will develop rabies even in the absence of treatment. The likelihood of clinical disease depends on the severity of the bite, the intrinsic ability of certain animals to transmit virus, and the protective effect of clothing (119).

Infected individuals usually develop a week-long prodrome of fever, malaise, and headache. Approximately 50% report abnormal sensation at the site of the bite. The prodrome is followed by the onset of signs and symptoms of neurologic disease. In the encephalitic form of rabies, early signs include periods of hyperactivity, seizures, hallucinations, and disorientation accompanied by hydrophobia and aerophobia leading to coma and death within 1 week without supportive therapy. With intensive therapy, the illness may last 3–4 weeks before death (122,123). Approximately 20% of individuals have a paralytic illness that may be confused with the Guillain-Barré syndrome or complications of rabies vaccine, but progresses to coma and death within days to weeks of onset (122–124).

### *Diagnosis*

The history of being bitten by a potentially rabid animal is useful in suspecting the diagnosis. However, it must be noted that exposure to the rabid animal may be relatively remote in time and that six of the nine most recent cases of rabies diagnosed in the United States have had no history of such a bite. The other three cases were imported from countries with endemic rabies in domestic animals (125).

In the absence of a history of exposure, the diagnosis may be difficult. In fact, for recent United States cases, rabies has often not been suspected, and the diagnosis has been made postmortem or by inadvertent transmission of rabies through organ transplantation (123). Fluorescent antibody staining of brain biopsy material is the most definitive means of diagnosis, but occasionally rabies virus antigen can be detected in corneal scrapings or in hair follicles, since virus is transported not only to but also from infected cells by axonal transport (123,126–128). The CSF is frequently abnormal, and antibody to rabies virus may be detectable (122). Appearance of antibody in the serum is useful diagnostically if the patient has not received rabies virus vaccine or antiserum earlier as prophylactic therapy.

### *Prevention/Therapy*

A number of effective rabies vaccines have been developed and are usually used as part of a regimen of postexposure prophylaxis. Use and availability vary in different geographic regions. The least expensive, effective vaccine is the Semple vaccine, a phenol-inactivated suspension of neural tissue from mature animals (goats, sheep, rabbits) infected with rabies virus. This vaccine dates in principle from the time of Pasteur. However, Semple vaccine has a significant incidence of neurologic complications due to the induction of an autoimmune response to myelin (129,130). Neurologic complications of rabies vaccine have been partially avoided in Latin America by use of a vaccine prepared from the unmyelinated brains of suckling mice (131). Both of these neural tissue-derived vaccines are given as a course of 14–21 daily subcutaneous injections. More recently, effective tissue-culture-derived vaccines prepared in human or rhesus monkey cells have been developed. These vaccines produce good immunity and are safe enough to be given for preexposure prophylaxis.

For preexposure immunization, human diploid cell vaccine (HDCV) is administered either intradermally (0.1 ml) or intramuscularly (1 ml) in a series of three injections (day 0, 7, and 21 or 28) to individuals planning to live in areas of endemic rabies in domestic animals and to persons (veterinarians, wildlife management personnel, etc.) with occupational exposure to animals (132,133). Antibody responses may be reduced when immunization is administered simultaneously with chloroquine for prophylaxis of malaria (134). Postexposure treatment of two 1.0 ml intramuscular booster doses (day 0 and 3) is still necessary if the immunized individual has contact with a rabid animal (135).

Postexposure prophylaxis of an unimmunized individual must include administration of vaccine (HDCV) intramuscularly into the deltoid region on day 0, 3, 7, 14, and 28), thorough cleansing of the wound with soap and water, and administration of rabies immune globulin (20 IU/kg). If possible, half of the immune serum should be infiltrated around the wound and half given intramuscularly into the gluteal region. Decision on the need for therapy is based on the type of animal exposure (Table 5). Postexposure prophylaxis should be administered as soon as possible after contact with a potentially rabid animal, but since the latent period can be prolonged, no time prior to the onset of symptoms should be considered too late for institution of treatment (133,136,137).

Once neurological symptoms have appeared, no intervention has been demonstrated to be of use. Trials of prolonged supportive therapy, interferon, and ribavirin have all failed to demonstrate any effect on the universally fatal outcome. (138; T. Hemachudha, unpublished observations). The few survivals have all been in individuals in whom postexposure prophylaxis was initiated prior to the onset of symptoms (122).

## Paramyxoviruses

The paramyxoviruses are enveloped, pleomorphic, negative-stranded RNA viruses. Two paramyxovirus infections are frequently associated with neurologic disease: mumps and measles. Primary infection is in the upper respiratory tract, with subsequent spread to draining lymph nodes followed by viremia. Mumps virus infects a variety of target organs, including glandular epithelium and the CNS (139). Measles virus in the blood seeds lymphoid tissue, the skin, and liver, but rarely the CNS (140).

### *Mumps Virus*

Prior to the development and widespread use of the live attenuated mumps virus vac-

**TABLE 5.** *Guidelines for postexposure rabies prophylaxis*

| Animal | Condition of animal | Treatment |
|---|---|---|
| Dog or cat | Healthy and available for 10-day observation | None, unless animal develops rabies |
| | Rabid or suspected rabid | Rabies immune globulin and human diploid cell vaccine |
| | Unknown or escaped | Consult public health officials in local area regarding risk |
| Skunk, bat, fox, racoon, coyote, bob cat, or other carnivae | Regard as rabid until proven negative by laboratory tests | Rabies immune globulin and human diploid cell vaccine |
| Livestock, rodents, and largomorphs | Consider individually. Public health officials should be consulted. Bites of squirrels, hamsters, guinea pigs, gerbils, chipmunks, rats, mice, rabbits, and horses almost never call for anti-rabies prophylaxis. | |

cine (introduced in 1967), mumps was one of the most common causes of viral meningoencephalitis (141). CNS disease usually follows parotitis by 3–10 days and is a relatively frequent complication of mumps. The virus has a predilection for ependymal cells and invades the CNS by infecting choroidal epithelial cells (139,142). Of infected individuals, 10% have clinical signs of meningitis and a CSF pleocytosis is present in an additional 50% (138).

Most cases of mumps meningitis and meningoencephalitis resolve without sequelae. However, mumps is a recognized cause of acquired hydrocephalus (143) and neurosensory deafness (144). Occasional cases are fatal (145). The virus can be cultured from the CSF during acute disease where it is present in desquamated choroidal and ependymal cells (142,144,146). CSF abnormalities may be prolonged, and hypoglycorrhacia may occur (147,148). Symptoms due to the glandular infection usually make the diagnosis relatively straightforward, but CNS disease can occur in the absence of parotitis, requiring virus isolation or serology for diagnosis (146,149). Intrathecal synthesis of antibody has been demonstrated (50). Prevention is by administration of the attenuated mumps virus vaccine. There is no proven effective therapy.

### *Measles*

Acute measles is not associated with virus infection of the CNS (140), even though postinfectious encephalomyelitis, an autoimmune disease, is relatively common (114,150,151) and is discussed later in this chapter. In persons with compromised cellular immunity, a subacute encephalitis may complicate measles (152). Measles inclusion body encephalitis usually appears within a few weeks of the primary infection, is slowly progressive over months, and is due to uncontrolled replication of measles virus in the CNS.

Subacute sclerosing panencephalitis (SSPE) is a rare late complication of measles. SSPE presents an average of 7–10 years after the original measles virus infection and usually occurs in individuals contracting measles at an early age (greater than 50% under the age of 2 years). SSPE occurs three times more often in males and is more common among children of rural origin (32,153–155). Typically, the first evidence of this afebrile disease is a decline in school performance. This is followed by the appearance of myoclonic jerks and frank dementia, progressing to coma and death in 1–3 years. Virus replication is defective (155,156), but viral antigen can be demonstrated in neurons and virus can occasionally be recovered by cocultivation (155–157). The state and location of the virus during the several year incubation period is unknown. Disease may progress rapidly to death over a few months or may stabilize for many years with or without treatment.

The incidence of SSPE has diminished markedly with the introduction of immunization for measles and does not appear to be a complication of the live virus vaccine (153,154). The diagnosis of SSPE is made by a compatible clinical picture and the presence of markedly elevated measles virus antibody in serum and CSF (46). Therapy is difficult to evaluate because of the rarity of the disease. Numerous drugs, including bromodeoxyuridine, iododeoxyuridine, azaguanine, amantadine, interferon, ether, isoprinosine, ribavirin, transfer factor, and inosiplex, have been tried, with only anecdotal uncorroborated reports of short-term benefit (158,159).

### **Arenaviruses**

The arenaviruses are enveloped viruses with segmented single-stranded negative-sense RNA. Viruses of this group usually infect their natural hosts in early life and induce life-long persistent infections with continuous release of infectious virus (156).

Essentially all of the pathogenic human arenaviruses have rodents as their natural hosts and reservoirs (160). The geographic distribution of each virus is distinct (160), and many of these agents are discussed in Chapter 18. The four most important human pathogens are lymphocytic choriomeningitis (LCM), lassa, Junin, and Machupo viruses. All have the potential to produce neurological complications late in infection. Analogous to the studies of experimental LCM virus infection of mice (161), many of the neurologic complications may be due to immunopathologic reactions to viral infection.

### Clinical Features

Lymphocytic choriomeningitis virus is found as an endemic infection of *Mus musculus* in focal areas of the Americas and Europe (160). Hamsters kept as pets (162) or for research purposes (163) may also be infected. The virus is shed in the urine of infected animals, and human infections are most common in the winter, when mice are more likely to be indoors. The incubation period of 5–10 days is followed by the onset of a flu-like febrile illness accompanied by leukopenia and thrombocytopenia. Neurologic disease, usually aseptic meningitis or meningoencephalitis, is a late manifestation of a typically biphasic illness and begins with the acute onset of headache, renewed fever, meningismus, and mental status changes. Recovery is slow with persistent pleocytosis, but is usually complete (32,163).

Lassa virus is found in West Africa where the rodent reservoir is *Mastomys natalensis,* and human infection is most common during the dry season. The virus can also be transmitted person to person (160). The incubation period is 3–16 days. The ratio of illness to infection ranges from 9% to 26%. In the general population, the case fatality rate is approximately 5% (164). Early symptoms are nonspecific and include fever, chills, myalgias, diarrhea, and pharyngitis. During the second week, a fulminant picture of hemorrhagic shock may appear (160). Of hospitalized cases, 17% die (165). Neurologic involvement other than acute mental status changes is primarily manifest by unilateral or bilateral eighth nerve deafness of unknown pathogenesis, which occurs in 4% of survivors. (157).

Junin and Machupo viruses, the causes of Argentine and Bolivian hemorrhagic fevers, respectively, are natural infections of *Calomys,* a small rodent (160). Argentine hemorrhagic fever occurs primarily in rural farm workers with occupational, presumably aerosol, exposure to *C. musculinis,* an inhabitant of corn and soybean fields. Bolivian hemorrhagic fever is acquired in houses, the habitat of *C. callosus*. Neurologic disease occurs in approximately 20% of individuals with clinically evident Junin virus infection. Neurological involvement during the acute phase of the disease is characterized by irritability, gait abnormalities, and tremor. The 25% mortality is decreased by treatment with immune plasma, but 11% of these patients develop a late neurologic syndrome of vertigo, oculomotor palsies, and cerebellar ataxia 2–3 weeks later. Human and animal studies both suggest that late neurologic disease is more common in individuals treated with antiviral serum. It is possible that early treatment with antibody promotes the establishment of persistent CNS infection (166–168).

### Therapy

Immune serum is effective therapy in clinical trials of Junin (166) but not lassa virus infection (169). Ribavirin has proven efficacious in the treatment of systemic lassa fever. Using a 10 day intravenous (IV) regimen of a 2-gm loading dose followed by 1 gm every 6 hrs for 4 days, and 0.5 gm every 8 hr for 6 days, mortality for high-risk patients was reduced from 76% to 9% when treatment was begun within 6 days of onset

(169). There are no published studies on treatment of lymphocytic choriomeningitis or Machupo virus infections of humans, but primate studies suggest that ribavirin is effective for treatment of the acute manifestations of Machupo and Junin virus infections but, like immune serum, does not prevent the late neurologic disease (Chapter 18).

## Retroviruses

Retroviruses are enveloped positive-stranded RNA viruses that are able to "reverse transcribe" their plus-stranded genomic RNA into DNA. Double-stranded copies of viral DNA are integrated into host DNA, producing a latent infection. Two human retroviruses, human immunodeficiency virus (HIV) and human lymphotropic virus type I (HTLV-I) are associated with neurologic disease in humans (170–175). For both, the latent period between infection and the onset of neurologic disease can be months to years. HIV belongs to the lentivirus group of nononcogenic retroviruses, whereas HTLV-I is oncogenic and causes an adult T-cell leukemia as well as neurologic disease (172,176). Transmission of either virus requires intimate contact between individuals or exposure to infected blood products. Geographic distribution of HIV is becoming worldwide, spreading out from several high incidence foci in the United States and Africa. HTLV-I infection is regionally distributed with the highest rates of seropositivity in southern Japan and the Caribbean and isolated foci identified in South America and Africa (177,178).

### *Clinical Features*

#### *Human Immunodeficiency Virus*

Neurologic disease in those infected with HIV is frequent (estimated at > 90% by the time of death) (179) and may be the presenting manifestation of infection (180,181). A wide variety of neurologic abnormalities may occur at different stages of HIV infection (175) (Fig. 2). Early in infection, some individuals develop an aseptic meningitis syndrome and others an asymptomatic mononuclear pleocytosis (170,171,182–184). Cognitive dysfunction at this stage is rare, although acute, self-limited meningoencephalitis does occur in association with a generalized infectious mononucleosis-type picture (182,184). After infection is established, but before the onset of immune deficiency, acute and chronic demyelinating polyneuropathies occur. These inflammatory polyneuropathies are likely to be immune-mediated and linked to the generalized immune dysfunction induced by HIV infection (181). Later, additional manifestations of neurologic disease (sensory neuropathy, encephalopathy, myelopathy) become apparent, usually coincident with evidence of immunodeficiency. Sensory neuropathy presenting as painful acral dysesthesias and paresthesias occurs in up to 30% (170,171). Acquired immune deficiency syndromes (AIDS) encephalopathy has a gradual onset, beginning with difficulty performing complicated tasks, and progressing to memory loss, apathy, and dementia and is a common complication late in disease (171,185). Myelopathy is well-described, but less common (172,186,187). CNS dysfunction is frequent in children with HIV infection, with acquired microcephaly, cognitive deficits, and bilateral pyramidal tract signs most common. Deterioration is usually subacute, but steadily progressive (188,189).

The pathogenesis of HIV-induced neurologic disease remains unclear since the role of the virus in the production of dementia, hypomyelination, vacuolar myelopathy, and sensory neuropathy has not yet been defined. Virus is frequently found in the CNS, but primarily in macrophages rather than in neural cells (190,191). Virus isolated from the CSF (192,193) can infect glial cells in culture (194,195) and may be biologically

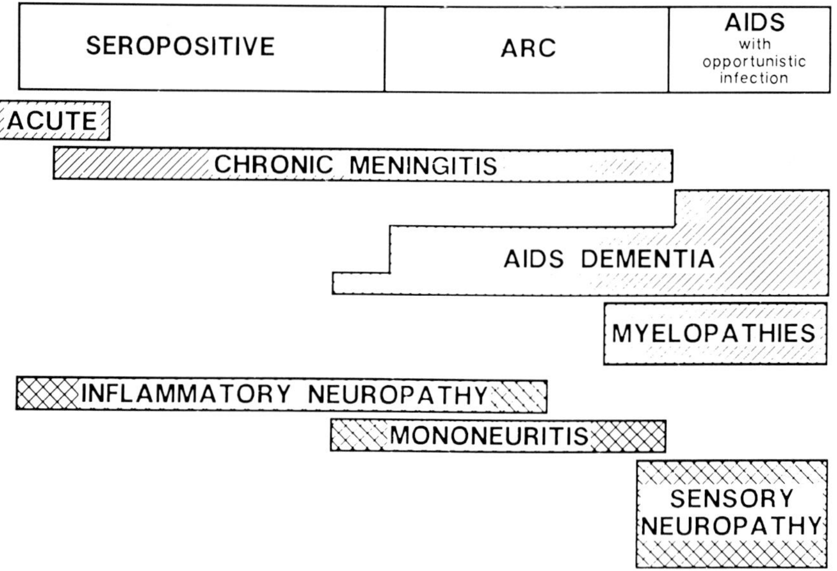


**FIG. 2.** Diagramatic representation of the neurologic diseases occurring in association with various stages of HIV infection. (From Johnson et al., ref. 175, with permission.)

distinct from virus isolated from blood (196).

### *Human T Lymphotropic Virus-I*

Infection with HTLV-I is strongly associated with the development of spastic paraparesis [termed "HTLV-I-associated myelopathy" (HAM) in Japan and "tropical spastic paraparesis" (TSP) elsewhere] (173,174,177). HTLV-I infection is also associated with chronic lymphocytosis and T-cell malignancy (176). Susceptibility to the neurologic disease is probably genetically linked (197) and may be more common when infection is acquired from blood transfusion (198). HTLV-I causes neurologic disease localized clinically and pathologically, primarily to the spinal cord. The onset of this symmetrical, upper motor neuron disorder is subacute, and the primary early symptoms are difficulty in walking and difficulty with urination. Sensory complaints are secondary or nonexistent. The disease progresses over months, with increasing spastic paralysis, and then stabilizes. Lower extremities are affected primarily, with usual sparing of the arms (165,166,190). Abnormal multilobulated T cells are present in the CSF as well as the blood (174,199). Virus has been isolated from the CSF (200), but has not yet been localized in tissue.

### ***Diagnosis***

Both HIV and HTLV-I can be cultured from CSF and blood of affected patients (192,193,200). A mononuclear CSF pleocytosis is common early in infection, but is usually absent late in disease (170,181–183). Intrathecal synthesis of antiviral antibody is often demonstrable late in both of these infectious processes (51,52). Neurologic disease due to treatable opportunistic infections, particularly cryptococcus and toxoplasma, should be ruled out in those with HIV infection (170,171,184).

### *Therapy*

Treatment of HIV- and HTLV-I-associated neurologic disease is under active investigation. Spastic paraparesis induced by HTLV-I shows some improvement with steroid treatment (173). This may be secondary to the effect of steroids on spasticity or may suggest an autoimmune component to the disease (197). Azidothymidine (AZT) is currently being evaluated as treatment for the neurologic manifestations of both HIV and HTLV-I infection. Effective penetration of the thymidine analogs, such as AZT, into the CNS has not been established. Like thymidine, these drugs have no affinity for the nucleoside transport systems located within the blood-brain barrier (22) but are effectively transported into the CSF, however, they do not equilibrate with brain interstitial fluid (23,24,201) (Table 1). Early data, however, suggest neurologic improvement in HIV-infected children treated intravenously with AZT (24) and mixed results with oral AZT therapy in HIV-infected adults with a variety of neurologic complications (23,202,203). Acute and chronic inflammatory neuropathies usually respond to conventional treatment with plasmapheresis (181,204).

## Herpesviruses

The herpesviruses are large, enveloped, double-stranded DNA viruses. Hundreds of species are known, and seven of these cause disease in humans. All of the human herpesviruses, except the newly described human herpesvirus-6, have been recognized as at least occasional causes of CNS disease, ranging from benign aseptic meningitis to fatal encephalitis. All of the herpesviruses establish latent, usually asymptomatic, infections after the primary infection (205). CNS disease can occur either during the primary or reactivated infection. HSV type 1 (HSV-1) is most often latent in sensory neurons of the trigeminal ganglion. The latent state of HSV-1 is probably in the form of episomal DNA and is associated with the expression of an immediate early gene "anti-sense" transcript not found during active infection (206,207). HSV-2 is usually latent in sensory neurons of the sacral ganglia. VZV is latent in multiple sensory ganglia but probably in the supporting satellite cells rather than the neurons themselves. Epstein-Barr virus (EBV) is latent in B lymphocytes (205). The site of cytomegalovirus (CMV) latency has not been established unequivocally (205).

### *Clinical Features*

#### *HSV*

Even though HSV-1 and HSV-2 are regularly found latent in sensory ganglia, symptomatic CNS infection is unusual. Encephalitis occurs as a consequence of perinatal infection with either virus and during primary or reactivated HSV-1 infection later in life (208,210). In adults, HSV-2 infection is most often associated with aseptic meningitis, but has caused significant encephalitis in immunocompromised individuals (211,212). HSV-1 is occasionally associated with meningitis. (210,213).

*Neonatal Infection.* Infants may be exposed to HSV at the time of birth or earlier if there is premature rupture of the membranes. HSV-induced disease in the newborn is most likely to occur when the mother contracts a primary HSV infection during pregnancy, exposing the infant to infectious virus in the absence of maternal antibody (214,215). The incubation period is typically 1–3 weeks. The most frequent initial manifestations of infection are lethargy, failure to feed, skin lesions, and fever (216,217). Nearly 50% of infants with neonatal HSV infection are premature (216). HSV-2 causes more severe disease than HSV-1. In neonatal infection with HSV-2, there is a higher frequency of seizures, more profound CSF abnormalities, and more frequent evidence of damage on computerized tomographic (CT) scanning of the brain (217).

*Diagnosis.* Cesarian section birth can prevent exposure of the infant to an HSV-infected genital tract, but maternal infection is usually asymptomatic and therefore unknown to mother and physician alike. Furthermore, most infected mothers do not provide a history of genital herpes, and cultures taken during gestation do not predict shedding at the time of delivery. Therefore, neonatal exposure to HSV is frequently not predictable or preventable (218). Fortunately, few exposed infants develop disease, but HSV must be considered in the differential diagnosis of illness in the first weeks of life regardless of the risk factors identified (218). The diagnosis of HSV infection is most frequently made in an ill infant by culturing skin lesions, but in some cases brain biopsy may be necessary (219). The CSF typically has a mononuclear pleocytosis, red blood cells, and increased protein. Admission electroencephalogram (EEG) is usually abnormal, whereas the CT scan is usually normal. The CT scan usually becomes abnormal during the course of encephalitis induced by HSV-2 but not necessarily during HSV-1-induced CNS disease (217).

*Therapy.* In the untreated neonate, the mortality of disseminated or CNS HSV infection is 74%. Of the survivors, 50% have significant residual morbidity (220). Children with delayed antibody synthesis and HSV-2 infection have the poorest prognosis. Both vidarabine and acyclovir (ACV) are effective treatments and cannot be distinguished (220,221). Recommended treatment with vidarabine is 30 mg/kg/day over 12 hr for 10 days and with ACV is 10 mg/kg every 8 hr for 10 days. Latent infection of the CNS may be established in some children despite treatment, resulting in recurrent reactivation and continued neurologic deterioration (222); therefore, longer antiviral therapy may be necessary.

*Encephalitis.* HSV encephalitis is the most common form of fatal endemic encephalitis in the United States (223). It occurs equally in both sexes and at all times of the year. Over 95% of cases are caused by infection with HSV-1 (210). Encephalitis may be a manifestation of primary infection (most common in children and young adults) or reactivated infection (most common in older adults) (210). There is no evidence for point source outbreaks of encephalitis due to more virulent strains of HSV (224,225). Virus isolated from a peripheral site may or may not be the same strain as found in brain of that individual (226). The route by which the virus enters the CNS is not yet clear, but the consistency with which infection localizes to the temporal lobe suggests that entry is by a neural route rather than from the blood. Encephalitis may be preceded by a nonspecific prodrome of fever and malaise. The onset of headache may be acute or subacute and accompanied by behavioral abnormalities, fever, focal or generalized seizures, and lethargy. Focal temporal lobe signs are common. The disease progresses to coma over days to weeks. There is a 70% mortality, and an additional 20% are left with severe neurologic residua. These problems include speech and cognitive deficits, seizures, paralysis, and ataxia.

*Diagnosis.* Temporal lobe localization of disease is an important diagnostic clue and is often demonstrated earliest by the EEG (227). Brain scan and magnetic resonance imaging (MRI) scan are often positive earlier than an enhanced CT scan (228,229). Previous history of herpes labialis or isolation of HSV from the oropharynx is not helpful (230). Early CSF may appear normal, but later a mononuclear pleocytosis with or without red blood cells (RBCs) is the rule. Protein is often elevated (48). Virus is rarely recovered from the CSF but can be recovered from the brain (210). Once temporal lobe localization is established, the involved area should be biopsied for definitive diagnosis. The biopsy should be subjected to routine pathologic examination and immunocytochemical staining for HSV antigen, and cultured for virus. Of these, culture is the most sensitive means of detecting infection (210).

Although the need for biopsy before treatment remains a subject of discussion (231,232), definitive diagnosis is important. The response to therapy is often slow, and the patient may continue to deteriorate even with appropriate treatment. Uncertainty about the diagnosis may encourage addition of other unnecessary therapeutic modalities or delay appropriate treatment for one of the many diseases that can mimic HSV-encephalitis and are not optimally treated with ACV (233). The need for a noninvasive diagnostic test is great, and there is some promise for the development and use of tests to detect HSV-related antigens in the CSF of infected individuals (234). CSF antibody levels rise during infection, but too late to be diagnostically useful (48).

*Therapy.* Treatment with vidarabine (15 mg/kg/day for 10 days) decreases the overall mortality from 70% to 30–40% at 1 month and 40–50% at 6 months (233,235). Treatment with ACV (10 mg/kg every 8 hr for 10 days) is more effective than vidarabine, decreasing overall mortality to 13% at 1 month and 28% at 6 months, with approximately 50% of survivors returning to normal function (235,236). The earlier treatment is begun in the course of the disease, the better the outcome (230,233,235). Additional prognostic indicators are the age of the patient (with younger patients doing significantly better), level of consciousness (233,235), and the amount of virus present in the biopsied brain (210). To balance the need for a biopsy-proven diagnosis and the need to begin therapy as soon as possible, it is reasonable to begin ACV when the diagnosis is suspected and while arranging for the biopsy to be done (preferably within the first 24 hr of presumptive treatment). The optimal duration of therapy has not been established. Controlled treatment trials have used 10 days. However, several patients have been reported to relapse after completing this course (237–239), and future trials will use a 14-day treatment period (240). Animal studies using combined vidarabine and ACV show enhanced antiviral activity compared to either drug alone, but controlled data from patients are not yet available (241).

*Meningitis.* Genital infection with HSV-2 has been associated with sacral radiculopathy and urinary retention (242), with meningitis (207), and infrequently with encephalitis (210,212). HSV-1 occasionally causes meningitis (213). Treatment with ACV is reasonable, but most patients recover uneventfully without therapy.

### *VZV*

A wide variety of neurologic complications has been reported in association with VZV infection. CNS complications occur in the setting of advanced age and immunosuppression, and in apparently normal individuals. Complications occur both during varicella (primary VZV infection) and in conjunction with herpes zoster or shingles (reactivated VZV infection) (243,244).

*Varicella.* The most common neurologic complication of varicella is cerebellar ataxia. This disease has a benign course and is thought to be immunologically mediated rather than the result of direct VZV infection of the CNS (244). A small number of individuals develop meningoencephalitis associated with altered consciousness, seizures, and motor deficits. Many of these cases are examples of postinfectious encephalomyelitis, an immune-mediated disease (245), but a few cases are due to direct virus invasion of the CNS (246). Cases of acute transverse myelitis of uncertain pathogenesis have also been described after varicella (247).

*Zoster.* During zoster or shingles, caused by reactivation of VZV from its latent state in one or more sensory ganglia, a number of neurological complications have been recognized. These include paralysis anatomically associated with anterior horn cells near the reactivated sensory ganglion (248), generalized meningoencephalitis (249), cerebral arteritis (250,251), and post herpetic neuralgia (252). In addition, a mononuclear pleocytosis is common in individuals with uncomplicated disease (253). Segmental zoster paresis is associated most frequently with lesions of the C5 and C6 dermatomes, probably because of their more important motor innervation compared with the thoracic dermatomes. Paresis is flaccid, sudden in onset, and occurs at the time of the rash. There is usually significant recovery.

Zoster meningoencephalomyelitis occurs almost exclusively in the elderly or immunocompromised host in association with cutaneous dissemination of virus (243). Affected individuals have the sudden onset of headache, fever, and/or hallucinations followed by obtundation. Seizures are relatively unusual, even though focal neurologic deficits are frequent. Mild to moderate pleocytosis and an elevated protein level are common CSF findings. The EEG is usually abnormal but nonfocal.

Granulomatous angiitis has been described in VZV infections both as part of the syndrome of ophthalmic zoster and contralateral hemiparesis, suggesting contiguous spread of virus to the CNS (250) and as generalized CNS involvement in the immunosuppressed patient (251). This complication usually appears weeks to months after the dermatomal eruption and follows a waxing and waning course. Angiography shows segmental narrowing of involved arteries. Pathologic examination shows infarction, granulomatous arteritis, and virus in vessels and brain (253,254).

The most common neurologic complication of shingles is postherpetic neuralgia. Pain in the involved dermatome is essentially universal during the early phases of the disease, often beginning before the appearance of the rash. Pain gradually subsides over weeks to months in the majority of individuals and is completely resolved in 80% by 1 year. However, in a small proportion of individuals, mostly those over 60 years of age with severe zoster, the pain does not subside and can be debilitating (252). This is not due to continued virus replication in the sensory ganglion, but rather to the inflammation and damage resulting from the acute phases of infection.

Two neurologic syndromes have also been attributed to VZV infection but occur without recent dermatomal evidence of virus reactivation: multifocal leukoencephalitis (255,256) and acute retinal necrosis (257). Multifocal VZV leukoencephalitis is a demyelinating disease that has been described only in immunocompromised patients. The disease has a subacute onset with progressive multifocal motor, sensory, and cognitive defects similar both clinically and pathologically to progressive multifocal leukoencephalopathy (PML) due to JC virus infection. VZV can be demonstrated in the brain parenchyma (255,256).

Acute retinal necrosis occurs primarily in previously healthy adults but probably in immunocompromised individuals as well (258). The disease presents with decreased vision, pain, and erythema in the involved eye, may spread to the other eye (36%), and progresses to blindness in over 70%. A few patients have a history of shingles within the previous 3 months (259), but many do not (257,260). Eye pathology shows necrotizing retinitis, retinal arteritis, and optic neuropathy. VZV antigens have been detected in the involved tissue, and VZV has been cultured from the vitreous humor in at least one case (260).

### *Therapy*

Treatment of immunocompromised patients with dermatomal zoster early in disease with interferon-α, vidarabine, or ACV can prevent visceral spread of infection (261–263). There is no controlled data on treatment of VZV-induced disease already localized to the nervous system. For complications likely to be due to direct virus infection of the CNS, ACV therapy at a dose of 500 mg/M$^2$ body surface area every 8 hr is generally accepted and has been reported to be efficacious in acute retinal necrosis (258,259,264). The incidence of postherpetic neuralgia may be decreased with antiviral therapy (261,262,265).

The role of steroids is controversial. One study has shown decreased time with pain in a small number of elderly patients treated with systemic steroids during acute disease (266), but there is also an increased likelihood of disseminated disease in patients taking steroids. Patients with post-herpetic neuralgia whose pain is not controlled with mild analgesics such as aspirin or tylenol can usually be effectively managed with a combination of aneleptics (diphenylhydantoin or tegretol) and tricyclic antidepressants titrated to full therapeutic doses (267,268). Narcotic analgesics are often not useful and should be avoided because of the problem of addiction in patients with chronic pain.

### *EBV*

EBV can cause meningoencephalitis as well as a variety of other neurologic problems as part of infectious mononucleosis (269–271). Less than 1% of cases of infectious mononucleosis are complicated by overt neurologic problems, but CSF abnormalities occur in up to 25% (272). Neurological problems that include Guillain-Barré syndrome, Bell's palsy, encephalitis, cerebellar ataxia, and myelitis usually occur 1–3 weeks after the onset of mononucleosis in immunologically normal individuals and may be the only manifestation of EBV infection (272,273). Complete recovery is the rule, but occasional fatalities have been reported (271). The clinical picture usually suggests meningitis or a diffuse meningoencephalitis, but occasionally the disease is focal or recurrent (274). An undetermined proportion of this neurologic disease is autoimmune [postinfectious encephalomyelitis (269) or Guillain-Barré syndrome (273)], but there is also disease due to direct virus invasion of the CNS since virus has occasionally been recovered from brain and from CSF (270). Although ACV has had limited use in EBV-induced infections (275), treatment for CNS disease has not been established.

### *CMV*

CMV is an uncommon, but reported, cause of meningoencephalitis in immunologically normal individuals (276,277) and has emerged as a significant cause of CNS disease in patients with immunosuppression related to organ transplantation or HIV infection (277–280). Acute CMV mononucleosis complicated by meningoencephalitis presents with headache, progressing over several days to confusion, disorientation, and seizures. Aseptic meningitis due to CMV has also been reported (277). Infants with congenital cytomegalic inclusion body disease may have microcephaly, seizures, growth retardation, chorioretinitis, and intracerebral calcifications (277). Immunosuppressed adults with CMV infection of the CNS present in a subacute fashion with confusion, disorientation, and myelopathy. Multiple glial nodules with cytomegalic cells are seen on pathology. Ganciclovir (DHPG) has been used successfully at a usual dose of 5 mg/kg every 12 hr for treatment of CMV retinitis (281), but its efficacy for meningoencephalitis has not been established.

### *Herpes B Virus*

Herpes B virus (HBV) (*Herpesvirus simiae*) is a benign, latent infection in macaques analogous to HSV infection in humans. The virus may be transmitted by the bite of an asymptomatic infected monkey and cause fatal encephalitis in humans (282,283). Of the 22 reported cases of symptomatic human infection, 20 have resulted in encephalitis, and 15 of these patients have died (284). Symptoms of HBV disease usually appear within 1 month of exposure and typically begin with vesicular skin lesions near the site of virus inoculation. This is followed by local neurologic symptoms (numbness, dysesthesies) and encephalitis (284). The most important control measures involve use of proper precautions when handling primates, particularly macaques, and their tissues. These precautions include use of protective clothing and proper methods of restraint (282). Viral replication is inhibited by ACV *in vitro* and *in vivo* (285), and early use in human infection has been associated with recovery (283).

### PML (JC Virus)

JC virus, a papovavirus, causes progressive multifocal leukoencephalopathy (PML), a noninflammatory demyelinating disease (286). Primary JC virus infection usually occurs in childhood and has not yet been associated with a disease entity (287). Virus appears to remain latent in the kidney and possibly the bone marrow but has not been found in brain in the absence of CNS disease (288,289). It appears most likely that the virus is reactivated and spreads to the CNS in infected B lymphocytes (288), concomitant with immunosuppressive disease or therapy. Asymptomatic urinary excretion is relatively common in immunosuppressed patients, whereas CNS disease remains rare (290). The lesions in the brain are multifocal demyelinating lesions caused by infection and lysis of oligodendroglial cells (291). Onset of PML is insidious and presents initially with impaired speech, vision, and mental function, without fever or headaches. CSF is often normal or may have an elevated protein. Progressive mental deterioration results in paralysis, blindness, and eventually, death within months. There is no established treatment.

### Unconventional Agents

Kuru, a neurological disease recognized only in the Fore people of New Guinea and now declining in incidence, and Creutzfeldt-Jacob disease, a sporadic disease found worldwide, are both caused by spongioform encephalopathy agents (292). The nature of the infectious agent remains unclear, but infectivity is postulated to be closely associated with an altered cellular protein (293). Kuru presents with motor incoordination, tremor, and ataxia, progressing to incapacitation and death within months after onset (292). The disease can be transmitted by several routes of inoculation to primates (294,295) and is thought to be transmitted within the Fore people by ceremonies of ritual cannibalism (292). Creutzfeldt-Jacob is an afebrile disease presenting as a presenile dementia characterized by deteriorating mental status, myoclonus, normal CSF, and a progressive decline to death within months. The disease has been transmitted to primates (295) and accidentally to humans through infected tissues and contaminated surgical instruments (296–298). The natural mode of spread is unknown, but person-to-person transfer appears to be unusual or nonexistent. The diagnosis is based on clinical features or brain biopsy. There is no known therapy.

## IMMUNE-MEDIATED CNS DISEASES RELATED TO VIRAL INFECTION OR IMMUNIZATION

A number of CNS diseases occur in association with viral infections and vaccines but are not clearly related to virus replication within the nervous system. Some have been shown to be immune-mediated, and for others the pathogenesis remains unclear.

### Post-Rabies Vaccine Encephalomyelitis

Rabies vaccine prepared from the neural tissue of mature animals has been associated with "neuroparalytic accidents" since shortly after its introduction by Pasteur in 1885. Because of low cost and good efficacy, phenol-inactivated neural tissue (Semple) vaccines continue to be the primary means of rabies immunization in much of the world. Neurologic complications occur in approximately 1 in 300 recipients and are more frequent in those who have received prior rabies immunization (129). Initial symptoms of fever, headache, and myalgia usually occur 6–14 days after the initiation of immunization. Neurologic signs usually appear within 1 week after the prodromal symptoms. Disease may be manifested as meningitis, altered consciousness, motor, or sensory deficits, or as a peripheral neuropathy resembling the Guillain-Barré syndrome. In most patients, the disease is monophasic, but occasionally it is progressive or relapsing (129). Treatment with steroids appears to be beneficial, and most patients improve within a week and go on to complete recovery. The reported mortality rate varies from 0% to 18%, with the highest rate being among patients developing the Guillain-Barré syndrome.

CSF examination shows a moderate mononuclear pleocytosis and increased protein. Myelin basic protein is present in the CSF of patients with encephalitis or myelitis, but not in patients with meningitis or peripheral neuritis (130). This demyelinating disease is similar in pathology and pathogenesis to experimental autoimmune encephalomyelitis (EAE). Of patients with major neurologic complications, 75% have high levels of antibody to myelin basic protein, the primary encephalitogen in EAE (130). The problem of CNS complications is circumvented by the use of rabies vaccine made in suckling mouse brain (131), eggs, or tissue culture cells (human diploid or Vero cell vaccine) (132–136). This disease is postulated to be the human equivalent of EAE.

### Postinfectious Encephalomyelitis

A disease clinically and pathologically similar to postrabies vaccine encephalomyelitis occurs in 1 in 1,000 cases of measles and less frequently after other viral exanthems and nonviral infectious diseases (114). The disease has an abrupt onset of fever and obtundation and is frequently associated with seizures and multifocal neurologic signs. Postinfectious encephalomyelitis characteristically occurs 4–8 days after the onset of the rash in measles. The disease has a monophasic course over 10–20 days in the majority of cases. The mortality is approximately 10–20%. The majority of the surviving patients have neurologic sequelae. The CSF usually has a mild mononuclear pleocytosis, modest protein elevation, and presence of myelin basic protein, but may be completely normal (151). The pathologic changes of inflammation and perivenular demyelination are remarkably similar to those seen in rabies vaccine complications and EAE (114). The autoimmune hypothesis is supported by the lack of demonstrable viral antigen or nucleic acid in the CNS (299), lack of a local antibody response to the virus, and the presence of an immune response to myelin basic protein (151). There is no recognized treatment.

### Guillain-Barré Syndrome

The Guillain-Barré syndrome is an acute monophasic inflammatory demyelinating polyneuropathy that occurs most often after infection (300). CMV is the virus that is most frequently associated with the Guillain-Barré syndrome (301), but several other viruses, including HIV and EBV, have been frequently linked to the onset of this disease (181,273). The disease presents with symmetrical paralysis usually within 1–4 weeks of the onset of the acute illness and is thought to be immunologically mediated (300). Plasmapheresis instituted early in the course of disease significantly improves outcome (302).

### Multiple Sclerosis

Multiple sclerosis has often been postulated to be caused by a virus based on epidemiologic considerations. Over the years, a large number of viruses have been implicated at one time or another, either by reports of isolation from brain or by increased amounts of antibody in serum or CSF, as the etiologic agent for this demyelinating disease (303). So far, none has been confirmed. Numerous abnormalities of immune regulation and a genetic susceptibility linked to the histocompatibility leukocyte antigen (HLA) locus have been documented. (304). Although the etiology and pathogenesis of this remitting and relapsing inflammatory demyelinating disease remain elusive, current thinking favors the possibility of a viral infection initiating an autoimmune process in a genetically susceptible individual.

## ACKNOWLEDGMENT

Work from my laboratory was supported by the National Multiple Sclerosis Society and grant AI23047 from the National Institutes of Health. Manuscript preparation by Linda Kelly is gratefully acknowledged.

## REFERENCES

1. Ehrlich P. Zur therapeutischen Bedeutung der substituirenden Schwefelsauregruppe. *Ther Monatsh* 1887;1:88–90.
2. Reese TS, Karnovsky MJ. Fine structural localization of a blood-brain barrier to exogenous peroxidase. *J Cell Biol* 1967;34:207–17.
3. Brightman MW, Reese TS. Junctions between intimately apposed cell membranes in the vertebrate brain. *J Cell Biol* 1969;40:648–77.
4. Goldstein GW, Betz AL. Blood vessels and the blood-brain barrier. In: Asbury AK, McKhann GM, McDonald WI, eds. *Diseases of the nervous system*. Philadelphia: W.B. Saunders, 1986:172–84.
5. Pardridge WM, Oldendorf WH, Cancilla P, Frank HJL. Blood-brain barrier: interface between internal medicine and the brain. *Ann Intern Med* 1986;105:82–95.
6. Helmer ME. Adhesive protein receptors on hematopoietic cells. *Immunol Today* 1988;9:109–13.
7. Friedemann U. Permeability of the blood-brain barrier to neurotropic viruses. *Arch Pathol* 1943;35:912–31.
8. Brightman MW, Klatzo I, Olsson Y, Reese TS. The blood-brain barrier to proteins under normal and pathological conditions. *J Neurol Sci* 1970;10:215–39.
9. Maxwell DS, Pease DC. The electron microscopy of the choroid plexus. *J Biophys Biochem Cytol* 1956;2:467–81.
10. Van Deurs B, Koehler JK. Tight junctions in the choroid plexus epithelium: a freeze-fracture study including complementary replicas. *J Cell Biol* 1979;80:662–73.
11. Felgenhauer K. Protein size and cerebrospinal fluid composition. *Klin Wochenschr* 1974;52:1158–64.
12. Griffin DE, Giffels J. Study of protein characteristics that influence entry into cerebrospinal fluid of normal mice and mice with encephalitis. *J Clin Invest* 1982;70:289–95.
13. Brightman MW. The intracerebral movement of proteins injected into blood and cerebrospinal fluid of mice. *Prog Brain Res* 1967;29:19–37.
14. Collins JM, Dedrick RL. Distributed model for drug delivery to CSF and brain tissue. *Am J Physiol* 1983;245:R303–10.
15. Benet LZ, Sheiner LB. Pharmacokinetics. The dynamics of drug absorption, distribution, and elimination. In: Gilman AG, Goodman LS, Rall TW, Murad F, eds. *The pharmacological basis of therapeutics*. New York: Macmillan Publishing Co., 1985:3–34.
16. Kalaria RN, Harik SI. Nucleoside transporter of cerebral microvessels and choroid plexus. *J Neurochem* 1986;47:1849–56.
17. Cornford EM, Oldendorf WH. Independent blood-brain barrier transport systems for nucleic acid precursors. *Biochem Biophys Acta* 1975;394:211–9.
18. Whitley RJ, Blum MR, Barton N, de Miranda P. Pharmacokinetics of acyclovir in humans following intravenous administration. *Am J Med* 1982;73(suppl):165–71.
19. Blum MR, Liao SHT, de Miranda P. Overview of acyclovir pharmacokinetic disposition in adults and children. *Am J Med* 1982; 73(suppl):186–92.
20. Spector R. Transport of amantadine and rimantadine through the blood-brain barrier. *J Pharmacol Exp Ther* 1988;244:516–9.
21. Norris SM, Mandell GL. Tables of antimicrobial agent pharmacology. In: Mandell GL, Douglas Jr RG, Bennett JE, eds. *Principles and practice of infectious diseases*. 2nd ed. New York: John Wiley & Sons, 1985:308–32.
22. Terasaki T, Pardridge WM. Restricted transport of 3′ azido-3′-deoxythymidine and dideoxynucleosides through the blood-brain barrier. *J Infect Dis* 1988;158:630–2.
23. Klecker Jr RW, Collins JM, Yarchoan R, Thomas R, Jenkins JF, Broder S, Myers CE. Plasma and cerebrospinal fluid pharmacokinetics of 3′-azido-3′-deoxythymidine: a novel pyrimidine analog with potential application for the treatment of patients with AIDS and related diseases. *Clin Pharmacol Ther* 1987;41:407–12.
24. Pizzo PA, Eddy J. Falloon J, et al. Effect of continuous intravenous infusion of zidovudine (AZT) in children with symptomatic HIV infection. *N Engl J Med* 1988;319:889–96.
25. Fletcher C, Sawchuk R, Chinnock B, de Mi-

randa P, Balfour Jr HH. Human pharmacokinetics of the anti-viral drug DHPG. *Clin Pharmacol Ther* 1986;40:281–6.
26. Emodi G, Just M, Hernandez R, Hirt HR. Circulating interferon in man after administration of exogenous human leukocyte interferon. *JNCI* 1975;54:1045–9.
27. Ferrar EA, Oishi JS, Wannemacher Jr RW, Stephen EL. Plasma disappearance, urine excretion, and tissue distribution of ribivirin in rats and rhesus monkeys. *Antimicrob Agents Chemother* 1981;19:1042–9.
28. Roberts RB, Laskin OL. Phase I clinical studies of ribavirin in high risk patients for the acquired immunosuppression syndrome. In: Smith RA, ed. *HIV and other highly pathogenic viruses*. New York: Academic Press, 1988:95–112.
29. Crumpacker C, Bubley G, Lucey D, Hussey D, Connor J. Ribavirin enters cerebrospinal fluid. *Lancet* 1986;2:45–6.
30. Whitley R, Alford C, Hess F, Buchanan R. Vidarabine: a preliminary review of its pharmacological properites and therapeutic use. *Drugs* 1980;20:267–82.
31. Shope TC, Kauffman RE, Bowman D, Marcus EL. Pharmacokinetics of vidarabine in the treatment of infants and children with infections due to herpesviruses. *J Infect Dis* 1983;148:721–5.
32. Johnson RT. *Viral infections of the nervous system*. New York: Raven Press, 1982.
33. Friedman HM, Macarak EJ, MacGregor RR, Wolfe J, Kefalides NA. Virus infection of endothelial cells. *J Infect Dis* 1981;143:266–73.
34. Mims CA. *The pathogenesis of infectious diseases*. 2nd ed. New York: Academic Press, 1982.
35. Hirsch RL. The complement system: its importance in the host response to viral infection. *Microbiol Rev* 1982;46:71–85.
36. Griffin JW, Watson DF. Axonal transport in neurological disease. *Ann Neurol* 1988;23:3–13.
37. Murphy FA. Rabies pathogenesis: a brief review. *Arch Virol* 1977;54:279.
38. Baringer JR. Herpes simplex virus infection of nervous tissue in animals and man. *Prog Med Virol* 1975;20:1–26.
39. Monath TP, Cropp CP, Harrison AK. Mode of entry of a neurotropic arbovirus into the central nervous system. Reinvestigation of old controversy. *Lab Invest* 1983;48:399–410.
40. Winkler WG, Fashinall TR, Leffingwell L, Howard P, Conomy JP. Airborne rabies transmission in a laboratory worker. *JAMA* 1973;226:1219–21.
41. Griffin DE, Hess JL, Moench TR. Immune response in the central nervous system. *Toxicol Pathol* 1987;15:294–302.
42. Tourtelotte WW. On cerebrospinal fluid immunogloblin quotients in multiple sclerosis and other diseases: a review and a new formula to estimate the amount of IgG synthesis per day by the central nervous system. *J Neurol Sci* 1970;10:279–304.
43. Kabat EA, Moore DH, Landow H. An electrophoretic study of the protein components in cerebrospinal fluid and their relationship to the serum proteins. *J Clin Invest* 1942;21:571–7.
44. Ganrot K, Laurell CB. Measurement of IgG and albumin content of cerebrospinal fluid, and its interpretation. *Clin Chem* 1974;20:571–3.
45. Eickhoff K, Heipertz R. Discrimination of elevated immunoglobulin concentrations in CSF due to inflammatory reaction of the central nervous system and blood-brain-barrier dysfunction. *Acta Neurol Scand* 1977; 56:475–82.
46. Tourtellotte WW, Ma BI, Brandes DB, Walsh MJ, Porvin AR. Quantification of de novo central nervous system IgG measles antibody synthesis in SSPE. *Ann Neurol* 1981;9:551–6.
47. Hovi T, Stenvik M, Kinnunen E. Diagnosis of poliomyelitis by demonstration of intrathecal synthesis of neutralizing antibodies. *J Infect Dis* 1986;153:998–9.
48. Koskiniemi M, Vaheri A, Taskinen E. Cerebrospinal fluid alterations in herpes simplex virus encephalitis. *Rev Infect Dis* 1984;6:608–17.
49. Vartdal F, Vandvik B, Norrby E. Intrathecal synthesis of virus-specific oligoclonal IgG, IgA and IgM antibodies in a case of varicella zoster meningoencephalitis. *J Neurol Sci* 1982;57:121–32.
50. Vandvik B, Nilsen RE, Vartdal F, Norrby E. Mumps meningitis: specific and nonspecific antibody responses in the central nervous system. *Acta Neurol Scand* 1982;65:468–87.
51. Gessain A, Caudie, C, Gout O, et al. Intrathecal synthesis of antibodies to human T lymphotropic virus type I and the presence of IgG oligoclonal bands in the cerebrospinal fluid of patients with endemic tropical spastic paraparesis. *J Infect Dis* 1988;157:1226–34.
52. Resnick L, diMarzo-Veronese F, Schupbach J, et al. Intra-blood-brain-barrier synthesis of HTLV-III-specific IgG in patients with neurologic symptoms associated with AIDS or AIDS-related complex. *N Engl J Med* 1985;313:1498–1504.
53. Melnick JL. Enteroviruses: polioviruses, coxsackie viruses, echoviruses and newer enteroviruses. In: Fields BN, eds. *Virology*. New York: Raven Press, 1985:739–94.
54. Modlin JF. Poliovirus. In: Mandell GL, Douglas Jr RG, Bennett JE, eds. *Principles and practice of infectious diseases*. 2nd ed. New York: John Wiley & Sons, 1985:806–14.
55. Modlin JF. Coxsackievirus and echovirus. In: Mandell GL, Douglas Jr RG, Bennett JE, ed. *Principles and practice of infectious diseases*. 2nd ed. New York: John Wiley & Sons, 1985:914–925.
56. Enders JF, Weller TH, Robbins FC. Cultivation of the Lansing strain of poliomyelitis virus in cultures of various human embryonic tissues. *Science* 1949;109:85.
57. Bodian D, Morgan IM, Howe HA. Differentiation of types of poliomyelitis viruses: III. The grouping of fourteen strains into three basic immunological types. *Am J Hyg* 1949;49:234–45.
58. Howe HA, Bodian D. Poliomyelitis in the

chimpanzee: a clinical-pathological study. *J Exp Med* 1941;69:149–81.

59. Sabin AB, Ward R. The natural history of poliomyelitis: I. Distribution of virus in nervous and non-nervous tissues. *J Exp Med* 1941;73:771–93.
60. Bodian D. Pathogenesis of poliomyelitis in normal and passively immunized primates after virus feeding. *Federation Proceedings* 1952; 11:462.
61. Horstmann DM, McCollum RW. Poliomyelitis virus in human blood during the "minor illness" and the asymptomatic infection. *Proc Soc Exp Biol Med* 1953;82:434.
62. Centers for Disease Control. Poliomyelitis—United States, 1975–1984. *Morb Mort Weekly Report* 1986;35:180–2.
63. Nathanson N. Epidemiologic agents of poliomyelitis eradication. *Rev Infect Dis* 1984; 6:S308–12.
64. Moore M. Enteroviral disease in the United States, 1970–1979. *J Infect Dis* 1982;146:103–8.
65. Modlin JF. Perinatal echovirus infection: insights from a literature review of 61 cases of serious infection and 16 outbreaks in nurseries. *Rev Infect Dis* 1986;8:918–26.
66. Kaplan MH, Klein SW, McPhee J, Harper RG. Group B coxsackie virus infections in infants younger than three months of age. *Rev Infect Dis* 1983;5:1019–32.
67. Hammond GW, MacDougall BK, Plummer F, Sekla LH. Encephalitis during the prodromal stage of acute hepatitis A. *Can Med Assoc J* 1982;126:269–70.
68. Hodges JR. Hepatitis A and meningoencephalitis. *J Neurol* 1987;234:364.
69. Melnick JL. Enterovirus type 71 infections: a varied clinical pattern sometimes mimicking paralytic poliomyelitis. *Rev Infect Dis* 1984;6:S387–90.
70. McKinney Jr RE, Katz SL, Wilfert CM. Chronic enteroviral meningoencephalitis in agammaglobulinemic patients. *Rev. Infect Dis* 1987;9:334–56.
71. Horstmann DM, Quinn TC, Robbins FC. International symposium on poliomyelitis control. *Rev. Infect Dis* 1984;6:S301–600.
72. Fox JP. Modes of action of poliovirus vaccines and relation to resulting immunity *Rev Infect Dis* 1984;6:S352–5.
73. Immunization Practices Advisory Committee. Poliomyelitis prevention: enhanced-potency inactivated poliomyelitis vaccine—supplementary statement. *Morb Mort Weekly Report* 1987;36:795–8.
74. Minor PD, John A, Ferguson, M, Icenogle JP. Antigenic and molecular evolution of the vaccine strain of type 3 poliovirus during the period of excretion by a primary vaccinee. *J Gen Virol* 1986;67:693–706.
75. WHO Consultative Group. The relation between acute persisting spinal paralysis and poliomyelitis vaccine—results of a ten-year enquiry. *Bull WHO* 1982;60:231–42.
76. Robinson WS. Hepatitis A virus. In: Mandell GL, Douglas Jr RG, Bennett JE, eds. *Principles and practice of infectious diseases*. New York: John Wiley & Sons, 1985:829–40.
77. Mease PJ, Ochs HD, Wedgwood RJ. Successful treatment of echovirus meningoencephalitis and myositis-fascitis with intravenous immune globulin therapy in a patient with X-linked agammaglobulinemia. *N Engl J Med* 1981;304:1278–81.
78. Erlendsson K, Swartz T, Dwyer JM. Successful reversal of echovirus encephalitis in X-linked hypogammaglobulinemia by intraventricular administration of immunoglobulin. *N Engl J Med* 1985;312:351–3.
79. Johnson RT. Arboviral encephalitis. In: Warren KS, Mahmoud AAF, eds. *Tropical and geographical medicine*. 2nd ed. New York: McGraw Hill (in press).
80. Griffin DE. Alphavirus pathogenesis and immunity. In: Schlesinger S, Schlesinger MJ, eds. *The togaviridae and flaviviridae*. New York: Plenum Publ. Corp., 1986:209–49.
81. Russell PK. Alphavirus (Eastern, Western, and Venezuelan equine encephalitis). In: Mandell GL, Douglas Jr RG, Bennett JE, eds. *Principles and practice of infectious diseases*, 2nd ed. New York: John Wiley, 1985:917–20.
82. Farber S, Hill A, Connerly ML, Dingle JH. Encephalitis in infants and children caused by the virus of the Eastern variety of equine encephalitis. *JAMA* 1940;114:1725–31.
83. Centers for Disease Control. Arboviral infections of the central nervous system—United States, 1987. *Morb Mort Weekly Report* 1988;37:506–15.
84. Kokernot RH, Shinefield HR, Longshore WA. The 1952 outbreak of encephalitis in California. *Calif Med* 1953;79:73–7.
85. Lennette EH, Koprowski H. Human infection with Venezuelan equine encephalomyelitis virus: a report on eight cases of infection acquired in the laboratory. *JAMA* 1943;123:1088–95.
86. Ehrenkranz NJ, Ventura AK. Venezuelan equine encephalitis virus infection in man. *Annu Rev Med* 1974;25:9–14.
87. Schlesinger S, Schlesinger MJ, eds. *The togaviridae and flaviviridae*. New York: Plenum Publ. Corp., 1986.
88. Monath TP. Flaviviruses. In: Fields BN, Knipe DM, Chanock RM, Melnick JL, Roizman B, Shope RE, eds. *Virology*. New York: Raven Press, 1985:955–1104.
89. Umenai T, Krzysko R, Bektimirov TA, Assaad FA. Japanese encephalitis: current worldwide status. *Bull WHO* 1985;63:625–31.
90. Sabin AB. Epidemic encephalitis in military personnel. *JAMA* 1947;133:281–93.
91. Dickerson RB, Newton JR, Hansen JE. Diagnosis and immediate prognosis of Japanese B encephalitis. *Am J Med* 1952;12:277–88.
92. Kokernot RH, Hayes J, Will RL, Tempelis CH, Chan DHM, Radivojivic B. Arbovirus studies in the Ohio-Mississippi basin, 1964–1967. II. St. Louis encephalitis virus. *Am J Trop Med Hyg* 1969;18:750–61.

93. Tsai TF, Canfield MA, Reed CM, et al. Epidemiological aspects of a St. Louis encephalitis outbreak in Harris County, Texas, 1986. *J Infect Dis* 1988;157:351–6.
94. Southern PM, Smith JW, Luby JP, Barnett JA, Sanford JP. Clinical and laboratory features of epidemic St. Louis encephalitis. *Ann Intern Med* 1969;71:681–90.
95. White MG, Carter NW, Rector FC, Seldin DW. Pathophysiology of epidemic St. Louis encephalitis. I. Inappropriate secretion of antidiuretic hormone. *Ann Intern Med* 1969;71:691–702.
96. Smorodintsev AA. Tick-borne spring-summer encephalitis. *Prog Med Virol* 1958;1:210–48.
97. Grascenkov NK. Tick-borne encephalitis in the USSR. *Bull WHO* 1964;30:187–96.
98. Asher DM. Chronic encephalitis. In: Boese A, ed. *Search for the cause of multiple sclerosis and other chronic diseases of the central nervous system*. Weinhem: Verlag Chemie, 1980:272–9.
99. Blaskovic D. The public health importance of tick-borne encephalitis in Europe. *Bull WHO* 1967;1:5–13.
100. Cruse RP, Rothner AD, Erenberg G, Calisher CH. Central European tick-borne encephalitis: an Ohio case with a history of foreign travel. *Am J Dis Child* 1979;133:1070–71.
101. Shope RE. Bunyaviruses. In: Fields BN, Knipe DM, Chanock RM, Melnick JL, Roizman B, Shope RE, eds. *Virology*. New York: Raven Press, 1985:1055–82.
102. Parkin WE, Hammon WMD, Sather GE. Review of current epidemiological literature on viruses of the California arbovirus group. *Am J Trop Med Hyg* 1972;21:964–78.
103. Johnson KP, Lepow ML, Johnson RT. California encephalitis. I. Clinical and epidemiological studies. *Neurology* 1969;18:250–4.
104. Centers for Disease Control. Arboviral infections of the central nervous system—United States, 1986. *Morb Mort Weekly Report* 1987;36:450–5.
105. Centers for Disease Control. Update: *Aedes albopictus* infestation—United States. *Morb Mort Weekly Report* 1987;35:769–73.
106. Centers for Disease Control. La Crosse encephalitis in West Virginia. *Morb Mort Weekly Report* 1988;37:79–82.
107. Van Velden DJ, Meyer JD, Oliver J, Gear JHS, McIntosh B. Rift Valley fever affecting humans in South Africa: a clinico-pathological study. *S Afr Med J* 1977;51:867–71.
108. Burke DS, Nisalak A, Ussery MA, Laorakpongse T, Clantavibul S. Kinetics of Japanese encephalitis virus immunoglobulin M and G antibodies in human serum and cerebrospinal fluid. *J Infect Dis* 1985;151:1093–9.
109. Hofmann H, Frisch-Niggemeyer W, Heinz F, Kunz Ch. Immunoglobulins to tick-borne encephalitis in the cerebrospinal fluid of man. *J Med Virol* 1979;4:241–5.
110. Hoke CH, Nisalak A, Sangawhipa N, et al. Protection against Japanese encephalitis by inactivated vaccines. *N Engl J Med* 1988;319:608–14.
111. Kunz Ch, Hofmann H, Heinz FX, Dippe H. Efficacy of vaccination against tick-borne encephalitis (TBE). *Wien Klin Wochenschr* 1980;92:890.
112. Randall R, Gibbs CJ, Aulisio CG, Binn LN, Harrison VR. The development of a formalin-killed Rift Valley fever vaccine for use in man. *J Immunol* 1962;89:660–71.
113. Glukhov BN, Jerusalimsky AP, Canter VM, Salganik RI. Ribonuclease treatment of tick-borne encephalitis. *Arch Neurol* 1976;33:598–603.
114. Johnson RT, Griffin DE, Gendelman HE. Postinfectious encephalomyelitis. *Semin Neurol* 1985;5:180–90.
115. Alford Jr CA. Rubella. In: Remington JS, Klein JO, eds. *Infectious diseases of the fetus and newborn infant*. Philadelphia: WB Saunders, 1976:71–106.
116. Townsend JJ, Baringer JR, Wolinsky JS, et al. Progressive rubella panencephalitis: late onset after congenital rubella. *N Engl J Med* 1975;292:990–3.
117. Weil ML, Itabashi HH, Cremer NE, Oshiro LS, Lennette EH, Carnay L. Chronic progressive panencephalitis due to rubella virus simulating subacute sclerosing panencephalitis. *N Engl J Med* 1975;292:994–8.
118. Wolinsky JS, Dau PC, Buimovici-Klein, et al. Progressive rubella panencephalitis: immunovirological studies and results of isoprinosine therapy. *Clin Exp Immunol* 1979;35:397–404.
119. Baer GM. Rabies virus. Fields BN, ed. In: *Virology*. New York: Raven Press, 1985:1133–56.
120. Murphy FA, Bauer SP, Harrison AK, et al. Comparative pathogenesis of rabies and rabies-like viruses: viral infection and transit from inoculation site to the central nervous system. *Lab Invest* 1973;28:361.
121. Iwasaki Y, Liu D-S, Yamamoto T, Konno H. On the replication and spread of rabies virus in the human central nervous system. *J Neuropathol Exp Neurol* 1985;44:185–95.
122. Bernard KW, Hattwick MAW. Rabies virus. In: Mandell GL, Douglas RG Jr, Bennett JE, eds. *Principles and infectious diseases*. 2nd ed. New York: John Wiley & Sons, 1985:897–909.
123. Anderson LJ, Nicholson KG, Tauxe RV, Winkler WG. Human rabies in the United States, 1960–1979: epidemiology, diagnosis and prevention. *Ann Intern Med* 1984;100:728–35.
124. Hemachudha T, Phanthumchinda K, Phanuphak P, Manutsathit S. Myoedema as a clinical sign in paralytic rabies. *Lancet* 1987;1:1210.
125. Centers for Disease Control. Human rabies—California, 1987. *Morb Mort Weekly Report* 1988;37:305–8.
126. Larghi OP, Gonzalez E, Held JR. Evaluation of the corneal test as a laboratory method for rabies diagnosis. *Appl Microbiol* 1973;25:187–9.
127. Bryceson ADM, Greenwood BM, Warrell DA, et al. Demonstration during life of rabies antigen in humans. *J Infect Dis* 1975;131:71–4.
128. Blenden DC, Creech W, Torres-Anjel MJ. Use of immunofluorescence examination to detect rabies virus antigen in the skin of humans with

clinical encephalitis. *J Infect Dis* 1986;154:698–701.

129. Hemachudha T, Phanuphak P, Johnson RT, Griffin DE, Ratanavongsiri J, Siriprasomsup W. Neurological complications of Semple type rabies vaccine: clinical and immunological studies. *Neurology* 1987;37:550–6.
130. Hemachudha T, Griffin DE, Giffels JJ, Johnson RT, Moser AB, Phanuphak P. Myelin basic protein as an encephalitogen in encephalomyelitis and polyneuritis following rabies vaccination. *N Engl J Med* 1987;316:369–74.
131. Fuenzalida, E, Palacios R. Rabies vaccine prepared from brains of infected suckling mice. *Boletino Instituto Bacteriologico Chile* 1955;8:3–10.
132. Immunization Practices Advisory Committee. Rabies prevention: supplementary statement on the preexposure use of human diploid cell rabies vaccine by the intradermal route. *Morb Mort Weekly Report* 1986;35:767–8.
133. Center for Disease Control. Rabies vaccine, adsorbed: a new rabies vaccine for use in humans. *Morb Mort Weekly Report* 1988;37:217–23.
134. Pappaioanou M, Fishbein DB, Dreeson DW, et al. Antibody response to preexposure human diploid-cell rabies vaccine given concurrently with chloroquine. *N Engl J Med* 1986;314:280–4.
135. Centers for Disease control. Human rabies—Kenya. *Morb Mort Weekly Report* 1983;32:494–5.
136. Immunization Practices Advisory Committee. Rabies prevention—United States, 1984. *Morb Mort Weekly Report* 1984;33:393–402.
137. Baer GM, Fishbein DB. Rabies post-exposure prophylaxis. *N Engl J Med* 1987;316:1270–2.
138. Merigan TC, Bar GM, Winkler WG, et al. Human leukocyte interferon administration to patients with symptomatic and suspected rabies. *Ann Neurol* 1984;16:82–7.
139. Wolinsky JS, Server AC. Mumps virus. In: Fields BN, ed. *Virology*. New York: Raven Press, 1985:1255–84.
140. Moench TR, Griffin DE, Obriecht CR, Vaisberg AJ, Johnson RT. Acute measles in patients with and without neurological involvement: distribution of measles virus antigen and RNA. *J Infect Dis* 1988;158:433–42.
141. Meyer HM, Johnson RT, Crawford IP, et al. Central nervous system syndromes of "viral" etiology: a study of 713 cases. *Am J Med* 1960;29:334–47.
142. Herndon RM, Johnson RT, Davis LE, Descalzi LR. Ependymitis in mumps virus meningitis. *Arch Neurol* 1974;30:475–9.
143. Timmons GD, Johnson KP. Aqueductal stenosis and hydrocephalus after mumps encephalitis. *N Engl J Med* 1970;283:1505–7.
144. Centers for Disease Control. Mumps surveillance. January 1977–December 1982. Atlanta, Georgia: United States Department Health and Human Services, Public Health Service, 1984.
145. Bistrian B, Phillips CA, Kaye IS. Fatal mumps meningoencephalitis: isolation of virus pre-mortem and post-mortem. *JAMA* 1972;222:478–9.
146. McLean DM, Bach RD, Larke RPB, McNaughton GA. Mumps meningoencephalitis, Toronto, 1963. *Can Med Assoc J* 1964; 90:458–62.
147. Wilfert CM. Mumps meningoencephalitis with low cerebrospinal fluid glucose, prolonged pleocytosis and elevation of protein. *N Engl J Med* 1969;280:855–9.
148. Azimi PH, Shaban S, Hilty MD, Haynes RE. Mumps meningoencephalitis: Prolonged abnormality of cerebrospinal fluid. *JAMA* 1975;234:1161–2.
149. Kilham L. Mumps meningoencephalitis with and without parotitis. *Am J Dis Child* 1949;78:324–33.
150. Miller DL. Frequency of complications of measles, 1963. *Br Med J* 1964;2:75–8.
151. Johnson RT, Griffin DE, Hirsch RL, et al. Measles encephalomyelitis—clinical and immunologic studies. *N Engl J Med* 1984;310:137–41.
152. Roos RP, Graves MC, Wollmann RL, Chilcote RR, Nixon J. Immunologic and virologic studies of measles inclusion body encephalitis in an immunosuppressed host: the relationship to subacute sclerosing panencephalitis. *Neurology* 1981;31:1263–70.
153. Modlin JF, Jabbour JT, Witte JJ, Halsey NA. Epidemiologic studies of measles, measles vaccine, and subacute sclerosing encephalitis. *Pediatrics* 1977;59:505–12.
154. Zilber N, Rannon L, Alter M, Kahana E. Measles, measles vaccination, and risk of subacute sclerosing panencephalitis (SSPE). *Neurology* 1983;33:2558–2564.
155. ter Meulen V, Carter MJ. Measles virus persistency and disease. *Prog Med Virol* 1984;30:44–61.
156. Kristensson K, Norrby E. Persistence of RNA viruses in the central nervous system. *Annu Rev Microbiol* 1986;40:159–84.
157. Horta-Barbosa L, Fucillo DA, Sever JL. Subacute sclerosing panencephalitis: Isolation of measles virus from a brain biopsy. *Nature* 1969;221:974.
158. Lehrich JR. Measles-like virus (subacute sclerosing panencephalitis). In: Mandell GL, Douglas Jr RG, Bennett JE, eds. *Principles and practice of infectious disease*. New York: John Wiley & Sons, 1985:1034–7.
159. Griffith JF, Ch'ien LT. Viral infections of the central nervous system. In: Galasso GJ. Merigan TC, Buchanan RA, eds. *Antiviral agents and viral diseases of man*. 2nd ed. New York: Raven Press, 1984:399–432.
160. Johnson KM. Lymphocytic choriomeningitis virus, lassa virus, tacaribe group of viruses and hemorrhagic fevers. In: Mandell GL, Douglas Jr RG, Bennett JE, eds. *Principles and practice of infectious diseases*. New York: John Wiley & Sons, 1985:909–14.
161. Buchmeier MJ, Welsh RM, Dutko FJ, Oldstone MBA. The virology and immunobiology of lymphocytic choriomeningitis virus infection. *Adv Immunol* 1980;30:275–331.

162. Hirsch MS, et al. Lymphocytic-choriomeningitis virus infection traced to a pet hamster. *N Engl J Med* 1974;291:610–2.
163. Vanzee BE, Douglas Jr RG, Betts RF, Bauman AW, Fraser DW, Hinman AR. Lymphocytic choriomeningitis in university hospital personnel. *Am J Med* 1975;58:803–9.
164. McCormick JB, Webb PA, Krebs JW, Johnson KM, Smith ES. A prospective study of the epidemiology and ecology of lassa fever. *J Infect Dis* 1987;155:437–44.
165. McCormick JB, King IJ, Webb, PA, et al. A case control study of the clinical diagnosis and course of lassa fever. *J Infect Dis* 1987;155:445–55.
166. Maiztegui JI, Fernandez NJ, de Damilano AJ. Efficacy of immune plasma in treatment of Argentine haemorrhagic fever and association between treatment and a late neurological syndrome. *Lancet* 1979;2:1216–7.
167. Kenyon RH, Green DE, Eddy GA, Peters CJ. Treatment of Junin virus-infected guinea pigs with immune serum: development of late neurological disease. *J Med Virol* 1986;20:207–18.
168. Eddy GA, Wagner FS, Scott SK, Mahlandt BJ. Protection of monkeys against Machupo virus by the passive administration of Bolivian hemorrhagic fever immunoglobulin (human origin) *Bull WHO* 1975;52:723–6.
169. McCormick JB, King IJ, Webb PA, et al. Lassa fever: effective therapy with ribavirin. *N Engl J Med* 1986; 314:20–6.
170. McArthur JC. Neurologic manifestations of human immunodeficiency virus infection. *Medicine* 1987;66:407–37.
171. Elder GA, Sever JL. Neurologic disorders associated with AIDS retroviral infection. *Rev Infect Dis* 1988;10:286–302.
172. Johnson RT, McArthur JC. Myelopathies and retroviral infections. *Ann Neurol* 1987;21:113–6.
173. Osame M, Matsumoto M, Usuku K, et al. Chronic progressive myelopathy associated with elevated antibodies to human T-lymphotropic virus type I and adult T-cell leukemia-like cells. *Ann Neurol* 1987;21:117–22.
174. Vernant JC, Maurs L, Gessain A, et al. Endemic tropical spastic paraparesis associated with human T-lymphotropic virus type I: a clinical and seroepidemiological study of 25 cases. *Ann Neurol* 1987;21:123–30.
175. Johnson RT, McArthur JC, Narayan O. The neurobiology of human immunodeficiency virus infections. *FASEB J* 1989;2:2970–81.
176. Murphy EL, Blattner WA. HTLV-I associated leukemia: a model for chronic retroviral diseases. *Ann Neurol* 1988;23 (suppl):S174–80.
177. Roman GC. The neuroepidemiology of tropical spastic paraparesis. *Ann Neurol* 1988;23 (suppl):S113–20.
178. Hinuma Y, Komoda H, Chosa T, et al. Antibodies to adult T-cell leukemia-virus-associated antigen (ATLA) in sera from patients with ATL and controls in Japan: a nationwide sero-epidemiologic study. *Int J Cancer* 1982;29:631–5.
179. Jordan BD, Navia BA, Petito C, Cho E-S, Price RW. Neurological syndromes complicating AIDS. *Front Radiat Ther Oncol* 1985;19:82–7.
180. Navia BA, Price RW. The acquired immunodeficiency syndrome dementia complex as the presenting or sole manifestation of human immunodeficiency virus infection. *Arch Neurol* 1987;44:65–9.
181. Cornblath DR, McArthur JC, Kennedy PGE, Witte AS, Griffin JW. Inflammatory demyelinating peripheral neuropathies associated with human T-cell lymphotropic virus type III infection. *Ann Neurol* 1987;21:32–40.
182. Hollander H, Stringari S. Human immunodeficiency virus-associated meningitis. *Am J Med* 1987;83:813–6.
183. Appleman ME, Marshall DW, Brey RL, et al. Cerebrospinal fluid abnormalities in patients without AIDS who are seropositive for the human immunodeficiency virus. *J Infect Dis* 1988;158:193–9.
184. Hollander H. Cerebrospinal fluid normalities and abnormalities in individuals infected with human immunodeficiency virus. *J Infect Dis* 1988;158:855–8.
185. Navia BA, Jordan BD, Price RW. The AIDS dementia complex: I. clinical features. *Ann Neurol* 1986;19:517–24.
186. Rance NE, McArthur JC, Cornblath DR, Landstrom DL, Griffin JW, Price DL. Gracile tract degeneration in patients with sensory neuropathy and AIDS. *Neurology* 1988;38:265–71.
187. Petito CK, Navia BA, Cho ES, Jordan BP, George DC, Price RW. Vacuolar myelopathy pathologically resembling subacute combined degeneration in patients with the acquired immunodeficiency syndrome. *N Engl J Med* 1985;312:874–9.
188. Epstein LG, Sharer LR, Oleske JM, et al. Neurologic manifestations of human immunodeficiency virus infection in children. *Pediatrics* 1986;78:678–87.
189. Belman AL, Diamond G, Dickson D, et al. Pediatric acquired immunodeficiency syndrome: Neurologic syndromes: *Am J Dis Child* 1988;142:29–35.
190. Keonig S, Gendelman HE, Orenstein JM, et al. Detection of AIDS virus in macrophages in brain tissue from AIDS patients with encephalopathy. *Science* 1986;233:1089–93.
191. Gabuzda DH, Ho DD, de la Monte SM, Hirsch MS, Rota TR, Sobel RA. Immunohistochemical identification of HTLV-III antigens in brains of patients with AIDS. *Ann Neurol* 1986;20:289–95.
192. Ho DD, Rota TR, Schooley RT, et al. Isolation of HTLV-III from cerebrospinal fluid and neural tissues of patients with neurologic syndromes related to the acquired immunodeficiency syndrome. *N Engl J Med* 1985;313:1493–7.
193. Hollander H, Levy JA. Neurologic abnormalities and recovery of human immunodeficiency virus from cerebrospinal fluid. *Ann Intern Med* 1987;106:692–5.
194. Chiodi F, Fuerstenberg S, Gidlund M, Asjo B,

Fenjo EM. Infection of brain derived cells with the human immunodeficiency virus. *J Virol* 1987;61:1244–47.
195. Cheng-Mayer C, Rutka JT, Rosenblum ML, McHugh T, Stites DP, Levy JA. Human immunodeficiency virus can productively infect cultured human glial cells. *Proc Natl Acad Sci USA* 1987;84:3526–30.
196. Cheng-Mayer C, Levy JA. Distinct biological and serological properties of human immunodeficiency viruses from the brain. *Ann Neurol* 1988;23(suppl):S58–61.
197. Ujsuku K, Sonoda S, Osame M, et al. HLA haplotype-linked high immune responsiveness against HTLV-I in HTLV-I-associated myelopathy: comparison with adult T-cell leukemia/lymphoma. *Ann Neurol* 1988;23(suppl):S143–50.
198. Osame M, Izumo S, Igata A, et al. Blood transfusion and HTLV-I associated myelopathy. *Lancet* 1986;2:104.
199. Johnson RT, Griffin DE, Arregui A, et al. Spastic paraparesis and HTLV-1 infection in Peru. *Ann Neurol* 1988;23(suppl):S151–5.
200. Jackson S, Raine CS, Mingioli ES, McFarlin DE. Isolation of an HTLV-1 like retrovirus from patients with tropical spastic paraparesis. *Nature* 1988;331:540–3.
201. Spector R, Berlinger WG. Localization and mechanism of thymidine transport in the central nervous system. *J Neurochem* 1982;39:837–41.
202. Fiala M, Cone LA, Cohen N, et al. Responses of neurologic complications of AIDS to 3′-azido-3′-deoxythymidine and 9-(1,3 dihydroxy-2-propoxymethyl) guanine. I. Clinical features. *Rev Infect Dis* 1988;10:250–6.
203. Schmitt FA, Bigley JW, McKinnis R, Logue PE, Evans RW, Drucker JL, AZT Collaborative Working Group. Neuropsychological outcome of zidovudine (AZT) treatment of patients with AIDS and AIDS-related complex. *N Engl J Med* 1988;319:1573–8.
204. Cornblath DR. Treatment of the neuromuscular complications of human immunodeficiency virus infection. *Ann Neurol* 1988;23(suppl)S88–91.
205. Jordan MC, Jordan GW, Stevens JG, Miller G. Latent herpesviruses of humans. *Ann Intern Med* 1984;100:866–80.
206. Stevens JG, Haar L, Porter DD, Cook ML, Wagner EK. Prominance of the herpes simplex virus latency-associated transcript in trigeminal ganglia from seropositive humans. *J Infect Dis* 1988;158:117–23.
207. Croen KD, Ostrove JM, Dragovic LJ, Smialek JE, Straus SE. Latent herpes simplex virus in human trigeminal ganglia: detection of an immediate early gene "anti-sense" transcript by *in situ* hybridization. *N Engl J Med* 1987;317:1427–32.
208. Craig CP, Nahmias AJ. Different patterns of neurologic involvement with herpes simplex virus types 1 and 2: isolation of herpes simplex virus type 2 from the buffy coat of two adults with meningitis. *J Infect Dis* 1973;127:365–72.
209. Nahmias AJ, Josey WE. Herpes simplex viruses 1 and 2. In: Evans AS, ed. *Viral infections of humans: epidemiology and control.* 2nd ed. New York: Plenum Medical Book Co., 1982:351–72.
210. Nahmias AJ, Whitley RJ, Visintine AN, Takei Y, Alford Jr CA, and the Collaborative Antiviral Study Group. Herpes simplex virus encephalitis. Laboratory evaluations and their diagnostic significance. *J Infect Dis* 1982;145:829–36.
211. Linneman CC, First MR, Alvira MM, Alexander JW, Schiff GM. Herpesvirus hominis type 2 meningoencephalitis following renal transplantation. *Am J Med* 1976;61:703–8.
212. Dix RP, Waitzman DM, Follansbee S, et al. Herpes simplex virus type 2 encephalitis in two homosexual men with persistent lymphadenopathy. *Ann Neurol* 1985;17:203–6.
213. Heller M, Dix RD, Baringer JR, Schachter J, Conte Jr JE. Herpetic proctitis and meningitis: recovery of two strains of herpes simplex type 1 from cerebrospinal fluid. *J Infect Dis* 1982;146:584–8.
214. Prober OG, Sullender WM, Yasukawa LL, Au DS, Yeager AS, Arvin AM. Low risk of herpes simplex virus infections in neonates exposed to the virus at the time of vaginal delivery to mothers with recurrent genital herpes simplex virus infections *N Engl J Med* 1987;316:240–4.
215. Brown ZA, Vontver LA, Benedetti J, Critchlow CW, Sells CJ, Berry S, Corey L. Effects on infants of a first episode of genital herpes during pregnancy. *N Engl J Med* 1987;317:1246–51.
216. Whitley RJ, Nahmias AJ, Visintine AM, Fleming CL, Alford CA. The natural history of herpes simplex virus infection of mother and newborn. *Pediatrics* 1980;66:489–94.
217. Corey L. Stone EF, Whitley RJ, Mohan K. Difference between herpes simplex virus type 1 and type 2 neonatal encephalitis in neurological outcome. *Lancet* 1988;1:1–4.
218. Prober CG, Hensleigh PA, Boucher FD, Yasukawa LL, Au DS, Arvin AM. Use of routine viral cultures at delivery to identify neonates exposed to herpes simplex virus. *N Engl J Med* 1988;318:887–91.
219. Nahmias AJ, Visintine AM. Herpes simplex. In: Remington JS, Klein JO, eds. *Infectious diseases of the fetus and newborn infant.* Philadelphia: WB Saunders Co., 1976:156–90.
220. Whitley RJ, Arvin A, Corey L, et al. *Vidarabine versus acyclovir therapy of neonatal herpes simplex infections.* Washington, D.C.: Society for Pediatric Research, 1986.
221. Whitley RJ, Nahmias AJ, Soong S-J, Galasso GG, Fleming CL, Alford CA. Vidarabine therapy of neonatal herpes simplex infection. *Pediatrics* 1980;66:498–501.
222. Gutman LT, Wilfert CM, Eppes S. Herpes simplex virus encephalitis in children: analysis of cerebrospinal fluid and progressive neuro-

developmental deterioration. *J Infect Dis* 1986;154:415–21.
223. Olson LC, Buescher EL, Artenstein MS, et al. Herpes virus infections of the human central nervous system. *N Engl J Med* 1967;227:1271–77.
224. Hammer SM, Buchman TG, D'Angelo LJ, Karchmer AW, Roizman B, Hirsch MS. Temporal clusters of herpes simplex encephalitis: investigation by restriction endonuclease cleavage of viral DNA. *J Infect Dis* 1980;141:436–40.
225. Landry ML, Berkovits IV, Summers WP, Booss J, Hsiung GD, Summers WC. Herpes simplex encephalitis: analysis of a cluster of cases by restriction endonuclease mapping of virus isolates. *Neurology* 1983;33:831–5.
226. Whitley R, Lakeman AD, Nahmias A, Roizman B. DNA restriction-enzyme analysis of herpes simplex virus isolates obtained from patients with encephalitis. *N Engl J Med* 1982;307:1060–2.
227. Whitley RJ, Soong S-J, Linneman Jr C, Liu C, Pazin G, Alford CA, NIAID Collaborative Antiviral Study Group. Herpes simplex: clinical assessment. *JAMA* 1982;247:317–20.
228. Neils EW, Lukin R, Tomsick TA, Tew JM. Magnetic resonance imaging and computerized tomography scanning of herpes simplex encephalitis. *J Neurosurg* 1987;67:592–4.
229. Schroth G, Gawehn J, Thron A, Vallbracht A, Voigt K. Early diagnosis of herpes simplex encephalitis by MRI *Neurology* 1987;37:179–83.
230. Whitley RJ, Soong S-J, Dolin R, Galasso CJ, Chien LT, Alford Jr CA, Collaborative Study Group. Adenine arabinoside therapy of biopsy-proved herpes simplex encephalitis. *N Engl J Med* 1977;297:289–94.
231. Hanley DF, Johnson RT, Whitley RJ. Yes, brain biopsy should be a prerequisite for herpes simplex encephalitis treatment. *Arch Neurol* 1987;44:1289–90.
232. Fishman RA. No, brain biopsy need not be done in every patient suspected of having herpes simplex encephalitis. *Arch Neurol* 1987;44:1291–2.
233. Whitley RJ, Soong S-J, Hirsch MS, et al. Herpes simplex encephalitis: vidarabine therapy and diagnostic problems. *N Engl J Med* 1981;304:313–8.
234. Lakeman FD, Koga J, Whitley RJ. Detection of antigen to herpes simplex virus in cerebrospinal fluid from patients with herpes simplex encephalitis. *J Infect Dis* 1987;155:1172–8.
235. Whitley RJ, Alford CA, Hirsch MS, et al. Vidarabine versus acyclovir therapy in herpes simplex encephalitis. *N Engl J Med* 1986;314:144–9.
236. Skoldenberg B, Alestig K, Burman L, et al. Acyclovir versus vidarabine in herpes simplex encephalitis. Randomised multicenter study in consecutive Swedish patients. *Lancet* 1984;2:707–11.
237. Dix RD, Baringer JR, Panitch HS, Rosenberg SH, Hagedorn J, Whaley J. Recurrent herpes simplex encephalitis: recovery of virus after ara-A treatment. *Ann Neurol* 1983;196–200.
238. Van Landingham KE, Marsteller HB, Ross GW, Hayden FG. Relapse of herpes simplex encephalitis after conventional acyclovir therapy. *JAMA* 1988;259:1051–3.
239. Rothman AL, Cheeseman SH, Lehrman SN, Cederbaum A, Glew RH. Herpes simplex encephalitis in a patient with lymphoma: relapse following acyclovir therapy. *JAMA* 1988;259:1056–7.
240. Whitley RJ. Editorial: the frustrations of treating herpes simplex virus infections of the central nervous system. *JAMA* 1988;259:1067.
241. Park N-H, Callahan JG, Pavon-Langston D. Effect of combined acyclovir and vidarabine on infection with herpes simplex virus *in vitro* and *in vivo*. *J Infect Dis* 1984;149:757–62.
242. Samaransinghe PL, Oates JK, Mac Lennan IPB. Herpetic proctitis and sacral radiculomyelopathy—a hazard for homosexual men. *Br Med J* 1979;2:365–6.
243. Jemsek J, Greenberg SB, Taber L, Harvey D, Gershon A, Couch RB. Herpes zoster-associated encephalitis: clinicopathologic report of 12 cases and review of the literature. *Medicine* 1983;62:81–7.
244. Johnson R, Milbourn PD. Central nervous system manifestations of chickenpox. *Can Med Assoc J* 1970;102:831–4.
245. Shope TC. Chickenpox encephalitis and encephalopathy: evidence for differing pathogenesis. *Yale J Biol Med* 1982;55:321–7.
246. Takashima S, Becker LE. Neuropathology of fatal varicella. *Arch Pathol Lab Med* 1979;103:209–13.
247. McCarthy JT, Amer J. Post varicella acute transverse myelitis: a case presentation and review of the literature. *Pediatrics* 1978;62:202–4.
248. Weiss S, Streifler M, Weiser HJ. Motor lesions in herpes zoster: incidence and special feature. *Eur Neurol* 1975;13:332–8.
249. Peterson LR, Ferguson RM. Fatal central nervous system infection with varicella zoster virus in renal transplant recipients. *Transplantation* 1984;37:366–8.
250. Gilbert GJ. Herpes zoster ophthalmicus and delayed contralateral hemiparesis: relationship of the syndrome to central nervous system granulomatous angiitis. *JAMA* 1979;229:302–304.
251. Rosenblum WI, Hadfield MG. Granulomatous angiitis of the nervous system in cases of herpes zoster and lymphosarcoma. *Neurology* 1972;22:348–54.
252. Ragozzino MW, Melton LJ, Kurland LT, Chu CP, Perry HO. Population-based study of herpes zoster and its sequelae. *Medicine* 1982;61:310–6.
253. Linnemann CC, Alvira MM. Pathogenesis of varicella-zoster angiitis in the CNS. *Arch Neurol* 1980;37:239–40.
254. Reyes MG, Fresco R, Chokroverty S, Salud EQ. Virus like particles in granulomatous an-

giitis of the central nervous system. *Neurology* 1976;26:797–9.
255. Morgello S, Block GA, Price RW, Petito CK. Varicella-zoster virus leukoencephalitis and cerebral vasculopathy. *Arch Pathol Lab Med* 1988;112:1873–7.
256. Horten B, Price RW, Jimenez D. Multifocal varicella-zoster virus leukoencephalitis temporally remote from herpes zoster. *Ann Neurol* 1981;9:251–66.
257. Fisher JP, Lewis ML, Blumenkranz M, et al. The acute retinal necrosis syndrome. Part 1: clinical manifestations. *Ophthalmology* 1982;89:1309–16.
258. Jabs DA, Schachat AP, Liss R, Knox DL, Michels RG. Presumed varicella zoster retinitis in immunocompromised patients. *Retina* 1987;7:9–13.
259. Browning DJ, Blumenkranz MS, Culbertson WW, et al. Association of varicella zoster dermatitis with acute retinal necrosis syndrome. *Ophthalmology* 1987;94:602–6.
260. Culbertson WW, Blumenkranz MS, Pepose JS, Stewart JA, Curtin VT. Varicella zoster virus is a cause of the acute retinal necrosis syndrome. *Ophthalmology* 1986;93:559–69.
261. Merigan TC, Rand KH, Pollard RB, Adballah PS, Jordan GW, Fried RP. Human leukocyte interferon for the treatment of herpes zoster in patients with cancer. *N Engl J Med* 1978;298:981–7.
262. Whitley RJ, Soong S-J, Dolin R, et al. Early vidarabine therapy to control the complications of herpes zoster in immunosuppressed patients. *N Engl J Med* 1982;307:971–5.
263. Balfour Jr HH, Bean B, Laskin OL, et al. Acyclovir halts progression of herpes zoster in immunocompromised patients. *N Engl J Med* 1983;308:1448–53.
264. Blumenkranz MS, Culbertson WW, Clarkson JG, Dix R. Treatment of the acute retinal necrosis syndrome with intravenous acyclovir. *Ophthalmology* 1986;93:296–300.
265. Sklar SH, Blue WT, Alexander EJ, Bodian CA. Herpes zoster: the treatment and prevention of neuralgia with adenosine monophosphate. *JAMA* 1985;253:1427–30.
266. Eaglstein WH, Katz R, Brown JA. The effects of early corticosteroid therapy on the skin eruption and pain of herpes zoster. *JAMA* 1970;211:1681–3.
267. Gerson GR, Jones RB, Luscombe DK. Studies on the concomitant use of carbamazepine and clomipramine for the relief of post-herpetic neuralgia. *Postgrad Med J* 1977;53(suppl 4):104–9.
268. Watson CP, Evans RJ, Reed K, Merskey H, Goldsmith L, Warsh J. Amitriptyline versus placebo in post herpetic neuralgia. *Neurology* 1982;32:671–3.
269. Ambler M, Stoll J, Tzamaloukas A, Albala MM. Focal encephalomyelitis in infectious mononucleosis: a report with pathological description. *Ann Intern Med* 1971;75:579–83.
270. Halsted CC, Chang RS. Infectious mononucleosis and encephalitis: recovery of EB virus from spinal fluid. *Pediatrics* 1979;64:257–9.
271. Schooley RT, Dolin R. Epstein-Barr virus. In: Mandell GL, Douglas Jr RG, Bennett JE, eds. *Principles and practice of infectious diseases.* New York: John Wiley & Sons, 1985:971–82.
272. Silverstein A, Steinberg G, Nathanson M. Nervous system involvement in infectious mononucleosis: the heralding and/or major manifestation. *Arch Neurol* 1972;26:353–8.
273. Grose C, Henle W, Henle G, Feorino PM. Primary Epstein-Barr virus infections in acute neurologic diseases. *N Engl J Med* 1975;292:392–5.
274. Graman PS. Mollaret's meningitis associated with acute Epstein-Barr virus mononucleosis. *Arch Neurol* 1987;44:1204–5.
275. Andersson J, Britton S, Ernberg I, et al. Effect of acyclovir on infectious mononucleosis: a double-blind, placebo-controlled study. *J Infect Dis* 1986;153:283–90.
276. Phillips CA, Fanning WL, Gump DW, Phillips CF. Cytomegalovirus encephalitis in immunologically normal adults: successful treatment with vidarabine. *JAMA* 1977;238:2299–300.
277. Bale Jr JF. Human cytomegalovirus infection and disorders of the nervous system. *Arch Neurol* 1984;41:310–20.
278. Dorfman LJ. Cytomegalovirus encephalitis in adults. *Neurology* 1973;23:136.
279. Morgello S, Cho ES, Nielsen S, Devinsky O, Petito CK. Cytomegalovirus encephalitis in patients with acquired immunodeficiency syndrome: an autopsy study of 30 cases and a review of the literature. *Hum Pathol* 1987;18:289–97.
280. Masdeu JC, Small CB, Weiss L, Elkin CM, Llena J, Mesa-Tejada R. Multifocal cytomegalovirus encephalitis in AIDS. *Ann Neurol* 1988;23:97–9.
281. Buhles WC, Mastre BJ, Tinker AJ, Strand V, Koretz SH, Syntex Collaborative Ganciclovir Treatment Study Group. *Rev Infect Dis* 1988;10:S495–506.
282. Palmer AE. B virus *Herpesvirus simiae:* historical perspective. *J Med Primatol* 1987;16:99–130.
283. Centers for Disease Control. B-virus infection in humans—Pensacola, Florida. *Morb Mort Weekly Report* 1987;36:289–96.
284. Centers for Disease Control. Guidelines for prevention of *Herpesvirus simiae* (B virus) infection in monkey handlers. *Morb Mort Weekly Report* 1987;36:680–9.
285. Boulter EA, Thorton B, Bauer DJ, Byer A. Successful treatment of experimental B virus (Herpesvirus simiae) infection with acyclovir. *Br Med J* 1980;280:681–3.
286. Padgett BL, Walker DL, ZuRhein GM, Hodach AE, Chou SM. JC papovavirus in progressive multifocal leukoencephalopathy. *J Infect Dis* 1976;133:686–90.
287. Padgett BL, Walker DL. Prevalence of antibodies in human sera against JC virus, an isolate from a case of progressive multifocal leukoence-

phalopathy. *J Infect Dis* 1973;127: 467–70.
288. Houff SA, Major EO, Katz DA, et al. Involvement of JC virus-infected mononuclear cells from the bone marrow and spleen in the pathogenesis of progressive multifocal leukoencephalopathy. *N Engl J Med* 1988;318: 301–5.
289. Grinnell BW, Padgett BL, Walker DL. Distribution of nonintegrated DNA from JC papovavirus in organs of patients with progressive multifocal leukoencephalopathy. *J Infect Dis* 1983;147:669–75.
290. Hogan TF, Borden EC, McBain JA, Padgett BL, Walker DL. Human polyomavirus infections with JC virus and BK virus in renal transplant patients. *Ann Intern Med* 1980; 92:373–8.
291. Walker DL Progressive multifocal leukoencephalopathy: an opportunistic viral infection of the central nervous system. In: Vinkin PU, Bruyn GW, eds. *Handbook of clinical neurology*, vol. 34. Amsterdam: Elsevier, 1978:307–29.
292. Gajdusek DC. Unconventional viruses and the origin and disappearance of kuru. *Science* 1977;197:943–60.
293. Prusiner SB. Prions and neurodegenerative diseases. *N Engl J Med* 1987;317:1571–81.
294. Gajdusek DC, Gibbs Jr CJ, Alpers M. Transmission and passage of experimental "kuru" to chimpanzees. *Science* 1967;155:212–4.
295. Gibbs Jr CJ, Amyx HL, Bacote A, Masters CL, Gajdusek DC. Oral transmission of Kuru, Creutzfeldt-Jakob disease and scrapie to nonhuman primates. *J Infect Dis* 1980;142:205–8.
296. Duffy P, Wolf J, Collins G, DeVoe AG, Streeten B, Cowen D. Person-to-person transmission of Creutzfeldt-Jakob disease. *N Engl J Med* 1974;290:692–3.
297. Bernoulli C, Siegfried J, Baumgartner G, et al. Danger of accidental person-to-person transmission of Creutzfeldt-Jakob disease by surgery. *Lancet* 1977;1:478–9.
298. Brown P, Gajdusek DC, Gibbs CJ, Asher DM. Potential epidemic of Creutzfedlt-Jakob disease from human growth hormone therapy. *N Engl J Med* 1985;313:728–30.
299. Gendelman H, Wolinsky JS, Johnson RT, Pressman NJ, Pezeshkpour GH, Poisset GF. Measles encephalitis: lack of evidence of viral invasion of the central nervous system and quantitative study of the nature of demyelination. *Ann Neurol* 1984;15:353–60.
300. Server AC, Johnson RT. Guillain Barré syndrome. In: Remington JS, Swartz MN, eds. *Current clinical topics in infectious diseases. Vol. 3.* New York: McGraw Hill Book Co., 1982:74–96.
301. Dowling P, Menonna J, Cook S. Cytomegalovirus complement fixation antibody in Guillain-Barré syndrome. *Neurology* 1977;27:1153–6.
302. Guillain-Barré Syndrome Study Group. Plasmapheresis and acute Guillain-Barré syndrome. *Neurology* 1985;35:1096–104.
303. Johnson RT. Viral aspects of multiple sclerosis. In: Koetsier JC, ed. *Handbook of clinical neurology: demyelinating diseases. Vol. 3.* Elsevier Science Publishers, 1985:3319–36.
304. McFarlin DE, McFarland HF. Multiple sclerosis. *N Engl J Med* 1982;307:1183–8.
305. Centers for Disease Control. Arboviral infections of the central nervous system—United States, 1985. *Morb Mort Weekly Report* 1986;35:341–50.

*Antiviral Agents and Viral Diseases of Man, 3rd Edition,*
edited by G. J. Galasso, R. J. Whitley, and
T. C. Merigan, Raven Press, Ltd., New York © 1990.

# 14

# Chronic Intrauterine and Perinatal Infections

Ann M. Arvin and *Charles A. Alford, Jr.

*Department of Pediatrics, Stanford University, Palo Alto, California 94305, and *Department of Pediatrics, University of Alabama in Birmingham, Birmingham, Alabama 35294*



Stimulated by the findings encountered during the rubella pandemic of the middle 1960s, researchers have focused considerable attention on viral infections acquired during pregnancy and in the immediate perinatal period. (1–4). Because two hosts (mother and fetus or infant) must be considered in the intrauterine and perinatal infections, unique theoretical and practical problems in the control of these entities are encountered. Among the viruses, three agents—rubella virus, cytomegaloviruses (CMV), and herpes simplex viruses (HSV)—have received intense scrutiny. Varicella-zoster virus (VZV), another human herpes virus, can also cause intrauterine or perinatal infections. Transmission of the human immunodeficiency virus (HIV) to the fetus and newborn has become one of the most serious and tragic consequences of the acquired immunodeficiency syndromes (AIDS) epidemic. Each of these viruses can produce a wide range of disease in the fetus and newborn, from subclinical presentation to fulminant neonatal disease. Infection with many of these agents in the pregnant woman is often difficult or nearly impossible to diagnose clinically. To compound the problem, these agents can cause chronic or recurrent infection (reactivation of latent virus or reinfection) in both mothers and infants. Clearly, they pose special therapeutic problems, whether one is considering prophylaxis (5) or treatment of established disease.

In this section, the infections produced by rubella virus, CMV, HSV, VZV, and HIV will be discussed with regard to characteristics of the viruses in relation to epidemiology, pathology, and natural history of infection in mother and infant in order to bring into perspective the special problems posed by intrauterine and perinatal infections.

## RUBELLA

Rubella is a mild exanthematous disease most commonly observed in young schoolage children, but it often occurs in young adults as well.

It was not until the latter half of the nineteenth century that rubella was distinguished from measles and scarlet fever. Originally it was named "Rotheln." In 1866, Dr. Veale succeeded in changing the name to rubella because it was short and euphonious (6). The important association linking rubella with the appearance of congenital anomalies, particularly cataracts and cardiac lesions, was made in 1941 by Sir Norman Gregg, an Australian ophthalmologist (7).

The viral nature of rubella had been postulated as early as 1914 on the basis of transmission studies in monkeys (8), and this was reinforced in 1938 by similar studies in humans (9). However, the agent itself was not isolated in cell culture until 1962 with the independent and simultaneous studies of Weller and Neva (10) and Parkman et al. (11). This discovery paved the way for accurate determination of the epidemiology of the disease and made available biologic tools for study of the virus. But, most important, it provided a foundation for vaccine development.

### The Virus

Rubella virus is generally spherical in shape: earlier reports of pleomorphism probably resulted from methods employed in purification (12–16). The virus particle is 60–70 nm in diameter, with a dense central nucleoid measuring 30 nm in diameter. The central nucleoid is surrounded by a 10-nm-thick single-layered envelope acquired during budding of the virus into cytoplasmic vesicles or through the plasma membrane (17). Surface spikes with knobbed ends that are 6 nm in length have been reported (12).

Wild virus contains a 40S single-stranded RNA with a 5′ cap structure and a 3′ poly (A) tract (18) (molecular weight, $3 \times 10^6$), which is infectious. DNA has not been detected in wild virus preparations, but after prolonged growth in tissue culture, 21 cells, viral variants, recombinants between rubella, and an intrinsic retrovirus have been detected that contain DNA, invert transcriptase, and DNA-directed DNA polymerase (19–23). Recombinants such as these, if naturally occurring, could account in part for the unusual persistence of this virus in certain humans, but the development of temperature-sensitive mutants and defective particles devoid of DNA could also contribute to persistence (24,25).

The rubella virus envelope contains lipids that are essential for infectivity (26,27). Rubella is heat-labile and has a half-life of 1 hr at 57°C (28). However, in the presence of protein—i.e., 1% serum or albumin—infectivity is maintained for a week or more at 4°C and indefinitely at −60°C. Storage at freezer temperatures of −10–−20°C should be avoided because of rapid loss of infectivity (28,29). Rubella virus can also be stabilized against heat inactivation by the addition of $MgSO_4$ to virus suspensions. Thus, suspect material to be examined virologically should be transported to distant laboratories packed in ice rather than frozen, with the addition of stabilizer if possible. Infectivity is also rapidly lost at pH levels below 6.8 or above 8.1, or in the presence of ultraviolet light, lipid-active solvents, or other chemicals (28,30–32). Infectivity of rubella in cell culture is inhibited by 1-adamantanamine (33–35).

Originally, three structural polypeptides with estimated molecular weights of 62,500, 47,500, and 35,000 daltons were identified by Vaheri and Hovi (36), who designated them VP1, VP2, and VP3, respectively. Subsequently, using different methodologies for virus purification and different electrophoretic techniques, up to 12 polypeptides have been identified in rubella-infected cells (12,37–39). The purified virus contains two envelope glycoproteins, E1 and E2, and one internal RNA associated capsid protein, C (18,40). These proteins are cleavage products of a 110,000 $M_r$ precursor translated from an mRNA representing one-third of the genome (12,32). The nucleocapsid capsomere consists of two disulfide-linked dimers of the C polypeptide (41).

Rubella has been classified as a member of the Togavirus family (genus *Rubivirus*) (42). Only one immunologically distinct type has been described, and no serologic relationship exists between rubella and other known viruses. Minor biologic differences in different strains of rubella virus as identified by infectivity neutralization and by detecting strain-specific epitopes in the E2 protein (41,43) are not reflected in antigenic differences as assessed by serologic reactions (12,37,44,45). Thus, differences in the immune response following immunization with the various vaccines now in use are not due to major differences in the viral strain but rather due to modification of the viruses during their attenuation in cell culture. The variation in the virulence of rubella epidemics does not appear to be dependent on viral strain.

The antigenic composition of rubella has been reviewed by Vesikari (39). Rubella virus has a hemagglutinin (HA) associated with the envelope (46,47). Antibodies to the E1 glycoprotein inhibit HA, and at least one neutralization epitope is within this E1 protein (18,40,41). The specific inhibition of HA by serum antibodies forms the basis for the hemagglutination inhibition (HI) test to measure humoral immunity. This antigen can agglutinate a variety of red blood cells. Fowl erythrocytes (newborn chick, adult goose, or pigeon) and human group O erythrocytes have been most extensively employed in the HI test. Rubella hemagglutination is unique in its dependency on $Ca^{2-}$ ions in order to attach to red blood cell receptors (48,49). After extraction from infected cells, rubella hemagglutination is stable for months at −20°C, for several weeks at 4°C, and overnight at 37°C, but is destroyed within minutes by heating at 56°C (46,48). Cells and serum both contain β-lipoproteins that inhibit rubella hemagglutination (30,48,50). Before performing the HI antibody test, care must be taken to remove these inhibitors from both the antigen and the serum; otherwise low-level false positive reactions will result, causing great confusion regarding the true immunologic status of the patient (32). This problem has prompted the recent development of many other serologic tests with sensitivity that is more specific but equal to or greater than the HI test for measuring rubella antibody. There are three complement-fixing antigens, two associated with the viral envelope and one with the nucleoprotein core, which provoke antibody production following infection and can be detected by serologic testing (39,51,52). A variety of precipitin antigens has been serologically demonstrated; two of these, the θ and ι antigens, are associated with the viral envelope and core, respectively (53–55). Platelet-agglutinating antigens are also associated with both the envelope and the nucleoprotein (52,56). Antibody directed against rubella antigens can also be measured by neutralization (32), passive hemagglutination (57–59), radial hemolysis (60–63), radioimmunoassay (RIA) (64–66), immunofluorescence (IF) (67,68), and enzyme-linked immunoassay (ELISA) (52,69). Immunoglobulin (lg) class-specific antibody can be measured in most of the serologic systems, either on whole serum (RIA, ELISA) or, preferably, following Ig class-specific separation in most tests (70–76).

Rubella replicates in a variety of cell culture systems, primary cell strains, and cell lines (32). As a generalization, rubella grown in primary cell cultures (human, simian, bovine, rabbit, canine, or duck) produces interference to superinfection by a wide variety of viruses but no cytopathic effect (CPE) (77). In contrast, cytopathology of widely varying natures results from infection of cell lines (hamster, rabbit, simian, and human). Generally, primary cells, especially monkey kidney, have proven superior for isolation of virus from human material, whereas cell lines have proven better for antigen production because of the higher virus yields. The mechanism of rubella-induced interference in cell culture is not completely understood. Although interferon production has been described after rubella infection of cell cultures, in most cases interference appears to be an intrinsic phenomenon (78–82).

Although rubella virus will replicate in primates and various small laboratory animals, the ferret is by far the most useful of the small laboratory animals in rubella studies (83). Ferret kits are highly sensitive to subcutaneous and particularly to intracerebral inoculations. Virus has been recovered from the heart, liver, spleen, lung, brain, eye, blood, and urine for a month or longer after inoculation, and both neutralizing and complement fixation (CF) antibodies develop (83). Ferret kits inoculated at birth develop corneal clouding. Virus appears in the fetal ferrets after inoculation of the pregnant animals.

## Epidemiology

Rubella is worldwide in distribution and has a seasonal pattern of epidemicity (spring). Humans are believed to be the only host. Therefore, continual cycling among humans is believed to be necessary to maintain the virus in nature (84). Congenitally infected infants who continue to shed virus for months after birth probably assist in maintaining the virus in the community during endemic periods (85). More important, the infected newborn represents a particular hazard for pregnant medical personnel and for spread of virus in obstetrical units (86–88).

Prior to mass immunization in the United States, epidemics occurred at 6–9-year intervals, with pandemics appearing at 10–30-year intervals, peaking and abating over 3–4 years (84). The causes of these epidemiologic patterns have been the subject of considerable interest over the years. Two of the more common explanations concern climate and increased biologic virulence of newly emerging viral strains. Neither alone nor together can they convincingly explain the peculiar epidemiology of rubella (44,84).

Attack rates are undoubtedly dependent upon the number of susceptible individuals, which varies widely between different countries and even between different locations within a single country. In closed populations, such as military recruit camps, boarding homes, schools, and the like, rubella virus seems to continually circulate infecting nearly all the susceptible individuals (84,89,90). Such settings represent another means whereby the virus may survive between epidemics. Reinfection is also more common in these closed settings than in the open population (91,92).

In most of the world, excluding those areas practicing mass immunization, rubella is typically a childhood disease that is most prevalent in the 5–14-year age group (84,85). The incidence increases slowly for the first 4 years, rises steeply between 5 and 14 years, peaks around age 35, and then levels off and actually decreases. In developed countries, the incidence of infection never reaches 100% before age 40; in fact, 5–20% of most persons between 15 and 35 years of age remain susceptible (84,85). The rate of susceptibility during the childbearing years remains the same for the United States in spite of the current practice of immunizing all children (93). Indeed, in the United States rubella now occurs most commonly in the 15–30-year age group, and small epidemics continue to occur in high schools, colleges, hospitals, and other settings where young adults live and work in close proximity (5,93,94). In certain tropical areas, there is an increased susceptibility (25–70%) during the childbearing years for reasons that are unknown, whereas in other developing nations rubella virus infects 95% or more of the population before puberty, resulting in a high level of seroimmunity during the childbearing years (95,96).

## Maternal Infection

### *Viral and Clinical Events*

The most saliant of the clinical and virologic features of rubella are depicted in Fig. 1. By the time the disease becomes clinically apparent, some 14–21 days (mean, 18 days) following exposure, excretion of virus (mainly from the nasopharynx, but also from other sites such as kidney, conjunctivae, etc.) has already been occurring for approximately 1 week. Multiple organ involvement probably is the result of viremic seeding (97–100). Virus excretion is most profound and prolonged from pharyngeal secretions, where shedding generally continues for 2 weeks and in rare cases as long as 5 weeks. Viral shedding from other sites is neither as consistent nor as prolonged. Knowledge of the duration of excretion is crucial in determining risk following exposure to an index case when viral isolation is being attempted for diagnosis.

Because rubella is a systemic infection, viremia is a consistent feature that is usually demonstrable when excretion begins from the pharynx. It is terminated when serum antibodies appear, some 14–18 days after acquisition of the infection

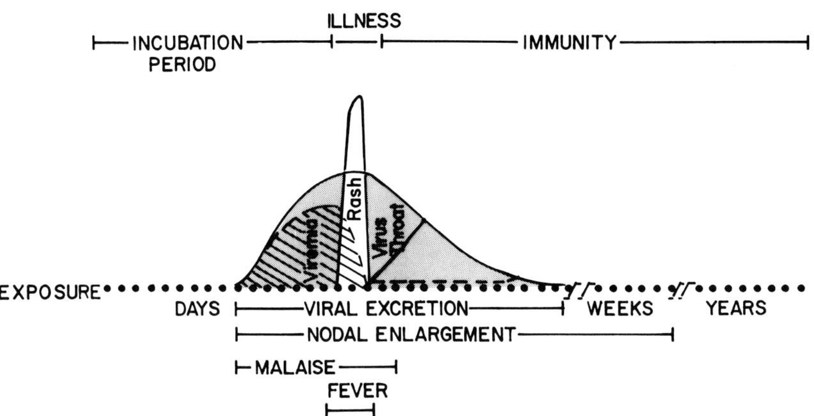


**FIG. 1.** Relationships among virus excretion, clinical findings, and antibody response in postnatally acquired rubella. (From Alford and Griffiths, ref. 168, with permission.)

(97,99,100). The viremic phase is responsible for placental infection of susceptible pregnant women, and it leads to fetal infection (101). Presumably, there is multiple maternal organ system involvement, with minimal or no impairment of function, except for the relatively common arthralgia and arthritis component of synovial infection or the rare encephalitic or thrombocytopenic syndromes (99,102,104). Virus is present in exanthematous lesions; whether this is because of epidermal replication or vascular replication or both is unclear (103). These findings translate into a clinical picture that is characteristic but not pathognomonic: fever, 3-day rash, and postauricular and suboccipital adenopathy found in approximately 50% of infected women. A presumptive clinical diagnosis can be considered only during epidemic periods, because other viral infections may mimic rubella. Definitive assessment should include appropriate serologic evaluation, a mandatory procedure should therapeutic abortion be under consideration.

### *Immunologic Events*

#### *Humoral Immune Response*

Since viral replication is widespread throughout the body at least 1 week before illness begins, specific antibodies can be detected in the serum during the disease or occasionally even before. The standard method for detecting rubella antibodies is by HI, but this test is plagued by false-positive and false-negative results. The HI technique has been exhaustively compared with a variety of other methods for measuring rubella antibody responses (105,106), including neutralization (107–109), RIA (66,73), ELISA (69,110–112), IF (113), passive hemagglutination (60,62,63). CF (114), and precipitation assays (114). The kinetics of the immune response to acute rubella infection detected by these various serological assays are depicted in Fig. 2. In general, three distinct patterns of reactivity can be discerned. Antibodies of IgG class measured by HI, neutralization, IF, single radial hemolysis, RIA,

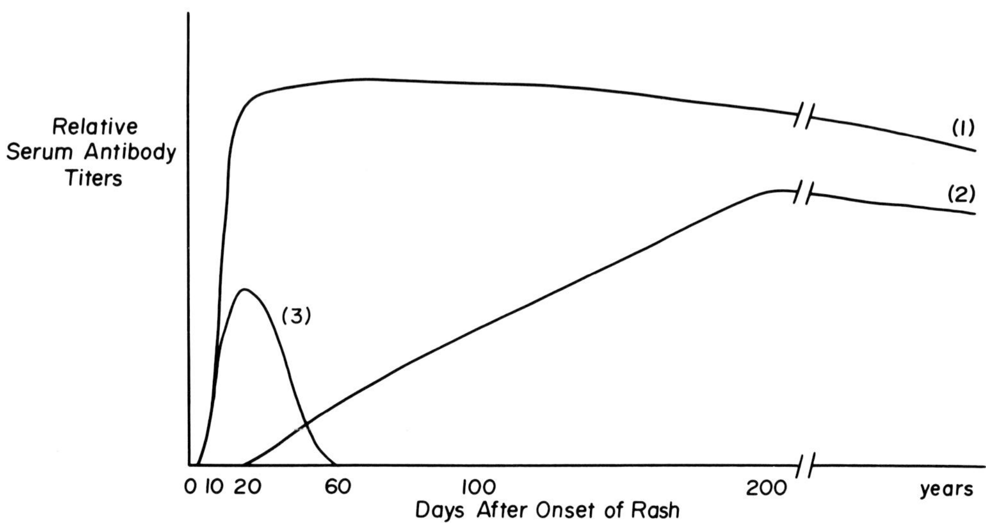


**FIG. 2.** Schematic representation of the humoral immune response to rubella infection detected by different serological assays. Pattern 1, antibodies of IgG class detected by HI, neutralization, IF, single radial hemolysis, RIA, ELISA, or θ precipitins. Pattern 2, IgG antibodies detected by passive hemagglutination. Pattern 3, antibodies of IgM class detected by HI, IF, RIA, or ELISA. (From Alford and Griffiths, ref. 168, with permission.)

ELISA, or θ precipitation follow the first pattern (59,76,108,114,115). Such antibodies usually become detectable 5–15 days after the onset of the rash, although they may appear earlier and, in the occasional patient, may even be present 1 or 2 days before the rash appears. The antibodies rapidly increase in titer to reach peak values at 15–30 days and then gradually decline over a period of years to a constant titer, which varies from person to person. In some patients with low levels of residual antibody, a second exposure to rubella virus may lead to low-grade reinfection of the pharynx; a booster antibody response can then be detected with any of these assays. This rapidly terminates the new infection, and viremic spread is not thought to occur. Reinfections should not, therefore, represent a threat to the fetus, because placental exposure to the virus should be minimal or nonexistent.

A second pattern of immune response (Fig. 2) to rubella infection is produced when IgG antibodies are measured by passive hemagglutination (PHA). The peak titer of these antibodies is similar to that measured by HI, but the PHA antibodies are relatively delayed in appearance and rise only slowly to their maximal titers (59,115). They first become detectable 15–50 days after the onset of the rash, and often take 200 days to reach peak titers. The antibodies probably persist for life, and booster responses may be seen with reinfection.

A third distinct pattern of antibody production is represented in Fig. 2 by the IgM class immune response. This class of specific antibody can be measured by HI, IF, RIA, or ELISA (59,64,68,74,116) Commercial ELISA methods for rubella IgM have proved reliable but the problem of false positive results has not been eliminated (117,118). If the apparent selective reactivity of IgM with the E1 protein is confirmed, monoclonal antibodies or purified protein antigens may be used to enhance specificity (119,120). IgM antibodies first become detectable 5–10 days after the onset of the rash, rise rapidly to peak values at approximately 20 days, and then decline so rapidly that they have usually disappeared by 50 days (59,76,116), although, in a few patients, low levels may persist for up to 1 year (70,121). The booster IgG antibody response to reinfection noted above does not involve the IgM class of antibody, so that the presence of high-titer IgM antibodies indicates recent primary infection with rubella. The more sensitive techniques, such as RIA or ELISA, may occasionally detect low levels of specific IgM antibodies in some patients with reinfections (122).

The kinetics of the immune response to rubella infection detected by other serological assays are not as distinct as the three patterns just described, and marked variability between patients has been noted. CF antibodies or ι precipitins are not present in the first 10 days after the rash and rise slowly to peak at 30–90 days (114). CF antibodies persist for several years in one-third of patients and may reappear during reinfections. Precipitins do not persist for more than a few months and do not usually reappear with reinfections. Antibodies of IgA class appear within 10 days but may then disappear within 20 days in some patients or may persist for several years in others (72,116,123). IgA antibodies react predominantly within the C protein (18).

### *Cellular Immune Response*

Cellular immunity to rubella virus has been measured by lymphocyte transformation response (124–127), secretion of interferon (128), secretion of macrophage migration inhibitory factor (129), induction of delayed hypersensitivity to skin testing (128), or the release of lymphokines by cultured lymphocytes (130,131). Peripheral blood lymphocytes from seropositive individuals respond better in each of these tests than do lymphocytes from uninfected people, showing that these assays can be considered to measure parameters of the cellular immune response to rubella virus. The results from other studies that have used $^{51}Cr$ microcytotoxicity assays are difficult to interpret, since syngeneic cell lines were not used (132).

In the first weeks after natural rubella infection, some degree of lymphocyte suppression may occur, but this phenomenon is only transient (130,133). Generally, cell-mediated immune responses precede the appearance of humoral immunity by 1 week, reach a peak value at the same time as the antibody response, and subsequently persist for many months or years, whether measured by migration inhibitory factor (128), lymphokine release (131), interferon secretion (128), or lymphocyte transformation (128).

#### *Local Immune Response*

The local antibody response at the portal of entry in the nasopharynx is essentially IgA in character; low levels of short-lived IgG antibody are rarely detectable in nasopharyngeal secretions. The nasopharyngeal IgA antibody persists at appreciable levels for at least 1 year after infection. Its persistence apparently minimizes the tendency for reinfection after natural rubella infection; the lack of a local IgA nasopharyngeal response after systemic immunization with certain of the live vaccines probably plays a key role in the increased incidence of reinfection after vaccination (65,134,135). Local antibody levels tend to be higher in individuals resistant to challenge with live virus, but no particular titer of antibody can be associated with complete protection (135).

A cell-mediated immune response in tonsillar cells has been detected by lymphocyte transformation and secretion of migration inhibitory factor following both natural rubella and intranasal challenge with live RA-27 vaccine (136).

### Congenital Infection

#### *Virologic Events*

Some of the more important sequential virologic and immunologic changes that accompany congenital infection are summarized in Fig. 3. The feature of chronicity clearly distinguishes congenital infection from postnatal infection (85,101,137–139). During the period of maternal viremia, the placenta may become infected and then seed the developing fetus. Virus can persist in the placenta for months, but it is cleared or markedly reduced during late gestation, and thus recovery of virus from the placenta at birth is uncommon (140). In contrast, once fetal infection occurs, virus persists throughout gestation and for weeks postnatally in the great majority of infants. Rubella can infect one fetal organ or many, resulting in a newborn who excretes virus from multiple sites: pharynx, urine, conjunctivae, feces, cerebrospinal fluid (CSF), bone marrow, and circulating white blood cells. As in postnatally acquired infections, pharyngeal shedding of virus is most common, prolonged, and intense; thus, this site is best for attempting virus isolation. Conjunctival swabs and CSF provide high yields of virus in the presence of manifest disease; virus may persist in these sites for longer periods (3,141,142). Because virus shedding from peripheral sites diminishes with time, an attempt should be made to isolate virus as soon as possible after delivery.

Infection of the fetus is not inevitable following maternal rubella. Transmission of virus *in utero* and virulence of the fetal infection are dependent on gestational age at the time of maternal infection (137,143,144). *In utero* transmission occurs in 80% or more with maternal infection in the first 12 weeks of gestation, declines to a low of 25% between 23 to 26 weeks (145,146), and then rises again to 70% or more in later gestation. Intrauterine transmission of rubella

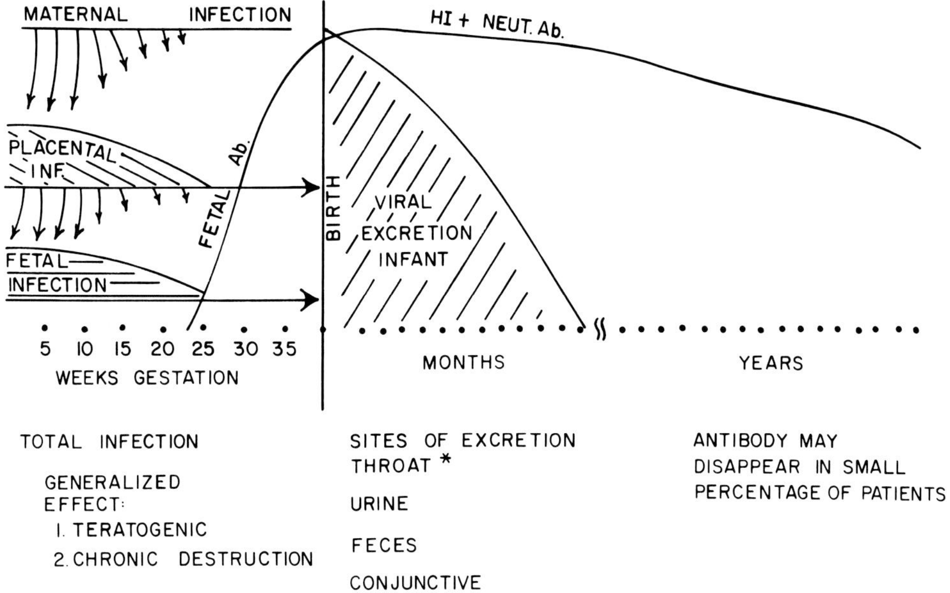


**FIG. 3.** Summary of virologic and serological parameters of congenitally acquired rubella. (From Alford et al., ref. 741, with permission.)

was originally thought to be confined to the first half of gestation, because overt fetal damage results mainly from maternal rubella in the first 20 weeks of gestation, with the most florid disease occurring in the first 8–10 weeks. Because fetal infection is not inevitable, new methods of virologic diagnosis are being evaluated, such as chronic biopsy to detect rubella virus RNA. However, the limited clinical experience and potential for laboratory artifact do not permit their application in practice (147).

### *Immunologic Events*

#### *Humoral Immune Response*

Since two humoral immune mechanisms, placental and fetal, develop *in utero,* they must both be considered in judging the host response of any intrauterine infection (148). In congenital rubella, this consideration is complicated by the fact that both the placenta and the fetus almost always become chronically infected in their earliest formative states (101). There is a potential danger, then, of interference with the normal sequence of events that leads to final maturation of either the placental transfer mechanisms for shunting maternal antibody or the ability of the fetus to manufacture antibody.

Placental transfer mechanisms mature normally in spite of chronic rubella infection (149). However, even under normal circumstances, they are incipient during the first half of gestation and only minimal amounts of maternal antibody are available to combat the spread of virus (150–153). The summary data in Fig. 4 depict this condition. From a practical standpoint, only IgG maternal antibodies are normally transferred by the placenta, but these are not transferred in substantial amounts until approximately 16–20 weeks of gestation. Levels of antibody in the fetal blood prior to that are only 5–10% of those in maternal serum with or without rubella infection

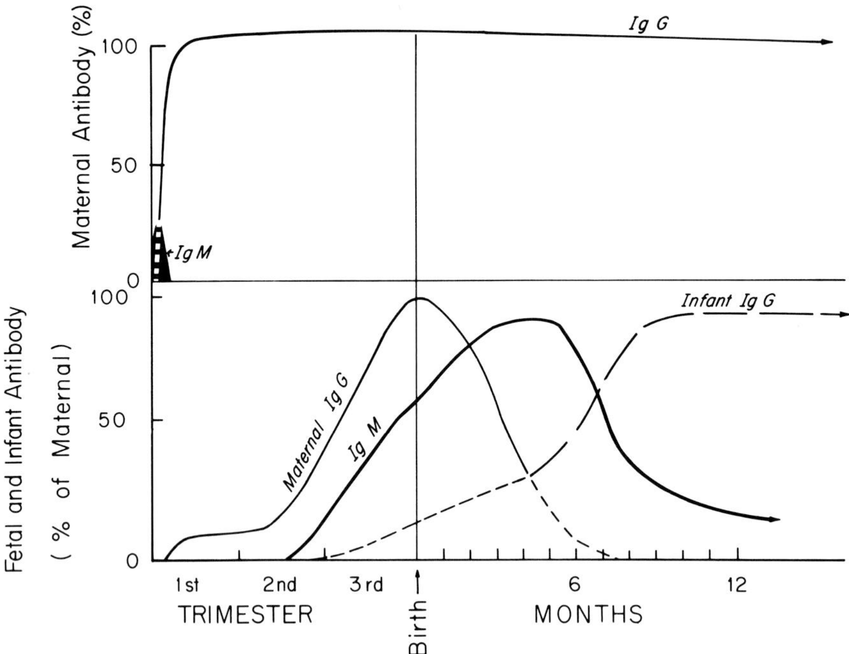


**FIG. 4.** Comparative immunoglobulin class rubella neutralizing and HI antibody responses in the mother, fetus, and infant following early gestational acquisition of infection. (From Alford, ref. 720, with permission.)

(150). This situation remains critical for many weeks after viral invasion of the conceptus. The placental transfer mechanisms mature rapidly around midgestation (152). Thus, IgG maternal antibodies are actively but belatedly transported to the infected fetus. By the time of delivery, levels of IgG rubella antibodies in cord sera are equal to or greater than those in the maternal sera, whether the infant is prematurely born or not (Fig. 4). In fact, the dominant antibody present at delivery of rubella-infected infants is maternal IgG rubella antibody (149). This, of course, complicates serologic diagnosis of congenital rubella, since most (85%) normal babics arc also born with comparable levels of maternally derived antibody.

The early development of the fetal humoral immune system, like that of the placenta, is also normally too slow to combat spread of virus properly. Cells with membrane-bound immunoglobulins of all three major classes, IgM, IgG, and IgA, appear in the fetus as early as 9–11 weeks of gestation (153). This antibody represents the early acquisition of receptor or recognition sites for antigen. Even cytoplasmic antibody production, although relatively delayed, begins at approximately 15–19 weeks of gestation (153).

During the early preparatory period, however, the functions of the B cells or those of other immune cells or substances with which they must interact are deficient or else antibody is removed by immune complex formation. Thus, circulating fetal antibody levels remain low in spite of high levels of rubella virus, whereas in the mothcr a prompt scrum antibody rcsponsc is elicited (Fig. 4) (149). Perhaps the poor fetal and placental immune responses contribute to much increased virulence of the early intrauterine infection in comparison to the later transmission (144).

The fetal humoral immune mechanisms mature sufficiently so that a serum antibody response usually can be elicited beginning around mid-gestation. Specific fetal IgM antibody is detectable about this time, leading to attempts at prenatal diagnosis by fetoscopy and serum sampling. Unfortunately, IgM antibodies are produced with subclinical infection, and affected infants have been born who had no rubella IgM by prenatal diagnosis (154–156). IgM may constitute a major or at least a significant portion of the pool of antibody in cord sera (149,157,158). If the antigenic stimulus is sufficient, usually with very severe infections, fetal IgA antibody may also be present at birth, but it is far less common than fetal IgM and is always present in lesser amounts (157). Probably, fetal IgG antibody production is also stimulated, but the fetus's contribution of this antibody type is buried in the large pool of maternal IgG and is therefore difficult to demonstrate (Fig. 4).

After birth, the infected infant may continue to manufacture IgM antibody for 6 months or even longer (68), whereas IgG antibodies are produced for years, if not for life, in most cases (68,159). An analysis of the specificity of IgG antibodies for rubella virus proteins indicated that infants with congenital rubella had decreased antibodies to E1 and C proteins (160).

### *Cellular Immune Response*

Like the B cells, the cells necessary to elicit a cellular immune response (T cell, macrophages, etc.) develop certain of their functions early in gestation (161,162). However, their intrauterine development with respect to rubella infection is virtually unknown because of the impossibility of specimen collection. The cellular immune response of the infected fetus has, therefore, often been inferred from studies in infected infants and children, leading to controversial interpretations. Retarded development of the thymus has been reported and lymphocyte depletion is also seen, but this defect may be the result of stress rather than a direct viral effect (163).

Buimovici-Klein et al. (173) showed that lymphocytes from older children and adolescents with congenital rubella (expanded syndrome) had no or very poor lymphocyte proliferative response with markedly reduced interferon and migration inhibitory factor production (164). These defects were greater in those children initially infected in the first 8 weeks of gestation than in those infected later and, obviously, had persisted for many years after viral excretion had ceased. The cellular immune defects then do not appear to be responsible for the viral persistence in early life but rather appear to be another anomaly associated with the acquisition of infection during the period of embryogenesis (164). Whether the cellular immune defects are related to the severity of the infection is yet to be determined, but the results with regard to gestational age suggest that they might be, since earlier acquisition of infection is known to be associated with a more severe form of disease.

A deficiency of the lymphocytes from infected children to specifically kill rubella-infected cells in a cytotoxicity assay has also been demonstrated, but the results are suspect, since syngeneic target cells were not employed and these responses are known to be human leukocyte antigen (HLA) restricted (165).

It has long been suggested that the human conceptus is deficient in its interferon response to viral infections, including rubella, but this evidence has been derived from indirect studies using *in vitro* cell systems or animal models. However, interferon has been demonstrated in rubella-infected human embryos that appeared to be specifically stimulated by the virus (166). The interferon was found as early as 7 weeks of gestation and as long as 12 weeks after cessation of symptoms in the mothers. Consequently, it can be stated that the human fetus and placenta, when stimulated by chronic infection, have the capacity to manufacture interferon early in gestation, but the actual quantitative responsiveness of the fetus as compared to the adult has not yet been assessed. The interferon has been characterized as acid-labile interferon-α (167).

### Clinical Findings and Outcome

Following the original observations of Gregg, the congenital rubella syndrome was most often identified as a combination of defects involving the heart, eye, and ear. However, after the extensive studies during the middle 1960s employing both virologic and serologic methods of assessment, the pathologic potential was seen to be greatly expanded, as shown in Table 1 (138,168). Since the mid 1960s, many investigators have contributed to the ever increasing number of clinical findings associated with congenital rubella. The manifestations have been reviewed in detail, along with an extensive reference list (168). Therefore, only pertinent summary data and references will be given here. Rubella can infect one fetal organ or virtually all of them; once established, the virus can persist for long periods of time (101). Thus, congenital rubella infection must be viewed as chronic, with a wide range of potential pathological injuries (168,169). In fact, silent infection is the most common form of disease (144). It is clear that many important rubella defects are overlooked in the early months of life, but other defects may be progressive in as-

**TABLE 1.** *Summary of clinical findings and their estimated frequencies of occurrence in young symptomatic infants with congenitally acquired rubella*

| Clinical findings | Frequency (%) | Clinical findings | Frequency (%) |
|---|---|---|---|
| Prematurity | <20 | Cardiovascular | |
| Intrauterine growth retardation | 51–75 | Pulmonary arterial hypoplasia | 51–75 |
| Extrauterine growth retardation | 21–50 | Patent ductus arteriosus | 21–50 |
| Hepatosplenomegaly | 51–75 | Myocardial necrosis | <20 |
| Jaundice (regurgitative) | <20 | Coarctation of aortic isthmus | <20 |
| Hepatitis | Rare | Interventricular septal | Rare |
| Immunologic dyscrasias | Rare | Others | Rare |
| Chromosomal abnormalities | Unknown | Hematologic | |
| Interstitial pneumonitis (acute, subacute, chronic) | 21–50 | Anemia | <20 |
| Bony radiolucencies | 21–50 | Thrombocytopenia c/s purpura | 21–50 |
| Malformations | 51–75 | Dermal erythropoiesis (blueberry muffin syndrome) | <20 |
| CNS | | Leukopenia | <20 |
| Encephalitis (active) | 21–50 | Adenopathies | 21–50 |
| Microcephaly | Rare | Genitourinary | |
| Brain calcification | Rare | Undescended testicle | <20 |
| Bulging fontanelle | <20 | Polycystic kidney | Rare |
| Neurological deficit | <20 | Bilobed kidney with reduplication ureter | Rare |
| Retinopathy | 21–50 | Unilateral renal agenesis | Rare |
| Cataracts | 21–50 | Renal artery stenosis with hypertension | Rare |
| Cloudy cornea | Rare | Hydroureter and hydronephrosis | Rare |
| Glaucoma | Rare | Bone | |
| Microphthalmia | <20 | Micrognathia | <20 |
| Hearing deficits (severe) | 21–50 | Extremities | Rare |
| Peripheral | | | |
| Central | | | |

c/s, with or without.

sociation with prolonged viral replication (170,171).

Even among symptomatic newborns, the range of disease is wide (Table 1). The prominent defects include cataracts and cardiac malformations, particularly those involving the pulmonary arterial tree, the ductus arteriosus or the aortic isthmus, or both. These cardiac lesions are the most obvious consequence of the arteritis caused by rubella infection of the fetus, which produces intimal thickening and stenosis (169). Although gross anatomic defects may occur in other organ systems, they are relatively rare and are often overlooked in the young infant (168).

Other defects that are encountered more commonly than the gross anatomic abnormalities include intrauterine and extrauterine growth retardation, hepatosplenomegaly, thrombocytopenia with purpura, prematurity, adenopathy, encephalitis, retinopathy, deafness, interstitial pneumonitis, and bony radiolucencies (138,168). The rubella syndrome, as expressed in the newborn, should now be expanded to include combinations of these findings, in addition to the so-called teratogenic effects.

The salt-and-pepper retinopathy, the discrete bluish-red lesions of dermal erythopoiesis, the disproportionately elevated protein to cell ratio of active encephalitis, the findings of glaucoma, cataracts, corneal clouding, bony radiolucencies, and characteristic heart lesions (peripheral pulmonic stenosis and ductal lesions), and the appearance of a myocardial infarction pattern on the electrocardiogram (EKG) (secondary to myocardial lesions) all lend a degree of specificity to the clinical diagnosis (138,168).

Certain defects carry a poor prognosis for survival. These include severe prematurity, severe cardiac lesions resulting in early heart failure, rapidly progressive hepatitis, persistent meningoencephalitis (104), and fulminant interstitial pneumonitis, among others. Serial assessment for immunologic debility is necessary early in life because humoral defects may be masked by the presence of maternal immunoglobulin. Even definitive eye lesions such as cataracts may not become apparent until months after birth. Thus, the prognosis must be guarded in the early months of life.

On the other hand, many of the lesions of congenital rubella are self-limiting and relatively harmless. Hepatosplenomegaly, anemia, thrombocytopenia, leukopenia, dermal erythropoiesis, and bony radiolucencies are all examples. These lesions are more important from a diagnostic standpoint than from a prognostic standpoint (138,168). The retinopathy of congenital rubella, which was previously believed to be completely benign, has recently been associated with later occurrence of visual difficulties due to subretinal neovascularization.

Some lesions of congenital rubella are missed in the first year of life because of the difficulties involved in their detection or because of their progressive nature (169,170,172,173). Included among these are hearing defects (peripheral or central), psychomotor defects, and language defects (176). Hearing defects are frequently associated with impaired language development and may lead to a false impression of mental retardation (172,174,175). Appropriate hearing aids, speech therapy, and special education are frequently required for such children, especially if hearing and psychomotor problems coexist. Sensorineural hearing loss can develop as a delayed consequence of congenital rubella (172). Serial psychological and perceptual testing should be performed beginning as soon as feasible after birth and continuing throughout childhood.

Genitourinary and bony abnormalities are easily overlooked in infancy. Certain of these lesions may require early surgical intervention in order to avoid eventual debilitation or even death. An increased incidence of frank diabetes mellitus has been found in children and adults with congenital rubella, probably caused by viral damage to the pancreas, and other endocrinopathies have been encountered, including thyroid disease and growth hormone deficiency (169,176,179). Progressive vascular effects such as arterial sclerosis and systemic hypertension secondary to renal disease cause late manifestations of congenital rubella. Likewise, autism and other psychiatric difficulties have been reported as late sequelae (169). Of particular concern regarding possible chronicity or reactivation are reports of the occurrence of a slowly progressive disease resembling subacute sclerosing panencephalitis during the second decade of life in a few children with congenital rubella. Rubella virus was recovered from the brain in one instance; elevated serum and CSF rubella antibodies, along with increased amounts of protein and gammaglobulin, were detected in the CSF in all instances. Although it is rare, this syndrome focuses attention on the need for better understanding of the dynamic interactions between host and virus in congenitally acquired rubella infections (180,182).

## Prevention

### *Active Immunization*

Currently, the only realistic approach to the problem of congenital rubella is prophylactic control through the use of active immunization. But the problem is unique in that protection is aimed at future fetuses, rather than at individuals who receive the vaccine (183,185). The current immunization program in the United States is based on the concept of developing a high level of herd immunity among children, who in the past were the primary source of virus in the population. Susceptible women of childbearing age would presumably be protected from exposure to virus because its circulation in the general population would be greatly reduced. In recent years, however, rubella has been most prevalent in persons over 15 years of age, since they have not received vaccine (which was initially licensed in 1969) and their level of susceptibility to rubella has not changed over the years (185). Active immunization of children is still recommended by the Advisory Committee on Immunization Practices of the United States Public Health Service and the Infectious Disease Committee of the American Academy of Pediatrics (186,188). In the United States, over 100 million doses of live rubella vaccine have been administered to date, mostly to children, with acceptable degrees of safety and early postvaccination immunity (189). Rubella vaccine can be given in combination with other live vaccines (measles, mumps) with the same immunogenicity as when given alone (190,191). Presently, vaccine is being given initially at 15 months of age in combination with other live vaccines, but it can be safely administered to all older age groups. The advisory committees are now recommending immunization of susceptible nonpregnant women of childbearing age with the warning to avoid pregnancy for 3 months following vaccination (186,187). This policy should be encouraged in all settings providing care for young women, including colleges and other schools, the military, hospitals and other health-care facilities, family planning clinics, physicians' offices, and the like. Unless this approach is combined with childhood immunization, it will take 10–30 years to achieve full immunity among women of childbearing age (192). Vaccination of susceptible young adult males has also been recommended particularly in high-risk settings such as the military, health care facilities, and schools. The vaccine is contraindicated in pregnancy or in individuals allergic to neomycin or with altered immunity or severe febrile illnesses (186,187).

Rubella virus was initially attenuated for use as a vaccine by passing it 77 times in green monkey kidney cells (193). These strains are referred to as high-passage virus ($HPV_{77}$), but to avoid preparation of the final product in monkey kidney cells, which are often contaminated by latent viruses, they were further passed in duck embryo ($HPV_{77}DE$) or dog kidney ($HPV_{77}DK$) cells (183,184). After original isolation in monkey kidney cells, the Cendehill strain was passaged 51 times in primary cultures of rabbit kidney cells for final attenuation. The RA-27 strain was adapted through low passage in WI-38 human diploid lung fibroblasts (194,195). Rubella rapidly loses its immunogenic properties during the course of passage *in vitro* so that only limited attenuation with respect to virulence can be achieved. Thus, all the presently available live vaccines produce a modified form of the natural disease in a rather high proportion of vaccines (183,184).

Since the natural disease itself is mild, the side effects of the vaccines are minimal and usually well tolerated by recipients (183). Arthralgia and, occasionally, frank arthritis are the most distressing reactions. Although fairly common in children, the incidence, severity, and persistence of joint involvement increase rather strikingly in individuals 10 years of age and older (109,196). The same is also true for fever, lymphadenopathy, and rash (183,184). All of these symptoms, if they occur, are usually short-lived; occasionally, however, joint symptoms may persist for longer (weeks to years), especially in adults (109,197–198). Most of the adverse reactions to rubella vaccine occur between 7 and 30 days after administration, but others may not appear for 4–7 weeks (188,200,201). Vaccine recipients should be advised of these possibilities.

The HPV and Cendehill vaccines had to be administered subcutaneously to be effective. During attenuation in nonhuman cells the viruses lose their capacity to infect the nasopharynx by direct inoculation (184). Of necessity then, the natural route of infection was bypassed and local respiratory tract immunity failed to develop. After subcutaneous administration, however, vaccine virus eventually replicates in the nasopharynx just as the wild virus does (195,202). This feature originally caused great concern because of the possibility that the vaccine virus might be transmitted to susceptible individuals in the general population. However, both the level and persistence of virus in the nasopharynx are markedly reduced and communicability is exceedingly rare, if indeed it exists at all (203–208). This feature is also true for RA-27 vaccine given subcutaneously (195). The RA-27 vaccine retains its ability to infect the nasopharynx by direct inoculation and therefore can stimulate local respiratory tract immunity as well as systemic immunity, like natural rubella infection (195). With nasopharyngeal inoculation, however, pharyngeal shedding of virus is more intense, closely resembling that seen following natural infection (209,211). Whether the increased viral excretion could lead to communicability is unknown but is of sufficient concern that RA-27 vaccine is licensed for subcutaneous use only.

All of the vaccine viruses can infect the human product of conception and can apparently produce fetal damage (212–214). They are thought to be considerably less virulent than wild virus in this regard (212). The Centers for Disease Control (CDC) register to monitor the risks to the fetus of exposure to rubella vaccine virus includes 170 susceptible women given RA 27/3 vaccine (215). Fifty-five of these women received the vaccine during the highest risk period for fetal defects, defined as 1 week before to 4 weeks after conception. No infants with congenital rubella syndrome have been identified after maternal vaccination despite the fact that 1–2% of these infants have serologic evidence of infection (216). Inadvertent rubella vaccination is not an indication to consider therapeutic abortion. Nevertheless care should be taken to avoid giving the vaccine to pregnant women, nor is it wise for vaccine recipients to become pregnant for 3 months following immunization (183,212). Rubella immunity should be determined by serologic testing before immunizing adult females if possible, but this approach is not considered to be essential (186,217).

The greatest concern about the rubella immunization program as presently structured in the United States arises from the reduced immunogenicity of the attenuated viruses (84). The antibody response that follows vaccine infection is qualitatively and quantitatively deficient compared to that of natural infection, particularly so with the HPV and Cendehill vaccines (84,218,219). However, the immune response and protection resulting from immunization with the RA-27 vaccine more closely resemble those following natural infection (220–227).

Waning of immunity is a feature of natural rubella infection. It may be accompanied by reinfection, which in the vast majority of cases is clinically silent and accompanied by an anamnestic antibody response and much abbreviated viral replication (84,91,92,228,229). In natural rubella, this occurs in only 1–3% of the population. A less sturdy barrier to reinfection is provided by live vaccine, especially so with the HPV and Cendehill strains. In fact, in military recruits, reinfection was found to be 10-fold higher in those with vaccine immunity ($HPV_{77}DE$) than in those with natural immunity (91). Since vaccine immunity can be bolstered by repeat exposure to wild virus, the mass immunization of children is a deterrant to maintaining long-lasting immunity, which is needed to protect women throughout their childbearing years. The use of the RA-27 vaccine should minimize the potential problems associated with waning immunity. Obviously, the crucial concern about rubella reinfection is whether a period of viremia occurs, and if so, whether the product of conception is at risk. A few case reports suggest that maternal reinfection can lead to fetal involvement, but the results of these reports are debatable (190,230–236). In recent cases comprising experience with nine mothers who had low levels of IgM consistent with rubella reinfection after immunization, one infant had intrauterine rubella but had no sequelae, whereas the others escaped infection (237,238). Even subclinical infection must be exceedingly rare considering the intense attention focused on solving this problem over the years. Clearly, reinfection will never pose the public health hazard that natural infection imposes on unimmunized or poorly immunized populations.

Immunization failures can also result from improper handling and/or administration of the vaccines (primary vaccine failures), and this defect is quite disturbing in mass immunization programs. Between this problem and waning immunity (secondary vaccine failures), anywhere from 2% to 36% vaccine failures have been documented in different populations (230,239–246). Improper immunization practices appear to be more important since vaccine failures have occurred much less often in small-scale, investigator-directed studies (122,247–250).

The concept of protecting women by producing a high level of immunity in children has been challenged (251,252). This problem was first reported in military populations, in whom rates of immunity as high as 86% failed to reduce spread of rubella to virtually all susceptible recruits (91). A similar situation has been reported in other populations, including open ones (190,228,253). Nevertheless, mass immunization of children in the United States has apparently had a salient effect. There have been no large-scale epidemics of rubella since 1964–1965. In addition, both maternal and congenital rubella appear to be decreasing (186,192). However, the continued occurrence of rubella in young unimmunized women indicates the need for vaccination of this group, as outlined by the advisory committees on immunization practices (see beginning of this section).

In England, mass immunization of children was deemed unnecessary and vaccination was provided for young adolescent and immediate postpartum females (254). The idea was to immunize at least 90% of the women at risk and simultaneously provide a higher level of immunity throughout the childbearing ages. These programs have not been entirely successful due to the inability to immunize a sufficient proportion of the female population (255–258). With this immunization approach, large-scale epidemics continue to occur and the incidence of congenital rubella has not declined significantly since the introduction of vaccines. Because of these problems, the targeted vaccine approach has been controversial, and only time will determine whether this or the mass immunization approach is better.

### *Passive Immunization*

The value of passive immunization in the control of rubella is questionable (138,259). Brody (259) reported that large doses of γ-globulin may have some efficacy as prophylaxis. Extensive virus replication is demonstrable a week or more before symptoms appear, and surely initial replication must begin even earlier. Indeed, fetal infection has occurred in many circumstances in which γ-globulin has been given to the mother in what was believed to be adequate amounts soon after exposure (138). In addition, the amount of antirubella antibody in commercial γ-globulin preparations is variable and unpredictable; specific hyperimmune globulin preparations are not readily available (260,261). Another disadvantage of γ-globulin is that it may reduce clinical findings without eliminating virus replication. Thus clinical clues may be masked without adequate protection of the fetus.

### *Chemotherapy*

Currently there is no effective drug therapy for rubella. Amantadine hydrochloride will reduce the replication of rubella virus *in vitro,* and therefore it has theoretical possibilities as a chemotherapeutic agent. However, its use has been confined to two infants who were severely damaged as a result of congenital infection. Virus excretion was reduced somewhat while the drug was being administered; clinical benefit was questionable, and virus excretion continued after administration of the drug was stopped (262). This limited experience with the use of amantadine does not permit determination of any role it might play in the treatment of rubella.

## CMV

CMVs are ubiquitous agents in nature, and they are the most common causes of human intrauterine and perinatal infection. Characteristically, CMV infections in both mother and baby, whether infected *in utero* or later, are asymptomatic. In a small percentage of congenitally acquired infections, the infection is virulent, with multiple organ involvement that is most prevalent in the central nervous (CNS) and reticuloendothelial system. However, a significant percentage of infants born with subclinical CMV infection may develop more subtle forms of perceptual and CNS pathology later in life, either as a result of damage incurred *in utero* that has been overlooked or because of persistence of infection for long periods postnatally. The clinical silence of CMV infections and their tendency to be chronic and recurrent (reactivation or reinfection or both) have posed major problems with regard to understanding the true public health significance of these infections (263).

### The Virus

CMV is the largest member of the human herpesvirus family. Physically, CMV is approximately 200 nm in diameter, making it one of the largest animal viruses. The virus consists of a 64-nm core containing the viral DNA enclosed by a 110-nm icosahedral capsid made up of 162 capsomeres (264,265). The complete particle is enclosed by an envelope consisting of at least 25–30 virion-encoded proteins and glycoproteins (266–268).

The linear double-stranded DNA of CMV is approximately 240 kilobases (kb) in size, making it approximately 50% larger than the genome of herpes simplex virus (HSV) (269–271). The CMV genome is similar to that of HSV in that it has unique long and short sequences, both of which are bounded by homologous repetitive sequences; it can assume four isomeric forms (269–272).

The size of the CMV genome would suggest that virus can encode a myriad of proteins. Approximately 33 structural proteins and an unknown number of infected cell proteins are encoded by the virus (266–268). The icosahedral structure surrounding the virion core contains two major structural proteins, the major and minor capsid protein, with molecular weights of 150 kilodaltons (kd) and 34 kd, respectively (266–268). Outside the virion capsid, two matrix proteins of 68 kd and 72 kd form a bridge between the capsid and virion envelope. The 68-kd matrix protein represents the most abundant protein in the virion (267,268). An additional 200-kd protein is also proposed to be located between the virion capsid and envelope (273). The CMV envelope is a complex structure and consists of at least six glycoproteins (267), three of which are found in abundance (267,273). The glycoproteins with apparent molecular weights of 140 kd, 62 kd, and 57 kd are the major protein constituents of the envelope (267,273). It is believed these glycoproteins express antigenic sites for neutralizing antibodies. A number of other proteins found in lesser abundance than the proteins discussed above have been described; however, their functional and structural role in CMV is unknown. The so called dense body of CMV probably represents a defective particle of CMV containing most, if not all, of the virion structural proteins yet lacking viral DNA (267,268).

The replication of CMV seems much akin to the better studied HSV, in that CMV has a temporally controlled replication regulated by different segments of its genome (274). Following adsorption, possibly through specific cell surface receptors, the virus uncoats within the cytoplasm and the nucleocapsids then proceed rapidly into the nucleus (275). Shortly thereafter, viral specific RNA can be found, indicating a rapid expression of the viral genome (276,277). Viral nucleic acid replication probably begins as early as 12 hr postinfection (278); however, it is readily detectable at 24–36 hr postinfection (278). Infectious particles are released approximately 72 hr after infection (279). The replicative cycle has been divided into three time periods; immediate early, early, and late, based on the appearance of different classes of CMV specific proteins during those time periods and the sensitivity of protein expression during these time periods to different pharmacologic agents (279,280,281).

The detection of CMV infection in humans has utilized both serologic and viral isolation procedures, and more recently methods of molecular biology (281). Hybridization methods, using cloned viral DNA, are not as sensitive as viral culture but are specific and can be performed rapidly (283–285). Traditional methods of histologic examination of tissue specimens remain a valuable technique for identification of acute infection with CMV (286). Viral isolation remains the standard method of documenting CMV infection. The shell vial culture method with immunoperoxidase staining for early viral proteins provides a rapid method for detecting infectious virus in clinical specimens (287).

Successful *in vitro* propagation of CMV has generally been limited to homologous fibroblast cells. In infected monolayers fixed with Bouin's solution and stained with hematoxylin-eosin, cell enlargement or rounding (strain-dependent) or both are visualized within 6 hr after infection (288). By 24 hr, the nucleus is eccentrically placed, with prominent nucleoli. An eosinophilic paranuclear inclusion develops, and cell enlargement is more apparent. Between 48 and 72 hr after infection, an irregular skein-like basophilic nuclear inclusion appears. The cytoplasm stains more basophilic, and the eosinophilic paranuclear inclusion is more prominent. Multinucleated cells can be seen with the inclusion-bearing nuclei arranged concentrically around the large eosinophilic inclusion (286).

Clinical specimens containing human CMV produce a characteristic CPE within hours or weeks following inoculation, depending on the amount of virus present in the preparations (286). Initially, the CPE effect consists of small round or elongated foci of enlarged refractile cells. Most clinical isolates produce early and marked cell rounding. Often, the affected cells have brownish refractile granules. Spread of infection in the monolayers usually is quite slow, involving adjacent cells first. Thus, foci gradually enlarge, often with central degeneration. Satellite foci usually form, but unless the inoculum is quite large, the initial infection rarely progresses to involve the entire monolayer. This slowly developing process may last for several weeks or months. When there are large quantities of CMV in the inoculum, generalized cell rounding may appear within 24 hr, but progression slows with passage.

A variety of serologic assays have been used to document serologic evidence of CMV infection. The CF test is probably one of the more commonly used serologic tests in the diagnosis of CMV infection (286). Both glycine extract (GE) and freeze-thaw (FT) preparation of CF antigen have been utilized. However, it has been suggested that the GE antigen provides more reproducible results (290). Pereria et al. have shown the GE extract of infected fibroblasts contains an abundance of a 66-kd and 50-kd glycoprotein that comigrated with structural glycoproteins of CMV on polyacrylamide gels (290). In addition, these investigators demonstrated a strong host response to these glycoproteins within the CF antigen (290). Seroconversion can be readily demonstrated using the CF test, but waning of CF antibody titers with time has made this test of questionable value as an epidemiological tool (291,292) and for the demonstration of host immunity (293).

IF is another technique widely used to detect both IgG and IgM antibodies to CMV. A variety of antigenic sources have been used including acetone-fixed infected fibroblasts, and nuclei of infected fibroblast and viable infected cells (286,289). A potential disadvantage of the IF assay is the ability of CMV to induce a cytoplasmic crystallizable fragment (Fc) receptor for human immunoglobulins (294–297). As a result, false-positive reactions can occur unless positive reactions are restricted to nuclear fluorescence. The technique of anticomplementary IF (ACIF), which is read as nuclear fluorescence, is a particularly sensitive and specific test for antibodies to CMV (298,299). In addition, these techniques of IF can be utilized to detect the early antigens of CMV (293).

Although rarely used in routine diagnostic serology, neutralization of CMV utilizing a plaque reduction assay remains a highly sensitive and specific method for the determination serologic reactivity to CMV (286). Other less commonly used methods, including indirect hemagglutination (286) and immune adherence hemagglutination, have proven useful in seroepidemiological studies of CMV (285,300,301).

More recently, sensitive RIAs, have been utilized to detect IgM antibodies to CMV in the cord serum of congenitally infected babies as well as the seroconversion of renal transplant patients with primary CMV (302,303). These methods are extremely sensitive but technically demanding and, therefore, are used primarily for seroepidemiological studies. Enzyme-linked immunoassays (EIA) are now being utilized in the diagnostic serology studies of CMV infections. Furthermore, EIA have been automated, thus allowing the processing of large numbers of clinical specimens (304).

Recently, the use of restriction endonucleases to characterize the genome of CMV have been particularly useful in the study of the epidemiology of CMV. Although there appears to be an approximate 80% homology between the genomes of a large number of CMV isolates (305), sufficient differences exist between strains of CMV to allow restriction endonuclease analysis to distinguish between different isolates of CMV (306).

## Epidemiology

Natural infection by CMV is species-specific. Humans are believed to be the only reservoir for human CMV, and transmission occurs by direct or indirect person-to-person contact. Because of the liability of CMV to various environmental factors, close or even intimate contact is believed to be required for horizontal spread (307). Sources of virus include oropharyngeal secretions, urine, cervical and vaginal excretions, spermatic fluids, breast milk, and blood (308–311). Spread in the larger population is enhanced by the prolonged duration of communicability in various infected populations. Virus excretion has persisted following congenital infection for as long as 8 years and commonly for 4 years; the same is true for the perinatally (natal) and early postnatally acquired infections (293,312). In fact, prolonged replication of CMV can follow primary infection in children and adults, and recurrences (either reactivations of latent infections or reinfections) are associated with intermittent shedding of CMV in a significant proportion of seropositive young adults (310,313,314).

As monitored by congenital involvement, CMV infection in women does not manifest seasonal occurrence (315). However, ill-defined socioeconomic factors do predispose to higher infection rates, both by vertical (intrauterine) transmission and by horizontal (extrauterine) transmission (315–318). Hygiene alone cannot explain the higher infection rates; rather, the closeness of contacts within population groups appears to be more important. Very high rates of infection among children have been recorded in isolated locations such as New Guinea and certain Pacific islands, as well as crowded areas of Africa, the Orient, and the Middle East, irrespective of hygienic practices (315,316). In the United States, black and Indian populations acquire CMV infections earlier in life than white middle-income groups (315–319). Whether or not there is racial predilection remains to be determined, but this seems doubtful on the basis of current knowledge.

There is also compelling evidence that CMV can be spread through venereal routes (320). In some populations there is a burst of infection with the advent of puberty. Infection rates as assessed by antibody status are much increased in promiscuous populations, especially so in young male homosexuals; genital shedding of virus is also markedly increased in these populations, including the frequency and amount of virus shed (300,309,316,317,321).

Between 0.5% and 2.2% (average, 1%) of infant populations are infected *in utero* (317). Another 8–60% become infected during the first 6 months of life as a result of natal or breast milk transmissions, with the latter being the most important source in breast feeding populations (308,310,317). Transmission among toddlers is exceptionally high in day-care centers and boarding schools (322). After infancy in most developed countries, infection rates increase slowly until the age of entry into school, at which time they rise more rapidly; 40–80% of children are infected by the age of puberty (315,316). In other areas of the world, 90–100% of a population may be infected during childhood even as early as 6 years of age (307,315,316). Clearly, then, there is a wide range of susceptibility (70% to less than 5%) to primary CMV infection during the childbearing years (316). Thus, the relative proportions of primary and recurrent infection in pregnant populations are highly variable, not only between but within countries (317). Primary infection during pregnancy is more common in younger women from the higher socioeconomic sector, while recurrent infection occurs more often in lower socioeconomic groups (317,318). CMV seropositivity in pregnancy correlates with socioculture variables, such as birth outside North America, and with sexual and reproductive history, such as greater total numbers of partners, first pregnancy at younger than 15 years, and multigravidity (323). Age is also an important determinant for recurrent infection, in the genital and urinary tracts of women and the injury tract of homosexual males (321,324). Although rates of seropositivity increase with age, there is a steady decline in virus excretion from puberty to age 30, when recurrent infection either ceases or is strikingly reduced.

Oral and respiratory spread are the dominant routes of transmission during childhood (325) and probably adulthood as well.

Day care center transmission has emerged as a new source of maternal infection (326–329). Investigations of nosocomial transmission in hospital settings and of acquisition by personnel in medical and educational occupations have demonstrated low rates of transmission (330,331). Restriction endonuclease analysis of strains from individuals thought to have occupation-related infection have proved other sources of CMV (332). Transmission among hospitalized patients is also low, including infants and children (333–337). The survival of CMV on toys and hands is presumed to lead to the increased rates of transmission in day care centers that care for young children as well as the fact that children are in day care before being toilet-trained (338,339). Transmission between infected and susceptible toddlers who then bring the virus into the household creates the opportunity for transmission to parents (340,345). This problem is clearly just as common in day care centers caring for healthy children as in centers for children with physical or developmental disabilities (346).

## Maternal Infection

### *Symptomatic Primary CMV Infection*

Whether primary or recurrent, CMV infection is subclinical in the vast majority of cases (317–319). However, in rare instances with natural primary infection, a heterophil-negative mononucleosis develops and a similar condition may follow transfusion of large quantities of blood or blood products (312,347–349). Some of the salient features of this syndrome are depicted in Fig. 5. The incubation period has not been precisely defined, but it is believed to be relatively long, on the order of 4–8 weeks (310,349).

The CMV mononucleosis is heralded by abrupt onset of spiking fever (temperature up to 40°C or 104°F) that persists from 2–6 weeks and occasionally longer (Fig. 5). Constitutional symptoms (malaise, chills, myalgia) are relatively common, but they are mild, as is sore throat accompanied by minimal pharyngeal erythema. Short-lived (hours to 2 days) and spotty rubelliform rash may appear that can be worsened or precipitated by ampicillin. Leukocytosis with relative and absolute lymphocytosis is the rule. Atypical lymphocytes (10–34%) appear early in the course of infection; they subside with the symptoms, as do liver-enzyme elevations, which occur early in the course of infection. However, lymphocytosis may persist for many months (347–349).

Although the disease is generally mild and is often overlooked, CMV mononucleosis can be more severe, with a protracted course and varying degrees of prostration. Frank hepatitis, pneumonia, polyneuritis, and other CNS complications and gastrointestinal involvements are uncommon features (350–357).

Symptomatic primary infection is undoubtedly generalized, but the portal of entry for CMV is poorly defined. Viremia is detectable for a few weeks to a few months (313,324,358). The polymorphonuclear leukocyte is the main source of CMV in the blood, but monocytes and occasionally T lymphocytes may harbor CMV in a form as yet undefined (358–362). Virus is consistently recovered from urine of symptomatic patients and commonly recovered from the pharynx, at least with onset of disease, and viruria may be persistent or intermittent for

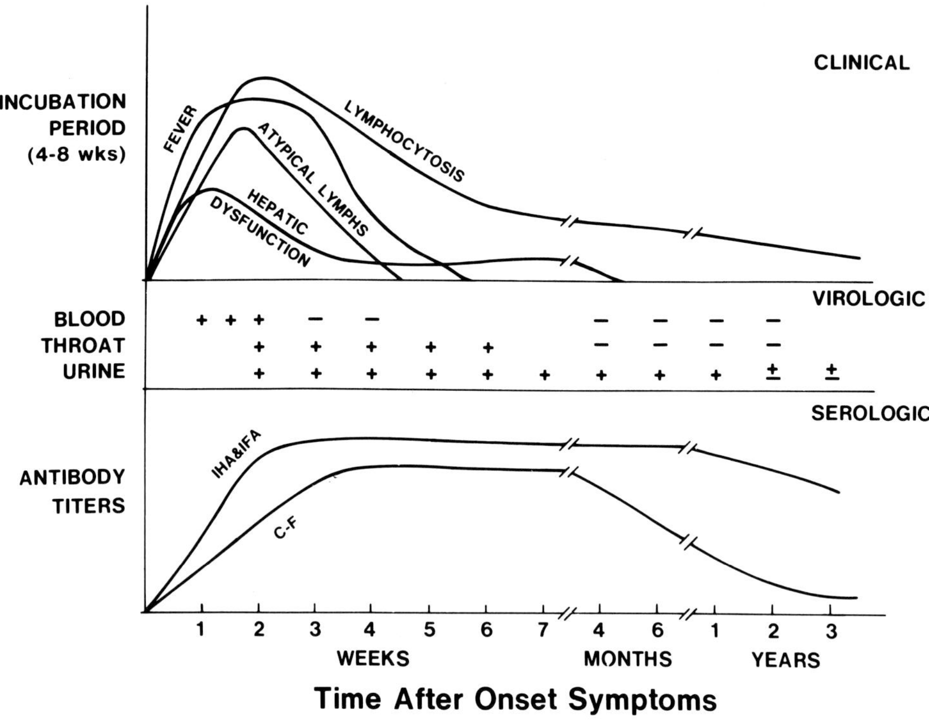


**FIG. 5.** Findings of symptomatic primary CMV infection in normal hosts (mononucleosis syndrome). Constructed from data in refs. 7–9 and 23. (From Alford et al., ref. 379, with permission.)

a year or more after symptoms disappear (348,349). Virus isolation is helpful, but it is not a conclusive diagnostic aid for primary infection, since asymptomatic individuals also can excrete CMV from multiple sites as a result of reactivation of virus (302,317). Conversely, CMV can be difficult to isolate from individuals with asymptomatic primary CMV infection (363). Consequently, demonstration of seroconversion is generally considered the best means of proving primary involvement.

### *Humoral and Cellular Immune Responses with Primary CMV Infection*

CMV antibodies can be detected by a number of different serologic assays, as outlined in the section on the virus. IgM and IgG class-specific antibodies can be determined by indirect fluorescence antibody (IFA), RIA, ELISA, and anticomplement immunofluorescence (ACIF). For the detection of IgM antibodies, these tests yield differing degrees of sensitivity and specificity, with the RIA giving the best results. Seroconversion can be demonstrated by any of the previously mentioned techniques. However, low-level seroconversion (titers of <8–16) in the CF test using crude antigens does not always mean primary infection, since levels may fluctuate in this range in individuals who have had prior CMV infection (289,293).

IgM antibodies peak during the early course of infection and tend to disappear 12–16 weeks following onset of subclinical infection, but may persist for longer periods with symptomatic infections (302,364). Unfortunately, not all women with primary CMV infection during pregnancy develop

IgM antibodies (365). Among 49 women, 73% had CMV IgM antibodies and 69% transmitted CMV to their infants *in utero* but the rate of transmission was 54% among those who had no detectable virus-specific IgM response (337). Except for neutralizing and perhaps IgG ELISA antibodies, other IgG antibodies peak during the first month to 6 weeks after onset of infection; the former two may not peak for 2–3 months after onset (347,366,367). The kinetics of the antibody responses over long term have not been well established due to difficulties in case-finding and follow-up. Indirect evidence indicates that most IgG antibodies, although they may wane to differing degrees, tend to persist for many years after initial infection. Booster antibody responses, including the IgM varieties, are unusual with recurrent infection in the normal host but are detected with greater frequency in the immunosuppressed individuals, probably due to increased antigenic load (303).

Cell-mediated immunity, unlike antibody responses, is depressed with symptomatic primary infections. T-cell dysfunctions appear to be the major problem (358). The peripheral blood monocytes respond (blastogenesis) poorly to mitogens, to CMV-specific antigens, and to antigens of other herpesviruses during the acute phase of illness (357–362,368). The responses recover slowly at variable rates during convalescence. With mononucleosis, there is also diminished cytotoxic ability of these cells (369). Activated (OKIa) cytotoxic suppressor (OKT8) cells increase strikingly during the disease, whereas helper inducer (OKT4) cells are slightly diminished, resulting in a reversal of the normal ratio of these cell types (370). The atypical lymphocytes that characterize the mononucleosis appear to be activated cytotoxic suppressor cells. It is believed that this defect predisposed patients with symptomatic primary CMV infection to superinfection, more commonly seen in immunosuppressed than normal individuals. In this way, CMV could play a role in the acute immunodeficiency disease, as it apparently does in transplant patients. Preliminary evidence suggests that the functions of B cell, polymorphonuclear leukocytes, and NK cells remain intact during symptomatic infections but these cell types have not been studied as extensively as the T cells (368, 371,372). Whether cell-mediated immunity is as depressed with primary subclinical CMV infection has not been established, but indirect evidence suggests that it may be less striking.

### *Asymptomatic CMV Infection*

Asymptomatic CMV infection has been best defined in young pregnant women, obviously because of interest in determining its role in intrauterine transmission. It is clear that subclinical infection is common during pregnancy (314,318,319,373,374). In different populations, primary subclinical infection has varied from 0.7% to 4% (average 2%) per annum in susceptible (seronegative) pregnant women (317,318,375–377). Because of greater susceptibility, younger women from middle to high income groups have a greater incidence of primary infections, as do women with at least one child in the home, due to greater exposure (317,378).

Recurrent CMV infections, which in normal people are virtually always subclinical, are far more common than primary infection in most adult populations because of the high rates of acquisition of primary infection during childhood and adolescence (317,318,379). Because the reactivation of latent CMV infection is not associated with a change in antibody status in normal hosts with recurrent CMV infections, this expression of infection can be detected only by mass screening for virus excretion. Reinfection may occur in immune persons because of antigenic and genetic disparity among CMV strains (305,306). Restriction enzyme analysis of viral DNA indicates that exogenous reinfection is common in women who have a high probability of exposure to CMV (380).

Molecular epidemiologic studies using restriction enzyme analysis of viral DNA suggests that reactivation or persistence of virus is more common than reinfection (306). Evidence for reinfection has been detected only in the genital tract of men and women with the possibility of coinfection in semen of male homosexuals (306,381). With recurrent infection, virus in intermittently excreted from multiple sites. Cervical shedding has varied from 3% to 18% (average 9%), urinary excretion has been detected in from 3% to 9% (average 3.5%), and pharyngeal shedding in 1–2% (average 1.8%) (310,317). In postpartal women, the breast is the most common site of reactivation, varying from 14% to 27% of the total population (308,311,317). Of seropositive women, 30% or more can intermittently excrete CMV into breast milk during the first year after delivery, most commonly between 2 and 4 months postpartum.

Gestation and age both have profound effects on reactivation of CMV. During the first trimester of pregnancy, both genital and urinary excretion of CMV are infrequent (316,317). However, shedding from both sites increases progressively, reaching high levels by term. Previously, this effect was believed to be due to progressive reactivation of CMV with advancing gestation (310,319). However, in one comparative study, the rate of cervical shedding of CMV in a comparable nonpregnant population proved to be 10%, a baseline incidence similar to that seen at term but significantly higher than that observed in the first trimester of pregnancy (314). Age has the opposite influence on reactivation of CMV. In both genital and urinary tract of females, reactivation diminishes steadily from puberty to age 30, after which viral excretion from these sites is very infrequent (323).

Vertical (*in utero*) transmission of CMV can result from primary or recurrent maternal infection (317,318). The latter is more prevalent in highly immune and lower socioeconomic populations because of intrauterine transmission with reactivated CMV infections (318,382). The ability to vertically transmit virus in the face of substantial maternal immunity accounts for the inordinately high rates of congenital CMV infection observed throughout the world (316). The maternal source of virus for this type of transmission is unknown, but latently infected white blood cells or endometrium are believed to be the most likely sources. On a worldwide basis, intrauterine transmission with recurrent maternal CMV is more common than vertical transmission with primary maternal infection (317). In one geographic setting, namely Birmingham, Alabama, the rate of congenital infection among the low income, highly immune (85% seropositive) group was 1.9%, whereas it was only 0.6% in the less immune (60% seropositive) higher income group (318). In the former population recurrent maternal CMV was responsible for most of the congenital infection, whereas in the latter primary and recurrent maternal infections were equally responsible.

Even with primary maternal CMV infection, intrauterine infection is not inevitable: it occurs in approximately 40% of the cases (317,318). Although not yet proven the most likely sequence of events is placental infection from maternal viremia or leucoviremia with subsequent spread to the fetus. Despite viremia, it is clear that infection can terminate in the placenta, but the factors that lead to *in utero* transmission of virus or the lack of it with primary maternal infection remain unknown (274,317,383,384). The rates of transmission are equivalent for primary infections during the first and second half of gestation, but the risk of sequelae is clearly related to maternal infection in early pregnancy. None of 26 infants born to mothers with infection at 23–40 weeks had significant handicaps compared to 5 of 33 infants (29%) of those whose mothers acquired CMV infection between 4 and 22 weeks of gestation (382). The risk of primary CMV infection in pregnant adolescents was 1% and was associated with a 50% risk of intrauterine infection (384). In assessing the risks of primary maternal CMV infection, it is important to emphasize that the most likely outcome is the birth of a healthy infant (385). Assuming a 50% risk of transmission and a 20% risk sequelae, 1 in 10 infants will be affected.

The fetal infection is most often subclinical with either reactivated or primary maternal infections (317,318,386). Maternal immunity does, however, modify virulence of the fetal infection (318). Following transmission with primary maternal infection, 10% or less of the infected infants have clinically evident disease during the neonatal period, whereas cytomegalic inclusion disease is exceedingly rare following transmission with recurrent maternal infection. The role of these two types of maternal infection as regards development of subtle late-appearing defects such as deafness is yet to be determined. Such defects have been observed following both types of maternal infection (317,318,387). Given the low frequency of such disabilities and the fact that most series evaluated children who had asymptomatic CMV at birth without knowledge of the type of maternal infection, it is likely that the morbidity observed is usually a result of primary maternal infection.

**Pathogenesis and Pathology**

Having gained access to the fetus, CMV can invade and replicate in virtually every organ, demonstrating a particular affinity for epithelial cells (263). Occasionally, typical intranuclear inclusions are recognized in vascular endothelium, which may be especially susceptible if undergoing rapid proliferation (263). The typical pathological sequence is cytolysis with focal necrosis and resultant inflammatory response (mainly mononuclear). The degree of the inflammatory response may be related to the gestational age at the time of the viral invasion, with lesser responses for infections occurring in the first half of gestation (388). Healing may occur, accompanied by fibrosis and occasionally calcification (brain and liver), or there may be restoration of normal structure in the continuing presence of infected cells. In newborns with lethal disease, retardation of intrauterine growth has been related to reductions in absolute numbers of cells in various organs, as opposed to diminution in cell size (389).

An immune response by the fetus is evidenced by the presence of elevated IgM levels and specific CMV IgM antibody in cord serum (390–393). IgG antibody, predominantly maternally derived, typically is present in substantial amounts at birth, having been progressively acquired by the fetus since midgestation. However, whatever defenses are marshaled appear inadequate, since viral replication and excretion persist throughout intrauterine life and long into extrauterine life. It is clear that such chronicity is not the result of development of antigenic tolerance *in utero,* since the production of specific antibody occurs for years, if not for life. Furthermore, acquisition of infection in adulthood also results in prolonged viruria (313). CMV infection may manifest as a chronic process with intermittent excretion in addition to latency with periodic activation (394). Given this circumstance, the potential for low-grade continued tissue injury is increased (293,395). Tissue tropism or local immune defenses or both may have significance with regard to sequelae.

Excessive production of IgM and IgG in the presence of high levels of virus replication during the early postnatal course of congenitally acquired CMV infection has suggested the possibility of immune complex formation and deposition as another cause of tissue damage (395). Recent evidence has suggested the presence of circulating immune complexes and rheumatoid factor in a significant proportion of young infants with congenital CMV infection (396,397). Preliminary results have suggested that heavy complexes (>19 S) that can be deposited in tissues are formed during symptomatic congenital infection, whereas lighter complexes (<19 S) circulate in the subclinical form. Exactly what the pathological potential for these complexes might be is currently unknown, but they serve to emphasize the possible role of immunologically mediated pathology, in addition to that resulting from viral cytolysis. Definition of specific mediators of pathology and their relative importance is critical for future therapeutic considerations.

### Congenital Infection

The spectrum of disease secondary to fetal infection is quite broad, with a marked skew toward asymptomatic infection at birth. Exact figures are unavailable, but a reasonable estimate of subclinical infection would be 90–95% of the total (374,395,398–400). For those with manifest neonatal illness, stigmata may range from isolated organ system involvement to multiple organ system dysfunction with life-threatening potential (392). Classically, the sick infant presents with hepatosplenomegaly, hyperbilirubinemia (usually direct), thrombocytopenia with petechiae and occasionally purpura, intrauterine growth retardation, and encephalitis with or without microcephaly (Table 2) (392,401,402). For the most part the extraneural pathology is self-limited, with the occasional exception of protracted hepatitis; however, pneumonitis and myocarditis (rarely), severe thrombocytopenia purpura (occasionally), and disseminated intravascular coagulopathy (commonly) possess life-threatening potential. This last process should be excluded in any infant with evidence of a bleeding dyscrasia (including petechiae), since early therapy may significantly improve the outcome. Fulminating encephalitis also may be incompatible with survival. In the debilitated infant, secondary bacterial infection is a frequent cause of death.

In lieu of microcephaly, neonatal CNS involvement may manifest as seizures, apnea, or focal neurologic signs (Table 2).

**TABLE 2.** *Clinical findings in infants with symptomatic congenital CMV infection*

| Clinical findings | Frequency (%) |
|---|---|
| Intrauterine death | Rare |
| Prematurity | Unknown |
| Intrauterine growth retardation | 21–50 |
| Reticuloendothelial system | |
| Hepatitis | 51–75 |
| Direct hyperbilirubinemia | 51–75 |
| Hemolytic and other anemias | 21–50 |
| Petechiae-ecchymoses | 76–100 |
| Disseminated intravascular coagulopathy | Rare |
| Hepatosplenomegaly | 76–100 |
| Adenopathies | Unknown |
| CNS | |
| Encephalitis | 51–75 |
| Microcephaly | 21–50 |
| Hydrocephalus | Rare |
| Intracranial calcifications | 21–50 |
| Eye, chorioretinitis | 9–20 |
| Congenital malformations | |
| Inguinal hernias | 21–50 |
| First branchial arch derivatives | 9–20 |
| Others | Rare |
| Myocarditis | Rare |
| Pneumonitis | 9–20 |
| Bone, vertical radiolucency | Rare |
| Sequelae | |
| Psychomotor retardation | 51–75 |
| Hearing loss | 21–50 |
| Visual impairment | 0–20 |

Even with CNS involvement, CSF changes including only protein elevations are observed in about 40% of cases (392). Other laboratory abnormalities include: increased cord serum IgM (>20 mg/100 ml) 85%, atypical lymphocytosis (≥5%) 80%, elevated SGOT (>80 μU/ml) 61%, and thrombocytopenia (<100,000 platelets/mm$^3$) 60% of cases. It is obvious that considerable clinical overlap exists between CMV infection and the other chronic intrauterine infections, and this necessitates laboratory confirmation of diagnosis in all cases.

The teratogenic potential of CMV has been discussed in an excellent review (403). Defects in virtually every organ system have been associated with intrauterine infection; however, for most anomalies only one or two case reports exist, and this

**TABLE 3.** *Outcome of infants and children presenting with symptomatic and asymptomatic congenital CMV infection*

| Complications | Symptomatic (%) | Asymptomatic (%) |
|---|---|---|
| Fatal | 20 | 0 |
| Psychomotor retardation or neuromuscular disorder | 70 | 2–7 |
| Hearing loss | 50 | 10 |
| Bilateral | 25 | 5 |
| Unilateral | 25 | 5 |
| Chorioretinitis or optic atrophy | 14 | 1 |
| Learning disability | 20 | 4 |
| Dental defects | 33 | 3 |
| Total, with one or more complications | 90–95 | 5–15 |

makes it virtually impossible to demonstrate a statistically valid cause-and-effect relationship. Exceptions to this observation include inguinal hernia in males and possibly first-arch abnormalities, both of which are relatively frequent (401).

Outcome of congenital CMV infection, which is clinically evident in the neonatal period, is summarized in Table 3 (392,404). Overt neonatal disease is usually but not inevitably a harbinger of later CNS and perceptual dysfunction (401,402). Apparently, extraneural organs are spared chronic morbidity, with the possible exception of the liver, despite the fact that virus replication continues in the kidney for years. Microcephaly that is present at birth or that develops within the first year of life is usually but not inevitably associated with significant mental disability (392,401). The distribution of intelligence and developmental test scores is bimodal in children with symptomatic CMV at birth (404). In the group with severe deficits, associated findings were microcephaly, chorioretinitis, and neurologic impairment evident in the first year of life. The severity of reticuloendothelial disease in the newborn period and hearing loss as an isolated deficit were not predictive of low intelligence. Pathologic conditions in brain and perceptual organs may manifest as mental retardation, spastic diplegia, seizures, optic atrophy, blindness, and sensorineural deafness, alone or in combination. Such defects may also develop in children without any evidence of CNS involvement at birth.

It is now clear that congenital CMV infection that is subclinical in the early months of life may result in significant late-appearing sequelae (Table 3) (395). Sensorineural hearing loss has been detected in 10% or so of infants born with subclinical infection. Considering the frequency of this infection (0.5–2.2% of live births), CMV may be one of the leading causes of deafness (317,379). Besides being late-appearing, auditory defects may also be progressive, although the numbers of such cases have not yet been determined (405). Children with asymptomatic CMV infection at birth who do not have hearing loss are not at increased risk for mental impairment. (406,407). Chorioretinitis is a rare late-appearing defect. A dental anomaly that can result in loss of the temporary tooth has been described in a significant number of infants with symptomatic and subclinical infection. Apparently this defect results from an enamel abnormality (317,408).

### Perinatal Infection

CMV infection acquired at or around the time of delivery is much more common than congenital CMV infection. Since these perinatal infections are chronic, like the congenital infection, they carry the potential for developing insidious disease (293,317,379). However, to date perinatal infection acquired through contact with infected cervical secretions or breast milk (409), the two most common sources for perinatal transmission, has been associated with little morbidity, except for the occurrence of penumonitis in young infants (410,411). Since most of these perinatal acquisitions are caused by reactivated maternal infection, the presence of transplacental maternal antibody apparently protects from disease, even though it does not stop transmission in 50% of the cases (412). Nevertheless, the small premature infant who is born with a reduced complement of maternal antibody could conceivably be in jeopardy from those maternally acquired perinatal infections (413).

Perinatal infection can also be acquired through transfusion of blood or blood products that contain white blood cells and has been obtained from CMV seropositive donors (412,414). Infection is dependent upon the number and volume of the transfusions and the number of donors. Occurrence of CMV-related disease is dependent upon the antibody status of the infant at the time of transfusion, gestational age, and preexisting illness. In general, seropositive infants, although not protected from infection, are protected from disease, with the possible exception of very small prematures. Here the situation is similar to the maternally acquired perinatal infections. However, the seronegative infant who is infected by blood transfusion may develop an illness characterized by the development of shock-like symptoms accompanied by a gray pallor, respiratory distress, and variable involvement of the reticuloendothelial system similar to that seen with milder forms of congenital infection (412), although generally self-limited death rates as high at 20% have been reported. This form of perinatal CMV infection is most severe in small premature infants who have or are recovering from pulmonary hyaline membrane or other debilitating diseases. Whether infants chronically infected by transfusions will develop late-appearing sequelae is yet to be determined but a distinct possibility. There is theoretical concern that seronegative infants who acquire CMV infection through banked breast milk or by nosocomial sources might also be in jeopardy for developing CMV-related disease similar to that acquired by transfusions (378).

### Diagnosis

The diagnosis of congenital infection is best confirmed by isolation of the virus, preferably during the first few days of life (289,392,415). Acquisition of virus at or near the time of delivery may result in shedding as early as 3 weeks and frequently by 8 weeks, thereby rendering this assay less specific for intrauterine infection with advancing age of the patient (286,289,293,310). The preferred source in the attempt to isolate virus is urine, although virus can be isolated from the throat and in symptomatic infants from conjunctival and rectal swabs, as well as from white blood cells. Transportation of specimens is best accomplished by packing them in wet ice. Because of marked loss of infectivity, freezing should be avoided (286). Inoculated cultures should be observed for 4 weeks, even though most will demonstrate CPEs within 7 days (286). Virus can also be demonstrated in urine by electron microscopy (EM), preferably employing the pseudoreplica technique, and CMV antigens can be detected in urine using ELISA technology (289,393). These techniques have differing sensitivities and specificities (varying from 50% to 90%), depending primarily on the amount of virus in the urine specimen (289). Various components of CMV can also be demonstrated in tissues and cells using fluorescent, radioactive, and hybridization techniques (393).

Cytologic examination of the urine sediment for inclusion-bearing cells should not be relied upon because of the high rate of false negatives, even among infants with classical disease (263). The presence of large intranuclear inclusion-bearing cells is presumptive evidence of infection, especially in the neonatal period; thereafter, similar cells may be shed secondary to adenovirus and other virus infections, which results in loss of specificity.

### *Humoral Immune Response of Congenital and Perinatal Infections*

The situation with regard to the humoral immune response with congenital CMV infection is similar to that associated with congenital rubella. Both transplacental transfer of maternal IgG antibodies and fetal production of IgM occur during pregnancy, so that at delivery the amount of antibody in the cord and maternal sera are equivalent when measured by standard serologic methods. As the maternal antibody, which is the major component in cord serum, declines, the infant begins to produce IgG antibody and continues to produce IgM antibody for weeks to months after delivery. After a slight drop during the first few months of life due to the catabolism of maternal antibody, the infant's IgG antibody response is maintained for years, if not for life, in association with the prolonged replication of virus. The antibody responses with the perinatally acquired infections are similar to those of the congenital infection except for a slightly longer catabolic period for maternal antibody before the infant first becomes infected, usually between 1 and 4 months postnatally depending upon the source of the infection. These sequential antibody responses as measured by different serologic tests in the congenital and perinatal infections, have been described in detail elsewhere (286).

In the past, serologic diagnosis of intrauterine was dependent on the demonstration of persistent antibody for the infant 6 months to 1 year after birth, as with other congenital infections such as rubella. However, the recognition of high rates of perinatally acquired infection, plus the presence of maternal antibody in the vast majority of cases, means that sequential monitoring of antibody as a precise diagnostic approach for congenital infection is virtually impossible (298). Persistence of antibody in the infant born with clinically apparent infection is presumptive evidence for intrauterine acquisition. But because of the poor prognosis of this variety of CMV infection as opposed to subclinical forms, proper diagnosis by viral isolation soon after delivery is much preferred.

Serologic diagnosis of congenital CMV infection can best be accomplished by detection of fetal IgM antibody in cord serum or early neonatal serum, thus obviating the need for sequential monitoring for total antibody. In the past IgM antibody to CMV was measured almost exclusively by IFA methods (391,393). The usefulness of these methods was limited because of problems of sensitivity and specificity which have not yet been resolved. It is clear that rheumatoid factor (IgM antibody directed against maternal IgG) can give false-positive reactions in the IgM IFA test, and rheumatoid factor is produced in a fairly high percentage of patients with subclinical CMV infections as well as patients with symptomatic congenital CMV infections (393,396). Therefore, serum should be examined for rheumatoid factor; if present, rheumatoid factor should be removed before testing for IgM antibodies. Recently CMV IgM antibody has been measured using ELISA and RIA methods. Both appear to be superior to the IgM IFA test, particularly the RIA approach which in one study yielded excellent results as regards sensitivity and specificity (390). Nevertheless, detection of IgM antibodies in cord or neonatal sera, in contrast to sera from children and adults, poses technical difficulties that seem to be related to the large quantities of maternal IgG antibody (390). Methods that eliminate or reduce IgG from cord sera or separate the IgM as a first step appear superior for detection of IgM antibody to those that employ untreated sera. Nevertheless, specific IgM antibodies are detected by IgM ELISA in only approximately half of infants with congenital CMV infections (324,365,416). Testing for CMV IgM antibodies in cord blood must be done by RIA to be reliable (417). Although other methods provide reproducible results under research conditions, their standardization is difficult to maintain (418). There are nonspecific findings that are useful in defining infants at high risk for congenital CMV infection, especially those neonates with clinically evident disease. These include the presence of elevated serum IgM, rheumatoid factor in cord or neonatal serum, and atypical lymphocytosis (392,393). Even with these abnormalities the diagnosis must be specifically confirmed by virologic or serologic means (289,393).

Because of all the complications of serological diagnosis of congenital infection, virus isolation from urine in the first week of life remains the best way to prove intrauterine involvement (289). The virus in urine has sufficiently high titer and is sufficiently stable at 4°C so that shipment to distant virology laboratories should pose no problem, provided that sterility is maintained (393). Proving intrauterine infection, especially in suspect infants, is of paramount importance because of associated developmental difficulties.

#### Cellular Immune Response

Abnormalities in cell-mediated immunity differ in infants and children with chronic congenital and perinatal infection from those observed in adults with CMV mononucleosis. Only one defect has been consistently observed in the chronically infected infants and children, and that is an inability of their lymphocytes to proliferate *in vitro* when challenged with CMV antigens (419–422). This defect is more profound than that seen in adults with mononucleosis and in contrast persists for many years whether the infections are symptomatic or asymptomatic in infancy (420). This inability in antigen recognition appears to be CMV-specific, occurs in the presence of normal numbers of B and T cells, including a normal ratio of T-cell subsets and a normal blastogenic response to mitogens (420). Natural killer cell activity appears to be relatively normal, but cytotoxic functions of the lymphocytes have not been adequately examined due to technical difficulties. After years antigenic recognition recovers and correlates with cessation or a reduction in viral excretion, but not with the presence or absence of disease (420).

## Therapy

### Prophylaxis

#### Active Immunization

Because CMV infection is silent in the adult female population, and because of the need to protect future fetuses, vaccination with live virus, as practiced with rubella, is the main focus of attention currently (423). Two "attenuated" strains of CMV (AD169 and Towne) have been administered to a limited number of human volunteers, both normal persons and renal transplant recipients (424–429). In all seronegative individuals, the vaccines produce a self-limited local reaction with erythema, induration, and pain at the injection site that lasts for a week or more and appears to be associated with local replication of the virus (423). In normal persons the vaccines are immunogenic as regards the development of antibody and lymphocyte blastogenic responses to CMV antigens (Towne, laboratory, and wild strains of CMV) at least for 2-year intervals (423). Antibody responses appear to wane more rapidly than with natural infection. Protection against reinfection when rechallenged with vaccine virus occurs in most but not all cases. Reactivation of the vaccine virus has not been detected to date in limited follow-up studies.

In renal transplant recipients, the Towne vaccine, although equally reactogenic, is less immunogenic with respect to both antibody and cellular immune responses (423). It does not afford protection against reinfection in the high-risk seronegative recipients who receive kidneys from seropositive donors, but again reactivation of vaccine virus has not been detected in the short follow-up studies (430). Preliminary results from the transplant studies suggest that the Towne vaccine may protect from the development of severe disease, although it has no effect on occurrence of milder disease or reinfection (431). In view of the need, these trials are laudable, and their results are encouraging. However because of the many gaps in our knowledge of the virus and the natural history of CMV infections, the concept of live CMV vaccination has become controversial (424,432–435).

Perhaps the most difficult issue to be resolved is the potential oncogenicity of CMV. *In vitro* CMV can stimulate cell metabolism and transform various cell types, including human, which in turn are malignant when transplanted in appropriate animal models. The transforming ability is associated with the genome of the virus, and these oncogenic properties are not necessarily attenuated with the vaccine strains (436,437). In addition the CMV genome has been associated with malignant tumors in humans, but whether CMV is the provocative agent, a cocarcinogen, or simply a natural latent inhabitant is unknown (413,438). Whether large-scale vaccination might enhance the putative oncogenicity of CMV is a major concern and one that is difficult to resolve. It should be emphasized, however, that the great majority of the world's population will eventually be naturally infected by CMV, and there is no indication that attenuated strains are more oncogenic than the many genetic variants of wild viruses.

Certain features of the natural history of CMV infection have presented conceptual difficulties about the value of active immunization as a strategy for reducing the morbidity of intrauterine CMV infections. Primary maternal infection is the major determinant of intrauterine fetal damage, although not of transmission of the virus (386,425). However, on a worldwide basis recurrent maternal infection, probably due mostly to reactivation of latent virus in immune women, is the major cause of intrauterine CMV infection (439). The public health significance of recurrent maternal infection in terms of late-appearing sequelae still requires further investigation (439). Surely factors other than the nature of the maternal infection, such as gestational influences, dictate whether or not an infant born with subclinical congenital CMV infection will develop sensorineural hearing loss or other CNS difficulties long after birth. Nevertheless, the accumulating data suggesting that infant defects following recurrent maternal CMV infection are uncommon (101) and the identification of a high rate of CMV acquisition among seronegative mothers with children in day care centers provide new impetus for developing vaccine programs for control of CMV infection (430,440,441).

To date, the possibility of using killed CMV vaccines or the more sophisticated subunit vaccines has received little serious consideration. But if molecular studies of CMV continue to expand at their present rate, a killed product might assume greater significance as a prophylactic agent in order to overcome some of the difficulties hampering live-vaccine testing (423).

### *Passive Immunization*

The role of antibody in the control of CMV infection is incompletely understood. Although it does not seem to block reactivation or perhaps reinfection, it may ameliorate the virulence of the infection. Maternal antibody reduces or eliminates the illness associated with transfusion-acquired CMV in infants (412,442). It is doubtful, however, that administration of antibody would be useful with clinically apparent congenital infection, since organ damage and extensive viral replication are present at the time of delivery. In any event, passive immunization has not been tried for the control of congenital or perinatal CMV infection.

### *Prophylaxis for Transfusion-Acquired CMV Infection*

Since blood from seropositive donors contains latently infected white blood cells, which can transmit infection in an unpredictable manner, the use of blood from seronegative donors has been advocated for treatment of infants, especially prematures who will require frequent or large volume transfusions (412,443). This approach eliminates transfusion-acquired CMV infection but has not been generally accepted because of practical considerations, such as the need to screen donors for CMV antibody and the reduction in acceptable donors. More recently, frozen deglycerolated red blood cells have been employed with good success rate in limited trials (444,446). Saline-washed red blood cells were not effective in reducing the risk of CMV transmission to seronegative infants (447). Clearly, when white blood cell transfusions are deemed necessary the blood should be obtained from seronegative donors, most particularly when debilitated small premature infants are the recipients.

## *Therapy*

### *Interferon*

Leukocyte interferon or interferon for (mechanism of action, see Chapter 2) stimulators have been administered to infants with symptomatic congenital CMV infections. This approach is based on findings that infected infants have no demonstrable circulating interferon and that they exhibit decreased *in vitro* production of interferon in response to viral challenge (448). Interferon inducers (measles virus and pyran copolymer) were given to four infants, with no apparent success (449,450). High-dose leukocyte interferon ($1.5–10 \times 10^5$ reference units) was given to 9 infants with congenital CMV infection, either as single doses or in repeat courses (7–10 days). The effect on viral excretion was highly variable. In two infants viruria was suppressed for months; in four infants interferon failed to alter virus excretion; and in three infants it produced transitory effects (451,452). Because of the spectrum of the disease and lack of controls, it is difficult to determine if this therapeutic approach has any clinical value. The adverse side effects of highdose leukocyte interferon include poor weight gain, transient elevation of aspartate aminotransferase (AST), and fever (451). Perhaps as the purity and potency of interferon preparations improve, some value in the treatment of certain forms of congenital CMV infection will emerge, but the problems that will be discussed in relation to drug therapy remain and must eventually be answered.

### *Chemotherapy*

Drugs have also been tried for treatment of congenital CMV infection. No effective therapy has been identified, but these clinical trials provide insights into the problems associated with assessment of drug effects on chronic congenital infection.

Treatment of subclinical intrauterine CMV infection is not justifiable at this time because of incomplete definition of its outcome; thus chemotherapeutic trials have been confined to intrauterine infections that have been symptomatic at birth or shortly thereafter (389,453–465). In these trials, treatment was administered after the fact, since the infections had begun at some unknown time *in utero,* and multiple organ system disease of a highly variable nature had already become well established. In addition to transfer factor, the drugs employed were 5-iodo-2′-deoxyuridine (IDU), 5-fluoro-2′-deoxyuridine, cytosine arabinoside (ara-C), vidarabine (adenine arabinoside; ara-A), and 9-(2-hydroxyethoxymethyl) guanine [acyclovir (ACV)]. Each of these compounds given in wide ranging doses in limited uncontrolled trials seemingly caused transitory and highly variable reductions in urinary virus excretion in most cases, with some reduction in pharyngeal shedding and leukoviremia. It appears that ara-C may have eliminated viruria in two instances (457,462). With IDU and ara-C, this apparent unpredictable reduction in viral replication occurred in the face of bone marrow and other forms of toxicity, with dose-related manifestations varying from subclinical to severe. This combination of events is not surprising, since each of the compounds affects both viral DNA metabolism and cellular DNA metabolism to different degrees and by different mechanisms. The use of toxic or potentially toxic compounds was justified on the grounds that symptomatic congenital CMV infection often results in prolonged illness in early life as well as debilitating permanent brain, eye, and auditory damage. The hope was to eliminate virus replication and thereby lessen the organ damage that continues in early postnatal life, thus achieving improved outcome with time. Instead, the antiviral effect was most often transitory, and with severe disease it was inadequate to reverse lethality in some cases (454,455,464). It was impossible to prove any clinical efficacy in these studies because of the enormous spectrum of disease resulting from intrauterine CMV infection and the unpredictable nature of its progression. From the standpoint of a possible clinical antiviral effect, such results remain dubious at best.

Clearly, pathogenesis and outcome with respect to presenting symptoms must be better defined before large-scale control studies can be justified in the attempt to determine if any antiviral agents, such as ganciclovir (DHPG), can be of clinical benefit. Of particular importance with regard to pathogenesis is the need to understand the pathological potential of the persistent virus replication in relation to immunologically mediated damage. Trying to estimate, during the newborn period, future damage from a preexisting fetal infection, especially when the brain and perceptual organs are involved, will pose a major hurdle. This is why, of course, there is currently greater emphasis on the prophylactic approach (423).

## HSV

The first description of herpetic disease dates to ancient Roman times, when an association between mouth sores and fever was recognized and reported (466). It was not until the eighteenth century that genital disease with lesions quite similar to those previously reported for the mouth and lip was elucidated and considered to be caused by the same infectious agent, called herpes (467). In 1921, Lipschutz proposed that herpes of the genitalia and herpes of the mouth were caused by different viral agents (468). Four decades passed before the antigenic differences between HSV type 1 (HSV-1) and HSV type 2 (HSV-2) were delineated (469). Use of virus isolation and typing techniques led to further definition of the disease states associated with HSV-1 and HSV-2 and demonstration that the route of transmission was primarily via respiratory secretions for HSV-1 and by venereal contact for HSV-2. The innumerable genetic variants of wild HSV-1 and 2 allow for reinfection as well as reactivation of latent virus as a cause for recurrent HSV infections in humans (470–472).

Neonatal herpes has attracted particular attention because of its mortality and morbidity which was reported in the middle 1930s nearly simultaneously by Hass (473) and Batignani (474). The finding that most cases of neonatal herpes are caused by HSV-2 provided support for the theory of acquisition occurring at the time of delivery from infected maternal genital secretions.

For discussion of the herpetic agents, see Chapter 11.

### Epidemiology

HSV-1 and HSV-2 can be distinguished on genetic, biologic, antigenic, and epidemiologic grounds (475). Both types are spread by close personal contact. HSV-1 usually infects the oropharynx, is most often acquired in early childhood, and the infection rate is increased among those in lower socioeconomic classes (298,476,477). In lower income groups more than 75% of individuals become infected by adulthood, in contrast to 50% or fewer among the more affluent (475). On the other hand, HSV-2 is usually transmitted venereally, infecting the genitalia, and therefore it most often becomes evident with onset of sexual activity. Recently, HSV-2 infections have been recognized in younger children as a result of child abuse. The frequency of HSV-2 antibody among adults from lower socioeconomic groups ranges between 20% and 60% (298,475,477). Recent seroprevalence studies indicate rates of at least 20% among higher socioeconomic groups as well (478).

Genital infection during pregnancy is quite common (479–481). Prospective cytologic and virologic screening of gravidas in the lower socioeconomic groups has revealed an incidence of 1% when sampling is carried out at any time during pregnancy. Fortunately, however, at or near term the rate is less, ranging from 1 in 250 to 1 in 1,000 (298,482). Rates of genital herpes in higher-income groups have been estimated to be 1 in 1,000 for the whole of gestation. However, routine surveillance cultures taken on the day of delivery demonstrated a rate of asymptomatic excretion of the virus that was approximately 0.2% among women of both lower and higher socioeconomic status (476).

Because of its rarity, large-scale studies to define the incidence of neonatal herpes in different populations has not been undertaken. Consequently, data on the prevalence of this infection are quite variable (380). Nahmias in Atlanta has observed rates varying from 1 per 2,000 to 1 per 7,500 live births (average 1 per 4,000) between 1976 and 1980 (479,483). Certainly neonatal herpes is much less prevalent than genital herpes, probably due to the fact that virus is not often present in the genital area at or around the time of delivery (484). Nevertheless, neonatal herpes appears to be on the increase paralleling the increase in genital herpes.

### Maternal Infection

Although HSV-2 is the resident pathogen in the genital tract by virtue of its venereal transmission, HSV-1 can infect the genital tract. Nevertheless, most recurrent genital herpes is caused by HSV-2. Around 20% of neonatal herpes is now caused by HSV-1, most (but not all) of which is likely transmitted from the genital tract (479,485,486). Both HSV-1 and HSV-2 produce latent infections with well-defined reactivation cycles; thus genital involvement during gestation may represent either primary or recurrent attacks (299,479). Although subclinical disease is more likely with recurrences, unrecognized infection is also common on first exposure to HSV (298,475,481). One explanation is possible amelioration caused by cross-reacting immunologic effects of previous HSV-1 infection (477,487). Using new methods that establish past HSV-2 infection by the detection of antibodies to HSV-2 proteins with type specific epitopes, such as glycoprotein G, it is apparent that the majority of infected adults have had asymptomatic or unrecognized HSV-2 (488,490). Distinguishing between the primary and the recurrent genital herpes during pregnancy is not merely an academic exercise; the primary infection persists for longer intervals and is associated with higher levels of virus production, and therefore it poses greater risk for intrapartum transmission (469,479).

Primary infections may also be associated with fetal loss early in pregnancy and with a syndrome of intrauterine growth retardation in late gestation (491). The symptomalogy of the primary, initial, and recurrent HSV infection is discussed in detail in Chapter 11.

The gravida with symptomatic lesions should be diagnosed by viral culture. Definitive diagnosis by viral isolation in cell culture is relatively rapid (requiring 24–96 hr) and specific. The development of satisfactory transportation media at ambient temperature facilitates the handling of clinical specimens (492). In addition, a rapid and type-specific test for HSV in cell scrapings has been devised employing direct immunofluorescence staining (493). Confirmation of infection by serological means is not a practical or necessary approach for most clinical purposes. Its main value is for differentiation between primary infection and recurrent infection by seroconversion if the individual does not have crossreactive antibodies because of previous HSV-1 infection.

### Pathogenesis and Routes of Transmission

Factors favoring intrapartum transmission include the presence of clinically overt genital lesions associated with primary infection and prolonged rupture of membranes. An increase in the quantity of virus inoculated probably accounts for the greater risk of neonatal disease. Cervical infection is typical of primary disease and much less like with recurrences. It is apparent that some women experience primary infection around the time of delivery that remains asymptomatic but leads to neonatal illness (478,494). In the case of primary infection, an absence of passively transferred maternal antibody or low levels of such antibody may contribute to the establishment and dissemination of infection once exposure occurs (495,496). If membrane rupture occurs, infection may ascend rapidly, a point of some importance when considering cesarean section. Fetal infection increases following rupture of membranes for 6 hr or longer, whereas abdominal delivery within 4 hr has been shown to decrease the risk of transmission (479). After delivery, the onset of illness can occur at any time during the first month of life; however, the average is 6 days, and this further suggests that most transmission occurs near the time of delivery rather than later.

The initial estimated risk of neonatal herpes when genital lesions are present at delivery was 40% (482). However, long-term surveillance data gathered by the same investigators indicate a much lower frequency. In the later studies the incidence of clinically apparent genital infection was 1 per 1,000 deliveries, whereas neonatal disease occurred in only 1 in 7,500 live births over a 9-year interval (479). Recently, the attack rate for neonatal herpes among infants exposed to recurrent maternal infection was calculated as a theoretical maximum of 8% (496). The possibility that inapparent or atypical neonatal infection went undetected could offer a partial explanation for this discrepancy, but subclinical neonatal infection has not been encountered very often. The follow-up of exposed infants by immunologic screening after 1 year failed to identify any cases of subclinical infection (496).

Neonatal transmission rates attending asymptomatic maternal genital infection at term have not yet been ascertained. However, the clinical experience documents that most infants with neonatal herpes are born to mothers who have no history of genital herpes or of contact with a sexual partner who has genital herpes (494,497). The routine surveillance of all deliveries for asymptomatic HSJ excretion indicates that the frequency of reactivation at delivery is the same, i.e., approximately 1%, whether or not the mother has ever had symptomatic disease (478). In fact, only one of 14 women whose delivery cultures were positive had known genital herpes, whereas 12 women had antibodies to HSV-2 glycoprotein G, consistent with silent past infection. These infants, had transplacentally acquired antibodies to HSV just as infants of mothers with known recurrent disease and none developed neonate herpes. In contrast, one of two infants whose mothers had asymptomatic primary HSV-2 had invasive HSV-2 infection in the newborn period (478).

Fetal infection antedating the immediate perinatal period is believed to be rare. Only a few cases have been described in which such presenting signs at birth as microcephaly, intracranial calcifications, and chorioretinitis suggested chronic intrauterine infection (479,498). In one of these cases, serological and clinical evidence of primary maternal HSV-2 infection was obtained, thus suggesting a bloodborne transplacental route of spread to the fetus (499). All of the cases identified in a recent series were caused by HSV-2 (504). It has not yet been determined if transplacental transmission is associated only with primary maternal infection or if local genital recurrences may spread directly to the conceptus with membranes intact. Regardless, powerful inherent protective mechanisms must be operative, considering the extraordinary rarity of transplacental infection (479). These mechanisms might include a low incidence of primary HSV infection during pregnancy, the probable absence of overt viremia attending recurrences, a barrier effect of the fetal membranes and placenta, and the relatively high rate of previous HSV-1 infection, which provides some maternal and fetal cross-immunologic protection.

Postnatal transmission from other infected infants or nursery personnel may occur; currently this means a spread is believed to be rare (485,486,500–503). Recently, HSV-2 infection was documented in a 42-day-old infant indirectly exposed in the nursery, by means of shared nursing personnel, to two other newborns with HSV-2 infection. Furthermore, the increasing incidence of HSV-1 being recognized in infected newborns (20% of total cases definitively studied), as compared with HSV-1 genital infections in mothers (9%), suggests the possibility of postnatal acquisition (479). Transmission from a father to an infant has been documented by restriction endonuclease analysis of the viral isolation (503). However, in view of the common occurrence of recurrent oral herpes in nursery personnel (estimated at 1% per week) and in the general population, the apparent low rate of postnatal acquisition is somewhat surprising (506). Protection occurring from passively acquired maternal antibody (HSV-1 or HSV-2 or both) and awareness of the infectious nature of their lesions among nursery personnel may offer a partial explanation for this apparent paradox (479).

## Perinatal Infection

### *Pathology, Pathogenesis, and Immunology*

Since HSV shuts down cellular metabolism, it results in cell death and tissue necrosis. The cell pathology of neonatal herpes is characterized by clumping of nuclear chromatin and formation of intranuclear eosinophilic inclusion bodies (507). Because of cell fusion, multinucleated giant cells are characteristic. An inflammatory response characterized by lymphocytes, plasma cells, and histiocytes is usually but not invariably present in visceral lesions and surrounding smaller blood vessels. Areas of hemorrhagic infarction are common; thus vasculitis may be an additional and important mechanism of tissue injury.

The infected cells produce large numbers of infectious and defective particles, which can spread to distant cells in the extracellular milieu. HSV can also spread rapidly to contiguous uninfected cells by virtue of its capacity to cause cell fusion, and by this route the virus can avoid extracellular immune attack.

Following direct exposure the neonatal

host may limit the infection to the portal of entry (i.e., skin, mouth, or eye) by mechanisms unknown or may suffer a disseminated process if initial defenses are inadequate for whatever reasons (479,487). In the latter case, hematogenous spread occurs. Whether blood-borne virus has an intracellular or extracellular residence is unknown, but is of considerable interest in view of the inability of passively transferred maternal antibody to block this occurrence uniformly (508). In addition to viremia, it is conceivable that virus may spread by a neurogenic route from the peripheral to the central nervous system (487). Such a phenomenon could explain the occurrence of localized central nervous system involvement in the absence of other apparent organ system disease, much like the occurrence of herpes encephalitis in older individuals.

Following the initial infection, infants may have recrudescent skin or corneal lesions caused by reactivation of virus that is latent in the sensory ganglion (475,509). However, the appearance of skin lesions in new sites suggests an alternative mechanism, such as chronically infected lymphocytes that periodically seed the integument (479).

Clearly, neonatal herpes is much more fulminant than most other forms of viral perinatal infections (479). It has been estimated that severe disease occurs 250 times for every subclinical infection, in contrast, for instance, to congenital CMV infection where severe disease occurs in no more than 10% of cases. The virulence factors for neonatal HSV are unknown. Certainly, HSV is more acutely cytolytic than the other herpesviruses of humans, but this characteristic cannot explain the striking differences between the severity of the infection in neonates and that occurring in other age groups.

The neonatal infection more closely resembles the infection as expressed in severely immunocompromised debilitated individuals. This resemblance has lead to the belief that some aspects of the neonate's immune mechanism are lacking (479). Whatever the deficiencies are, they must be specific for HSV, since the human fetus and newborn have far better control over most other intrauterine and perinatal infections. A number of possible deficiencies have been suggested. The humoral immune response with neonatal herpes appears to be intact and generally resembles the response described for perinatal CMV infection. Infected newborns are able to produce specific IgM antibodies within 1–3 weeks after the onset of infection; the IgM response increases for 2–3 months, and lower levels may be detectable for upwards of a year (510). However, IgM herpes antibodies appear to be less effective at neutralization than the IgA and IgG classes, which appear somewhat later after initiation of infection.

Several defects in nonspecific or specific cellular immune mechanisms have been found in the human and other newborn animals that might contribute to the virulence of neonatal herpes, especially when taken in combination (511,520). Antibody-dependent cellular cytotoxicity (ADCC) is operative in aborting HSV infections *in vitro*. Both K cells and leukocytes mediate ADCC *in vitro*. K cells in the newborn appear to be reduced in number, and the functional capacity of leukocytes to mediate ADCC is diminished. The macrophages of newborn mice appear to be less able to limit dissemination of HSV than adult macrophages, and they are more easily infected by HSV. Natural killer cells, which appear to play a role in controlling HSV infection, are reduced in the newborn and less responsive to interferon induction than the adult counterparts. Finally, the capacity of the infected newborn to develop T lymphocytes that recognize HSV antigens is poor. Failure to acquire helper T lymphocytes specific for HSV is likely to interfere with the host response in several ways, including the production of lymphokines such as interleukin 2 (521) and interferon-$\gamma$, and the clonal expansion of cytotoxic T lymphocytes.

### *Clinical Findings and Outcome*

For prognostic, therapeutic, and pathogenetic considerations, sick infants may be divided into two groups, those with disseminated disease and those with localized disease, based on the extent of involvement (479,497,508). In the disseminated form the illness usually commences within the first week of life with some combination of the following findings: constitutional signs and symptoms, irritability or seizures, respiratory distress, jaundice, petechiae or ecchymoses, a shock-like syndrome, and vesicular exanthem. Infants with disseminated infection are more likely to be premature than would be expected for the general population of newborns. The vesicular rash, which is of major importance because of its diagnostic specificity, unfortunately occurs as the presenting sign in only a small number of infants with disseminated infection; however, vesicles subsequently appear in almost 50% of infants who do not receive antiviral therapy. In the absence of this dermatologic manifestation, a clinical diagnosis becomes exceedingly difficult because of the similarity between the clinical findings of neonatal herpes and those of other severe infectious and noninfectious diseases of the newborn.

CNS involvement occurs in more than 50% of infants with disseminated disease; it commonly manifests with seizures or irritability or both, occasionally associated with bulging fontanelle, opisthotonos, and pyramidal tract signs. CSF abnormalities typically consist of moderate pleocytosis (50–200 WBCs/mm$^3$) and disproportionate elevations in protein levels (500–1,000 mg/dl). Virus is relatively commonly isolated from the CSF with disseminated infection. Brain damage is the apparent cause of death in two-thirds of such patients.

In disseminated infections with or without evident CNS involvement malfunctions of the hematopoietic, reticuloendothelial, and pulmonary systems are the prominent features of neonatal herpes. Of particular concern are pneumonia (522,523) and bleeding diatheses. In the absence of rapidly progressive CNS disease, pulmonary disease accounts for half of all deaths, whereas a shocklike syndrome often associated with severe metabolic acidosis and disseminated intravascular coagulopathy is the lethal insult in the remainder. Extensive hepatitis is common, adding to the coagulation disorder and infection of the adrenal cortex may potentiate shock. The mortality of disseminated infection with or without CNS disease is approximately 75% or greater. Death usually supervenes during the first 2 weeks following onset of symptoms (average 1 week) but may occur in a few days or up to 1 month in a few cases (508).

Between 30 and 60% of infected newborns will manifest disease in the CNS, eye, skin, or oral cavity without evidence of visceral involvement (479). Localized CNS disease usually presents after the first week of life, typically with a brief fever that may be low grade, lethargy, and poor feeding, in a previously healthy term infant. The illness progresses within 24–48 hr to the onset of seizures and other neurologic signs. Some of these infants have herpetic skin vesicles at the onset of their CNS symptoms or have had such lesions during the first week or two of life, but many infants with neonatal HSV encephalitis have no mucocutaneous infection (524,525). The virus is rarely isolated from the CSF, in spite of CSF abnormalities including pleocytosis. (WBCs 20–200 or higher), elevated protein, and excess RBCs in the absence of a traumatic tap. EEG abnormalities are also common (526). The CT scan may not be abnormal for several days after symptoms appear (527). Without antiviral therapy, a fatal outcome can be expected in approximately 50% of newborns with localized CNS infection, and residual brain damage can be expected in a high proportion of survivors. With localized CNS disease, death occurs later than with disseminated infection, usually between 1 and 2 months.

Ocular involvement, which is uncommon

as a primary manifestation of neonatal herpes, may be present as conjunctivitis, keratoconjunctivitis, chorioretinitis, and rarely uveitis (479). Blindness can result, and recurrences are common. The ocular involvement is seen more commonly with the localized CNS form than with the disseminated form of disease.

Infection clinically limited to the skin was observed in approximately 10% of cases of neonatal herpes described before the use of antiviral agents. At least 75% of infants who presented with mucocutaneous lesions only developed progressive infection (479,497,508). The typical skin lesions are discrete vesicles on erythematous bases varying from 1 mm to 1 cm in diameter; clusters of lesions are common. The presenting parts at delivery (i.e., scalp and buttocks, as well as the extremities) are most frequently involved, although eruptions may occur anywhere. Vesicles rapidly ulcerate, thereby lessening their diagnostic specificity.

The prognosis for survivors with encephalitis, following either disseminated or localized CNS disease, is bleak (479,497,508). Psychomotor retardation, often severe, develops in 50 to 75% of such patients, occasionally in association with microcephaly, hydraencephaly, or porencephalic cysts. Brain damage may also supervene in those without clinically manifest CNS disease, although less often. Ocular infection may result in visual handicap as a result of corneal scarring, chorioretinitis, cataracts, or optic atrophy (one case reported). Localized skin, disease which does not seem to progress is usually benign. A unique feature of skin, oral, and corneal infection is a tendency for frequent recurrences. Reappearances of skin lesions at the same sites, and less frequently at new sites, have been observed for as long as 5 years after onset of the illness. A few infants have an insidious form of neonatal herpes in which the CNS involvement is acutely subclinical, including absence of CSF abnormalities, but that may result in severe brain damage or eye involvement at a later date (479,508).

### *Diagnosis*

Diagnosis of neonatal herpes is difficult unless skin, oral, or corneal lesions are present. Even with these lesions, the diagnosis of neonatal herpes is often not entertained because of a low index of suspicion (528) and delays created by the observation of gram-positive bacteria, which may be present with gram stain of an herpetic lesion. This infection can resemble almost any serious disease of the newborn according to presentation and progression. Because therapy is now available, every effort should be made to prove the diagnosis by rapid diagnostic methods such as direct IF of cells scraped from a suspicious lesion and by the definitive procedure of viral culture. The laboratory evaluation should be pursued regardless of a failure to elicit a history of genital herpes in the mother or her sexual partners. Examination of the mother and viral cultures of the maternal genital tract are useful for the diagnosis of primary maternal HSV since lesions may have appeared subsequent to the delivery and viral cultures are usually positive for more than 1 or 2 weeks in this circumstance.

In the past, cytological examination of cells obtained from skin or mucous membrane lesions was advocated for the diagnosis of HSV infection. This method is not reliable enough as a diagnostic procedure for the life-threatening disease caused by HSV in the newborn period. Direct IF with HSV-specific antiserum, along with viral culture to confirm the results of the IF stain, is the optimal approach.

Virus isolation is the definitive diagnostic method. Obviously, visible lesions, especially skin lesions, are the preferred sites for isolation attempts (479,497,508). However, additional material from throat, stool, conjunctivae, urine, and CSF should be sampled to assess the extent of infection. These sites, especially the oropharynx, should be cultured in suspect infants without external lesions. HSV grows readily in many cell culture systems, and therefore most virology laboratories can provide this diagnostic service. The type (HSV-1 or HSV-2) of the infecting strain can be determined from the cell culture and is important for epidemiologic and pathogenetic considerations (469). Biopsy specimens can be tested IF and immunoperoxidase techniques, which is necessary to diagnose HSV encephalitis in the absence of mucocutaneous lesions. Herpes viral particles can be demonstrated by EM, preferably by the pseudoreplica method (479,529).

Diagnosis of neonatal herpes by classical serologic means is complicated in many cases by the presence of maternally transferred IgG antibody that masks the infant's own antibody response (479,530). In the absence of postnatally acquired HSV infection the persistence of HSV antibody throughout the first year of life is good presumptive evidence of neonatal herpes. Only in those instances in which the mother, in the absence of prior HSV-1 infection, acquires primary genital infection late in gestation, before significant transfer of antibody to the fetus occurs, can an early diagnostic rise in antibody be demonstrated. Even in this instance the delay in the infant's response will make this laboratory aid less rapid and thus less useful than those previously discussed. Type-specific antibody responses can be determined in specialized research laboratories, but even these methods are not useful for the diagnosis of neonatal HSV in the newborn because of the delay of several weeks that is required to document the response. Some infants fail to develop antibodies to HSV-2 glycoprotein G-2 despite extensive HSV-2 encephalitis (490). Persistence of HSV-2 antibody into the latter half of the first year can confirm the diagnosis of neonatal herpes, since the risk of infection with HSV-2 during that time period is essentially nil. In fact, demonstration of HSV-2 antibody at any time before the onset of sexual activity constitutes good presumptive evidence of perinatal acquisition. However this finding is not definitive evidence of neonatal infection, since HSV-2 infection has been documented in children as a result of contact with infected adults (531). Multiple serologic tests are available: CF, passive hemagglutination, neutralization, IF, RIA, and ELISA assays (530,532,533). Analysis of the infant's IgM-specific antibody response is another serological means of establishing the diagnosis (510,530), but testing by research laboratories with expertise using this technique is required; the IgM response is not detected soon enough to allow early antiviral therapy. Clearly virus isolation is the preferred means of proving neonatal herpes.

### *Chemotherapy*

The chances for successful antiviral therapy should be greater in neonatal HSV infection than in CMV and rubella infections simply because the disease is generally acquired intrapartum, and therefore treatment can theoretically be instituted early in the course of the disease, providing the infection is diagnosed quickly.

Four purine and pyrimidine nucleosides have been employed for the treatment of neonatal herpes. These include IDU, ara-C, adenine arabinoside (vidarabine) and ACV. The former two drugs were tried in uncontrolled and therefore uninterpretable trials as regards their efficacy (534–540). Both IDU and ara-C, are toxic by virtue of their adverse effect on cellular DNA metabolism, and consequently neither is currently considered useful therapeutic modalities for the treatment of neonatal herpes. In contrast, the earlier encouraging results regarding the potential usefulness of vidarabine, and more recently of ACV, have been confirmed in large scale multiinstitution control trials sponsored by the National Institute of Allergy and Infectious Disease (NIAID) (508,541). With vidarabine treatment overall mortality of neonatal herpes can be reduced from 75% to 40% over a 2-year period (508). Outcome was clearly related to the form of the infection under therapy. Vidarabine treatment is most effective in babies with insidious brain and/or eye involvement who appear during early life to have only localized skin infection. Because of this effect and the fact that infants who present with apparent localized disease can rapidly progress to a more malignant form of infection, vidarabine (or ACV) should be used in all infants from whom virus has been recovered, regardless of site or symptomatology. With localized CNS disease with or without superficial involvement, both mortality and morbidity were significantly improved by vidarabine in comparison with outcome with disseminated herpes (508,542). Although mortality is improved with treatment of disseminated herpes, the overall outcome is still dismal. It is noteworthy that disease can progress from milder to more severe forms during the course of therapy. For prognostic reasons then, it is important to appropriately monitor the patient frequently for evidence of brain and visceral (hepatitis, pneumonia, and bleeding) disorders. To properly monitor for progress, laboratory (including CSF examinations) and other diagnostic aids are required to identify subclinical involvement of organ systems. Early therapy and good supportive care are essential, since death usually occurs during the first and second week after onset of disease, mostly from pneumonia and/or hemorrhage and brain damage. Because of all of these problems, the suspect neonate should be referred to centers with experience in diagnosing and managing these seriously ill newborns.

Vidarabine is given intravenously in doses from 15–30 mg/kg·day over a 12-hr period for 14 days or even longer without significant toxicity (508,542). It is, however, a relatively insoluble drug, and concentrations should not exceed 0.5 mg/ml in the intravenous fluid. There are apparent cases of recurrent or recrudescent infection, especially in the CNS, following 14 days of drug administration. In such circumstances, repeat therapy is advisable, although every effort should be made to prove that the recurrence is due to HSV rather than some other complication, such as bacterial infection or simply the result of severe brain damage.

ACV, the latest antiherpetic compound to reach clinical trials in humans, is more HSV-specific by virtue of interactions with HSV thymidine kinase and DNA polymerase with minimal reactions with the cellular counterparts (544). Its therapeutic index for treatment of HSV infections is therefore better. During pharmacokinetic and uncontrolled clinical trials, ACV was administered to infants with neonatal herpes at various stages of the infection and at varying doses (465,545–551).

The Collaborative NIAID Antiviral Study Group has compared the efficacy of vidarabine and ACV in a large-scale controlled trial.

In the course of this study, 92 infants received vidarabine and 104 infants were given ACV (552). The demographic characteristics with respect to sex, race, gestational age, age at enrollment, duration of disease prior to entry, virus type, and maternal characteristics were comparable between the two treatment groups. When the populations were analyzed according to disease category, the only difference noted was a mortality rate of 65% among infants with disseminated infection who received ACV compared to a 42% mortality rate for those given vidarabine ($p = 0.03$); nevertheless, the long-term outcome for patients in this disease category was not related to the specific antiviral drug. The overall mortality for disseminated neonatal herpes remains very high despite antiviral therapy. In contrast to older children and adults who have HSV-1 encephalitis (Chapter 8), the response to therapy with vidarabine was equivalent to that observed among infants receiving ACV for HSV encephalitis in the newborn period, with mortality rates of 18% and 15%, respectively. Other factors that correlated with adverse outcome in infants with disseminated and CNS infections included a diminished level of consciousness, the development of HSV pneumonitis, prolonged seizures and the absence of CSF pleocytosis in the presence of brain infection. CNS infection caused by HSV-2 also has a worse prognosis than CNS disease caused by HSV-1 (553). The optimal response to antiviral therapy was observed among infants treated for localized skin, eye, or mouth infection in the newborn period, with no cases of obvious progression occurring while the infants were receiving vidarabine or ACV at 30 mg/kg/day, no fatalities and normal assessments at 12 months in 93% of vidarabine recipients and 96% of ACV treated infants. However, an important clinical observation was that the small percentage of infants with neurologic sequelae were those who had frequent recurrences of mucocutaneous lesions during the first 6 months of life. Only 68% of children who had three or more recurrences during this period were normal at 1-year follow-up. The risk of late sequelae in this disease category was also linked to virus type; all infants with HSV-1 infection had a normal neurologic examination at 1 year compared to only 76% of those with HSV-2 infection. These cases appear to result from a gradual progression of CNS disease, whereas some infants have also been described who presented with severe acute HSV encephalitis several weeks after completing a course of vidarabine or ACV for localized mucocutaneous disease in the newborn period (554,555).

Based upon the findings of Collaborative Antiviral Study Group comparative trial, new protocols are being designed to evaluate the efficacy of higher doses of ACV compared to vidarabine and of prolonging the course of treatment to 21 days for infants with disseminated or CNS disease. The efficacy of suppressive therapy with oral ACV suspension to prevent mucocutaneous recurrences will also be investigated as a means of reducing the risk of late sequelae among infants with localized skin, eye or mouth disease in the newborn period.

Attention must be directed to the treatment of ocular involvement should it be present or supervene during the course of the neonatal infection. Preparations containing antiviral compounds are available for local application. Those include 5-iodo-2′-deoxyuridine, ACV, adenine arabinoside, and trifluorothymidine (TFT). The reader is referred to the section on the treatment of ocular HSV infection for more details concerning their use (Chapter 6). Whether they should be used prophylactically in the case where contiguous spread from skin to eye seems imminent is an interesting question but one that has not been adequately addressed. Topical therapy may be used as an adjunct to intravenous antiviral therapy of neonatal herpes, but it must not be considered to be a substitute for the systemic treatment of these infections.

When using the currently available antiherpetic drugs evidence of toxicity should be sought, including bone marrow suppression, hepatic and renal dysfunctions, and CNS disturbances. This is especially important in the presence of dehydration, and primary renal or hepatic dysfunction. In these situations, doses of the drugs should be altered accordingly. Although very little toxicity has been encountered to date in treating neonatal herpes with vidarabine or ACV, the possibility, among others, of CNS disturbances with vidarabine or renal dysfunctions with ACV is real (544,556–558). In addition, allergic reactions may occur, especially with the ophthalmic preparations. Strains of HSV resistant to the drug being employed may emerge during or after therapy, but the clinical significance of this phenomenon is unknown, and HSV strains isolated from recurrent lesions in infants with neonatal infection have remained sensitive to ACV *in vitro*.

Other therapeutic approaches, including hyperimmune globulin, Bacille Calmette Guerin (BCG), hyperthermia, interferon, and interferon inducers, have been entertained, but there are as yet no data regarding their potential usefulness (479).

### Prevention

Active prevention of this infection by immunization of susceptible women is desirable and currently under consideration using virus manipulated in the laboratory to reduce virulence and latency without loss of immunogenicity. Approaches to active immunization must be pursued, but the failure of past HSV-1 infection to prevent HSV-2 infection despite extensive antigenic homologies suggests that this objective will be difficult to achieve (559). Immunization, even if successful, will not solve the problem of potential infection of the infants of the substantial portion of women of childbearing age who have already had symptomatic or asymptomatic genital HSV infection.

It is clear that therapeutic abortion in early pregnancy as a preventive measure for transplacental infection in cases of primary or recurrent maternal genital or nongenital herpes is contraindicated because of the extreme rarity of congenital herpes.

The only preventive approach for neonatal herpes is cesarean section to avoid ascending and natal infection from the maternal genital tract. However, this approach is fraught with confusion and controversy because of the lack of knowledge concerning the natural history of HSV genital infection in relation to transmission to the newborn and fails to prevent transmission in some infants despite delivery with apparently intact membranes. Since most infants with neonatal herpes are born to women with no prior knowledge of genital infection, cesarean section cannot prevent the majority of transmissions to the newborn. Past definitions of women considered to be at higher risk for transmitting HSV to the neonate, including women with clinically evident genital herpes at any time during pregnancy, women with a prior history confirmed or highly suggestive of genital herpes, and women who have had sexual relations with a male who has genital herpes, either before or during pregnancy have proved inadequate for identifying more than 80% of women with active HSV infection at delivery (478). Serial virologic monitoring beginning at 34 weeks of gestation or even sooner (479), which was advocated for groups considered to be at high risk, failed to predict the infant's risk of exposure to HSV at delivery (554). The likelihood of asymptomatic excretion at delivery could not be related to the clinical pattern of disease since the frequency was the equivalent between women who had no clinical recurrences and those who had one or more episodes during the gestation. The conclusion from this prospective study is that cesarean delivery is not warranted routinely even if the mother has known genital herpes and has had recurrences during pregnancy, assuming that she is asymptomatic at the onset of labor. The low frequency of silent infection on the day of delivery (1–2%) taken in conjunction with the low attack rate for exposed infants of mothers with past infection (approximately 5%) produces a risk that is comparable to the complication rate associated with cesarean delivery.

Another approach to prevention that could be considered is the administration of suppressive antiviral therapy to the pregnant woman during late gestation (525). Oral ACV may be valuable for this purpose, but careful studies are required to demonstrate its safety and efficacy. Preliminary evidence suggests that the dosage may need to be increased during pregnancy to achieve plasma concentrations of the drug comparable to those in nonpregnant adults given 200 mg three times daily as prophylaxis. The identification of a high-risk population for the initial evaluation of this preventive measure is suggested by the morbidity described among infants of mothers with primary genital HSV late in pregnancy (491). Meanwhile, the administration of intravenous ACV is clearly indicated for the few instances when maternal HSV infection becomes disseminated during pregnancy because of the risk to the mother and because the threat to the viability of the fetus from maternal morbidity outweighs the risk of adverse effects from the drug (560–562).

Routine surveillance cultures taken at delivery could be used to identify infants who were exposed to HSV. Although this strategy does not prevent the exposure of the infant, it allows the immediate initiation of antiviral therapy if symptoms appear. However, the cost of this approach, applied universally, does not appear to be justified (478). Delivery cultures done among women with a past history of genital herpes or serologic evidence of HSV-2 infection might be warranted, but infants exposed to primary maternal HSV in late pregnancy who are at the highest risk for acquiring neonatal herpes would not be identified by this procedure. Even if the exposure of an infant is detected, the use of antiviral agents as prophylaxis cannot be undertaken without specific evidence of its value. Given the usual circumstance of exposure to recurrent maternal infection and the low attack rate in these infants, it would be necessary to treat approximately 100 infants to provide possible benefit to five infants. Because of the poor absorption of oral ACV (563) and the lack of a suspension formulation, the drug would have to be given intravenously. The optimal duration of administration is unknown, but the use of a chemotherapeutic agent as prophylaxis would probably require giving the drug through the expected period of risk which, in the case of neonatal herpes, extends for at least 3 weeks after birth. Most importantly, it is far from predictable that antiviral drug prophylaxis will demonstrate any efficacy for neonatal exposure to HSV. Fatal infections have been observed despite the initiation of intravenous vidarabine or ACV beginning less than 48 hr after birth, at the time that maternal infection was documented (491,564). Because of the low attack rate, a large-scale clinical investigation will be needed to address this issue. Theoretically, infants exposed to HSV at delivery who lack HSV antibodies might benefit from passive antibody prophylaxis. However, most of these infants are born to mothers with primary infections at delivery, which are difficult to identify in a timely manner, and no high titer preparation of HSV $\gamma$-globulin is available.

In summary, without a rapid and sensitive laboratory method to detect silent maternal HSV infection at the onset of labor, most exposures of infants to HSV cannot be prevented. Unfortunately, the enzyme immunoassays for detecting HSV antigens and the IF method for identifying infected cells have no value for demonstrating asymptomatic infection. Therefore, reducing the morbidity and mortality of neonatal herpes requires early antiviral therapy, which means that pediatricians must maintain a high index of suspicion for HSV infections in the newborn and pursue the laboratory diagnosis immediately in suspected cases.

## VZV

### Epidemiology

VZV is an unusual cause of perinatal infection in the United States and Europe because more than 90% of women of childbearing age who live in temperate climates have had varicella in childhood. In one study of 30,000 pregnancies, the incidence of varicella was 0.7 per 1,000 (567). However, certain population groups, especially women who were born in tropical areas, are likely to be susceptible to varicella into the adult years. For example, 16% of Puerto

Rican women of childbearing age in New York had no antibodies to VZV (568).

### Maternal Infection

#### *Clinical Manifestations of Maternal VZV Infection*

Although most women with varicella during pregnancy have an uncomplicated clinical course, varicella pneumonia and other manifestations of visceral dissemination have been described with primary VZV infection during pregnancy (569–571). Whether morbidity is more common in pregnant women than among other adults with varicella cannot be established from the literature. Some retrospective series have reported maternal mortality rates as high as 41% (572), but in a prospective study of 150 cases one pregnant woman had fatal infection (0.7%) (573). In our experience, varicella pneumonia occurred in 9.3% of women with varicella during pregnancy, and the frequency of fatal infection was 2.4% (574). Maternal varicella during the second or third trimester was associated with premature labor in 9.3% of patients and premature delivery in 4.7% of cases. If the maternal infection is severe, especially when complicated by varicella pneumonia, fetal death or fetal loss from premature delivery can occur even if the mother escapes fatal infection. Spontaneous abortion was noted in 4 of 35 pregnancies (575) in which the mother had varicella in the first trimester and in 5 of 32 pregnancies in another series (576). Progressive varicella in pregnancy, associated with varicella pneumonia, which in our experience has occurred most often in later gestation infections, should be treated with intravenous ACV in order to reduce the risk of severe or fatal maternal varicella.

Herpes zoster, caused by the reactivation of latent VZV, occurs during pregnancy but has not been associated with significant maternal morbidity or mortality or with adverse effects upon the pregnancy. Most cases of herpes zoster occur in late gestation. Although some cutaneous lesions may appear outside of the primary dermatome, antiviral therapy for the mother is rarely needed for recurrent VZV infection in pregnancy.

#### *Mechanism of Transmission to the Fetus*

Both a primary and a secondary viremic phase is necessary to account for the clinical manifestations of varicella (575) and viremia has been demonstrated in otherwise healthy subjects with primary VZV infection. Therefore, the virus can be presumed to cross the placenta as a consequence of maternal viremia. The viremia of VZV in healthy individuals is associated with mononuclear cells, which indicates that the transplacental transfer of peripheral blood mononuclear cells from the mother to the fetus is required for viral transmission. The low frequency with which VZV infects peripheral blood mononuclear cells and the relative resistance of these cells to viral replication probably protects the fetus from infection in most circumstances (578). The fact that infectious virus is not recovered from peripheral blood mononuclear cells of healthy individuals with herpes zoster explains the observation that fetal complications from recurrent maternal VZV infections are difficult to document (574,575).

#### *Prevention*

Whether the fetus can be protected from VZV infection by the administration of varicella-zoster immune globulin (VZIG) to the susceptible pregnant woman who has been exposed to VZV is unknown. If symptomatic maternal infection is prevented, as it was in seven reported cases, it is reasonable to assume that the risk of maternal viremia is also reduced or eliminated (575). Although the recommendation is controversial, our experience suggests that VZIG prophylaxis should be considered if the mother is proved to be susceptible by a sensitive serologic test for VZV antibodies, such as IF or ELISA, in order to modify the severity of the maternal infection. The CF method is not reliable for establishing VZV immunity. In practice, it is unusual to identify a close exposure and establish the susceptibility of the mother soon enough to provide effective prophylaxis, since VZIG must be given within 72–96 hr after the exposure.

The prevention of varicella during pregnancy is likely to be one of the primary benefits from the administration of the live attenuated varicella vaccine to susceptible adults (579). The serologic evaluation of women of childbearing age for VZV susceptibility and active immunization before pregnancy should reduce the maternal and fetal complications of varicella.

### Intrauterine Infection

#### *Risk of Fetal Infection*

The accumulated clinical experience indicates that VZV transmission to the fetus does occur in some cases of primary VZV infection during pregnancy (569,574,580–584). The congenital varicella syndrome is a unique constellation of findings now associated with maternal varicella during pregnancy on epidemiologic grounds and, in a few cases, by serologic methods (585,586). Based upon the limited data available, anomalies that are attributable to intrauterine infection with VZV are present at birth in fewer than 5% of infants born to mothers who have had varicella during pregnancy (574–576). Most cases have followed maternal infection in the first trimester, but one case of an infant with mild limb damage occurred after maternal varicella at 28 weeks of gestation (587).

Asymptomatic intrauterine VZV infection can follow maternal varicella during pregnancy. Some infants who have had exposure to maternal varicella have immunologic evidence of intrauterine infection based on the persistence of VZV antibodies and the detection of cellular immunity to VZV in the absence of any signs of the congenital varicella syndrome (574). By immunologic criteria, 12.5% of asymptomatic infants had subclinical intrauterine VZV infection. In other cases, the transmission of the virus to the infant *in utero* is established by the development of herpes zoster during infancy without a preceding episode of varicella (574,588). Using immunologic measures and the later occurrence of herpes zoster as markers of intrauterine infection, VZV appears to reach the fetus during maternal infection in the second and third trimesters with approximately the same frequency as in the first trimester, but the consequences of transmission later in gestation are minimal (574).

Herpes zoster, due to the reactivation of latent VZV during pregnancy, has not been associated with the classic features of the congenital varicella syndrome. Other etiologies have not been excluded conclusively in the few reported instances of fetal pathology attributed to recurrent maternal VZV infection.

#### *Clinical and Pathologic Manifestations in the Newborn*

The clinical features of varicella embryopathy include cutaneous ulceration or cicatricial scarring in a focal or dermatomal distribution, limb hypoplasia and rudimentary digits, and paralysis with limb atrophy; other common findings include cataracts, microophthalmia and other eye pathology, microcephaly secondary to cortical atrophy, chorioretinitis, hydronephrosis and hydroureter, and esophageal dysfunction with gastroesophageal reflux (569,570,580,584). The unusual cutaneous defects, limb atrophy, and evidence of autonomic dysfunction distinguish the congenital varicella syndrome from other viral embryopathies. The findings in cases following maternal infection during the second trimester have been limited more exclusively to ocular defects (577). Death in infancy is common due to the damage to the CNS and the autonomic disorders, especially severe gastroesophageal reflux, which causes recurrent aspiration pneumonia.

Many of the characteristic findings of the congenital varicella syndrome are consistent with a pathologic process in which the neurotropic potential of the virus is expressed. For example, microcephaly is a predictable consequence of intrauterine encephalitis with necrosis and denervation caused by destruction of neuronal cells in the spinal ganglia could produce hypoplasia of the developing limb. Autopsy of severely affected infants has demonstrated necrotizing encephalomyelitis and, in one case, extensive scarring within the dorsal ganglia (586). Other findings, such as pancreatic and adrenal scarring and calcifications of the lungs, liver, and spleen probably represent the residuae of disseminated visceral infection *in utero* (584).

The diagnosis of the congenital varicella syndrome is made by the observation of the characteristic anomalies in the context of maternal varicella during pregnancy, which, in contrast to rubella or primary CMV infection, is easily established from the clinical history. Although VZV IgM titers have been recommended for diagnosing intrauterine VZV infection (589), it is obvious that affected infants do not produce VZV IgM antibodies reliably (572), as is typical for most intrauterine viral infections. In addition, VZV IgM antibody assays are technically difficult to perform with accuracy. Virologic diagnosis is hampered by the fact that infectious virus cannot be recovered by the time the infant is born. Viral cultures of fetal tissue after therapeutic abortion of pregnancies complicated by maternal varicella have not yielded VZV, but the low incidence of fetal infection may account for this observation.

Prenatal diagnosis is difficult because of the unpredictable nature of the fetal immune response, although infection of the fetus was established in one instance by the detection of VZV IgM antibodies in serum obtained by cordocentesis (582). There is no evidence that amniotic fluid cultures would yield infectious virus even if the fetus were infected. Parents should be counseled about the low risk of fetal damage even with maternal varicella during the first trimester and advised that this risk is comparable to the risk of fetal malformation with any pregnancy. Serial evaluation by ultrasound later in pregnancy may provide some reassurance that microcephaly and limb defects have not occurred (584).

## Perinatal Infection

### *Transmission to the Newborn*

Infants born to mothers who acquire varicella late in gestation may develop clinical signs of varicella (569,581,583,590). In most instances, transmission of the virus is attributable to the secondary phase of viremia in the mother (577). If the maternal infection occurs in the last few weeks of pregnancy, the infant may be asymptomatic or may have cutaneous varicella lesions at or shortly after birth. These infants who have acquired VZV transplacentally rarely develop complications from the infection. In contrast, infants who are born within 4 days after or 48 hr before the onset of maternal varicella are at risk for fatal varicella. The attack rate for perinatal infection under these circumstances was approximately 20%, and the incidence of fatal infection was 30% among cases (590). These infants are delivered prior to the transmission of maternal VZV antibodies across the placenta; they become infected with VZV either transplacentally, as a consequence of maternal viremia, or by exposure to maternal cutaneous lesions at delivery or in the perinatal period.

Infants who are exposed to varicella by nonmaternal contacts rarely develop severe varicella. Although other children in the household may have varicella, the infant is usually protected by transplacentally acquired VZV antibodies (568). The infant whose mother has never had varicella may be the exception, but this circumstance, like maternal varicella during pregnancy, is rare because of the high prevalence of VZV immunity among adult women. Neonatal varicella is not always prevented by transplacental antibodies judging from two infants who developed mild symptoms after household exposure despite maternal immunity to VZV (591). High-risk, hospitalized infants have occasionally developed varicella after nosocomial exposure to a caretaker with varicella. Symptomatic varicella occurred in two infants despite the persistence of passive antibodies to VZV (592).

Infants whose mothers develop herpes zoster late in pregnancy or immediately postpartum are not at risk for serious illness. The primary concern in these cases arises when the zosteriform eruption is in the lumbosacral dermatomes since the rash is caused by HSV in as many as 15% of patients with apparent herpes zoster in this distribution (593).

### *Clinical and Pathologic Manifestations in the Infant*

Infants at risk for serious varicella are well until after the first 5–10 days at age (583,590,593). The infection begins with the typical cutaneous exanthem. The diagnosis is usually obvious because of the characteristic vesicular lesions and the recognition of recent maternal varicella. The clinical diagnosis can be confirmed by viral culture of the lesions or by direct immunofluorescence stain of cells from the base of the cutaneous lesion using VZV specific antibody. Progressive cutaneous infection is associated with lifethreatening illness resulting from VZV pneumonia, encephalitis, hepatitis, and bleeding diathesis. Varicella in these infants resembles disseminated varicella in other immunocompromised populations (see Chapter 7).

### *Management of Perinatal VZV Exposure and Infection*

Passive antibody administration, given as VZIG, is recommended for infants with perinatal exposure to maternal varicella. VZIG should be given to the infant immediately after birth if the mother has acute varicella with onset less than 4 days before delivery or if the mother develops varicella within 48 hr.

Perinatal VZV infection in infants in the group identified as high-risk, i.e., those with a late onset of symptoms, who were born to mothers with illness beginning 4 days before or within 48 hours after delivery, should be treated with intravenous ACV (10 mg/kg/dose every 8 hr) if the infant did not receive VZIG prophylaxis. Although the clinical experience with ACV treatment of infants with perinatal varicella is limited, the drug prevents progressive VZV infection among other immunodeficient patients (see Chapter 7). Its safety is established from its use in infants with neonatal HSV infection.

Infants in the high-risk group who have received VZIG should be observed carefully since cases of progressive varicella have been observed despite prophylaxis (594–596). Intravenous ACV is indicated for these infants if extensive skin lesions appear or if there is clinical or laboratory evidence of visceral dissemination. Any infant who develops varicella should also be monitored clinically despite being in a low-risk group since a few of these infants have developed disseminated varicella (597).

No intervention is required for infants exposed to maternal herpes zoster because these infants can be predicted to have transplacentally acquired antibodies to VZV (598).

## HIV

The cause of the current epidemic of AIDS has been identified as a human retrovirus, originally designated the lymphadenopathy associated virus (LAV) or human T-cell leukemia virus III (HTLV-III) and now referred to as HIV. Although none of the first 1,000 cases of AIDS in the United States occurred among children (599), the possibilities of transfusion acquired infection in infants and of transmission from mothers to infants were considered early in the course of the epidemic and probable cases were soon identified (600–605). It is now apparent that many children, including infants, were placed at risk for AIDS because they received blood products from donors infected with HIV. That maternal HIV infection is, in fact, transmissable to the fetus or to the infant in the perinatal period has proved to be a tragic consequence of the AIDS epidemic (Table 4).

**TABLE 4.** *Differences between perinatal and adult infections with HIV*

| |
|---|
| Clinical presentation |
| Enhanced susceptibility to bacterial infection |
| Delayed psychomotor development |
| Lymphoid interstitial pneumonitis |
| Parotitis |
| More diverse manifestations of AIDS-related complex |
| Differential diagnosis |
| Primary congenital immunodeficiency disorders |
| Other intrauterine and perinatal infections |
| Laboratory evaluation |
| Diagnostic problem caused by transplacental transfer of maternal HIV antibodies |
| Better preservation of T-lymphocyte numbers and function |
| Earlier loss of B-lymphocyte function |
| Management issues |
| Appropriate immunizations |
| Intravenous γ-globulin |
| Need to evaluate antiviral agents without proved infection |
| Psychosocial problems |
| Limited parental resources |
| Foster care and day care placement |
| Delays in adoption |

### The Virus

Aspects of the molecular virology of HIV are discussed in Chapter 15. From the perspective of perinatal infection, one characteristic of the virus that probably facilitates its transmission to the fetus is its persistence in peripheral blood mononuclear cells. Since the placenta does not provide a barrier against the transfer of some circulating maternal lymphocytes and monocytes into the fetal circulation, the virus may be transported in such cells to the fetus. The CD4 surface receptor for the virus is expressed on fetal lymphocytes, providing the usual target cell for HIV. Other important target cell types, including macrophages, brain macrophages and parenchymal cells, and endothelium are susceptible to HIV infection in the fetus and newborn as in the older child or adult. Although maternal antibodies with HIV neutralizing activity should be transmitted along with infectious virus, the presence of these antibodies does not prevent progression of AIDS in older patients and is probably not sufficient to prevent the acquisition of perinatal infection. The ability of infectious virus to persist at mucosal surfaces and in secretions provides the circumstance for its potential transmission to the infant at the time of delivery. Leakage of maternal blood into the fetal circulation during labor and delivery could also result in the direct inoculation of the infant with HIV-infected maternal mononuclear cells or with cell-free virus, since infectious virus has been detected in plasma (606).

### Epidemiology

Among the cases of pediatric AIDS reported to the Centers for Disease Control (CDC) between 1982 and 1985, approximately 1% of individuals with symptomatic HIV infections were younger than 13 years old and 79% of these infections were attributed to vertical transmission from mothers with HIV infection (607). In retrospect, the acquisition of infection by this route probably occurred in the United States as early as 1973 (601). The absolute number of pediatric AIDS cases remains low, at 501 cases in June, 1987 (608). However, this figure underestimates the number of children in the United States who have HIV infection because reporting is voluntary and because, during most of this period, cases were identified by the CDC definition of unexplained cellular immunodeficiency as indicated by the diagnosis of an opportunistic infection, Kaposi sarcoma, non-Hodgkins lymphoma, or primary lymphoma of the brain. Less specific diseases occurring in children who have a positive laboratory test for HIV infection are now included (609) (Table 5), but the statistics still reflect only symptomatic cases and as few as 48% of symptomatic children fulfill the revised CDC criteria (610).

The first cases of transfusion-related AIDS in infants were described in 1983 (602,604). Infants exposed to infected blood products seem to be at significantly higher risk of HIV transmission than older children and adults (611,612). Based upon epidemiologic data, the incidence of transfusion-associated AIDS is estimated to be sixfold higher for infants than adults. For example, all of nine newborns who were exposed to infected plasma from a single donor developed laboratory evidence of HIV infection or signs of AIDS or AIDS-related complex (ARC) (613). The routine screening of blood products has essentially eliminated this source of perinatal HIV infection, but children continue to be identified who have HIV infection resulting from transfusions given in the newborn period as many as 7 years earlier. Before the role of transfusion in AIDS epidemiology was known, our experience and that at other centers suggests that infants were probably protected from exposure to HIV-infected blood because of the practice of using blood products from CMV seronegative donors (614).

As in the regions of Africa where HIV is endemic, most infections among children in the United States are acquired from infected mothers (615,616). Therefore, the epidemiology of perinatal HIV parallels the pattern of HIV infection in women of childbearing age. The devastating effects of vertical transmission in other areas of the world is apparent from the observation that at least 98% of children requiring hospitalization in Central Africa had complications of HIV infection (617). The primary risk factors for HIV infection among women in the United States include intravenous drug abuse, prostitution, or sexual contact with partner who acquired HIV as a result of drug abuse or bisexual contact. In the CDC survey, a history of intravenous drug abuse by the mother or her sexual partner was identified in 74% of mothers of HIV-infected infants (607). In another cohort, one

**TABLE 5.** *Classification of HIV infection in children younger than 13 years old*

| Major group | Clinical status | Subclass |
|---|---|---|
| Class P-0 | Indeterminate infection | |
| Class P-1 | Asymptomatic infection | A. Normal immune function |
| | | B. Abnormal immune function |
| | | C. Immune function not tested |
| Class P-2 | Symptomatic infection | A. Nonspecific findings |
| | | B. Progressive neurologic disease |
| | | C. Lymphoid interstitial pneumonia |
| | | D. Secondary infectious disease |
| | | E. Secondary cancers |
| | | F. Other diseases possibly caused by HIV infection |

Data from ref. 609.

or both parents of 76% of infants with presumed vertically transmitted AIDS abused intravenous drugs (618). Other sources of maternal HIV infection include birth in countries where heterosexual transmission of HIV is common, e.g., Haiti (619) and Africa, exposure to blood products prior to the advent of HIV screening, or sexual contact with a partner who has HIV acquired from blood products. Although a specific risk factor may not be noted initially, a source can be identified for almost all pediatric AIDS cases. When infections acquired from blood products are excluded, the distribution of cases in male and female infants is equivalent, with a ratio of approximately 1:1.

The geographic distribution of perinatal HIV in the United States, in which 75% of cases have been reported from New York, New Jersey, and Florida, reflects the higher prevalence of HIV infections related to illicit drug use by young adults in the urban areas of these states (620). That black and Hispanic infants among children with perinatally acquired AIDS account for 91% of cases is due to the higher risk of HIV infection among adults in these population groups, which is also attributable to drug abuse. Among women with AIDS, 87% are black or Hispanic. For unexplained reasons, the risk of heterosexual transmission of HIV from men with hemophilia does not appear to be high (621); only 0.6% of 530 infants born to such couples from 1979 to 1985 developed HIV infection (622).

Recent surveillance studies indicate that the prevalence of HIV infection in individuals with a history of intravenous drug abuse has increased steadily in the geographic areas where most pediatric AIDS cases have been identified (623). The number of pediatric AIDS cases has risen in parallel, with 2.3 times as many cases in 1985 than in 1984 (607). HIV infection associated with drug abuse has continued to spread in urban areas of the United States. Although heterosexual transmission accounts for relatively few cases of AIDS in the United States at present (624), the number of cases due to this source is increasing (625). The fact that 30–50% of women have been infected by heterosexual contact (626) suggests that the population of infants at risk for intrauterine or perinatal HIV transmission will continue to expand (Table 6). In Massachusetts, 2.1 per 1000 infants were born to mothers with HIV antibody (627). Generalizing to the whole population, the

**TABLE 6.** *HIV antibody prevalence in women of reproductive age, 1984–1987[a]*

| State | City/region | Type of clinic | Number tested | Percent positive |
|---|---|---|---|---|
| Alabama | Montgomery | Family planning | 694 | 0.3 |
| California | Alameda County | Premarital | 377 | 0.5 |
| | Los Angeles | Delivery | 500 | 0.4 |
| | Long Beach | Prenatal | 277 | 0.0 |
| Florida | Jacksonville | Prenatal | 299 | 0.7 |
| Illinois | Chicago | Pregnant drug user | 150 | 10.7 |
| Massachusetts | Statewide | Newborn | 30,708 | 0.2 |
| Maryland | Baltimore | Delivery | 678 | 0.7 |
| | Baltimore | High risk prenatal | 115 | 29.6 |
| | Baltimore | Family planning | 693 | 0.9 |
| Michigan | Detroit | Pregnant drug user | 170 | 9.4 |
| North Carolina | Statewide | Prenatal | 200 | 0.0 |
| | Statewide | Family planning | 200 | 0.0 |
| New York | Bronx | Hospital | 820 | 2.4 |
| | Brooklyn | Delivery | 602 | 2.0 |
| | New York City | Delivery | 1,192 | 2.3 |
| Pennsylvania | Pittsburgh | Family planning | 191 | 0.0 |
| Wisconsin | Central | Prenatal | 1,000 | 0.0 |
| Puerto Rico | | Prenatal | 2,633 | 1.7 |

[a]Including surveys in which at least 150 individuals were tested.
Data from ref. 624.

birth of 1,620–4,860 HIV exposed infants was predicted for each year after 1987. In specific urban areas, such as New York, the rate is estimated to be 20 infants per 1,000 live births (628). The prevalence rates of HIV seropositivity among intravenous drug abusers in European cities is comparable to that observed in New York, and cases of perinatal HIV have resulted (625,629).

## Maternal Infection

### *Identification of Pregnancies at Risk*

HIV antibody screening of pregnant women at risk for HIV infection should be carried out as early in the pregnancy as possible. The high-risk pregnancy is identified by ascertaining the maternal history of intravenous drug abuse, prostitution, sexual contact with a partner who is at risk because of drug abuse, bisexual contact or exposure to blood products, maternal exposure to blood products especially before 1984 when routine HIV screening was introduced, or maternal country of origin in a geographic region where HIV is prevalent. However, the limitations of voluntary testing based on active case finding and self-identification by mothers at risk must be recognized (630) so that a high index of suspicion for HIV infection is maintained if an infant presents with compatible symptoms.

### *Routes of Transmission to the Fetus or Newborn*

The potential mechanisms for the transmission of HIV from mother to infant include transplacental transmission with infection of the fetus *in utero,* inoculation of the infant during labor and delivery as a result of contact with vaginal secretions or maternal blood, and postpartum acquisition from breast milk. Because of the limitations of diagnostic methods, the usual distinction between viral infections acquired *in utero* and those transmitted at delivery or in the newborn period cannot be made. Until infections caused by each type of exposure can be differentiated, all maternally derived HIV infections are referred to as "perinatal" HIV infections.

The evidence for intrauterine infection consists of reports of HIV isolation from two fetuses of 15 and 20 weeks' gestation (631,632) and from the cord blood of some infants (633,634). Although the possible contamination of the samples by maternal blood cannot be excluded, these cases suggest the transplacental transmission of the virus. HIV has also been cultured from amniotic fluid (635). One premature infant who died 3 weeks after birth had HIV antigens detected in thymic tissue (636). By analogy with other perinatal infections, such as hepatitis B, the fact that some infants develop HIV infection in spite of cesarean delivery does not prove transplacental transmission because exposure to maternal blood is not prevented. The syndrome of HIV embryopathy implies intrauterine infection, but the opinions of pediatricians caring for children with perinatal HIV infections at different centers concerning the occurrence of such a syndrome is variable (637–640). Since these infants are usually born to mothers who have abused drugs during pregnancy, who are at risk for other infections complicating pregnancy, such as CMV and syphilis, and whose prenatal care is limited, many factors other than HIV infection may affect fetal development. Some infants born to HIV-infected women have microcephaly at birth, but it is difficult to attribute this finding to HIV unequivocally in the context of other prenatal risk factors. Microcephaly demonstrated several months after birth cannot be taken as proof of intrauterine infection because some infants with HIV develop microcephaly postnatally. Intrauterine growth retardation is not a constant finding in infants born to HIV seropositive mothers (639) and, when present, also has many possible etiologies. The documentation of craniofacial dysmorphism provides the focus of disagreement about the HIV embryopathy syndrome. The characteristic findings enumerated by Marion et al. (638) are a prominent box-like forehead, a flattened nasal bridge, a well-formed philtrum and upper vermilion border, and eye findings, including hypertelorism, obliquity of the eye, long palpebral fissures and blue sclera. However, normal standards are not available for determining hypertelorism in black and Hispanic children, and, by comparison with measurements of healthy black and Hispanic children, palpebral fissure length was not increased in infants with HIV infection (637). Blue sclera are also common in normal infants and obliquity of eyes is common in nonwhite children. Recently, Qazi et al. (639) have described identical twin girls both of whom had the craniofacial findings that have been described in infants with AIDS and only one of whom was infected; these features were often observed in a control population of uninfected black and Hispanic infants.

The potential for infection of the infant during vaginal delivery arises from the fact that more than 50% of women with HIV infection have infectious virus in cervical and vaginal secretions (641,642). Cervical cultures were intermittently positive in a cohort of HIV-infected women who had sequential cultures (643). If most perinatal HIV infection is due to exposure at delivery, the usual brief interval from birth to the onset of symptoms in infants implies a much shorter incubation period in infants than is observed among older children and adults. Nevertheless, HIV infections acquired from transfusion in the neonatal period have a short incubation period in many cases (619,644). The dilemma concerning the specific risks of intrauterine and peripartum infection will remain unresolved until better methods of intrauterine diagnosis become available and more experience with the examination of fetal tissue by *in situ* hybridization or by immunologic staining for viral antigens is accumulated. Ultimately, the relative risks may not be determined until an intervention is devised that will prevent peripartum acquisition, allowing the attribution of the residual cases to intrauterine infection, as has occurred with the successful prophylaxis of infants against exposure to hepatitis B at delivery.

The transmission of HIV postpartum by breast milk was established in a unique circumstance in which a mother became infected from a transfusion after delivery and her infant acquired HIV infection after 6 weeks of breast feeding (645). HIV has been isolated from the breast milk of infected mothers (646).

Because of the potential for a long incubation period in some infants, the frequency of perinatal transmission of HIV from infected mothers to their infants is just being defined. The available information demonstrates that although transmission is very likely, it does not always occur. Discordance in the acquisition of HIV has been reported in monozygotic and dizygotic twins. Even the previous birth of an infected child does not lead to an inevitable risk of infection among subsequent infants. However, in one study, 65% of 20 infants born to mothers who had already had one child with AIDS had serologic evidence of HIV infection, with or without clinical signs within several months after birth (647). The relationship between the stage of the maternal infection and the risk of transmission is uncertain. In many instances, the diagnosis of HIV infection in an infant is the first indication of probable maternal HIV infection in a mother who is asymptomatic. Infected infants have been born to mothers with normal immunologic parameters (627,648). Conversely, some infants of mothers who have frank AIDS during pregnancy appear to escape infection. It is obvious that the maternal infection need not be primary during the pregnancy to allow transmission of the virus to the fetus or newborn. However, the usual analysis of the relative risks of intrauterine and peripartum viral transmission in terms of whether the maternal infection during pregnancy was primary, or preceded the pregnancy, cannot be made from current data about HIV.

### *Other Consequences of HIV Infection During Pregnancy*

Despite the potential effects of pregnancy upon the immune system of the mother, a specific effect of pregnancy upon the course of maternal HIV infection has not been documented. Pregnancies have been uncomplicated despite significant abnormalities of maternal T-lymphocyte numbers and function (608,647,649,650). In one series, 12 of 15 mothers who were asymptomatic at the birth of an affected infant progressed to AIDS or ARC during an average surveillance of 30 months (range 8–47 months) (647). Since all of these women had immunologic abnormalities associated with HIV infection at the time of delivery, the subsequent attack rate for HIV disease is not unexpected in an adult population (651). A number of women have been described whose HIV infection has remained asymptomatic despite multiple pregnancies over a several year period.

Although some cohort studies suggest an increased incidence of prematurity among infants born to HIV-infected mothers (639), this finding has not been uniform and, because of confounding clinical variables in these high-risk mothers, is not known to be caused by maternal HIV infection. Similarly, there is no specific evidence that the frequency of spontaneous abortion is higher for pregnancies complicated by HIV infection.

Maternal HIV infection could potentiate the transmission of other pathogens to the fetus *in utero* or at delivery. However, it is difficult to establish a specific role for HIV-related immunosuppression in enhancing the risks because these women are likely to be exposed to other pathogens from the same high-risk circumstances that led to HIV infection. Nevertheless, optimal management of pregnancies complicated by HIV infection will require an aggressive effort to determine whether the understanding of the common intrauterine and perinatal pathogens must be revised for this population. For example, recurrent as well as primary infections with CMV or toxoplasmosis may produce fetal damage, the frequency of asymptomatic genital HSV reactivation at delivery may be increased, or the potential for the transplacental transmission of other pathogens, such as toxoplasmosis, EBV and VZV, may be enhanced in the context of maternal HIV infection (652).

## Intrauterine and/or Perinatal Infection

In general, the clinical and pathologic manifestations of HIV infection observed in infants as in older patients, derive from three potential sources, including the destruction of cells infected by HIV because of virus-induced or immune-mediated cell lysis; the disruption of cell and organ function by secondary pathogens, and immune-mediated damage related to inflammation, autoantibody production, and immune complex formation (608,640,653). Although AIDS is recognizable in infants by the characteristics familiar from adult disease, the concept of AIDS-related complex is less useful because the potential manifestations of symptomatic HIV infection in the absence of the complete immunodeficiency syndrome are much more variable in infants (608,653).

With intensive surveillance for maternal infection during pregnancy, many infants who are asymptomatic at birth, but who are at risk for HIV infection, are being identified. Information about the patterns of clinical outcome among these infants remains fragmentary. However, the current experience suggests that most children with HIV infection contracted *in utero* or in the perinatal period will develop clinical manifestations of immunodeficiency during the first or second year of life. In the initial phase of the epidemic, the mean age at the time of diagnosis of perinatally acquired HIV infection was 17 months, with a range of 1–86 months, although the onset of symptoms was likely to have preceded the diagnosis by several months (607). Of infected infants, 82% were diagnosed by 3 years.

At birth, infants born to HIV-infected mothers may have intrauterine growth retardation and often exhibit signs of maternal alcohol or drug abuse, but there are no pathognomonic clinical manifestations associated with HIV infection in the newborn. Among infants who develop symptoms of HIV infection within the first few months of life, the most consistent clinical features are failure to thrive, chronic interstitial pneumonitis, and hepatosplenomegaly. Other abnormalities that are often apparent on physical examination include diffuse adenopathy, persistent thrush, protracted or recurrent diarrhea, and various secondary infections (654,655).

Clinically, many of the obvious manifestations of disease in children with HIV infection result from opportunistic infections. Infants with AIDS develop invasive infections caused by the same pathogens encountered among older children and adults, such as *Candida* species, *Pneumocystis carinii,* and atypical mycobacteria. Localized and disseminated herpes viral infections caused by CMV, HSV, VZV, and EBV are observed in infants with HIV infection (655). Intrauterine or perinatally acquired CMV can cause pneumonitis, chorioretinitis, hepatitis, and enterocolitis in infants, as in adults with AIDS. Infants with AIDS are more susceptible than adults to pyogenic infections including otitis media, mastoiditis, sinusitis, lymphadenitis, pneumonia, septicemia, and meningitis (619,650,656,657). Serious bacterial infection is observed even if other symptoms of HIV infection are minimal. Susceptibility to invasive bacterial disease, especially caused by encapsulated organisms, is probably related to the failure to produce antibodies against specific antigens despite the usual finding of hypergammaglobulinemia in infants and children with AIDS (658). The most frequent bacterial pathogens isolated from patients with bacteremia are *Streptococcus pneumoniae, Haemophilus influenzae* type b, *Salmonella sp* and other enteric gram-negative organisms (619,650,657) (Table 7). Staphylococcal soft tissue infections and *E. coli* urinary tract infections are also common (619). Relapsing disease due to some of the enteric bacterial pathogens, as well as to cryptosporidium, accounts in part for the chronic diarrhea observed in many infants with HIV infection.

The hematologic abnormalities associated with AIDS in infants are variable, but anemia and thrombocytopenia are common features. Anemia may be related to chronic secondary infections, nutritional deficien-

**TABLE 7.** *Bacteriologically confirmed infections in HIV-infected children*

| | All sites | Blood cultures |
|---|---|---|
| Gram positive organisms | | |
| *Staphylococcus epidermidis* | 26 | 1 |
| *Streptococcus viridans* | 18 | 2 |
| *Staphylococcus aureus* | 15 | 2 |
| *Streptococcus pneumoniae* | 14 | 11 |
| Enterococcus | 13 | 2 |
| Streptococcus group A | 4 | 1 |
| Streptococcus group B | 1 | 1 |
| Gram negative organisms | | |
| *Escherichia coli* | 31 | 1 |
| *Pseudomonas aeruginosa* | 8 | 2 |
| Other pseudomonas | 7 | |
| *Enterobacter spp.* | 7 | 2 |
| *Proteus mirabilis* | 6 | |
| *Klebsiella spp.* | 11 | 2 |
| *Salmonella enteritidis* | 6 | |
| *Haemophilus influenzae* | 5 | |

Data from Krasinski et al., ref. 630.

cies that are aggravated by chronic diarrhea or autoantibody production. Severe hemolytic anemia has been encountered (640). In addition to lymphopenia and altered T4/T8 lymphocyte ratios, some infants with AIDS have pancytopenia with absolute neutrophil counts less than 500 (659–662). Petechiae and ecchymoses resulting from thrombocytopenia constituted the initial manifestation of HIV infection, appearing at 8–9 months of age, in three infants with transfusion-acquired disease (663). Neutropenia and thrombocytopenia have been demonstrated to be immune mediated in some cases.

Although many infants with AIDS have hypergammaglobulinemia, some infants who have panhypogammaglobulinemia have been described. (644,664). Three of 12 infants with transfusion acquired HIV had severe panhypogammaglobulinemia associated with significantly lower absolute numbers and percentages of T-helper cells (644).

Diffuse lymphadenopathy is associated with follicular hyperplasia demonstrated by lymph node biopsy, with progression to atrophy of lymphatic cells also noted (608). The thymus may be visible on chest x-ray in infants with AIDS, but thymic biopsies demonstrated pathologic changes described as involution, thymic dysplasia, or thymitis (665). Parotitis, a manifestation of AIDS noted in children which is unusual among adults, is characterized by lymphocytic infiltration of the salivary gland tissue (640).

The pulmonary manifestations of HIV infection in young children resemble those in adults with AIDS, with *Pneumocystis carinii* being the prominent cause of acute interstitial pneumonitis. However, infants and children also have the unique syndromes of lymphoid interstitial pneumonitis, pulmonary lymphoid hyerplasia, and desquamative interstitial pneumonia (666–668). Lymphoid interstitial pneumonitis is associated with diffuse infiltrates of the alveolar septae and peribronchiolar regions, composed of lymphocytes, plasma cells, and immunoblasts. HIV RNA was detected in lung tissue from one child with lymphoid interstitial pneumonitis (666). Eight children whose pulmonary disease was investigated by lung biopsy had *Pneumocystis carinii* pneumonia, whereas six patients had pulmonary lymphoid hyperplasia (668). The clinical differences noted between these two patient groups included fever, tachypnea, and more severe hypoxemia in those with pneumocytis pneumonia compared to a more chronic process, with digital clubbing, in those with pulmonary lymphoid hyperplasia. Patients in the latter group were older, typically had extensive lymphadenopathy and parotid gland swelling, and had laboratory evidence of persistent EBV infection as well as elevated serum immunoglobulins. The chest x-rays of these patients showed a nodular pattern extending to the periphery of the lungs, often associated with hilar and mediastinal adenopathy. The pathologic examination of lung tissue showed aggregates of mononuclear cells, especially T8+ (cytotoxic/suppressor) T lymphocytes and plasma cells located around bronchiolar mucosal epithelium with some large nodules containing a germinal center and a thick-walled venule. Interstitial infiltrates with widening of the alveolar septae and alveolar cell hyperplasia was also seen. EBV DNA was detected by Southern blot analysis in lung tissue from four of five patients evaluated. The prognosis for survival was significantly better in patients with pulmonary lymphoid hyperplasia than those with *Pneumocystis carinii* pneumonia. Desquamative interstitial pneumonitis, which is the least common type of interstitial pneumonitis described in children with HIV infection, emphasizes the histologic observation of intraalveolar collections of mononuclear cells and cuboidal metaplasia of the alveolar epithelial cells. Finally, infants with HIV infection, like those with primary congenital immunodeficiency may have persistent infections with parainfluenza 3 or respiratory syncytial viruses (RSVs) (669).

Progressive neurologic disease has emerged

as one of the major clinical forms of HIV infection in infancy (670–674). Neurologic findings developed in 28 of 36 infants, 26 of whom were born to infected mothers and 98 of whom had transfusion-related HIV acquired in the newborn period, during a mean surveillance period of 19 months (673). Progressive encephalopathy was the most common syndrome in this cohort, with signs appearing between 2 months and 5 years of age. The average age at onset among those with apparent *in utero* or peripartum exposure was 18 months but extended to 5 years even in this subpopulation. Affected infants demonstrate delayed development with perceptual motor deficits or loss of developmental milestones, impaired brain growth, hypotonia, pyramidal tract signs, and ataxia (670) (Table 8). Seizures occur in some cases, but there is no specific pattern of EEG abnormalities (674). Impaired brain growth can be documented as secondary microcephaly or by CT brain scan, which shows cortical atrophy with enlargement of the subarachnoid spaces and ventricles. In one series, bilaterally symmetrical calcifications in the basal ganglia appeared on sequential CT scans from five children. Despite their neurologic manifestations, the majority of these patients had normal CSF findings. In later phases, the signs evolve to spastic quadriparesis and pseudobulbar palsy with dysphagia and dysarthria. Progressive encephalopathy is a specific risk factor, independent of other clinical variables, for fatal HIV infection (673). Histologically, brain tissue from these children demonstrates inflammatory cell infiltrates consisting of microglia, lymphocytes, plasma cells, mononuclear cells, and multinucleated giant cells, most prominently involving the basal ganglia and brain stem. Other findings include perivascular calcifications and reactive astrocytosis in the white matter. In some cases, localized HIV antibody synthesis was demonstrated in CSF, and there is some evidence for a correlation between HIV antigen in the CSF and progressive encephalopathy (675). In one instructive case, HIV DNA sequences were detected in brain tissue from an infant with progressive encephalopathy whose serum was persistently negative for HIV antibodies (676). The failure to identify opportunistic organisms in brain tissue from many infants with progressive encephalopathy suggests that HIV infection is the direct cause of this manifestation of perinatal HIV disease (670,677).

**TABLE 8.** *Neurologic manifestations in population of 68 infants and children with HIV infection*

| | Number of patients with abnormality during the clinical course of HIV infection |
|---|---|
| Microcephaly | |
| Acquired (≤2%) | 34 |
| Head circumference (10–25%) | 12 |
| Early developmental history | |
| Normal | 34 |
| Mild delays | 16 |
| Moderate to severe | 14 |
| Cognitive deficits | |
| Borderline to mild | 19 |
| Moderate to profound | 19 |
| Pyramidal tract signs | |
| Bilateral | 52 |
| Progressive | 25 |
| Ataxia | 6 |
| Seizures | 6 |
| CNS infection with conventional pathogens | 10 |

Data from Belman et al., ref. 670.

Chronic active hepatitis was demonstrated by liver biopsy in three children who had elevated transaminases as well as hepatomegaly (610). Pathologic changes included hyperplasia of the sinusoidal lining cells, lymphocytic infiltrates with necrosis, and portal fibrosis.

Mucocutaneous lesions are most often related to candidiasis, bacterial cellulitis, or herpes simplex in infants with AIDS, but unusual clinical syndromes such as noma, which is a necrotizing gingivostomatitis, and acrodermatitis enteropathica have been observed. (667,678,679).

Severe cardiac involvement, associated with myocardial dysfunction, congestive heart failure, and pericardial effusions, has been described in infants with perinatal HIV infection (680–682).

Although Kaposi's sarcoma was noted in some of the earliest cases of perinatal HIV infection (619), malignancies have not been a prominent finding in infants with AIDS. Primary lymphoma of the brain and Burkitt lymphoma related to EBV have been reported (683–685,718). Infiltrates of B lymphocytes of polyclonal origin, some of which contain EBV gene sequences, are noted in many tissues from young children with AIDS, but the significance of this finding is uncertain.

### *Laboratory Diagnosis*

In the newborn infant, nonspecific findings such as signs of drug withdrawal or intrauterine growth retardation, in conjunction with a maternal history suggesting risk, provide a sufficient indication for HIV testing of the mother. HIV evaluation is also indicated for any infant who presents with unexplained failure to thrive, hepatosplenomegaly, chronic diarrhea, or other evidence of immunodeficiency. The differential diagnosis of HIV infection requires an assessment for other congenital infections and the exclusion of congenital immunodeficiency disorders. The evaluation for congenital infections must be interpreted with the knowledge that infants of HIV-infected mothers are also at risk for other intrauterine and perinatal infections, especially CMV, toxoplasmosis, syphilis, and hepatitis B (686). The availability of specific methods for viral diagnosis of HIV, applied to samples from the mother as well as the infant, has eliminated some of the uncertainty encountered in differentiating the initial cases of perinatal HIV infection from the primary congenital immunodeficiencies (687). In situations in which samples are not available from the mother and samples from the infant are not diagnostic, severe combined immunodeficiency, DiGeorge syndrome, Wiskott-Aldrich syndrome, ataxia telangiectasia, graft versus host disease, agammaglobulinemia, and hypogammaglobulinemia with elevated IgM must be considered (640,659).

The serologic evaluation of high-risk mothers and their infants for HIV infection is done using the standard ELISA methods, with positive results confirmed by Western blot. The evidence suggests that the IgG antibody response to HIV is diminished in infected infants and children, with negative ELISA titers and weaker or absent antibodies against specific polypeptides of HIV on Western blot than are detectable in maternal serum (688,689). The interval required before serologic testing of the infant can confirm the diagnosis of HIV infection is prolonged because transplacentally acquired IgG antibodies against HIV antigens can persist for as long as 15 months after birth. Conversely, in infants with hypogammaglobulinemia whose transplacentally acquired HIV antibodies have disappeared, the suppression of immunoglobin production in the infant can obscure the diagnosis of HIV infection. The potential loss of HIV antibodies with disease progression complicates the serologic diagnosis of HIV infection in infants in whom the diagnosis is considered late in the clinical course (612). Unfortunately, methods for detecting IgM antibodies to HIV antigens are problematic for technical reasons. In addition, whether the infected infant will produce HIV-specific IgM antibodies is uncertain, and the timing or persistence of the response is unpredictable in those who do (690). In one infant followed closely from birth, the synthesis of IgG against HIV proteins, p55 and p66, was demonstrated by Western blot, but IgM antibodies never appeared. The appearance of new bands using

Western blots to compare maternal serum and sequential infant sera permitted the early confirmation of perinatal infection (688). Occasionally, the presence of HIV antibodies in serum from an infant may not indicate exposure to maternal infection, as was true in our experience with several infants whose HIV antibodies were traced to the administration of a preparation of hepatitis B immune globulin that contained HIV antibodies and in a reported case (691). The available preparations of intravenous γ-globulin and immune serum globulins no longer contain HIV antibodies.

Infants may have HIV infection proved by viral culture of peripheral blood mononuclear cells or secretions or by HIV core antigen (p24) detection without having measurable HIV antibodies in serum (620,692). Conversely, the experience in infants parallels the diagnostic problems encountered in adult patients with AIDS or ARC whose cultures may be negative despite serologic evidence of HIV infection. The sensitivity of cultures for HIV may be enhanced by assays for p24 antigen or *in situ* hybridization in addition to reverse transcriptase (693). For example, infection was diagnosed in one infant by culturing peripheral blood mononuclear cells taken 24 hr after birth with phytohemagglutinin and Il-2 for 3 days and then with Il-2 for 7 and 14 days before examination for HIV by *in situ* hybridization (694). Amplification of HIV sequences by polymerase chain reaction may prove useful to enhance HIV detection in infants. HIV core antigen detection methods applied directly to plasma or secretions do not appear to be very reliable for diagnosing HIV infection in infants. HIV antigen has been detected in CSF from children with progressive encephalopathy (675), and it may be measured more readily in advanced disease (693).

As was anticipated from the evaluation of adult patients, the immunologic investigations of the first infants with suspected AIDS revealed progressive lymphopenia with an absolute decrease in helper T lymphocytes (CD4+), reversed helper/suppressor (CD4+/CD8+) ratios, and diminished lymphoproliferative responses to mitogens, antigens, and alloantigens in some patients (650,655,658). In general, T-cell function tends to deteriorate later in children than in adults, whereas B cell function tends to deteriorate earlier. Young children who have HIV-related disease, including opportunistic infections, are less likely to have a total lymphocyte count of <1,500/μl than adults, and T4/T8 ratios are greater than 1.0 in up to 15% of pediatric cases (610,655,695). Within the first 6 months of life, normal infants have higher T-cell ratios, which may account for the better preservation of ratios in HIV-infected infants under 6 months of age (608). The clinical experience demonstrates that infants and young children with minimal laboratory abnormalities of T- and B-lymphocyte numbers and function can develop life-threatening secondary infections, and infants whose T-helper/suppressor ratios were never abnormal have died from HIV infection (659). The immunologic evaluation of infants at risk for HIV infection is further complicated by the observation of persistent lymphocyte abnormalities in infants born to drug-abusing mothers who do not have HIV infection (696).

Defective *in vitro* B-lymphocyte responses to pokeweed mitogen and Staphylococcus Cowan A strain are observed in young children with AIDS despite normal or elevated numbers of circulating B lymphocytes (660,697,698). Altered B-lymphocyte function is intrinsic and is not attributable only to the lack of effective helper T-lymphocyte function (655); it may be related to chronic EBV infection in some cases. Infants with HIV infection often have hypergammaglobulinemia involving all immunoglobulin classes. However, the humoral immune responses to specific antigens as demonstrated after immunization with pneumococcal vaccine, tetanus toxoid, and other immunogens is impaired *in vivo*. Failure to demonstrate switching from

IgM to IgG antibody production after *in vivo* exposure to antigen is also observed (697).

Deficiencies in the production of lymphokines, including interferon-α and interferon-γ, and of thymulin have been noted in children with AIDS (659,699) as has impaired NK cell cytoxicity (697).

### Prognosis

The prognosis of infants with AIDS is very poor, characterized in many cases by a fatal outcome within months (618). For example, among 64 cases of AIDS in children, 59 of which were presumed to be vertically transmitted, the median survival time from the time of diagnosis was slightly less than 3 months (618) (Fig. 6). Of the children, 75% were dead within 1 year of diagnosis. Considering perinatal infections only, the CDC survey noted a median survival 6.5 months after diagnosis, which was significantly shorter the the median survival of 19.7 months in older children (607). Infants with symptomatic AIDS, particularly those who have *Pneumocystitis carinii* pneumonia usually have a fulminant course, and children younger than 1 year are more likely to develop this complication (72%) than older children (38%) (607). The average survival among infants diagnosed at more than 1 year was 22 months.

The loss of *in vitro* responses to the B-cell mitogens has been described as an early marker of immunologic failure and risk of progressive disease (659,698). In one cohort of infants with perinatal HIV infection whose symptoms appeared at an average of 6 months, the absence of antigen-induced lymphocyte proliferation *in vitro* and skin test anergy at diagnosis correlated with rapidly progressive and fatal disease (610). These infants were more likely to have frequent opportunistic infections, failure to thrive, and neurologic disease, and were less likely to have lymphoid interstitial pneumonitis.

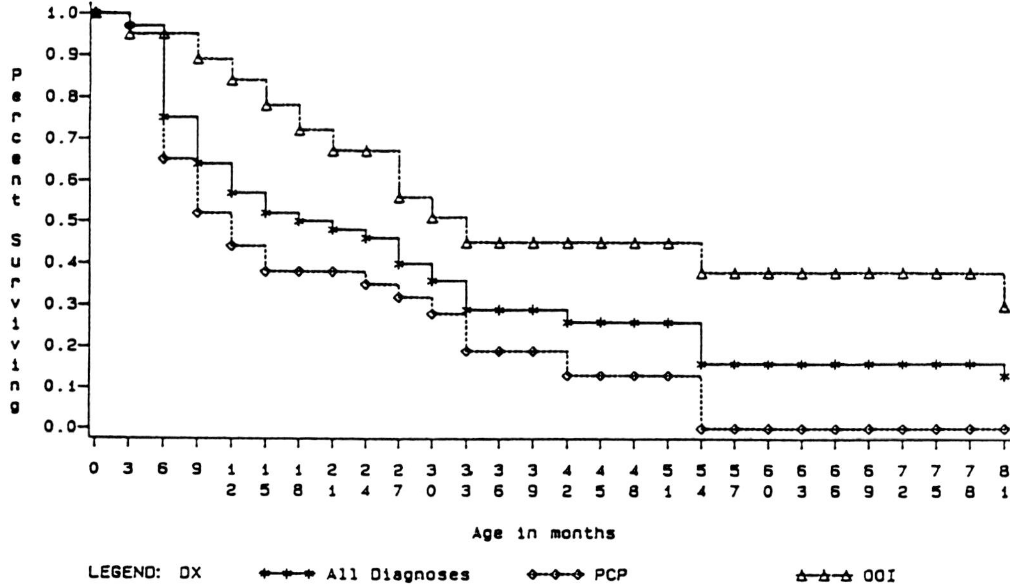


**FIG. 6.** Survival from birth of 59 children with vertically transmitted AIDS: New York City, 1979 through May 1985. DX, diagnosis; *asterisk*, all diagnoses combined (all AIDS-related infections); *open triangle, non-Pneumocystis* pneumonia infections, or simply other opportunistic infections (OOI); *open diamond*, children with a diagnosis of *P. carinii* pneumonia (PCP).

In a cohort of 12 infants with exposure to HIV by transfusion from an infected donor, four infants were described who had illnesses typically found in infants with HIV infection but who subsequently become asymptomatic. The interpretation of this experience is limited by the fact that these infants had been followed for only 2–2.5 years (644). Although some infants may exhibit periods of relative well-being after the onset of symptomatic disease, it is unlikely that reversal to asymptomatic infection will be common.

The attempt to relate the prognosis of asymptomatic or symptomatic infants to markers of immunity directed against specific HIV antigens has not yielded definitive information. Antibodies to gp110 were noted in serum from all of the infants described by Blanche et al. (629), but those who lacked proliferative responses and who had severe disease usually lacked or lost antibodies to p18 and p25. In one series of infants with AIDS and progressive encephalopathy, the absence of neutralizing antibodies against HIV correlated with an accelerated clinical course (700).

## Clinical Management

Because of the anticipated high attack rate and the fact that active infection of the infant often cannot be proved or excluded until after the first year of life, all exposed infants should have sequential clinical and laboratory evaluations to diagnose HIV infection and to identify and treat infections that are secondary to the progressive immunodeficiency caused by HIV (654).

The high attack rate for HIV infection in exposed infants, the fulminant course of the disease in most infants, and the possibility that infections due to perinatal exposure might be preventable creates a critical need to evaluate specific antiviral drugs in this population. In order to determine whether the natural history of perinatal HIV infection can be altered, intervention must begin immediately after birth, which, because of the limitations of diagnostic methods and the objective of preventing infection, necessitates treating infants who do not have proved HIV infection. At present, older children have participated in clinical trials of AZT therapy for AIDS, but its evaluation in infants has just entered phase I pharmacokinetic and tolerance studies. Infants with HIV infection who were treated with intravenous or oral ribavirin demonstrated no change in clinical or immunologic status (701). Because of the possible benefit of intravenous γ-globulin in infants and young children with AIDS, it will be important to evaluate the response to antiviral agents given alone or in conjunction with passive antibody administration. Clinical investigations of the potential value of combination therapy with specific antiviral agents such as AZT and dideoxycitidine or of immunomodulators, such as interleukin 2, in combination with AZT have not been undertaken in children.

The susceptibility of infants with HIV infection to *Pneumocystis carinii* pneumonia warrants prophylaxis and trimethoprim sulfamethoxazole. The prophylactic administration of intravenous γ-globulin to infants with symptomatic HIV infection is controversial. It has been recommended because of the known deficiencies of B-lymphocyte function in infants with AIDS and the clinical evidence that this approach reduces the frequency of bacterial infections among children with congenital immunodeficiencies (702). In uncontrolled experiences, similar benefits have been described for infants with AIDS or ARC (703). Improvements in laboratory parameters, including less severe CD4+ lymphopenia, a decrease of circulating immune complexes, improved lymphocyte responses to mitogens, and normalization of suppressor cell function have been described among treated infants (704). Intravenous γ-globulin has been given to these patients at a maintenance dose of 200–500 mg/kg every two weeks of 400–500 mg/kg every month (702).

Passive antibody prophylaxis for known exposures to VZV is necessary, but failures in protection should be anticipated. Intravenous ACV therapy is indicated for acute VZV and HSV infections. Some infants with HIV complicated by recurrent herpes may benefit from suppressive therapy with oral ACV. The exposure of HIV-infected infants to blood products from CMV immune donors should be avoided. Despite precautions about blood exposure, many of these infants will have maternally acquired CMV infections. Although CMV pneumonitis, retinitis, and enterocolitis in infants with HIV infection might respond to ganciclovir therapy, experience with this drug in infants and young children is quite limited (705).

The relative efficacy of hepatitis B immune globulin and vaccine in preventing hepatitis B among infants with HIV remains to be determined, but passive and active prophylaxis should be given at birth if the mother is positive for hepatitis B surface antigen. Despite the potential deficiencies in response to tetanus toxoid and diphtheria antigens, infants with possible or proved HIV infection should receive the usual childhood immunizations with diphtheria-pertussis-tetanus vaccine (DPT), but the inactivated polio vaccine must be substituted for oral polio vaccine. The administration of the live measles-mumps-rubella vaccine has been recommended for asymptomatic infants, but this recommendation remains controversial (695,704,707). The observation that 60% of children who received measles-mumps-rubella (MMR) vaccine before the diagnosis of HIV infection had antibody responses constitutes the argument in favor of giving the live vaccine (708). However, the response to measles immunization in these children is unpredictable, and the risk of exposure in some communities can be judged to be very low. Hemophilus influenza B vaccine should be given, but the response to the capsular polysaccharide of hemophilus influenza B is likely to be impaired (709).

Other general measures in the care of these infants include the suppression of oral candidiasis by chronic therapy with clotrimazole or ketoconazole, the use of irradiated blood products to reduce the risk of graft versus host disease, and maintenance of a protected environment during hospitalizations to reduce the risk of nosocomial infections.

The administration of steroids to infants with HIV infection has generally been avoided. Nevertheless, severe thrombocytopenia resolved in three infants who were treated with corticosteroids before the diagnosis of HIV infection was made, and no adverse effects were attributable to drug-induced immunosuppression (663). Improvement of lymphoid interstitial pneumonitis has also been described in children given prednisone and intravenous $\gamma$-globulin (710).

### Prevention

Since most cases of HIV acquired in the perinatal period result from exposure to infected mothers, the prevention of AIDS in adults should reduce the risk to infants (711). Counselling services and testing for antibody to HIV should be offered to pregnant women and women who may become pregnant who belong to population groups at high risk for HIV infection. Women identified as being infected with HIV should be advised to postpone pregnancy until more is known about the specific risk factors relating to the vertical transmission of HIV. Infected women who are already pregnant should be informed of the evidence that *in utero* or peripartum transmission is common, that transmission is not preventable, and that transmission appears to carry a high risk of symptomatic disease in the infant. If maternal HIV infection is diagnosed early in the pregnancy, some mothers may choose to terminate the pregnancy by therapeutic abortion. At present, this decision must be made with the knowledge that the information about risks is based upon limited data. If the pregnancy is continued, the current recommendation is to deliver the infant vaginally, assuming that there are no other indications for cesarean delivery. Women with HIV infection should be advised against breastfeeding to avoid postnatal transmission to a child who may have escaped infection *in utero* or at delivery.

Transfusion-related, perinatally acquired AIDS is now of much less concern than vertical transmission of HIV. The current policy of screening all donors and blood products for antibody to HIV and excluding all seropositive donors should eliminate almost all cases of perinatal transfusion-related infection. Nevertheless, careful criteria establishing the indications for the administration of blood products to neonates should be maintained (712).

There is no evidence that infants are at increased risk for household transmission when the infected contact is not the mother or for nosocomial acquisition in neonatal nurseries (685,713,714). General guidelines for daycare and foster care for infants and children with HIV infection have been designed to minimize the risks of exposure of the immunocompromised child to infectious agents and of care givers to potentially infected body fluids (715–717). One foster parent, who had eczema, has acquired infection from an infected infant (605), but transmission to hospital personnel caring for infected infants has not been documented.

## ACKNOWLEDGMENT

This work is supported in part by a NIAID contract NO1-A1-12667, by NICHD program project grant HD10699, and by National Institutes of Health General Clinical Research Center Grant 5-MO1-RR32. The investigations of HSV at Stanford are supported by NICHD R01-16080 and by the Valley Foundation, San Jose, California.

## REFERENCES

1. Charles D, Finland M, eds. *Obstetric and perinatal infections*. Philadelphia: Lea and Febiger, 1973.
2. Krugman S, and Gershon AA, eds. *Infections of the fetus and the newborn infant. vol. 3*. New York: Alan R. Liss, 1975.
3. Monif GRG, ed. *Infectious diseases in obstetrics and gynecology*. New York: Harper and Row, 1974.
4. Remington JS, Klein JO. *Infectious diseases of the fetus and the newborn infant*. 2nd ed. Philadelphia: W.B. Saunders, 1983.
5. Preblud SR, Gross F, Halsey NA. Assessment of susceptibility to measles and rubella. *JAMA* 1982;247:1134.
6. Veale H. History of an epidemic of Rotheln, with observations on its pathology. *Edinburgh Med J* 1866;12:404–14.
7. Gregg NM. Congenital cataract following German measles in the mother. *Trans Ophthalmol Soc Aust (BMA)* 1942;3:35–46.
8. Hess AF. German measles (rubella): an experimental study. *Arch Intern Med* 1914;13:913–6.
9. Hiro Y, Tasaka S. Die Rotheln sind eine Viruskrankheit. *Monatsschr Kinderheilkd* 1938; 76:328–32.
10. Weller TH, Neva FA. Propagation in tissue culture of cytopathic agents from patients with rubella-like illness. *Proc Soc Exp Biol Med* 1962;111:215–25.
11. Parkman PD, Buescher EL, Artenstein, MS. Recovery of rubella virus from army recruits. *Proc Soc Exp Med* 1964;111:225–30.
12. Bardeletti G, Kessler N, Aymard-Henry M. Morphology, biochemical analysis and neuraminidase activity of rubella virus. *Arch Virol* 1975;40:175.
13. Bardeletti G, Tektoff J, Gautheron D. Rubella virus maturation and production in two host cell systems. *Intervirology* 1979;11:97.
14. Best JM, Banatvala JE, Almeida JD, Waterson AP. Morphological characteristics of rubella virus. *Lancet* 1967;2:237.
15. Murphy FA, Halonen PE, Harrison, AK. Electron microscopy of the development of rubella virus in BHK-21 cells. *J Virol* 1968;2:1223.
16. Oshiro LS, Schmidt NJ, Lennette EH. Electron microscopic studies of rubella virus. *J Gen Virol* 1969;5:205.
17. von Bonsdorff CH, Vaheri A. Growth of rubella virus in BHK21 cells: Electron microscopy of morphogenesis. *J Gen Virol* 1969;5:47.
18. Pettersson RF, Oker-Blom C, Kalkkinen N, et al. Molecular and antigenic characteristics and synthesis of rubella virus structural proteins. *Rev Infect Dis* 1985;7:S140–63.
19. Sato M, Maeda N, Shirasuna K, et al. Presence of DNA in rubella variant with DNA polymerase activity. *Arch Virol* 1979;61:251.
20. Sato M, Maeda N, Urade M, et al. Persistent infection of primary human cell cultures with rubella variant carrying DNA polymerase activity. *Arch Virol* 1978;56:181.

21. Sato M, Tanaka H, Yamada T, Yamamoto N. Persistent infection of BHK21/WI-2 cells with rubella virus and characterization of rubella variants. *Arch Virol* 1977;54:333.
22. Sato M, Urade M, Maeda N, et al. Isolation and characterization of a new rubella variant with DNA polymerase activity. *Arch Virol* 1978;59:89.
23. Sato M, Yamada T, Yamamoto K, Yamamoto N. Evidence for hybrid formation between rubella virus and a latent virus of BHK21/WI-2 cells. *Virology* 1976;69:692.
24. Mifune K, Matsuo S. Some properties of temperature-sensitive mutant of rubella virus defective in the induction of interference to Newcastle disease virus. *Virology* 1975;63:278.
25. Norval M. Mechanism of persistence of rubella virus in LLC-MK2 cells. *J Gen Virol* 1979; 43:289.
26. Bardeletti G, Gautheron DC. Phospholipid and cholesterol composition of rubella virus and its host cell BHK21 grown in suspension cultures. *Arch Virol* 1978;52:19.
27. Voiland A, Bardeletti G. Fatty acid composition of rubella virus and BHK21/13S infected cells. *Arch Virol.* 1980;64:319.
28. Parkman PD, Buescher EL, Artenstein MS, McCown JM, Mundon FK, Druzd AD. Studies of rubella. I. Properties of the virus. *J Immunol* 1964;93:595.
29. McCarthy K, Taylor-Robinson CH. Rubella. *Br Med Bull* 1967;23:185.
30. Chagnon A, Laflamme P. Effect of acidity on rubella virus. *Can J Microbiol* 1964;10:501.
31. Fabiyi A, Sever JL, Ratner N, Caplan G. Rubella virus. Growth characteristics and stability of infectious virus and complement-fixing antigen. *Proc Soc Exp Biol Med* 1966;122:392.
32. Herrmann KL. Rubella virus. In: Lennette EH, Schmidt NJ, eds. *Diagnostic procedures for viral, rickettsial and chlamydial infections.* Washington, D.C.: American Public Health Association, 1979:725–66.
33. Cochron KW, Maassab HF. Inhibition of rubella virus by 1-adamantanamine hydrochloride. *Federation Proceedings* 1964;23:387.
34. Oxford JS, Schild GC. *In vitro* inhibition of rubella virus by 1-adamantanamine hydrochloride. *Arch Gesamte Virusforsch* 1965;17:313.
35. Plotkin SA. Inhibition of rubella virus by amantadine. *Arch Gesamte Virusforsch* 1965;16:438.
36. Vaheri A, Hovi T. Structural proteins and subunits of rubella virus. *J Virol* 1972;9:10.
37. Chantler JK. Rubella virus: intracellular polypeptide synthesis. *Virology* 1979;98:275.
38. Liebhaber H, Gross PA. The structural proteins of rubella virus. *Virology* 1972;47:684.
39. Vesikari T. Immune response in rubella infection. *Scand J Infect Dis* 1972;(suppl 4):1.
40. Waxham MN, Wolinsky JS. Immunochemical identification of rubella virus hemagglutinin. *Virology* 1983;126:194.
41. Dorsett PH, Miller DC, Green KY, Byrd FI. Structure and function of the rubella virus proteins *Rev Infect Dis* 1985;7:S150.
42. Fenner F. The classification and nomenclature of viruses. *Intervirology* 1976;6:1.
43. Gould J, Butler M. Differentiation of rubella virus strains by neutralization kinetics. *J Gen Virol* 1980;49:423.
44. Best JM, Banatvala JE. Studies on rubella virus strain variation by kinetic hemagglutination-inhibition tests. *J Gen Virol* 1970;9:215.
45. Fogel A, Plotkin SA. Markers or rubella virus strains in RK13 culture. *J Virol* 1969;3:157.
46. Halonen PE, Ryan JM, Stewart JA. Rubella hemagglutinin prepared with alkaline extraction of virus grown in suspension culture of BHK-21 cells. *Proc Soc Exp Biol Med* 1967; 125:162.
47. Schmidt NJ, Dennis J, Lennette EH. Rubella virus hemagglutination with a wide variety of erythrocyte species. *Appl Environ Microbiol* 1968;16:469.
48. Furukawa T, Plotkin SA, Sedwick WD, Profeta MD. Studies on hemagglutination by rubella virus. *Proc Soc Exp Biol Med* 1967;126:745.
49. Liebhaber H. Measurement of rubella antibody by hemagglutination inhibition. I. Variables affecting rubella hemagglutination. *J Immunol* 1970;104:818.
50. Blom H, Haukenes G. Identification of nonspecific serum inhibitors of rubella virus hemagglutination. *Med Microbiol Immunol* 1974; 159:271.
51. Schmidt NJ, Lennette EH. Rubella complement-fixing antigens derived from the fluid and cellular phases of infected BHK-21 cells: extraction of cell-associated antigen with alkaline buffers. *J Immunol* 1966;97:815.
52. Vaheri A, Vesikari T. Small size rubella virus antigens and soluble immune complexes, analysis by the platelet aggregation technique. *Arch Gesamte Virusforsch* 1971;35:10.
53. LeBouvier GL. Precipitinogens of rubella virus infected cells. *Proc Soc Exp Biol Med* 1969; 130:51.
54. Salmi AA Gel precipitation reactions between alkaline extracted rubella antigens and human sera. *Acta Pathol Microbiol Scand* 1969;76:271.
55. Schmidt NJ, Styk B. Immunodiffusion reactions with rubella antigens. *J Immunol* 1968; 101:210.
56. Penttinen K, Myllyla G. Interaction of human blood platelets, viruses, and antibodies. I. Platelet aggregation test with microequipment. *Ann Med Exp Biol Fenn* 1968;46:188.
57. Birch CJ, Glaun BP, Hunt V, Irving LG, Gust ID. Comparison of passive haemagglutination and haemagglutination-inhibition techniques for detection of antibodies to rubella virus. *J Clin Pathol* 1979;32:128.
58. Kilgore JM. Clinical evaluation of a rubella passive hemagglutination test system. *J Med Virol* 1979;3:231.
59. Meurman OH. Antibody responses in patients with rubella infection determined by passive hemagglutination, hemagglutination inhibition, complement fixation, and solid-phase radioimmunoassay tests. *Infect Immun* 1978;19:369.

60. Gee B, Jordan BE, Mortimer PP. An assessment of radial haemolysis in the detection of rubella antibody. *J Clin Pathol* 1978;31:35.
61. Harnett GB, Palmer CA, Mackay-Scollay EM. Single-radial-hemolysis test for the assay of rubella antibody in antenatal, vaccinated, and rubella virus-infected patients. *J Infect Dis* 1979;140:937.
62. Russell SM, Benjamin SR, Briggs, M, Jenkins M, Mortimer PP, Payne SB. Evaluation of the single radial haemolysis (SRH) technique for rubella antibody measurement. *J Clin Pathol* 1978;31:521.
63. Shafi MS, Jordan SM, Mortimer PP. Experience with radial haemolysis for rubella antibody screening. *J Med Microbiol* 1978;12:131.
64. Meurman OH, Viljanen MK, Granfors K. Solid-phase radioimmunoassay of rubella virus immunoglobulin M antibodies: comparison with sucrose density gradient centrifugation test. *J Clin Microbiol* 1977;5:257.
65. Ogra PL, Kerr-Grant D, Umana G, Dzierba J, Weintraub D. Antibody response in serum and nasopharynx after naturally acquired and vaccine-induced infection with rubella virus. *N Engl J Med* 1971;285:1333.
66. Sugishita C, O'Shea S, Best JM, Banatvala JE. Rubella serology by solid-phase radioimmunoassay: its potential for screening programmes. *Clin Exp Immunol* 1978;31:50.
67. Brown GC, Maassab HF, Veronelli JA, Francis TJ Jr. Rubella antibodies in human serum. Detection by the indirect fluorescent-antibody technic. *Science* 1964;145:943.
68. Cradock-Watson JE, Ridehalgh MKS, Pattison JR, Anderson MJ, Kangro HO. Comparison of immunofluorescence and radioimmunoassay for detecting IgM antibody in infants with the congenital rubella syndrome. *J Hyg (Camb)* 1979;83:413.
69. Cleary TJ, Cid A, Ellis B, et al. A direct enzyme-linked immunosorbent assay (ELISA) for detection of antibodies for rubella virus in human sera. *Res Commun Chem Pathol Pharmacol* 1978;19:281.
70. Caul EO, Hobbs SJ, Roberts PC, Clarke SKR. Evaluation of a simplified sucrose gradient method for the detection of rubella-specific IgM in routine diagnostic practice *J Med Virol* 1978;2:153.
71. Frisch-Niggemeyer W. Rapid separation of immunoglobulin M from immunoglobulin G antibodies for reliable diagnosis of recent rubella infections. *J Clin Microbiol* 1975;2:377.
72. Halonen P, Meurman O, Matikainen M-T, Torfason E, Bennich H. IgA antibody response in acute rubella determined by solid-phase radioimmunoassay. *J Hyg (Camb)* 1979;83:69.
73. Kangro HO, Pattison JR, Heath RB. The detection of rubella-specific IgM antibodies by radioimmunoassay. *Br J Exp Pathol* 1978;59:577.
74. Leinikki PO, Shekarchi I, Dorsett P, Sever JL. Determination of virus-specific IgM antibodies by using ELISA: Elimination of false-positive results with protein A-sepharose absorption and subsequent IgM antibody assay. *J Lab Clin Med* 1978;92:849.
75. Pattison JR, Jackson CM, Hiscock JA. Cradock-Watson JE, Ridehalgh KS. Comparison of methods for detecting specific IgM antibody in infants with congenital rubella. *J Med Microbiol* 1978;11:411.
76. Vejtorp M, Fanoe E, Leerhoy J. Diagnosis of postnatal rubella by the enzyme-linked immunosorbent assay for rubella IgM and IgG antibodies. *Acta Pathol Microbiol Scand* 1979; 87:155.
77. Parkman PD, Meyer HM, Kirschstein RL, Hopps HE. Attenuated rubella virus. I. Development and laboratory characterization. *N Engl J Med* 1966;275:569.
78. Desmyter J, DeSomer P, Rawls WE, Melnick JL. The mechanism of rubella virus interference. In: *International Symposium on Rubella Viruses* New York: S. Karger. 1969:139–48.
79. Kleiman MB, Carver DH. Failure of the RA 27/3 strain of rubella virus to induce intrinsic interference. *J Gen Virol* 1977;36:335.
80. Marcus PI, Carver DH. Hemadsorption-negative plaque test: New assay for rubella virus revealing a unique interference. *Science* 1965; 149:983.
81. Marcus PI, Carver DH. Intrinsic interference: A new type of viral interference. *J Virol* 1967;1:334.
82. Wong KT, Baron S, Ward TG. Rubella virus: role of interferon during infection of African green monkey kidney tissue cultures. *J Immunol* 1967;99:1140.
83. Fabiyi A, Gitnick GL, Sever JL. Chronic rubella virus infection in the ferret (*Mustela putorius fero*) puppy. *Proc Soc Exp Biol Med* 1967;125:766.
84. Horstmann DM. Rubella: the challenge of its control. *J Infect Dis* 1971;123:640–54.
85. Weller TH, Alford CA Jr, Neva FA. Changing epidemiologic concepts of rubella, with particular reference to unique characteristics of the congenital infection. *Yale J Biol Med* 1965; 37:455–72.
86. Carne S, Dewhurst CJ, Hurley R. Rubella epidemic in a maternity unit. *Br Med J* 1973;1:444.
87. McLaughlin MC, Gold LH. The New York rubella incident: a case for changing hospital policy regarding rubella testing and immunization. *Am J Public Health* 1979;79:287.
88. Polk BF, White JA, DeGirolami PC, Modlin JF. An outbreak of rubella among hospital personnel. *N Engl J Med* 1980;303:541.
89. Gremillion DH, Gengler RE, Lathrop GD. Epidemic rubella in military recruits. *South Med J* 1978;71:932.
90. Horstmann DM. Rubella and the rubella syndrome. New epidemiologic and virologic observations. *Calif Med* 1965;102:397.
91. Horstmann DM, Liebhaber H, LeBouvier GL, Rosenberg DA, Halstead SB. Rubella. Reinfection of vaccinated and naturally immune persons exposed in an epidemic. *N Engl J Med* 1970;283:771.

92. Wilkins J, Leedom JM, Portnoy B, Salvatore MA. Reinfection with rubella virus despite live vaccine-induced immunity. *Am J Dis Child.* 1969;118:275.
93. Bader H, Bonin P. Rubella in Seattle–King County Washington. *Am J Public Health* 1977; 67:1087.
94. Strassburg MA, Stephenson TG, Habel LA, Fannin SL. Rubella in hospital employees. *Infect Control* 1984;5:123.
95. Dowdle WR, Ferreira W, Gomes LFD, et al. WHO collaborative study on the sero-epidemiology of rubella in Caribbean and Middle and South American populations in 1968. *Bull WHO* 1970;42:419–22.
96. Rawls, WE, Melnick JL, Bradstreet CMP, et al. WHO collaborative study on the sero-epidemiology of rubella. *Bull WHO* 1967;37:79–88.
97. Cooper LZ. Rubella. A preventable cause of birth defects. In: Bergsma D, ed. *Birth defects original articles series,* vol. 4, no. 23. New York: National Foundation-March of Dimes, 1978.
98. Green RH, Balsame MR, Giles JP, Krugman S, Mirick GS. Studies of the natural history and prevention of rubella. *Am J Dis Child* 1965;110:348.
99. Krugman S, Katz SL. Rubella (German measles). In: Krugman S, Katz SL, eds. *Infectious diseases of children.* 7th ed. St. Louis: C.V. Mosby Company, 1981:315–31.
100. Sever JL, Brody JA, Schiff GM, McAlister R, Cutting R. Rubella epidemic on St. Paul Island in the Pribilofs, 1963. II. Clinical and laboratory findings for the intensive study population. *JAMA* 1965;191:88.
101. Alford CA, Neva FA, Weller TH. Virologic and serologic studies on human products of conception after maternal rubella. *N Engl J Med* 1964;271:125.
102. Hildebrandt HM, Maassab HF. Rubella synovitis in a 1-year-old patient. *N Engl J Med* 1966;274:1428.
103. Heggie AD. Pathogenesis of the rubella exanthem. Isolation of rubella virus from the skin. *N Engl J Med* 1971;285:664–6.
104. Waxham MN, Wolinsky JS. Rubella virus and its effects on the central nervous system. *Neurol Clin* 1984;2:367.
105. Enders G, Knotek F, Pacher U. Comparison of various serological methods and diagnostic kits for the detection of acute, recent, and previous rubella infection, vaccination, and congenital infections. *J Med Virol* 1985;16:219.
106. Forsgren M. Standardization of techniques and reagents for the study of rubella antibody. *Rev Infect Dis* 1985;7:S129.
107. Horstmann DM. Serologic responses after primary infection and after reinfection with rubella virus. In: Friedman H, Prier JE, eds. *Rubella.* Springfield: Charles C Thomas, 1973:84–93.
108. Lennette EH, Schmidt NJ. Neutralization fluorescent antibody and complement fixation tests for rubella. In: Friedman H, Prier JE, eds. *Rubella.* Springfield: Charles C Thomas. 1973:18–32.
109. Lerman SJ, Nankervis GA, Heggie AD, Gold E. Immunologic response, virus excretion, and joint reactions with rubella vaccine. A study of adolescent girls and young women given live attenuated virus vaccine (HPV-77:DE-5). *Ann Intern Med* 1971;74:67.
110. Bidwell D, Chantler SM, Morgan-Capner P, Pattison JR. Further investigation of the specificity and sensitivity of ELISA for rubella antibody screening. *J Clin Pathol* 1980;33:200.
111. Morgan-Capner P, Pullen HJM, Pattison JR, Bidwell DE, Bartlett A, Voller A. A comparison of three tests for rubella antibody screening. *J Clin Pathol* 1979;32:542.
112. Vejtorp M. Enzyme-linked immunosorbent assay for determination of rubella IgG antibodies. *Acta Pathol Microbiol Scand* 1978;86:387.
113. Deibel R, D'Areangelio D, Ducharme CP, and Schryner GD. Assay of rubella antibody by passive hemagglutination and by a modified indirect immunofluorescent test. *Infection* 1980;8 (suppl 3):5255.
114. Cappel R, Schluederberg A, Horstmann DM. Large scale production of rubella precipitinogens and their use in the diagnostic laboratory. *J Clin Microbiol* 1975;1:201.
115. Deibel R, D'Areangelis D, Ducharme CP, Schryner GD. Assay of rubella antibody by passive hemagglutination and by a modified indirect immunofluorescent test. *Infection* 1980;8(suppl 3):S255.
116. Pattison JR, Mace JE. Elution patterns of rubella IgM, IgA, and IgG antibodies from a dextran and an agarose gel. *J Clin Pathol* 1975;28:670.
117. Best JM, Palmer SJ, Morgan-Capner P, Hodgson J. A comparison of Rubazyme-M and MACRIA for the detection of rubella-specific IgM. *J Virol Methods* 1984;8:99.
118. Chernesky MA, Wyman L, Mahony JB, et al. Clinical evaluation of the sensitivity and specificity of a commercially available enzyme immunoassay for detection of rubella virus-specific immunoglobulin M. *J Clin Microbiol* 1984;20:400.
119. Gerna I, Zannino M, Revello MG, Petruzzelli E, Dovis M. Development and evaluation of a capture enzyme-linked immunosorbent assay for determination of rubella immunoglobulin M using monoclonal antibodies. *J Clin Microbiol* 1987;25:1033.
120. Ho-Terry L, Cohen A. Radioimmunoassay for antibodies to rubella virus and its ribonucleoprotein component. *J Med Microbiol* 1979;12:441.
121. Pattison JR, Dane DS, Mace JE. The persistence of specific IgM after natural infection with rubella virus. *Lancet* 1975;1:185.
122. McDonald H, Tobin JOH, Cradock-Watson JE, Lomax J, Bourne MS. Antibody titers in women six to eight years after the administration of RA27/3 and Cendehill rubella vaccines. *J Hyg (Camb)* 1978;80:337.

123. Hornsleth A, Leerhoy J, Grauballe P, Spang-gaard H. Persistence of rubellavirus-specific immunoglobulin M and immunoglobulin A antibodies: Investigation of successive serum samples with lowered immunoglobulin G concentration. *Infect Immun* 1975;11:804.
124. McMorrow L, Vesikari T, Wolman SR, Giles JP, Cooper LZ. Suppression of response of lymphocytes to phytohemagglutinin in rubella. *J Infect Dis* 1974;130:464.
125. Rossier E, Phipps PH, Polley JR, Webb T. Absence of cell-mediated immunity to rubella virus 5 years after rubella vaccination. *Can Med Assoc J* 1977;116:481.
126. Smith KA, Chess L, Mardiney MR Jr. The relationship between rubella hemagglutination inhibitin antibody (HIA) and rubella induced *in vitro* lymphocyte titrated thymidine incorporation. *Cell Immunol* 1973;8:321.
127. Buimovici-Klein E, Cooper LZ. Cell-mediated immune response in rubella infections. *Rev Infect Dis* 1985;7:S123.
128. Bouimovici-Klein E, Weiss KE, Cooper LZ. Interferon production in lymphocyte cultures after rubella infection in humans. *J Infect Dis* 1977;135:380.
129. Honeyman MC, Forrest JM, Dorman DC. Cell-mediated immune response following natural rubella and rubella vaccination. *Clin Exp Immunol* 1974;17:665.
130. Kanra GY, Vesikari T. Cytotoxic activity against rubella-infected cells in the supernatants of human lymphocyte cultures stimulated by rubella virus. *Clin Exp Immunol* 1975;19:17.
131. Vesikari T, Kanra TY, Buimovici-Klein E, Cooper LZ. Cell-mediated immunity in rubella assayed by cytotoxicity of supernatants from rubella virus-stimulated human lymphocyte cultures. *Clin Exp Immunol* 1975;19:33.
132. Steele RW, Hensen SA, Vincent MM, Fuccillo DA, and Bellanti JA. Development of specific cellular and humoral immune responses in children immunized with liver rubella virus vaccine. *J Infect Dis* 1974;130:449.
133. Ganguly R, Cusumano CL, Waldman RH. Suppression of cell-mediated immunity after infection with attenuated rubella virus. *Infect Immun* 1976;13:464.
134. Ogra PL, Kerr-Grant D, Umana G, Dzierba J, Weintraub D. Antibody response in serum and nasopharynx after naturally acquired and vaccine-induced infection with rubella virus. *N Engl J Med* 1971;285:1333.
135. Harcourt GC, Best JM, Banatvala JE. Rubella-specific serum and nasopharyngeal antibodies in volunteers with naturally acquired and vaccine-induced immunity after intranasal challenge. *J Infect Dis* 1980;142:145.
136. Morag A, Morag B, Bernstein JM, Beutner K, Ogra PL. In vitro correlates of cell-mediated immunity in human tonsils after natural or induced rubella virus infection. *J Infect Dis* 1975;131:409.
137. Alford CA Jr. Congenital rubella: a view of the virologic and serologic phenomena occurring after maternal rubella in the first trimester. *South Med J* 1966;59:745.
138. Krugman S. Rubella symposium. *Am J Dis Child* 1965;110:345–476.
139. Rudolph AJ, Yow MD, Phillips A, Desmond MM, Blattner RJ, and Melnick JL. Transplacental rubella infection in newly born infants. *JAMA* 1965;191:843.
140. Catalano LW Jr, Fuccillo DA, Traub R, Sever JL. Isolation of rubella virus from placentas and throat cultures of infants. A prospective study after the 1964–65 epidemic. *Obstet Gynecol* 1971;38:6.
141. Desmond MM, Wilson GS, Melnick JL, et al. Congenital rubella encephalitis. *J Pediatr* 1967;71:311.
142. Menser MA, Harley JD, Herzberg R, Dorman DC, Murphy AM. Persistence of virus in lens for three years after prenatal rubella. *Lancet* 1967;2:387.
143. Cradock-Watson JE, Ridehalgh MKS, Anderson MJ, Pattison JR. Outcome of asymptomatic infection with rubella virus during pregnancy. *J Hyg (Camb)* 1981;87:147–54.
144. Miller E, Cradock-Watson JE, Pollock TM. Consequences of confirmed maternal rubella at successive stages of pregnancy. *Lancet* 1982; 2:781–4.
145. Grillner L, Forsgren M, Barr B, Bottiger M, Danielsson L, De Verdier C. Outcome of rubella during pregnancy with special reference to the 17th-24th weeks of gestation. *Scand J Infect Dis* 1983;15:321.
146. Munro ND, Sheppard S, Smithells RW, Holzel H, Jones G. Temporal relations between maternal rubella and congenital defects. *Lancet* 1987;2:201.
147. Terry GM, Ho-Terry L, Warren RC, Rodeck CH, Cohen A, Rees KR. First trimester prenatal diagnosis of congenital rubella: a laboratory investigation. *Br Med J* 1986;292:930.
148. Alford CA Jr. Immunoglobulin determinations in the diagnosis of fetal infection. *Pediatr Clin N Am* 1971;18:99.
149. Alford CA Jr. Studies on antibody in congenital rubella infections. I. Physicochemical and immunologic investigations of rubella-neutralizing antibody. *Am J Dis Child* 1965;110:455.
150. Alford CA Jr, Blankenship WJ, Straumfjord JV, Cassady G. The diagnostic significance of IgM-globulin elevations in newborn infants with chronic intrauterine infections. In: Bergsma D, ed. *Birth Defects—original article series*, vol. 4 no. 5. New York: National Foundation-March of Dimes, 1968.
151. Gitlin D. The differentiation and maturation of specific immune mechanisms. *Acta Paediatr Scand* [*Suppl*] 1967;172:60.
152. Gitlin D, Biasucci A. Development of gamma G, gamma A, beta, IC-beta IA, CI esterase inhibitor, ceruloplasmin, transferrin, hemopexin, haptoglobin, fibrinogen, plasminogen, alpha 1-antitrypsin, orosomucoid, beta-lipoprotein, alpha 2-macroglobulin, and prealbumin in the human conceptus. *J Clin Invest* 1969;48:1433.

153. Lawton AR, Self KS, Royal SA, Cooper MD. Ontogeny of lymphocytes in the human fetus. *Clin Immunol Immunopathol* 1972;1:104.
154. Morgan-Capner P, Rodeck CH, Nicolaides KH, Cradock-Watson JE. Prenatal detection of rubella-specific IgM in fetal sera. *Prenat Diagn* 1985;5:21.
155. Daffos F, Forestier F, Grangeot-Keros L, Pavlovsky MC. Gradual appearance of total IgM in fetal serum during the second trimester of pregnancy. Application to the prenatal diagnosis of fetal infections [Letter]. *Ann Biol Clin (Paris)* 1984;42:135.
156. Enders G, Jonatha W. Prenatal diagnosis of intrauterine rubella. *Infection* 1987;15:162.
157. Cradock-Watson JE, Ridehalgh MKS, Chantler S. Specific immunoglobulin in infants with the congenital rubella syndrome. *J Hyg (Camb)* 1976;76:109.
158. Vesikari T, Vaheri A, Pettay O, Kunnas M. Congenital rubella: Immune response of the neonate and diagnosis by demonstration of specific IgM antibodies. *J Pediatr* 1969;75:658.
159. Alford CA Jr. Fetal antibody in the diagnosis of chronic intra-uterine infections. In: Thalhammer O, ed. *Prenatal Infections*. Stuttgart: Georg Thieme Verlag, 1971:53–69.
160. de Mazancourt A, Waxham MN, Nicolas JC, Wolinsky JS. Antibody response to the rubella virus structural proteins in infants with the congenital rubella syndrome. *J Med Virol* 1986;19:111.
161. Cooper MD, Dayton DH. *Development of host defenses*. New York: Raven Press, 1977.
162. Miller ME. *Host defenses in the human neonate (Monographs in Neonatology)*. New York: Grune and Stratton, 1978.
163. Berry CL, Thompson EN. Clinicopathological study of thymic dysplasia. *Arch Dis Child* 1968;43:579.
164. Buimovici-Klein E, Lang PB, Ziring PR, Cooper LZ. Impaired cell-mediated immune response in patients with congenital rubella: correlation with gestational age at time of infection. *Pediatrics* 1979;64:620.
165. Fuccillo DA, Steele RW, Hensen SA, Vincent MM, Hardy JB, and Bellanti JA. Impaired cellular immunity to rubella virus in congenital rubella. *Infect Immun* 1974;9:81.
166. Alford CA Jr. Production of interferon-like substance by the rubella-infected human conceptus. Program and Abstracts, American Pediatric Society and Society of Pediatric Research Meeting, Atlantic City, April 29–May 2, 1970, p. 203.
167. Lebon P, Daffos F, Checoury A, Grangeot-Keros L, Forestier F, Toublanc JE. Presence of an acid-labile alpha-interferon in sera from fetuses and children with congenital rubella. *J Clin Microbiol* 1985;21:775–8.
168. Alford CA, Griffiths PD. Rubella. In: Remington JS, Klein JO, eds. *Infectious diseases of the fetus and newborn infant*. 2nd ed. Philadelphia: W.B. Saunders Co., 1983;69–103.
169. Cooper LZ. Congenital rubella in the United States. In: Krugman S, Gershon AA, eds. *Infections of the fetus and the newborn infant* New York: Alan R. Liss, 1975:1–22.
170. Peckham CS. Clinical and laboratory study of children exposed in utero to maternal rubella. *Arch Dis Child* 1972;47:571.
171. Sheridan MD. Final report of a prospective study of children whose mothers had rubella in early pregnancy. *Br Med J* 1964;2:536.
172. Desmond ME, Fisher ES, Vorderman AL, et al. The longitudinal course of congenital rubella encephalitis in nonretarded children. *J Pediatr* 1978;93:584.
173. Sever JL, South MA, Shaver K. *Delayed manifestations of congenital rubella. Rev Infect Dis* 1985;7:S164.
174. Rossi M, Ferlito A, Plidoro F. Maternal rubella and hearing impairment in children. *J Laryngol Otol* 1981;94:281.
175. Weinberger MM, Maslund MW, Asbed R, Sever JL. Congenital rubella presenting as retarded language development. *Am J Dis Child* 1970;120:125.
176. Hanid TK. Hypothyroidism in congenital rubella. *Lancet* 1976;2:854.
177. Menser MA, Forrest JM, Bransby RD. Rubella infection and diabetes mellitus. *Lancet* 1978; 1:57.
178. Preece MA, Kearney PJ, Marshall WC. Growth hormone deficiency in congenital rubella. *Lancet* 1977;2:842.
179. Rayfield EJ, Seto Y. Viruses and the pathogenesis of diabetes mellitus. *Diabetes* 1978;27:1126.
180. Cremer NE, Oshiro LS, Weil ML, Lennette EH, Itabashi HH, Carnay L. Isolation of rubella virus from brain in chronic progressive panencephalitis. *J Gen Virol* 1975;29:143.
181. Vandvik B, Weil ML, Grandien M, Norrby E. Progressive rubella virus panencephalitis synthesis of oligoclonal virus-specific IgG antibodies and homogeneous free light chains in the central nervous system. *Acta Neurol Scand* 1978;57:53.
182. Wolinsky JS, Berg BO, Maitland CJ. Progressive rubella panencephalitis. *Arch Neurol* 1976;33:722.
183. Centers for Disease Control. Rubella surveillance. January, 1976–December, 1978. 1980.
184. Krugman S. *Proceedings of the International Conference on Rubella Immunization, Am J Dis Child* 1969;118.
185. Meyer HM, Hopps HE, Parkman PD. Appraisal and reappraisal of viral vaccines. *Adv Int Med* 1980;25:533.
186. Centers for Disease Control. Rubella prevention. *MMWR* 1981;30:37.
187. Committee on Infectious Diseases. Rubella. In: Klein JO, ed. *Report of the Committee on Infectious Diseases*. Evanston, Illinois: American Academy of Pediatrics, 1982:231–5.
188. Modlin JF, Brandling-Bennett AD, Witte JJ, Campbell CC, Meyers JD. A review of five years' experience with rubella vaccine in the United States. *Pediatrics* 1975;55:20.
189. Krugman S. Rubella immunization: present sta-

tus and future perspectives. *Pediatrics* 1980; 65:1174.
190. Schwarz AJF, Jackson JR, Ehrenkranz NJ, Ventura A, Schiff GM, Walters VW. Clinical evaluation of a new measles-mumps-rubella trivalent vaccine. *Am J Dis Child* 1975;129: 1403.
191. Weibel RE, Buynak EB, McLean AA, Hilleman MR. Long-term follow-up for immunity after monovalent or combined live measles, mumps, and rubella virus vaccines. *Pediatrics* 1975;56:380.
192. Bart KJ, Orenstein WA, Preblud SR, Hinman AR, Lewis FL, Williams NM. Elimination of rubella and congenital rubella from the United States. *Pediatr Infect Dis* 1985;4:14.
193. Meyer HM Jr, Parkman PD, Panos T. Attenuated rubella virus. II. Production of an experimental live-virus vaccine and clinical trial. *N Engl J Med* 1966;275:575.
194. Ingalls TH, Plotkin SA, Pilbrook FR, Thompson RF. Immunization of school children with rubella (RA 27/3) vaccine. *Lancet* 1970;1:99.
195. Plotkin SA, Farquhar JD, Ogra PL. Immunologic properties of RA 27/3 rubella virus vaccine. A comparison with strains presently licensed in the United States. *JAMA* 1973; 225:585.
196. Weibel RE, Stokes J, Buynak EB, Hilleman MR. Influence of age on clinical response to HPV-77 duck rubella vaccine. *JAMA* 1972; 222:805.
197. Spruance SL, Klock LE, Bailey A, Ward JR, and Smith CB. Recurrent joint symptoms in children vaccinated with HPV-77:DK-12 rubella vaccine. *J Pediatr* 1972;80:413.
198. Thompson GR, Weiss JJ, Eloise MI, Shillis JL, Brockett RG. Intermittent arthritis following rubella vaccination: a 3-year follow-up. *Am J Dis Child* 1973;125:526.
199. Tingle AJ, Chantler JK, Pot KH, Paty DW, Ford DK. Postpartum rubella immunization: association with development of prolonged arthritis, neurological sequelae, and chronic rubella viremia. *J Infect Dis* 1985;152:606.
200. Schaffner W, Fleet WF, Kilroy AW, Lefkowitz LB, Herrmann KL, Thompson J, Karzn DT. Polyneuropathy following rubella immunization. A follow-up study and review of the problem. *Am J Dis Child* 1974;127:684.
201. Spruance SL, Metcalf R, Smith CB, Griffiths MM, Ward JR. Chronic arthropathy associated with rubella vaccination. *Arthritis Rheum* 1977; 20:741.
202. Meyer HM, Parkman PD. Rubella vaccination: a review of practical experience. *JAMA* 1971; 215:613.
203. Fleet WF, Shaffner W, Lefkowitz KB, Murphy GD, Karzon DT. Exposure of susceptible teachers to rubella virus. *Am J Dis Child* 1972;123:28.
204. Halstead SB, Diwan AR. Failure to transmit rubella virus vaccine: a close contact study in adults *JAMA* 1971;215:634.
205. Plotkin JA, Farquhar JD, Katz M. Attenuation of RA 27/3 rubella virus with WI-38 human diploid cells. *Am J Dis Child* 1969;118:78.
206. Scott HD, Byrnes EB. Exposure of susceptible pregnant women to rubella vaccines: serologic findings during the Rhode Island immunization campaign. *JAMA* 1971;215:609.
207. Swidi S, Naficy K. Subcutaneous and intranasal administration of RA 27/3, alone and in conjunction with live attenuated measles vaccines. *Am J Dis Child* 1969;118:2092.
208. Wilkins J, Leedom JM, Salvatore MA, Portnoy B. Transmission of rubella vaccine virus from vaccines to contacts. *Calif Med* 1971;115:16.
209. Banatvala JE, Best JM, O'Shea S, Harcourt GC. Rubella immunity gap: is intranasal vaccination the answer? *Lancet* 1979;i:970.
210. Philbrook RF, Ingalls TH. Risk of contact infection after intranasal rubella vaccination. *Lancet* 1980;i:147.
211. Taylor-Robinson CH, Mallinson H. Risk of contact infection after intranasal rubella vaccination. *Lancet* 1979;ii:1128.
212. Modlin JF, Herrmann KL, Brandling-Bennett AD, Eddins DL, Hayden GF. Risk of congenital abnormality after inadvertent rubella vaccination of pregnant women. *N Engl J Med* 1976;294:972.
213. Phillips CA, Maeck JVS, Rogers WA, Savel H. Intrauterine rubella infection following immunization with rubella vaccine. *JAMA* 1970; 213:624.
214. Vaheri A, Vesikari T, Oker-Blom N, et al. Transmission of attenuated rubella vaccines to the human fetus. A preliminary report. *Am J Dis Child* 1969;118:243.
215. Rubella vaccination during pregnancy—United States, 1971–1986. *MMWR* 1987;36:457–61.
216. Preblud SR, Williams NM. Fetal risk associated with rubella vaccine: implications for vaccination of susceptible women. *Obstet Gynecol* 1985;66:121.
217. Shlian DM. Screening and immunization of rubella-susceptible women: Experience in a large, prepaid medical group. *JAMA* 1978;240:662.
218. Meyer HM Jr, Parkman PD, Hobbins TE, et al. Attenuated rubella viruses. Laboratory and clinical characteristics. *Am J Dis Child* 1969;118:155.
219. Schmidt NJ, Lennette EH. Complement-fixing and fluorescent antibody responses to an attenuated rubella virus vaccine. *Am J Epidemiol* 1970;91:351.
220. Balfour HH, Groth KE, Edelman CK. RA 27/3 rubella vaccine: a four-year follow-up. *Am J Dis Child* 1980;134:350.
221. Black FL, Lamm SH, Emmons JE, Pinheiro FP. Durability of antibody titers induced by RA 27/3 rubella virus vaccine. *J Infect Dis* 1978;137:322.
222. Grillner L. Neutralizing antibodies after rubella vaccination of newly delivered women: a comparison between three vaccines. *Scand J Infect Dis* 1975;7:169.
223. Grillner L. Immunity to intranasal challenge with rubella virus two years after vaccination:

comparison of three vaccines. *J Infect Dis* 1976;133:637.
224. Heigl Z, Wasserman J, Forsgren M. *In vitro* lymphocyte reactivity to rubella antigen following vaccination. *Scand J Infect Dis* 1980;12:13.
225. LeBouvier GL, Plotkin SA. Precipitin responses to rubella vaccine RA 27/3. *J Infect Dis* 1971;123:220.
226. Liebhaber H, Ingalls TH, LeBouvier GL, Horstmann DM. Vaccination with RA 27/3 rubella vaccine. *Am J Dis Child* 1972;123:133.
227. Van Rooyen CE, Ozere RL, Perlin I, Faulkner RS. A trial of rubella RA 27/3 vaccine. *Can J Public Health* 1977;68:375.
228. Abrutyn E, Herrman KL, Karchmer AW, Friedman JP, Page E, White JJ. Rubella vaccine comparative study. Nine-month follow-up and serologic response to natural challenge *Am J Dis Child* 1970;120:129.
229. Brody JA. The infectiousness of rubella and the possibility of reinfection. *Am J Public Health* 1966;56:1082.
230. Balfour HH Jr, Amren DP. Rubella vaccine (HPV77 DE5 strain) fails to sustain antibody titres. *Lancet* 1977;2:1130.
231. Boué A, Nicholas A, Montagnon C. Reinfection with rubella in pregnant women. *Lancet* 1971;2:1251.
232. Eilard T, Strannegard O. Rubella reinfection in pregnancy followed by transmission to the fetus. *J Infect Dis* 1974;129:594.
233. Forsgren M, Carlstrom G, Strangert K. Congenital rubella after maternal reinfection. *Scand J Infect Dis* 1979;11:81.
234. Haukenes G, Haram KO. Clinical rubella after reinfection. *N Engl J Med* 1970;287:1204.
235. Northrop RL, Gardner WM, Geittman WF. Rubella reinfection during early pregnancy. *Obstet Gynecol* 1972;39:524.
236. Snijder JAM, Schroder FF, Hoekstra JH. Importance of IgM determination in cord blood in cases of suspected rubella infection. *Br Med J* 1977;1:23.
237. Forsgren M, Soren L. Subclinical rubella reinfection in vaccinated women with rubella-specific IgM response during pregnancy *Scand J Infect Dis* 1985;17:337.
238. Morgan-Capner P, Hodgson J, Hambling MH, et al. Detection of rubella specific IgM in subclinical reinfection in pregnancy. *Lancet* 1985;1:244.
239. Balfour HH Jr, Amren DP. Rubella, measles and mumps antibodies following vaccination of children. *Am J Dis Child* 1978;132:573.
240. Gringras M. Follow-up study of rubella vaccination in general practice. *Br Med J* 1980; 280:18.
241. Hough JC, Walker RB, Brough JW. Rubella seroconversion following immunization in a rural practice. *J Fam Pract* 1979;9:587.
244. Lawless MR, Abramson JS, Harlan JE, Kelsey DS. Rubella susceptibility in sixth graders: effectiveness of current immunization practice. *Pediatrics* 1980;65:1086.
245. Lawless MR, Abramson JS, Harlan JE, Kelsey DS. Rubella susceptibility in sixth graders: effectiveness of current immunization practice. *Pediatrics* 1980;65:1086.
246. Raugh JL, Schiff GM, Johnson LB. Follow-up studies of rubella vaccines at adolescence. *J Pediatr* 1975;86:13.
247. Herrmann KL, Halstead SB, Brandling-Bennett AD, Witte JJ, Wiebenga NH, Eddins, DL. Rubella immunization. Persistence of antibody four years after a large-scale field trial. *JAMA* 1976;235:2201.
248. Hillary IB, Griffith AH. Persistence of antibody 10 years after vaccination with Wistar RA 27/3 strain live attenuated rubella vaccine. *Br Med J* 1980;2:1580.
249. Just M, Berger-Hernandez R, Burgin-Wolff A. Serum antibodies 9 years after Cendehill rubella immunization. *Lancet* 1977;2:1349.
250. Schiff GM, Raug JL, Rotte T. Rubella vaccine evaluation in a public school system. *Am J Dis Child* 1969;118:203.
251. Fulginiti VA. Controversies in current immunization policy and practices: one physician's viewpoint. *Curr Prob Pediatr* 1976;6:3.
252. Siegel M. Unresolved issues in the first five years of the rubella immunization program. *Am J Obstet Gynecol* 1976;124:327.
253. Klock LE, Rachelefsky GS. Failure of rubella herd immunity during an epidemic. *N Engl J Med* 1973;288:69.
254. Dudgeon JA. Measles and rubella vaccines. *Arch Dis Child* 1977;52:907.
255. Clarke M, Boustred J, Schild GC, et al. Effect of rubella vaccination programme on serological status of young adults in United Kingdom. *Lancet* 1979;1:1224.
256. Goldwater PH, Quiney JR, Banatvala JE. Maternal rubella at St. Thomas' hospital: Is there a need to change British vaccination policy? *Lancet* 1978;2:1298.
257. Peckham CS, Marshall WC, Dudgeon JA. Rubella vaccination of schoolgirls: factors affecting vaccine uptake. *Br Med J* 1977;1:760.
258. Dudgeon JA. Selective immunization: protection of the individual. *Rev Infect Dis* 1985;7:S185.
259. Brody JA, Sever JL, Schiff GM. Prevention of rubella by gamma globulin during an epidemic in Barrow, Alaska, in 1964. *N Engl J Med* 1965;272:127.
260. Schiff GM, Sever JL, Huebner RJ. Rubella virus. Neutralizing antibody in commercial gamma globulin *Science* 1963;142:58.
261. Urquhart GED, Crawford RJ, Wallace J. Trial of high-titre human rubella immunoglobulin. *Br Med J* 1978;2:1331.
262. Plotkin SA, Klaus RM, Whitely JA. Hypogammaglobulinemia in an infant with congenital rubella syndrome: failure of 1-adamantanamine to stop virus excretion. *J Pediatr* 1966;69:1085.
263. Weller TH. The cytomegaloviruses: ubiquitous agents with protein clinical manifestations. *N Engl J Med* 1971;285:203–4, 267–74.
264. Smith JD, de Harven E. Herpes simplex virus

and human cytomegalovirus replication in WI-38 cells: I. Sequence of viral replication. *J Virol* 1973;12:919–30.
265. Wright HT, Jr, Goodheart CR, Lielausis A. Human cytomegalovirus. Morphology by negative staining. *Virology* 1964;23:419–24.
266. Sarov I, Abady I. The morphogenesis of human cytomegalovirus. Isolation and polypeptide characterization of cytomegalovirus and dense bodies. *Virology* 1975;66:464–473.
267. Stinski MF. Human cytomegalovirus: glycoproteins associated with virions and dense bodies. *J Virol* 1976;19:594–609.
268. Stinski MF. Synthesis of proteins and glycoproteins in cells infected with human cytomegalovirus. *J Virol* 1977;23:751–67.
269. DeMarchi JM, Blankenship ML, Brown GD, Kaplan AS. Size and complexity of human cytomegalovirus DNA. *Virology* 1978;89:643–6.
270. Geelen JLMC, Walig C, Wertheim P, Vander NJ. Human cytomegalovirus DNA. I. Molecular weight and infectivity. *J Virol* 1978;26:813–6.
271. Kilpatrick BA, Huang ES. Human cytomegalovirus genome: partial denaturation map and organization of genome sequences. *J Virol* 1977;24:261–76.
272. LeFemina RL, Hayward GS. Structural organization of the DNA molecules from human cytomegalovirus. In: Jarrisch R, Fields, BN, Fox CF, eds. *Animal virus genetics*. New York: Academic Press, 1980.
273. Gibson W. Protein counterparts of human and simian cytomegaloviruses. *Virology* 1983; 128:391–406.
274. Roizman B, Furlong D. The replication of herpesviruses. In: Fraenkel-Conrat H, Wagner RR, eds. *Comprehensive Virology, vol. 3*. New York: Plenum Press, 1974;229–403.
275. Smith JD, de Harven E. Herpes simplex virus and human cytomegalovirus replication in WI-38 cells. II. An ultrastructural study of viral penetration. *J Virol* 1974;14:945–56.
276. DeMarchi JM, Schmidt CA, Kaplan AS. Patterns of transcription of human cytomegalovirus in permissively infected cells. *J Virol* 1980;35:277–86.
277. Wather MW, Stinski MF. Temporal patterns of human cytomegalovirus transcription: mapping of the viral RNAs synthesized at immediate early, early and late times after infection. *J Virol* 1982;41:462–77.
278. Stinski MF. Sequence of protein synthesis in cells infected with human cytomegalovirus: early and late virus-induced polypeptides. *J Virol* 1978;26:686–701.
279. McAllister RM, Straw RM, Filbert JE, Goodheart CR. Human cytomegalovirus. Cytochemical observations of intranuclear lesion development correlated with viral synthesis and release. *Virology* 1963;19:521.
280. Stinski MF, Thomson DR, Steinberg RM, Goldstein LC. Organization and expression of the immediate early genes of human cytomegalovirus. *J Virol.* 1983;456:1–14.
281. Stinski MF, Thomson DR, Wathen MW. Structure and function of the cytomegalovirus genome. In: Nahmias A, Dowdle A, Schinazi R, eds. *The human herpesviruses*. New York: Elsevier Press, 1981:72–84.
282. Chou S, Merrigan T. Rapid detection and quantitation of human cytomegalovirus in urine through DNA hybridization. *N Engl J Med* 1983;308:921–25.
283. Schuster V, Matz B, Wiegand H, Traub B, Kampa D, Neumann-Haefelin D. Detection of human cytomegalovirus in urine by DNA-DNA and RNA-DNA hybridization. *J Infect Dis* 1986;154:309.
284. Buffone GJ, Schimborg CM, Demmler GJ, Wilson DR, and Darlington GJ. Detection of cytomegalovirus in urine by nonisotopic DNA hybridization. *J Infect Dis* 1986;154:163.
285. Spector SA, Rua JA, Spector DH, and McMilland R. Detection of human cytomegalovirus in clinical specimens by DNA-DNA hybridization. *J Infect Dis* 1984;150:121.
286. Reynolds DW, Stagno S, Alford CA. Laboratory diagnosis of cytomegalovirus infections. In: Lennette EH, Schmidt NJ, eds. *Diagnostic procedures for viral, rickettsial and chlamydial infections*. Washington, D.C.: American Public Health Association, 1979:399–439.
287. Gleavens CA, Smith TF, Shuster EA, Pearson GR. Comparison of standard tube and shell vial cell culture techniques for the detection of cytomegalovirus in clinical specimens. *J Clin Microbiol* 1985;21:217.
288. Kanich RE, Craighead JE. Human cytomegalovirus infection of cultured fibroblasts: II. viral replicative sequence of a wild and an adapted strain. *Lab Invest* 1972;27:273–82.
289. Stagno S, Pass RF, Reynolds DW, Alford CA. Diagnosis of cytomegalovirus infections. In: Nahmias A, Dowdle W, Schinazi R, eds. *The human herpesvirus*. New York: Elsevier Press, 1981:363–73.
290. Pereria L, Hoffman M, Cremer N. Electrophoretic analysis of polypeptides immune precipitated from cytomegalovirus-infected cell extracts by human sera. *Infect Immun.* 1982; 36:933–42.
291. Spencer ES. Clinical aspects of cytomegalovirus infection in kidney-graft recipients. *Scand J Infect Dis* 1974;6:315–23.
292. Waner JL, Weller TH, Kevy SV. Patterns of cytomegalovirus complement-fixing antibody activity: a longitudinal study of blood donors. *J Infect Dis* 1973;127:538–43.
293. Stagno S, Reynolds DW, Tsiantos A, Fuccillo DA, Long W, Alford CA. Comparative serial virologic and serologic studies of symptomatic and subclinical congenitally and natally acquired cytomegalovirus infections. *J Infect Dis* 1975;132:568–77.
294. Furukawa T, Hornberger E, Sakuma S, Plotkin SA. Demonstration of immunoglobulin G receptors induced by human cytomegalovirus. *J Clin Microbiol* 1975;2:332–6.
295. Keller R, Peitchel R, Goldman JN. An Fc re-

ceptor induced in cytomegalovirus-infected human fibroblasts. *J Immunol* 1976;116:772–7.
296. Rahman AA, Teschner M, Sethi KK, Brandis H. Appearance of IgG (Fc) receptor(s) on cultured human fibroblasts infected with human cytomegalovirus. *J Immunol* 1976;117:253–8.
297. Westmoreland D, St. Jeor S, Rapp F. The development of cytomegalovirus-infected cells of binding affinity for normal human immunoglobulin. *J Immunol* 1976;116:1566–70.
298. Rawls WE, Campione-Piccardo J. Epidemiology of herpes simplex virus type 1 and type 2 infections. In: Nahmias A, Dowdle W, Schinazi R, eds. *The human herpesviruses: an interdisciplinary perspective.* New York: Elsevier North Holland, 1981:137.
299. Reeves WC, Corey L, Adams HG, Vontver LA, Holmes KK. Risk of recurrence after first episodes of genital herpes: relation to HSV type and antibody response. *N Engl J Med* 1981;305:315.
300. Jordan MC, Rousseau WE, Noble GR, Stewart JA. Chin TDY. Association of cervical cytomegalovirus with venereal disease. *N Engl J Med* 1973;288:932–4.
301. Yeager AS. Improved indirect hemagglutination test for cytomegalovirus using human 0 erythrocytes in lysine. *J Clin Microbiol* 1979;10:64–8.
302. Griffiths PD, Stagno S, Pass RF, Smith RJ, Alford CA. Infection with cytomegalovirus during pregnancy: Specific IgM antibodies as a marker of recent primary infection *J Infect Dis* 1982;145:647–53.
303. Pass RF, Griffiths PD, August AM. Antibody response to cytomegalovirus after renal transplantation: comparison of patients with primary and recurrent infections. *J Infect Dis* 1983;147:40–6.
304. Yolken RH, Stopa PJ. Comparison of seven enzyme immunoassay systems for measurement of cytomegalovirus. *J Clin Microbiol* 1980;11:546–51.
305. Huang ES, Kilpatrick BA, Huang YT, Pagano JS. Detection of human cytomegalovirus and analysis of strain variation. *Yale J Biol Med* 1976;49:29.
306. Huang ES, Alford CA, Reynolds DW, Stagno S, Pass RF. Molecular epidemiology of cytomegalovirus infection in women and their infants. *N Engl J Med* 1980;303:958–62.
307. Lang DJ. The epidemiology of cytomegalovirus infections: Interpretations of recent observations. In: Krugman S, Gershon AA, eds. *Infections of the fetus and the newborn infant, vol. 3.* New York: Alan R. Liss, 1975:35–45.
308. Hayes K, Danks DM, Gibas H, Jack I. Cytomegalovirus in human milk. *N Engl J Med* 1972;287:177–8.
309. Lang DJ, Krummer JF. Cytomegalovirus in semen: observations in selected populations. *J Infect Dis* 1975;132:472–3.
310. Reynolds DW, Stagno S, Hosty TS, Tiller M, Alford CA, Jr. Maternal cytomegalovirus excretion and perinatal infection. *N Engl J Med* 1973;289:1–5.
311. Stagno S, Reynolds DW, Pass RF, Alford CA. Breast milk and the risk of cytomegalovirus infection. *N Engl J Med* 1979;302:1073–6.
312. Kumar ML, Nankervis GA, Gold E. Inapparent congenital cytomegalovirus infection: a follow-up study. *N Engl J Med* 1973;288:1370–2.
313. Klemola E, von Essen R, Wager O. Cytomegalovirus mononucleosis in previously healthy individuals. *Ann Intern Med* 1969;71:11–19.
314. Stagno S, Reynolds D, Tsiantos A, Fuccillo DA, Smith R, Tiller M, Alford CA Jr. Cervical cytomegalovirus excretion in pregnant and nonpregnant women: suppression in early gestation. *J Infect Dis* 1975;131:522–7.
315. Gold E, Nankervis GA. Cytomegalovirus. In: Evans AS, ed. *Viral infections of humans epidemiology and control.* New York: Plenum Medical Book Company, 1982;167–86.
316. Alford CA, Stagno S, Pass RF, Huang ES. Epidemiology of cytomegalovirus. In: Nahmias A, Dowdle W, Schinazi R, eds. *The human herpesviruses: an interdisciplinary perspective.* New York: Elsevier Press, 1981:159–171.
317. Stagno S, Pass RF, Dworsky ME, Alford CA. Maternal cytomegalovirus infection and perinatal transmission. In: Knox GE, ed. *Clinical obstetrics and gynecology.* Philadelphia: Lippincott Co., 1982:563–76.
318. Stagno S, Pass RF, Dworsky ME, et al. Congenital cytomegalovirus infection: the relative importance of primary and recurrent maternal infection. *N Engl J Med* 1982;306:945–9.
319. Montgomery R, Youngblood L, Medearis DN Jr. Recovery of cytomegalovirus from the cervix in pregnancy. *Pediatrics* 1972;49:524–31.
320. Handsfield HH, Chandler SH, Caine VA, et al. Cytomegalovirus infection in sex partners: evidence for sexual transmission. *J Infect Dis* 1985;151:344.
321. Drew WL, Mintz L, Miner RC, Sands M, Ketterer B. Prevalence of cytomegalovirus infection in homosexual men. *J Infect Dis* 1981;143:188–92.
322. Pass RF, August AM, Dworsky ME, Reynolds DW. Cytomegalovirus infection in a day care center. *Pediatr Res* 1982;16:248A.
323. Chandler SH, Alexander ER, Holmes KK. Epidemiology of cytomegaloviral infection in a heterogeneous population of pregnant women. *J Infect Dis* 1985;152:249.
324. Knox GE, Pass RF, Reynolds DW, Stagno S, Alford CA. Comparative prevalence of subclinical cytomegalovirus and herpes simplex virus infections in the genital and urinary tracts of low income, urban females. *J Infect Dis* 1979;140:419–22.
325. Yow MD, White NH, Taber LH, Frank AL, Gruber WC, May RA, Norton HJ. Acquisition of cytomegalovirus infection from birth to 10 years: a longitudinal serologic study. *J Pediatr* 1987;110:37
326. Pass RF, Hutto C, Reynolds DW, Polhill RB.

Increased frequency of cytomegalovirus infection in children in group day care. *Pediatrics* 1984;74:121.
327. Pass RF, Kinney JS. Child care workers and children with congenital cytomegalovirus infection. *Pediatrics* 1985;75:971.
328. Hutto C, Ricks R, Garvie M, Pass RF. Epidemiology of cytomegalovirus infections in young children: day care vs. home care. *Pediatr Infect Dis* 1985;4:149.
329. Dworsky M, Lakeman A, Stagno S. Cytomegalovirus transmission within a family. *Pediatr Infect Dis* 1984;3:236.
330. Blackman JA, Murph JR, Bale JF Jr. Risk of cytomegalovirus infection among educators and health care personnel serving disabled children. *Pediatr Infect Dis J* 1987;6:725.
331. Dworsky ME, Welch K, Cassady G, Stagno S. Occupational risk for primary cytomegalovirus infection among pediatric health-care workers. *N Engl J Med* 1983;309:950.
332. Yow MD, Lakeman AD, Stagno S, Reynolds RB, Plavidal FJ. Use of restriction enzymes to investigate the source of a primary cytomegalovirus infection in a pediatric nurse. *Pediatrics* 1982;70:713.
333. Wilfert CM, Eng-Shang H, Stagno S. Restriction endonuclease analysis of cytomegalovirus deoxyribonucleic acid as an epidemiologic tool. *Pediatrics* 1982;70:717.
334. Plotkin SA. Cytomegalovirus in hospitals. *Pediatr Infect Dis* 1986;5:177.
335. Adler SP. Nosocomial transmission of cytomegalovirus. *Pediatr Infect Dis* 1986;5:239.
336. Adler SP, Baggett J, Wilson M, Lawrence L, McVoy M. Molecular epidemiology of cytomegalovirus in a nursery: lack of evidence for nosocomial transmission. *J Pediatr* 1986;108:117.
337. Demmler GJ, Yow MD, Spector SA, Reis SG, Brady MT, Anderson DC, Tabler LH. Nosocomial cytomegalovirus infections within two hospitals caring for infants and children. *J Infect Dis* 1987;156:9.
338. Hutto C, Little EA, Ricks R, Lee JD, Pass RF. Isolation of cytomegalovirus from toys and hands in a day care center. *J Infect Dis* 1986;154:527.
339. Schupfer PC, Murph JR, Bale JF. Survival of cytomegalovirus in paper diapers and saliva. *Pediatr Infect Dis* 1986;5:677.
340. Adler SP. Molecular epidemiology of cytomegalovirus: evidence for viral transmission to parents from children infected at a day care center. *Pediatr Infect Dis* 1986;3:315.
341. Pass RF, Hutto C, Ricks R, Cloud GA. Increased rate of cytomegalovirus infection among parents of children attending day-care centers. *N Engl J Med* 1986;314:1414.
342. Taber LH, Frank AL, Yow MD, Bagley A. Acquisition of cytomegaloviral infections in families with young children: a serologic study. *J Infect Dis* 1985;151:948.
343. Adler SP. The molecular epidemiology of cytomegalovirus transmission among children attending a day care center. *J Infect Dis* 1985;152:760.
344. Murph JR, Bale JF Jr, Murray JC, Stinski MF, Perlman S. Cytomegalovirus transmission in a Midwest day care center: possible relationship to child care practices. *J. Pediatr* 1986;109:35.
345. Grillner L, Strangert K. Restriction endonuclease analysis of cytomegalovirus DNA from strains isolated in day care centers. *Pediatr Infect Dis* 1986;5:184.
346. Jones LA, Duke-Duncan PM, Yeager AS. Cytomegaloviral infections in infant-toddler centers: centers for the developmentally delayed versus regular day care. *J Infect Dis* 1985;151:953.
347. Jordan MC, Rousseau WE, Stewart JA, Noble GR, Chin TDY. Spontaneous cytomegalovirus mononucleosis. *Ann Intern Med* 1973;79:153–60.
348. Klemola E. Cytomegalovirus infection in previously healthy adults. *Ann Intern Med* 1973; 79:267–8.
349. Lang DJ, Hanshaw JB. Cytomegalovirus infection and the postperfusion syndrome: recognition of primary infections in four patients. *N Engl J Med* 1969;280:1145–9.
350. Dent DM, Duys PJ, Bird AR, Birkenstock WE. Cytomegalic virus infection of bowel in adults. *S Afr Med J* 1975;49:669–72.
351. Duchowny M, Caplan L, Siber G. Cytomegalovirus infection of adult nervous system. *Ann Neurol.* 1979;5:458–61.
352. Hanshaw JB, Betts RF, Simon G, Boynton RC. Acquired cytomegalovirus infection. *N Engl J Med* 1965;272:602–9.
353. Horwitz CA, Burke D, Grimes P, Tombers J. Hepatic function in mononucleosis induced by Epstein-Barr virus and cytomegalovirus. *Clin Chem* 1980;26:243–6.
354. Kabins S, Keller R, Peitchel R, Ali MA. Acute and idiopathic polyneuritis caused by cytomegalovirus. *Arch Intern Med* 1976;136:100–1.
355. Schmitz H, Enders G. Cytomegalovirus as a frequent cause of Guillian-Barre syndrome. *J Med Virol* 1977;1:21–7.
356. Spiegel JS, Schwabe AD. Disseminated cytomegalovirus infection with gastrointestinal involvement. *Am J Gastroenterol* 1980;73:37–44.
357. Stern H. Isolation of cytomegalovirus and clinical manifestations of infection. *Br Med J* 1968;1:665–9.
358. Rinaldo CR Jr, Black PH, Hirsch MS. Virus-leukocyte interactions in cytomegalovirus mononucleosis. *J Infect Dis* 1977;136:667–78.
359. Carney WP, Hirsch MS. Mechanisms of immunosuppression in cytomegalovirus mononucleosis. II. Virus-monocyte interactions. *J Infect Dis* 1981;144:47–54.
360. Fiala M, Payne JE, Berne TV, et al. Epidemiology of cytomegalovirus infection after transplantation and immunosuppression. *J Infect Dis* 1975;132:421–33.
361. Garrett HM. Isolation of human cytomegalovirus from peripheral blood T cells of renal transplant patients. *J Lab Clin Med* 1982;99:92–7.

362. Rinaldo CR Jr, Carney WP, Richter BS, Black PH, Hirsch MS. Mechanisms of immunosuppression in cytomegalovirus mononucleosis. *J Infect Dis* 1980;141:488–95.
363. Demmler GJ, O'Neil GW, O'Neil JH, Spector SA, Brady MT, Yow MD. Transmission of cytomegalovirus from husband to wife. *J Infect Dis* 1986;154:545–6.
364. Horwitz CA, Henle W, Henle G. Diagnostic aspects of the cytomegalovirus mononucleosis syndrome in previously healthy persons. *Postgrad Med* 1979;66:153–8.
365. Ahlfors K, Forsgren M, Ivarsson S-A, Harris S, Svanberg L. Congenital cytomegalovirus infection: on the relation between type and time of maternal infection and infant's symptoms. *Scand J Infect Dis* 1983;15:129–38.
366. Andersen HK. Complement-fixing and virus-neutralizing antibodies in cytomegalovirus infection as measured against homologous and heterologous antigen. *Acta Pathol Microbiol Scand* 1970;78:504–8.
367. Spencer ES, Andersen HK. The development of immunofluorescent antibodies as compared with complement-fixing and virus-neutralizing antibodies in human cytomegalovirus infection. *Scand J Infect Dis* 1972;4:109–12.
368. Levin MJ, Rinaldo CR Jr, Leary PL, Zaia JA, Hirsch MS. Immune response to herpes virus antigens in adults with acute cytomegalovirus mononucleosis. *J Infect Dis* 1979;140:851–7.
369. Carney WP, Iacoviello V, Hirsch MS. Functional properties of T lymphocytes and their subsets in cytomegalovirus mononucleosis. *J Immunol* 1983;130:390–3.
370. Carney WP, Rubin RH, Hoffman RA, Hansen WP, Healey K, Hirsch MS. Analysis of T lymphocyte subsets in cytomegalovirus mononucleosis. *J Immunol* 1981;126:2114–6.
371. Rinaldo CR Jr, Stossel TP, Black PH, Hirsch MS. Leukocyte function during cytomegalovirus mononucleosis. *Clin Immunol Immunopathol* 1979;12:331–4.
372. Schooley RT, Hirsch MS, Colvin RB, et al. Association of herpesgroup virus infections with T-lymphocyte subset alterations, glomerulopathy, and opportunistic infections following renal transplantation. *N Engl J Med* 1983;308:307–13.
373. Numazaki Y, Yano N, Morizuka T, Takai S, Ishida N. Primary infection with human cytomegalovirus: virus isolation from healthy infants and pregnant women. *Am J Epidemiol* 1970;91:410–7.
374. Stern H, Tucker SM. Prospective study of cytomegalovirus infection in pregnancy. *Br Med J* 1973;2:268–70.
375. Ahlfors K, Forsgren M, Ivarsson SA, Harris S, Svanberg L. Congenital cytomegalovirus infection: on the relation between type and time of maternal infection and infant's symptoms. *Scand J Infect Dis* 1983;15:129–38.
376. Grant S, Edmond E, Syme J. A prospective study of cytomegalovirus infection in pregnancy: I. Laboratory evidence of congenital infection following maternal primary and reactivated infection. *J Infect* 1981;3:24–31.
377. Griffiths PD, Campbell-Benzie A. A prospective study of cytomegalovirus infection in pregnant women. *Br J Obstet Gynaecol* 1980;87:308.
378. Dworsky M, Welch K, Stagno S, Cassady G. Occupational risk of seroconversion to cytomegalovirus (CMV) [Abstract]. *Pediatr Res* 1983;17:268A.
379. Alford CA, Stagno S, Pass RF. Natural history of perinatal cytomegaloviral infection. In: *Perinatal Infections*. Amsterdam: Excerpta Medica. 1980:125–47.
380. Chandler SH, Handsfield HH, McDougall J. Isolation of multiple strains of cytomegalovirus from women attending a clinic for sexually transmitted disease. *J Infect Dis* 1987;155:655.
381. Spector SA. Systemic infection with multiple strains of cytomegalovirus assessed by restriction enzyme digestion analyses. *Pediatr Res* 1982;16:1383.
382. Stagno S, Pass RF, Cloud G, et al. Incidence, transmission to fetus, and clinical outcome. *JAMA* 1986;256:1904.
383. Hayes K, Gibas H. Placental cytomegalovirus infection without fetal involvement following primary infection in pregnancy. *J Pediatr* 1971;79:401–5.
384. Kumar ML, Gold E, Jacobs IB, Ernhart CB, Nankervis GA. Primary cytomegalovirus infection in adolescent pregnancy. *Pediatrics* 1984;74:493.
385. Pass RF, Little EA, Stagno S, Britt WJ, Alford CA. Young children as a probable source of maternal and congenital cytomegalovirus infection. *N Engl J Med* 1987;316:1366.
386. Stagno S, Reynolds DW, Huang E-S, Thames SD, Smith RJ, Alford CA Jr. Congenital cytomegalovirus infection—occurrence in an immune population. *N Engl J Med* 1977;396:1254–8.
387. Ahlfors K, Harris S, Ivarsson S, Svanberg L. Secondary maternal cytomegalovirus infection causing symptomatic congenital infection. *N Engl J Med* 1973;305:284.
388. Benirschke K, Mendoza GR, Bazeley PL. Placental and fetal manifestations of cytomegalovirus infection. *Virchows Arch [Zellpathol]* 1974;16:121–39.
389. Thomas IT, Soothill JF, Hawkins GT, Marshall WC. *Lancet* 1977;2:1056.
390. Griffiths PD, Stagno S, Pass RF, Smith RJ, Alford CA. Congenital cytomegalovirus infection: diagnostic and prognostic significance of the detection of specific IgM antibodies in cord serum. *Pediatrics* 1982;69:544–9.
391. Hanshaw JB, Stanfield HJ, White CJ. Fluorescent-antibody test for cytomegalovirus macroglobulin. *N Engl J Med* 1968;279:566–70.
392. Pass RF, Stagno S, Myers GJ, Alford CA. Outcome of symptomatic congenital CMV infection: results of long-term longitudinal follow-up. *Pediatrics* 1980;66:758–62.
393. Stagno S, Pass RF, Reynolds DW, Moore M, Nahmias AJ, Alford CA. Comparative study of

diagnostic procedures for congenital cytomegalovirus infection. *Pediatrics* 1980;65:251–7.

392. Pass RF, Stagno S, Dworsky ME, Smith RJ, Alford CA. Excretion of cytomegalovirus in mothers. *J Infect Dis* 1982;146:1–6.
393. Reynolds DW, Stagno S, Stubbs KG, et al. Inapparent congenital cytomegalovirus infection with elevated cord IgM levels. *N Engl J Med* 1974;290:291–6.
396. Stagno S, Volanakis JE, Reynolds DW, Stroud R, Alford CA. Immune complexes in congenital and natal CMV infections of man. *J Clin Invest* 1977;60:838–45.
397. Stagno S, Volanakis J, Reynolds DW, Stroud R, Alford CA. Virus-host interactions in perinatally acquired cytomegalovirus infections of man: Comparative studies on antigenic load and immune complex formation. In: Cooper MD, Dayton DJ, eds. *Development of host diseases*. New York: Raven Press, 1977:237–50.
398. Hanshaw JB. Congenital cytomegalovirus infection: a fifteen year perspective. *J Infect Dis* 1971;123:555–61.
399. Melish ME, Hanshaw JB. Congenital cytomegalovirus infection: developmental progress of infants detected by routine screening. *Am J Dis Child* 1973;126:190–4.
400. Starr JG, Bart RD Jr, Gold E. Inapparent congenital cytomegalovirus infection: clinical and epidemiologic characteristics in early infancy. *N Engl J Med* 1970;282:1075–8.
401. McCracken GH Jr, Shinefield HR, Cobb K, Rausen AR, Dische R, Eichenwald HF. Congenital cytomegalic inclusion disease: longitudinal study of 20 patients. *Am J Dis Child* 1969;117:522–39.
402. Weller TH, Hanshaw JB. Virologic and clinical observations on cytomegalic inclusion disease. *N Engl J Med* 1962;266:1233–44.
403. Hanshaw JB. Developmental abnormalities associated with congenital cytomegalovirus infection. *Adv Teratol* 1970;4:64–93.
404. Conboy TJ, Pass RF, Stagno S, et al. Early clinical manifestations and intellectual outcome in children with symptomatic congenital cytomegalovirus infection. *J Pediatr* 1987;111:343–8.
405. Stagno S, Reynolds DW, Amos CS, Dahle AJ, McCollister FP, Mohindra I, Ermocilla R, Alford CA Jr. Auditory and visual defects resulting from symptomatic and subclinical congenital cytomegaloviral and toxoplasma infections. *Pediatrics* 1977;59:669–78.
406. Conboy TJ, Pass RF, Stagno S, Britt WJ, Alford CA, McFarland CE, Boll TJ. Intellectual development in school-aged children with asymptomatic congenital cytomegalovirus infection. *Pediatrics* 1986;77:801.
407. Kumar ML, Nankervis GA, Jacobs IB, Ernhart CB, Glasson CE, McMillan PM, Gold E. Congenital and postnatally acquired cytomegalovirus infections: long-term follow-up. *J Pediatr* 1984;104:674.
408. Stagno S, Pass RF, Thomas JP, Navia JM, Dworsky ME. Defects of tooth structure in congenital cytomegalovirus infection. *Pediatrics* 1982;69:646–8.
409. Dworsky M, Yow MD, Stagno S, Pass RF, Alford C. Cytomegalovirus infection of breast milk and transmission in infancy. *Pediatrics* 1983;72:295.
410. Stagno S, Brasfield DM, Brown MB, et al. Infant pneumonitis associated with cytomegalovirus, chlamydia, pneumocystis, and urea-plasma—a prospective study. *Pediatrics* 1981;68:322–9.
411. Kumar ML, Nankervis GA, Cooper AR, Gold E. Postnatally acquired cytomegalovirus infections in infants of CMV-excreting mothers. *J Pediatr* 1984;104:669.
412. Yeager AS, Grumet FC, Hafleigh EB, Arvin AM, Bradley JS, Prober CG. Prevention of transfusion-acquired cytomegalovirus infections in newborn infants. *J Pediatr* 1981;988:281–7.
413. Yeager AS, Palumbo PE, Malachowski N, Ariagno RL, Stevenson DK. Sequelae of maternally derived cytomegalovirus infections in premature infants. *J Pediatr* 1983;102:918.
414. Ballard RA, Drew WL, Hufnagle KG, Riedel PA. Acquired cytomegalovirus infection in preterm infants. *Am J Dis Child* 1979;133:482–5.
415. Hanshaw JB. Congenital cytomegalovirus infection: laboratory methods of detection. *J Pediatr* 1969;75:1179–85.
416. Stagno S, Tinker MK, Elrod C, Fuccillo DA, Cloud G, O'Beirne AJ. Immunoglobulin M antibodies detected by enzyme-linked immunosorbent assay and radioimmunoassay in the diagnosis of cytomegalovirus infections in pregnant women and newborn infants. *J Clin Microbiol* 1985;21:930.
417. Demmler GJ, Six HR, Hurst SM, Yow MD. Enzyme-linked immunosorbent assay for the detection of IgM-class antibodies to cytomegalovirus. *J Infect Dis* 1986;153:1152.
418. Ahlfors K, Forsgren M, Griffiths P, Nielsen CM. Comparison of four serological tests for the detection of specific immunoglobulin M in cord sera of infants congenitally infected with cytomegalovirus. *Scand J Infect Dis* 1987;19:303.
419. Gehrz RC, Knorr SO, Marker SC, Kalalis JM, Balfour HH Jr. Specific cell-mediated immune defect in active cytomegalovirus infection of young children and their mothers. *Lancet* 1977;2:844–7.
420. Pass RF, Stagno S, Britt WJ, Alford CA. Specific cell mediated immunity and the natural history of congenital infection with cytomegalovirus. *J Infect Dis* 1986;147:40–6.
421. Reynolds DW, Dean PH, Pass RF, Alford CA. Specific cell-mediated immunity in children with congenital and neonatal cytomegalovirus infection and their mothers. *J Infect Dis* 1979;140:493–9.
422. Starr SE, Tolpin MD, Friedman HM, Paucker K, Plotkin SA. Impaired cellular immunity to cytomegalovirus in congenitally infected children and their mothers. *J Infect Dis* 1979; 140:500–5.

423. Plotkin SA, Friedman HM, Starr SE, Arbeter AM, Furukawa T, Fleisher GR. Prevention and treatment of cytomegalovirus infection. In: Nahmias A, Dowdle W, Schinazi R, eds. *The human herpesviruses: an interdisciplinary perspective*. New York: Elsevier, 1981:403–413.
424. Editorial comments. Congenital cytomegalovirus infection—more problems. *Lancet* 1974;1:845–6.
425. Elck SD, Stern H. Development of a vaccine against mental retardation caused by cytomegalovirus infection *in utero*. *Lancet* 1974;1:1–4.
426. Just M, Burgin-Wolff A, Emodi G, Hernandez R. Immunization trials with live attenuated cytomegalovirus Towne 125. *Infection* 1975;3:111–4.
427. Neff BJ, Weibel RE, Buynak EB, McLean AA, Hilleman MR. Clinical and laboratory studies of live cytomegalovirus vaccine AD 169. *Proc Soc Exp Biol Med* 1979;160:32–7.
428. Plotkin SA, Farquhar J, Hornberger E. Clinical trials of immunization with the Towne 125 strain of human cytomegalovirus. *J Infect Dis* 1976;134:470–5.
429. Plotkin SA, Furukawa T, Zygraich N, Huygelen C. Candidate cytomegalovirus strain for human vaccination. *Infect Immun* 1975;12:521–7.
430. Plotkin SA, Huang E-S. Cytomegalovirus vaccine virus (Towne strain) does not induce latency. *J Infect Dis* 1985;152:395.
431. Plotkin SA. Personal communications, 1983.
432. Editorial comments. Cytomegalovirus in adults. *Lancet* 1977;2:541.
433. Marx JL. Cytomegalovirus: a major cause of birth defects. *Science* 1975;190:1184–6.
434. McDougall JK, Harnden DG. Vaccination against cytomegalovirus? *Lancet* 1974;1:135–6.
435. Pagano JS, Huang ES. Vaccination against cytomegalovirus? [Letter to the editor] *Lancet* 1974;1:316–7.
436. Albrecht T, Rapp F. Malignant transformation of hamster embryo fibroblasts following exposure to ultraviolet-irradiated human cytomegalovirus. *Virology* 1973;55:53–61.
437. St. Jeor SC, Albrecht TB, Funk FD, Rapp F. Stimulation of cellular DNA synthesis by human cytomegalovirus. *J Virol* 1974;13:353–362.
438. Lang DJ. Cytomegalovirus immunization: status, prospects, and problems. *Rev Infect Dis* 1980;2:449–58.
439. Alford CA, Stagno S, Reynolds DW, Dahle A, Amos C, Saxon S. Long-term mental and perceptual defects associated with silent intrauterine infections. In: Gluck L, ed. *Intrauterine asphyxia and the developing fetal brain*. Chicago: Year Book, 1977:377–93.
440. Plotkin SA, Weibel RE, Alpert G, et al. Resistance of seropositive volunteers to subcutaneous challenge with low-passage human cytomegalovirus *J Infect Dis* 1985;151:737.
441. Stern H. Live cytomegalovirus vaccination of healthy volunteers: eight-year follow-up studies. *Birth Defects* 1984;20:263.
442. Meyers JD, Lexzczynski J, Zaia JA, et al. Successful prevention of cytomegalovirus infection after marrow transplant with cytomegalovirus immune globulin. *Ann Intern Med* 1983;98:442–6.
443. Hersman J, Meyers JD, Thomas ED, Buckner CD, Clift R. The effect of granulocyte transfusions upon the incidence of cytomegalovirus infection after allogenic marrow transplantation. *Ann Intern Med* 1982;96:149–52.
444. Brady MT, Anderson DC, Milam JD, Hawkins EP, Yow MD, Speer ME, Seavy DE. Prevention of posttransfusion cytomegalovirus infection (PTCMV) in neonates by the use of frozen-washed red blood cells (FWRBC). *Pediatr Res* 1983;17:50A.
445. Tolkoff-Rubin N, Rubin RH, Keller EW, Baker GP, Stewart JA, Hirsch MS. Cytomegalovirus infection among dialysis patients and personnel. *Ann Intern Med* 1978;89:625–8.
446. Taylor BJ, Jacobs RF, Baker RL, Moses EB, McSwain BE, Shulman G. Frozen deglycerolyzed blood prevents transfusion-acquired cytomegalovirus infections in neonates. *Pediatr Infect Dis* 1986;5:188.
447. Demmler GJ, Brady MT, Bijou H, Speer ME, Milam JD, Hawkins EP, Anderson DC, Six H, Yow MD. Posttransfusion cytomegalovirus infection in neonates: role of saline-washed red blood cells. *J Pediatr* 1986;108:762.
448. Emodi G, Just M. Impaired interferon response of children with congenital cytomegalovirus disease. *Acta Paediatr Scand* 1974;63:183–7.
448. Falcoff E, Falcoff R, Foumier F, Chany C. Production en masse, purification partielle et caractérisation d'un interféron destiné a des essais thérapeutiques humains. *Ann Inst Pasteur (Paris)* 1966;111:562–84.
450. Glasgow LA, Hanshaw JB, Merigan TC, Petralli JK. Interferon and cytomegalovirus *in vivo* and *in vitro*. *Proc Soc Exp Biol Med* 1967;125:843–9.
451. Arvin AM, Yeager AS, Merigan TC. Effect of leukocyte interferon on urinary excretion of cytomegalovirus by infants. In: Merigan TC, ed. *Antivirals with clinical potential*. Chicago: University of Chicago Press, 1976:205–10.
452. Emodi G, O'Reilly R, Muller A, Everson LK, Binswanger U, Just M. Effect of human exogenous leukocyte interferon in cytomegalovirus infections. *J Infect Dis* 1976;133:A199–204.
453. Alford CA Jr. Summary of parenteral use of adenine arabinoside. In: Pavan-Langston D, Buchanan RA, Alford CA, eds. *Adenine arabinoside: an antiviral agent*. New York: Raven Press, 1975:287–91.
454. Baublis JV, Whitley RJ, Ch'ien LT, Alford CA Jr. Treatment of cytomegalovirus infection in infants and adults. In: Pavan-Langston D, Buchanan RA, Alford CA, eds. *Adenine arabinoside: an antiviral agent*. New York: Raven Press, 1975:247–60.
455. Ch'ien LT, Cannon NJ, Whitley RJ, et al. Effect of adenine arabinoside on cytomegalovirus infections. *J Infect Dis* 1974;130:32–9.
456. Conchie AF, Barton BW, Tobin JO. Congenital cytomegalovirus infection treated with idoxuridine. *Br Med J* 1968;4:162–3.

457. Emodi G, Sartorius J, Just M, Rohner F, Buhler U. Virus studies in the treatment of congenital cytomegalovirus infections by cytosine arabinoside. *Helv Pediatr Acta* 1972;27:557–64.
458. Kraybill EN, Sever JL, Avery GB, Movassaghi N. Experimental use of cytosine arabinoside in congenital cytomegalovirus infection. *J Pediatr* 1972;80:485–7.
459. Plotkin SA, Starr SE, Bryan CK. *In vitro* and *in vivo* responses at cytomegalovirus to acyclovir. *Am J Med* 1982;73:257–61.
460. McCracken GH Jr, Luby JP. Cytosine arabinoside in the treatment of congenital cytomegalic inclusion disease. *J Pediatr* 1972;80:488–95.
461. Plotkin SA, Starr SE, Bryan CK. *In vitro* and *in vivo* responses of cytomegalovirus to acyclovir. *Am J Med* 1982;73:257–61.
462. Plotkin SA, Stetler H. Treatment of congenital cytomegalic inclusion disease with antiviral agents. *Antimicrob Agents Chemother.* 1969;372–9.
463. Rytel MW, Aaberg TM, Dee TH, Heim LH. *Cell Immunol* 1975;19:8.
464. Whitley RJ, Ch'ien LT, Buchanan RA, Alford CA Jr. Studies on adenine arabinoside—a model for antiviral chemotherapeutics. In: Pollard M, ed. *Antiviral mechanisms—perspectives in virology, vol. 9.* New York: Academic Press, 1975;315–36.
465. Yeager AS. Use of acyclovir in premature and term neonates. *Am J Med* 1982;73:205–9.
466. Mettler C, ed. *History of medicine* Philadelphia: Blakiston, 1947:356.
467. Astruck J, ed. (1736): *De morbis venereis libri sex.* Paris: G. Cavelier, 1736:61–98.
468. Lipschutz B. Untersuchungen uber die Aetiologie der Krankheiten der Herpesgruppe (Herpes zoster, Herpes genitalis, Herpes febriles). *Arch Derm Syph* 1921;136:428–82.
469. Nahmias AJ, Dowdle W. Antigenic and biologic differences in *Herpesvirus hominis. Prog Med Virol* 1968;10:110–59.
470. Buchman T, Roizman B, Nahmias A. Demonstration of exogenous genital reinfection with herpes simplex virus type 2 by restriction endonuclease fingerprinting of viral DNA. *J Infect Dis* 1979;140:195.
471. Buchman TG, Roizman B, Nahmias AJ. Structure of herpes simplex virus DNA and application to molecular epidemiology. *Ann NY Acad Sci* 1980;354:279.
472. Halperin SA, Hendley JO, Nosal C, Roizman B. DNA fingerprinting in investigation of apparent nosocomial acquisition of neonatal herpes simplex. *J Pediatr* 1980;97:91.
473. Hass M. Hepato-adrenal necrosis with intranuclear inclusion bodies: report of a case. *Am J Pathol* 1935;11:127–42.
474. Batignani A. Conjunctivite da virus erpetico in neonato. *Bull Ocul* 1934;13:1217–20.
475. Nahmias A, Roizman B. Herpes simplex viruses. *N Engl J Med* 1973;289:667–74, 719–25, 781–9.
476. Nahmias AJ, Josey WE. Epidemiology of herpes simplex viruses 1 and 2. In: Evans A, ed. *Viral infections of humans. 2nd ed.* New York: Plenum Press, 1989:351.
477. Nahmias AJ, Josey WE, Naib ZM, Luce CR, Duffey A. Antibodies to *Herpesvirus hominis* types 1 and 2 in humans. I. Patients with genital herpetic infections. *Am J Epidemiol* 1970;91:539–47.
478. Prober CG, Hensleigh PA, Boucher FD, Yasukawa LL, Au DS, Arvin AM. Identification of neonates exposed to herpes simplex virus: the value of routine viral cultures at delivery. *N Engl J Med* 1988;318:887.
479. Nahmias AJ, Keyserling HL, Kerrick GM. Herpes simplex. In: Remington JS, ed. *Infectious diseases of the fetus and newborn infant.* Philadelphia: W.B. Saunders Co., 1983;636–78.
480. Tejani M, Klein SW, Kaplan M. Subclinical herpes simplex genitalis infections in the perinatal period. *Am J Obstet Gynecol* 1978;135:547.
481. Vontver LA, Hickok DE, Brown Z, Reid L, Corey L. Recurrent genital herpes simplex virus infection in pregnancy: infant outcome and frequency of asymptomatic recurrences. *Am J Obstet Gynecol* 1982;143:75.
482. Nahmias AJ, Josey WE, Naib ZM. Significance of herpes simplex virus infection during pregnancy. *Clin Obstet Gynecol* 1972;15:929–38.
483. Stagno S, Whitley RJ. Herpesvirus infections of pregnancy. Part II: herpes simplex virus and varicella-zoster virus infections. *N Engl J Med* 1985;313:1327.
484. Arvin AM, Yeager AS, Bruhn FW, Grossman M. Neonatal herpes simplex infection in the absence of mucocutaneous lesions. *J Pediatr* 1982;100:715.
485. Light IJ. Postnatal acquisition of herpes simplex virus by the newborn infant: a review of the literature. *Pediatrics* 1979;63:480.
486. Linnemann CC Jr, Light IJ, Buchman TG, Ballard JL. Transmission of herpes simplex virus type 1 in a nursery for the newborn: identification of viral isolates by DNA "fingerprinting." *Lancet* 1978;1:964.
487. Nahmias A, Alford C, Korones S. Infection of the newborn with *Herpesvirus hominis.* In: Schulman I, ed. *Advances in Pediatrics.* Chicago: Year Book Medical Publishers, 1970:185.
488. Lee FK, Coleman RM, Pereira L, Bailey PD, Tatsuno M, Nahmias AJ. Detection of herpes simplex virus type 2 specific antibody with glycoprotein G. *J Clin Microbiol* 1985;22:641.
489. Nahmias AJ, Keyserling H, Bain R. Prevalence of herpes simplex virus type-specific antibodies in a USA prepaid medical practice population [Abstract]. 6th International Society for STD Research.
490. Sullender WM, Yasukawa LL, Schwartz M, Pereira L, Hensleigh PA, Prober CG, Arvin AM. Type-specific antibodies to herpes simplex virus type 2 (HSV-2) glycoprotein G in pregnant women, infants exposed to maternal HSV-2 infection at delivery and infants with neonatal herpes. *J Infect Dis* 1988;157:164.
491. Brown ZA, Vontver LA, Benedetti J, et al.

Effects on infants of a first episode of genital herpes during pregnancy. *N Engl J Med* 1987;317:1246.

492. Nahmias AJ, Wickliffe C, Pipkin J, Leibovitz A, Hutton A. Transport media for herpes simplex virus types 1 and 2. *Appl Microbiol* 1971;22:451–4.
493. Rubin SJ, Wende RD, Rawls WE. Direct immunofluorescence test for the diagnosis of genital herpesvirus infections. *Appl Microbiol* 1973;26:373–6.
494. Yeager AS, Arvin AM. Reasons for the absence of a history of recurrent genital infections in mothers of neonates infected with herpes simplex virus. *Pediatrics* 1984;73:188.
495. Sullender WM, Miller JL, Yasukawa LL, et al. Humoral and cell-mediated immunity in neonates with herpes simplex virus infection. *J Infect Dis* 1987;155:28.
496. Prober CG, Sullender WM, Yasukawa LL, Au DS, Yeager AS, Arvin AM. Low risk of herpes simplex virus infections in neonates exposed to the virus at the time of vaginal delivery to mothers with recurrent genital herpes simplex virus infections. *N Engl J Med* 1987;316:240.
497. Whitley RJ, Nahmias AJ, Visintine AM, Fleming CL, Alford CA. The natural history of herpes simplex virus infection of mother and newborn. *Pediatrics* 1980;66:489–94.
498. Florman AL, Gershon AA, Blackett PR, Nahmias AJ. Intrauterine infection with herpes simplex virus. *JAMA* 1973;225:129–32.
499. South MA, Tompkins WAF, Morris CR, Rawls WE. Congenital malformations of the central nervous system associated with genital type (type 2) herpesvirus. *J Pediatr* 1969;75:13–8.
500. Dunkle LM, Schmidt RR, O'Connor DM. Neonatal herpes simplex infection possibly acquired via maternal breast milk. *Pediatrics* 1979;63:150.
501. Kibrick S. Herpes simplex virus in breast milk. *Pediatrics* 1979;64:390.
502. Ito T, Ono K. Neonatal herpes simplex: a newborn infected by a midwife. *Cutis* 1985;35:169.
503. Hammerberg O, Watts J, Chernesky M, Luchsinger I, Rawls W. An outbreak of herpes simplex virus type 1 in an intensive care nursery. *Pediatr Infect Dis* 1983;2:290.
504. Hutto C, Arvin A, Jacobs R, Steele R, Stagno S, Lyrene R, Willett L, Powell D, Andersen R, Werthammer J. Intrauterine herpes simplex virus infections. *J Pediatr* 1987;110:97.
505. Yeager AS, Ashley RL, Corey L. Transmission of herpes simplex virus from father to neonate. *J Pediatr* 1983;103:905.
507. Singer DB. Pathology of neonatal herpes simplex virus infection. In: Rosenberg HS, Bernstein J, eds. *Perspectives in pediatric pathology*. New York: Masson Pub., 1981:243.
508. Whitley RJ, Nahmias AJ, Soong S-J, Galasso GJ, Fleming CL, Alford CA. Vidarabine therapy of neonatal herpes simplex infection. *Pediatrics* 1980;66:495.
509. Barringer JR. Latency of herpes simplex and varicella-zoster viruses in the nervous system. In: Nehmias A, Dowdle W, Schinazi R, eds. *The human herpesviruses: an interdisciplinary perspective*. New York: Elsevier North Holland, 1981:202.
510. Nahmias A, Dowdle W, Josey W, Naib Z, Painter L, Luce C. Newborn infection with *Herpesvirus hominis* types 1 and 2. *J Pediatr* 1969;75:1194–203.
511. Hirsch MS, Zisman B, Allison AC. Macrophages and age-dependent resistance to herpes simplex virus in mice. *J Immunol* 1970;104:1160.
512. Kohl S, Frazier JJ, Greenberg SB, Pickering L, Loo LS. Interferon induction of natural killer cytotoxicity in human neonates. *J Pediatr* 1981;98:379.
513. Kohl S, Frazier JP, Pickering LK, Loo LS. Normal function of neonatal polymorphonuclear leukocytes in antibody-dependent cellular cytotoxicity to herpes simplex virus-infected cells. *J Pediatr* 1981;98:783.
514. Kohl S, Loo LS, Pickering LK. Protection of neonatal mice against herpes simplex viral infection by human antibody and leukocytes from adult, but not neonatal humans. *J Immunol* 1981;127:1273.
515. Kohl S, Shaban S, Starr S, Wood P, Nahmias A. Human neonatal and maternal monocyte-macrophage and lymphocyte mediated antibody dependent cytoxicity to herpes simplex infected cells. *J Pediatr* 1978;93:206.
516. Lopez C, Ryshke R, Bennett M. Marrow-dependent cells depleted by $^{89}$Sr mediated genetic resistance to herpes simplex virus type 1 infection in mice. *Infect Immun* 1980;28:1028.
517. Mintz H, Drew WL, Hoo R, Finley TN. Age-dependent resistance of human alveolar macrophages to herpes simplex virus. *Infect Immun* 1980;28:417.
518. Pass RF, Dworsky ME, Whitley RJ, August AM, Stagno S, Alford CA Jr. Specific lymphocyte blastogenic responses in children with cytomegalovirus and herpes simplex virus infections acquired early in infancy. *Infect Immun* 1981;34:166–70.
519. Starr SE, Karatela SA, Shore SL, Duffey A, Nahmias A. Stimulation of human lymphocytes by herpes simplex virus antigens. *Infect Immun* 1975;11:109.
520. Trofatter KF Jr, Daniels CA, Williams RJ Jr, Gall SA. Growth of type 2 herpes simplex virus in newborn and adult mononuclear leukocytes. *Intervirology* 1979;II:117.
521. Kohl S, Cox PA, Loo LS. Defective production of antibody to herpes simplex virus in neonates: defective production of T helper lymphokine and induction of suppression. *J Infect Dis* 1987;155:1179.
521. Greene GR, King D, Romansky SG, Marble RD. Primary herpes simplex pneumonia in a neonate. *Am J Dis Child* 1983;137:464.
523. Lissauer TJ, Shaw PJ, Underhill G. Neonatal herpes simplex pneumonia. *Arch Dis Child* 1984;59:668.

524. Amortegui AJ, Macpherson TA, Harger JH. A cluster of neonatal herpes simplex infections without mucocutaneous manifestations. *Pediatrics* 1984;73:194.
525. Brown Z, Coery L, Unadkat J, et al. Pharmacokinetics of ACV in the term human pregnancy and neonate. In: *Program and abstracts of the 27th Interscience Conference on Antimicrobial Agents and Chemotherapy, New York*. October 4–7, American Society for Microbiology 1987:298.
526. Mizrahi EM, Tharp BR. A unique electroencephalogram pattern in neonatal herpes simplex virus encephalitis. *Neurology* 31(2):164.
527. Noorbehesht B, Enzmann DR, Sullender W, Bradley JS, Arvin AM. Neonatal herpes simplex encephalitis: correlation of clinical and CT findings. *Radiology* 1987;162:813.
528. Sullivan-Bolyai JZ, Hull HF, Wilson C, Smith AL, Corey L. Presentation of neonatal herpes simplex virus infections: implications for a change in therapeutic strategy. *Pediatr Infect Dis* 1986;5:309.
529. Lee FK, Takei Y, Dannenbarger J, Visintine A, Whitley R, Nahmias A. Rapid detection of viruses in biopsy or autopsy specimens by the pseudoreplica method of electron microscopy. *Am J Surg Pathol* 1981;5:565.
530. Herrmann KL, Stewart JA. Diagnosis of herpes simplex virus type 1 and 2 infections. In: Nahmias A, Dowdle W, Schinazi R, eds. *The human herpesviruses: an interdisciplinary perspective*. New York: Elsevier, 1981:343–50.
531. Nahmias AJ, Dowdle WR, Naib ZM, Josey WE, Luce CF. Genital infection with *Herpesvirus hominis* types 1 and 2 in children. *Pediatrics* 1968;42:659–66.
532. Kalimo KOK, Martilla RJ, Granfors K, Vilijanen MK. Solid-phase radioimmunoassay of human immunoglobulin M and immunoglobulin G antibodies against herpes simplex virus type 1 capsid, envelope, and excreted antigens. *Infect Immun* 1976;15:883.
533. Kurtz JB. Specific IgG and IgM antibody responses in herpes simplex infections. *J Med Microbiol* 1974;7:333.
534. Charnock EL, Cramblett HG. 5-Iodo-2′-deoxyuridine in neonatal herpesvirus hominis encephalitis. *J Pediatr* 1970;76:459–63.
535. Chow AW, Ronald A, Fiala M, Hrynuik W, Weil ML, St. Geme J, Guze LB. Cytosine arabinoside therapy for herpes simplex encephalitis—clinical experience with six patients. *Antimicrob Agents Chemother* 1973;3:412–17.
536. Hanshaw JB. *Herpesvirus hominis* infections in the fetus and newborn. *Am J Dis Child* 1973;126:546–55.
537. Partridge JW, Mills RR. Systemic herpes simplex in a newborn treated with intravenous idoxuridine. *Arch Dis Child* 1968;43:377–381.
538. Pettay O, Leinikki P, Donner M, Lapinleimu K. Herpes simplex virus infection in the newborn. *Arch Dis Child* 1972;47:97–103.
539. Strawn EY, Scrimenti RJ. Intrauterine herpes simplex infection. *Am J Obstet Gynecol* 1973;115:581–2.
540. Tuffi GA, Nahmias A. Neonatal herpetic infection. *Am J Dis Child* 1969;118:909–14.
541. Ch'ien L, Whitley R, Nahmias A, et al. Antiviral chemotherapy and neonatal herpes simplex virus infection: A pilot study—experience with adenine arabinoside (ara-A). *Pediatrics* 1975;55:678-85.
542. Whitley RJ, Yeager A, Kartus P, et al. Neonatal herpes simplex virus infection: follow-up evaluation of vidarabine therapy. *Pediatrics* 72:778–85.
543. NIAID Antiviral Study Group. Personal observations.
544. King DH, Galasso G, eds. *Proceedings of a Symposium on Acyclovir.* New York: The American Journal of Medicine, Yorke Med. Group, 1982.
545. Blum, MR, Liao SHT, De Mirada P. Overview of acyclovir pharmacokinetic disposition in adults and children. *Am J Med* 1982;73:186–92.
546. Brunell PA. Prevention and treatment of neonatal herpes. *Pediatrics* 1980;66:806–8.
547. Gould JM, Chessells JM, Marshall WC, McKendrick GDW. Acyclovir in herpesvirus infections in children: experience in an open study with particular reference to safety. *J Infect* 1982;5:283–9.
548. Hintz M, Connor JD, Spector SA, et al. Neonatal acyclovir pharmokinetics in patients with herpes virus infections. *Am J Med* 1982;73:210–4.
549. Honig PJ, Brown D. Congenital herpes simplex virus infection initially resembling epidermolysis bullosa. *J Pediatr* 1982; 101:958–60.
550. Naib ZM, Nahmias AJ, Josey WE, Zaki SA. Relation of cytohistopathology of genital herpesvirus infection to cervical anaplasia. *Cancer Res* 1973;33:1452–63.
551. Spector SA, Hintz M, Connor JD, Quinn RP, Blum MR, Keeney RE. Single dose pharmacokinetic properties of acyclovir. *Antimicrob Agents Chemother* 1981;19:608–12.
552. Whitley RJ, et al. Comparison of vidarabine and acyclovir for the treatment of neonatal HSV infections (in preparation).
553. Corey L, Whitley RJ, Stone EF, Mohan K. Difference between herpes simplex virus type 1 and type 2 neonatal encephalitis in neurological outcome. *Lancet* 1988;i:1.
554. Arvin AM, Hensleigh PA, Prober CG, et al. Failure of antepartum maternal cultures to predict the infant's risk of exposure to herpes simplex virus at delivery. *N Engl J Med* 1986;315:796.
555. Dankner WM, Spector SA. Recurrent herpes simplex in a neonate. *Pediatr Infect Dis* 1986;5:582.
556. Marker SG, Howard RJ, Groth KE, Mastry AR, Simmons RL, Balfour HH. A trial of vidarabine for cytomegalovirus infection in renal transplant patients. *Arch Intern Med* 1980;140:1441–4.
557. Pavan-Langston C, Buchanan RA, Alford CA

Jr, eds. *Adenine arabinoside: an antiviral agent*. New York: Raven Press, 1975.
558. Sachs SL, Smith JL, Pollard RB, et al. Toxicity of vidarabine. *JAMA* 1979;241:28–9.
559. Ashley R, Mertz GJ, Corey L. Detection of asymptomatic herpes simplex virus infections after vaccination. *J Virol* 1987;61:264.
560. Cox SM, Phillips LE, DePaolo HD, Faro S. Treatment of disseminated herpes simplex virus in pregnancy with parenteral acyclovir. A case report. *J Reprod Med* 1986;31:1005.
561. Grover L, Kane J, Kravitz J, Cruz A. Systemic acyclovir in pregnancy: a case report. *Obstet Gynecol* 1985;65:284.
562. Lagrew DC Jr, Furlow TG, Hager WD, Yarrish RL. Disseminated herpes simplex virus infection in pregnancy. Successful treatment with acyclovir. *JAMA* 1984;252:2058.
563. Sullender WM, Arvin AM, Diaz PS, et al. Pharmacokinetics of acyclovir suspension in infants and children. *Antimicrob Agents Chemother* 1987;31:1722.
564. Feder HM JR. Disseminated herpes simplex infection in a neonate during prophylaxis with vidarabine. *JAMA* 1988;259:1054.
565. Sullivan-Bolyai J, Hull HF, Wilson C, Corey L. Neonatal herpes simplex virus infection in King County, Washington. Increasing incidence and epidemiologic correlates. *JAMA* 1983;250:3059.
566. Brown ZA, Ashley R, Douglas J, Keilly M, Corey L. Neonatal herpes simplex virus infection: relapse after initial therapy and transmission from a mother with an asymptomatic genital herpes infection and erythema multiforme. *Pediatr Infect Dis J* 1987;6:1057.
567. Sever J, White LR, Intrauterine viral infections. *Ann Rev Med* 1968;19:471.
568. Gershon AA, Raker R, Steinberg S, Topg-Olstien B, Drusin, L. Antibody to varicella-zoster virus in parturient women and their offspring during the first year of life. *Pediatrics* 1976;58:962.
569. Gershon AA. Varicella in mother and infant: problems old and new. In: Krugman S, Gershon AA, eds. *Infections of the fetus and newborn. Progress in clinical and biological research, vol. 3*. New York: Alan R. Liss, 1975:79.
570. Young NA, Gershon AA. Chickenpox, measles and mumps. In: Remington JS, Klein JO, eds. *Infections of the fetus and newborn infant*. Philadelphia: W.B. Saunders, 1983:375.
571. Brunell PA. Varicella-zoster infections in pregnancy. *JAMA* 1967;199:315.
572. Harris RE, Phoades ER. Varicella pneumonia complicating pregnancy: report of a case and review of the literature. *Obstet Gynecol* 1965;23:734.
573. Siegel M, Fuerst HT, Peress NS. Comparative fetal mortality in maternal virus diseases: a prospective study on rubella, measles, mumps, chickenpox, and hepatitis. *N Engl J Med* 1966;274:768.
574. Paryani SG, Arvin AM. Intrauterine infection with varicella-zoster virus after maternal varicella. *N Engl J Med* 1986;314:1542.
575. Enders G. Varicella-zoster virus infection in pregnancy. *Prog Med Virol* 1984;29:166.
576. Seigel M. Congenital malformations following chickenpox, measles, mumps and hepatitis. *JAMA* 1973;226:1521.
577. Grose C. Varicella-zoster virus: pathogenesis of the human disease, the virus and viral replication and the major viral glycoproteins and proteins. In: Hyman RW, ed. *Natural history of varicella-zoster virus*. Boca Raton: CRC Press, 1987:13.
578. Koropchak CM, Diaz PS, Arvin AM. Detection of varicella-zoster virus in tissue culture and in peripheral blood mononuclear cells by in situ hybridization with cloned fragments of VZV DNA. 12th International Herpesvirus Workshop, Philadelphia, 1987.
579. Gershon AA, Steinberg SP, LaRussa P, Ferrara A, Hammerschlag M, Gelb L, the NIAID Varicella Vaccine Collaborative Study Group. Immunization of healthy adults with live attenuated varicella vaccine. *J Infect Dis* 1988;158:132–7.
580. Borzyskowski M, Harris RF, Jones RWA. The congenital varicella syndrome. *Eur J Pediatr* 1981;137:335.
581. Brunell PA. Fetal and neonatal varicella-zoster infections. In: Amstey MS, ed. *Virus Infections in Pregnancy*. Orlando: Grune and Stratton, 1984.
582. Cuthbertson G, Weiner CP, Giller RH, Grose C. Prenatal diagnosis of second-trimester congenital varicella syndrome by virus-specific immunoglobulin M. *J Pediatr* 1987;111:592.
583. DeNicola LK, Hanshaw HB. Congenital and neonatal varicella. *J Pediatr* 1979;94:175.
584. Roberts, RM. The fetal varicella syndrome. In: *Birth defects encyclopedia*. New York: Alan R. Liss (in press).
585. Frey HM, Bialkin G, Gershon AA. Congenital varicella: case report of a serologically proved long term survivor. *Pediatrics* 1977;59:110.
586. Strabstein JC, Morris N, Larke RPB. Is there a congenital varicella syndrome? *J Pediatr* 1974;84:239.
587. Asha Bai PV, John TJ. Congenital skin ulcers following varicella in late pregnancy. *J Pediatr* 1981;98:71.
588. Brunell PA. Zoster in infancy: failure to maintain virus latency following intrauterine infection. *J Pediatr* 1981;98:71.
589. Alkalay AL, Pomerance JJ, Rimoin DL. Fetal varicella syndrome. *J Pediatr* 1987;111:320.
590. Myers JD. Congenital varicella in term infants: risk reconsidered. *J Infect Dis* 1974;129:215.
591. Readett MD, McGibbon C. Neonatal varicella. *Lancet* 1961;i:644.
592. Gustafson TL, Shehab Z, Brunell PA. Outbreak of varicella in a newborn intensive care nursery. *Am J Dis Child* 1984;138:548.
593. Prober CG, Arvin AM. Perinatal viral infections. *Eur J Clin Microbiol* 1987;6:245.

594. Bakshi SS, Miller TC, Kaplan M, Hammerschlag MR, Prince A, Gershon AA. Failure of varicella-zoster immunoglobulin in modification of severe congenital varicella. *Pediatr Infect Dis* 1986;5:699.
595. Bose B, Kerr M, Brookes E. Varicella zoster immunoglobulin to prevent neonatal chickenpox. *Lancet* 1986;i:449.
596. King SM, Gorensek M, Ford-Jones EL, Read SE. Fatal varicella-zoster infection in a newborn treated with varicella-zoster immunoglobulin. *Pediatr Infect Dis* 1986;5:588.
597. Rubin L, Leggiadro R, Elie MT, Lipsitz P. Disseminated varicella in a neonate: implications for immunoprophylaxis of neonates postnatally exposed to varicella. *Pediatr Infect Dis* 1986;5:1.
598. Arvin AM. Clinical manifestations of varicella and herpes zoster and the immune response to varicella-zoster virus. In: Hyman RW, ed. *Natural history of varicella-zoster virus*. Boca Raton: CRC Press, 1987:87–90.
599. Jaffe HW, Bregman DJ, Selik RM. Acquired immunodeficiency syndrome in the United States: the first 1,000 cases. *J Infect Dis* 1983;148:339.
600. Ammann AJ, Cowan MJ, Wara DW. Acquired immunodeficiency in an infant: possible transmission by means of blood product administration. *Lancet* 1983;i:956.
601. Cowan MJ, Hellmann D, Chudwin D, Wara DW, Chang RS, Ammann AJ. Maternal transmission of acquired immune deficiency syndrome. *Pediatrics* 1984;73:382.
602. Church JA, Isaacs H. Transfusion-associated acquired immune deficiency syndrome in infants. *J Pediatr* 1984;985:731.
603. DiNaria H, Courpotin C, Rouzioux C, et al. Transplacental transmission of human immunodeficiency virus. *Lancet* 1986;i:215.
604. Unexplained immunodeficiency and opportunistic infections in infants-New York, New Jersey, California. *MMWR* 1982;31:665.
605. Apparent transmission of HTLV-III/LAV from a child to a mother providing health care. *MMWR* 1986;35:75.
606. Zagury D, Fouchard M, Lol JC, et al. Detection of infectious HTLV-III/LAV virus in cell-free plasma from AIDS patients. *Lancet* 1985;ii:505.
607. Rogers MF, Thomas PA, Starcher ET, Noa MC, Bush TH, Jaffe HW. Acquired immunodeficiency syndrome in children: report of the Centers for Disease Control National Surveillance, 1982 to 1985. *Pediatrics* 1987;79:980.
608. Fallon J, Pizzo P. The acquired immunodeficiency syndrome in the infant. In: Remington J, Klein J, eds. *Infectious diseases of the fetus and newborn. 3rd ed.* Philadelphia: Saunders, Inc. (in press).
609. Classification system for human immunodeficiency virus (HIV) infection in children under 13 years of age. *MMWR* 1987;36:225.
610. Pahwa S, Kaplan M, Fikrig S, et al. Spectrum of human T-cell lymphotropic virus type III infection in children. Recognition of symptomatic, asymptomatic, and seronegative patients. *JAMA* 1986;255:222.
611. Hardy AM, Allen JR, Morgan WM, et al. The incidence rate of acquired immunodeficiency syndrome in selected populations. *JAMA* 1985; 253:215.
612. Rubinstein A. Pediatric AIDS. *Curr Probl Pediatr* 1986;16:361.
613. Lange JMA, van den Berg H, Dooren LJ, et al. HTLV-III/LAV infection in nine children infected by a single plasma donor: clinical outcome and recognition patterns of viral proteins. *J Infect Dis* 1986;154:171.
614. Brady MT, Ng A. Protection of neonates from transfusion associated AIDS by the use of CMV seronegative blood before availability of specific serologic tests for HTLV-III (HIV). *Am J Perinatol* 1987;4:305.
615. Mann JM, Francis H, Davachi F, et al. Risk factors for human immunodeficiency virus seropositivity among children 1-24 months old in Kinshasa, Zaire. *Lancet* 1986;ii:654.
616. Quinn TC, Mann JM, Curran JW, Piot P. AIDS in Africa: an epidemiologic paradigm. *Science* 1986;234:955.
617. Mann JM, Francis H, Davachi F, et al. Human immunodeficiency virus seroprevalence in pediatric patients 2 to 14 years of age at Mama Yemo Hospital, Kinshasa, Zaire. *Pediatrics* 1986;78:673.
618. Lampert R, Milberg J, O'Donnell R, et al. Life table analysis of children with acquired immunodeficiency syndrome. *Pediatr Infect Dis* 1986;5:374.
618. Scott GB, Buck BE, Letterman JG, et al. Acquired immunodeficiency syndrome in infants. *N Engl J Med* 1984;398:76.
620. Goetz DW, Hall SE, Harbison RW, Reid MJ. Pediatric acquired immunodeficiency syndrome with negative human immunodeficiency virus antibody response by enzyme-linked immunosorbent assay and Western blot. *Pediatrics* 1988;81:356.
621. Jason JM, McDougal JS, Dixon G, et al. HTLV-III/LAV antibody and immune status of household contacts and sexual partners of persons with hemophilia. *JAMA* 1986;255:212.
622. Hilgartner MW. Low risk of HIV infection in children of men with hemophilia. *N Engl J Med* 1986;315:969.
623. Oxtoby MJ, Rogers M, Thomas P. National trends in perinatally acquired AIDS. United States. In: *Abstracts of the Third International Conference on AIDS, June 1987*. Washington D.C.
624. Human immunodeficiency virus infection in the United States: a review of current knowledge. *MMWR* 1987;36:S6.
625. Friedland GH, Klein RS. Transmission of the human immunodeficiency virus. *N Engl J Med* 1987;317:1125.
626. Guinan ME, Harby A. Epidemiology of AIDS

in women in the United States: 1981 through 1986. *JAMA* 1987;257:2039.
627. Hoff R, Berard VP, Weiblen BJ, Mahoney-Trout L, Mitchell ML, Grady GF. Seroprevalence of human immunodeficiency virus among childbearing women. *N Engl J Med* 1988;318:525.
628. Landesman S, Minkoff H, Holman S, McCalla S, Sijin O. Serosurvey of human immunodeficiency virus infection in parturients. *JAMA* 1987; 258:2701.
629. Blanche S, Fischer A, Le Deist F, et al. LAV infections and the acquired immunodeficiency syndrome in infants. *Arch Fr Pediatr* 1986;43:87.
630. Krasinski K, Borkowsky W, Bebenroth D, Moore T. Failure of voluntary testing for human immunodeficiency virus to identify infected parturient women in a high-risk population. *N Engl J Med* 1988;318:185.
631. Jovaisas E, Koch MA, Schafer A, et al. LAV/HTLV-III in a 20 week fetus. *Lancet* 1985;ii:1129.
631. Sprecher S, Soumenkoff G, Puissant F. et al. Vertical transmission of HIV in 15 week old fetus. *Lancet* 1986;2:228.
633. Rubinstein A, Bernstein L. The epidemiology of pediatric acquired immunodeficiency syndrome. *Clin Immunol Immunopathol* 1986;40:115.
634. Schafer A, Jovaisas E, Stauber M, Lowenthal D, Koch MA. Proof of diaplacental transmission of HTLV III/LAV before the 20th week of pregnancy. *Geburtshilfe Frauenheilkd* 1986;46:88.
635. Laurence J. Tracking the transmission of HTLV-III infection. *Infect Med* 1986;3:348.
636. Lapointe N, Michand J, Pekovic D, Chausseau JP, Dupuy J-M. Transplacental transmission of HTLV-III virus. *N Engl J Med* 1985;312:1325.
637. Iosub S, Bamji M, Stone RK, Gromisch DS, Wasserman E. More on human immunodeficiency virus embryopathy. *Pediatrics* 1987;80:512.
638. Marion RW, Wiznia AA, Hutcheon G, Rubinstein A. Human T-cell lymphotropic virus type III (HTLV-III) embryopathy. A new dysmorphic syndrome associated with intrauterine HTLV-III infection. *Am J Dis Child* 1986;140:638.
639. Qazi QH, Sheikh TM, Fikrig S, Menikoff H. Lack of evidence for craniofacial dysmorphism in perinatal human immunodeficiency virus infection. *J Pediatr* 112:7.
640. Weintrub PS, Scott GB. Pediatric HIV infection. In: Mills J, Leoung G. Opportunistic infections in patients with the acquired immune deficiency syndrome. New York: Marcel Dekker, 1988.
641. Wofsy CB, Cohen JB, Hauer LB, et al. Isolation of AIDS associated retrovirus from genital secretions of women with antibodies to the virus. *Lancet* 1986;1:527.
642. Vogt MW, Witt DJ, Craven DE, Byington R, Crawford DF, Schooley RT, Hirsch MS. Isolation of HTLV-III/LAV from cervical secretions of women at risk for AIDS. *Lancet* 1986; 1:525.
643. Vogt MW, Witt DJ, Craven DE, et al. Isolation patterns of the human immunodeficiency virus from cervical secretions during the menstrual cycle of women at risk for the acquired immunodeficiency syndrome. *Ann Intern Med* 1987;106:380.
644. Saulsbury FT, Wykoff RF, Boyle RJ. Transfusion acquired human immunodeficiency virus infection in twelve neonates: epidemiologic, clinical and immunologic features. *Pediatr Infect Dis J* 1987;6:544.
645. Ziegler JB, Cooper DA, Johnson RO, et al. Postnatal transmission of AIDS-associated retrovirus from mother to infant. *Lancet* 1985;1:896.
646. Thiry L, Sprecher-Goldberger S, Jonckheer T, et al. Isolation of AIDS virus from cell-free breast milk of three healthy virus carriers. [Letter]. *Lancet* 1985;2:891.
647. Scott GB, Fischl MA, Klimas N, et al. Mothers of infants with the acquired immunodeficiency syndrome: evidence for both symptomatic and asymptomatic carriers. *JAMA* 1985;253:363.
648. Laurence J, Brun-Vezinet F, Schutzer SE, et al. Lymphadenopathy associated viral (LAV) antibody in AIDS: immune correlations and definition of a carrier state. *N Engl J Med* 1984;311:1269.
649. Rogers MF, Ewing EP Jr, Warfield D, Hardy AM, Emery DR, Wolf GC. Virologic studies of HTLV-III/LAV in pregnancy: case report of a woman with AIDS. *Obstet Gynecol* 1986;68:2S–6S.
650. Rubinstein A, Sisklick M, Gupta A, et al. Acquired immunodeficiency with reversed T4/T8 ratios in infants born to promiscuous and drug-addicted mothers. *JAMA* 1983;249:2350.
651. Bacchetti P, Osmond D, Chaisson RE et al. Survival patterns of the first 500 patients with AIDS in San Francisco. *J Infect Dis* 1988;157:1044.
652. Shanks GD, Redfield RR, Fischer GW. Toxoplasma encephalitis in an infant with acquired immunodeficiency syndrome. *Pediatr Infect Dis* 1987;6:70.
653. Prober CG, Arvin AM. Perinatal viral infections. *Eur J Clin Microbiol* 1987;6:245.
654. Rogers MF. AIDS in children: a review of the clinical, epidemiologic and public health aspects. *Pediatr Infect Dis* 1985;4:230.
655. Shannon KM, Ammann AJ. Acquired immune deficiency syndrome in childhood. *J Pediatr* 1985;106:332.
656. Bernstein LJ, Kriegler BZ, Novick B, et al. Bacterial infection in the acquired immunodeficiency syndrome of children. *Pediatr Infect Dis* 1985;4:472.
657. Krasinski K, Borkowsy W, Bonk S, Lawrence R, Chandwani S. Bacterial infections in human immunodeficiency virus-infected children *Pediatr Infect Dis J* 1988;7:323.
658. Ammann AJ, Schiffman G, Adams D, et al. B-cell immunodeficiency in acquired immune deficiency syndrome. *JAMA* 1984;251:1447.
659. Ammann AJ, Levy J. Laboratory investigation of pediatric acquired immunodeficiency syndrome. *Clin Immunol Immunopathol* 1986;40:122.
660. Bernstein LJ, Rubinstein A. Acquired immu-

nodeficiency syndrome in infants and children. *Prog Allergy* 1986;37:194–206.

661. McCance-Katz EG, Hoecker JL, Vitale NB. Severe neutropenia associated with anti-neutrophil antibody in a patient with acquired immunodeficiency syndrome-related complex. *Pediatr Infect Dis* 1987;6:417.
662. Wycoff RF, Pearl ER, Saulsbury FT. Immunologic dysfunction in infants infected through transfusion with HTLV-III. *N Engl J Med* 1985;312:294.
663. Saulsbury FT, Boyle RJ, Wykoff RF, Howard TH. Thrombocytopenia as the presenting manifestation of human T-lymphotropic virus type III infection in infants. *J Pediatr* 1986;109:30.
664. Maloney JM, Gyuill MF, Wray BB, Lobel SA, Ebbeling W. Pediatric acquired immune deficiency syndrome with panhypogammaglobulinemia. *J Pediatr* 1987;198:266.
665. Joshi VV, Oleske JM, Minnefor AB, et al. Pathologic pulmonary findings in children with the acquired immunodeficiency syndrome: a study of ten cases. *Hum Pathol* 1985;16:241.
666. Chayt KJ, Harper ME, Marselle LM, et al. Detection of HTLV-III RNA in lungs of patients with AIDS and pulmonary involvement. *JAMA* 1986;256:2356.
667. Laurence J. HIV infections in infants and children. *Infect Med* 1987;2:44.
668. Rubenstein A, Morecki R, Silverman B, et al. Pulmonary disease in children with acquired immune deficiency syndrome and AIDS-related complex. *J Pediatr* 1986;108:498.
669. Josephs S, Kim HW, Brandt CD, Parrott RH. Parainfluenza 3 virus and other common respiratory pathogens in children with human immunodeficiency virus infection. *Pediatr Infect Dis J* 1988;7:207.
670. Belman AL, Diamond G, Dickson D, et al. Pediatric acquired immunodeficiency syndrome: neurologic syndromes. *AJDC* 1988;142:29.
671. Belman AL, Horoupian D, Lantos G, et al. Calcification of the basal ganglia in infants and children with acquired immune deficiency syndrome (AIDS). *Neurology* 1986;36:1192–9.
672. Davis SL, Halsted CC, Levy N, Ellis W. Acquired immune deficiency syndrome presenting as progressive infantile encephalopathy. *J Pediatr* 1987;198:884.
673. Epstein LG, Sharer LR, Joshi VV. Progressive encephalopathy in children with acquired immune deficiency syndrome. *Ann Neurol* 1985;17:488.
674. Epstein LG, Sharer LR, Oleske JM, et al. Neurologic manifestations of human immunodeficiency virus infection in children. *Pediatrics* 1986;78:678.
675. Goudsmit J, de Wolf F, Paul DA, et al. Expression of human immunodeficiency virus antigen (HIV-Ag) in serum and cerebrospinal fluid during acute and chronic infection. *Lancet* 1986;ii:177.
676. Ragni MV, Urbach AH, Taylor S, et al. Isolation of human immunodeficiency virus and detection of HIV DNA sequences in the brain of an ELISA antibody-negative child with acquired immune deficiency syndrome and progressive encephalopathy. *J Pediatr* 1987;198:892.
677. Sharer LR, Epstein LG, Cho ES, et al. Pathologic features of AIDS encephalopathy in children: evidence for LAV/HTLV-III infection of brain. *Hum Pathol* 1986;17:271.
678. Rotbart HA, Levin MJ, Jones JF, et al. Noma in children with severe combined immunodeficiency. *J Pediatr* 1986;989:596.
679. Tong TK, Andrew LR, Albert A, Mickell JJ. Childhood acquired immune deficiency syndrome manifesting as acrodermatitis enteropathica. *J Pediatr* 1986;108:426.
680. Issenberg HJ, Charytan M, Rubenstein A. Cardiac involvement in children with acquired immune deficiency. *Am Heart J* 1985;198:798.
681. Sherron P, Pickoff AS, Ferrer PL, Tamer D, Scott GB. Echocardiographic evaluation of myocardial function in pediatric AIDS patients. *Am Heart J* 1985;198:798.
682. Steinherz LJ, Brochstein JA, Robins J. Cardiac involvement in congenital acquired immunodeficiency syndrome. *Am J Dis Child* 1986;140:1241.
683. Andiman W, Eastman R, Martin K, et al. Opportunistic lymphoproliferations associated with EBV/DNA in infants and children with AIDS. *Lancet* 1985;ii:1390.
684. Kamani N, Kennedy J, Brandsma J. Burkitt lymphoma in a child with human immunodeficiency virus infection. *J Pediatr* 1988;112:241.
685. Kapland JE, Oleske JM, Getchell JP, et al. Evidence against transmission of human T-lymphotropic virus/lymphadenopathy associated virus (HTLV-III/LAV) in families of children with the acquired immunodeficiency syndrome. *Pediatr Infect Dis* 1985;4:468.
686. Shannon K, Ball E, Wasserman RL, et al. Transfusion-associated cytomegalovirus infection and acquired immune deficiency syndrome in an infant. *J Pediatr* 1983;103:859.
687. Ammann AJ, Kaminsky L, Cowan M, Levy JA. Antibodies to AIDS associated retrovirus distinguish between pediatric primary and acquired immunodeficiency disease. *JAMA* 1985;253:3116.
688. Johnson JP, Nair P. Early diagnosis of HIV infection in the neonate. *N Engl J Med* 1987;316:273.
689. Martin K, Katz BZ, Miller G. AIDS and antibodies to human immunodeficiency virus (HIV) in children and their families. *J Infect Dis* 1987;155:54.
690. Pyun KH, Ochs HD, Dufford MTW, Wedgwood RJ. Perinatal infection with human immunodeficiency virus: specific antibody response by the neonate. *N Engl J Med* 1987;317:611.
691. Albershein SG, Smyth JA, Solimano A, Cook D. Passively acquired human immunodeficiency virus seropositivity in a neonate after hepatitis B immunoglobulin. *J Pediatr* 1988;112:915.
692. Borkowsky W, Krasinski K, Paul E, et al. Human immunodeficiency-virus infections in infants negative for anti-HIV by enzyme-linked immunoassay. *Lancet* 1987;i:1168.
693. Wittek AE, Phelan MA, Wells MA, et al. Detection of human immunodeficiency virus core

protein in plasma by enzyme immunoassay: association of antigenemia with symptomatic disease and T-helper cell depletion. *Ann Intern Med* 1987;107:286.
694. Harnish EG, Hammerberg O, Walker IR, Rosenthal KL. Early detection of HIV infection in a newborn. *N Engl J Med* 1987;316:272.
695. Pawha S. Human immunodeficiency virus infection in children: nature of immunodeficiency, clinical spectrum and management. *Pediatr Infect Dis J* 1988;7:S61.
696. Culver KW, Amman AJ, Partridge JC, Wong DF, Wara DW, Cowan MJ. Lymphocyte abnormalities in infants born to drug-abusing mothers. *Pediatrics* 1987;111:230.
697. Bernstein LJ, Ochs HD, Wedgwood RH, et al. Defective humoral immunity in pediatric acquired immune deficiency syndrome. *J Pediatr* 1985;987:352.
698. Pawha S, Fikrig S, Menez R, Pawha R. Pediatric acquired immunodeficiency syndrome; demonstration of B lymphocyte defects in vitro. *Diag Immunol* 1986;4:24.
699. Rubinstein A, Novick BE, Sicklick MJ, et al. Circulating thymulin and thymosin-alpha 1 activity in pediatric acquired immune deficiency syndrome: in vivo and in vitro studies. *J Pediatr* 1986;109:422.
700. Robert-Guroff M, Oleske JM, Connor EM, Epstein LG, Minnefor AB, Gallow RC. Relationship between HTLV-III neutraling antibody and clinical status of pediatric acquired immunodeficiency syndrome (AIDS) and AIDS-related complex cases. *Pediatr Res* 1987;21:547.
701. Blanche S, Fischer A, LeDeist F, et al. Ribavirin in HTLV-III/LAV infection of infants. *Lancet* 1986;i:863.
702. Ochs H. Intravenous immunoglobulin in the treatment and prevention of acute infections in pediatric acquired immunodeficiency syndrome patients. *Pediatr Infect Dis J* 1987;6:509.
703. Cavelli TA, Rubinstein A. Intravenous gammaglobulin in infant acquired immunodeficiency syndrome. *Pediatr Infect Dis* 1986;5:S207.
704. Gupta A, Novick BE, Rubinstein A. Restoration of suppressor T-cell functions in children with AIDS following intravenous gammaglobulin treatment. *Am J Dis Child* 1986;140:143.
705. Lim W, Kahn E, Gupta A, et al. Treatment of cytomegalovirus enterocolitis with ganciclovir in an infant with acquired immunodeficiency syndrome. *Pediatr Infect Dis J* 1988;7:354.
706. Immunization of children infected with human T-lymphotropic virus type III/lymphadenopathy-associated virus. *MMWR* 1986;35:595.
707. Immunization of children infected with human immunodeficiency virus—supplementary ACIP statement. *MMWR* 1988;37:181.
708. Measles in HIV-infected children, United States. *MMWR* 1988;37:183.
709. Borkowsky W, Steele CJ, Grubman S, Moore T, LaRussa P, Krasinksi K. Antibody responses to bacterial toxoids in children infected with human immunodeficiency virus. *J Pediatr* 1987;198:563.
710. Bernstein LH, Rubinstein A. Pulmonary lymphoid hyperplasia in children with AIDS: long-term effects of periodic intravenous gammaglobulin and corticosteroid treatment. *Pediatr Res* 1986;20:292A.
711. Recommendations for assisting in the prevention of perinatal transmission of human T-lymphotropic virus type III/Lymphadenopathy-associated virus and acquired immunodeficiency syndrome. *MMWR* 1985;34:721.
712. Ward JW, Holmberg SD, Allen JR, et al. Transmission of human immunodeficiency virus (HIV) by blood transfusion screened as negative for HIV antibody. *N Engl J Med* 1988;318:473.
713. Koenig RE, Gautier T, Levy JA. Unusual intrafamilial transmission of human immunodeficiency virus [Letter]. *Lancet* 1986;ii:627.
714. MacDonald KL, Danila RN, Osterholm MT. Infection with human T-lymphotropic virus type III/lymphadenopathy-associated virus: considerations for transmission in the child day care setting. *Rev Infect Dis* 1986;8:606.
715. Brunell PA, Daum RS, Giebink GS, et al. Committee on Infectious Diseases, American Academy of Pediatrics: health guidelines for the attendance in day-care and foster care settings of children infected with human immunodeficiency virus. *Pediatrics* 1987;79:466.
716. Church JA, Allen JR, Stiehm ER. New scarlet letter(s): pediatric AIDS. *Pediatrics* 1986;77:423.
717. Grossman M. Human immunodeficiency virus infections in children: public health and public policy issues. 1987;6:113.
718. Katz BZ, Andiman WA, Eastman R, Martin K, Miller G. Infection with two genotypes of Epstein-Barr virus in an infant with AIDS and lymphoma of the central nervous system. *J Infect Dis* (1986) 153:601.

*Antiviral Agents and Viral Diseases of Man, 3rd Edition,* edited by G. J. Galasso, R. J. Whitley, and T. C. Merigan, Raven Press, Ltd., New York 1990.

# 15

# HIV and Other Human Retroviruses

Douglas D. Richman

*Departments of Pathology and Medicine, University of California, San Diego, and Veterans Administration Medical Center, San Diego, California 92161*



Until 1980, no pathogenic human retroviruses had been isolated. Retroviruses were of great scientific interest because they were associated with malignancies in several animal species, they provided insight into the relationship of gene expression and neoplasia, and they utilized reverse transcription in their replication. The isolation of the first pathogenic human retrovirus, human T lymphotropic virus type 1 (HTLV-1), was reported in 1980 (1) almost coincident with the recognition of a new clinical syndrome, acquired immunodeficiency syndrome (AIDS) (2–5). The isolation and characterization of the human retrovirus that is the etiologic agent of AIDS, human immunodeficiency virus (HIV) (6–8), has in only a few years resulted in the most intensively investigated subject in the history of medicine.

The family *Retroviridae* includes many important agents of birds and mammals that share a number of common taxonomic features (9). Virions are enveloped and spherical (80–120 nm in diameter) with surface glycoprotein projections and an internal ribonucleoprotein complex. This complex includes a RNA-dependent DNA polymerase (reverse transcriptase) and a linear, positive sense single-stranded RNA genome composed of two identical subunits. The genomes of nondefective (replication competent) retroviruses are characterized by sequences at each end, designated long terminal repeats (LTRs), that flank three sets of structural genes that code for the core antigens (*gag* for group antigen), the reverse transcriptase/protease complex (*pol* for polymerase), and the envelope glycoproteins (*env*). In addition, all human retroviruses that have been identified also contain several genes that code for accessory proteins.

The *Retroviridae* consist of three subfamilies: the *Oncovirinae,* the *Spumavirinae,* and the *Lentivirinae.* The *Oncovirinae* (Greek, *oncos* = tumor) consist primarily of oncogenic viruses and include the widely investigated RNA tumor viruses of birds, rodents, and, more recently cats, ruminants, and lower primates (9). The first pathogenic human retrovirus isolates, HTLV-1 and HTLV-2, belong to the oncornavirus subfamily (1,10). The *Spumavirinae* (Latin, *spuma* = foamy) have been isolated, usually as contaminants of primary tissue culture in which these agents in duce a "foamy" degenerative cytopathology. Spumaviruses have been isolated from many species including humans, from which several serotypes have been identified since 1971 (11,12). Although foamy viruses, as they are commonly called, often cause persistent infection, they have not yet been associated with a distinct disease in any species, including humans.

The first recognized member of the *Lentivirinae* (Latin, *lenti* = slow) were the closely related agents of *visna* (wasting due to progressive neurologic impairment) and *maedi* (shortness of breath) that were characterized by an Icelandic veterinarian, Sigurdsson (13,14) as transmissible "slow" agents of disease in sheep. Lentiviruses have also been identified in goats, horses, bovines, cats, monkeys, and humans. These are not primarily transforming viruses, they often infect cells of the monocyte-macrophage series, and they are associated with chronic progressive degenerative disease of various target organ systems including the nervous system.

Although human viruses from each of these subfamilies have been identified, disease has been associated only with the oncornaviruses (HTLV-1 and HTLV-2) and the lentiviruses (HIV-1 and HIV-2). This chapter will focus primarily on the HIVs because the AIDS pandemic has focused attention on them as the most intensive targets for antiviral drug development. At least in the near future, antiviral treatment of infection with HTLV-1 and other members of the oncornavirus subfamily will represent the application of drugs developed against HIV to other retroviruses sharing common targets such as reverse transcriptases. Investigation of antivirals is merited for disease processes in which active replication of HTLV-1 is occurring, such as HTLV-1-associated myelopathy (HAM) (15–19). The chemotherapy of adult T-cell leukemia (ATL) secondary to HTLV-1 probably needs to be directed against malignantly transformed cells rather than against virus replication (20).

## CHARACTERISTICS OF HIV AND HTLV

### Virion Structure

Retroviruses are roughly spherical structures, approximately 100 nm in diameter (Figs. 1 and 2). Glycoprotein spikes project from the virion surface, anchored into an envelope consisting of a phospholipid bilayer derived from the host cell membrane.

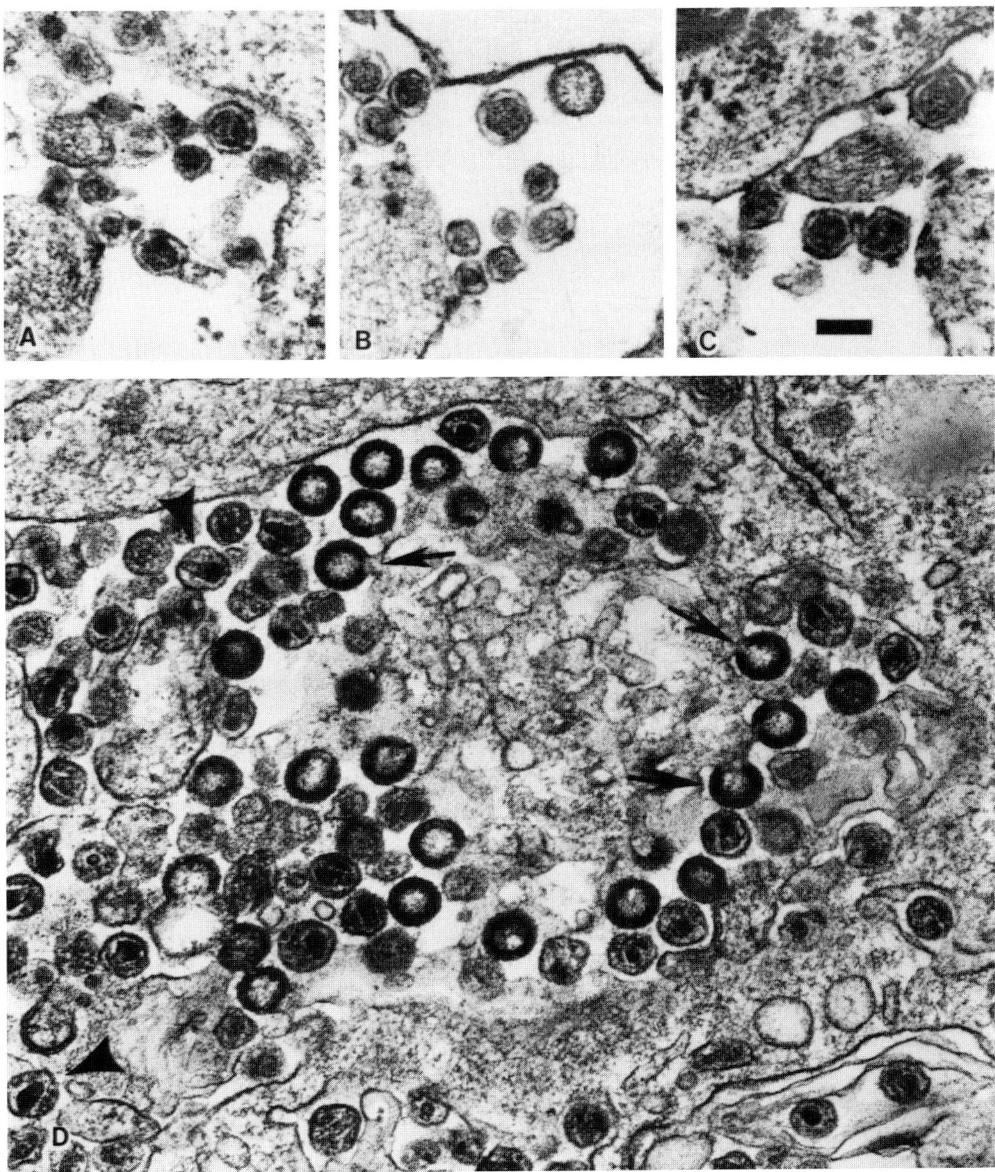


**FIG. 1.** Electron photomicrographs of human retroviruses. **A–C:** Electron photomicrographs of extracellular HTLV-1 virus particles produced by the chronically HTLV-1-infected T lymphoblastoid cell line, MT-2. The particles contain a condensed nucleoid surrounded by an outer membrane or envelope. The diameters of particles vary from 70 to 140 μm. Bar = 100 μm. × 95,000. **D:** Electron photomicrograph of HIV particles in a large intracytoplasmic vacuole of a cultured human peripheral blood macrophage, 10 days after viral inoculation. This intracytoplasmic vacuole contains numerous HIV particles at various stages of maturation. These include budding virions (*arrows*), numerous particles with immature or ring shaped nucleoids, and a few mature particles with condensed cylindrical nucleoids (*arrowheads*). Note that the budding and immature particles have very spherical envelopes, whereas the envelopes of the mature particles are irregular. The diameters of the particles vary from 90 to 120 μm. × 95,000. (Photomicrographs generously provided by Patrick Cleveland, Ph.D.)

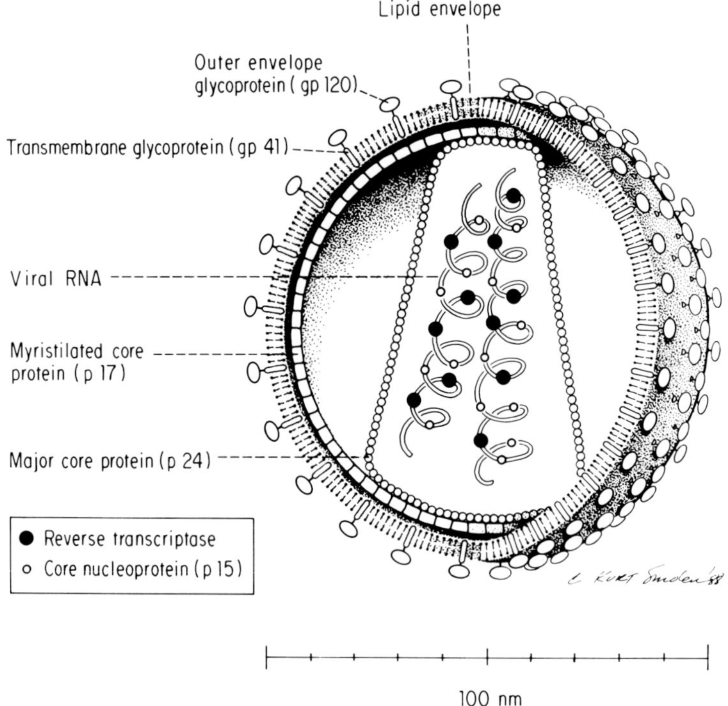


**FIG. 2.** Diagram of the structure of HIV showing the proposed location of the processed structural proteins of the virion.

As an enveloped virus, HIV is readily inactivated by detergents and soaps, or by organic solvents like ethanol, acetone, and phenol. It is also inactivated by 0.2% sodium hypochlorite, which is commonly available in household bleaches, by 1% glutaraldehyde for disinfection of medical instruments, or by heat (21–23). For example, infectious virus in serum is inactivated at 56°C for 60 min, which preserves antibody activity as measured by many immunoassays including commercial enzyme-linked immunosorbent assays (ELISA) (22–27).

With electron microscopy (EM), the inside of the virion contains an electron-dense cylindrical nucleoid consisting of the RNA genome and associated viral proteins (Figs. 1 and 2). The internal proteins include structural proteins of the gag family and the reverse transcriptase. Recently, a protein unique to HIV-2 and its close relative from macaques, simian immunodeficiency virus (SIV), has been identified and associated with the ribonucleoprotein structure (28). This protein (p16 in HIV-2) is a product of the open reading frame designated *vpx* or *sid*.

### Genome Organization and Virus Proteins

The genome of HIV is a single-stranded RNA that is approximately 9,200 bases long (Fig. 3). Two copies of this molecule, which is of the same polarity as messenger RNA, are present in each infectious virion. The RNA is converted by reverse transcription in the host cell into a double-stranded DNA provirus that for HIV-1 is approximately 9,750 base pairs long (Fig. 3). This elongation is accounted for by duplication of components of the long terminal repeats (LTRs) that flank the viral genome. The LTR regions define sites for circularization and chromosomal integration. The 5′-LTR also contains transcriptional regulatory se-

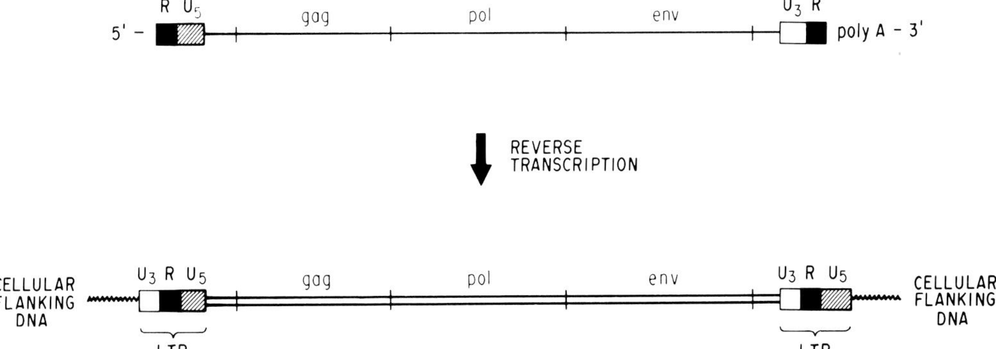


**FIG. 3.** Schematic representation of a single RNA genomic subunit and its reverse transcribed provirus. This is the general structure of all replication competent retroviruses including HIV and HTLV. The structural organization of the genome including the regulatory genes is depicted in Fig. 4. The provirus is represented as integrated into cellular sequences; however, closed circular (episomal) proviral forms are present in most, if not all, cells infected with HIV.

quences and the initiation site for transcription.

The LTR of HIV-1 consists of a 453-base-pair U3 region, a 98-base-pair R region and an 83-base-pair U5 region (29) (Fig. 3). The U3 and R regions contain multiple *cis*-acting elements that regulate proviral expression. These include a TATA box that is 27 base pairs upstream from the transcription initiation site. The TATA box in other eukaryotic transcription systems contributes to transcription initiation and promoter efficiency.

Upstream of this TATA box are several elements that bind cellular transcription factors that augment HIV transcription. These elements include three tandem, GC-rich sequences between −46 and −77 (+1 represents the U3/R junction or the base at which transcription is initiated) that bind the cellular protein Sp1 (30,31) and an enhancer element between −82 and −105 that is highly conserved with the sequence of the cellular binding site of the inducible transcription factor NF-κB (32–34). The NF-KB binding site in HIV was first found in the K light chain immunoglobulin enhancer in B cells and has been shown to bind NF-κB *in vitro* (34). Activation of T cells releases transcriptionally active NF-κB, which may induce the replication of HIV following T-cell activation. *Trans*-acting herpesvirus proteins such as the 110 kilodalton immediate early protein (ICP O) of herpes simplex virus (HSV) can interact with these sequences to enhance HIV transcription (35–39). Other sequences in the LTR almost certainly resemble other cellular regulatory elements, and these are being delineated (40). For example, the region −357 to −278 of the HIV LTR shares a sequence with a eukaryotic regulatory element that binds the nuclear activator protein-1 (AP-1). Both sequences bind the nuclear protein products of the proto-oncogenes c-*fos* and c-*jun* (41).

HIV, as well as the host cell, codes for a number of regulatory proteins that act in *trans* to regulate HIV-transcription. These proteins interact either directly or indirectly with elements that act in *cis* to control the quantity and relative ratios of viral proteins. These elements include the *tat* responsive region, termed the TAR, that is located between −17 and +44 and probably forms a hairpin loop structure in the RNA transcripts (32,42–44). This stem loop structure in the TAR region of RNA transcripts appears to terminate transcription in the absence of the tat protein. The rev (previously termed art or trs) 20-kilodalton protein appears to regulate cellular splicing

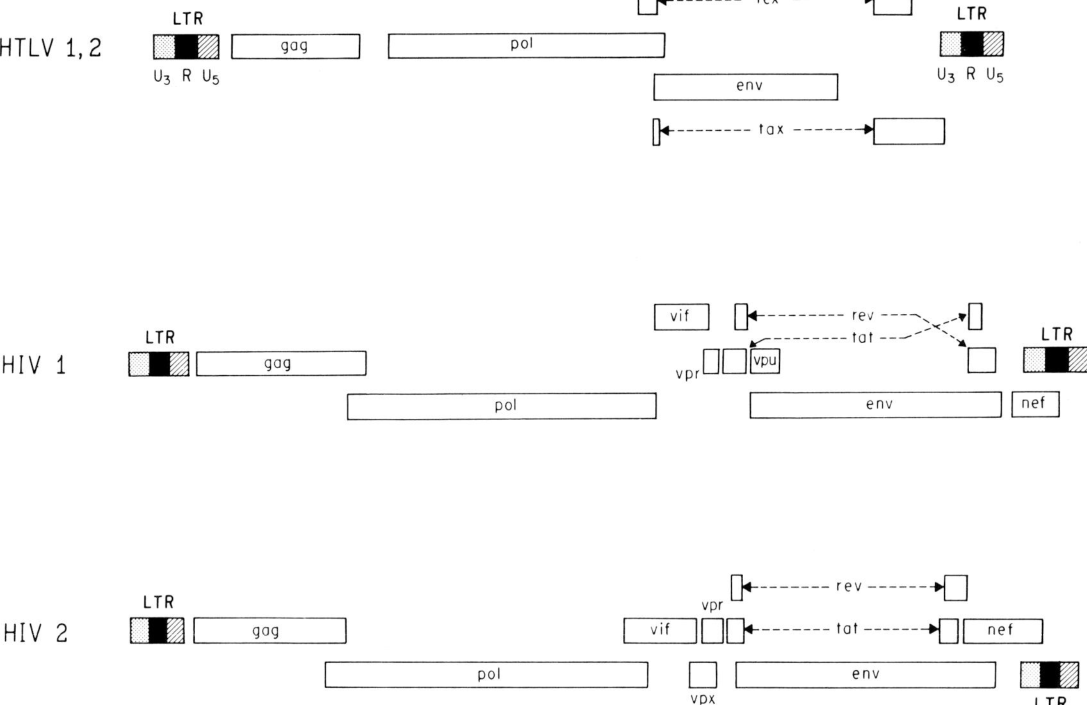


**FIG. 4.** Genome organization of the human retroviruses. The components of the LTRs are shaded. The open reading frames that encode viral proteins are depicted by unshaded boxes. The gene products and their functions are described in the text.

mechanisms by directly or indirectly interacting with *cis*-acting sequences in the *env* region (45). Cellular factors may also interact with these *cis*-acting elements (31,46,47).

The gene coding sequences lie between the LTR flanking regions (Fig. 4). The *gag* gene represents a single open reading frame that is translated into a polypeptide (p55) that is proteolytically cleaved into three proteins: p17, which is myristoylated and associates with the inner surface of the cell membrane; p24, which is phosphorylated and is the major core protein of the nucleocapsid; and p15 (48). The p15 gag product is further processed into a proline rich p9 and a nucleic acid binding p7. (By convention, p55, for example, designates a virion protein of 55 kilodaltons; gp designates a glycoprotein).

*Pol* overlaps *gag* and is translated from a different reading frame on the same messenger RNA (49). *Pol* codes for three known proteins: a protease, a reverse transcriptase/ribonuclease H complex, and an integrase/endonuclease. The 99 amino acid protease is coded for at the 5′ end of the *pol* gene and is required for viral infectivity, suggesting that it is a logical target for an antiviral agent (50–52). The 10,774-dalton protease is generated by an autocatalytic process from a pol precursor and is active as a dimer (50,51,53–55). It is an aspartic protease that recognizes certain amino acid sequences for endoproteolytic cleavage (56–60). The amino acid sequences recognized by the HIV protease have not yet been fully delineated. The identification of transition state analogs of these peptide sequences should provide the first leads for antiviral inhibitors of this enzyme. The crystal structure of the protease has been determined to 3A resolution, which should facilitate the design of inhibitors (61).

The reverse transcriptase/ribonuclease H complex consists of a heterodimer of a 66-kilodalton polypeptide and a 51-kilodalton polypeptide that represents the truncated amino portion of p66 (62–66). Functional domains of the reverse transcriptase enzyme have been identified by site-directed mutagenesis (63). The reverse transcriptase contains both RNA-dependent DNA polymerase and ribonuclease H activities, each located on different sites of the same protein. The reverse transcriptase is a $Mg^{2+}$-requiring polymerase that requires a double-stranded region as a primer to initiate DNA synthesis from a single-stranded RNA. This primer is a specific lysine tRNA that is complementary to the 5′ end of the virion RNA and is incorporated during virion assembly. The RNase H degrades the RNA from the RNA/DNA hybrids as a processive exonuclease to permit completion of the synthesis of the double-stranded DNA provirus (67). This enzyme does not degrade single-stranded or double-stranded RNA. The ribonuclease H activity resides in the carboxy terminus of the p66 polypeptide and may also exist as a free p15 derivative of p66 (67). In the cell, the *pol* gene products probably function in capsid structures rather than in free solution, as assays are performed in cell free experiments. The integrase/endonuclease has not undergone as complete characterization as the other pol protein products.

The *env* gene code for a highly glycosylated polyprotein (gp160) that is cleaved by a cellular serine protease into two virion glycoproteins, gp120 and gp41. The glycoprotein spike on the surface of the HIV virion and infected cells is a trimer of the more exposed gp120 component and the transmembrane gp41 component. The 480 amino acid surface glycoprotein, gp120, binds a domain at the amino end of CD4 with a very high binding affinity. CD4 is the principal, if not only, host cell receptor protein for HIV (68–71) and is present on the CD4 subset of T lymphocytes and many macrophage/monocyte cells. This mediation of binding to host cells represents a target for antiviral candidate compounds, like recombinant soluble CD4. Gp120 displays many epitopes for neutralizing antibodies; however, it also displays a remarkable hypervariability in many regions among different virus strains (72,73). This variability may contribute to the evasion of immune surveillance by the virus. The transmembrane glycoprotein, gp41, mediates membrane fusion, resulting in the virus uncoating process during entry and the formation of multinucleated giant cells, termed "syncytia." Of interest, the amino terminus of gp41 that is generated by the endoproteolytic cleavage shares sequence similarities with the fusion (F) glycoprotein of the *Paramyxoviridae* which are activated by a similar posttranslational cleavage event by host cell serine proteases to mediate similar fusion activity (74–77). Virus mutants that are not susceptible to the endoproteolytic cleavage of gp160 cannot mediate membrane fusion and remain noninfectious unless cleavage is performed (78).

The *gag, pol,* and *env* gene organization in the HIV genome has been preserved throughout the *Retroviridae.* The nucleotide sequences of HIV-1 and HIV-2 as well as HTLV-1 and HTLV-2, however, reveal additional open reading frames (79–86). These open reading frames represent genes that code accessory proteins (87). Several of these genes (*tat, rev, nef*) have been shown to regulate proviral expression, and the delineation of the functions of the others (*vif, vpr, vpu* in HIV-1; *vpx* in HIV-2) are being intensively investigated.

The 86 amino acid tat protein is the product of a doubly spliced messenger RNA that is coded for by two open reading frames, the first 5′ to *env* and the second overlapping gp41 but in a different reading frame (88,89). The tat protein localizes in the nucleus (90), and more recent evidence suggests nucleolar localization. Designated tat for *trans*-activation of transcription, this protein appears to act in *trans* to regulate both transcription and posttranscriptional processes (32,90–96). The tat protein functions as a dimer, with each p15 monomer containing seven cysteine residues, six of which are essential. Two molecules of zinc or cadmium are bound per dimer (97,98). Although such structures often represent DNA-binding regions in many proteins, they may serve to mediate dimerization of *tat* (97). Synthetic peptides of these structures form nonfunctional heterodimers with *tat* and have been proposed as models for tat inhibitory antiviral compounds (97). It has not been shown whether the action of *tat* depends upon interaction with viral nucleic acid, cellular nucleic acid, or cellular regulatory factors. Nevertheless, *tat* expression is essential for the replication of HIV (94,98–100), thus identifying another promising target for antiviral drugs.

A second regulatory gene is *rev* (regulator of expression of virion proteins, formerly designated *art* or *trs*). The *rev* gene is also doubly spliced and overlaps the *tat* exons but in different open reading frames, a testimony to genetic efficiency. The 116-amino-acid 20-kilodalton rev protein is located predominantly in the nucleus (101) and is phosphorylated on a serine residue (102). This protein appears to modulate the transcription of virion mRNA. Rev-minus mutants appear to accumulate messages for early accessory genes and fail to produce stable messages for the structural *gag, pol,* and *env* genes (94,98,103–106). There are at least four *cis*-acting repression sequences (*CRS*) in *env* that are present in introns of *tat* and *rev* and are conserved in HIV-1 and HIV-2 (45). These sequences, when present transcripts in the absence of the rev product in the nucleus, repress the expression of the corresponding gene products. These CRS rev-response elements, which have highly complex predicted secondary structure, prevent the transport of these transcripts from the nucleus to the cytoplasm, presumably permitting splicing to *CRS*-minus transcripts such as *tat* and *rev* (107). The expression of *rev* in the nucleus results in the transport of these unspliced *CRS*-containing transcripts to the cytoplasm where the mRNA for structural genes can be translated and the virion RNA can be encapsidated (107). A *cis*-acting antirepressive element (CAR) that helps mediate this response to *rev* has been mapped to the gp120 portion of *env* (45). These functions are necessary for viral replication (104,105); *rev* thus also represents a promising target for antiviral drugs. Of note, HTLV-1 and HTLV-2 have two regulatory genes, designated *tax* and *rex,* which appear to have actions analogous to *tat* and *rev,* although these genes display no homology and their mechanisms of action may be distinct.

HIV contains a third regulatory gene designated *nef* (negative factor). This gene was previously designated F or 3′ ORF because it is the most 3′-open reading frame of the HIV genome; it actually overlaps the 3′ LTR. *Nef* encodes a 27-kilodalton protein to which at least two-thirds of infected people can be shown to produce antibody (108). Nef-minus mutants replicate to higher titers than wild-type virus, suggesting a negative regulatory role (99). The nef protein appears to inhibit transcription from the LTR of HIV-1 (109), although it appears to localize in the cytoplasm (110). Characterization of the nef protein expressed in *Escherichia coli* indicates that it is a guanosine-triphosphate-(GTP)-binding protein, with GTPase activity resembling the p21 *ras* oncogene (111).

The function of other accessory genes is not yet clear; however, the existence of their protein products is indicated by the prevalence of specific antibodies in the sera of seropositive subjects to polypeptides expressed by recombinant DNA technology. *Vif* (virus infectivity factor) formerly termed *sor,* encodes a 23-kilodalton protein (112–115). Vif-deletion mutants produce virions that are poorly infectious (112,115). The extent of this impaired infectivity varies from cell to cell. There is no evidence as to whether or not the vif product is a virion protein. The designation vpr (viral protein

R) indicates an unknown function and an inevitable name change. *Vpr* encodes a 78-amino-acid protein to which at least one-third of seropositive subjects have detectable antibodies (116). A ninth gene has been identified for HIV-1 and HIV-2, but this differs for each. An 81-amino-acid, 16-kilodalton product of the *vpu* gene of HIV-1 is produced *in vivo,* as evidenced by measurable antibody responses in patients with AIDS (117,118). Deletion of this gene reduces the yield of progeny virions (118). It is of interest that not all published sequences of HIV-1 contain a functional *vpu* gene. The biologic significance of this observation is unclear. In HIV-2, *vpx* (viral protein X) or *sid* encodes a 16-kilodalton, apparently virion, RNA-binding protein to which many infected subjects possess antibody (28,119–121).

### Replication and Potential Sites for Specific Antiviral Therapy

Infection is initiated by the binding of gp120 on the surface of a virion or a virus-infected cell to the CD4 glycoprotein on the surface of susceptible host cells. This high-affinity interaction, which is amplified by the presence of multiple ligand-receptor pairs, can be blocked by monoclonal antibodies to the amino terminus of CD4 (68,69,71) or by soluble polypeptides containing the amino-terminal portion of CD4 (122–128). CD4 is present on a subset of T cells, many monocyte-macrophages, and Langerhan's cells. Controversy exists whether cells not expressing CD4 are permissive host cells. Expression of the CD4 receptor on HeLa cells by transfection or transfection of HIV proviruses into CD4 negative human (but not murine) cells indicates that CD4 alone can be a restricting factor for infection with HIV (70,129). CD4 negative monocyte-macrophages can readily propagate virus (130). It is not clear whether the absence of CD4 on these permissive cells demonstrates an alternative receptor or an insensitive assay for CD4.

After adsorption, penetration of the host cell membrane is mediated by fusion of virus envelope and host cell membrane, by the fusogenic gp41 (41). The mechanism for this process remains to be elucidated. This step results in release of the nucleoprotein complex into the cell cytoplasm where reverse transcription is activated. The generation of the double-stranded viral DNA is catalyzed by the reverse transcriptase/ribonuclease complex.

Complementarity between sequences 5′ to the transfer RNA (tRNA) binding site and the 3′ LTR permit circularization and duplication of LTR elements to occur during reverse transcription. The activated reverse transcriptase, RNase H, and virion RNA generate a double-stranded viral DNA that is circular and longer than the virion genome by the length of the duplicated U3 and U5 regions of the LTR. The double-stranded viral DNA then migrates to the nucleus by a mechanism that is not well understood. Some of these DNA molecules are then integrated into apparently random sites in the host genome by the third pol product, the integrase that is a DNA endonuclease. The integrated viral DNA, termed the "provirus," however, maintains its genome organization with the flanking LTRs (Fig. 3) by integrating at a defined site in the viral DNA. For every integrated provirus in the cell, there are many more free closed circular (episomal) and linear double-stranded forms of virus DNA. The replicative and pathogenetic roles of these episomal forms has not been defined. It is also unclear whether integration requires prior circularization, as had been believed (131).

The level of transcription of this viral DNA is largely determined by the relative levels of expression of cellular *trans*-acting factors that interact with the 5′-LTR. These include cellular factors that interact with the *cis*-acting enhancers, promoters, and other domains in the 5′-LTR, as well as with the newly synthesized viral regulatory proteins. All transcription is initiated in the 5′-LTR. Multiple transcripts have been mapped. These range in size from the full-length genomic transcripts necessary to assemble new progeny with complete virion RNAs to smaller transcripts that are generated by one or more steps, including splicing, presumably mediated by cellular mechanisms. The time courses and relative proportions of the synthesis of these different transcripts are still being defined. As described above, conversion from the transcription of messenger RNAs (mRNAs) for regulatory genes to those for structural genes is probably mediated by the rev protein.

After migration of these transcripts from the nucleus to the cytoplasm, cellular translational machinery synthesizes viral polypeptides. Many of these mRNAs, especially those for the structural genes of *gag, pol,* and *env,* yield polyproteins that are endoproteolytically cleaved by the viral protease into individual viral proteins, probably during the encapsidation/budding process. Other posttranslational modification of viral proteins include myristoylation of p17, glycosylation of the env protein products, and phosphorylation of the *rev* gene product.

The mechanisms of virion assembly and budding have not been elucidated; however, the precise molecular interactions of each of the virion components must define this process. The viral glycoprotein, gp160, contains several hydrophobic amino acid domains that anchor the newly synthesized env polypeptide into membrane of the endoplasmic reticulum during translation. The env polypeptide, always anchored in membrane, is glycosylated and cleaved as it is translated and then transported to the external cell membrane. The glycoprotein spikes associate, whereas cellular proteins are excluded, in the regions of cell membrane associated with the myristoylated, hydrophobic p17 protein that is assembling subjacent to the cell membrane in this region. Virion RNA and virion core proteins then assemble in the region of the newly budding virion. It is not known how these proteins assemble. Similarly, it remains to be clarified how two viral RNA subunits are selectively encapsidated with their complementary cellular tRNAs.

## PATHOGENESIS

### Host Cells

In one of the first descriptions of AIDS, the depletion of CD4 helper T cells was appreciated (2). It was soon demonstrated that HIV produced a cytolytic infection of lymphocytes *in vitro* in contrast to the lymphoproliferative response characteristic of HTLV-1 or HTLV-2 and other oncornaviruses (6,7). The identification of CD4 itself as the cellular receptor for HIV gp120 (68,69,71) explains the selective susceptibility of this subset of lymphocytes for infection with HIV, the continuing depletion of circulating CD4 helper T lymphocytes with progressive infection, and the characteristic array of opportunistic infections with endogenous flora that are prevented from proliferating by normal cellular immunity. Although these observations have been substantiated, the pathogenesis of HIV infection not surprisingly has proven to be more complex.

A balanced view of the pathogenesis of HIV infection must account for a number of observations: (a) the mechanism by which HIV replication kills cells has not been elucidated; (b) the infection of CD4 lymphocytes *in vitro* is not always immediately cytolytic; (c) alternative mechanisms of both killing and functional impairment of CD4 positive cells can be demonstrated *in vitro* without infecting CD4 cells themselves; and (d) cells other than CD4 helper T lymphocytes have been shown to be host cells for infection with HIV both *in vitro* and *in vivo*. Infection of monocyte-macrophages and perhaps other cells are a critical aspect of the pathogenesis of HIV infection.

How HIV kills CD4 lymphocytes is still debated. The intracellular accumulation of toxic complexes of CD4 and gp120 (71,132), the accumulation of toxic episomal DNA as occurs in oncornaviruses (133), and the parasitic competition for essential cellular functions (134) have all been proposed.

Many observers have proposed cytolysis of uninfected CD4 cells to explain depletion in HIV-infected subjects, because at any given time only approximately 1 in $10^5$ circulating lymphocytes expresses detectable viral antigen or nucleic acid (135). We do not know the proportion of infected cells at different stages of disease, the sensitivities of these assays, the life spans of infected cells detected with these assays, the life spans and numbers of infected cells not detected by these assays, the impact of HIV infection on stem cells or developing lymphocytes, or how well assays of circulating cells reflect pathology outside of the bloodstream. Consequently, the analysis of the mechanism of depletion is difficult.

As already described, *trans*-acting factors of viral and host origin can profoundly affect *cis*-acting regulatory elements in the virion LTR. This may account for the profound stimulation of virus replication upon activation of lymphocytes (136,137). It has thus been proposed that infection of a lymphocyte may not be lethal until that antigen-committed lymphocyte is activated by exposure to the specific antigen. This hypothesis would predict the progressive depletion of lymphocytes that recognize and suppress the normal flora by agents such as cytomegalovirus (CMV) or *Pneumocystis carinii*. It is also possible that coinfection of host cells with herpesviruses, such as CMV, that encode *trans*-acting proteins that interact with the LTR of HIV to stimulate transcription could activate HIV replication (35,36,38,138).

CD4 lymphocytes can be depleted *in vitro* without being primarily infected. Any cell that is infected with HIV and expressing gp120 on its surface has a high-affinity receptor for cells bearing CD4. Fusion of the membranes of the infected and uninfected CD4 cells results in a syncytium, a terminal event for the uninfected cell (139–141). It has also been proposed that viral components bound to uninfected cells, for example gp120 to CD4, could provide a target for antigen-specific cytolytic cells and antibody-dependent killing (142,143).

Additional potential pathogenetic mechanisms continue to be proposed (144,145). For example, the production of large quantities of recombinant tat protein has permitted the demonstration of uptake by uninfected cells of low concentrations (1 ug/ml) of cell-free protein that exert trans-activating activities upon these cells in culture (C. A. Rosen, unpublished observations). The release of tat protein from dying cells could theoretically affect the function or survival of uninfected cells. The pathogenicity of *tat* is also indicated by the development of dermal lesions resembling Kaposi's sarcoma in male mice trangenic for *tat*-1 (146).

The monocyte-macrophage and related cells are a critical component in the pathogenesis of HIV infection. The resemblance of lymphadenopathy-associated virus (LAV) to lentiviruses using EM was suggested in the first published report of an isolate of HIV (6). Soon, sequence homologies between HIV and animal lentivirus confirmed the relationship (147–150). For those familiar with the pathogenesis of animal lentiviruses (151–153), in which the macrophage is the primary host cell, the prospect that HIV might infect macrophages was a consideration at the outset, despite the intense focus on CD4 T lymphocytes. Retrovirus particles were observed with EM in the follicular dendritic cells and macrophages of lymph nodes from patients prior to the development of AIDS (154,155). Several investigators soon reported the isolation of HIV *in vitro* using macrophages from infected patients as inocula and macrophages from uninfected subjects as a permissive cell substrate (156–158).

Documentation of infection of the monocyte-macrophage *in vivo* soon followed. Macrophages in the alveoli (159), lymph nodes (160,161), and brain (162–166) were shown by immunoperoxidase staining and *in situ* DNA hybridization to be the most heavily infected cells in the body. In the central nervous system (CNS), a major target organ of HIV disease, the primary pathology seen is an increased mononuclear inflammatory infiltrate and occasional multinucleate giant cells (162). These inflammatory cells and the giant cells possess macrophage markers and are infected with HIV. No primary cell of the CNS such as neuronal cells has been consistently and definitively shown to be infected with HIV.

One of the most heavily infected cells of the body are Langerhan's cells (167,168). Langerhan's cells are antigen-presenting cells in the skin that express CD4, class II Ia antigens, and (Fc) receptors for immunoglobulin, thus sharing certain characteristics and functions of macrophages in the epidermis (169–171). These cells become progressively more depleted as infection progresses (172,173), and infection of them by HIV may have many consequences.

The macrophage and its relatives are a complex group of cells. They are heterogeneous with regard to surface antigen expression, levels of differentiation, and levels of activation (174–176). They migrate, undergo chemotaxis, kill microorganisms, present antigens to lymphocytes, and elaborate monokines that modulate many aspects of the immune system. Infection, of these cells or subsets of them, may have manifold consequences (177). HIV infection could have profound consequences on immune function in many ways. The elaboration of monokines or viral products in the brain could account for much of the neuropathology of HIV infection (178). The fact that infected macrophages can survive infection for months *in vitro* suggests that these cells may serve as a reservoir, contributing to the persistent chronic infection by HIV (130,179). Infected macrophages could contribute to the depletion of CD4 T lymphocytes by persistently elaborating viral progeny, or by fusing with and killing uninfected helper T cells via the gp120/CD4 interaction or via their role as antigen presenting cells to antigen-specific T lymphocytes (180).

Dissection of the role of HIV in the monocyte/macrophage group of cells *in vivo* will be difficult. As mentioned, these are a complex and heterogeneous group of cells. They propagate poorly or not at all *in vitro*. The studies conducted *in vitro* may not reflect all of the important cells or functions *in vivo*. In addition to the heterogeneity of host cells, it is becoming increasingly clear that HIV isolates are heterogeneous (or mixed) and that some isolates are more tropic for macrophages than lymphocytes or vice versa (130,181). These issues represent obstacles to aspects of pathogenesis that are clearly important in order to understand the disease and its treatment.

### Target Organ Systems

The primary target organ systems of HIV infection are the immune system and the nervous system. With CD4 helper T lymphocytes and monocyte-macrophages as the primary host cells of HIV infection, the impact on the immune system is not surprising, although the mechanisms of immunodeficiency require more definition, as already discussed. Pathologically, the organs of the reticuloendothelial system display lymphoid hyperplasia with enlarged, irregular secondary follicles and expanded germinal centers (182–185). Lymphoid depletion with involution of nodes and spleen is often associated with the progression of generalized lymphadenopathy to AIDS (184,186). Using immunohistochemical staining with monoclonal antibodies, much more viral antigen is seen in the large nodes with proliferating follicles than in the degenerating nodes (182). These nodes, as in the blood, display depleted CD4 lymphocytes and increased numbers of CD8 lymphocytes (185,186).

The chronic degenerative CNS disease seen in HIV infection (187–191) appears to be the consequence of infection of the macrophage that represents the principal infected cell in the brain (162–165,192–194). By analogy to other lentiviral encephalopathies, the infected macrophage may enter the CNS as a "Trojan horse," seeking to respond to low grade replication of CMV or *Toxoplasma* or to perform other duties only to establish a site for persistent infection and its consequences (151,153,157).

Virtually all organs have been involved with an opportunistic infection or malignancy resulting from AIDS; however, pathology has been documented in association with HIV infection itself, independent of opportunistic consequences in several organ systems other than the immune and nervous systems. A minority of patients with AIDS develop an unexplained cardiomyopathy (195–197), arthritis (198,199), nephropathy (200,201), myositis (76,202), dermatitis (203,204), gastric secretory failure (205), enteropathy (206), or endocrinopathies (207). It is the bone marrow, however, that is most consistently affected by HIV infection (208). As infection progresses to AIDS-related complex (ARC) and AIDS, the majority, if not all, individuals exhibit granulocytopenia and anemia (209). It is not clear whether HIV can directly affect marrow precursors or whether cytokines or immune responses elaborated by infected cells inhibit marrow function. Hematopoiesis *in vitro* is inhibited by serum from seropositive subjects (210,211). Nevertheless, it is clear that impaired marrow reserve can be clinically significant; for example, it may restrict the utility of chemotherapeutic agents. Thrombocytopenia may also be seen in patients infected with HIV (212–214). The mechanism in contrast to the myeloid and erythroid pathology is probably antibody mediated as in other forms of autoimmune thrombocytopenia (144,215–217).

## IMMUNE RESPONSE

Within days of exposure to HIV, viremia and p24 antigenemia can be documented. Within 1 or 2 weeks, the p24 antigenemia is no longer detectable and a series of humoral and cellular immune responses can be measured. This is the limited evidence of the role of immunity in dampening viral replication. The principal interest in characterizing the immune response, both the important viral antigens and the important humoral and cellular components, is to ascertain the protective elements that could help vaccine design. To date, such beneficial immunity has been difficult to document even in simian or other animal models of lentiviral immunodeficiency. The primary utility of assays of immune responses to HIV has been for epidemiology, natural history, and diagnosis.

Immunoglobulin M (IgM) antibodies to the major structural proteins (gag and env products) appear within days of infection and IgG antibodies within weeks. These IgM antibodies can be assessed by a number of methods including indirect immunofluorescence (IF), ELISA, and immunoblotting (218–220). Antibodies to the gag and env products occur almost universally in infected subjects, although antibody to p24 tends to disappear in a significant proportion of subjects as they progress to ARC and AIDS (221). Antibodies to reverse transcriptase and an epitope of gp41 are also common and may represent a favorable prognosis (222,223). A proportion, but not all subjects can be shown to produce antibodies to proteins of each of the accessory genes (*tat, rev, nef, vpu, vpx, vif*) (28,108,113,114,118–121,224–227) using immunoblotting with cell lysates as antigen or ELISA with recombinant expressed polypeptides as antigen. The biologic significance of these antibodies is unclear; however, the demonstration of these antibodies has been useful in confirming that putative open reading frames in the HIV genome actually code for true viral products.

Within months, neutralizing antibody can be measured (228,229). Several neutralizing epitopes have been mapped to gp120 and at least one to gp41 (230–235). Because HIV exhibits much genetic variation, especially in the "hypervariable" regions of gp120 (29,236–240), it will be important not only to measure these neutralizing antibodies against laboratory strains but to assess patients' responses to their own virus (241). The presence of genotypic mixtures and variation of isolates from an individual with time, as has been shown with animal lentivirus (242,243), further complicates these assessments (244–247). Antibody-mediated cellular cytotoxicity, like neutralizing antibodies, also appears early in seropositive subjects and persists throughout the duration of infection (248–250).

Cell-mediated immune responses also develop in infected subjects. Lymphoproliferation responses to gag and env epitopes have been demonstrated using recombinant proteins and synthetic oligopeptides (251–258). Utilizing vaccinia virus expression vectors to express antigens in histocompatible target cells, CD8 cytotoxic T-cell responses occur to *gag, env,* and *pol* gene products (254,259,260). All these responses appear to decline in intensity with disease progression, raising the issue of cause and effect. As with neutralizing epitopes, T-cell responses to epitopes of HIV can be restricted to a virus strain (142).

Not only have clear benefits been difficult to ascribe to the immune response, but allegations of adverse consequences have been made. In addition to failing to perform its duties as infection progresses, the immune system has been theorized to contribute to some of the pathology in HIV infection. Higher frequencies of certain adverse drug reactions that may be immunologically mediated have been described. These include dermatitis and drug reactions, especially to trimethoprim-sulfamethoxazole (261,262). Immune complexes are common, most likely consisting of p24 and its antibody, the consequences of which have not been well delineated (263,264). Polyclonal B cell activation with hypergammaglobulinemia is commonly seen in infected subjects (265). This may be associated with the presence of a lupus anticoagulant (266,267) or other autoantibodies (200). In addition, patients may develop a clinically significant idiopathic thrombocytopenic purpura, the pathogenesis of which is unclear, but which may be immunologically mediated. It has also been demonstrated *in vitro* that free gp120 bound to uninfected CD4 cells can provide a target for cytolytic T cells (142,268) and antibody-dependent cytotoxicity (143).

## CLINICAL MANIFESTATIONS

Infection with HIV is followed within 1–2 weeks by a nonspecific viral or mononucleosis-like syndrome characterized by fever, lymphadenopathy, pharyngitis, aseptic meningitis, and a mild erythematous macular exanthem (220,269–278). This syndrome, termed "primary HIV infection syndrome," may occur in a majority of individuals; however, its nonspecificity renders quantitation and characterization difficult. Resolution over days to a few weeks results in the most common condition associated with HIV infection, the asymptomatic carrier. Antibodies to HIV develop 2 weeks to 2 months after the onset of illness.

Asymptomatic individuals seropositive for HIV may maintain this status for a year to decades, and may transmit the virus by blood or genital secretions. During this asymptomatic state, circulating CD8 T-cell numbers may increase, CD4 T-cell numbers may plateau at a subnormal level or gradually decline, and subtle subclinical cognitive defects may develop (188). Asymptomatic seropositive individuals usually can be shown to have B-cell activation with increased immunoglobulin and autoantibody production as well as CD4 helper defects with specific recall antigens. Generalized lymphadenopathy may develop and persist for months to years. The development or presence of lymphadenopathy due to HIV infection has been shown to have little prognostic significance (279).

The continuing decline in immune function may first manifest itself clinically with infections such as thrush or herpes zoster, which in the correct epidemiological setting can suggest HIV infection but may occur in uninfected, healthy subjects. Nonspecific constitutional symptoms like fever, night sweats, weight loss, and diarrhea of undetermined etiology also may develop (228,280–284). These symptoms are components of ARC, a syndrome associated with progressive HIV infection not sufficiently specific to provide an etiologic diagnosis.

Attempts have been made to stage this progressive disease, on the basis of symptoms by the Centers for Disease Control (CDC) (285) or immunological status by the Walter Reed group (286). These are useful for the purposes of epidemiology and health policy planning; however, they provide little use at present for the management of individual patients (287).

The development of any of several opportunistic infections or malignancies (Table 1) in the absence of an alternative explanation (congenital immunodeficiency, transplantation, immunosuppressive chemotherapy) fulfills the diagnostic criteria for AIDS. Prior to the identification of HIV, an operational definition of AIDS for epidemiologic purposes was needed. Because the opportunistic complications associated with AIDS are so infrequent in normal hosts, this definition proved quite sensitive and specific. With time, minor modifications have been made, especially the inclusion of severe symptoms of ARC and encephalopathy as criteria sufficient to fulfill the diagnosis of AIDS. These modifications acknowledge the fact that ARC symptoms alone can be seriously debilitating or even lethal in the absence of an AIDS-defining opportunistic infection or malignancy and that encephalopathy and other CNS complications can develop concurrently or independently of the immunologic dysfunction in any given individuals (288).

The establishment of diagnostic criteria for the definition of AIDS, although critical for epidemiologic purposes, does not ad-

**TABLE 1.[a] AIDS Defining Conditions**

| AIDS-defining conditions |
|---|
| AIDS-defining conditions requiring no laboratory evidence of HIV infection (alternative causes of immunosuppression excluded) |
| Candidiasis: esophageal, bronchopulmonary |
| *Pneumocystis carinii*: pneumonia |
| *Toxoplasma gondii*: encephalitis |
| Cryptococcosis: extrapulmonary |
| CMV: any organ other than liver, spleen, and lymph node, especially retinitis |
| HSV: esophageal, mucocutaneous (>1 month) |
| *Mycobacterium avium* complex or *M. kansasii*: disseminated |
| Cryptosporidiosis: enteritis (>1 month) |
| Strongyloidiasis: gastrointestinal |
| Progressive multifocal leukoencephalopathy |
| Kaposi's sarcoma: affecting a patient <60 years of age |
| Lymphoma of the brain: primary, affecting a patient <60 years of age |
| AIDS-defining conditions requiring laboratory evidence of HIV infection |
| Coccidiomycosis: disseminated |
| Histoplasmosis: disseminated |
| Isosporiasis: enteritis (>1 month) |
| Mycobacteriosis (other than *M. tuberculosis*): disseminated |
| *M. tuberculosis*: extrapulmonary |
| Salmonella (nontyphoidal): recurrent septicemia |
| Encephalopathy or dementia |
| HIV wasting syndrome ("slim disease") |
| Kaposi's sarcoma at any age |
| Lymphomas of the brain, or other non-Hodgkins, non T-cell lymphomas in patients at any age |

[a]The criteria for pediatric AIDS are less sensitive and specific but also include lymphoid interstitial pneumonia and multiple or recurrent bacterial infections in a seropositive child.

Revised from Morbidity Mortality Weekly Reports, ref. 288.

dress two essential concepts. One is that HIV infection is a chronic, persistent, relentless infection that occurs in continuous real time, in some patients over a year or two, in others a decade or more. The abrupt presentation of an opportunistic infection does not reflect this continuous infectious process by HIV. The second concept is that opportunistic complications of HIV infection cannot be absolutely predicted by any marker of infection or immunodeficiency that we now can measure. Low CD4 T-lymphocyte enumeration, p24 antigenemia, high $\beta_2$ microglobulin levels have all been shown to be independently predictive of likelihood of progression; however, these are all statistical likelihoods (221,282,289–291). One patient may develop AIDS with over 400 CD4 lymphocytes/$mm^3$ of blood; another may remain asymptomatic for 2 years with 20 cells. Both of these concepts are critical in the evaluation of the clinical impact of antiviral drugs. Chemotherapy must be assessed with the perspective that HIV infection is persistent and progressive, that clinical end points are statistical likelihoods in any patient population, and, as a corollary, that no outcome can be confidently expected in any individual patient.

In the United States and many locations with similar populations, *Pneumocystis carinii* pneumonia (PCP) is the AIDS-defining opportunistic infection in over two-thirds and the most frequently diagnosed complication in patients with AIDS (292). In other populations, such as Haitians and Africans, tuberculosis, toxoplasmosis, and cryptosporidiosis are seen more frequently (293), reflecting the prevalence of these organisms in the premorbid population. For those surviving the AIDS-defining condition, relapse of that condition or the appearance of any or several of the others may occur within months or over a period of several years.

The medical community is becoming increasingly sophisticated and expert with regard to the diagnosis and treatment of AIDS-related opportunistic infections and malignancies. AZT and prophylaxis are also prolonging life in these patients. As the natural history of AIDS evolves, the relative likelihood of different conditions may change. As chemoprophylaxis and prompt diagnosis and treatment of opportunistic infections become more established, it is probable that malignancies or HIV encephalopathy may become more prevalent. The challenge is to improve the recognition and management of the AIDS-defining conditions and to appreciate the implications of this changing natural history for the design of clinical studies and the interpretation of treatment interventions.

## EPIDEMIOLOGY

The appreciation of the distinctive clinical syndromes of adult T-cell leukemia and AIDS, and the epidemiological characterization of these diseases preceded the isolation of HTLV-1 and HIV-1, respectively. The epidemiology of AIDS remains dependent upon identification and reporting the clinical syndrome rather than virologic markers. By mid-1988, approximately 250,000 cases of AIDS had occurred worldwide, 75,000 of which were identified in the United States. Over one-half of these individuals with AIDS had died (294). A total of 365,000 cases of AIDS, with 263,000 cumulative deaths, are projected in the United States alone by the year 1992 (295).

In contrast to the prevalence of AIDS, which requires reliable case recognition and reporting, the incidence of new infections is more difficult to ascertain. Serologic testing is a psychologically, socially, and politically charged subject, often requiring informed consent. Determining prevalence of infections requires selection of valid sample populations that reflect the real population. Incidence determinations require multiple tests at different intervals. These determinations are subject to population differences, geographic differences, and changing practices. Nevertheless, by mid-1988

1–1.5 million individuals were estimated to be infected with HIV-1 in the United States and 5–10 million worldwide (294).

Roughly 5% of antibody positive individuals will develop AIDS annually (294). Thus, approximately one-half of people infected with HIV will have developed AIDS after one decade. It is too early to know about the natural history of HIV infection for longer periods of infection. Intervention in the natural history of progression of HIV infection to disease will depend upon inroads in chemotherapy at least in the near future. Intervention in the transmission of HIV to uninfected individuals will depend upon education and behavioral modifications, unless and until a vaccine is developed.

Transmission of HIV requires contact with infected body substances (296). The virus is readily isolated from blood (both plasma and leukocytes), semen, cervicovaginal secretions, breast milk, and cerebrospinal fluid (CSF) (6,8,297–304). All but the last are relevant to transmission. The virus is infrequently detected in low titer in tears and saliva, which represent relatively unimportant sources of virus epidemiologically (305–307). With virus in these body substances, infection occurs via blood and sex. These facts were also known before the identification of HIV because of the epidemiologic resemblance of AIDS and hepatitis B.

The exchange of blood and blood products results in transmission to several high-risk groups: intravenous drug abusers, transfusion recipients, hemophiliacs, and the offspring of seropositive mothers (296). Transfusions of blood products from seropositive donors were infectious to 90–100% of recipients. Screening for antibody to HIV since 1985 in many countries has almost eliminated infection by transfusion or blood products such as factor VIII. AIDS is the leading killer of hemophiliacs and intravenous drug abusers. Intravenous drug abuse is now the leading cause of transmission of HIV (and HTLV) in the developed countries of the Western world (308). The rising relative importance of transmission by intravenous drug abuse and heterosexual contact are resulting in a rising frequency of pediatric AIDS. In the United States, these factors are resulting in blacks and Hispanics representing an increasing proportion of newly infected individuals.

Sexual transmission may occur from blood, semen, or cervicovaginal secretions. Anal receptive intercourse, by men or women, appears to provide the highest risk (309,310). Vaginal intercourse may also transmit infection (311). Rates of infection are higher in individuals with epithelial ulceration due to herpes simplex, syphilis, or chancroid (312). The role of other infections as cofactors of infection or disease has been postulated, especially for the herpesviruses, but not yet proven. Other factors such as virus titer in the inoculum, variation among virus strains, and immune and other susceptibility factors of the recipient and donor have all been proposed to affect the likelihood of transmission.

Of heterosexual partners of infected individuals, 10–70% are themselves seropositive. Symptomatic individuals are more likely to transmit infection than are asymptomatic individuals. The role of virus titer and isolate cytopathogenicity, both of which increase in patients as disease progresses, have not been well characterized regarding transmission, as have genetic or other factors in the recipient.

Contamination of the skin or mucous membranes with infected body or laboratory substances, especially when not intact because of inflammation or trauma, represent a small but definite risk of infection. This exposure, as well as needle sticks, represents a relatively rare but real occupational risk for health care workers (313–315) and laboratory workers (316). This risk and the demonstration that AZT therapy early in the course of animal retroviral infections can prevent the establishment of infection provide the rationale for drug intervention studies in individuals receiving needle sticks potentially contaminated with HIV (317). Nevertheless, the greatest single impact that can be made on the AIDS pandemic, in the absence of an effective vaccine, is the prevention of transmission by behavioral modification.

## DIAGNOSIS

The clinical diagnosis of AIDS and related HIV disease has been described above. The diagnosis of HIV infection in an individual, as with other viruses, is made by detecting a specific immune response or by detecting the presence of the virus itself. Detection of the presence of the virus in clinical specimens requires an assay for infectivity (virus isolation) or an assay for a viral component (detection of viral antigen or nucleic acid).

The standard method for detection of antibody to HIV has been with commercial kits licensed for blood banks. In the United States, these are indirect, solid-phase immunoassays that utilize partially purified, disrupted, inactivated preparations of HIV as antigen. These ELISAs are extremely sensitive and specific and have almost completely eliminated transmission of HIV via blood products. Since the first kits were licensed in March 1985, refinements have made these kits even more sensitive and specific. No single test is perfect however. Tubes may be mislabeled, transcription errors occur, and false-positive results occur in an extremely sensitive assay. Considering the tremendous psychological, social, economic, and medical consequences of a positive test when used to diagnose an individual rather than to dispose of a unit of blood, a number of steps must be in place to conduct a diagnostic test. Informed counseling should be available. A positive ELISA test must be repeated, starting with a repeat phlebotomy to rule out errors of labeling. A repeat positive ELISA test must be confirmed with one of a number of confirmatory assays such as a Western (immuno-) blot assay or IF assay to rule out a false-positive result. False-positive ELISA results can be due to antibodies in multiparous or multiply transfused individuals reacting to class-II HLA antigens from host cells used to propagate HIV (318–321), nonspecific adherence to the solid phase (especially with African sera) (322,323), and cross-reactions between antigens of HIV (especially gag and vif) and other antigens (114,324).

Confirmatory assays such as the Western blot and IF have further improved the dependability of serodiagnosis (325,326); nevertheless, they remain imperfect. For example, the Western blot is expensive, not standardized, and not objective for interpretation, and may yield indeterminant results (327). For example, a p24-only blot may reflect a true positive to p24 of HIV or reactivity with a class II HLA antigen or other nonviral antigen (324,328). Expert counseling must be available for each newly detected seropositive individual.

Improvements in immunoassays are continually being introduced, and the availability of recombinant polypeptides or synthetic oligopeptides as antigens may provide sufficient improvements in sensitivity and specificity to eliminate the need for confirmatory tests in the future (329–334).

ELISA tests and the various confirmatory tests turn positive within 2 weeks to 2 months (218,219,277,335,336). A small percentage of congenitally infected infants may not generate a measurable antibody response, and an occasional patient may progressively lose measurable antibodies (337,338). The concept of occasional patients with prolonged incubation periods in which they are infected, and perhaps infectious, but seronegative (339) remains an area of investigation and some controversy (340). The role of other assays for antibody such as neutralization, antibody-dependent cytotoxicity, subclass specific antibodies, p24, and other antigen-specific responses remains an important area of investigation;

however, it does not yet have a role in patient management.

Virus isolation has been performed from peripheral blood mononuclear cells, plasma, CSF, genital secretions, and other clinical materials. Isolation has been performed with primary human peripheral blood mononuclear cells, primary human monocyte macrophages, and various human cell lines. No drug has yet been definitely demonstrated to reduce isolation rates of HIV with any of these cells.

In contrast, circulating p24 antigen as assayed in a number of commercially available ELISA kits has been shown to diminish with therapy with a number of drugs (see below). Antigenemia occurs within days of infection and clears weeks later with the appearance of measurable antibody (221,277,341,342). Over a period of years, some patients may develop a diminution of measurable p24 antibody and an appearance of p24 antigenemia (153, 221,290,341,343). Of asymptomatic seropositive individuals, 8–10% will be p24 antigenemic. These individuals have a much higher likelihood of progressing to AIDS (290,344,345). Nevertheless, not all antigenemic asymptomatic patients will progress to AIDS within 2 years and not all individuals who develop AIDS are antigenemic. Approximately one-third of patients with ARC and one-half of patients with AIDS are antigenemic.

Although a negative prognostic sign, p24 antigenemia-like depressed CD4 lymphocyte counts, elevated β-microglobulinemia, and a number of other assays provide only statistical likelihoods for an individual patient (346). The p24 ELISA test has proven useful as a measure of antiviral activity in phase 1/phase 2 studies of investigational drugs. AZT reduces p24 antigenemia and has clinical benefit; several drugs without well-demonstrated clinical benefit (ribavirin, oral dextran sulfate, Ampligen, AL721, HPA23) have been shown not to reduce antigen levels. Nevertheless, not enough experience has been accrued to depend upon p24 antigenemia as a predictor of clinical utility of a candidate drug.

Assays for HIV-specific nucleic acid are still completely investigational. *In situ* cytohybridization has proven extremely useful for identifying infected cells in tissue; for example, macrophages in the brain (see above). HIV RNA sequences are much more prevalent than DNA sequences in peripheral blood and can be detected directly by blot hybridization (347). The development of the polymerase chain reaction to amplify target sequences was a revolutionary innovation for diagnosis (348,349). It has been successfully applied to the detection of the DNA and RNA in clinical material of both HIV (349–351) and HTLV-1 (18). This method and its derivatives will have a major impact on our understanding of the epidemiology and pathogenesis of retroviral infections. It may also prove valuable in monitoring antiviral therapy. By early 1989, however, technical development and methodologic validation should precede its use to generate definitive conclusions.

## COMPOUNDS WITH ANTIRETROVIRAL ACTIVITY *IN VITRO*

An effective antiretroviral drug was identified and licensed only 5 years after the first published description of AIDS and only 3 years after the isolation of the etiologic agent, HIV. The unprecedented speed of this medical achievement is gratifying. This drug, azidothymidine (AZT), is neither completely suppressive of disease nor free from toxicity. The impetus for more and better drugs is thus great. AZT and the majority of the first promising candidate compounds are nucleoside analogs. This situation is not surprising for a number of reasons. Because of the utility of nucleoside analogs for cancer chemotherapy and, of more importance (for medical virologists), for the therapy of herpesviruses in-

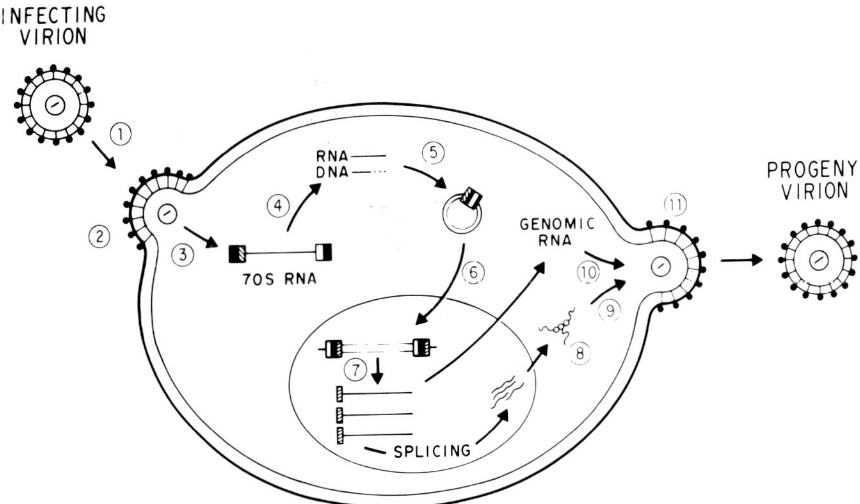


**FIG. 5.** Retroviral replication cycle and potential sites for specific antiviral therapy. Eleven arbitrarily identified steps in retroviral replication are diagrammed. Each virus-specific component of this cycle is a potential target for selective antiviral therapy. Some viral proteins may function at more than one step. For example, tat may regulate both transcription and translation. In addition, many steps involve the combined contribution of several viral proteins. The proposed targets of potential antiretroviral drugs are indicated in Table 1. ①, binding; ②, penetration; ③, uncoating; ④, reverse transcription; ⑤, circularization; ⑥, integration; ⑦, transcription; ⑧, translation; ⑨, post-translational processing; ⑩, assembly; ⑪, budding.

fections, large collections of such compounds and much expertise in nucleoside synthetic chemistry were already available. With the success of AZT, nucleosides will remain promising compounds among the candidate drugs. Nevertheless, the remarkably speedy advance in the understanding of the molecular biology of HIV has resulted in an extensive set of programs to identify compounds that interfere with each of the possible virus-specific targets in the replication of HIV (Fig. 5). These targets and the compounds that act on them will be identified. Those compounds not yet associated with a target will then be summarized.

### Compounds that Inhibit Binding and Penetration

The critical first step in the life cycle of HIV is the high-affinity binding of gp120, the surface glycoprotein on the virion or infected cells, to CD4. Compounds that specifically interfere with this interaction should inhibit infection. In fact, the inhibition of infection with monoclonal antibodies to CD4 was the first approach used to identify the host cell receptor for HIV (68,69,71). However, there are a number of theoretical objections to the consideration of antibodies or other ligands directed against CD4 as therapeutic agents. Because human retroviral infections are persistent, the ideal therapies should be administered chronically and orally. They should also penetrate the blood-brain barrier. Antibodies fail to fulfill these criteria. In addition, the target, CD4, is a specific host cell functional protein rather than a viral one.

The use of neutralizing antibodies against virion glycoproteins direct an intervention against the pathogen rather than the host cell. In general, neutralizing antibodies do not inhibit binding of the virus to the host cell. They more likely modify in the tertiary structure or encumber the glycoprotein to prevent it from mediating the penetration process. Plasma from seropositive donors has been administered to small numbers of patients with advanced AIDS with clearance of p24 antigenemia and enhancement of neutralizing and anti-p24 antibody levels (352,353). Further studies are needed to identify if this approach is antigen-specific and in fact beneficial, and if so, the mechanism of action. If beneficial effects could be confirmed, a possible role as intermittent therapy, induction for example, merits consideration. Another theoretical approach is the use of antiidiotype antibody to the CD4 binding site; this antibody binds to the reciprocal binding site on gp120 (354).

An alternative approach to inhibit the interaction between gp120 and CD4 is to use portions of the CD4 molecule that bind gp120. CD4 is a glycoprotein with a hydrophobic, membrane anchoring amino acid sequence at the carboxy terminus and a gp120 binding site at the amino terminus (355–357). The construction by recombinant DNA technology of expression vectors that encode and express a CD4 polypeptide truncated between these two sites results in a soluble secreted polypeptide that inhibits HIV-1 infectivity at approximately 10 μg/ml (122–126). Recombinant soluble CD4 blocks virus binding to CD4 positive cells (358,359) and may also prevent infection by virus already bound to cells. Shorter sequences of CD4 representing the gp120 binding site have been prepared by synthesis of oligopeptides. These also block infectivity, but 100-fold higher concentrations are required because the oligopeptides initially examined have lower binding affinities than the larger polypeptides (360). The first phase I studies of this theoretically intriguing approach were initiated in late 1988. Theoretical concerns about the ability of recombinant soluble CD4 to interfere with normal immune functions, to cross the blood-brain barrier, or to induce an antibody response have been raised but should not inhibit careful phase I studies.

This concept has been carried one step further by generating a recombinant human CD4-*Pseudomonas* exotoxin hybrid protein with the rationale of selectively targeting a lethal toxin to HIV-infected cells expressing gp120 (361). There are many steps between this theoretically elegant approach and therapeutic utility. Other modifications are also under investigation. For example, a chimeric molecule containing the amino terminal binding site of CD4 and the Fc end of the IgG heavy chain appears to retain the gp120 affinity of the former and the prolonged serum half-life of the latter (362).

A synthetic octapeptide, termed "peptide T"—four amino acids of the octapeptide are threonine (abbreviated T, hence peptide T) (363)—has been reported to block infectivity of HIV and binding between radiolabeled gp120 and CD4 in the 100 nM range (364). Several investigators have been unable to demonstrate antiviral activity with peptide T (365); nevertheless, further investigations, including phase I studies, have been initiated to assess the potential of this compound.

In addition to agents that inhibit specific, virally defined functions during the steps of binding and penetration, a class of compounds that act to block binding nonspecifically have been identified. It has been appreciated for decades that polycations can enhance viral infectivity *in vitro* and polyanions can inhibit infectivity of many viruses including retroviruses (366–369). Viruses and cells both have negatively charged surfaces resulting in mutual repulsion that can be neutralized by polycations and enhanced by polyanions. Dextran sulfate is a polysulfated polymer of glucose. Dextran sulfate blocks the binding of HIV-1 to CD4-positive target cells (358,359). The drug inhibits the expression of viral antigen and syncytium formation of HIV-1- and HIV-2-infected cells at concentrations between 1 and 10 μg/ml, whereas minimal cellular toxicity is seen at 1,000 μg/ml (358,359,370,371). Thus, dextran sulfate has an extremely high selectivity index (therapeutic ratio *in vitro*). Active preparations have contained approximately 18% sulfur by molecular weight. Removal of sulfate groups eliminates antiviral activity (122,358). A wide range of molecular weight species can be synthesized, and preparations represent a heterogeneous mixture of molecular weights. Preparations with a peak of 5,000 and 8,000 daltons appeared equally effective (371).

Other polyanionic compounds inhibit the replication of HIV *in vitro*. These include sulfated polysaccharides extracted from animal sources (heparin) (359,371–373), sea algae (374,375), and licorice (376). These compounds and dextran sulfate inhibit membrane fusion following contact between infected and uninfected cells in contrast to nucleoside analogs like AZT (376). It is possible that other nonpolymeric but large polyanionic compounds with antiretroviral activity may also belong in this class of compounds that act at an early step. Such compounds include aurintricarboxylic acid (372,373), Evan's Blue (372,373), and suramin, which is reviewed later. These compounds and the sulfated polymers inhibit the activity of cell-free reverse transcriptase (358,372–374,377). It is unlikely that such compounds traverse the cell membrane well. In addition, these compounds inhibit host cell DNA polymerase α equally well (358). Consequently, these compounds are likely to act at the surface interactions of virus, and cell enzyme inhibition is probably not relevant beyond the test tube. This conclusion is further supported by the observation that these sulfated polysaccharides are selective inhibitors of a wide range of enveloped DNA and RNA viruses (378).

## Compounds that Inhibit Reverse Transcriptase

Reverse transcriptase is an essential virion enzyme of all retroviruses found associated with the nucleocapsid in the virion. Inhibitors of this function in animal retroviruses were intensively investigated before the discovery of HIV [summarized in de Clercq (379)]. The first drugs to inhibit antiretroviral activity clinically belong to this class [AZT, dideoxycytidine (ddC), dideoxyadenosine (ddA), dideoxyinosine (ddI), foscarnet]. The nucleoside analogs will be reviewed first, followed by the other compounds in this class.

### *Nucleoside Analogs*

The art and science of synthesis of nucleoside analogs have flourished for decades in the occasionally successful search for anticancer and antiviral drugs. Most such syntheses are reported as accomplishments of organic chemistry but fail to result in a therapeutically useful compound. For example, Horwitz et al. in 1964 (380) and later Lin and Prusoff in 1978 (381) reported the synthesis of 3′-azido-3′-deoxythymidine (AZT), which failed to find a role in cancer chemotherapy. The synthesis of 2′,3′-dideoxynucleosides (382,383) resulted in the generation of reagents critical to the performance of the Sanger DNA sequencing technique (384). Nevertheless, with the experience in nucleoside synthesis and the success in identifying effective inhibitors of herpesvirus DNA polymerases (see Chapters 3, 4, and 8), reverse transcriptase was not surprisingly the first viral target for which an effective compound was identified. Dozens of nucleoside analogs have been shown to inhibit HIV *in vitro,* and many of these will undergo clinical trial. The first to be identified and reach clinical trial (AZT and the 2′,3′-dideoxynucleosides) will initially be described.

#### *AZT*

AZT is a white to off-white, odorless, bitter, crystalline solid with a molecular weight of 267.24 daltons. It is soluble to 25 mg/ml in water at 25°C. It has a $pK_a$ of 9.68, and is relatively stable in solution or at room temperature in crystalline form. AZT is a dideoxynucleoside analog of thymidine in which the 3′-hydroxyl (-OH) is replaced by an azido ($-N_3$) group (Fig. 6). Because the term "thymidine" designates a 2′-deoxynucleoside, the term "3′-deoxythymidine" or its derivatives designates a 2′,3′-dideoxynucleoside. The generic designation for AZT is zidovudine (occasionally abbreviated ZDV). This term conveys no information, whereas AZT or azidothymidine indicates the structure of the compound and represents the designation in common usage by patients, physicians, and researchers.

In 1985, Mitsuya et al. (385) reported that AZT inhibited the replication of HIV in peripheral blood mononuclear cells and several T-cell lines at concentrations of 1 μM, approximately 100-fold less than the toxic concentration for these cells. Many other groups have confirmed similar levels of efficacy and toxicity in human cells with one major exception. AZT at concentrations as low as 1–3 μM appears to be toxic *in vitro* to normal human granulocyte-macrophage progenitor cells (386). These concentrations approach the peak levels attained in serum. In addition, the replication of LAV in primary human macrophages appeared to be resistant to AZT and other dideoxynucleosides (347), whereas the macrophage-tropic Ba-L strain was shown to be fully sensitive by this same group and others (387).

Unlike the physiologic deoxynucleosides, which are transported across cell membranes, AZT appears to enter cells by nonfacilitated diffusion (388). The lipophilic 3′-azido group imparts this membrane permeability. Cellular thymidine kinase converts AZT into its monophosphate (389). Cellular thymidylate kinase converts the monophosphate into the diphosphate, which is further converted to the triphosphate (AZT-TP), the active antiviral compound, by other cellular enzymes (389). This anabolic phosphorylation of AZT, an inactive compound, to the active metabolite, AZT-TP, by host cell enzymes indicate potential host cell influences on antiviral activity. The predominance of AZT monophosphate (AZT-MP) in human cells exposed to AZT (389,390) suggests that thymidylate kinase is the rate-limiting enzyme in the synthesis of the active AZT-TP, which represents only approximately 1% of intracellular drug. AZT-MP presumably inhibits thymidylate kinase resulting in this anabolic block and also resulting in the inhibition of phosphorylation of thymidine in cells treated with AZT (389). This impact on intracellular nucleotide pools has consequences on cell toxicity and antagonism or synergy with other antiviral drugs (391,392). This block does not appear to occur in murine cells, in which AZT appears to be more effective both *in vitro* and *in vivo* (390,393,394).

AZT-TP, as an analog of thymidine triphosphate, inhibits the reverse transcriptase of HIV-1 and other lentiviruses *in vitro* (395). Inhibition of host cell DNA polymerases α and β is considerably weaker, presumably accounting for its therapeutic ratio (395). Of interest, inhibition by AZT of the DNA polymerase of many Gram-negative bacteria results in antibacterial activity (396). Bacterial resistance readily develops as a consequence of loss of thymidine kinase activity; nevertheless, toxicologic studies of AZT that were undertaken in animals would later prove time-saving in the development of AZT as an antiviral agent. Chain termination has been demonstrated with the *E. coli* DNA polymerase (396,397). Studies *in vitro* with reverse transcriptase and the synthetic template, poly (rA)-oligo$(dT)_{12-18}$, have demonstrated chain termination with AZT-TP (395). With the incorporation of AZT-TP, a 3′-OH group is no longer available to form a 3′-5 phosphodiester bond to permit the addition of another nucleotide triphosphate to the DNA chain. Such terminated chains have not been demonstrated in mammalian cells, suggesting that for retroviruses and eucar-

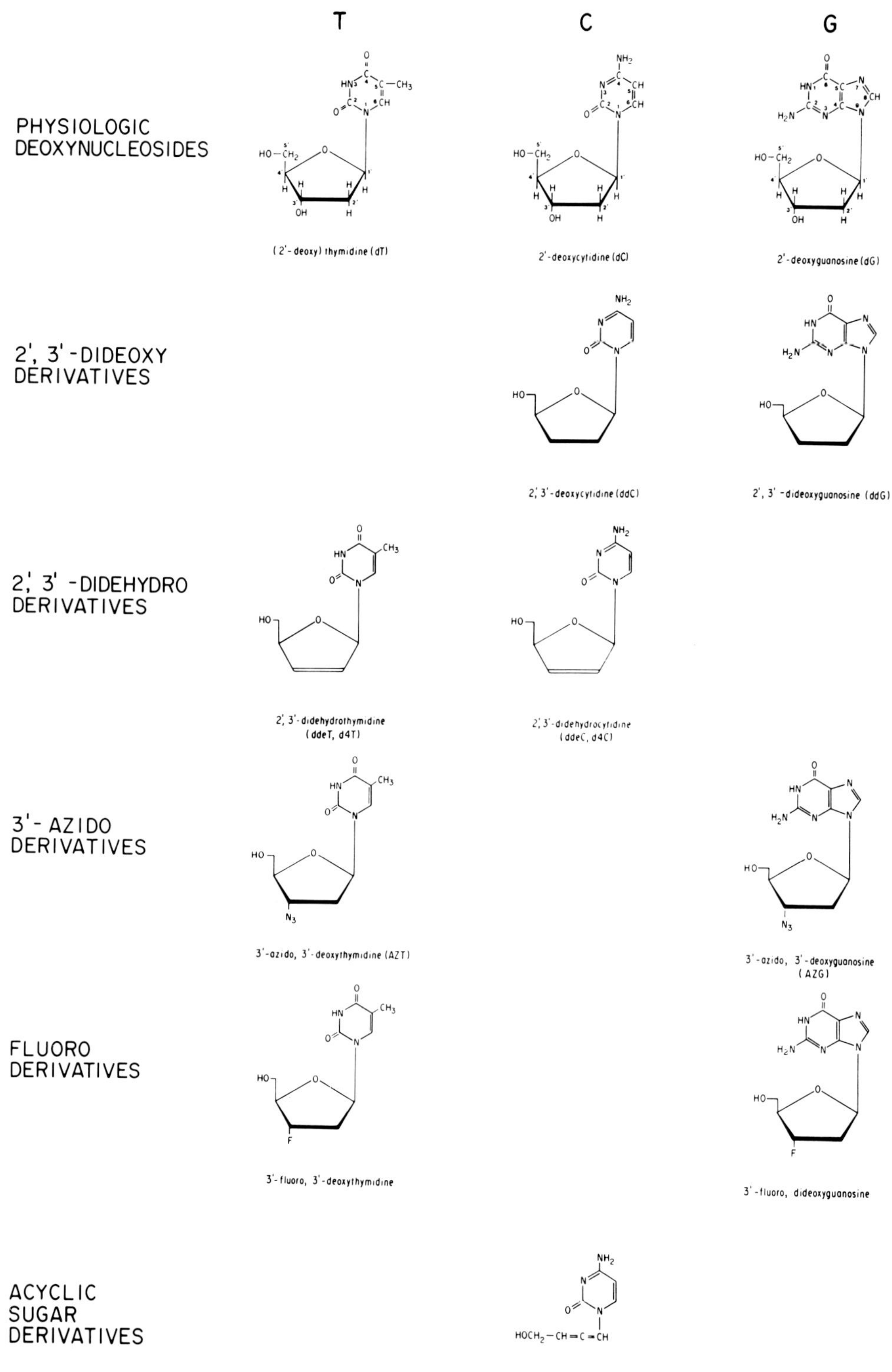


**FIG. 6.** Chemical structures of nucleoside analogs with selective antiretroviral activity. In the top row, the physiologic nucleosides are depicted with carbon and hydrogen atoms included. The carbon or nitrogen atoms in the ring structures are enumerated for the physiologic nucleosides and implied in the analog. Absent substrates have not been shown to be effective.

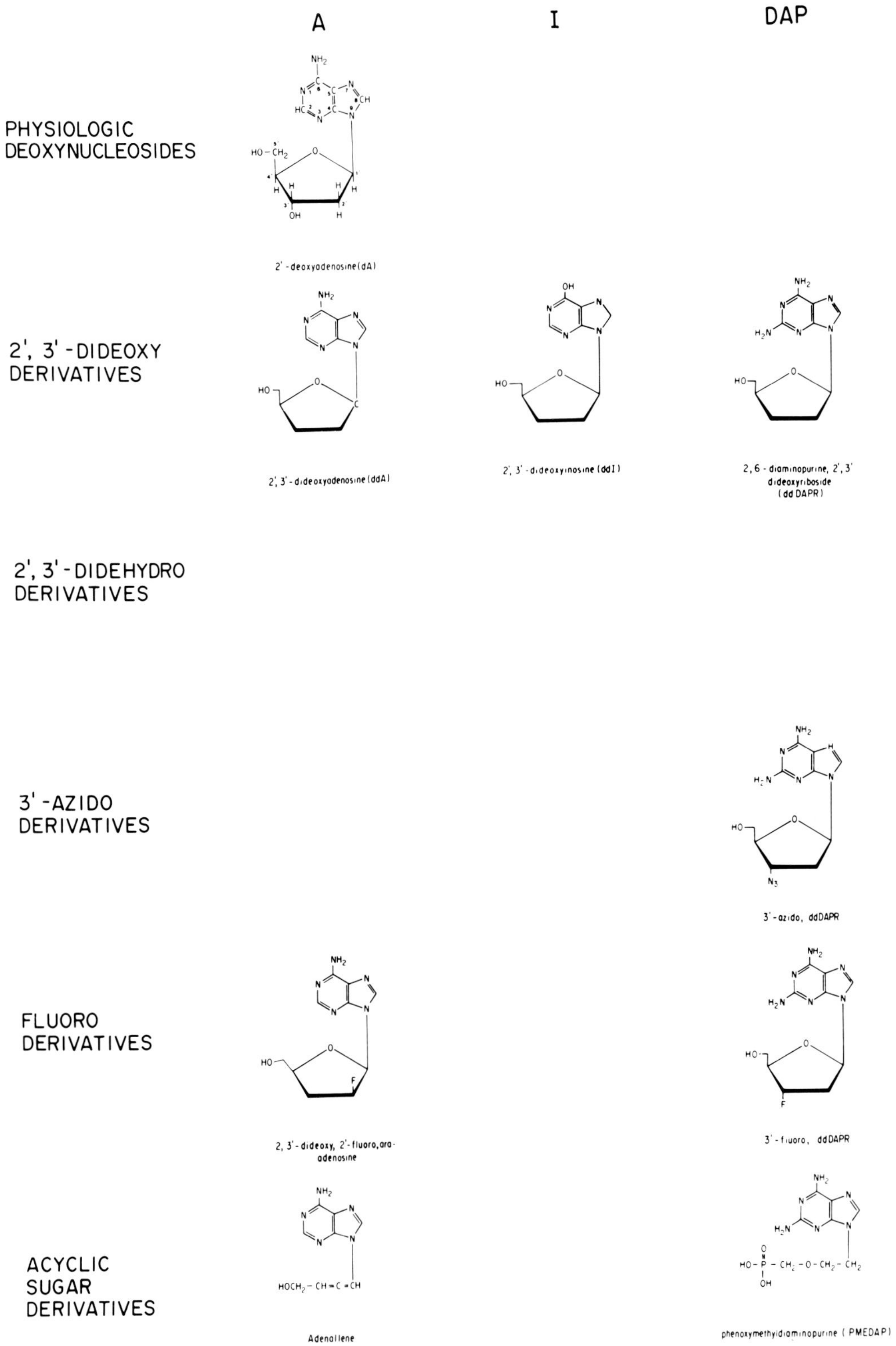

| | A | I | DAP |
|---|---|---|---|
| PHYSIOLOGIC DEOXYNUCLEOSIDES | 2'-deoxyadenosine (dA) | | |
| 2',3'-DIDEOXY DERIVATIVES | 2',3'-dideoxyadenosine (ddA) | 2',3'-dideoxyinosine (ddI) | 2,6-diaminopurine, 2',3' dideoxyriboside (dd DAPR) |
| 2',3'-DIDEHYDRO DERIVATIVES | | | |
| 3'-AZIDO DERIVATIVES | | | 3'-azido, ddDAPR |
| FLUORO DERIVATIVES | 2,3'-dideoxy, 2'-fluoro,ara-adenosine | | 3'-fluoro, ddDAPR |
| ACYCLIC SUGAR DERIVATIVES | Adenallene | | phenoxymethyldiaminopurine (PMEDAP) |

**FIG. 6.** *Continued.*

yotic cells AZT-TP may act more as a competitive enzyme inhibitor than a chain terminator (389). Thus, the relative importance of chain termination and competition with thymidine triphosphate as the mechanism of action of AZT-TP remains to be determined.

Addition of thymidine reverses both the efficacy and toxicity of AZT (385,398), indicating the competition of thymidine triphosphate and AZT-TP for viral and host DNA polymerases. The toxicity of AZT for human granulocyte progenitor cells *in vitro* occurs at concentrations of 1–5 μM, approximately 100-fold less than that required to produce toxicity in lymphoid cell lines (306). This hypersensitivity to the effects of AZT in marrow cells is reversed by uridine but not thymidine (398). Both the mechanisms and potential applications of this observation await future investigations.

The inhibition of reverse transcriptase prevents the normal production of viral products and cytopathology. This observation has been made with several laboratory strains of HIV-1 in peripheral blood mononuclear cells and in many continuous cell lines utilizing cytopathology, the production of reverse transcriptase in antigens, or even T-cell functions as end points. Despite the variation in assay systems, inhibition is observed at concentrations as low as 0.01–0.1 μM (347,385,398–401). Clinical isolates from patients never administered AZT display little variation in susceptibility to AZT (401). Other retroviruses examined to date also are inhibited by AZT *in vitro*. These include HTLV-1 (402), avian leukosis virus (403), several murine retroviruses (393,404), feline leukemia virus (317), and equine infectious anemia virus (393). No antiviral activity has been observed against a broad range of human viruses from other families with the exception of one of the human herpesviruses, EBV, for which the 50% effective dose ($ED_{50}$) appears to be between 1 and 10 μM (405).

Although AZT effectively inhibits the replication of HIV-1 initiated by cell-free virus, it does not inhibit virus production by chronically infected cells or transmission of infection to uninfected cells by syncytium formation (399,406,407). The viral progeny of infected cells that are chronically producing virus *in vitro*, even in the presence of high but nontoxic levels of AZT, remain sensitive to AZT.

In preclinical toxicologic studies, the median lethal dose of AZT in mice and rats is greater than 750 mg/kg intravenously and greater than 3000 mg/kg orally (408). The intravenous administration of up to 150 mg/kg per day of AZT for 4 weeks in rats and of up to 85 mg/kg per day for 2 weeks in dogs resulted in no recognized toxicity (408). Oral administration of 500 mg/kg AZT to beagle dogs produces vomiting and bloody stools. Oral administration of 30–100 mg/kg per day of AZT to mice, rats, or monkeys will produce a macrocytic anemia over a period of 1 month or more (394,408). Mutagenicity can be detected at 1,000 to 5,000 μg/ml in the L5178Y mouse lymphoma cell mutagenicity assay (408). Chromosomal aberrations in human lymphocytes cultured in 3 μg/ml AZT and transformation of T3 mouse cells in 0.5 μg/ml occur. No genetic toxicology has been documented in the bacterial mutagenicity assay (Ames test), the marrow cytogenetics of rats assay, or teratogenicity studies in rats and rabbits (408).

The expeditious introduction of AZT into clinical trials and the documentation of efficacy preceded the evaluation of AZT in animal models of retrovirus infection. As a consequence, the clinical experience with AZT is being used as the standard by which animal models are being validated rather than using animal models to validate the efficacy of a drug prior to clinical evaluation. A number of animal retroviral models for evaluation of antivirals have been developed, and additional models are certain to be developed. AZT administered intraperitoneally or in drinking water from the time of inoculation is effective in treating mice infected with the Rauscher murine leukemia virus complex as measured by spleen weight, infectious spleen cells, infectivity titers in plasma, or mortality (394). The injection of a murine type-C retrovirus (designated Cas-Br-E) into embryos produces a progressive neurologic disease in the newborns, which is inhibited by administering AZT in the drinking water of the pregnant mothers (409). This transplacental delivery of drug is encouraging for the potential in treating congenital HIV infection, as well as the treatment of CNS disease produced by retroviruses. AZT administered at the time of inoculation can prevent the establishment of infections with feline leukemia viruses (317), supporting the possible application to postexposure prophylaxis of health care workers.

### *2′,3′-Dideoxynucleosides*

Shortly after the documentation of the antiretroviral activity of AZT, Mitsuya and Broder (410) reported that the 2′,3′-dideoxynucleosides, ddC, dideoxyguanosine (ddG), ddA, and its deaminated metabolite ddI all inhibited HIV-1 *in vitro* (410). Of interest, dideoxythymidine (ddT), which is AZT without the 3′-azido group, was relatively impotent (410). These 2′,3′-dideoxynucleosides structurally are the physiologic deoxynucleosides, with the 3′-hydroxyl group removed from the sugar moiety (Fig. 6). Both ddA and ddI are approximately 10-fold less potent than AZT but exhibit little toxicity *in vitro* even at concentrations approaching 1,000 ug/ml. They, thus, have the highest selectivity index among these compounds *in vitro*. ddC was selected for the first clinical development for several reasons. It is more potent than AZT *in vitro*, with activity demonstrable at 0.01 μM or lower in some assay systems. It also is resistant to deamination (411,412) and acid-mediated hydrolysis of base from sugar. It is well absorbed from the gastrointestinal tract, had uncomplicated pharmacokinetics in pilot animal studies, and appeared nontoxic in animals (397,413).

The cellular metabolism of ddC appears even less complicated than AZT. It enters the cell by the nucleoside transport system and is anabolized to the triphosphate by deoxycytidine kinase and subsequent cellular enzymes in the phosphorylation of deoxycytidine (412,414–416). A higher proportion of intracellular nucleotide is ddC-TP, probably accounting for some of the greater potency when compared to AZT (411,417). In contrast to AZT, ddC is poorly phosphorylated by murine cells (390). The mouse may thus be a poor model to evaluate ddC. As with AZT, the physiologic nucleoside (deoxycytidine in the case of ddC) competes with both the efficacy and toxicity of ddC *in vitro* (415). The addition of thymidine to cells significantly enhances the phosphorylation of ddC, presumably by reducing the intracellular pools of cytidine deoxynucleotides (415). These observations point out the complex interactions of intracellular nucleotide pools and the potential for synergy or antagonism between combinations of nucleoside analogs which is well documented (391,392).

The triphosphate of ddC inhibits reverse transcriptase to confer its antiviral activity (419). Chain termination does occur *in vitro* (397). The selectivity of ddC is based on the lower susceptibility of human DNA polymerases α and β to ddC-TP (411,420). Of note, mitochondrial DNA polymerase γ is as sensitive as reverse transcriptase (411), perhaps accounting for the neurotoxicity seen with the drug.

The generation of active triphosphates from ddA and ddI are much more complicated than for AZT or ddC. Adenosine deaminase, which is abundant in serum and cells, rapidly deaminates ddA to ddI (421,422). Purine nucleoside phosphorylase converts ddI to the monophosphate (422). If deamination of ddA is prevented, ddA can be phosphorylated to ddA-monophosphate predominantly by deoxycytidine kinase as well as by adenosine kinase

(422,423); ddAMP is then readily deaminated to ddIMP (423). The active triphosphate is then generated by a series of enzymes steps that convert ddIMP to ddATP via ddAMP and ddADP (424). These pathways may thus be subject to variability among different cells (423) and to complex interactions with other nucleosides. As with AZT-TP and ddC-TP, ddA-TP then inhibits the activity of reverse transcriptase of HIV (397,419), other lentiviruses (393), and host cell DNA polymerases (420,421).

The animal toxicology of the 2′,3′-dideoxynucleosides has not been published; however, data have been presented to the Food and Drug Administration (FDA) for Investigational New Drug Applications. No toxicity of ddC is recognized in rodents with any single dose that can be administered or with oral drug at 1,000 mg/kg three times daily for 5 days or with peritoneal infusions of 47 mg/kg daily for 1 week. The only toxicity seen was some decrease in bone colony forming units when cultured *in vitro* from mice receiving the infusion. In dogs receiving constant intravenous infusions for 5 days, soft, blood-tinged stools became apparent when the dose attained was 3.53 mg/kg/hr. In dogs, oral or parenteral doses approaching 100 mg/kg daily for 4 weeks resulted in similar gastrointestinal toxicity and moderate thrombocytopenia and anemia. It must be remembered that nucleoside anabolism varies significantly among species with important implications of animal models both for efficacy and toxicity. Following the first clinical trials of ddC, high-dose oral administration of drug to *Cynomolgus* monkeys resulted in peripheral neuropathy (W. Soo, unpublished observations).

The pharmacokinetics of ddC in mouse, dog, and rhesus monkey indicate some species variation. Oral bioavailability is 100% in monkeys and dogs, but 30–50% in mice. The elimination half-life is 2 hr in monkey and dog but 1 hr in mouse. The total body clearance is 9.5–12 ml/min/kg in the monkey, 5–6 ml/min/kg in the dog, and 30–50 ml/min/kg in the mouse. Penetration of ddC into the CSF is 2–6% of the plasma level in dogs and monkeys.

Continuous intravenous infusions of ddA in dogs at 31 mg/kg/hr resulted in the steady state plasma levels of 1.5 μg/ml (6 μM) ddA and 25 μg/ml (95 μM) ddI. Not toxicity was observed for 10 days of infusion at these levels, which exceed the antiviral levels by at least an order of magnitude. Higher infusion levels produce hypotension and tachycardia.

ddA is deaminated completely to ddI in minutes in the dog and rat. In the dog, the elimination half-life of ddI is 73 min and the total body clearance is 4–5 ml/kg min. Orally administered ddA produces gastric irritation and undergoes hydrolysis to base and sugar unless it is administered with a buffer. Reliable oral bioavailability data will thus depend upon formulation; however, 30–50% of administered ddA or ddI appears to reach the circulation as ddI in various buffers. In rats and dogs, high oral doses of ddA yield a nephrotoxic catabolite generated in the gut. Because ddI and ddA appear to the interconverted by cellular metabolism and yield equivalent levels of the active ddA-triphosphate, of the two ddI has been selected for clinical evaluation.

### *Other Nucleosides*

AZT and the 2′,3′-dideoxynucleosides share the properties of being phosphorylated by host cell enzymes to generate a triphosphate metabolite that competes with a physiologic deoxyribonucleotide triphosphate for the retroviral reverse transcriptase. The analog's selectivity index is presumably conferred by the relative inhibition of the reverse transcriptase and host cell DNA polymerases, although other effects are certainly possible. The success of these analogs has prompted numerous efforts to screen every nucleoside known as well as any new one that could be synthesized for activity against HIV.

Dozens of nucleoside analogs have been shown to inhibit the replication of HIV selectively or as the triphosphate to inhibit reverse transcriptase activity *in vitro*. Many of these will be entering clinical trials. Most of those whose structures have been published are depicted in Fig. 6. Because assay systems for antiviral activity and cell toxicity vary with each investigator, strict comparisons are difficult.

Compounds with selective activity against HIV include the unsaturated 2′,3′-didehydro-derivatives of ddC and ddT termed "2′,3′-didehydrodideoxy cytosine" (ddeC, or d4C) and "2′,3′-didehydrodideoxy thymidine" (ddeT, or d4T) (377,425–429). The 2′,3′-didehydropurines are relatively ineffective (430–433); however, the carbocyclic equivalent of didehydroguanosine (Carbovir) has a promising selectivity index against HIV-1 *in vitro*. The 3′-azido derivatives of deoxyguanosine (AZG) and several pyrimidines, such as azidodeoxyuridine, are promising *in vitro* (430,434–436), as are the 3′ fluoro derivatives of ddT and ddG but not ddA or ddC (426,436–440). 2,6-Diaminopurine, 2′,3′-deoxyriboside, and its 3′ fluoro and 3′ azido derivatives are effective *in vitro* (433,437,441). Another effective derivative of this purine with an additional two-amino group is an acyclic derivative that has a phosphonylmethoxyethyl side chain instead of a sugar (PMEDADP) (442). Another series of compounds with an acyclic component instead of sugar are 9-(4,-hydroxy -1′,2′-butadienyl) adenine (termed "adenallene") and its cytosine equivalent (termed "cytallene") (443). 9-(2-phosphonylmethoxyethyl)adenine (PMEA) is the first of these acyclic nucleosides to be considered for clinical development (444). Analogous to acyclovir and its relatives (Chapter 4), these unsaturated acyclic compounds may structurally resemble a cyclic nucleoside and undergo phosphorylation at a site resembling the 5′ carbon. This speculation is under investigation.

Factors such as preclinical animal toxicology and constraints on synthesis of large quantities of compound may dictate which compounds progress to clinical trial. Additional studies, including structural studies of the triphosphates and reverse transcriptase, may help elucidate the critical structure/activity relationships that will help us to understand how certain analogs work and permit the design of additional, more effective, and less toxic compounds.

Properties in addition to antiviral activity may be incorporated into drug design. For example, one possible limitation of ddA and ddI are their susceptibility to gastric acid-catalyzed hydrolysis of the glycosidic bond. The derivative 2′-fluoro-ddA is more resistant to this acid catalyzed hydrolysis; however, most antiretroviral activity is lost (445). Its stereoisomer 2′-fluoro, ara-ddA is resistant to hydrolysis and retains antiretroviral activity comparable to ddA (445).

### *Foscarnet*

Foscarnet [phosphonoformate (PFA)] is a pyrophosphate analog that inhibits directly a broad range of DNA polymerases and to a certain extent influenza virus RNA polymerase (446). The compound has been most extensively examined for use for herpesvirus infections and is reviewed in detail in Chapter 8. Foscarnet was shown to inhibit the reverse transcriptase activity of all animal retroviruses examined with cell-free assays (447). One of the first retroviruses shown to be inhibited in culture by Foscarnet was the sheep lentivirus, visna (448).

The drug inhibits the replication of HIV-1 in several assay systems at concentrations of 100 μM or less, which are readily attainable clinically (449,450). The drug is relatively nontoxic *in vitro* at concentrations approaching 1,000 μM (449,450). Foscarnet inhibits reverse transcriptase at concentrations below 1 μM by a noncompetitive mechanism with respect to deoxynucleotide triphosphate substrates (449–452). The discrepancy between concentrations necessary to inhibit enzyme in cell-free assays and virus replication in cells is accounted for by the poor entry into cells of this highly charged molecule. In cell-free systems, cellular DNA polymerases α and β are orders of magnitude less sensitive to inhibition by Foscarnet than is the reverse transcriptase of HIV-1, supporting the possibility of a good therapeutic ratio (435). Several dozen pyrophosphate analogs have been synthesized and examined, and none has yet been found more promising *in vitro* than Foscarnet (451). With the encouraging results *in vitro* and clinical experience with Foscarnet for the treatment of herpesvirus infections, Foscarnet was an early candidate to enter clinical trials for infection with HIV.

### *Heteropolyanion-23*

Heteropolyanion-23 (HPA-23) is a complex compound with a molecular weight of 6,800, containing a core of tungsten and antimony, that was shown to inhibit the reverse transcriptase of murine oncornaviruses and to protect mice from mammary tumors (453,454). HPA-23 competitively inhibits the reverse transcriptase of HIV-1 at concentrations down to 0.1 μM (452,455). Less encouraging is the lack of selectivity of viral over cellular DNA polymerases (452). Little data regarding toxicology or pharmacokinetics appear to be available; nevertheless, clinical trials were initiated in 1983 (456).

### *Rifamycins*

In the 1970s, rifamycin compounds were demonstrated to inhibit the reverse transcriptase of animal retroviruses in cell-free systems; however, this occurred at concentrations exceeding those attainable clinically (457,458). Rifabutin, also known as ansamycin, was shown to inhibit the production of HIV-1 reverse transcriptase *in vitro* at concentrations between 1 and 10 μg/ml in one study (459) but to be inactive at these concentrations in another study (460). Although these concentrations exceed the peak concentrations readily attainable in serum, this observation and the experience with this drug in patients with AIDS for the therapy of mycobacterial infection prompted its evaluation as an antiretroviral. No selectivity of viral over cellular DNA polymerases was observed in cell-free assays.

### *Oligonucleotides*

Several oligonucleotides of various composition have been synthesized as potential antisense inhibitors of transcription or RNA processing (461–470). In addition, 2′,5′-oligoadenylates, which are induced by interferon to inhibit cap methylation of viral mRNA, have been shown to inhibit reverse transcriptase in cell-free systems (122). The activity of most of these oligonucleotides does not appear to be related to the specific sequence. Data are suggestive but not conclusive that these compounds compete with the virion RNA for the template-binding site of the reverse transcriptase (471). Because their size and charge impair entry into cells and because the synthesis of these compounds is difficult, they seem unlikely candidates for clinical use. Nevertheless, template-primer binding remains a theoretical target for therapy acting at reverse transcription. Oligonucleotides as inhibitors of transcription are reviewed below.

### *Other Reverse Transcriptase Inhibitors*

A number of compounds, including suramin, dextran sulfate, and sakyomicin A have been reported to inhibit reverse transcriptase in cell-free systems and to inhibit the replication of HIV (358,472–474). The concentrations required for enzyme inhibition exceed those for antiviral activity and are similar to concentrations that inhibit host cell polymerases. It is also unlikely that these compounds readily cross cell membranes. The triphosphates of dideoxynucleosides and Foscarnet inhibit reverse transcriptase in cell-free assays at concentrations lower than those required for the drug to inhibit replication in cell culture. Consequently, it is unlikely that reverse transcriptase is the target for the former group of compounds, which are considered elsewhere.

### Compounds that Inhibit Transcription and Translation

Viruses parasitize host cell machinery to transcribe their mRNA and to translate these messages into polypeptides. Consequently, to target virus-specific functions at these steps in replication is challenging. At least three approaches have been described: ribavirin, synthetic "antisense" oligonucleotides, and interferons. Interferons may act at several sites, and their clinical use will be considered with the biological response modifiers. They are discussed in detail in Chapter 9.

#### *Ribavirin*

Ribavirin [1-β-D-ribofuranosyl-1,2,4-triazole-3-carboxamide (Virazole)] is an analog of guanosine with a broad spectrum of antiviral activity. It may act by several possible mechanisms, including interference with the guanylation step required for 5′-capping of viral messenger RNA and inhibition of viral polymerase by ribavirin triphosphate (475,476). The preclinical information regarding ribavirin is summarized in detail in Chapter 3.

Ribavirin was one of the first drugs shown to inhibit the replication of HIV in cell culture (477). Concentrations of 50 μM or more, which exceed those attainable clinically, are necessary *in vitro* to inhibit HIV. Nevertheless, the documentation of activity against HIV *in vitro* and the successful experience with the treatment of Lassa fever (478) prompted clinical evaluation.

Ribavirin has several effects on host cell metabolism, including the perturbation of intracellular nucleotide pools, at least partially by the inhibition of inosine monophosphate dehydrogenase by ribavirin monophosphate (479). As a consequence, the purine deoxynucleotide triphosphates (dGTP and dATP) diminish intracellularly. In addition, ribavirin results in increased intracellular concentrations of thymidine triphosphate, which competes with AZT-TP and which inhibits phosphorylation of AZT (392,480). These perturbations in intracellular nucleotides result in a marked antagonism of the antiretroviral activity of AZT and other dideoxypyrimidines by ribavirin and enhancement of activity of dideoxypurines such as ddA and ddI (391,392).

#### *Synthetic Oligonucleotides*

In addition to targeting antivirals to virus-specific proteins, synthetic oligonucleotides of 14–30 base pairs in length have been investigated as "antisense" oligonucleotides, with the potential to hybridize with sequences of HIV messenger RNA, thereby interfering with transcription. Methylphosphonate, phosphorothioate, and other backbone derivatives have been generated to minimize nuclease sensitivity (461–463,465–468,470). Antiviral activity has been documented with such compounds; however, these activities are not always sequence specific, suggesting a number of possible mechanisms, including template primer-binding, to interfere with reverse transcriptase. The sequence nonspecific activity is seen only with the inhibition of acute infection *in vitro* (S. Broder, unpublished observations). Sequence specific activity has been shown at 1 μM with a 28-base phosphorothioate antisense analog against *rev* (*art*/*trs*) (466) and at 100 μM with the 8-base methyl phosphate antisense sequence of the *tat* first splice acceptor site (468). This sequence-specific activity can be observed both in acutely and chronically infected cells with the 28-base antisense rev compound. This theoretically interesting approach still requires much investigation to determine effective sequences, backbone composition, and drug delivery methods, as well as feasibility of economic scale-up of production. This approach will continue to be an active area of investigation (481).

A variant of this approach would be the delivery of sequence-specific RNA enzymes with endoribonuclease activities (482). These "ribozymes" have been identified for plant viroids and could theoretically be applied to any specific transcripts.

## Compounds that Inhibit Posttranslational Modification

Retroviral polypeptides are translated as polyproteins that are cleaved posttranslationally by a viral protease. Many proteins also undergo glycosylation, phosphorylation, or myristoylation by host enzymes. These types of posttranslational modifications have been approached as targets of antiviral therapy.

### *Protease Inhibitors*

As previously described, the protease of HIV-1 and other retroviruses cleaves viral polypeptides at well defined sites (50–52,483). Synthetic peptides of as few as six amino acids including pepstatin A can completely inhibit virus-specific proteolysis (57–59,435). Peptides do not permeate cell membranes; however, the availability of cell-free assays of the proteolytic activity of cloned and expressed viral protease should permit the screening of compounds that act on this target and the analysis of structure/activity relationships to design compounds with therapeutic potential.

### *Glycosylation Inhibitors*

The inhibition of glycosylation of the envelope glycoproteins could be expected to affect viral budding, release, binding, or penetration by fusion, all functions presumably mediated by the env products. Glycosylation inhibitors, typically 2-deoxy-D-glucose, have been examined for years with this target in mind (484). 2-Deoxy-D-glucose acts as a substrate for glycosylating enzymes and exerts some inhibition of the expression of HIV glycoproteins *in vitro* (485). Castanospermine is an alkaloid isolated from the seeds of an Australian chestnut tree, *Castanospermum australe,* that inhibits α-glucosidase I (486). 1-Deoxynojirimycin inhibits this same enzyme, and 1-deoxymannojirimycin inhibits mannosidase 1. Each of these enzymes trim *N*-linked glycan structures (487). These three compounds inhibit syncytium formation by HIV at concentrations above 50 μg/ml for castanospermine and at 1–10 μg/ml for the others. At these concentrations, glycosylation of envelope products is inhibited to impair their function (486,487). Whether compounds that inhibit host cell enzymes can effectively inhibit retroviral replication with acceptable toxicity *in vivo* remains to be determined. A series of the deoxynojirimycin compounds, which are glucose analogs, have been identified as effective antiretroviral compounds with *in vitro* assays. *N*-Butyl-deoxynojirimycin entered clinical investigation in early 1989.

## Compounds that Interact with the Virion Structure

The virus envelope is derived from the host cell membrane during the budding process. One would, thus, expect little antigenically or functionally in this phospholipid bilayer to represent a selective target. Nevertheless, several candidates have been proposed as potential antiretroviral agents that presumably would act upon the virus during budding or after release from the host cell.

AL721 is a mixture of neutral glycerides, phosphotidyl choline, and phosphatidylethanolamine in a 7:2:1 ratio that can extract cholesterol from cellular membranes (488). The published data regarding AL721 as an antiviral compound have been limited to a letter to the editor (489). A concentration of 100 μg/ml reduced the production of viral products by 50% in cultured, infected H9 cells, and 1,000 μg/ml reduced these products by >90%. These concentrations did not reduce cell numbers, but viability of cells was not assessed. A great deal of enthusiasm has been generated for the preparation of this compound by infected individuals; however, few scientific data are available about either the effects of this compound in infected cell cultures or the pharmacology of AL721. For example, 10–15 gr orally are recommended daily (489). It is unclear whether or not these lipids are absorbed from the gastrointestinal tract to remain associated and maintain their allegedly effective ratio in the circulation.

Amphotericin B and its water-soluble derivative amphotericin B methyl ester are polyene macrolide antifungal antibiotics that act on the basis of a greater affinity for ergosterol, a component of fungal membranes, than for cholesterol, which is in the membranes of mammalian cells and their viruses. Drug concentrations can be found in cell culture that inhibit replication of HIV and sustain cell viability (490). The amount of reduction observed is always less than 90% in contrast to nucleoside analogs, for example, where reduction can be measured in orders of magnitude.

In summary, compounds that act upon the viral envelope, including lipid solvents and detergents, may physically inactivate HIV. The critical issue for therapy is whether such an agent can be identified that selectively inactivates virus over host cells.

Hypericin and pseudohypericin are aromatic polycyclic diones extracted from the Saint Johnswort plant of the *Hypericum* family (491). These have antiviral activity against Friend murine leukemia virus *in vitro* and *in vivo* and have been proposed for evaluation against HIV (491). Preliminary data suggest that hypericin inactivates cell-free virus and has a prolonged plasma half-life in animals, adding to the interest in these compounds. "Health-food" stores sell preparations of St. Johnswort for infusions, which may permit endeavors of self-medication. The concentrations of hypericin and pseudohypericin are extremely low in these preparations, which also contain other toxic alkaloids.

## Compounds with an Undetermined Site of Action

### *Suramin*

Suramin is a complex polyanionic dye synthesized in 1920 at Bayer and used for decades for the therapy of African trypanosomiasis and onchocerciasis (492). Its mechanism of action for these infections has not been elucidated, although interaction with numerous proteins and cell function have been observed (492). In 1979, de Clercq demonstrated that at approximately 0.1 μM the drug inhibited the reverse transcriptases of several murine and avian retroviruses in cell-free assays (474). This observation was confirmed for the reverse transcriptase of HIV-1 (473,493). Derivatives of suramin and structurally similar dyes, such as Chicago sky blue, Congo red, direct yellow 50, and Evans blue have similar effects (372,373). In 1984, Mitsuya et al. (493) demonstrated that suramin, at concentrations of 10–50 μg/ml (7–35 μM), protected T cells *in vitro* from the infectivity and cytopathic effects (CPEs) of HIV (493). Cell toxicity was not apparent *in vitro* until concentrations of 100 μg/ml were attained, a relatively narrow margin of safety (493).

Of historic interest, this was the first compound reported to inhibit the replication of HIV. The related dyes were shown also to inhibit virus replication (372,373). Although suramin and the related dyes are potent enzyme inhibitors in cell-free assays, action at this site in infected cells has not been proven and a number of other mechanisms are possible (494). Regardless of the mechanism, these *in vitro* results led to studies showing effective antiviral effects in murine leukemia virus models (495) and to clinical trials.

### *Other Candidate Compounds*

Several other compounds have been reported to inhibit the replication of HIV *in vitro,* such as penicillamine, avarol, and avarone (496,497). Confirmation of the magnitude and selectivity of the effects are needed. Certain plant extracts have been reported to have antiretroviral activity as well. Glycyrrhizin, a structurally defined polycyclic extract of the licorice root, *Glycyrrhiza radix,* inhibits the replication of HIV *in vitro,* approaching concentrations of 1 mg/ml (498). Although these effective concentrations are not toxic *in vitro,* the low potency of this large molecule may not be therapeutically practical. Chemical congeners might merit investigation. Extracts of a large number of other Chinese medicinal herbs have been reported to have activity *in vitro* (499). Further studies, including purification and characterization of the active compounds, will be of interest.

Fusidic acid, which has been used as an antibacterial agent in Europe and Canada for years, was associated with dramatic clinical improvement in a patient with AIDS who was administered the drug for mycobacterial infection (500). This prompted an *in vitro* study showing reduced viral replication in the presence of fusidic acid (500), promoting much enthusiasm and further clinical trials (501). When *in vitro* assays of antiviral activity are conducted with controls for cell toxicity, all the antiviral effects can be attributed to cellular toxicity (502,503).

## CLINICAL STUDIES

Several of the drugs reviewed in the previous section have entered clinical trials. The experience in these studies will be summarized (Table 2); however, the use of these drugs in pediatric populations will be considered in Chapter 4.

### Suramin

Suramin was the first drug shown to inhibit HIV *in vitro* (493) and was soon evaluated clinically because it had undergone extensive prior clinical use in humans (492). With a newly developed high-performance liquid chromatography (HPLC) assay for suramin, the pharmacokinetics of suramin were evaluated in 10 patients with Kaposi's sarcoma or ARC (504). A total intravenous dose of 6.2 gr was administered over a 5-week period. The plasma half-life of the drug was approximately 7 weeks. The plasma level exceeded 100 μg/ml for 2 months. Of the drug, 99.7% is bound to

**TABLE 2.** *Antiretroviral drugs with documented sites of action*

| |
|---|
| Attachment/penetration |
| Dextran Sulfate |
| Soluble CD4 |
| Reverse transcription |
| Nucleoside analogs |
| Foscarnet |
| Template-binding oligonucleotides |
| HPA-23 |
| Rifabutin |
| Transcription |
| Ribavirin |
| Translation |
| Antisense oligonucleotides |
| Interferons? |
| Posttranslational processing |
| Glycosylation inhibitors |
| Protease inhibitors |
| Assembly/budding |
| Interferons? |

plasma proteins. Metabolites are not found in plasma (504). Almost all administered drug is ultimately excreted in the urine. In four of the patients, the ability to isolate virus appeared to diminish during peak plasma levels of the drug (505). Serum p24 antigenemia was not assessed. No significant clinical or immunological improvement was recognized. At least half of the subjects each experienced fever, rash, proteinuria, pyuria, and subclinical hepatitis as determined by aminotransferase elevations in serum (505).

Additional clinical trials were undertaken, which essentially confirmed and extended these clinical observations in over 100 total patients (506–508). Suramin sodium at 0.5, 1.0, or 1.5 gr/week for 6 weeks was followed by maintenance therapy of 0.5 or 1.0 gr weekly for 3–6 months in most cases. As with the preliminary study, virus isolations were unsuccessful from some patients administered suramin, but no clinical or immunological improvement was appreciated. In addition to the toxicity originally reported, a significant minority of patients experienced malaise, nausea, vomiting, neurologic symptoms (headache, metallic taste, parathesias, and peripheral neuropathy), neutropenia, and adrenal insufficiency. A more recent study of 10 patients with AIDS and p24 antigenemia, half of whom were administered suramin, could demonstrate no reduction in antigenemia (508). With the failure to observe benefit and the frequent occurrence of serious toxicity, suramin is no longer under active clinical investigation. Further clinical trials must probably await identification of compounds of this class of polyanionic dyes with a higher selectivity index.

## AZT

AZT was the first drug demonstrated to be clinically effective and licensed for use for the treatment of HIV infection. It was first administered to patients in 1985 within only 6 months of the demonstration of its efficacy *in vitro* (385). In a phase 1 dose escalation study in 19 adults with severe HIV infection (509), AZT was shown to be rapidly absorbed from the gastrointestinal tract with mean peak serum levels attained at approximately 1 hr. Dose-independent kinetics occurred at doses up to 10 mg/kg every 4 hr. Approximately 60% of ingested drug is bioavailable because of first passage glucuronidation by the liver (510). This glucuronidated metabolite has no apparent toxicity or antiviral activity and like AZT is excreted almost exclusively by the kidneys with a mean half-life of 1 hr. The mean peak serum concentration in an adult administered 200 mg is approximately 2–3 μM. Renal clearance of AZT is approximately 350 ml/min/70 kg, and total body clearance is approximately 1,900 ml/min/70 kg at doses up to 5 mg/kg (511). In patients with impaired renal function, the half-life of AZT is only slightly prolonged because of rapid hepatic glucuronidation. The glucuronide of AZT (GAZT) does accumulate in patients with reduced creatinine clearance (512). The toxicity of chronically elevated levels of GAZT is unknown. AZT penetrates into the CSF well, with CSF to plasma ratios of 50–100% at least 4 hr after the first dose (510). Semen concentrations of AZT ranged from 1.3- to 20-fold higher than serum when studied in six patients, suggesting pH-dependent trapping of AZT, which is a weak base ($pK_a$ = 9.68) (513).

In addition to pharmacokinetic data, the phase 1 study generated anecdotal evidence of some toxicity during the 6-week regimen (headaches and leukopenia), which was manageable. Therapeutic benefits were also suggested in several patients including weight gain, improved sense of well being, improved CD4 lymphocyte counts, and return of delayed type hypersensitivity skin test reactions. These observations prompted the design of a multicenter, randomized, placebo-controlled, double-blind study (514,515).

A total of 282 patients with either a first

episode of *Pneumocystis carinii* pneumonia diagnosed within 120 days or with advanced ARC were stratified according to CD4 lymphocyte counts and then randomly assigned to receive either placebo or 250 mg of AZT by mouth every 4 hr for 24 weeks. A total of 145 subjects receiving AZT and 137 receiving placebo entered the study between February and June of 1986. The study was terminated on September 18, 1986 by an independent monitoring board because 19 placebo recipients and one AZT recipient had died ($p < 0.001$). At that time, 27 subjects had completed 24 weeks of study, 152 had completed 16 weeks, and the remainder had completed at least 8 weeks. In addition to prolonged survival, AZT therapy reduced the frequency and severity of opportunistic infections, improved body weight, prevented deterioration of Karnofsky performance score, increased peripheral CD4 lymphocyte counts, and reversed skin test anergy in many patients. Of note, the rates of opportunistic infections in the AZT and placebo groups did not begin to diverge until after 6–8 weeks of therapy. The drug did not reduce the isolation rates of HIV from peripheral blood mononuclear cells; however, viral p24 antigenemia as measured by ELISA was significantly reduced by AZT therapy (514).

This reduction of p24 antigenemia with AZT administration and its rise following withdrawal of drug has been observed by several investigators (516–519). In some patients, the level of p24 antigenemia may increase although the patient continues to ingest drug. The mechanism by which this occurs is unknown. No systematic studies correlating dosing regimens and clearance of p24 antigenemia have yet been published. AZT also consistently has cleared p24 antigen from the CSF from a small number of patients (518–521), although the drug has no benefit on virus isolation (520).

The administration of AZT has been associated with the anecdotal reports of significant neurological improvement (522, 523). These observations have been supported by the analysis of the neuropsychological assessments of the subjects participating in the placebo-controlled study. AZT partially reversed and delayed further deterioration of cognitive dysfunction, utilizing tests of memory and attention, for example (524). No improvement was appreciated in measures of affective symptoms.

Thrombocytopenia may be another specific complication of HIV infection to respond to the administration of AZT. Although AZT is toxic to cells of the erythroid and granulocytic series, slight mean increases were observed in platelet counts in the phase II study (515). Several case reports have appeared describing significant improvements of thrombocytopenia associated with the administration of AZT (525,526). A prospective, placebo-controlled, blinded cross-over study of 10 patients with severe thrombocytopenia documented an impressive impact of AZT on this condition (527). Neither the mechanism of the thrombocytopenia nor how AZT reverses it has been elucidated.

Although significant clinical benefit has been documented with AZT, serious adverse clinical reactions occur, particularly bone marrow suppression (515). In the phase 2, placebo-controlled trial, nausea, myalgia, insomnia, and severe headaches were reported more frequently by recipients of AZT; macrocytosis developed within weeks in most of the AZT group. Anemia with hemoglobin levels below 7.5 gr/dl developed in 24% of AZT recipients and 4% of placebo recipients ($p < 0.001$). These patients have an increased requirement for transfusions with packed red blood cells. Macrocytosis developed within weeks in most of the AZT group. Of note, not all patients with macrocytosis developed anemia and not all episodes of anemia were not macrocytic. Erythropoietin levels are increased in the presence of red cell hypoplasia (528). Neutropenia (<500 cells/mm$^3$ millimeter) occurred in 15% of AZT recipients, as compared with 2% of placebo recipients ($p < 0.001$). Subjects who entered the study with low CD4 lymphocyte counts, low serum vitamin $B_{12}$ levels, anemia, or low neutrophil counts were more likely to have hematologic side effects. Prolonged marrow failure has been associated with AZT administration (479). Although marrow toxicity with AZT is more likely with more severe underlying disease, no absolute predictors of susceptibility to toxic side effects are available (515). Moreover, the underlying mechanism of marrow insufficiency in HIV infection remains obscure.

An apparent increased association of hematologic toxicity with acetominophen administration (515) may not hold up with further scrutiny. No other association of drug interactions was appreciated in the phase 2 study (515). Prolongation of the serum half-life of AZT due to administration of probenecid (529), quinine, and sulfamethoxisole have been documented. Ganciclovir (DHPG), a drug of great use for a number of patients with AIDS, has significant additive toxicity with AZT on granulocytes to the extent that the two drugs cannot be safely coadministered at full or even half doses (530). This toxicity cannot be accounted for by pharmacokinetic interaction; neither drug affects the excretion of the other (531).

Anecdotal reports of infrequent toxicities, e.g., seizures, have also been published. These reports are always difficult to interpret. Seizures occur in patients with AIDS, even in the absence of neuroradiological abnormalities that are suggestive of cerebral toxoplasmosis or malignancy. The question is whether AZT adds an additional, but small, risk for seizures. Although none of the original 282 study patients, 127 of whom received drug for more than 1 year, were reported with seizure, several case reports of seizures temporarily associated with administration of AZT were reported once thousands of patients were receiving drug (532,533). Whether to risk rechallenge with AZT following a seizure in a patient is a question for which the physician and patient must make a risk: benefit decision must be based upon judgment about the patients' prospects for prolonged therapy, marrow reserve, alternative etiologies of the seizure, and personal wishes. Other anecdotal reports such as post-AZT withdrawal meningitis have not yet been appreciated by others (D. Barry, unpublished observations). A myositis-like syndrome, characterized by parathesias, myalgias, muscle edema, muscle wasting, and elevations of serum lactate dehydrogenase and creatinine phosphokinase levels, has also been associated with prolonged AZT administration (534). A similar syndrome has also been described in one series of two and another series of 11 untreated patients infected with HIV (76,202). A case of nemaline rod myopathy in a patient with HIV infection has also been reported (535). The causal role of AZT in myopathy is thus difficult to assess. The ongoing large placebo controlled studies should provide useful information regarding this association.

AZT has now been administered to over 10,000 subjects, with many receiving drug for over 2 years. Some conclusions can be gleaned from this experience. The continued monitoring of the phase 2 study patients suggested continued benefit with prolonged therapy (536). Survival rates of patients treated with AZT were higher than those that might have been expected from previous experience with similar patients. Patients continued to experience episodes of opportunistic infections; however, these infections were either of decreased severity or were more responsive to conventional therapy. Hematologic toxicities continued to be the major laboratory abnormality associated with drug administration; however, new or more frequent toxicity was not observed with more prolonged therapy (536). Progressive bone marrow suppression did not appear to be associated with prolonged administration.

AZT was made available to 4,805 patients with a previous diagnosis of *Pneumocystis carinii* pneumonia, through a compassionate plea program (Treatment IND) following the termination of the placebo-controlled trial in late 1986. The analysis of this large experience with this prelicensure distribution program confirmed the positive association of survival and pretherapy clinical status as defined by hemoglobin level, functional status as measured by Karnofsky score, or stage of disease as measured by recency of first diagnosis of *Pneumocystis* pneumonia (537). A similar experience was reported in an open study of 365 French patients (538). These data indicate that delay of AZT administration in patients with AIDS is not in the best interests of the patient and that efforts are needed to document how much benefit derives with administration even earlier in the course of HIV infection.

The documentation of the emergence of AZT resistance in patients with AIDS or ARC raises new considerations in the use of the drug and for the design of new drug regimens (401). Little variation in AZT sensitivity was seen in isolates from patients never treated with AZT. No reduction in sensitivity was documented during the first 6 months of treatment. After 6 months, most isolates replicate in the presence of higher concentrations of AZT. Many isolates have more than 100-fold increases in resistance and replicate at drug concentrations not attainable with normal doses of drug. Although the emergence of resistance has not yet been demonstrated to be associated with diminished drug efficacy, this is a reasonable concern. The relative likelihood of the emergence of resistance in other patient populations, such as asymptomatic seropositive subjects, is under investigation. Cross-resistance to AZdU was documented but not to other nucleosides or other compounds. Drug combinations to reduce the likelihood of the emergence of resistance are thus a reasonable strategy for the future.

## Clinical Use of AZT

AZT prolongs survival and reduces morbidity. It is also expensive and potentially toxic. There is much to be learned about its proper use. The prudent physician must thus exercise judgement, monitor for toxicity, and appreciate his or her ignorance. The dose of AZT in the placebo controlled study was 250 mg every 4 hr. For the open label study, for subsequent studies and for licensing, the dose was changed to 200 mg every 4 hr to permit production of 100 mg capsules and easier dosage reduction for toxicity. No differences in rates of opportunistic infection or toxicity were appreciated between the 1,500 mg daily dose used in the placebo controlled study and the 1,200 mg daily dose used subsequintly (536).

The recent reports of preliminary results from three large multicenter studies of the National Institutes of Health AIDS Clinical Trials Group (ACTG) will have important implications for future use of AZT and other drugs. ACTG study 002 has shown that patients who were status-post *Pneumocystis carinii* pneumonia fared at least as well and with less toxicity when administered a lower dose regimen (100 mg orally evey 4 hr after 1 month of the original phase II full dose) than with the original regimen (250 mg orally every 4 hr).

ACTG study 016 has demonstrated that patients with 200 to 500 CD4 lymphocytes and a symptom of AIDS-related complex were less likely to experience disease progression if they were administered the licensed dose of 200 mg orally every 4 hr than a placebo.

ACTG study 019 demonstrated that asymptomatic seropositive subjects with less than 500 CD4 cells fared better when administered AZT than placebo. The reduction of progression to disease, when compared to placebo, was similar for subjects administered 300 mg or 100 mg orally 5 times daily; however, less toxicity was observed in the subjects receiving the lower dose. No benefit of AZT therapy could be discerned in subjects with more than 500 CD4 cells. Remarkably little toxicity was observed in the relatively well subjects in with ACTG 016 or 019.

The results of these trials will undergo more complete and careful analysis before additional conclusions can be drawn; nevertheless, it is probably reasonable to make several predictions. Both ACTG 002 and 019 suggested that AZT has been administered in doses that were too high and that less toxicity and perhaps longer and more sustained thereapy will be possible in the future with little if any loss of efficacy, with only 500 to 600 mg daily. This lower dosage will also benefit combination drug regimens. In addition, therapy of patients at earlier stages of infection will become standard practice. Even more certain is the prospect that in the field of chemotherapy of HIV our information base and practice will be rapidly changing.

Although suppression of p24 antigenemia has not been proven to correlate with clinical outcome, the return of p24 antigenemia within a week or two of significant reduction or withdrawal of AZT therapy would argue that AZT should be conceived of as a suppressive regimen (539). This problem raises the issue of the proper management of drug toxicity. Adverse reactions, including nausea, insomnia, and headaches, occur in many patients taking AZT. Most endure these symptoms because of the potential benefit and find that these reactions subside with time. Occasionally a patient will find the symptoms intolerable and elect to discontinue.

The management of hematologic toxicity is a more frequent problem. Many physicians treat anemia alone with packed red blood cell transfusions while maintaining the therapy with AZT. In the future much anemia may be ameliorated with erythropoietin therapy. Some patients can be sustained in this manner for long periods; for others anemia is the harbinger of granulocytopenia. If the packed blood cell requirement exceeds 4 units per month, dose reduction is probably indicated.

Granulocytopenia and the infrequent severe thrombocytopenia require dose reduction. Once again there are no data to argue a best method for dose reductions. The magnitude of fall from baseline and the rate of fall influence modification. One guideline is to reduce the dose from 100 mg every 4 hr if the neutrophil count falls below 800 cells/mm$^3$ or 50,000 platelets and to discontinue drug at 400 to 500 neutrophils or 25,000 platelets. This guideline is arbitrary and will probably change.

If a patient requires withdrawal of AZT on 2 or 3 occasions or it is apparent that the patient will not be able to sustain the regimen for the 6 to 8 weeks necessary to reduce the rate of opportunistic infection, then the potential harm, effort, and cost of further attempts to administer AZT should be avoided. Similarly, if the patient develops a serious opportunistic infection for which the treatment can improve the quality and duration of life (for example, ganciclovir for serious CMV retinitis or pyrimethamine for toxoplasmosis), then AZT should be discontinued rather than delay or interfere with indicated treatment.

In the absence of studies to support or question a particular approach to toxicity management, these recommendations are reasonable guidelines for managing the individual patient. Septic complications of granulocytopenia in patients who have received AZT are remarkably rare; nevertheless, embarking on a regimen of AZT should include a clear understanding between physician and patient that, with our current experience with the drug, a patient should have a complete blood count with differential at least monthly under the best of circumstances; usually more frequently and weekly if rapidly falling or significantly depressed blood cell counts are probable.

What can be done to reduce the likelihood of hematologic toxicity? Potentially toxic drugs should be avoided; however, as previously mentioned, other drugs which may cause granulocytopenia, such as ganciclovir or pyrimethamine, are clearly indicated and should take priority. Drugs that may prolong the half life of AZT, like probenecid, should be avoided. Although lower levels of serum vitamin $B_{12}$ levels were associated with more frequent hematologic toxicity (515), the co-administration of intramuscular vitamin $B_{12}$ with AZT, sufficient to elevate serum vitamin $B_{12}$ levels persistently, did not appear to diminish drug toxictiy (*unpublished observations*).

Other important unanswered questions are the role of additional antiviral drugs (acyclovir, interferons, foscarnet, ddC), additional immunomodulators (interleukin-2), other cytokines (GM-CSF, erythropoietin) or the interaction with other important drugs (antifolates, antimycobacterial drugs, acetominophen, opiates) or conditions (renal impairment, hepatic impairment) on AZT therapy. Studies to address these important questions are in progress.

The addition of acyclovir to AZT is of potential interest for two reasons. One group of investigators has observed some enhancement of inhibition of the repliction of HIV *in vitro* although acyclovir has no antiretroviral activity on its own (431). Secondly, acyclovir might be expected, as a prophylactic agent, to reduce the morbidity of herpes virus infections in patients with HIV infection. A pilot study has demonstrated independent pharmacokinetics of acyclovir and AZT (540). Larger studies to examine additional parameters like p24 antigenemia and viremia are in progress. A cooperative study of AZT with or without high dose acyclovir (800 mg orally every 6 hr) has been recently conducted by investigators from Europe and Australia (541). The data, which have not yet been fully analyzed or published, suggested that the combination regimen of AZT and high dose acyclovir in this high-risk population with AIDS resulted in less frequent episodes of infection with CMV or HSV and an attendant improved mortality rate. It will be important to analyze and confirm these encouraging results. *Pneumocystis carinii* pneumonia is the most frequent opportunistic cause of morbidity and mortality in HIV infected AIDS patients. The roles of systemic and aerosolized regimens of prophylaxis and their interaction with AZT are under active investigation in various patient populations.

### Dideoxycytidine

In phase 1 studies, ddC was administered at 0.03–0.25 mg/kg intravenously and then orally at 4- or 8-hr intervals (542). The peak concentration of ddC was roughly proportional to the administered dose, and a peak concentration of 0.5 μM was observed after a 1-hr infusion of 0.06 mg/kg. The plasma half-life was approximately 1–2 hr, with renal clearance accounting for drug elimination. Oral bioavailability was 70–80%. Concentrations of drug in the CSF were 9–37% of the concurrent plasma levels 2–3.5 hr after an intravenous infusion (542). No evidence of metabolism of ddC has been noted. Unfortunately, the reduction of doses with the appreciation of toxicity prevented the acquisition of additional pharmacokinetic data, because plasma levels are below the threshold of detection by current assay methods. The phase 1 studies also indicated that ddC decreased circulating p24 antigenemia as does AZT; however, it produced a moderate dermatitis and mucositis in the first few weeks of therapy and, more importantly, a severe peripheral neuropathy in the second or third month of therapy (542). A larger dose ranging study conducted by four cooperating NIH AIDS Clinical Treatment Groups was recently completed (543). At 0.06 and 0.03 mg/kg orally every 4 hr, a diffuse erythematous rash and aphthous stomatitis occurred in the first weeks on drug, which resolved without interruption of therapy. Hematologic toxicity was notably rare. Peripheral sensory neuropathy occurred in all patients at these doses, between the fourth and 14th week, and improved slowly in most patients after discontinuation of ddC. Serum p24 antigen fell significantly (>70% fall) in most patients during therapy. CD4 cell numbers tended to rise transiently on study; however, no clear difference in skin test positivity or rate of HIV isolation from blood coculture positivity was seen. At the 0.01 and 0.005 mg/kg orally every 4-hr dose levels, skin rash and aphthous stomatitis were mild or absent. Peripheral neuropathy, which occurred by week 12–14 in all patients on 0.01 mg/kg orally every 4 hr, was less severe and resolved more quickly than at higher doses. Significant suppression of serum p24 antigen was seen in many patients on the dose of 0.01 mg/kg orally every 4 hr.

Although these initial studies indicate that ddC may have a limited role as a single drug for the treatment of HIV infection, several encouraging observations prompt the evaluation of alternating regimens of ddC and AZT (542). First, ddC significantly reduced p24 antigenemia, an effect seen previously only with AZT. Second, ddC resulted in little hematologic toxicity. Thus, these two dideoxynucleosides with suppressive activity against p24 antigenemia have significant, but nonoverlapping, toxicities. These observations form the rationale for protocols with alternating regimens of AZT and ddC, with the hope of reducing toxicity and maintaining antiviral benefits.

### Foscarnet

A moderate amount of pharmacokinetic data and clinical experience have been acquired with the use of Foscarnet for herpesvirus infections (Chapter 3 and 4). More recent studies of Foscarnet in patients with AIDS suggests that this drug, like AZT and ddC, may have antiretroviral activity as measured by suppression of p24 antigenemia (544–546), but not reduction of ability to isolate virus from peripheral blood cells by culture (545). Foscarnet has been administered at 120–180 mg/day divided into two or three 1- to 2-hr infusions for up to 4 weeks or as a continuous infusion at 0.15 mg/kg/min for up to 21 days. The clinical experience in patients infected with HIV suggest the drug is relatively well tolerated; however, reversible renal dysfunction, thrombophlebitis at the infusion site, headaches, and anemia are associated with administration of Foscarnet (544,545). Further evaluation of this compound is warranted; however, it is not orally bioavailable, thus limiting its utility because of the requirement to administer the drug intravenously. Foscarnet is poorly soluble, and large doses are required because of its relatively low potency (274). Systemic therapy thus requires large doses of intravenous solution. Severe adverse interaction with pentamidine have been observed. In addition, Foscarnet stimulates the release of parathyroid hormone, and the resulting hyperphosphatemia raises concerns about chronic therapy. Additional investigation is needed to define more clearly the clinical role of Foscarnet.

### HPA-23

Few pharmacokinetic data are available with regard to HPA-23, although open administration to some patients was begun in 1983 (456). Reports of administration in 1985 to four patients (456) and in 1986 to 16 patients (547) indicated that thrombocytopenia and occasional elevations in serum aminotransferase were associated with drug administration. In a larger multicenter clinical trial in 69 patients with AIDS, the administration of HPA-23 at 1 mg/kg intravenously 5 days per week for 8 weeks was well tolerated; however, the 2-mg/kg dose was not tolerated in eight of 14 patients because of thrombocytopenia and elevated aminotransferases (548). No changes in immune function or clinical status were appreciated. P24 antigenemia was not assessed. The manufacturer of HPA-23 has apparently suspended further development of this compound.

### Rifabutin

Consistent with the *in vitro* observations (see above), no effects on viral or immunological endpoints were observed in a dose-escalating study of rifabutin in patients with AIDS or ARC (549).

### Ribavirin

A moderate amount of clinical experience with ribavirin had been accumulated before its consideration as an antiretroviral drug (Chapter 4). Nevertheless, its use to treat infection with HIV presented new considerations because of the potential for new or different toxicities with the background of HIV infection and because HIV infection requires chronic therapy. The most extensive prior experience with ribavirin was for acute infections, especially respiratory virus infections and Lassa fever.

Using a newly available radioimmunoassay (RIA), single-dose pharmacokinetics with oral or intravenous ribavirin at 600, 1,200, and 2,400 mg were conducted in asymptomatic men seropositive for HIV (550). Approximately one-half of orally administered drug is absorbed into the circulation. The most striking characteristic of the pharmacokinetics of ribavirin is its accumulation within erythrocytes. This results in a prolonged terminal phase half-life of 36 hr. This means that a steady state serum concentration will take days to attain and weeks to eliminate.

Two large randomized double-blind, placebo-controlled trials have been conducted with 600 and 800 mg daily oral doses of ribavirin, one in patients with lymphadenopathy and one in patients with ARC. These results have generated a great deal of publicity and controversy; however, the data were not yet published in a peer reviewed journal by late 1989. Consequently, definitive conclusions would be premature. Preliminary reports of these studies and a phase 1 study of 10 patients with AIDS (551) indicate that little toxicity occurs at these doses. Even with chronic administration, the only consistent toxic effect is a mild compensated anemia that reverses with discontinuation of drug. Suppression of p24 antigenemia has not been seen (518). The critical conclusions about clinical benefit await the published final analyses of the studies and additional studies that are in progress.

### Dextran Sulfate

A preparation of dextran sulfate has been used in Japan for decades as an oral agent for anticoagulation and lipid reduction. Few data are published regarding pharmacokinetics, efficacy, or toxicity. Nevertheless, the absence of appreciated toxicity in Japan, the remarkable selectivity index *in vitro* (358,359,370,371), and the ready availability of an inexpensive, well-characterized compound has prompted both controlled phase 1 investigations of oral drug and uncontrolled street use. The first phase 1 evaluation in 30 patients with AIDS or ARC indicated little evidence of efficacy or toxicity (552). A number of important questions need to be addressed. How much, if any, of this large, highly charged compound is absorbed from the gastrointestinal tract? What is the metabolism of the drug? What are the pharmacokinetics of the drug and its metabolic products? What are the efficacy and toxicity of the drug and its metabolic products? If no antiviral activity can be documented with oral drug or little absorption from the gastrointestinal tract, what results can be obtained with parenteral administration of dextran sulfate or drugs in its class of sulfated polysaccarides?

### AL721

One open study with eight seropositive subjects with lymphadenopathy who were administered 10 gr of AL721 twice daily for 18 weeks and later 15 gr twice daily could demonstrate no effects on p24 antigenemia, CD4 cell counts, or toxicity (553). A threefold reduction was seen in peak reverse transcriptase levels in the supernatants of cultures of some of these patients; however, this parameter has never been shown to quantitate viral load reliably. A second larger study with higher doses is in progress. Not surprisingly, hyperlipidemia does occur with ingestion of this quantity of lipid.

### Other Drugs

Inconclusive, small, open clinical studies with little encouragement to pursue further studies have also been reported with D-penicillamine (554) and lithium carbonate (555).

### Biological Response Modifiers

Biological response modifiers are the natural products of cells, or compounds that induce or interact with these products, to modulate immune responses, cell proliferation, cell differentiation, or cell metabolism. This class of materials is extensive and rapidly growing in number of identified compounds. For example, the macrophage alone has already been shown to secrete more than 100 molecular species, many of which have multiple activities, many of which interact with each other, many of which are also elaborated by other types of cells, and many of which have overlapping activities (176).

This class of compounds is of keen interest to those involved with the therapy of AIDS for several reasons. The interferons have long interested virologists because they induce antiviral effects in cells, as well as mediate metabolic and functional changes in cells of the immune system (Chapter 9). Other cytokines are of theoretical interest for the treatment of patients with HIV infection for at least two reasons. Agents such as granulocyte macrophage-colony stimulating factor (GM-CSF) and erythropoietin have been considered for the alleviation of hematologic suppression of HIV disease or hematotoxic drug therapy such as AZT or DHPG. Agents such as interleukin-2 have been proposed to help restore deficiencies of immunity.

Most of the experience with interferons in patients with AIDS has been in open trials for the treatment of Kaposi's sarcoma. These trials have utilized recombinant interferon-α or purified interferon-α prepared from lymphoblastoid cells (556–561). Tumor regression is seen in a minority of patients, with a greater likelihood of response in patients with higher CD4 lymphocyte counts. The dose-limiting toxicities of interferon (fever, chills, weakness, fatigue, anorexia, headache, myalgias, arthralgias leukopenia, and elevations of aminotransferase) occur in a small proportion of patients. It should be remembered that dose-limiting toxicity in oncologic practice may occur at much higher doses than would be tolerated for the suppression of chronic HIV infection. A similar uncontrolled experience with interferons β and γ has been generated with five patients with HTLV-1 associated adult T-cell leukemia (562).

The data regarding the use of interferon for the treatment of HIV infection, rather than its malignant complications, are much more limited. *In vitro* interferon-α, interferon-β, and interferon-γ all inhibit the replication of HIV both in T lymphoid cells (563–567) and in primary human macrophages (179). There is an unresolved conflict in data regarding whether or not interferon-γ is active *in vitro* against HIV in peripheral blood mononuclear cells (564,567). In addition, recombinant interferon-α synergistically inhibits HIV replication *in vitro* with two drugs that have antiretroviral activity *in vivo,* AZT (568) and Foscarnet (569). A randomized, double-blind, placebo-controlled trial of recombinant human interferon-$\alpha_{2a}$ in patients with AIDS was initiated before the recognition of AIDS as a retroviral disease (570). Randomization of 67 subjects to placebo, 3 million units, or 36 million units 3 times weekly for 12 weeks failed to demonstrate significant differences in tolerance, laboratory end points (p24, CD4 cell counts), or clinical status. The power of this study to detect a clinically relevant difference among the study arms of this study was inadequate because of the small number of study subjects and their heterogeneity. Several investigators have reported in abstract form that combined administration of AZT and recombinant or cell derived interferon-α for patients with Kaposi's sarcoma result in at least additive marrow toxicity manifested as leukopenia. In open studies, administration of interferon-α does appear to reduce p24 antigenemia (560,561,571). The critical first questions to be answered for HIV infection regard the dose-related effects of different interferon preparations on viral parameters, immune functions, and toxicity, and, secondarily, what effects are seen in combination with AZT.

Ampligen is a synthetic double-stranded RNA consisting of one strand of a homopolymer of inosine and its complement, a random copolymer of cytosine and uridine in a ratio of 12:1 (572). This mismatched double-stranded RNA [(formula: rIn · r($C_{12}$ · U)n] was designed as a less toxic interferon inducer than poly I · C because at the sites of U · I mismatch, there are structural changes that render ampligen susceptible to ribonucleases. Ampligen is a complex preparation with a mean length of 600 bases; however, there is a distribution of molecular sizes, with most molecules having overlapping unpaired single strands. Ampligen acts as an interferon inducer and may have other activities as well (573). *In vitro* it inhibits the replication of HIV-1 in a number of cell lines at concentrations of approximately 10 μg/ml, whereas little toxicity is recognized at 50 μg/ml (574,575). It also acts synergistically with AZT (572).

Some experience has been acquired with the administration of ampligen to animals and humans, primarily for tumor therapy (576–578). Intravenous administration of up to 450 mg twice weekly to patients with tumor appeared to be relatively nontoxic (578). Ampligen was administered to 10 patients infected with HIV ranging in severity from lymphadenopathy to AIDS (579). A dose of 200–250 mg intravenously for up to 18 weeks was associated with little toxicity and some claims of clinical and antiviral effects (579). Preliminary reports from several additional controlled and systematic studies that have been initiated indicate that little toxicity or efficacy can be documented.

Interleukin-2 is a T-cell-derived glycoprotein with many activities including the induction of T lymphocyte proliferation (580), a function critical for the culture systems used to isolate HTLV-1 and HIV (1,6,7). Deficient lymphocyte functions in assays such as *in vitro* natural killer (NK) cell function, can be restored by the addition of interleukin-2 (581,582). These observations and the ready availability of both purified natural and recombinant interleukin-2 have prompted several open trials in patients with AIDS. At doses up to 2,000,000 u/$m^2$/day intravenously, no clinical, virologic, or immunological benefits have been documented (583–586). Influenza-like symptoms and hypotension were observed in many patients receiving 1,000,000 units/$m^2$, or more (586). Although interleukin-2 therapy alone is unlikely to be useful, it is possible that immunological restoration in conjunction with antiviral drugs may have a role in the treatment of HIV infection.

Both HIV infection and its treatment can be toxic to the bone marrow (208,209,515). Cytokines important for the proliferation and differentiation of marrow precursors are potentially useful in overcoming the severe anemia or leukopenia. Several trials of the administration of recombinant GM-CSF to patients with AIDS have documented dramatic dose-dependent elevations of leukocyte counts primarily attributable to neutrophils, monocytes, and eosinophils within hours of initiating infusions, but the counts returned to baseline equally quickly (587). Low-grade fever, myalgia, bone pain, phlebitis, and flushing occur in some patients. The newly circulating cells appear functionally normal (588). No effects on erythroid or platelet elements were seen (587). Trials of erythropoietin, especially for the anemia associated with AZT administration, are also in progress.

A large number of biological response modifiers and "immunomodulating" compounds have been proposed for the therapy of HIV infection. Some of these are well characterized compounds; some have been systematically evaluated in clinical trials. None has yet been shown effective.

No efficacy was shown in small, open trials of cyclosporin (589), levamisole (590), thymopentin (591,592), and transplantations of thymic tissue (593). Investigators administering tranfer factor (not further characterized) or cyclosporin were encouraged by their trials, but no viral markers were tested (589,594). Lithium carbonate appeared ineffective but toxic (555).

A final class of compounds are those "immunomodulating" compounds, such as AS 101 (ammonium trichloro[dioxyethylene -0,0′-] tellurite) (595), diethyldithiocarbamate (DTC;Imuthiol) (597), Imreg-1, disulfiram, isoprinosine (598), thymostimulin (TP-1) (596), and methionine-enkephalin, that are represented by many abstracts at large clinical meetings. Critical interpretation of the merits of such compounds requires information about their composition and purity, well-designed systematic studies, scrutiny of the primary data, and statistical analysis. The importance of conclusions of benefit (or the lack of it) for a disease with the impact of AIDS requires that this information be available accurately and expeditiously. A report of a controlled trial of DTC claimed clinical benefit but no impact on p24 antigenemia (597). This study merits careful analysis of the primary data and confirmatory studies.

To ascribe potential utility to a biologic response modifier and then to assess it properly in clinical trials is even more complicated than for antiviral drugs. The experience with interleukin-2, which is a pure and molecularly defined material, documents several of the difficulties that arise between the production of cytokine preparations by recombinant DNA technology and the documentation of even a potential role in the therapy of disease. Cytokines are being identified, cloned, and expressed faster than their biologic roles can be documented. Should a function of a cytokine be identified *in vitro,* there is no guarantee that that function is biologically relevant. Most cytokines identified to date have a multiplicity of functions, often different ones on different cells, which may vary significantly depending on the presence of other cytokines and which may act in microenvironments based upon physical relationships of cells (599). Serum concentrations may be irrelevant to local concentrations. Cytokine actions may be more a function of changing levels or the presence of other cytokines (599,560) than the levels generated *in vitro* or in serum. Studies *in vitro* of biological response modifiers may thus be much less predictive of potential clinical effects than is obtained with antiviral drugs. Proper regimens of administration may be very difficult to ascertain. Further investigation including both laboratory-based studies and empirical trials will help to elucidate this complex and cloudy picture.

## REFERENCES

1. Poiesz BJ, Ruscetti FW, Mier JW, Woods AM, Gallo RC. Detection and isolation of type-C retrovirus particles from fresh and cultured lymphocytes of a patient with cutaneous T-cell lymphoma. *Proc Natl Acad Sci USA* 1980;77:7415–9.
2. Gottlieb MS, Schroff R, Schanker HM, et al. Pneumocystis carinii pneumonia and mucosal candidiasis in previously healthy homosexual men. *N Engl J Med* 1981;305:1425–31.
3. Masur H, Michelis MA, Greeme JB, et al. An outbreak of community-acquired *Pneumocystis carinii* pneumonia: initial manifestation of cel-

lular immune dysfunction. *N Engl J Med* 1981;305:1431–8.
4. Siegal FP, Lopez C, Hammer FS, et al. Severe acquired immunodeficiency in male homosexuals manifested by chronic perianal ulcerative herpes simplex lesions. *N Engl J Med* 1981;305:1439–44.
5. Hymes KB, Cheung T, Greene JB, et al. Kaposi's sarcoma in homosexual men: a report of eight cases. *Lancet* 1981;ii:598–600.
6. Barre-Sinoussi F, Chermann JC, Jey R, et al. Isolation of a T-lymphotropic retrovirus from a patient at risk for acquired immune deficiency syndrome (AIDS). *Science* 1983;220:868–71.
7. Popovic M, Sarngadharan MG, Read E, Gallo RC. Detection, isolation and continuous production of cytopathic retroviruses (HTLV-III) from patients with AIDS and pre-AIDS. *Science* 1984;224:497–500.
8. Levy JA, Hoffman AD, Kramer AD, et al. Isolation of lymphocytopathic retrovirus from San Francisco patients with AIDS. *Science* 1984;225:840–2.
9. Teich N. Taxonomy of retroviruses. In: Weiss R, Teich N, Varmus H, Coffin J, eds. *RNA tumor viruses.* 2nd ed. Cold Spring Harbor, New York: Cold Spring Harbor Laboratory, 1984:25–208.
10. Kalyanamaran VS, Sarngadharan MG, Robert-Guroff M, et al. A new subtype of human T-cell leukemia virus (HTLV-II) associated with a T-cell variant of hairy cell leukemia. *Science* 1982;218:571–5.
11. Achong BG, Mansell PWA, Epstein MA, Clifford P. An unusual virus in cultures from a human nasopharyngeal carcinoma. *JNCL* 1971;46:299–307.
12. Maurer B, Bannert H, Daral G, Flugel RM. Analysis of the primary structure of the long terminal repeat and the *gag* and *pol* genes of the human spumaretrovirus. *J Virol* 1988;62:1590–7.
13. Sigurdsson B. Maedi, a slow progressive pneumonia of sheep: an epizoological and pathological study. *Br Vet J* 1954;110:225–70.
14. Sigurdsson B. Rida, a chronic encephalitis of sheep: with general remarks on infections which develop slowly and some of their special characteristics. *Br Vet J* 1954;110:341–54.
15. Osame M, Matsumoto M, Usuku K, et al. Chronic progressive myelopathy associated with elevated antibodies to human T-lymphotropic virus type I and adult T-cell leukemialike cells. *Ann Neurol* 1987;21:117–22.
16. Vernant JC, Maurs L, Gessain A, et al. Endemic tropical spastic paraparesis associated with human T-lymphotropic virus type I: a clinical seroepidemiological study of 25 cases. *Ann Neurol* 1987;21:123–30.
17. Jacobson S, Raine CS, Mingioli ES, McFarlin DE. Isolation of an HTLV-1 like retrovirus from patients with tropical spastic paraparesis. *Nature* 1988;331:540–3.
18. Bhagavati S, Ehrlich G, Kula RW, et al. Detection of human T-cell lymphoma/leukemia virus type I DNA and antigen in spinal fluid and blood of patients with chronic progressive myelopathy. *N Engl J Med* 1988;318:1141–7.
19. Newton M, Miller D, Rudge P, et al. Antibody to human T-lymphotropic virus type 1 in West-Indian-born UK residents with spastic paraparesis. *Lancet* 1987;i:415–6.
20. Rosenblatt JD, Chen ISY, Wachsman W. Infection with HTLV-I and HTLV-II: evolving concepts. *Semin Hematol* 1988;25:230–46.
21. Spire B, Montagnier L, Barre-Sinoussi F, Chermann JC. Inactivation of lymphadenopathy associated virus by chemical disinfectants. *Lancet* 1984;ii:899–901.
22. Resnick L, Veren K, Salahuddin SZ, Tondreau S, Markham PD. Stability and inactivation of HTLV-III/LAV under clinical and laboratory environments. *JAMA* 1988;255:1887–91.
23. Martin LS, McDougal JS, Loskoski SL. Disinfection and inactivation of the human T lymphotropic virus type III/lymphadenopathy-associated virus. *J Infect Dis* 1985;152:400–3.
24. Spire B, Dormont D, Barre-Sinoussi F, Montagnier L, Chermann JC. Inactivation of lymphadenopathy-associated virus by heat, gamma rays, and ultraviolet light. *Lancet* 1985;1:188–9.
25. Markowski MA, Coard JG, Griffin B, Mayo DR. Effect of 10 minutes heat treatment on HIV antibody testing from alternate testing sites. *Diagn Microbiol Infect Dis* 1988;9:225–30.
26. Harada S, Yoshiyama H, Yamamoto N. Effect of heat and fresh human serum on the infectivity of human T-cell lymphotropic virus type III evaluated with new bioassay systems. *J Clin Microbiol*1985;22:908–11.
27. McDougal JS, Martin LS, Cort SP, Mozen M, Heldebrandt CM, Evatt BL. Thermal inactivation of the acquired immunodeficiency syndrome virus, human T lymphotropic virus III/lymphadenopathy-associated virus, with special reference to antihemophilic factor. *J Clin Invest* 1985;76:875–7.
28. Henderson LE, Sowder RC, Copeland TD, Benveniste RE, Oroszlan S. Isolation and characterization of a novel protein (X-ORF Product) from SIV and HIV-2. *Science* 1988; 241:199–201.
29. Starcich BR, Hahn BH, Shaw GM, et al. Identification and characterization of conserved and variable regions in the envelope gene of HTLV-III/LAV, the retrovirus of AIDS. *Cell* 1986;45:637–48.
30. Jones KA, Kadonaga JT, Luciw PA, Tjian R. Activation of the AIDS retrovirus promoter by the cellular transcription factor, Spl. *Science* 1986;232:755–9.
31. Garcia JA, Wu FK, Mitsuyasu R, Gaynor RB. Interactions of cellular proteins involved in the transcriptional regulation of the human immunodeficiency virus. *EMBO J* 1987;6:3761.
32. Rosen CA, Sodroski JG, Haseltine WA. Loca-

tion of cis-acting regulator sequences in the T-cell lymphotropic virus type III (HTLV-III/LAV) long terminal repeat. *Cell* 1985;41:813–23.

33. Kaufman JD, Roderiquex VG, Bushar G, Biri C, Norcross MA. Phorbol ester enhances human immunodeficiency virus-promoted gene expression and acts on a repeated 10-base pair functional enhancer element. *Mol Cell Biol* 1987;7:3759.
34. Nabel G, Baltimore D. An inducible transcription factor activates expression of human immunodeficiency virus in T cells. *Nature* 1987;326:711–3.
35. Mosca JD, Bednarik DP, Raj NBK, Rosen CA, Sodroski JG, Haseltine WA. Herpes simplex virus type-1 can reactivate transcription of latent human immunodeficiency virus. *Nature* 1987;325:67–70.
36. Mosca JD, Bednarik DP, Raj NBK, Rosen CA, Sodroski JG. Activation of human immunodeficiency virus by herpesvirus infection: identification of a region within the long terminal repeat that responds to a trans-acting factor encoded by herpes simplex virus 1. *Science* 1988;84:7408–12.
37. Davis MG, Kenney SC, Kamine J, Pagano JS, Huang E-S. Immediate-early gene region of human cytomegalovirus trans-activates the promoter of human immunodeficiency virus. *Proc Natl Acad Sci USA* 1987;84:8642–6.
38. Rando RF, Pellett PE, Luciw PA, Bohan CA, Srinivasan A. Transactivation of human immunodeficiency virus by herpesvirus. *Oncogene* 1987;1:13–18.
39. Ostrove JM, Leonard J, Weck LE, Rabson A, Gendelman HE. Activation of the human immunodeficiency virus by herpes simplex virus type 1. *J Virol* 1987;61:3726–32.
40. Bohnlein E, Lowenthal JW, Siekevitz M, Ballard DW, Franza BR, Greene WC. The same inducible nuclear proteins regulates mitogen activation of both the interleukin-2 receptor-alpha gene and type 1 HIV. *Cell* 1988;53:827–36.
41. Franza Jr BR, Rauscher III FJ, Josephs SF, Curran T. The fos complex and fos-related antigens recognized sequence elements that contain AP-1 binding sites. *Science* 1988;239:1150–3.
42. Okamoto T, Wong-Staal F. Demonstration of virus-specific transcriptional activator(s) in cells infected with HTLV-III by an *in vitro* cell-free system. *Cell* 1986;47:29–35.
43. Feng S, Holland EC. HIV-1 tat trans-activation requires the loop sequence within tar. *Nature* 1988;334:165–7.
44. Hauber J, Cullen BR. Mutational analysis of the trans-activation-responsive region of the human immunodeficiency virus type 1 long terminal repeat. *J Virol* 1988;62:673–9.
45. Rosen CA, Terwilliger E, Dayton AI, Sodroski JG, Haseltine WA. Intragenic cis-acting art responsive sequences of the human immunodeficiency virus. *Proc Natl Acad Sci USA* 1988;85:2071–5.
46. Maio JJ, Brown FL. Regulation of expression driven by human immunodeficiency virus type 1 and human T-cell leukemia virus type 1 long terminal repeats in pluripotential human embryonic cells. *J Virol* 1988;62:1398–407.
47. Valerie K, Delers A, Bruck C, et al. Activation of human immunodeficiency virus type 1 by DNA damage in human cells. *Nature* 1988;333:78–81.
48. Veronese FD, Copeland TD, Oroszlan S, Gallo RC, Sarngadharan MG. Biochemical and immunological analysis of human immunodeficiency virus *gag* gene products p17 and p24. *J Virol* 1988;62:795–801.
49. Jacks T, Power MD, Masiarz FR, Luciw PA, Barr PJ, Varmus HE. Characterization of ribosomal frameshifting in HIV-1 gag-pol expression. *Nature* 1988;331:280–5.
50. Nutt RF, Brady SF, Darke PL, et al. Chemical synthesis and enzymatic activity of a 99-residue peptide with a sequence proposed for the human immunodeficiency virus protease. *Proc Natl Acad Sci USA* 1988;85:7129–33.
51. Hansen J, Billich S, Schulze T, Sukrow S, Moelling K. Partial purification and substrate analysis of bacterially expressed HIV protease by means of monoclonal antibody. *EMBO J* 1988;7:1785–91.
52. Kohl NE, Emini EA, Schleif WA, et al. Active human immunodeficiency virus protease is required for viral infectivity. *Proc Natl Acad Sci USA* 1988;85:4686–90.
53. Lillehoj EP, Salazar FHR, Mervis RJ, et al. Purification and structural characterization of the putative gag-pol protease of human immunodeficiency virus. *J Virol* 1988;62:3053–8.
54. Mous J, Heimer EP, Le Grice SFJ. Processing protease and reverse transcriptase from human immunodeficiency virus type I polyprotein in *Escherichia coli*. *J Virol* 1988;62:1433–6.
55. Debouck C, Gorniak JG, Strickler JE, Meek TD, Metcalf BW, Rosenberg M. Human immunodeficiency virus protease expressed in *Escherichia coli* exhibits autoprocessing and specific maturation of the gag precursor. *Proc Natl Acad Sci USA* 1987;84:8903–6.
56. Le Grice SFJ, Mills J, Mous J. Active site mutagenesis of the AIDS virus protease and its alleviation by trans complementation. *EMBO J* 1988;7:2547–53.
57. Katoh I, Yasunaga T, Ikawa Y, Yoshinaka Y. Inhibition of retroviral protease activity by an aspartyl proteinase inhibitor. *Nature* 1987;329:654–6.
58. Schneider J, Kent SBH. Enzymatic activity of a synthetic 99 residue protein corresponding to the putative HIV-1 protease. *Cell* 1988;54:363–8.
59. Seelmeier S, Schmidt H, Turk V, Von der Helm K. Human immunodeficiency virus has an aspartic-type protease that can be inhibited

by pepstatin A. *Proc Natl Acad Sci USA* 1988;85:6612–6.
60. Weber IT, Miller M, Jaskolski M, Leis J, Skalka AM, Wlodawer A. Molecular modeling of the HIV-1 protease and its substrate binding site [Abstract]. *Science* 1989;243:928–31.
61. Navia MA, Fitzgerald PMD, McKeever BM, et al. Three-dimensional structure of aspartyl protease from human immunodeficiency virus HIV-1. *Nature* 1989;337:615–20.
62. Farmerie WG, Loeb DD, Casavant NC, Hutchison III CA, Edgell MH, Swanstrom R. Expression and processing of the AIDS virus reverse transcriptase in *Escherichia coli*. *Science* 1987; 236:305–8.
63. Larder BA, Purifoy DJM, Powell KL, Darby G. Site-specific mutagenesis of AIDS virus reverse transcriptase. *Nature* 1987;327:716–8.
64. Hansen J, Schulze T, Moelling K. RNase H activity associated with bacterially expressed reverse transcriptase of human T-cell lymphotropic virus III/lymphadenopathy-associated virus. *J Biol Chem* 1987;262:12393–6.
65. Tanese N, Sodroski J, Haseltine WA, Goff SP. Expression of reverse transcriptase activity of human T-lymphotropic virus type III (HTLV-III/LAV) in *Escherichia coli*. *J Virol* 1986; 59:743–5.
66. Veronese FD, Copeland TD, DeVico AL, et al. Characterization of highly immunogenic p66/p51 as the reverse transcriptase of HTLV-III/LAV. *Science* 1986;231:1289–91.
67. Hansen J, Schulze T, Mellert W, Moelling K. Identification and characterization of HIV-specific RNase H by monoclonal antibody. *EMBO J* 1988;7:239–43.
68. Dalgleish AG, Beverly PCL, Clapham PR, Crawford DH, Greaves MF, Weiss RA. The CD4 (T4) antigen is an essential component of the receptor of the AIDS retrovirus. *Nature* 1984;312:763–7.
69. Klatzmann D, Champagne E, Chamaret S, et al. T-lymphocyte T4 molecule behaves as the receptor for human retroviruses LAV. *Nature* 1984;312:767–8.
70. Maddon PJ, Dalgleish AG, McDougal JS, Clapham PR, Weiss RA, Axel R. The T4 gene encodes the AIDS virus receptor and is expressed in the immune system and the brain. *Cell* 1986;47:333–48.
71. McDougal JS, Kennedy MS, Sligh JM, Cort SP, Mawle A, Nicholson JKA. Binding of HTLV-III/LAV to T4+ T cells by a complex of the 110K viral protein and the T4 molecule. *Science* 1986;231:382–5.
72. Modrow S, Hahn BH, Shaw GM, Gallo RC, Wong-Staal F, Wolf H. Computer-assisted analysis of envelope protein sequences of seven human immunodeficiency virus isolates: prediction of antigenic epitopes in conserved and variable regions. *J Virol* 1987;61:570–8.
73. Gurgo C, Guo HG, Franchini G, et al. Envelope sequences of two new United States HIV-1 isolates. *Virology* 1988;164:531–6.
74. Scheid A, Choppin PW. Protease activation mutants of Sendai virus. Activation of biological properties by specific proteases. *Virology* 1976;69:265–77.
75. White J, Kielian M, Helenius A. Membrane fusions proteins of enveloped animal viruses. *Q Rev Biophys* 1983;16:151–95.
76. Gonzales MF, Olney RK, So YT, et al. Subacute structural myopathy associated with human immunodeficiency virus infection. *Arch Neurol* 1988;45:585–7.
77. Gonzalez-Scarano F, Waxham MN, Ross AM, Hoxie JA. Sequence similarities between human immunodeficiency virus gp41 and paramyxovirus fusion proteins. *AIDS Res Hum Retroviruses* 1987;3:245–52.
78. McCune JM, Rabin LB, Feinberg MB, et al. Endoproteolytic cleavage of gp160 is required for the activation of human immunodeficiency virus. *Cell* 1988;53:55–67.
79. Guyader M, Emerman M, Sonigo P, Clavel F, Monagnier L, Alizon M. Genome organization and transactivation of the human immunodeficiency virus type 2. *Nature* 1987;326:662–9.
80. Muesing MA, Smith DH, Cabradilla CD, Benton CV, Lasky LA, Capon DJ. Nucleic acid structure and expression of the human AIDS/lymphadenopathy retrovirus. *Nature* 1985; 313:450–8.
81. Sanchez-Pescador R, Power MD, Barr PJ, et al. Nucleotide sequence and expression of an AIDS-associated retrovirus (ARV-2). *Science* 1985;227:484–92.
82. Ratner L, Haseltine W, Patarca R, et al. Complete nucleotide sequence of the AIDS virus, HTLV-III. *Nature* 1985;313:277–84.
83. Wain-Hobson S, Sonigo P, Danos O, Cole S, Alizon M. Nucleotide sequence of the AIDS virus, LAV. *Cell* 1985;40:9–17.
84. Seiki M, Hattori S, Hirayama Y, Yoshida M. Human adult T-cell leukemia virus: Complete nucleotide sequences of the provirus genome integrated in leukemia cell DNA. *Proc Natl Acad Sci USA* 1983;80:3618–22.
85. Haseltine WA, Sodroski J, Patarca R, Briggs D, Perkins D, Wong-Staal F. Structure at 3′ terminal region of type II human T-lymphotropic virus: evidence for new coding region. *Science* 1984;225:419–21.
86. Shimotohno K, Wachsman W, Takahashi Y, et al. Nucleotide sequence of the 3′ region of an infectious human T-cell leukemia virus type II genome. *Proc Natl Acad Sci USA* 1984; 81:6657–61.
87. Gallo R, Wong-Staal F, Montagnier L, Haseltine WA, Yoshida M. HIV/HTLV gene nomenclature. *Nature* 1988;333:504.
88. Arya SK, Gua C, Josephs SF, Wong-Staal F. Transactivator gene of human T-lymphotropic virus type III (HTLV-III). *Science* 1985; 229:69–73.
89. Sodroski J, Patarca R, Rosen C, Wong-Staal F, Haseltine W. Location of the *trans*-activating region of the genome of human T-cell lymphotropic virus type III. *Science* 1985;229:74–7.
90. Hauber J, Perkins A, Heimer EP, Cullen BR.

*Trans*-activation of human immunodeficiency virus gene expression is mediated by nuclear events. *Proc Natl Acad Sci USA* 1987;84: 6364–8.

91. Peterlin M, Luciw P, Barr P, Waler M. Elevated levels of mRNA can account for the *trans*-activation of human immunodeficiency virus. *Proc Natl Acad Sci USA* 1986;83:9734–8.
92. Cullen BR. Transactivation of human immunodeficiency virus occurs via a bimodal mechanism. *Cell* 1986;46:973–82.
93. Kao SY, Calma AF, Luciw PA, Peterlin BM. Anti-termination of transcription within the long terminal repeat of HIV-1 by *tat* gene product. *Nature* 1987;330:489–93.
94. Feinberg MB, Jarrett RF, Aldavini A, Gallo RC, Wong-Staal F. HTLV-III expression and production involve complex regulation at the levels of splicing and translation of viral mRNA. *Cell* 1986;46:807–17.
95. Muesing MA, Smith DH, Capon DJ. Regulation of mRNA accumulation by a human immunodeficiency virus *trans*-activator protein. *Cell* 1987;48:691–701.
96. Wright CM, Felber BK, Paskalis H, Pavlakis GN. Expression and characterization of the *trans*-activator of HTLVB-III/LAV virus. *Science* 1986;234:988–9.
97. Frankel AD, Bredt DS, Pabo CO. Tat protein from human immunodeficiency virus forms a metal-linked dimer. *Science* 1988;240:70–3.
98. Sadaie MR, Benter T, Wong-Staal F. Site directed mutagenesis of two trans-regulatory genes (*tat*-iii, *trs*) of HIV-1. *Science* 1988; 239:910–3.
99. Fisher AG, Ratner L, Mitsuya H, et al. Infectious mutants of HTLV-III with changes in the 3′ region and markedly reduced cytopathic effects. *Science* 1986;233:655–9.
100. Dayton AI, Sodroski JG, Rosen CA, Goh WE, Haseltine WA. The trans-activator gene of the human T cell lymphotropic virus type III is required for replication. *Cell* 1986;44:941–7.
101. Cullen BR, Hauber J, Campbell K, Sodroski JG, Haseltine WA, Rosen CA. Subcellular localization of the human immunodeficiency virus trans-acting *art* gene product. *J Virol* 1988;62:2498–501.
102. Hauber J, Bouvier M, Malim MH, Cullen BR. Phosphorylation of the *rev* gene product of human immunodeficiency virus type 1. *J Virol* 1988;62:4801–4.
103. Knight DM, Flomerfelt FA, Ghrayeb J. Expression of the art/trs protein of HIV and study of its role in viral envelope synthesis. *Science* 1987;236:837–40.
104. Sodroski J, Goh WC, Rosen CA, Dayton A, Terwilliger E, Haseltine WA. A second post-transcriptional trans-activator gene required for HTLV-III replication. *Nature* 1986;321: 412–7.
105. Terwilliger E, Burghoff R, Sia R, Sodroski J, Haseltine W, Rosen C. The *art* gene product of the human immunodeficiency virus is required for replication. *J Virol* 1988;62:655–8.
106. Malim MH, Hauber J, Fenrick R, Cullen BR. Immunodeficiency virus rev trans-activator modulates the expression of the viral regulatory genes. *Nature* 1988;335:181–3.
107. Malim MH, Hauber J, Le S-Y, Maizel JV, Cullen BR. The HIV-1 rev trans-activator acts through a structured target sequence to activate nuclear export of unspliced viral mRNA. *Nature* 1989;338:254–7.
108. Franchini G, Robert-Guroff M, Wong-Staal F, et al. Expression of the protein encoded by the 3′ open reading frame of human T-cell lymphotropic virus type III in bacteria: demonstration of its immunoreactivity with human sera. *Proc Natl Acad Sci USA* 1986;83:5282–5.
109. Ahmad N, Venkatesan S. *Nef* protein of HIV-1 is a transcriptional repressor of HIV-1 LTR. *Science* 1988;241:1481–5.
110. Franchini G, Robert-Guroff M, Ghrayeb J, Chang NT, Wong-Staal F. Cytoplasmic localization of the HTLV-III 3′ ORF protein in cultured T cells. *Virology* 1986;155:593–9.
111. Guy B, Kieny MP, Reviere Y, et al. HIV F/3′ orf encodes a phosphorylase GTP-binding protein resembling an oncogene product. *Nature* 1987;330:266–9.
112. Strebel K, Daugherty D, Clouse K, Cohen D, Folks T, Martin MA. The HIV 'A' (*sor*) gene product is essential for virus infectivity. *Nature* 1987;328;728–30.
113. Kan GC, Franchini G, Wong-Staal F, et al. Identification of HTLV-III/LAV *sor* gene product and detection of antibodies in human sera. *Science* 1986;231:1553–5.
114. Franchini G, Robert-Guroff M, Aldovini A, Kan NC, Wong-Staal F. Spectrum of natural antibodies against five HTLV-III antigens in infected individuals: correlation of antibody prevalence with clinical studies. *Blood* 1987; 69:437–41.
115. Fisher AG, Ensoli B, Ivanoff L, et al. The *sor* gene of HIV-1 is required for efficient virus transmission in vitro. *Science* 1987;237:888–93.
116. Wong-Staal F, Chanda PK, Ghrayeb J. Human immunodeficiency virus: the eighth gene. *AIDS Res Hum Retroviruses* 1987;3:33–9.
117. Cohen EA, Terwilliger EF, Sodroski JG, Haseltine WA. Identification of a protein encoded by the *vpu* gene of HIV-1. *Nature* 1988; 334:532–4.
118. Strebel K, Klimkait T, Martin MA. A novel gene of HIV-1, *vpu*, and its 16-kilodalton product. *Science* 1988;241:1221–23.
119. Franchini G, Rusche JR, O'Keeffe TJ, Wong-Staal F. The human immunodeficiency virus type 2 (HIV-2) contains a novel gene encoding a 16 kD protein associated with mature virions. *AIDS Res Hum Retroviruses* 1988;4:243.
120. Kappes JC, Morrow CD, Lee SW, et al. Identification of a novel retroviral gene unique to human immunodeficiency virus type 2 and simian immunodeficiency virus SIVmac. *J Virol* 1988;62:3501–5.
121. Yu XF, Ito S, Essex M, Lee TH. A naturally

immunogenic virion-associated protein specific for HIV-2 and SIV. *Nature* 1988;335:262–5.
122. Bertonis JM, Meier W, Johnson VA, et al. HIV infection is blocked *in vitro* by recombinant soluble CD4. *Nature* 1988;331:76–8.
123. Hussey RE, Richardson NE, Kowalski M, et al. A soluble CD4 protein selectively inhibits HIV replication and syncytium formation. *Nature* 1988;331:78–81.
124. Deen KC, McDougal JS, Inacker R, et al. A soluble form of CD4 (T4) protein inhibits AIDS virus infection. *Nature* 1988;331:82–4.
125. Traunecker A, Luke W, Karjalainen K. Soluble CD4 molecules neutralize human immunodeficiency virus type 1. *Nature* 1988;331:84–6.
126. Smith DH, Byrn RA, Marster SA, Gregory T, Groopmen JE, Capon DJ. Blocking of HIV-1 infectivity by a soluble, secreted form of the CD4 antigen. *Science* 1987;238:1704–7.
127. Peterson A, Seed B. Genetic analysis of monoclonal antibody and HIV binding sites on the human lymphocyte antigen CD4. *Cell* 1988; 54:65–72.
128. Clayton LK, Hussey RE, Steinbrich R, Ramachandran H, Husain Y, Reinherz EL. Substitution of murine for human CD4 residues identifies amino acids critical for HIV-gp 120 binding. *Nature* 1988;335:363–6.
129. Chesebro B, Wehrly K. Development of a sensitive quantitative focal assay for human immunodeficiency virus infectivity. *J Virol* 1988;62:3779–88.
130. Gendelman HE, Orenstein JM, Martin MA, et al. Efficient isolation and propagation of human immunodeficiency virus on recombinant colony-stimulating factor 1-treated monocytes. *J Exp Med* 1988;167:1428–41.
131. Fujiwara T, Mizuuchi K. Retroviral DNA integration: structure of an integration intermediate. *Cell* 1988;54:497–504.
132. Hoxie JA, Alpers JE, Rackowski J, et al. Alterations in T4(CD4) protein and mRNA synthesis in cells infected with HIV. *Science* 1986;234:1123–7.
133. Keshet E, Temin HM. Cell killing by spleen necrosis virus is correlated with a transient accumulation of spleen necrosis virus DNA. *J Virol* 1979;31:376–86.
134. Somasundaran M, Robinson HL. A major mechanism of human immunodeficiency virus-induced cell killing does not involve cell fusion. *J Virol* 1987;61:3114–9.
135. Harper ME, Marselle LM, Gallo RC, Wong-Staal F. Detection of lymphocytes expressing human T-lymphotropic virus type III in lymph nodes and peripheral blood from infected individuals by *in situ* hybridization. *Proc Natl Acad Sci USA* 1986;83:772–6.
136. Zagury D, Bernard J, Leonard R, et al. Long-term cultures of HTLV-III infected T cells: a model of cytopathology of T-cell depletion in AIDS. *Science* 1986;231:850–3.
137. Margolick JB, Volkman SJ, Folks TM, et al. Amplification of HTLV-III/LAV infection by antigen-induced activation of T cells and direct suppression by virus of lymphocyte blastogenic responses. *J Immunol* 1987;138:1719–23.
138. Gendelman HE, Phelps W, Feigenbaum L, et al. *Trans*-activation of the human immunodeficiency virus long terminal repeat sequence by DNA viruses. *Proc Natl Acad Sci USA* 1986;83:9759–63.
139. Sodroski J, Goh WC, Rosen C, Campbell K, Haseltine WA. Role of the HTLV-III/LAV envelope in syncytium formation and cytopathicity. *Nature* 1986;322:470–4.
140. Yoffe B, Lewis DE, Petrie BL, et al. Fusion as a mediator of cytolysis in mixtures of uninfected CD4+ lymphocytes and cells infected by human immunodeficiency virus. *Proc Natl Acad Sci USA* 1987;84:1429–33.
141. Lifson JD, Reyes GR, McGrath MS, et al. AIDS retrovirus induced cytopathology: giant cell formation and involvement of CD4 antigen. *Science* 1986;232:1123–7.
142. Siliciano RF, Lawton T, Knall C, et al. Analysis of host-virus interactions in AIDS with anti-gp120 T cell clones: effect of HIV sequence variation and a mechanism for CD4+ cell depletion. *Cell* 1988;54:561–75.
143. Lyerly HK, Matthews TJ, Langlois AJ, Bolognesi DP, Weinhold KJ. Human T-cell lymphotropic virus III beta glycoprotein (gp120) bound to CD4 determinants on normal lymphocytes and expressed by infected cells serves as target for immune attack. *Proc Natl Acad Sci USA* 1987;84:4601–5.
144. Stricker RB, McHugh TM, Moody DJ, et al. An AIDS-related cytotoxic autoantibody reacts with a specific antigen on stimulated CD4 T cells. *Nature* 1987;327:710–3.
145. Shearer GM. AIDS: an autoimmune pathologic model for the destruction of a subset of helper T lymphocytes. *Mt Sinai J Med (NY)* 1986; 53:609–15.
146. Vogel J, Hinrichs SH, Reynolds RK, Luciw PA, Jay G. The HIV *tat* gene induces dermal lesions resembling Kaposi's sarcoma in transgenic mice. *Nature* 1988;335:606–11.
147. Gonda MA, Wong-Staal F, Gallo RC, Clements JE, Narayan O, Gilden RV. Sequence homology and morphologic similarity of HTLV-III and visna virus, a pathogenic lentivirus. *Science* 1985;227:173–7.
148. Sonigo P, Alizon M, Staskus K, et al. Nucleotide sequence of the visna lentivirus: relationship to the AIDS virus. *Cell* 1985;42:369–82.
149. Stephens RM, Casey JW, Rice NR. Equine infectious anemia virus *gag* and *pol* genes: relatedness to visna and AIDS virus. *Science* 1986;231:589–94.
150. Chiu I-M, Yaniv A, Dahlberg JE, et al. Nucleotide sequence evidence for relationship of AIDS retrovirus to lentiviruses. *Nature* 1985; 317:366–8.
151. Haase AT. Pathogenesis of lentivirus infections. *Nature* 1986;332:130–6.
152. Narayan O, Wolinsky JS, Clements JE, Strandberg JD, Griffin DE, Cork LC. Slow virus replication: the role of macrophages in the persis-

tent and expression of visna viruses of sheep and goats. *J Gen Virol* 1982;59:345–56.

153. Pederson C, Nielsen CM, Vestergaard BF, Gerstoft J, Krogsgaard K, Nielsen JO. Temporal relation of antigenaemia and loss of antibodies to core antigens to development of clinical disease in HIV infection. *Br Med J* 1987;295: 567–9.
154. Gyorkey F, Melnick JL, Sinkovics JG, Gyorkey P. Retrovirus resembling HTLV in macrophages of patients with AIDS. *Lancet* 1985;i:106.
155. Armstrong JA, Horne J. Follicular dendritic cells and virus-like particles in AIDS-related lymphadenopathy. *Lancet* 1984;ii:370–2.
156. Gartner S, Markovits P, Markovitz DM, Kaplan MH, Gallo RC, Popovic M. The role of mononuclear phagocytes in HTLV-III/LAV infection. *Science* 1986;233:215–9.
157. Ho DD, Rota TR, Hirsch MS. Infection of monocyte/macrophages by human T lymphotropic virus type III. *J Clin Invest* 1986; 77:1712–5.
158. Salahuddin SZ, Rose RM, Groopman JE, Markham PD, Gallo RC. Human T lymphotropic virus type III infection of human alveolar macrophages. *Blood* 1986;68:281–4.
159. Chayt KJ, Harper ME, Marselle LM, et al. Detection of HTLV-III RNA in lungs of patients with AIDS and pulmonary involvement. *JAMA* 1986;256:2356–9.
160. Ward JM, O'Leary TJ, Baskin GB, et al. Immunohistochemical localization of human and simian immunodeficiency virus antigens in fixed tissue sections. *Am J Pathol* 1987; 127:199–205.
161. Le Tourneau A, Audouin J, Diebold J, Marche C, Tricottet V, Reynes M. LAV-like viral particles in lymph node germinal centers in patients with the persistent lymphadenopathy syndrome and the acquired immunodeficiency syndrome-related complex: an ultrastructural study of 30 cases. *Hum Pathol* 1986;17:1047–53.
162. Wiley CA, Schrier RD, Nelson JA, Lampert PW, Oldstone MBA. Cellular localization of human immunodeficiency virus infection within the brains of acquired immune deficiency syndrome patients. *Proc Natl Acad Sci USA* 1986;83:7089–93.
163. Gabuzda DH, de la Monte SM, Ho DD, Hirsch MS, Rota TR, Sobel RA. Immunohistochemical identification of HTLV-III antigen in brains of patients with AIDS. *Ann Neurol* 1986; 20:289–95.
164. Stoler MH, Eskin TA, Benn S, Angerer RC, Angerer LM. Human T-cell lymphotropic virus type III infection of the central nervous system. A preliminary *in situ* analysis. *JAMA* 1986;256:2360–4.
165. Koenig S, Gendelman HE, Orenstein JM, et al. Detection of AIDS virus in macrophages in brain tissue from AIDS patients with encephalopathy. *Science* 1986;233:1089–93.
166. Gartner S, Markovits D, Markovitz DM, Betts RF, Popovic M. Virus isolation from and identification of HTLV-III/LAV-producing cells in brain tissue from a patient with AIDS. *JAMA* 1986;256:2365–71.
167. Tschachler E, Groh V, Popovic M, et al. Epidermal Langerhans cells—a target for HTLV-III/LAV infection. *J Invest Dermatol* 1987; 88:233–7.
168. Rappersberger K, Gartner S, Schenk P, et al. Langerhans' cells are an actual site of HIV-1 replication. *Intervirology* 1988;29:185–94.
169. Wood GS, Warner NL, Warnke RA. Anti-leu-3/T4 antibodies react with cells of monocyte/macrophage and Langerhans lineage. *J Immunol* 1983;131:212–6.
170. Groh V, Tani M, Harrer A, Wolff AB, Stingl G. Leu-3/T4 expression on epidermal Langerhans cells in normal and diseased skin. *J Invest Dermatol* 1986;86:115–20.
171. Wolf K, Stingl G. The Langerhans cell. *J Invest Dermatol* 1983;80:17s–21s.
172. Belisto DV, Sanchez MR, Baker RL, Valentine F, Thorbecke GJ. Reduced Langerhans' cell Ia antigen and ATPase activity in patients with the acquired immunodeficiency syndrome. *N Engl J Med* 1984;20:1279–82.
173. Dreno B, Milpied B, Bignon JD, Stalder JF, Litoux P. Prognostic value of Langerhans cells in the epidermis of HIV patients. *Br J Dermatol* 1988;118:481–6.
174. Unanue ER, Allen PM. The basis for the immunoregulatory role of macrophages and other accessory cells. *Science* 1987;236:551–7.
175. Haas JG, Riethmuller G, Ziegler-Heitbrock WL. Monocyte phenotype and function in patients with the acquired immunodeficiency syndrome (AIDS) and AIDS-related disorders. *Scand J Immunol* 1987;26:371–9.
176. Nathan CF. Secretory products of macrophages. *J Clin Invest* 1987;79;319–26.
177. Roy S, Wainberg MA. Role of the mononuclear phagocyte system in the development of acquired immunodeficiency syndrome (AIDS). *J Leukocyte Biol* 1988;43:91–7.
178. Brenneman DE, Westbrook GL, Fitzgerald SP, et al. Neuronal cell killing by the envelope protein of HIV and its prevention by vasoactive intestinal peptide. *Nature* 1988;335:639–42.
179. Kornbluth RS, Oh PS, Munis JR, Cleveland PH, Richman DD. Interferons and bacterial lipopolysaccharide protect macrophages from productive infection by HIV *in vitro*. *J Exp Med* 1989;169:1137–51.
180. Pauza CD. HIV persistence in monocytes leads to pathogenesis and AIDS. *Cell Immunol* 1988;112:414–24.
181. Koyanagi Y, Miles S, Mitsuyasu RT, Merrill JE, Vinters HV, Chen ISY. Dual infection of the central nervous system by AIDS viruses with distinct cellular tropisms. *Science* 1987; 236:819–22.
182. Tenner-Racz K, Racz P, Dietrich M, et al. Monoclonal antibodies to human immunodeficiency virus: Their relation to the patterns of lymph node changes in persistent generalized

lymphadenopathy and AIDS. *AIDS* 1987;2:95–104.
183. O'Murchadha MT, Wolf BC, Neiman RS. The histologic features of hyperplastic lymphadenopathy in AIDS-related complex are nonspecific. *Am J Surg* 1987;11:94–9.
184. Diebold J, Marche CL, Audouin J, et al. Lymph node modification in patients with the acquired immunodeficiency syndrome (AIDS) or with AIDS-related complex (ARC). *Pathol Res Pract* 1985;180:590–611.
185. Garcia CF, Lifson JD, Engleman EG, et al. The immunohistology of persistent generalized lymphadenopathy syndrome (PGL). *Am J Clin Pathol* 1986;86:706–15.
186. Biberfeld P, Porwit-Ksiazek A, Bottiger B, et al. Immunohistology of lymph nodes in HTLV-III infected homosexuals with persistent adenopathy or AIDS. *Cancer Res* 1985; 45(suppl):4665s–70s.
187. McArthur JC. Neurologic manifestations of AIDS. *Medicine* 1987;66:407–37.
188. Grant I, Atkinson JH, Hesselink JR, et al. Evidence for early central nervous system involvement in the acquired immunodeficiency syndrome (AIDS) and other human immunodeficiency virus (HIV) infections. *Ann Intern Med* 1987;107:828–36.
189. Jarvik JG, Hesselink JR, Kennedy C, et al. Acquired immunodeficiency syndrome magnetic resonance patterns of brain involvement with pathologic correlation. *Arch Neurol* 1988; 45:731–8.
190. Navia BA, Cho E-S, Petito CK, Price RW. The AIDS dementia complex: II. neuropathology. *Ann Neurol* 1986;19:525–35.
191. Navia BA, Jordan BD, Price RW. The AIDS dementia complex: I. clinical features. *Ann Neurol* 1986;19:517–24.
192. Epstein LG, Sharer LR, Cho E-S, Myenhofer M, Navia BA, Price RW. HTLV-III/LAV-like retrovirus particles in the brains of patients with AIDS encephalopathy. *AIDS Res* 1984; 14:447–54.
193. Popovic M, Mellert W, Erfle V, Gartner S. Role of mononuclear phagocytes and accessory cells in human immunodeficiency virus type I infection of the brain. *Ann Neurol* 1988; 23(suppl):S74–7.
194. Vazeux R, Brousse N, Jarry A, et al. AIDS subacute encephalitis: identification of HIV-infected cells. *Am J Pathol* 1987;126:403–10.
195. Kaminski HJ, Katzman M, Wiest PM, et al. Cardiomyopathy associated with the acquired immune deficiency syndrome. *Journal of Acquired Immune Deficiency Syndromes* 1988; 2:105–10.
196. Roldan EO, Moskowitz L, Hensley GT. Pathology of the heart in acquired immunodeficiency syndrome. *Arch Pathol Lab Med* 1987;111:943–6.
197. Cohen IS, Anderson DW, Virmani R, et al. Congestive cardiomyopathy in association with the acquired immunodeficiency syndrome. *N Engl J Med* 1986;315:628–30.
198. Rynes RI, Goldenberg DL, Digiacomo R, Olson R, Hussain M, Veazey J. Acquired immunodeficiency syndrome-associated arthritis. *Am J Med* 1988;84:810–6.
199. Winchester R, Bernstein DH, Fischer HD, et al. The co-occurrence of Reiter's syndrome and acquired immunodeficiency. *Ann Intern Med* 1987;106:19–26.
200. Rao TK, Friedman EA, Nicastri AD. The types of renal disease in the acquired immunodeficiency syndrome. *N Engl J Med* 1987; 316:1062–8.
201. Pardo V, Aldana M, Colton RM, et al. Glomerular lesions in the acquired immunodeficiency syndrome. *Ann Intern Med* 1984;101:429–34.
202. Simpson DM, Bender AN. Human immunodeficiency virus-associated myopathy: analysis of 11 patients. *Ann Neurol* 1988;24:79–84.
203. Goodman DS, Teplitz ED, Wishner A, et al. Prevalence of cutaneous disease in patients with acquired immunodeficiency syndrome (AIDS) or AIDS-related complex. *J Am Acad Dermatol* 1987;17:210–20.
204. Sindrup JH, Lisby G, Weismann K. Skin manifestations in AIDS, HIV infection, and AIDS-related complex. *Int J Dermatol* 1987;26:267–72.
205. Lake-Bakaar G, Quadros E, Beidas S, et al. Gastric secretory failure in patients with the acquired immunodeficiency syndrome (AIDS). *Ann Intern Med* 1988;109:502–4.
206. Kotler DP, Gaetz HP, Lange M, Klein EB, Holt PR. Enteropathy associated with the acquired immunodeficiency syndrome. *Ann Intern Med* 1984;101:421–8.
207. Dobs AS, Dempsey MA, Ladenson PW, Polk BF. Endocrine disorders in men infected with human immunodeficiency virus. *Am J Med* 1988;84:611–5.
208. Zon LI, Groopman JE. Hematologic manifestations of the human immune deficiency virus (HIV). *Semin Hematol* 1988;25:208–18.
209. Spivak JL, Bender BS, Quinn TC. Hematologic abnormalities in the acquired immunodeficiency syndrome. *Am J Med* 1984;77:224–8.
210. Donahue RE, Honson MM, Zon LI, Clark SC, Groopman JE. Suppression of *in vitro* haematopoiesis following human immunodeficiency virus infection. *Nature* 1987;326:200–3.
211. Stella CC, Ganser A, Hoelzer D. Defective *in vitro* growth of the hemopoietic progenitor cells in the acquired immunodeficiency syndrome. *J Clin Invest* 1987;80:286–93.
212. Morris L, Distenfeld A, Amorosi E, et al. Autoimmune thrombocytopenic purpura in homosexual men. *Ann Intern Med* 1982;96:714–7.
213. Walsh C, Krigel R, Lennette E, et al. Thrombocytopenia in homosexual men. *Ann Intern Med* 1985;103:542.
214. Abrams DI, Kiprov DD, Goedert JJ, et al. Antibodies to human T-lymphotropic virus type III and development of the acquired immunodeficiency syndrome in homosexual men presenting with immune thrombocytopenia. *Ann Intern Med* 1986;104:47.

215. Walsh CM, Nardi NA, Karpatkin S. On the mechanism of thrombocytopenia purpura in sexually active homosexual men. *N Engl J Med* 1984;311:635.
216. Yu J-R, Lennette ET, Karpatkin S. Anti-F(ab′)2 antibodies in thrombocytopenic patients at risk for acquired immunodeficiency syndrome. *J Clin Invest* 1986;77:1756–61.
217. McGrath KM, Spelman D, Barnett M, et al. Spectrum of HTLV-III infection in a hemophilic cohort treated with blood products from a single manufacturer. *Am J Hematol* 1986;23:239–45.
218. Cooper DA, Imrie AA, Penny R. Antibody response to human immunodeficiency virus after primary infection. *J Infect Dis* 1987;155:1113–8.
219. Gaines H, von Sydow M, Parry JV, et al. Rapid communication: detection of immunoglobulin M antibody in primary human immunodeficiency virus infection. *AIDS Res Hum Retroviruses* 1988;2:11–6.
220. Lange JMA, Parry JV, De Wolf F, Mortimer PP, Goudsmit J. Diagnostic value of specific IgM antibodies in primary HIV infection. *AIDS Res Hum Retroviruses* 1988;2:31–6.
221. Allain JP, Laurian Y, Paul DA, et al. Long-term evaluation of HIV antigen and antibodies to p24 and gp41 in patients with hemophilia. *N Engl J Med* 1987;317:1114–21.
222. Klasse PJ, Pipkorn R, Blomberg J. Presence of antibodies to a putatively immunosuppressive part of human immunodeficiency virus (HIV) envelope glycoprotein gp41 is strongly associated with health among HIV-positive subjects. *Proc Natl Acad Sci USA* 1988;85:5225–9.
223. Sano K, Lee MH, Morales F, et al. Antibody that inhibits human immunodeficiency virus reverse transcriptase and association with inability to isolate virus. *J Clin Microbiol* 1987;25:2415–7.
224. Goh WC, Sodroski JG, Rosen CA, Haseltine WA. Expression of the *art* gene protein of HTLV-III/LAV in bacteria. *J Virol* 1987; 61:633–7.
225. Barone AD, Silva JJ, Ho DD, Gallo RC, Wong-Staal W, Chang NT. Reactivity of *E. coli*-derived *trans*-activating protein of human T lymphotropic virus type III with sera from patients with acquired immune deficiency syndrome. *J Immunol* 1986;137:669–73.
226. Aldovini A, Debouck C, Feinberg MB, Rosenberg M, Arya SK, Wong-Staal F. Synthesis of the complete trans-activation gene product of human T-lymphotropic virus type II in *Escherichia coli:* demonstration of immunogenicity *in vivo* and expression *in vitro*. *Proc Natl Acad Sci USA* 1986;83:6672–6.
227. Arya SK, Gallo RC. Three novel genes of human T-lymphotropic virus type III: immune reactivity of their products with sera from acquired immune deficiency syndrome patients. *Proc Natl Acad Sci USA* 1986;83:2209–13.
228. Clapham P, Nagy K, Weiss R. Pseudotypes of human T-cell leukemia virus types 1 and 2: neutralization by patients' sera. *Proc Natl Acad Sci USA* 1984;81:2886–9.
229. Robert-Guroff M, Brown M, Gallo RC. HTLV-III-neutralizing antibodies in patients with AIDS and AIDS-related complex. *Nature* 1985; 316:72–4.
230. Chanh TC, Dreesman GR, Kanda P, et al. Induction of anti-HIV neutralizing antibodies by synthetic peptides. *EMBO J* 1986;5:3065–71.
231. Ho DD, Sarngadharan MG, Hirsch MS, et al. Human immunodeficiency virus neutralizing antibodies recognize several conserved domains on the envelope glycoproteins. *J Virol* 1987;61:2024–8.
232. Ho DD, Kaplan JC, Rackauskas IE, Gurney ME. Second conserved domain of gp120 is important for HIV infectivity and antibody neutralization. *Science* 1988;239:1021–3.
233. Kennedy RC, Dreesman GR, Chanh TC, et al. Use of a resin-bound synthetic peptide for identifying a neutralizing antigenic determinat associated with the human immunodeficiency virus envelope. *J Biol Chem* 1987;262:5769–74.
234. Linsley PS, Ledbetter JA, Kinney-Thomas E, Hu S-L. Effects of anti-gp120 monoclonal antibodies on CD4 receptor binding by the env protein of human immunodeficiency virus type 1. *J Virol* 1988;62:3695–702.
235. Putney SD, Matthews TJ, Robey WG, et al. HTLV-III/LAV neutralizing antibodies to an *E. coli*-produced fragment of the virus envelope. *Science* 1986;234:1392–5.
236. Wong-Staal F, Shaw FM, Hahn BH, et al. Genomic diversity of human T-lymphotropic virus type III (HTLV-III). *Science* 1985;229:759–62.
237. Cloyd MW, Holt MJ. Heterogeneity of human immunodeficiency virus cell-associated antigens and demonstration of virus type specificities of the human antibody responses. *Virology* 1987;161:286–92.
238. Looney DJ, Fisher AG, Putney DS, et al. Type-restricted neutralization of molecular clones of human immunodeficiency virus. *Science* 1988;241:357–9.
239. Prince AM, Pascual D, Kosolapov LB, Kurokawa D, Baker L, Rubinstein P. Prevalence, clinical significance, and strain specificity of neutralizing antibody to the human immunodeficiency virus. *J Infect Dis* 1987;156:268–72.
240. Weiss RA, Clapham PR, Weber JN, Dalgleish AG, Lasky LA, Berman PW. Variable and conserved neutralization antigens of human immunodeficiency virus. *Nature* 1986;324:572–5.
241. Nara PL, Robey WG, Pyle SW, et al. Purified envelope glycoproteins from human immunodeficiency virus type 1 variants induce individual, type-specific neutralizing antibodies. *J Virol* 1988;62:2622–8.
242. Montelaro RC, Parekh B, Orrego A, Issel CJ. Antigenic variation during persistent infection by equine infectious anemia virus, a retrovirus. *J Biol Chem* 1984;259:10539–44.
243. Clements JE, Pedersen FS, Narayan O, Haseltine WA. Genomic changes associated with antigenic variation of visna virus during per-

sistent infection. *Proc Natl Acad Sci USA* 1980;77:4454–8.
244. Yoshiyama H, Kobayashi N, Matsui T, et al. Transmission and genetic shift of human immunodeficiency virus (HIV) *in vivo*. *J Mol Biol Chem* 1987;4:385–96.
245. Saag MS, Hahn BH, Gibbons J, et al. Extensive variation of human immunodeficiency virus type-1 *in vivo*. *Nature* 1988;334:440–4.
246. Fisher AG, Ensoli B, Looney D, et al. Biologically diverse molecular variants within a single HIV-1 isolate. *Science* 1988;334:444–7.
247. Hahn BH, Shaw GM, Taylor ME, et al. Genetic variation in HTLV-III/LAV over time in patients with AIDS or at risk for AIDS. *Science* 1986;232:1548–33.
248. Blumberg RS, Paradis TJ, Hartshorn KL, et al. Antibody-dependent cell-mediated cytotoxicity against cells infected with the human immunodeficiency virus. *J Infect Dis* 1987; 156:878–84.
249. Rook AH, Lance HC, Folks T, et al. Sera from HTLV-III/LAV antibody positive individuals mediate antibody-dependent cellular cytotoxicity against HTLV-III/LAV-infected T cells. *J Immunol* 1987;138:1064–7.
250. Ljunggren K, Bottiger B, Biberfeld G, Karlson A, Fenyo EM, Jondal M. Antibody-dependent cellular cytotoxicity-inducing antibodies against human immunodeficiency virus. *J Immunol* 1987;139:2273–7.
251. Berzofsky JA, Bensussan A, Cease KP, et al. Antigenic peptides recognized by T lymphocytes from AIDS viral envelope-immune humans. *Nature* 1988;334:706–8.
252. Ahearne PM, Matthews TJ, Lyerly HK, White GC, Bolognesi DP, Weinhold KJ. Cellular immune response to viral peptides in patients exposed to HIV. *AIDS Res Hum Retroviruses* 1988;4:259.
253. Schnittman SM, Lane HC, Higgins SE, et al. Direct polyclonal activation of human B lymphocytes by the acquired immune deficiency syndrome virus. *Science* 1986;233:1084–6.
254. Nixon DF, Townsend ARM, Elvin JG, Rizza CR, Gallwey J, McMichael AJ. HIV-1 gag-specific cytotoxic T lymphocytes defined with recombinant vaccinia virus and synthetic peptides. *Nature* 1988;336:484–6.
255. Plata F, Autran B, Martins LP, et al. AIDS virus-specific cytotoxic T lymphocytes in lung disorders. *Nature* 1987;328:348–51.
256. Schrier RD, Gnann Jr JW, Landes R, et al. T cell recognition of HIV synthetic peptides in natural infection. *J Immunol* 1989;142:1166–76.
257. Wahren B, Morfeldt-Mansson L, Biberfeld G, et al. Characteristics of the specific cell-mediated immune response in human immunodeficiency virus infection. *J Virol* 1987;61: 2017–23.
258. Weinhold KJ, Matthews TJ, Ahearne PM, et al. Cellular anti-gp120 cytolytic reactivities in HIV-1 seropositive individuals. *Lancet* 1988; i:902–4.
259. Walker BD, Chakrabarti S, Moss B, et al. HIV-specific cytotoxic T lymphocytes in seropositive individuals. *Nature* 1987;328:345–8.
260. Walker BD, Flexner C, Paradis TJ, et al. HIV-1 reverse transcriptase is a target for cytotoxic T lymphocytes in infected individuals. *Science* 1988;240:64–6.
261. Gordin FM, Simon GL, Wofsy CB, Mills J. Adverse reations to trimethoprim-sulfamethoxazole in patients with the acquired immunodeficiency syndrome. *Ann Intern Med* 1984;100:495–9.
262. Kovacs JA, Hiemenz JW, Macher AM, et al. Pneumocystis carinii pneumonia: a comparison between patients with the acquired immunodeficiency syndrome and patients with other immunodeficiencies. *Ann Intern Med* 1984;100:663–71.
263. Schupbach J, Sarngadharan MG, Blayney DW, Kalyanaraman VS, Bunn PA, Gallo RC. Demonstration of viral antigen p24 in circulating immune complexes of two patients with human T-cell leukaemia/lymphoma virus (HTLV) positive lymphoma. *Lancet* 1987;i:302–4.
264. McDougal JS, Hubbard M, Nicholson JKA, et al. Immune complexes in the acquired immunodeficiency syndrome (AIDS): relationship to disease manifestation, risk group, and immunologic defect. *J Clin Immunol* 1985;5:130–8.
265. Lane HC, Masur H, Edgar LC, Whalen G, Rook AH, Fauci AS. Abnormalities of B-cell activation and immunoregulation in patients with the acquired immunodeficiency syndrome. *N Engl J Med* 1983;309:453–8.
266. Bloom EJ, Abrams DI, Rodgers G. Lupus anticoagulant in the acquired immunodeficiency syndrome. *JAMA* 1986;256:491–3.
267. Cohen AJ, Philips TM, Kessler CM. Circulating coagulation inhibitors in the acquired immunodeficiency syndrome. *Ann Intern Med* 1986;104:175–80.
268. Lanzavecchia A, Roosnek E, Gregory T, Berman P, Abrignani S. T cells can present antigens such as HIV gp120 targeted to their own surface molecules. *Nature* 1988;334:530–2.
269. Cooper DA, Maclean P, Gold J, et al. Acute AIDS retrovirus infection: Definition of a clinical illness associated with seroconversion. *Lancet* 1985;i:537–40.
270. Ho DD, Sarngadharan MG, Resnick L, et al. Primary human T-lymphotropic virus type III infection. *Ann Intern Med* 1985;103:880–3.
271. Tucker J, Ludlam CA, Craig A, et al. HTLV-III infection associated with glandular-fever-like illness in a haemophiliac. *Lancet* 1985;i:585.
272. Feorino PM, Kalyanaraman VS, Haverkos HW, et al. Lymphadenopathy associated with virus infection of a blood donor-recipient pair with acquired immunodeficiency syndrome. *Science* 1984;225:69.
273. Needlestick transmission of HTLV-III from a patient infected in Africa. *Lancet* 1984;ii:1376.
274. Sjovall J, Karlsson A, Ogenstad S, Sandstrom E, Saarimaki M. Pharmacokinetics and absorption of foscarnet after intravenous and oral administration to patients with human immu-

nodeficiency virus. *Clin Pharmacol Ther* 1988; 44:65–73.
275. Fox R, Eldred LJ, Fuchs EJ, et al. Clinical manifestations of actue infection with human immunodeficiency virus in a cohort of gay men. *AIDS Res Hum Retroviruses* 1987;1:35–8.
276. Colebunders R, Greenberg AE, Francis H, et al. Short communication: acute HIV illness following blood transfusion in three African children. *AIDS Res Hum Retroviruses* 1988;2: 125–8.
277. Kessler HA, Blaauw B, Spear J, et al. Diagnosis of human immunodeficiency virus infection in seronegative homosexuals presenting with an acute viral syndrome. *JAMA* 1987;258:1196–202.
278. Valle S-L. Febrile pharyngitis as the primary sign of HIV infection in a cluster of cases linked by sexual contact. *Scand J Infect Dis* 1988;19:13–7.
279. Lang W, Anderson RE, Perkins H, et al. Clinical, immunologic, and serologic findings in men at risk for acquired immunodeficiency syndrome. *JAMA* 1987;257:326–30.
280. Mathur-Wagh U, Spigland I, Sacks HS, et al. Longitudinal study of persistent generalized lymphadenopathy in homosexual men: Relation to acquired immunodeficiency syndrome. *Lancet* 1984;i:1033–8.
281. Metroka CD, Cunningham-Rundles S, Pollack MS, et al. Generalized lymphadenopathy in homosexual men. *Ann Intern Med* 1983;99:585–91.
282. Kaslow RA, Phair JP, Friedman HB, et al. Infection with the human immunodeficiency virus: clinical manifestations and their relationship to immune deficiency. *Ann Intern Med* 1987;107:474–80.
283. Howard J, Sattler F, Mahon R, et al. Clinical features of 100 human immunodeficiency virus antibody-positive individuals from an alternate test site. *Arch Intern Med* 1987;147:2131–3.
284. Abrams DI, Lewis BJ, Beckstead JH, et al. Persistent diffuse lymphadenopathy in homosexual men: endpoint or prodrome?. *Ann Intern Med* 1984;100:801–8.
285. Centers for Disease Control. Classification system for human T-lymphotropic virus type III/ lymphadenopathy-associated virus infections. *MMWR* 1986;35:334–9.
286. Redfield RR, Wright DC, Tramont EC. The Walter Reed Staging Classification for HTLV-III LAV infection. *N Engl J Med* 1986;314:131–2.
287. MacDonell KB, Chmiel JS, Goldsmith J, et al. Prognostic usefulness of the Walter Reed Staging classification for HIV infection. *Journal of Acquired Immune Deficiency Syndromes* 1988; 1:367–74.
288. Centers for Disease Control. Revision of the CDC surveillance case definition for acquired immunodeficiency syndrome. *MMWR* 1987; 36:35–95.
289. Goedert JJ, Biggar RJ, Melbye M, et al. Effect of T4 counts and cofactors on the incidence of AIDS in homosexual men infected with human immunodeficiency virus. *JAMA* 1987;257:331–4.
290. Lange JM, Paul DA, Huisman HG, et al. Persistent HIV antigenemia and decline of HIV core antibodies associated with the transition to AIDS. *Br Med J* 1986;293:1459–62.
291. Lacey CJM, Forbes MA, Waugh MA, Cooper EH, Hambling MH. Serum beta$_2$-microglobulin and human immunodeficiency virus infection. *AIDS Res Hum Retroviruses* 1987;1:123–7.
292. Centers for Disease Control. Update: acquired immunodeficiency syndrome—United States. *MMWR* 1986;35:17.
293. Quinn TC, Mann JM, Curran JW, Piot P. AIDS in Africa: an epidemiologic paradigm. *Science* 1986;234:955–63.
294. Curran JW, Jaffe HW, Hardy AM, Morgan WM, Selik RM, Dondero TJ. Epidemiology of HIV infection and AIDS in the United States. *Science* 1988;239:610–6.
295. Centers for Disease Control. Quarterly report to the domestic policy council on the prevalence and rate of spread of HIV and AIDS—United States. *MMWR* 1988;37:551–9.
296. Friedland GH, Klein RS. Transmission of the human immunodeficiency virus. *N Engl J Med* 1987;317:1125–35.
297. Pomerantz RJ, de la Monte S, Donegan SP, et al. Human immunodeficiency virus (HIV) infection of the uterine cervix. *Ann Intern Med* 1988;108:321–7.
298. Wofsy C, Cohen J, Hauer L, et al. Isolation of AIDS-associated retrovirus from genital secretions of women with antibodies to the virus. *Lancet* 1986;i:527–9.
299. Gallo RC, Salahuddin SZ, Popovic M, et al. Frequent detection and isolation of cytopathic retroviruses (HTLV-III) from patients with AIDS and at risk for AIDS. *Science* 1984; 224:500–3.
300. Zagury D, Leibowitch J, Bernard J, et al. HTLV-III in cells cultured from semen of two patients with AIDS. *Science* 1984;226:449–51.
301. Ho DD, Schooley RT, Rota TR, et al. HTLV-III in the semen and blood of a healthy homosexual man. *Science* 1984;226:451–3.
302. Ho DD, Rota TR, Schooley RT, et al. Isolation of HLTV-III from cerebrospinal fluid and neural tissues of patients with neurologic syndromes related to the acquired immunodeficiency syndrome. *N Engl J Med* 1985;313:1493–7.
303. Thiry L, Sprecher-Goldberger S, Jonckheer T, et al. Isolation of AIDS virus from cell-free breast milk of three healthy virus carriers [letter]. *Lancet* 1985;ii:891.
304. Vogt MW, Witt DJ, Craven DE, et al. Isolation of HTLV-III/LAV from cervical secretions of women at risk for AIDS. *Lancet* 1986;i:525–7.
305. Ho DD, Byington RE, Schooley RT, et al. Infrequency of isolation of HTLV-III virus from saliva in AIDS. *N Engl J Med* 1985;313:1606.
306. Fujikawa LS, Palestine AG, Nussenblatt RB, Salahuddin SZ, Masur H, Gallo RC. Isolation of human T-lymphotropic virus type III from

the tears of a patient with the acquired immunodeficiency syndrome. *Lancet* 1985;ii:529–30.
307. Groopman JE, Salahuddin SZ, Sarngadharan MG, et al. HTLV-III in saliva of people with AIDS-related complex and healthy homosexual men at risk for AIDS. *Science* 1984;226:447–8.
308. Des Jarlais DC, Friedman SR. HIV infection among intravenous drug users: epidemiology and risk reduction. *AIDS Res Hum Retroviruses* 1987;1:67–76.
309. Chmiel JS, Detels R, Kaslow RA, et al. Factors associated with prevalent human immunodeficiency virus (HIV) infection in the multicenter AIDS cohort study. *Am J Epidemiol* 1987;126:568–76.
310. Winklestein W, Lyman DM, Padian N, et al. Sexual practices and risk of infection by the human immunodeficiency virus. *JAMA* 1987;257:321–5.
311. Fischl MA, Dickinson GM, Scott GB, Kimas N, Fletcher MA, Parks W. Evaluation of heterosexual partners, children, and household contacts of adults with AIDS. *JAMA* 1987; 257:640–4.
312. Greenblatt RM, Lukehart SA, Plummer FA, et al. Genital ulceration as a risk factor for human immunodeficiency virus infection. *AIDS Res Hum Retroviruses* 1988;2:47–50.
313. Gerberding JL, Bryant-LeBlanc CE, Nelson K, et al. Risk of transmitting the human immunodeficiency virus, cytomegalovirus, and hepatitis B virus to health care workers exposed to patients with AIDS and AIDS-related conditions. *J Infect Dis* 1987;156:1–8.
314. Centers for Disease Control. Update: acquired immunodeficiency syndrome and human immunodeficiency virus infection among health-care workers. *MMWR* 1988;37:229–39.
315. Centers for Disease Control. Human immunodeficiency virus infections in health-care workers exposed to blood of infected patients. *MMWR* 1987;36:285–9.
316. Weiss SH, Goedert JJ, Gartner S, et al. Risk of human immunodeficiency virus (HIV-1) infection among laboratory workers. *Science* 1988;239:68–71.
317. Tavares L, Roneker C, Johnston K, Nusinoff-Lehrman S, de Noronha F. 3′-Azido-3′-deoxythymidine in feline leukemia virus-infected cats: a model for therapy and prophylaxis of AIDS. *Cancer Res* 1987;47:3190–4.
318. Weiss SH, Mann DL, Murray C, et al. HLA-DR antibodies and HTLV-III antibody ELISA testing. *Lancet* 1985;2:157–60.
319. Sayer MH, Beatty PG, Hensen JA. HLA antibodies as a cause of false-positive reactions in screening enzyme immunoassays for antibodies to human T-lymphotropic virus type III. *Transfusion* 1986;26:113–8.
320. Henderson LE, Sowder R, Copeland TD, et al. Direct identification of class II histocompatibility DR proteins in preparations of human T-cell lymphotropic virus type III. *J Virol* 1987;61:629–32.
321. Kuhnl P, Seidl S, Holzberger G. HLA DR4 antibodies cause positive HTLV-III antibody ELISA results. *Lancet* 1985;i:1222–5.
322. Biggar RJ, Gigase PL, Melbeye M, et al. Elisa HTLV retrovirus antibody reactivity associated with malaria and immunocomplexes in healthy Africans. *Lancet* 1985;ii:520–21.
323. Schupbach J, Tanner M. Specificity of human immnodeficiency virus(LAV/HTLV-III)-reactive antibodies Africa sera from southeastern Tanzania. *Acta Chem Scand [B]* 1986;43:195–9.
324. Tribe DE, Reed DL, Lindell RP, et al. Antibodies reactive with human immunodeficiency virus gag-coded antigens (gag reactive only) are a major cause of enzyme-linked immunosorbent assay reactivity in a blood donor population. *J Clin Microbiol* 1988;26:641–7.
325. Burke DS, Brundage JF, Redfield RR, et al. Measurement of the false positive rate in a screening program for human immunodeficiency virus infections. *N Engl J Med* 1988; 319:961–4.
326. Gallo D, Diggs JL, Shell GR, Dailey PJ, Hoffman MN, Riggs JL. Comparison of detection of antibody to the acquired immune deficiency syndrome virus by enzyme immunoassay, immunofluorescence, and western blot methods. *J Clin Microbiol* 1986;23:1049–51.
327. Centers for Disease Control. Update: serologic testing for antibody to human immunodefiency virus. *MMWR* 1988;36:833–40.
328. Saag MS, Britz J. Asymptomatic blood donor with a false positive HTLV-III Western blot. *N Engl J Med* 1986;314:118
329. Chiodi F, von Gegerfeldt A, Albert J, et al. Site-directed ELISA with synthetic peptides representing the HIV transmembrane glycoprotein. *J Med Virol* 1987;23:1–9.
330. Dawson GJ, Heller JS, Wood CA, et al. Reliable detection of individuals seropositive for the human immunodeficiency virus (HIV) by competitive immunoassays using *Escherichia coli*–expressed HIV structural proteins. *J Infect Dis* 1988;157:149–55.
331. Gnann Jr JW, McCormick JB, Mitchell S, Nelson JA, Oldstone MBA. Synthetic peptide immunoassay distinguishes HIV type 1 and HIV type 2 infections. *Science* 1987;237:1346–9.
332. Thorn RM, Beltz GA, Hung C-H, Fallis BF, Winkle S, Cheng K-L, Marciani DJ. Enzyme immunoassay using a novel recombinant polypeptide to detect human immunodeficiency virus env antibody. *J Clin Microbiol* 1987;25:1207–12.
333. Smith RS, Naso RB, Rosen J, et al. Antibody to synthetic oligopeptide in subjects at risk for human immunodeficiency virus infection. *J Clin Microbiol* 1987;25:1498–504.
334. Shoeman RL, Young D, Pottathil R, et al. Comparison of recombinant human immunodeficiency virus gag precursor and gag/env fusion proteins and a synthetic env peptide as diagnostic reagents. *Anal Biochem* 1987;161: 370–9.
335. Joller-Jemelka HI, Joller PW, Muller F, Schup-

bach J, Grob PJ. Anti-HIV IgM analysis during early manifestations of HIV infections. *AIDS Res Hum Retroviruses* 1987;1:45–7.
336. Saah AJ, Farzadegan H, Fox R, et al. Detection of early antibodies in human immunodeficiency virus infection by enzyme-linked immunosorbent assay, western blot, and radioimmunoprecipitation. *J Clin Microbiol* 1987; 25:1605–10.
337. Pan L-Z, Cheng-Mayer C, Levy JA. Patterns of antibody response in individuals infected with the human immunodeficiency virus. *J Infect Dis* 1987;155:626–30.
338. Farzadegan H, Polis MA, Wolinsky SM, et al. Loss of human immunodeficiency virus type 1 (HIV-1) antibodies with evidence of viral infection in asymptomatic homosexual men. *Ann Intern Med* 1988;108:785–90.
339. Ranki A, Krohn M, Allain J-P. Long latency precedes overt seroconversion in sexually transmitted human immunodeficiency virus infection. *Lancet* 1987;ii:589–90.
340. Albert J, Pehrson PO, Schulman S, et al. HIV isolation and antigen detection in infected individuals and their seronegative sexual partners. *AIDS Res Hum Retroviruses* 1988;2:107–11.
341. Goudsmit J, Paul DA, Lange JM, et al. Expression of human immunodeficiency virus antigen (HIV-Ag) in serum and cerebrospinal fluid during acute and chronic infection. *Lancet* 1986;ii:177–80.
342. von Sydow M, Gaines H, Sonnerborg A, Forsgren M, Pehrson PO, Strannegard O. Antigen detection in primary HIV infection. *Br Med J* 1988;296:238–40.
343. Weber JN, Weiss RA, Roberts C, et al. Human immunodeficiency virus infection in two cohorts of homosexual men: neutralizing sera and association of anti-gag antibody with prognosis. *Lancet* 1987;i:119–22.
344. De Wolf F, Goudsmit J, Paul DA, et al. Risk of AIDS related complex and AIDS in homosexual men with persistent HIV antigenaemia. *Br Med J* 1987;293:569–72.
345. Mayer KH, Falk LA, Paul DA, et al. Correlation of enzyme-linked immunosorbent assays for serum human immunodeficiency virus antigen and antibodies to recombinant viral proteins with subsequent clinical outcomes in a cohort of asymptomatic homosexual men. *Am J Med* 1987;83:208–12.
346. Moss AR, Bacchetti P, Osmond D, et al. Seropositivity for HIV and the development of AIDS or AIDS related condition: three year follow up of the San Francisco General Hospital cohort. *Br Med J* 1988;296:745–50.
347. Richman DD, Kornbluth RS, Carson DA. Failure of dideoxynucleosides to inhibit human immunodeficiency virus replication in cultured human macrophages. *J Exp Med* 1987; 166:1144–9.
348. Saiki RK, Scharf S, Faloona F, et al. Enzymatic amplification of β-globin genomic sequences and restriction site analysis for diagnosis of sickle cell anemia. *Science* 1985; 230:1350–4.
349. Guatelli JC, Gingeras TR, Richman DD. Nucleic acid amplification *in vitro:* The detection of sequences with low copy numbers and the application to the diagnosis of HIV-1 infection. *Clin Microbiol Rev* 1989;2:217–26.
350. Hart C, Spira T, Moore J, et al. Direct detection of HIV RNA expression in seropositive subjects. *Lancet* 1988;ii:596–9.
351. Murakawa GJ, Zaia JA, Spallone PA, et al. Direct detection of HIV-1 RNA from AIDS and ARC patient samples. *DNA* 1988;7:287–95.
352. Jackson GG, Rubenis M, Knigge M, et al. Passive immunoneutralization of human immunodeficiency virus in patients with advanced AIDS. *Lancet* 1988;ii:647–52.
353. Karpas A, Hill F, Youle M, et al. Effects of passive immunization in patients with the acquired immunodeficiency syndrome-related complex and acquired immunodeficiency syndrome. *Proc Natl Acad Sci USA* 1988;85:9234–7.
354. Dalgleish AG, Kennedy RC, Chanh TC, et al. Therapeutic strategies against HIV based on the CD4 molecule: monoclonal antibody therapy, soluble CD4 and anti-idiotype vaccines. *IVth International Conference on AIDS, Stockholm, Sweden,* 1988.
355. Richardson NE, Brown NR, Hussey RE, et al. Binding site for human immunodeficiency virus coat protein gp120 is located in the NH2-terminal region of T4 (CD4) and requires the intact variable-region-like domain. *Proc Natl Acad Sci USA* 1988;85:6102–6.
356. Landau NR, Warton M, Littman DR. The envelope glycoprotein of the human immunodeficiency virus binds to the immunoglobulin-like domain of CD4. *Nature* 1988;334:159–62.
357. Jameson BA, Rao PE, Kong LI, et al. Location and chemical synthesis of a binding site for HIV-1 on the CD4 protein. *Science* 1988;240:1335–9.
358. Mitsuya H, Looney DJ, Kuno S, Ueno R, Wong-Staal W, Broder S. Dextran sulfate suppression of viruses in the HIV family: inhibition of virion binding to CD4+ cells. *Science* 1988;240:646–8.
359. Baba M, Pauwels R, Balzarini J, Arnout J, Desmyter J, De Clercq E. Mechanism of inhibitory effect of dextran sulfate and heparin on replication of human immunodeficiency virus *in vitro. Proc Natl Acad Sci USA* 1988;85:6132–6.
360. Lifson JD, Hwang KM, Nara PL, et al. Synthetic CD4 peptide derivatives that inhibit HIV infection and cytopathicity. *Science* 1988;241: 712–6.
361. Chaudhary VK, Mizukami T, Fuerst TR, et al. Selective killing of HIV-infected cells by recombinant human CD4-pseudomonas exotoxin in hybrid protein. *Nature* 1988;335:369–72.
362. Capon DJ, Chamow SM, Mordenti J, et al. Designing CD4 immunoadhesins for AIDS therapy. *Nature* 1989;337:525–31.
363. Pert CB, Ruff MR, Ruscetti F, Farrar WL, Hill

JM. HIV receptor in brain and deduced peptides that block viral infectivity. In : Bridge TP, Mirsky AF, Goodwin FK, eds. *Psychological, neuropsychiatric, and substance abuse aspects of AIDS*. New York: Raven Press, 1988:73–83.
364. Pert CB, Hill JM, Ruff MR, et al. Octapeptides deduced from the neuropeptide receptor like pattern of antigen T4 in brain potently inhibit human immunodeficiency virus receptor binding and T-cell infectivity. *Proc Natl Acad Sci USA* 1986;83:9254–8.
365. Barnes DH. Debate of potential AIDS drug. *Science* 1987;237:128–30.
366. Toyoshima K, Vogt PK. Enhancement and inhibition of avian sarcoma viruses by polycations and polyanions. *Virology* 1969;384:414–26.
367. Takemoto KK, Spicer SS. Effects of natural and synthetic sulfated polysaccharides on viruses and cells. *Ann NY Acad Sci* 1965; 130:365–73.
368. De Somer P, De Clercq E, Billiau A, Schonne E, Claesen M. Antiviral activity of polyacrylic acid polymethacrylic acids. I. Mode of action *in vitro*. *J Virol* 1968;2:878–85.
369. Toyoshima K, Vogt PK. Enhancement and inhibition of avian sarcoma viruses by polycations and polyanions. *Virology* 1969;38:414–26.
370. Ueno R, Kuno S. Dextran sulfate, a potent anti-HIV agent *in vitro* having synergism with zidovudine [Letter]. *Lancet* 1987;i:1379.
371. Ito M, Baba M, Sato A, Pauwels R, De Clercq E, Shigeta S. Inhibitory effect of dextran sulfate and heparin on the replication of human immunodeficiency virus (HIV) *in vitro*. *Antiviral Res* 1987;7:361–7.
372. Balzarini J, Mitsuya H, De Clercq E, Broder S. Aurintricarboxylic acid and Evans Blue represent two different classes of anionic compounds which selectively inhibit the cytopathogenicity of human T-cell lymphotropic virus type III/lymphadenopathy-associated virus. *Biochem Biophys Res Commun* 1986; 136:64–71.
373. Balzarini J, Mitsuya H, De Clercq E, Broder S. Comparative inhibitory effects of suramin and other selected compounds on the infectivity and replication of human T-cell lymphotropic virus (HTLV-III)/lymphadenopathy-associated virus (LAV). *Int J Cancer* 1986;37:451–7.
374. Nakashima H, Kido Y, Kobayashi N, et al. Purification and characterization of an avian myeloblastosis and human immunodeficiency virus reverse transcriptase inhibitor, sulfated polysaccharides extracted from sea algae. *Antimicrob Agents Chemother* 1987;31:1524–8.
375. Yoshida O, Nakashima H, Yoshida T, et al. Sulfation of the immunomodulating polysaccharide lentinan: a novel strategy for antivirals to human immunodeficiency virus (HIV). *Biochem Pharmacol* 1988;37:2887–981.
376. Tochikura TS, Nakashima H, Tanabe A, Yamamoto N. Human immunodeficiency virus (HIV)-induced cell fusion: quantification and its application for the simple and rapid screening of anti-HIV substances *in vitro*. *Virology* 1988;164:542–6.
377. Chu CK, Schinazi RF, Arnold BH, et al. Comparative activity of 2′,3′-saturated and unsaturated pyrimidine and purine nucleosides against human immunodeficiency virus type 1 in peripheral blood mononuclear cells. *Biochem Pharmacol* 1988;37:3543–8.
378. Baba M, Snoeck R, Pauwels R, De Clercq E. Sulfated polysaccharides are potent and selective inhibitors of various enveloped viruses, including herpes simplex virus, cytomegalovirus, vesicular stomatitis virus, and human immunodeficiency virus. *Antimicrob Agents Chemother* 1988;32:1742–5.
379. De Clercq E. Chemotherapeutic approaches to the treatment of the acquired immune deficiency syndrome (AIDS). *J Med Chem* 1986;29:1561–9.
380. Horwitz JP, Chua J, Noel M. Nucleosides. V. The monomesylates of 1-(2′-deoxy-β-D-lyxofuranosyl) thymine. *J Org Chem* 1964;29:2076–8.
381. Lin TS, Prusoff WH. Synthesis and biological activity of several amino analogues of thymidine. *J Med Chem* 1978;21:109–12.
382. Robins MJ, Robins RK. The synthesis of 2′,3′-dideoxyadenosine from 2′-deoxyadenosine. *J Am Chem Soc* 1964;86:3585–6.
383. Horwitz JP, Chua J, Noel M, Donatti JT. Nucleosides. XI. 2′,3′-Dideoxycytidine. *J Org Chem* 1967;32:817–8.
384. Sanger F, Nicklen S, Coulson AR. DNA sequencing with chain-terminating inhibitors. *Proc Natl Acad Sci USA* 1987;74:5463–7.
385. Mitsuya H, Weinhold KJ, Furman PA, StClair MH, et al. 3′-Azido-3′-deoxythymidine (BW A509U): an antiviral agent that inhibits the infectivity and cytopathic effect of human T-lymphotropic virus type III/lynphadenopathy-associated virus *in vitro*. *Proc Natl Acad Sci USA* 1985;82:7096–100.
386. Sommadossi JP, Carlisle R. Toxicity of 3′-azido-3′-deoxythymidine and 9-(1,3-dihydroxy -2-propoxymethyl)guanine for normal human hematopoietic progenitor cells *in vitro*. *Antimicrob Agents Chemother* 1987;31:452–4.
387. Perno C-F, Yarchoan R, Cooney DA, et al. Inhibition of human immunodeficiency virus (HIV-1/HTLV-IIIBa-L) replication in fresh and cultured human peripheral blood monocytes/ macrophages by azidothymidine and related 2′,3′-dideoxynucleosides. *J Exp Med* 1988; 168:1111–25.
388. Zimmerman TP, Mahony WB, Prus KL. 3′-azido-3′-deoxythymidine. *J Biol Chem* 1987; 262:5748–54.
389. Furman PH, Fyfe JA, StClair MH, et al. Phosphorylation of 3′-azido-3′-deoxythymidine and selective interaction of the 5′-triphosphate with human immunodeficiency virus reverse transcriptase. *Proc Natl Acad Sci USA* 1986;83:8333–7.

390. Balzarini J, Pauwels R, Baba M, et al. The *in vitro* and *in vivo* anti-retrovirus activity, and intracellular metabolism of 3′-azido-2′,3′-dideoxythymidine and 2′,3′-dideoxycytidine are highly dependent on the cell species. *Biochem Pharmacol* 1988:37:897–903.
391. Baba M, Pauwels R, Balzarini J, Herdewijn P, De Clercq E, Desmyter J. Ribavirin antagonizes inhibitory effects of pyrimidine 2′,3′-Dideoxynucleosides but enhances inhibitory effects of purine 2′,3′-dideoxynucleosides on replication of human immunodeficiency virus *in vitro*. *Antimicrob Agents Chemother* 1987; 31:1613–7.
392. Vogt MW, Hartshorn KL, Furman PA, et al. Ribavirin antagonizes the effect of azidothymidine on HIV replication. *Science* 1987;235:1376–9.
393. Dahlberg JE, Mitsuya H, Blam SB, Broder S, Aaronson SA. Broad spectrum antiretroviral activity of 2′,3′-dideoxynucleosides. *Proc Natl Acad Sci USA* 1987;84:2469–73.
394. Ruprecht RM, O'Brien LG, Rossoni LD, Nusinoff-Lehrman S. Suppression of mouse viremia and retroviral disease by 3′-azido-3′deoxythymidine. *Nature* 1986;323:467–9.
395. StClair MH, Richards CA, Spector T, et al. 3′-azido-3′-Deoxythymidine triphosphate as an inhibitor and substrate of purified human immunodeficiency virus reverse transcriptase. *Antimicrob Agents Chemother* 1987;31:1972–7.
396. Elwell LP, Ferone R, Freeman GA, et al. Antibacterial activity and mechanism of action of 3′-azido-3′-deoxythymidine (BW A509U). *Antimicrob Agents Chemother* 1987;31:274–80.
397. Mitsuya H, Jarrett RF, Matsukura M, et al. Long-term inhibition of human T-lymphotropic virus type III/lymphadenopathy-associated virus (human immunodeficiency virus) DNA synthesis and RNA expression in T cells protected by 2′,3′-dideoxynucleosides *in vitro*. *Proc Natl Acad Sci USA* 1987;84:2033–7.
398. Sommadossi JP, Carlisle R, Schinazi RF, Zhou Z. Uridine reverses the toxicity of 3′-azido-3′-deoxythymidine in normal human granulocyte-macrophage progenitor cells *in vitro* without impairment of antiretroviral activity. *Antimicrob Agents Chemother* 1988;32:997–1001.
399. Nakashima H, Matsui T, Harada S, et al. Inhibition of replication and cytopathic effect of human T cell lymphotropic virus type III/lymphadenopathy-associated virus by 3′-azido-3′-deoxythymidine in vitro. *Antimicrob Agents Chemother* 1986;30:933–7.
400. Lyerly HK, Cohen OJ, Weinhold KJ. Transmission of HIV by antigen presenting cells during T-cell activation: prevention by 3′-azido-3′-deoxythymidine. *AIDS Res Hum Retroviruses* 1987;3:87–94.
401. Larder BA, Darby G, Richman DD. HIV with reduced sensitivity to zidovudine isolated during prolonged therapy. *Science* 1989;243: 1731–4.
402. Matsushita S, Mitsuya H, Reitz MS, Broder S. Pharmacological inhibition of *in vitro* infectivity of human T lymphotropic virus type 1. *J Clin Invest* 1987;80:394–400.
403. Olsen JC, Furman P, Fyfe JA, Swanstrom R. 3′-azido-3′-deoxythymidine inhibits the replication of avian leukosis virus. *J Virol* 1987; 61:2800–6.
404. Ostertag W, Roesler G, Krieg CJ, et al. Induction of endogenous virus and of thymidine kinase by bromodeoxyuridine in cell cultures transformed by Friend virus. *Proc Natl Acad Sci USA* 1974;71:4980–5.
405. Lin JC, Zhang ZX, Smith MC, Biron K, Pagano JS. Anti-human immunodeficiency virus agent 3′-azido-3′-deoxythymidine inhibits replication of Epstein-Barr virus. *Antimicrob Agents Chemother* 1988;32:265–7.
406. Smith MS, Brian EL, Pagano JS. Resumption of virus production after human immunodeficiency virus infection of T lymphocytes in the presence of azidothymidine. *J Virol* 1987;61:3769–73.
407. Nakashima H, Tochikura T, Kobayashi N, Matsude A, Ueda T, Yamamoto N. Effect of 3′-azido-2′,3′-dideoxythymidine (AZT) and neutralizing antibody on human immunodeficiency virus (HIV)-induced cytopathic effects: implication of giant cell formation for the spread of virus *in vivo*. *Virology* 1987;159:169–73.
408. Ayers KM. Preclinical toxicology of zidovudine. *Am J Med* 1988;85:186–8.
409. Sharpe AH, Jaenisch R, Ruprecht RM. Retroviruses and mouse embryos: a rapid model for neurovirulence and transplacental antiviral therapy. *Science* 1987;236:1671–4.
410. Mitsuya H, Broder S. Inhibition of the in vitro infectivity and cytopathic effect of human T-lymphotrophic virus type III/lymphadenopathy-associated virus (HTLV-III/LAV) by 2′,3′-dideoxynucleosides. *Proc Natl Acad Sci USA* 1986;83:1911–5.
411. Starnes MC, Cheng YC. Cellular metabolism of 2′,3′-dideoxycytidine, a compound active against human immunodeficiency virus in vitro. *J Biol Chem* 1987;262:988–91.
412. Cooney DA, Dalal M, Mitsuya H, et al. Initial studies on the cellular pharmacology of 2′,3′-dideoxycytidine, an inhibitor of HTLV-III infectivity. *Biochem Pharmacol* 1986;35:2065–8.
413. Mitsuya H, Broder S. Strategies for antiviral therapy in AIDS. *Nature* 1987;325(6107):773–8.
414. Eriksson B, Vrang L, Bazin H, Chattopadhyaya J, Oberg B. Different patterns of inhibition of avian myeloblastosis virus reverse transcriptase activity by 3′-azido-3′-deoxythymidine 5′-triphosphate and its threo isomer. *Antimicrob Agents Chemother* 1987;31:600–4.
415. Balzarini J, Cooney DA, Dalal M, et al. 2′,3′-Dideoxycytidine: regulation of its metabolism and anti-retroviral potency by natural pyrimidine nucleosides and by inhibitors of pyrimidine nucleotide synthesis. *Mol Pharmacol* 1987;32:798–806.
416. Ullman B, Coons T, Rockwell S, McCartan K. Genetic analysis of 2′,3′-dideoxycytidine in-

corporation into cultured human T lymphoblasts. *J Biol Chem* 1988;263:12391–6.
417. Hao Z, Cooney DA, Hartman NR, et al. Factors determining the activity of 2′,3′-dideoxynucleosides in suppressing human immunodeficiency virus *in vitro*. *Mol Pharmacol* 1988;34:431–5.
418. Hirsch MS, Kaplan JC. Prospects of therapy for infections with human T-lymphotropic virus type III. *Ann Intern Med* 1985;103:750–5.
419. Chen MS, Oshana SC. Inhibition of HIV reverse transcriptase by 2′,3′-dideoxynucleoside triphosphates. *Biochem Pharmacol* 1987;36: 4361–2.
420. Wagar MA, Evans MJ, Manly KF, Hughes RG, Huberman JA. Effects of 2′,3′-dideoxynucleosides on mammalian cells and viruses. *J Cell Physiol* 1984;121:402–8.
421. Montefiori DC, Mitchell WM. Infection of the HTLV-II-bearing T-cell line C3 with HTLV-III/LAV is highly permissive and lytic. *Virology* 1986;155:726–31.
422. Cooney DA, Ahluwalia G, Mitsuya H, et al. Initial studies on the cellular pharmacology of 2′,3′-dideoxyadenosine, an inhibitor of HTLV-III infectivity. *Biochem Pharmacol* 1987;36: 1765–8.
423. Carson DA, Haertle T, Wasson DB, Richman DD. Biochemical genetic analysis of 2′,3′-dideoxyadenosine metabolism in human T lymphocytes. *Biochem Biophys Res Commun* 1988;151:788–93.
424. Ahluwalia G, Cooney DA, Mitsuya H, et al. Initial studies on the cellular pharmacology of 2′,3′-dideoxyinosine, an inhibitor of HIV infectivity. *Biochem Pharmacol* 1987;36:3797–800.
425. Lin TS, Schinazi RF, Chem MS, Kinney-Thomas E, Prusoff WH. Antiviral activity of 2′,3′-dideoxycytidin-2′-ene (2′,3′-dideoxy-2′,3′-didehydrocytidine) against human immunodeficiency virus *in vitro*. *Biochem Pharmacol* 1987;36:311–6.
426. Matthes E, Lehmann Ch, Scholz D, et al. Inhibition of HIV-associated reverse transcriptase by sugar-modified derivatives of thymidine 5′-triphosphate in comparison to cellular DNA polymerases alpha and beta. *Biochem Biophys Res Commun* 1987;1:78–85.
427. Balzarini J, Pauwels R, Herdewijn P, et al. Potent and selective anti-HTLV-III/LAV activity of 2′,3′-dideoxycytidinene, the 2′,3′-unsaturated derivative of 2′,3′-dideoxycytidine. *Biochem Biophys Res Commun* 1986;140:735–42.
428. Lin TS, Schinazi RF, Prusoff WH. Potent and selective *in vitro* activity of 3′-deoxythymidin-2′-ene (3′-deoxy-2′,3′-didehydrothymidine) against human immunodeficiency virus. *Biochem Pharmacol* 1987;36:2713–8.
429. Hamamoto Y, Nakashima H, Matsui T, Matsuda A, Ueda T, Yamamoto N. Inhibitory effect of 2′,3′-didehydro-2′,3′-dideoxynucleosides on infectivity, cytopathic effects, and replication of human immunodeficiency virus. *Antimicrob Agents Chemother* 1987;31:907–10.
430. Baba M, Pauwels R, Balzarini J, Herdewijn P, De Clercq E. Selective inhibition of human immunodeficiency virus (HIV) by 3′-azido-2′,3′-dideoxyguanosine *in vitro*. *Biochem Biophys Res Commun* 1987;145:1080–6.
431. Mitsuya H, Matsukura M, Broder S. Rapid *in vitro* systems for assessing activity of agents against HTLV-III/LAV. In: Broder S, ed. *AIDS: modern concepts and therapeutic challenges*. New York: Marcel Dekker, Inc. 1987:303–33.
432. Baba M, Pauwels R, Herdewijn P, De Clercq E, Desmyter J, Vandeputte M. Both 2′,3′-dideoxythymidine and its 2′,3′-unsaturated derivative (2′,3′-dideoxythymidinene) are potent and selective inhibitors of human immunodeficiency virus replication in vitro. *Biochem Biophys Res Commun* 1987;142:128–34.
433. Balzarini J, Pauwels R, Baba M, et al. The 2′,3′-dideoxyriboside of 2,6-diaminopurine selectively inhibits human immunodeficiency virus (HIV) replication *in vitro*. *Biochem Biophys Res Commun* 1987;145:269–76.
434. Lin TS, Chen MS, McLaren C, Gao YS, Ghazzouli I, Prusoff WH. Synthesis and antiviral activity of various 3′-azido, 3′-amino, 2′,3′-unsaturated and 2′,3′-dideoxy analogues of pyrimidine deoxyribonucleosides against retroviruses. *J Med Chem* 1987;30:440–4.
435. Lin TS, Guo JY, Schinazi RF, Chu CK, Xiang JN, Prusoff WH. Synthesis and antiviral activity of various 3′-azido analogues of pyrimidine deoxyribonucleosides against human immunodeficiency virus (HIV-1, HTLV-III/LAV). *J Med Chem* 1988;31:336–40.
436. Balzarini J, Baba M, Pauwels R, Herdewijm P, De Clercq E. Anti-retrovirus activity of 3′-fluor-and 3′azido-substituted pyrimidine 2′,3′-dideoxynucleoside analogues. *Biochem Pharmacol* 1988;37:2847–56.
437. Balzarini J, Baba M, Pauwels R, et al. Potent and selective activity of 3′-azido-2,6 diaminopurine -2′,3′-dideoxyriboside, 3′-fluoro-2,6-diaminopurine-2′,3′-dideoxyriboside, and 3′-fluoro-2′,3′-dideoxyguanosine against human immunodeficiency virus *Mol Pharmacol* 1988; 33:243–9.
438. Herdewijn P, Pauwels R, Baba M, Balzarini J, De Clercq E. Synthesis and anti-HIV activity of various 2′-and 3′-substituted 2′,3′-dideoxyadenosines: a structure-activity analysis *J Med Chem* 1987;30:2131–7.
439. Herdewijn P, Balzarini J, Baba M, et al. Synthesis and anti-HIV acitivity of different sugar-modified pyrimidine and purine nucleosides. *J Med Chem* 1988;31:2040–8.
440. Matthew E, Lehmann C, Scholz D, Rosenthal HA, Langen P. Phosphorylation, anti-HIV activity and cytotoxicity of 3′-fluorothymidine. *Biochem Biophys Res Commun* 1988;153: 825–31.
441. Balzarini J, Robins MJ, Zou RM, Herdewijn P, De Clercq E. The 2′,3′-dideoxyriboside of 2,6-diaminopurine and its 2′,3′-didehydro derivative inhibit the deamination of 2′,3′-dideox-

yadenosine, an inhibitor of human immunodeficiency virus (HIV) replication. *Biochem Biophys Res Commun* 1987;145:277–83.

442. Pauwels R, Balzarini J, Schols D, et al. Phosphonylmethoxyethyl purine derivatives, a new class of anti-human immunodeficiency virus agents. *Antimicrob Agents Chemother* 1988; 32:1025–30.
443. Hayashi S, Phadtare S, Zemlicka J, Matsukura M, Mitsuya H, Broder S. Adenallene and cytallene: Acyclic nucleoside analogues that inhibit replication and cytopathic effect of human immunodeficiency virus in vitro. *Proc Natl Acad Sci USA* 1988;85:6127–31.
444. Balzarini J, Naesens L, Herdewijn P, et al. Marked in vivo antiretrovirus activity of 9-(2-phosphonylmethoxy-ethyl) adenine, a selective anti-human immunodeficiency virus agents. *Proc Natl Acad Sci USA* 1989;86:332–6.
445. Marquez VE, Tseng CK-H, Kelley JA, et al. 2′,3′-Dideoxy-2′-fluoro-ARA-A. An acid-stable purine nucleoside active against human immunodeficiency virus (HIV). *Biochem Pharmacol* 1987;36:2719–22.
446. Oberg B. Antiviral effects of phosphonoformate (PFA, Foscarnet Sodium). *Pharmacol Ther* 1983;19:387–415.
447. Sundquist B, Oberg B. Phosphonoformate inhibits reverse transcriptase. *J Gen Virol* 1979; 45:273–81.
448. Sundquist B, Larner E. Phosphonoformate inhibition of visna virus replication. *J Virol* 1979;30:847–51.
449. Sandstrom EG, Kaplan JC, Byington RE, Hirsch MS. Inhibition of human T-cell lymphotropic virus type III *in vitro* by phosphonoformate. *Lancet* 1985;i:1480–2.
450. Sarin PS, Taguchi Y, Sun D, Thornton A, Gallo RC, Oberg B. Inhibition of HTLV-III/LAV replication by foscarnet. *Biochem Biophys Res Commun* 1985;34:4075–9.
451. Vrang L, Oberg B. PPi analogs as inhibitors of human T-lymphotropic virus type III reverse transcriptase. *Antimicrob Agents Chemother* 1986;29:867–72.
452. Wondrak EM, Lower J, Kurth R. Inhibition of HIV-1 RNA-dependent DNA polymerase and cellular DNA polymerases alpha, beta and lambda by phosphonoformic acid and other drugs. *J Antimicrob Chemother* 1988;21:151–61.
453. Chermann JC, Sinoussi FC, Jasmin C. Inhibition of RNA-dependent DNA polymerase of murine oncornaviruses by ammonium-5-tungsto-2-antimoniate. *Biochem Biophys Res Commun* 1975;65:1229–36.
454. Lidereau R, Bouchet C, Barre-Sinoussi F, Saracino R, Chermann JC. Inhibition of spontaneously occurring mammary tumors in the mouse by tungstoantimoniate. *Curr Chemother* 1977;2:1323–5.
455. Dormont D, Spire B, Barre-Sinoussi F, Montagnier L, Chermann JC. Inhibition of RNA-dependent DNA polymerases of AIDS and SAIDS retroviruses by HPA-23 (ammonium-21-tungsto-9-antimoniate). *Ann Inst Pasteur/Virol* 1985;136:75–83.
456. Rozenbaum W, Dormont D, Spire B, et al. Antimoniotungstate (HPA 23) treatment of three patients with AIDS and one with prodrome [Letter]. *Lancet* 1985;i:450–1.
457. Gurgo C, Ray R, Green M. Rifamycin derivatives strongly inhibiting RNA-DNA polymerase (reverse transcriptase) of murine sarcoma viruses. *JNCI* 1972;49:61–79.
458. Wu AM, Gallo RC. Interaction between murine type-C virus RNA-directed DNA polymerase and rifamycin derivatives. *Biochim Biophys Acta* 1974;240:419–36.
459. Anand R, Moore J, Feorino P, Curran J, Srinivasan A. Rifabutine inhibits HTLV-III. *Lancet* 1986;i:97–8.
460. Birch C, Tachedjian G, Lucas CR, Gust I. *In vitro* effectiveness of a combination of zidovudine and ansamycin against human immunodeficiency virus. *J Infect Dis* 1988;158:895.
461. Zamecnik PC, Stephenson ML. Inhibition of Rous sarcoma virus replication and cell transformation by a specific oligodeoxynucleotide. *Proc Natl Acad Sci USA* 1978;75:280–4.
462. Agris CH, Blake KR, Miller PS, Reddy MP, Ts'o PO. Inhibition of vesicular stomatitis virus protein synthesis and infection by sequence-specific oligodeoxyribonucleoside methylphosphonates. *Biochemistry* 1986;25:6268–75.
463. Zamecnik PC, Goodchild J, Taguchi Y, Sarin PS. Inhibition of replication and expression of human T-cell lymphotropic virus type III in cultured cells by exogenous synthetic oligonucleotides complementary to viral RNA. *Proc Natl Acad Sci USA* 1986;83:4143–6.
464. Miller PS, Ts'o POP. A new approach to chemotherapy based on molecular biology and nucleic acid chemistry: Matagen (masking tape for gene expression). *Anti-Cancer Design* 1987;2:117–28.
465. Lemaitre M, Bayard B, Lebleu B. Specific antiviral activity of a poly(L-lysine)-conjugated oligodeoxyribonucleotide sequence complementary to vesicular stomatitis virus N protein mRNA initiation site. *Proc Natl Acad Sci USA* 1987;84:648–52.
466. Matsukura M, Shinozuka K, Zon G, et al. Phosphorothioate analogs of oligodeoxynucleotides: inhibitors of replication and cytopathic effects of human immunodeficiency virus. *Proc Natl Acad Sci USA* 1987;84:7706–10.
467. Goodchild J, Agrawal S, Civeira MP, Sarin PS, Sun D, Zamecnik PC. Inhibition of human immunodeficiency virus replication by antisense oligodeoxynucleotides. *Proc Natl Acad Sci USA* 1988;85:5507–11.
468. Zaia JA, Rossi JJ, Murakawa GJ, et al. Inhibition of human immunodeficiency virus by using an oligonucleoside methylphosphonate targeted to the *tat*-3 gene. *J Virol* 1988;62:3914–7.
469. Agrawal S, Goodchild J, Civeira MP, Thornton AH, Sarin PS, Zamecnik PC. Oligodeoxynucleoside phosphoramidates and phosphorothioates as inhibitors of human immunodefi-

ciency virus. *Proc Natl Acad Sci USA* 1988; 85:7079–83.
470. Sarin PS, Agrawal S, Civeira MP, Goodchild J, Ikeuchi T, Zamecnik PC. Inhibition of acquired immunodeficiency syndrome virus by oligodeoxynucleoside methylphosphonates. *Proc Natl Acad Sci USA* 1988;85:7448–51.
471. Liu DK, Owens GF. Inhibition of viral reverse transcriptase by 2′,5′-oligoadenylates. *Biochem Biophys Res Commun* 1987;145: 291–7.
472. Tanaka N, Okabe T, Take Y, et al. Inhibition by sakyomicin A of avian myeloblastosis virus reverse transcriptase and proliferation of AIDS-associated virus (HTLV-III/LAV). *Jpn J Cancer Res* 1986;77:324–6.
473. Jentsch KD, Hunsmann G, Hartmann H, Nickel P. Inhibition of human immunodeficiency virus type 1 reverse transcriptase by suramin-related compounds. *J Gen Virol* 1987; 68:2183–92.
474. De Clercq E. Suramin: a potent inhibitor of the reverse transcriptase of RNA tumor viruses. *Cancer Letter* 1979;8:9–22.
475. Smith RA and Kirkpatrick W. *Ribavirin: a broad spectrum antiviral agent*. New York: Academic Press, 1980.
476. Goswami DB, Borek E, Sharma OK, Fujitaki J, Smith RA. The broad spectrum antiviral agent ribavirin inhibits capping of RNA. *Biochem Biophys Res Commun* 1979;89:830–6.
477. McCormick JB, Getchell JP, Mitchell SW, Hicks DR. Ribavirin suppresses replication of lymphadenopathy-associated virus in cultures of human adult T lymphocytes. *Lancet* 1984; ii:1367–9.
478. McCormick JB, King IJ, Webb PA, et al. Lassa fever: effective therapy with ribavirin. *N Engl J Med* 1986;314:20–6.
479. Streeter DF, Witkowski JT, Khare GP, et al. Mechanism of action of 1-beta-delta-ribofuranosyl-1,2,4-triazole-3-carboxamide(Virazole), a new broad-spectrum antiviral agent. *Proc Natl Acad Sci USA* 1973;20:1174–8.
480. Fyfe JA, Furman P, Vogt M, Sherman P. Mechanism of ribavirin antagonism of anti-HIV activity of azidothymidine. A. *IVth International Conference on AIDS, Stockholm, Sweden*, 1988.
481. Stein CA, Cohen JS. Oligodeoxynucleotides as inhibitors of gene expression: a review. *Cancer Res* 1988;48:2659–68.
482. Haseloff J, Gerlach WL. Simple RNA enzymes with new and highly specific endoribonuclease activities. *Nature* 1988;334:585–91.
483. Kotler M, Katz RA, Danho W, Leis J, Skalka AM. Synthetic peptides as substrates and inhibitors of a retroviral protease. *Proc Natl Acad Sci USA* 1988;85:4185–9.
484. Blough HA, Ray EK. Glucose analogues in the chemotherapy of herpesvirus infections. *Pharmacol Ther* 1988;10:669–81.
485. Blough HA, Pauwels R, De Clercq E, Cogniaux J, Sprecher-Goldberger S, Thiry L. Glycosylation inhibitors block the expression of LAV/HTLV-III (HIV) glycoproteins. *Biochem Biophys Res Commun* 1986;141:33–8.
486. Walker BD, Kowalski M, Goh WC, et al. Inhibition of human immunodeficiency virus syncytium formation and virus replication by castanospermine. *Proc Natl Acad Sci USA* 1987;84:8120–4.
487. Gruters RA, Neefjes JJ, Tersmette M, et al. Interference with HIV-induced syncytium formation and viral infectivity by inhibitors of trimming glucosidase. *Nature* 1987;350:74–7.
488. Lyte M, Shinitzky M. A special lipid mixture for membrane fluidization. *Biochim Biophys Acta* 1958;812:133–8.
489. Sarin PS, Gallo RC, Scheer DI, Crews F, Lippa AS. Effects of a novel compound (AL 721) on HTLV-III infectivity in vitro. *N Engl J Med* 1985;313:1289–90.
490. Schaffner CP, Plescia OJ, Pontani D, et al. Anti-viral activity of amphotericin B methyl ester:inhibition of HTLV-III replication in cell culture. *Biochem Pharmacol* 1986;35:4110–3.
491. Meruelo D, Lavie F, Lavie D. Therapeutic agents with dramatic antiretroviral activity and little toxicity at effective doses: aromatic polycyclic diones hypericin and pseudohypericin. *Proc Natl Acad Sci USA* 1988;85:5230–4.
492. Hawking F. Suramin: with special reference to onchocerciasis. In: S Garatini, F Hawking, Goldin, A, Kopin IJ, eds. *Advances in Pharmacology and Chemotherapy*. 15th ed. New York: Academic Press, 1978:289–322.
493. Mitsuya H, Popovic M, Yarchoan R, Matsushita S, Gallo RC, Broder S. Suramin protection of T cells *in vitro* against infectivity and cytopathic effect of HTLV-III. *Science* 1984;226:172–4.
494. De Clercq E. Suramin in the treatment of AIDS: mechanism of action. *Antiviral Res* 1987;7:1–10. [Published erratum appears in *Antiviral Res* 1987;7(3):185.]
495. Ruprecht RM, Rossoni LD, Haseltine WA, Broder S. Suppression of retroviral propagation and disease by suramin in murine systems. *Proc Natl Acad Sci USA* 1985;82:7733–7.
496. Sarin PS, Sun D, Thorton A, Muller WEG. Inhibition of replication of the etiologic agent of acquired immunodeficiency syndrome (human T-lymphotropic retrovirus/lymphadenopathy-associated virus) by avarol and avarone. *JNCI* 1987;78:663–6.
497. Chandra P, Sarin PS. Selective inhibition of replication of the AIDS-associated virus HTLV-III/LAV by synthetic D-penicillamine. *Arzneimittelforschung* 1988;36:184–6.
498. Ito M, Nakashima H, Baba M, et al. Inhibitory effect of glycyrrhizin on the in vitro infectivity and cytopathic activity of the human immunodeficiency virus [HIV(HTLV-III/LAV)]. *Antiviral Res* 1987; 7:127–37.
499. Chang RS, Yeung HW. Inhibition of growth of human immunodeficiency virus *in vitro* by crude extracts of Chinese medicinal herbs. *Antiviral Res* 1988;9:163–76.
500. Faber V, Dalgleish AG, Newell A, Malkovsky

M. Inhibition of HIV replication *in vitro* by fusidic acid. *Lancet* 1987;i:827–8.
501. Barnes DM. "On the shelf" AIDS drug in clinical trial. *Science* 1987;238:276–6.
502. Richman DD, Mitsuya H, Broder S, Hostetler KY. Fusidic acid, HIV, and host cell toxicity. *Lancet* 1988;i:1051–2.
503. Lloyd G, Atkinson T, Sutton PM. Effect of bile salts and of fusidic acid on HIV-1 infection of cultured cells. *Lancet* 1988;i:1418–21.
504. Collins JM, Klecker Jr KW, Yarchoan R, et al. Clinical pharmacokinetics of suramin in patients with HTLV-III/LAV infection. *J Clin Pharmacol* 1986;26:22–6.
505. Broder S, Yarchoan R, Collins JM, et al. Effects of suramin on HTLV-III/LAV infection presenting as Kaposi's sarcoma or AIDS-related complex: clinical pharmacology and suppression of virus replication *in vivo*. *Lancet* 1985;ii:627–30.
506. Levine AM, Gill PS, Cohen J, et al. Suramin antiviral therapy in the acquired immunodeficiency syndrome: clinical, immunological and virologic results. *Ann Intern Med* 1988;105: 32–7.
507. Cheson BD, Levine A, Mildvan D, et al. Suramin therapy in AIDS and related diseases. Initital report of the US suramin working group. *JAMA* 1987;258:1347–51.
508. Schattenkerk JKME, Danner SA, Paul DA, et al. Persistence of human immunodeficiency virus antigenemia in patients with the acquired immunodeficiency syndrome treated with a reverse transcriptase inhibitor, suramin. *Arch Intern Med* 1988;148:209–11.
509. Yarchoan R, Lyerly HK, Weinhold KJ, et al. Administration of 3′-azido-3′deoxythymidine, an inhibitor of HTLV-III/LAV replication, to patients with AIDS or AIDS-related complex. *Lancet* 1986;i:575–80.
510. Klecker Jr KW, Collins JM, Yarchoan R, et al. Plasma and cerebrospinal fluid pharmacokinetics of 3′-azido-3′-deoxythymidine: a novel pyrimidine analog with potential application for the treatment of patients with AIDS and related diseases. *Clin Pharmacol Ther* 1987;41:407–12.
511. Blum MR, Liao SHT, Good SS, de Miranda P. Pharmacokinetics and bioavailability of zidovudine in humans. *Am J Med* 1988;85:189–94.
512. Pioger JC, Taburet AM, Fillastre JP, Singlas E. Pharmacokinetics of zidovudine (AZT) and its glucuronide in healthy volunteers and in uremic patients. A. *28th ICAAC, Los Angeles, California, June*, 1988.
513. Henry K, Chinnock BJ, Quinn RP, et al. Concurrent zidovudine levels in semen and serum determined by radioimmunoassay in patients with AIDS or AIDS-related complex. *JAMA* 1988;259:3023–6.
514. Fischl MA, Richman DD, Grieco MH, et al. The efficacy of azidothymidine (AZT) in the treatment of patients with AIDS and AIDS-related complex. A double-blind, placebo-controlled trial. *N Engl J Med* 1987;317:185–91.
515. Richman DD, Fischl MA, Grieco MH, et al. The toxicity of azidothymidine (AZT) in the treatment of patients with AIDS and AIDS-related complex. A double-blind, placebo-controlled trial. *N Engl J Med* 1987;317:192–7.
516. Pizzo PA, Eddy J, Falloon J, et al. Effect of continuous intravenous infusion of ziodvudine (AZT) in children with symptomatic HIV infection. *N Engl J Med* 1988;319:889–96.
517. Jackson GG, Paul DA, Falk LA, et al. Human immunodeficiency virus (HIV) antigenemia (p24) in the acquired immunodeficiency syndrome (AIDS) and the effect of treatment with zidovudine (AZT). *Ann Intern Med* 1988; 108:175–80.
518. Spector SA, Kennedy C, McCutchan JA, et al. Antiviral effect of zidovudine and ribavirin in clinical trials. *J Infect Dis* 1989;159:822–9.
519. De Wolf F, Goudsmit J, De Gans J, et al. Effect of zidovudine on serum human immunodeficiency virus antigen levels in symptom-free subjects. *Lancet* 1988;i:373–6.
520. Kennedy CJ, Teschke RS, Hesselink J, et al. Clinical evaluation of the central nervous system in HIV infected patients on azidothymidine (AZT) [Abstract]. *III International Conference on AIDS, Washington, D.C., June*, 1987.
521. De Gans J, Lange JMA, Derix MMA, et al. Decline of HIV antigen levels in cerebrospinal fluid during treatment with low-dose zidovudine. *AIDS Res Hum Retroviruses* 1988;2:37–40.
522. Fiala M, Cone LA, Cohen N, et al. Responses of neurologic complications of AIDS to 3′-azido-3′deoxythymidine and 9-(1,3-dihydroxy-2-propoxymethyl) guanine. I. Clinical features. *J Infect Dis* 1988;2:250–256.
523. Yarchoan R, Berg G, Brouwers P, et al. Response of human-immunodeficiency-virus-associated neurological disease to 3′-azido-3′-deoxythymidine. *Lancet* 1987;i:132–5.
524. Schmitt FA, Bigley JW, McKinnis R, et al. Neuropsychological outcome of zidovudine (AZT) treatment of patients with AIDS and AIDS-related complex. *N Engl J Med* 1988; 319:1573–8.
525. Hymes KB, Greene JB, Karpatkin S. The effect of azidothymidine on HIV-related thrombocytopenia. *N Engl J Med* 1988;318:516–7.
526. Gottlieb MS, Wolfe PR, Chafey S. Case report: response to AIDS-related thrombocytopenia to intravenous and oral azidothymidine (3′-azido-3′-deoxythymidine). *AIDS Res Hum Retroviruses* 1987;3:109–14.
527. Swiss Group for Clinical Studies on AIDS. Zidovudine for the treatment of HIV-associated thrombocytopenia: a placebo-controlled prospective study. *Ann Intern Med* 1988;109:718–21.
528. Walker RE, Parker RI, Kovacs JA, et al. Anemia and erythropoiesis in patients with the acquired immunodeficiency syndrome (AIDS) and Kaposi Sarcoma tested with zidovudine. *Ann Intern Med* 1988;108:372–6.
529. de Miranda P, Good SS, Blum MR, et al. The effect of probenecid on the pharmacokinet-

ic disposition of azidothymidine (AZT) [Abstract]. *II International Conference on AIDS, Paris, France* 1986;

530. Hochster H, Dieterich D, Laverty M, et al. Toxicity of coadministered AZT and ganciclovir (DHPG) for CMV infection (AIDS Treatment Evaluation Units 004) [Abstract] *IVth International Conference on AIDS, Stockholm, Sweden, June,* 1988.
531. Hochster H, Liebes L, Conner J, Reichman R, Richman DD. Pharmacokinetics of combined AZT and DHPG (Ganciclover). Results of a multicenter phase I study (ACTG/004). [Abstract] *28th Interscience Conference on Artimicrobial Agents and Chemotherapy, Los Angeles, October,* 1988.
532. Hagler DN, Frame PT. Azidothymidine neurotoxicity. *Lancet* 1986;ii:1392–3.
533. Harris PJ, Caceres C. Azidothymidine in the treatment of AIDS. *N Engl J Med* 1988; 318:250.
534. Bessen LJ, Greene JB, Louie E, Seitzman P, Weinberg H. Severe polymyositis-like syndrome associated with zidovudine therapy of AIDS and ARC. *N Engl J Med* 1988;318:708.
535. Dalakas MC, Pezeshkpour GH, Flaherty M. Progressive nemaline (ROD) myopathy associated with HIV infection. *N Engl J Med* 1987;317:1602–3.
536. Richman DD, Andrews J, AZT Collaborative Working Group. Results of continued monitoring of participants in the placebo-controlled trial of zidovudine for serious human immunodeficiency virus infection. *Am J Med* 1988; 85:208–13.
537. Creagh-Kirk T, Doi E, Andrews S, Nusinoff-Lehrman S, Tilson H, Barry D. Survival experience among patients with acquired immunodeficiency syndrome receiving zidovudine therapy. *JAMA* 1988;260:3009–15.
538. Dournon E, Rozenbaum W, Michon C, et al. Effects of zidovudine in 365 consecutive patients with AIDS or AIDS-related complex. *Lancet* 1988;i:1297–302.
539. Spear JM, Benson CA, Pottage Jr JC, Paul DA, Landay AL, Kessler HA. Rapid rebound of serum human immunodeficiency virus antigen after discontinuing zidovudine therapy. *J Infect Dis* 1988;158:1132–3.
540. Surbone A, Yarchoan R, McAtee N, et al. Treatment of the acquired immunodeficiency syndrome (AIDS) and AIDS-related complex with a regimen of 3′-azido-2′,3′-dideoxythymidine (azidothymidine or zidovudine) and acyclovir. *Ann Intern Med* 1988;108:534–40.
541. Fiddian AP, European/Australian Collaborative Study Group. Zidovudine plus or minus acyclovir in patients with AIDS or ARC [Abstract]. *28th ICAAC, Los Angeles, California, June,* 1988.
542. Yarchoan R, Thomas RV, Allain JP, et al. Phase studies of 2′,3′-dideoxycytidine in severe human immunodeficiency virus infection as a single agent and alternating with zidovudine (AZT). *Lancet* 1988;i:76–81.
543. Merigan TC, Skowron G, Bozzette S, et al. Circulating p24 antigen levels and responses to dideoxycytidine in human immunodeficiency virus (HIV) infection. *Ann Intern Med* 1989;110:189–94.
544. Bergadahl S, Sonnerborg A, Larsson A, Strannegard O. Declining levels of HIV p24 antigen in serum during treatment with foscarnet. *Lancet* 1988;i:1052.
545. Gaub J, Pedersen C, Poulsen AG, et al. The effect of foscarnet (Phosphonoformate) on human immunodeficiency virus isolation, T-cell subsets and lymphocyte function in AIDS patients. *AIDS Res Hum Retroviruses* 1987;1:27–33.
546. Jacobson MA, Crowe S, Levy J, et al. Effect of foscarnet therapy on infection with human immunodeficiency virus in patients with AIDS. *J Infect Dis* 1988;158:862–5.
547. Buimovici-Klein E, Ong KR, Lange M, et al. Reverse transcriptase activity (RTA) in lymphocyte cultures of AIDS patients treated with HPA-23. *AIDS Res Hum Retroviruses* 1986;2:279–83.
548. Moskovitz BL, The HPA-23 Cooperative Study Group. Clinical trial of tolerance of HPA-23 in patients with acquired immune deficiency syndrome. *Antimicrob Agents Chemother* 1988;32:1300–03.
549. Torseth J, Bhatia G, Harkonen S, et al. Evaluation of the antiviral effect of rifabutin in AIDS-related complex. *J Infect Dis* 159:1115–8.
550. Laskin OC, Longstreth JA, Hart CC, et al. Ribavirin disposition in high risk patients for acquired immunodeficiency syndrome. *Clin Pharmacol Ther* 1987;41:546–55.
551. Crumpacker C, Heagy W, Bubley G, et al. Ribavirin treatment of the acquired immunodeficiency syndrome (AIDS) and the acquired immunodeficiency syndrome related complex (ARC) *Ann Intern Med* 1987;107:664–74.
552. Abrams DI, Kuno S, Wong R, et al. Oral dextran sulfate (UA001) in the treatment of the acquired immunodeficiency syndrome (AIDS) and AIDS-related complex. *Ann Intern Med* 1989;110:183–8.
553. Grieco MH, Lange M, Buimovici-Klein E, et al. Open study of AL-721 treatment if HIV-infected subjects with generalized lymphadenopathy syndrome: an eight week open trial and follow-up. *Antiviral Res* 1988;9:177–90.
554. Schulof RS, Scheib RG, Parenti DM, et al. Treatment of HTLV-III/LAV-infected patients with D-penicillamine. *Arzneimittelforschung* 1986;36:1531–4.
555. Parenti DM, Simon GL, Scheib RG, et al. Effect of lithium carbonate in HIV-infected patients with immune dysfunction. *Journal of Acquired Immune Deficiency Syndromes* 1988;1:119–24.
556. Groopman JE, Gottlieb MS, Goodman J, et al. Recombinant alpha-2 interferon therapy for Kaposi's sarcoma assoicated with the acquired

immunodeficiency syndrome. *Ann Intern Med* 1984;100:671–6.

557. Krown SD, Real FX, Cunningham-Rundles S, et al. Preliminary observations on the effect of recombinant leukocyte A interferon in homosexual men with Kaposi's Sarcoma. *N Engl J Med* 1983;308:1071–6.
558. Volberding P. Therapy of Kaposi's Sarcoma in AIDS. *Semin Oncol* 1984;11:60–7.
559. Rios A, Mansell PWA, Newell GR, Reuben JM, Hersh EM, Gutterman JU. Treatment of acquired immunodeficiency syndrome-related Kapoi's sarcoma with lymphoblastoid interferon. *J Clin Oncol* 1985;3:506–12.
560. De Wit R, Boucher CA, Veenhof KH, Schattenkerk JKME, Bakker PJ, Danner SA. Clinical and virological effects of high-dose recombinant interferon-alpha in disseminated AIDS-related Kaposi's Sarcoma. *Lancet* 1988;ii: 1214–7.
561. Lane HC, Feinberg J, Davey V, et al. Anti-retroviral effects of interferon-alpha in AIDS-associated Kaposi's sarcoma. *Lancet* 1988; ii:1218–22.
562. Tamura K, Makino S, Araki Y, Imamura T, Seita M. Recombinant interferon beta and gamma in the treatment of adult T-cell leukemia. *Cancer* 1987;59:1059–62.
563. Ho DD, Hartshorn KL, Rota TR, et al. Recombinant human interferon alpha-A suppresses HTLV-III replication *in vitro*. *Lancet* 1985; i:602–4.
564. Hartshorn KL, Neumeyer D, Vogt MW, Schooley RT, Hirsch MS. Activity of interferons alpha, beta, and gamma against human immunodeficiency virus replication *in vitro*. *AIDS Res Hum Retroviruses* 1987;3:125–33.
565. Nakashima H, Yoshida T, Harada S, Yammamoto N. Recombinant human interferon gamma suppresses HTLV-III replication *in vitro*. *Int J Cancer* 1986;38:433–6.
566. Yamamoto JK, Barre-Sinoussi F, Bolton V, Pedersen NC, Gardner MB. Human alpha- and beta-interferon but not gamma- suppress the *in vitro* replication of LAV, HTLV-III, and ARV-2.. *J Interferon Res* 1986;6:143–52.
567. Wong GHW, Krowka JF, Stites DP, Goeddel DV. In vitro anti-human immunodeficiency virus activities of tumor necrosis factor-alpha and interferon-lambda. *J Immunol* 1988; 140:120–4.
568. Hartshorn KL, Vogt MW, Chou TC, et al. Synergistic inhibition of human immunodeficiency virus *in vitro* by azidothymidine and recombinant alpha A interferon. Antimicrob Agents Chemother 1987;31:168–72.
569. Hartshorn KL, Sandstrom EF, Neumeyer D, et al. Synergistic inhibition of human T-cell lymphotropic virus type III replication *in vitro* by phosphonoformate and recombinant alpha-A interferon. *Antimicrob Agents Chemother* 1986; 30:189–91.
570. Interferon Alpha Study Group. A randomized placebo-controlled trial of recombinant human interferon alpha 2a in patients with AIDS. *Journal of Acquired Immune Deficiency Syndromes* 1988;1:111–8.
571. Brook MG, Gor D, Forster SM, Harris W, Jeffries DJ, Thomas HC. Short communication suppression of HIV p24 antigen and induction of HIV anti-p24 antibody by alpha interferon in patients with chronic hepatitis B. *AIDS Res Hum Retroviruses* 1988;2:391–3.
572. Mitchell WM, Montefiori DC, Robinson Jr WE, Strayer DR, Carter WA. Mismatched double-stranded RNA (ampligen) reduces concentration of zidovudine (azidothymidine) required for *in vitro* inhibition of human immunodeficiency virus. *Lancet* 1987;i:890–2.
573. Herberman RB, Pinsky CM. Polyribonucleotides for cancer therapy: summary and recommendations for further research. *J Biol Response Mod* 1985;4:680–4.
574. Montefiori DC, Mitchell WM. Antiviral activity of mismatched double-stranded RNA against human immunodeficiency virus in vitro. *Proc Natl Acad Sci* 1987;84:2985–9.
575. Montefiori DC, Robinson Jr WE, Mitchell WM. Mismatched dsRNA (ampligen) induces protection against genomic variants of the human immunodeficiency virus type 1 (HIV-1) in a multiplicity of target cells. *Antiviral Res* 1988;9:47–56.
576. Carter WA, O'Malley J. An integrated and comparative study of the antiviral effects and other biological properaties of the polyinosine polycytidylic acid duplex and its mismatched analogues. *Mol Pharmacol* 1976;12:440–53.
577. Carter WA, Strayer DR, Hubbell HR, Brodsky I. Preclinical studies with ampligen (Mismatched double-stranded RNA). *J Biol Response Mod* 1985;4:495–502.
578. Brodsky I, Strayer DR, Kruger LJ, Carter WA. Clinical studies with ampligen (mismatched double-stranded RNA). *J Biol Response Mod* 1985;4:669–75.
579. Carter WA, Strayer DR, Brodsky I, et al. Clinical, immunological, and virological effects of ampligen, a mismatched double-stranded RNA, in patients with AIDS or AIDS-related complex. *Lancet* 1987;i:1286–92.
580. Smith KA. Interleukin-2: inception, impact and implications. *Science* 1988;240:1169–76.
581. Ciobanu N, Kruger G, Welte K. Defective T cell response to PHA and mitogenic monoclonal antibodies in male homosexuals with acquired immunodeficiency syndrome and its in vitro corrections by interleukin 2. *J Clin Immunol* 1983;3:332–40.
582. Rook AH, Masur H, Lane HC, et al. Interleukin-2 enhances the depressed natural killer and cytomegalovirus-specific cytotoxic activities of lymphocytes from patients with the acquired immune deficiency syndrome. *J Clin Invest* 1983;72:398–403.
583. Lane HC, Siegel JP, Rook AH, et al. Use of interleukin-2 in patients with acquired immunodeficiency syndrome. *J Biol Resp Mod* 1984;3:512–6.
584. Mertelsmann R, Welta K, Sternberg C, et al.

Treatment of immunodeficiency with interleukin-2: initial exploration. *J Biol Resp Mod* 1984;3:483–90.

585. Ernst M, Kern P, Flad HD, Ulmer AJ. Effects of systemic in vivo interleukin-2 (IL-2) reconstitution in patients with acquired immune deficiency syndrome (AIDS) and AIDS-related complex (ARC) on phenotypes and functions of peripheral blood mononuclear cells (PBMC). *J Clin Immunol* 1986;6:170–81.
586. Volberding P, Moody DJ, Beardslee D, Bradley EC, Wofsy CB. Therapy of acquired immune deficiency syndrome with recombinant interleukin-2. *AIDS Res Hum Retroviruses* 1987; 3:115–24.
587. Groopmen JE, Mitsuyasu RT, DeLeo MJ, Oette DH, Golde DW. Effect of recombinant human granulocyte-macrophage colony-stimulating factor on myelopoiesis in the acquired immunodeficiency syndrome. *N Engl J Med* 1987;317:593–8.
588. Baldwin GC, Gasson JC, Quan SG, et al. Granulocyte-macrophage colony-stimulating factor enhances neutrophil function in acquired immunodeficiency syndrome patients. *Proc Natl Acad Sci USA* 1988;85:2763–6.
589. Andrieu JM, Even P, Venet A, et al. Effects of Cyclosporin on T-cell subsets in human immunodeficiency virus disease. *Clin Immunol Immunopathol* 1988;146:181–98.
590. Surapaneni N, Raghunathan R, Beall GN, Daniel K, Mundy TM. Levamisole, immunostimulation, and the acquired immunodeficiency syndrome [Letter]. *Ann Intern Med* 1985; 102:137.
591. Clumeck N, Cran S, Van de Perre P, Mascart-Lemone F, Duchateau J, Bolla K. Thymopentin treatment in AIDS and pre-AIDS patients. *Surv Immunol Res* 1985;4(suppl I):58–62.
592. Clumeck N, Van de Perre P, Mascart-Lemone F, Cran S, Bolla K, Duchateau J. Preliminary results on clinical and immunological effects of thymopentin in AIDS. *Int J Clin Pharmacol Res* 1984;IV:459–63.
593. Dwyer JM, Wood CC, McNamara J, Kinder B. Transplantation of thymic tissue into patients with AIDS. *Arch Intern Med* 1987;147:513–7.
594. Carey JT, Lederman MM, Toossi Z, et al. Augmentation of skin test reactivity and lymphocyte blastogenesis in patients with AIDS treated with transfer factor. *JAMA* 1987; 257:651–5.
595. Sredni B, Caspi RR, Klein A, et al. A new immunomodulating compound (AS-101) with potential therapeutic application. *Nature* 1987;330:173–6.
596. Palmisano L, Chisesi T, Galli M, et al. Thymostimulin treatment in AIDS-related complex. *Clin Immunol Immunopathol* 1988; 47:253–61.
597. Lang JM, Trepo C, Kirstetter M, et al. Randomised, double-blind, placebo-controlled trial of ditiocarb sodium (Imuthiol) in human immunodeficiency virus infection. *Lancet* 1988; ii:702–5.
598. Glasky AJ, Gordon JF. Isoprinosine (Isoprine Pranobex BAN, INPX) in the treatment of AIDS and other acquired immunodeficiencies of clinical importance. *Cancer Detect Prev Suppl* 1987;1:597–609.
599. Miyajima A, Miyatake S, Schreurs J, et al. Coordinate regulation of immune and inflammatory responses by T cell-derived lymphokines. *FASEB J* 1988;2:2462–73.
600. Belosevic M, Davis CE, Meltzer MS, Nacy Ca. Regulation of activated macrophage antimicrobial activities. *J Immunol* 1988;141:890–6.

*Antiviral Agents and Viral Diseases of Man, 3rd Edition,*
edited by G. J. Galasso, R. J. Whitley, and
T. C. Merigan, Raven Press, Ltd., New York 1990.

# 16

# Epstein-Barr Virus and Human Herpesvirus Type 6

Stephen E. Straus

*Laboratory of Clinical Investigation, National Institute of Allergy and Infectious Diseases, National Institutes of Health, Bethesda, Maryland 20892*



The Epstein-Barr virus (EBV) and human herpesvirus type 6 (HHV-6) are notably lymphotropic. All human herpesviruses infect and replicate within lymphocytes to some extent, but EBV and HHV-6 do so efficiently. Most importantly, the pathogenesis and host responses to infection with EBV (and, perhaps, with HHV-6, as well) are more dependent upon lymphocytic infection than is evident with the other human herpesviruses. Curiously, the adaptation of these viruses to lymphocytes may have exacted some biological toll, for neither EBV nor HHV-6 can be readily grown in the variety of epithelial or fibroblastic cells that so readily support the replication of the other human herpesviruses; herpes simplex viruses 1 and 2 (HSV-1, HSV-2), varicella-zoster virus (VZV), and cytomegalovirus (CMV). It is these features which EBV and HHV6 share that suggest their joint description in this chapter.

## EBV

### History

In 1958, Burkitt (1), a British surgeon working in East Africa, described a common lymphoma of young children. The remarkable geographical distribution of the tumor suggested an exogenous cause. An intense effort to discern a viral etiology led to the cultivation of explanted tumor cells and the subsequent recognition of a novel herpesvirus named after two of its discoverers, Epstein and Barr (2).

Working in Philadelphia, Henle and Henle (3) found that these tumor cells contain antigens which react in immunofluorescence (IF) assays with antibodies present in virtually all sera of African Burkitt's lymphoma patients, and commonly in the sera of healthy persons as well. The fortuitous observation in 1967 of a primary serologic response to these antigens in the course of a heterophile-positive illness led to a series of seroepidemiologic studies proving that EBV is the predominant cause of acute infectious mononucleosis (4–6).

By the early 1970s, means of recovering virus from the saliva by cord blood transformation and the detection of viral nucleic acids in both Burkitt's tumor and in nasopharyngeal carcinoma tissues had been reported (7,8). In subsequent years, EBV was increasingly recognized as a cause of B-cell lymphoproliferative diseases, first in young boys with an X-linked disorder, and later in transplant recipients and other immunodeficient individuals, including acquired immune deficiency syndromes (AIDS) patients (9–11).

By the mid 1980s, EBV was linked to a variety of other severe and chronic illnesses. Its association with certain disorders, such as a rare progressive mononucleosis-like syndrome and oral hairy leukoplakia in AIDS patients appears to be valid (12–14). The suggestion that EBV is a major cause of chronic fatigue has not withstood scrutiny (15).

## Description of Agent

### *Virus Biology*

This lymphotropic agent is, from a molecular standpoint, among the best understood of human herpesviruses, but among the least understood with regard to its pathobiology (16–18). EBV has the classic structure of herpesviruses, viz., its double-stranded DNA genome is contained within an icosapentahedral nucleocapsid, which, in turn, is surrounded by a lipid envelope studded with viral glycoproteins. An amorphous tegument protein occupies the space between the envelope and the nucleocapsid (Table 1).

**TABLE 1.** *Structural features of human lymphotropic herpesviruses*

| | EBV | HHV-6 |
|---|---|---|
| Virion components | | |
| Virion diameter | 120 nm | 160–200 nm |
| Capsid diameter | 80 nm | 95–105 nm |
| Capsid symmetry | Icosahedral | Icosahedral |
| Capsomere number | 162 | 162 |
| Lipid envelope | Yes | Yes |
| Genome | | |
| Size (kilobases) | 175 | 168–172 |
| G + C percent content | 59 | 42–44 |
| Isomeric forms | No | No |

The entire genome has been sequenced, and many of its RNA products have been identified and characterized (19,20). The genome comprises approximately 175,000 pairs of bases distributed among five unique stretches of sequence that are flanked by tandem repeat elements (Fig. 1). Within virus particles, the genome is linear, but in latently infected B lymphocytes, the genome is circularized by fusion of the terminal repeats (21).

Transcription of the more than 60 EBV RNAs is a highly coordinated process (Fig. 1). Shortly after infection, only a restricted number of "early" genes are active. Most of these appear to regulate viral latency or facilitate DNA synthesis. Among the early RNA products are at least five EBV nuclear antigens (EBNAs 1–5), the latent membrane protein (LMP), at least two early antigens (EAs), and the viral DNA polymerase (22). EBV has recently been shown to possess a gene that encodes thymidine kinase as well (23).

Following replication of the genome, many other genes are transcribed, ones that primarily encode viral structural components. The most abundant EBV protein detected within virus-producing cells is the viral capsid antigen (VCA). VCA was the protein detected by the Henles in Burkitt's tumor cells (3).

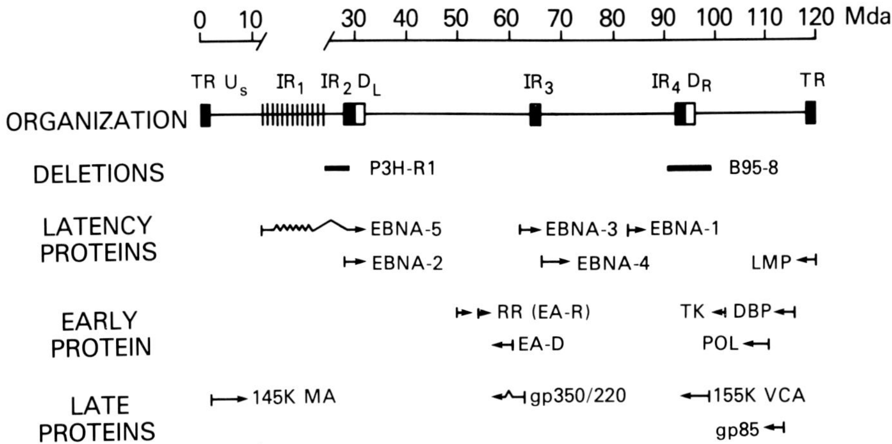


**FIG. 1.** Structure, organization, and expression of the EBV genome. Sequences that are deleted in strains P3H-R1 and B95-8 are shown as *heavy lines.* The location, directionality, and splicing of selected transcripts are indicated. EA-D, diffuse early antigen; RR, ribonucleotide reductase; TK, thymidine kinase; POL, polymerase; MA, membrane antigen; gp, glycoprotein; EBNA, EBV nuclear antigen.

Embedded within the virion envelope and within the membrane of virus-producing cells is a series of EBV proteins that are collectively called "membrane antigens" (MAs). Three MAs, of 350 kd (kilodaltons), 220 kd, and 85 kd in size, are glycosylated (24). Antibodies to these three antigens are neutralizing. The 350-kd and 220-kd MAs are encoded by the same gene, are responsible for binding to cellular receptors for EBV, and are the primary candidates for recombinant vaccines (see below) (25).

### *Virus Strains*

Two closely-related families of EBV strains are recognized. None of the strains are sufficiently different from the others to be considered individual types of EBV. The prototypical strains are B95-8 and the HR-1 subline of the P3J virus (P3-HR1). These strains differ by deletions and rearrangements of small portions of their genomes, sufficient to confer unique biological attributes on each. Specifically, B95-8 virus transforms B cells; P3-HR1 does not. P3-HR1 superinfection will activate the replication of latent B95-8 within B cells. All EBV clinical isolates resemble these prototypical strains to varying degrees, being likely to generate progeny virus and lyse B cells (P3-HR1-like) or being strictly transforming (like B95-8) (26). There is no definite clinical consequence of being infected with viruses of one or the other class, but there are reports of chronic infections being associated with the more lytic strains of EBV (27).

Recently, EBV strains have also been distinguished by the variant of EBNA-2 protein that they express (28). Most Western isolates represent the EBNA-2A variant and efficiently transform B cells. Most African isolates transform B cells inefficiently and express the EBNA-2B variant protein. It is unknown whether the presence of either variant correlates with a virus' propensity for inducing clinical disease.

### *Sites of Infection*

Among the human herpesviruses, EBV is remarkable for its ability to infect and immortalize B lymphocytes (29). These cells possess the specific CR2 receptor for C3d

(25). Because EBV has been identified in the salivary gland, in exfoliated oral and genital epithelial cells, in the tongue, in nasopharyngeal carcinoma tissues, and in T-cell lymphomas (7,11,30–33), cells other than B cells must possess the CR2 receptor at some point in their developmental cycles or EBV can enter some cells by alternative mechanisms. Cells known to lack the CR2 receptor are capable of supporting EBV replication. For example, EBV multiplies efficiently in T lymphocytes that are transfected with EBV DNA (34).

### *Patterns of Infection*

EBV exhibits at least two distinct patterns of infection. Productive replication occurs in differentiated epithelium and leads to release of progeny virions. Saliva is the major site from which cell-free virus can be recovered (7,30). Most or all viral genes participate in the productive replicative cycle. Cells that are producing virus express viral EA, VCA, and MA, and contain numerous linear copies of the genome.

A very small proportion (usually <0.1%) of EBV-infected B lymphocytes are also virus-producers. Most B cells host a latent infectious cycle in which the virus transforms a number of morphologic properties and the growth pattern of the cells, such that they are activated and immortalized (29). This latent replicative process involves the transcription of at least eight viral genes, including those encoding the EBNAs 1–5, a leader protein and LMP (35). Two small RNAs (EBERs) of unknown function are also transcribed. In latently infected B cells, the EBV genome persists as one or many copies of an autonomously replicating circular episome (21).

Studies of cells transfected with individual EBV genes have elucidated the roles they play in the initiation and maintenance of virus latency. For example, EBNA-1 appears responsible for replicating the episomal (circular) genome (36). EBNA-2 initiates growth transformation (37). LMP confers B cells with many features of the transformed state including increased proliferation and adhesion (38).

The ability of EBV to transform cells *in vitro* is relevant to EBV-associated diseases. In marmosets and in humans, EBV-infected B cells with the transformed phenotype can be found in certain malignant lymphomas. The paradigm for this is African Burkitt's lymphoma. It is not certain what role EBV plays in these lymphomas because virtually identical, but EBV-negative lymphomas occur frequently. The favored hypothesis is the EBV-transformed cells proliferate more quickly, thereby affording greater opportunities for outgrowth of clones of cells in which other, more relevant, transforming events have occurred (39).

### *Reactivation*

As indicated, the predominant source of infectious virus is the salivary gland. Some believe that EBV is constantly shed into the lumen of the gland, in essence serving as a permanent reservoir of virus available to infect lymphocytes in transit through the oropharynx (40). Others suggest that constraints upon virus replication, which maintain its latency in the gland, are only intermittently released, permitting periodic reactivation.

What the actual constraints upon virus reactivation are, and what, in turn, permits it, are general questions of great importance with all herpesviruses. Parts of the answers to these questions exist for EBV. Miller et al. (41) have proven that a specific EBV gene is capable of inducing the reactivation of latent virus. This gene is expressed in heterogeneously rearranged defective (*het*) DNA present in stocks of P3-HR1 virus.

With standard techniques for detecting immortalizing EBV, the saliva of normal seropositive persons is found to contain virus on at least 15% of attempts. This shedding rate and the titer of virus recovered rises inversely with cellular immune competence (30). In patients with AIDS or recent bone marrow transplants, most cultures are positive (42). As with other herpesviruses, then, the likelihood of EBVs reactivation is strongly influenced by immunoregulatory mechanisms (43).

## Epidemiology

### *Seroprevalence*

EBV infection is ubiquitous (Fig. 2) (44). As revealed by the percentage of individuals seropositive for immunoglobulin G (IgG) antibodies to EBV VCA, nearly all life-long residents of developing nations are infected during early childhood. In industrialized nations, exposure to the virus is often delayed. Upon entry to university, only about one-half of American students are seropositive (5,6).

Studies of seroconversion to EBV among college students were instrumental in proving that this virus causes acute infectious mononucleosis (5). For example, retrospective serologic assessments of students entering Yale revealed that one-half to three-fourths of first-year students were susceptible to EBV (6). During college, approximately 13% of susceptibles seroconverted to EBV each academic year. Approximately one-third of these primary infections resulted in mononucleosis; the remainder seroconverted asymptomatically.

### *Transmission*

Several studies implicated intimate exchange of saliva as a leading factor in the transmission of EBV in adolescents (45,46). A similar route of transmission is probably operative in other age groups.

Evans (46) surveyed students with acute infectious mononucleosis or other illnesses

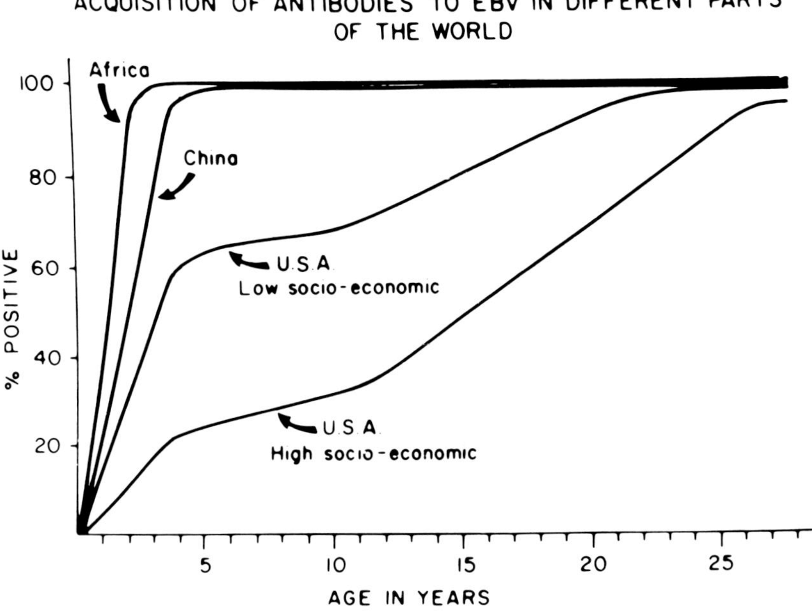


**FIG. 2.** Seroepidemiologic patterns of acquisition of EBV in different parts of the world and among various socioeconomic groups in the United States. (From Fleischer and Straus, ref. 44, with permission.)

at the University of Wisconsin infirmary. He noted that a significantly high proportion of students with mononucleosis reported intimate kissing within 60 days prior to illness than did students with other acute problems.

Several studies, however, showed that EBV is not very contagious. Nye and Lambert (47) found that only 19% of susceptible family members seroconverted within 6 months of the index case. More casual contacts than those which occur among family members are even less likely to permit EBV transmission. Storrie (48) showed that no susceptible members of a submarine crew seroconverted, despite continuous duty for over 2 months with two shipmates with mononucleosis.

In sexually active individuals, other mechanisms besides exchange of saliva must also be considered. Sixbey showed EBV in exfoliated vaginal-cervical cells, suggesting the possibility of sexual transmission (11). This will be difficult to prove, however, because saliva is also exchanged routinely between sexual partners.

### *Incubation Period*

From studies of case contacts, the incubation period of acute infectious mononucleosis has been determined to be 4–6 weeks (45).

## Diagnosis

### *Serodiagnosis*

The diagnosis of an EBV infection is usually confirmed serologically (Table 2) (49,50). Most often, heterophile antibody responses are used to assess mononucleosis-like syndromes. Heterophile antibodies are IgM molecules directed at red blood cell antigens of sheep, horse, or beef and not against EBV proteins. The classical method of detecting heterophile antibodies was described by Paul and Bunnell (51). First, the serum is adsorbed with an extract of guinea pig kidney to remove cross-reacting Forssman antibody and serum sickness antibodies. It is then incubated with sheep, beef, horse, or certain other animal erythrocytes. The titer reported is the highest dilution at which the cells are agglutinated. In the proper clinical setting, a heterophile titer of 1:56 or greater correlates extremely well with acute infectious mononucleosis.

Despite the nonspecificity of heterophile antibodies, their detection is very useful. Approximately 85% of sera from patients with fever, lymphadenopathy, pharyngitis, and greater than 10% atypical lymphocytes are heterophile-positive at some point during the course of illness. Over 90% of heterophile-positive infections are caused by EBV (52). The remainder are associated

**TABLE 2.** *Serologic responses to patients with EBV-associated diseases*[a]

| Condition | Anti-VCA | | | Anti-EA | | Anti-EBNA | Heterophile (IgM) |
|---|---|---|---|---|---|---|---|
| | IgM | IgG | IgA | D | R | | |
| Uninfected | – | – | – | – | – | – | – |
| Infectious mononucleosis | + | ++ | ± | + | – | – | + |
| Convalescent | – | + | – | – | ± | + | ± |
| Past infection | – | + | – | – | – | + | – |
| Chronic infection | – | +++ | ± | ++ | ++ | ± | – |
| Reactivation with immunodeficiency | – | ++ | ± | + | + | ± | – |
| Burkitt's lymphoma | – | +++ | – | ± | ++ | + | – |
| Nasopharyngeal carcinoma | – | +++ | + | ++ | ± | + | – |

[a]Based upon Okano et al., ref. 50.

with CMV, hepatitis B virus (HBV), *Toxoplasma gondii,* or any of a variety of other agents. Ultimately, however, the definitive implication of EBV in any illness rests upon virus-specific serologic tests (50,53). All classical EBV serologic tests rely upon IF techniques. Acute EBV infection is accompanied by the appearance of IgM antibodies to VCA, typically with titers in the range of 1:40–1:320. These antibodies persist for several weeks to months and have not been shown convincingly to reappear with chronic or reactivation disease.

IgG anti-VCA antibodies rise rapidly, peak in titer in several weeks (typically 1:160–1:1,280), and persist at a reduced titers for life (typically 1:40–1:320). Higher VCA-IgG titers are maintained in immunocompromised patients and in others with any of a variety of chronic or recurrent disease states. Titers as high as 1:40,960 have been seen in patients with chronic EBV infection (12,13,54).

Antibodies to EBV EA are operationally distinguished into those of the diffuse (EA-D) or restricted (EA-R) types, depending upon the distribution of antigen in fixed, IF-stained cells. Antibodies to EA-D are detectable shortly after the onset of acute infectious mononucleosis in 70–80% of patients. These antibodies wane and are supplanted in some persons by anti-EA-R, which persists in low titer for 1–4 years (55). Anti-EA-D or EA-R reappear with virus reactivation in immunodeficient patients (54). Their titers can be exceedingly high (1:1,280–1:10,240) in EBV-associated malignancies and in chronic EBV infection (12,13).

Antibodies to EBNAs are detected by an anticomplement immunofluorescence assay (56). Anti-EBNA responses emerge relatively late in the course of infection but persist for life. The presence of EBNA antibodies in an acute phase serum specimen is presumptive evidence against there being an ongoing primary EBV infection (53). Antibodies to all EBNA proteins or to just one of them, EBNA-1, can fail to appear or wane in patients with cellular immune deficiency (57).

### *Virus Isolation*

To recover virus, filtered saliva is inoculated onto cord blood lymphocytes (7,58). Cultures are examined for up to 6 weeks, during which time outgrowth of transformed B cells become apparent as floating aggregates of lymphocytes in a background of degenerating, uninfected cells. Virus presence in the cells is routinely confirmed by IF staining for EBNA.

Salivary shedding is nearly universal during acute infectious mononucleosis and persists at a slowly decreasing rate over a period of many months; approximately 50% of cultures are positive at 6 months after the onset of illness (59). Ultimately, at least 15% of saliva specimens from EBV seropositives can be found to contain virus. Thus, virus recovery is not diagnostic of recent infection, but its absence suggests that an alternative diagnosis might be entertained.

### *Nucleic Acid Hybridization*

Nucleic acid hybridization by either the Southern or *in situ* techniques are helpful in the evaluation of certain EBV-associated disorders (11,14,33). In normal seropositive persons, the proportion of cells that contain EBV is so low (less than 1 out of $10^5$ B cells) that Southern hybridization of DNA extracted from tissue biopsies should be negative, even if heavily infiltrated with lymphocytes. Similarly, only rare cells from normal persons reveal viral sequences upon *in situ* hybridization. In contrast, EBV-associated tumors and organs infiltrated with infected cells contain abundant viral DNA and selected viral RNAs and are positive by either hybridization technique. Although DNA spot (dot-blot, slot-blot) hybridizations have been used successfully, their greater propensity for false-positive reactions relative to Southern hybridization limits their general appeal (60).

## Clinical Manifestations

### *Asymptomatic Infection*

Primary EBV infections that occur early or late in life are nearly always asymptomatic. In adolescents or young adults, one-half to one-third of infections are asymptomatic (6,61). In the normal host, virus reactivation is also asymptomatic or at least has not been associated with a distinct clinical syndrome. Patients with cellular immune deficiency experience symptomatic reactivation infections.

### *Acute Infectious Mononucleosis*

The paradigm for EBV-induced illness is acute infectious mononucleosis, a syndrome characterized by fever, lymphadenopathy, pharyngitis, and a wide range of other clinical and laboratory findings (Tables 3 and 4) (62). Complications of acute infectious mononucleosis are recognized to involve nearly every organ system (Table 5). The diagnosis of acute infectious mononucleosis requires, in addition to typical signs and symptoms, circulating atypical lymphocytes and heterophile antibodies. The quantities required of each have been arbitrarily set, largely for clinical research purposes. Most authorities require that there be an absolute lymphocytosis with at least 10% of lymphocytes being atypical and that the heterophile antibodies be detectable by commercial slide kits (or within an appropriate pattern and titer by the Paul-Bunnell test). These stringent requirements correlate best with primary EBV infection. Unfortunately, they exclude many cases that are also EBV-induced (52).

**TABLE 3.** *Clinical features of acute infectious mononucleosis*[a]

| Feature | Percent |
|---|---|
| Symptoms | |
| Sore throat | 70–88 |
| Malaise | 43–76 |
| Headache | 37–55 |
| Anorexia | 10–27 |
| Myalgias | 12–22 |
| Chills | 9–18 |
| Nausea | 2–17 |
| Gastrointestinal discomfort | 2–14 |
| Others | ≤5 |
| Signs | |
| Lymphadenopathy | 93–100 |
| Pharyngitis | 69–91 |
| Fever | 63–100 |
| Splenomegaly | 50–63 |
| Hepatomegaly | 6–14 |
| Palatal enanthem | 5–13 |
| Jaundice | 4–10 |
| Rash | 0–15 |

[a]Adapted from Schooley and Dolin, ref. 133.

**TABLE 4.** *Laboratory features of acute infectious mononucleosis*

| Feature | Percent[a] |
|---|---|
| Hematologic | |
| Atypical lymphocytes (>20%) | 70–100 |
| Mild neutropenia | 20–50 |
| Mild thrombocytopenia | 35–60 |
| Autoimmune hemolytic anemia | 2–3 |
| Chemical | |
| Mild hepatitis | 50–100 |
| Mild hyperbilirubinemia | 30–50 |
| Serologic | |
| EBV seroconversion | 85–90 |
| Heterophile antibodies (≥1:56) | 75–90 |

[a]The percentage of certain features vary even more widely with age.

Classical infectious mononucleosis, in which these stringent criteria are met, is primarily a disease of adolescents. It is observed infrequently in young children or the elderly (63–65). The rarity of the syndrome in the elderly is explicable by the small reservoir of susceptibles that remain beyond middle age. That infectious mononucleosis is uncommon in children speaks more to the differences in potential outcome upon exposure to EBV with maturation.

During childhood, EBV is apparently met with a prompt and measured host response, one that is sufficient to resolve the

**TABLE 5.** *Complications of acute infectious mononucleosis*

| |
|---|
| Hematologic |
| Autoimmune hemolytic anemia, thrombocytopenia, hemorrhage, neutropenia, agranulocytosis, aplastic anemia |
| Neuropsychiatric |
| Meiningoencephalitis, encephalitis, cerebellitis, seizures, cranial nerve palsies, mononeuritis multiplex, Guillain-Barré syndrome, transverse myelitis, psychosis |
| Respiratory |
| Airway obstruction, interstitial pneumonia |
| Other |
| Ampicillin sensitivity, acute hepatitis, splenic rupture, myocarditis, pericarditis, pancreatitis, parotitis, nephritis, erythema multiforme, erythema nodosum |

infection with few, if any, recognizable symptoms. In adolescents, host responses to infection are often excessive. In fact, most of the clinical and laboratory manifestations of acute infectious mononucleosis can be attributed to these immunopathologic responses (43). For example, EBV activates B cells, induces their proliferation, and stimulates a polyclonal antibody response. In infectious mononucleosis, autoantibodies and other nonspecific antibodies including the heterophile ones can be detected. Furthermore, the atypical lymphocytes and lymphoid organ infiltration largely reflects the vigorous proliferation of reactive T lymphocytes, rather than infected B cells (66). Most, if not all, of the clinical complications of acute infectious mononucleosis seen in the normal host (Table 5) are also considered to be immunologically mediated. This is true of the cranial nerve palsies, Guillain-Barré syndrome, and other neurologic problems, as well as the hematologic events seen during mononucleosis.

Other infections can produce mononucleosis-like illnesses, presumably by provoking similar immunopathologic processes (52). The less the illness resembles classical heterophile-positive mononucleosis, the lower the likelihood that EBV is the etiologic agent. As indicated below, HHV-6 may also be a cause of mononucleosis-like illness.

There have been reports of second or multiple episodes of infectious mononucleosis (67). Most were published before the availability of EBV-specific serologic testing. It is likely that these were instances of sequential infections with different agents, each of which can provide clinically similar lymphadenopathic illnesses. The possibility that these could represent reactivation EBV infections should not be totally dismissed, however. They do occur in the immune deficient host, and reactivation infections are hallmarks of other human herpesviruses (68).

### *EBV-Associated Malignancies*

The soft tissue tumor recognized by Burkitt (1) in Ugandan children is a unique lymphoma that has a predilection for the jaw and viscera. At least 95% of tumors from endemic (African) cases are EBV-positive (61). Less than 20% of sporadic cases, such as those in the United States, are EBV-associated. That percentage has increased with the emergence of AIDS. A notable and possibly essential pathophysiologic feature of Burkitt's lymphoma is the occurrence of translocations of portions of chromosome 8 onto the arms of other chromosomes, so as to move endogenous growth regulatory genes, such as c-*myc*, adjacent to immunoglobulin genes (69).

Nasopharyngeal carcinoma is also EBV-associated. It is the most prevalent tumor in males in parts of China, Southeast Asia, and North Africa. Epidemiologic studies linked disease risk with genetic factors and with exposure to a wide variety of environmental cocarcinogens such as the phorbal esters (61). The tumor cells contain EBV, but apparently lack receptors for the virus; thus, the route of infection of these tumor cells remains undefined.

It is noteworthy that levels of antibodies

to EBV, particularly the IgA anti-VCA, correlate with tumor burden and progression of the nasopharyngeal tumor (70). This has not been shown for Burkitt's tumor. The difference may reflect the biology of EBV in each instance. Productive replication, hence the quantity of VCA synthesized and presented at the mucosal surface for humoral immune response, is greater in nasopharyngeal carcinoma cells than in B lymphocytes.

A variety of much rarer human cancers has been associated with EBV as well. The problem of assuming viral carcinogenesis is even greater with these tumors than with Burkitt's lymphoma and nasopharyngeal carcinoma. Included are a few salivary tumors, malignant thymomas, and squamous tumors of the head, neck, and lung (71).

### *EBV-Associated Disorders in Immunodeficient Patients*

Patients with congenital cellular immunodeficiency syndromes suffer severe primary or reactivation infections with EBV, ones that are manifested as polyclonal or monoclonal B cell lymphoproliferative disorders. Those at risk include patients with ataxia-telangiectasia, Wiskott-Aldrich syndrome, severe combined immunodeficiency, common variable immunodeficiency, and the Chediak-Higashi syndrome (50).

A unique subset of patients known to be congenitally at risk of severe EBV infection are males with the X-linked lymphoproliferative syndrome (XLPS) (9,72,73). Prior to EBV infection, these boys appear normal. Of these, 60–70% succumb in a matter of weeks to fulminant mononucleosis. Unlike the situation with acute mononucleosis, in which T cells proliferate excessively, the acute XLPS response involves a totally unbridled polyclonal B-cell expansion. It appears as if there were absolutely no cellular immune response to infection; in fact, profound T-cell and natural killer (NK) cell deficiencies have been observed (73). Major viscera are infiltrated in XLPS with EBV-containing cells. Replacement of the normal marrow architecture leads to a precipitous decline in blood elements other than lymphocytes. Death is usually attributable to secondary bacterial sepsis or hemorrhage.

The survivors of acute EBV infection acquire a spectrum of chronic or progressive complications including hypo- or hypergammaglobulinemia, bone marrow aplasia, or B-cell lymphomas. The pathogenetic mechanisms underlying these late complications are not understood. Purtilo (74) proposed that they reflect a spectrum of residual immune abnormalities resulting in slowly progressive or smoldering illness due to either excessive suppressor (antiproliferative) or inadequate suppressor (B-cell proliferative) responses.

Transplant recipients, patients with AIDS, and, to a lesser extent, patients with Sjogren's syndrome or other collagen-vascular diseases experience more severe EBV infections than normals; at times, reactivation infections in patients such as these are also symptomatic. Two EBV-associated syndromes that present in this setting are noteworthy.

The first involves B-cell proliferation (10). The proliferative response is usually polyclonal initially. The features of the process may resemble infectious mononucleosis for the presence of fever, lymphadenopathy, and hepatosplenomegaly. Heterophile antibodies and atypical lymphocytes are usually absent, however (68). With time, progressively fewer EBV-transformed clones are evident in these patients, until but a few or one clone may dominate the tumor masses (75). The net result is that EBV-associated non-Hodgkins B cell lymphomas, including Burkitt's lymphoma, occur at greatly increased rates in these patients.

AIDS patients experience another remarkable EBV-associated disorder, known as "oral hairy leukoplakia," whose lesions are characterized by exophytic proliferation of the buccal and lingual epithelium. EBV actively replicates in these tissues (14). That the leukoplakia remits during acyclovir (ACV) treatment indicates a primary role for EBV in its pathogenesis (76). The leukoplakia is usually indolent or slowly progressive and causes no symptoms. The importance of this syndrome is to distinguish it from other oral lesions. Moreover, it is a unique model of an EBV infectious process in which productive virus replication predominates. Molecular analyses of hairy leukoplakia tissues showed that all of the EBV genomes detectable within them are in the linear conformation.

### *Chronic Mononucleosis*

This is a rare, heterogeneous syndrome that should not be confused with the mild fatigue or adenopathy that often persists for several weeks after acute mononucleosis (12,13,57). Most patients are boys with no family history to suggest XLPS and nothing to indicate prior immune impairment. Examination reveals recurring or chronic fevers, weight loss, lymphadenopathy, hepatosplenomegaly, interstitial pneumonia, and/or uveitis. Some patients demonstrate thrombocytopenia, hemolytic anemia, leukopenia, mild hepatitis, hypo- or hypergammaglobulinemia, and indolent B- or T-cell lymphoproliferation. From the limited experience with the syndrome, its long-term prognosis seems very bad, with most patients succumbing to bacterial sepsis or other opportunistic infections.

The diagnosis of chronic mononucleosis is difficult to confirm. A series of criteria for the syndrome was recently proposed (Table 6). They are designed to recognize abnormal serologic responses to EBV as well as evidence of ongoing virus replication within involved tissues. As indicated above, given the universal persistence of virus within seropositive individuals, proof that EBV infection is more active than normal is difficult.

**TABLE 6.** *Suggested criteria for diagnosing chronic mononucleosis*

| |
|---|
| Severe illness of greater than six months' duration that |
| Began as primary EBV infection, *or* |
| Is associated with grossly abnormal EBV antibody titers (IgG to VCA ≥ 1:5120; antibody to EA ≥ 1:640; or antibody to EBNA < 1:2) |
| **and** |
| Histological evidence of major organ involvement, such as |
| Interstitial pneumonia |
| Hypoplasia of some bone marrow elements |
| Uveitis |
| Lymphadenitis |
| Persistent hepatitis |
| Splenomegaly |
| **and** |
| Detection of increased quantities of EBV in affected tissues by |
| Anticomplementary immunofluorescence for EBNA, *or* |
| Nucleic acid hybridization |

EA, early antigens, EBNA, Epstein-Barr nuclear antigens.

Adapted from Straus, ref. 13.

### *Chronic Fatigue Syndrome*

Within the past several years, a syndrome of debilitating fatigue has been associated with EBV infection (13,15). Some cases are precipitated by acute infectious mononucleosis. Still others show elevated EBV-specific antibody titers (77–79). The epidemiology and pathogenesis of the chronic fatigue syndrome remain obscure. Recent work has indicated that a similar syndrome can be precipitated by other infections including influenza, hepatitis, and brucellosis (80). Mild cellular immune alterations have been noted in many patients, particularly reductions in number and function of natural killer cells (81). None of these immune differences, however, are proven to correlate with disease severity. Neuropsychiatric abnormalities are common as well in chronic fatigue syndrome patients. Whether these represent risk factors for, or consequences of, the syndrome is not known. The combined data argue strongly against EBV being a major factor in the pathogenesis of the syndrome (15,82).

## Treatment

### *General Considerations*

Acute infectious mononucleosis is treated with rest, hydration, antipyretics, and symptomatic care. Contact sports should be avoided for fear of rupturing an enlarged spleen. Activities are tempered in accord with the symptoms and only gradually resumed as convalescence proceeds. Most students with acute infectious mononucleosis can return to school in less than 3–4 weeks.

More substantive supportive measures are needed to manage major complications of acute infectious mononucleosis. These include tracheostomy for acute airway obstruction, transfusions for severe hemolysis, and anticonvulsants for seizures. Coincident group A β-hemolytic streptococcal pharyngitis is common; penicillin or erythromycin treatment is warranted. Ampicillin is to be avoided because of the 80% incidence of transient rash (83). Major bacterial superinfections are only seen in the rare instances of agranulocytosis and require parenteral antibiotics (84).

### *Corticosteroids*

Corticosteroids are widely used in the treatment of acute infectious mononucleosis. A high-dose, rapidly-tapering course of prednisone seems useful in the management of impending airway obstruction and acute hemolysis. Controlled trials revealed that corticosteroids speed defervescence and resolution of pharyngitis (85,86). Despite these data, their use is not universally accepted. It is felt that the palliative effects of corticosteroids could give a false sense of well-being and encourage a return to full activity before it is appropriate. There is also a general concern about treating a viral infection with an immunosuppressive agent. To address some of these concerns, a study comparing ACV with ACV plus corticosteroids has begun in Sweden (87).

**TABLE 7.** *Antiviral drugs that inhibit EBV DNA replication*

| Drug | $ED_{50}$ (μg/ml) |
|---|---|
| Foscarnet | 125 |
| Acyclovir | 0.5 |
| Bromovinyldeoxyuridine | 0.06 |
| Ganciclovir | 0.05 |
| Fluoromethylarabinosyluridine | 0.006 |
| Fluoroiodoarabiniosylcytidine | 0.005 |
| Fluoroiodoarabinosyluridine | 0.005 |

Effective dose that inhibits viral DNA replication by 50%.

### *Antiviral Therapy*

EBV replication is effectively inhibited *in vitro* by a number of nucleoside analogs including ACV and ganciclovir (DHPG), as well as the interferons (Table 7) (88–91). Controlled studies in acute infectious mononucleosis have only been undertaken with ACV (59,92). In acute infectious mononucleosis, ACV markedly reduces the rates of salivary shedding of virus. The effect, however, is transient; once treatment is completed, high rates of shedding resume (Table 8). Little or no symptomatic improvement can be attributed to ACV.

**TABLE 8.** *Proportion of patients with acute infectious mononucleosis with positive oropharyngeal cultures for EBV*

| Day | Placebo | ACV |
|---|---|---|
| 0 | 15/16 | 14/15 |
| 3–4 | 14/16 | 0/14[a] |
| 7 | 16/16 | 1/15[a] |
| 28 | 13/15 | 12/14 |
| 180 | 9/16 | 8/15 |

[a]Difference with respect to placebo group is significant ($p < 0.001$).
Modified from Andersson, ref. 59.

ACV and other agents have been used compassionately in severe EBV-associated disorders. In XLPS patients, they appear to be of no benefit (93). Anecdotal reports cite temporary remissions of chronic EBV infection and of polyclonal B-cell proliferative disorders in transplant recipients treated with ACV (12,75).

The one EBV-associated disorder in which a role for antiviral therapy seems proven is oral hairy leukoplakia (Table 9). Intravenous and oral ACV and an oral acyclovir pro-drug (6-deoxyacyclovir) each induce marked remissions in hairy leukoplakia lesions (76,94). The lesion often recurs after completion of therapy.

### *Prospects for Control and Prevention*

The ability of ACV to ameliorate oral hairy leukoplakia and to reduce virus shedding in acute infectious mononucleosis verifies the antiviral potency of this drug. The inability, in turn, of ACV to ameliorate B-cell proliferative disorders, or even the symptoms of acute infectious mononucleosis, has major implications for control of EBV-associated disease.

First, it is evident that the existing classes of drug can only inhibit replication of EBV that is dependent upon the viral DNA-dependent DNA polymerase; in other words, the pool of linear genomes. Since persistence and replication of circular forms of the genome are dependent on cellular enzymes, situations in which the expression of these forms of the genome contributes to disease pathogenesis cannot be expected to respond to existing drugs (95). Other antiviral strategies are required.

Second, the lack of symptomatic improvement of acute infectious mononucleosis with ACV is in accord with the notion that they are, at least in part, immunopathologically mediated. As expected, EBV-associated disorders reflect an imbalance between host and virus. Ultimately, control of EBV infection is going to have to depend upon the judicious selection of antiviral agents in some settings and immunoactive agents in others. Unfortunately, most immunoactive agents are too nonspecific; others are better able to suppress, rather than stimulate, host responses (96,97). Nonetheless, serious attention needs to be given to controlled exploration of these agents, alone or in combination with antiviral drugs.

Prospects are better for prevention of EBV infection (98). Multiple vaccine strategies are currently being explored. Inactivated EBV has been shown to induce neutralizing antibodies in experimental animals

**TABLE 9.** *Results of ACV trials for the treatment of oral hairy leukoplakia*

| Regimen | Virologic response | Clinical response | Posttreatment relapse | Reference |
|---|---|---|---|---|
| ACV 800 mg p.o., q.i.d., 20 days | 3/5 studied | 3/6 complete<br>2/6 partial<br>1/6 no change | 5/5 | 76 |
| No treatment | Not studied | 6/7 no change<br>1/7 progression | — | |
| ACV 7.5 mg/kg, i.v. q 8 hr, 7 days | Not studied | 2/2 complete | 2/2 | 134 |
| ACV 200 mg, p.o., 5/day | Not studied | 2/2 no change | — | |
| ACV 400 mg, p.o., 5/day | Not studied | 2/2 complete | — | |
| Vitamin A acid, 0.1%, topical, b.i.d., 10 days | Not studied | 2/2 complete | 2/2 | |
| ACV 800 mg, p.o., q.i.d., 14 days | Not studied | 9/9 complete | 4/9 | 135 |

(99). Major immunogenic envelope proteins of EBV (gp350/220) have been cloned and expressed in yeast and mammalian cell lines (100). When given directly or when incorporated into immune-stimulating complexes (ISCOMs), these recombinant glycoproteins induce effective immunity to EBV in cotton-top tamarin monkeys (101,102). The vaccinated animals exhibit a significantly reduced incidence of EBV-induced lymphomas.

The gene encoding these EBV glycoproteins has also been cloned into heterologous live carrier viruses. Lowe et al. (103) showed that the EBV 350-kilodalton (kd) glycoprotein is synthesized in cells infected with the live Oka-strain varicella virus vaccine into which the EBV gene was inserted. Similarly, Morgan et al. (104) inserted the gp350 gene into vaccinia and induced immunity in cotton-top tamarins sufficient to resist lymphomagenic doses of EBV (104).

Now that a vaccine is feasible, the questions of whom to vaccinate and when to do so loom larger. There is no great impetus at present to explore universal vaccination as a means of preventing acute infectious mononucleosis. Third world populations at risk for EBV-associated malignancies should be the first targets of controlled vaccine trials. Although such studies would need to be very large and take many years before evidence of efficacy could be obtained, their ultimate impact on world health is great.

## HHV-6

The discovery of HHV-6, also known as "human B lymphotropic herpesvirus" (HBLV), was reported in 1986 by Salahuddin et al. (105). Extensive morphologic, serologic, and biochemical studies showed it to be a unique and ubiquitous human lymphotropic herpesvirus (106–109). Knowledge regarding HHV-6 is emerging rapidly: much of it remains unpublished.

### Description of the Agent

#### *Structure*

Table 1 compares the structural features of HHV-6 with those of EBV, the other human lymphotropic herpesvirus (109–111). In all regards, it is a typical herpesvirus (Fig. 3). The HHV-6 genome is approximately 170,000 base pairs in size and it has a relatively low guanine plus cytosine (G + C) percent content, estimated to be 42–44%. Endonuclease analyses have thus far failed to demonstrate submolar bands, implying that the HHV-6 genome lacks large inverted repeat elements seen in HSV and VZV DNAs (112). Restriction fragment polymorphisms distinguish diverse clinical isolates of HHV-6, much as they do with the other herpesviruses.

Part of the proof that HHV-6 is a previously unrecognized virus is that its DNA showed no major homology to the known human and animal herpesviruses (106,112). But it does have partial homology to human CMV and to the avian Marek's disease virus (113,114). Portions of the HHV-6 genome have been molecularly cloned and sequenced. The distribution and organization of genes within these regions are most similar to that of CMV (R. Honess, unpublished observations, 1988).

Polyacrylamide gel electrophoresis (PAGE) and Western blot analyses reveal that major antigens of HHV-6 include proteins of 200 kd, 120 kd, 80 kd, 72 kd, 30 kd, and 19 kd in size (112). Proteins that project outward from the virion envelope have been detected by immune electron microscopy (IEM), but their nature and glycosylation patterns remain undefined (109,110).

#### *Cultivation*

HHV-6 was initially recognized by its ability to induce the appearance of intranuclear and intracytoplasmic inclusions in large multinucleated refractile cells in

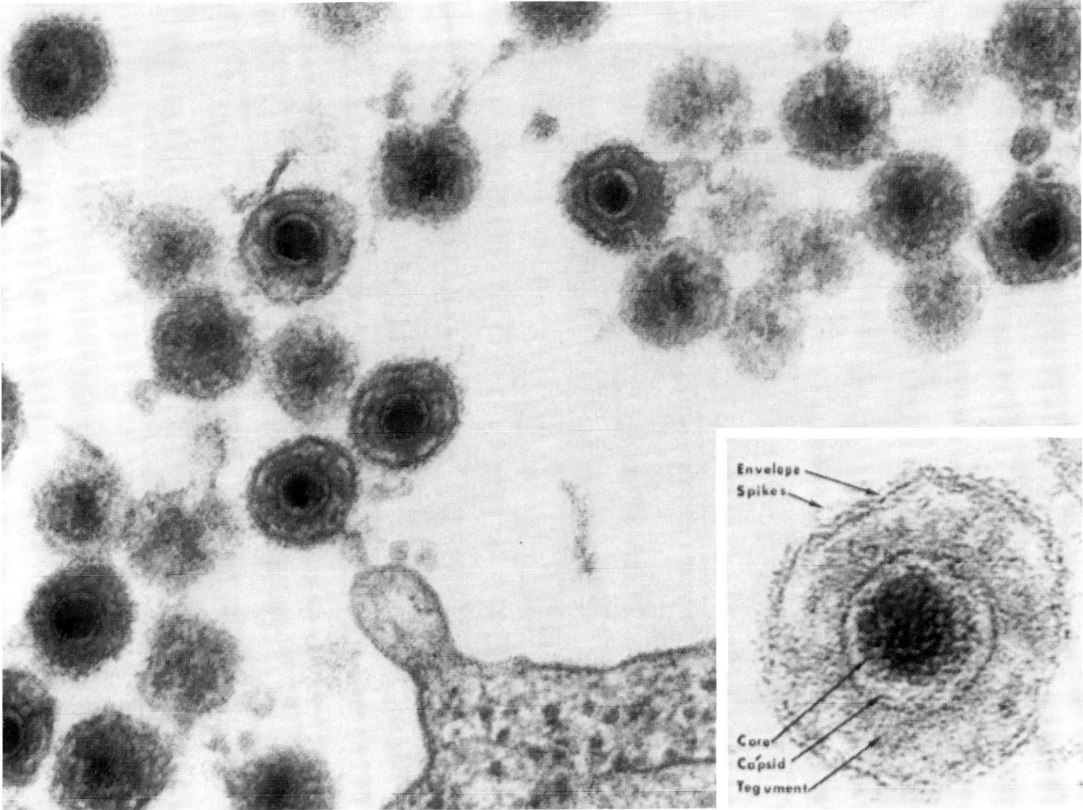


**FIG. 3.** EMs of HHV-6 particles from cultured mononuclear cells. The *insert* shows a higher magnification of a single particle and its components. (From Ablashi et al., ref. 109, with permission.)

cultures of peripheral blood lymphocytes (105). These infected cells survive in culture for 15–20 days. In contrast to EBV-infected lymphocytes, HHV-6-infected cells are lysed rather than immortalized.

HHV-6 is fastidious. It is recovered directly by culturing peripheral blood mononuclear cells or by cocultivating them with cord blood cells. In either case, the cultures must be stimulated with phytohemagglutinin (105,107,108). Virus is further passaged into mitogen-stimulated cord blood cells. Isolation of HHV-6 is confirmed by indirect IF microscopy using standardized antisera or by Southern blot hybridization using virus-specific genomic clones (106).

The B-cell tropism of HHV-6 was appreciated first, hence its original name, "HBLV." HHV-6 was then found to replicate in cells of diverse origins including T lymphocytes, megakaryocytes, macrophages, monocytes, and human embryonic glial and embryonic lung cells (109,115–118).

It is now appreciated that most HHV-6 infected cells bear T-cell markers. B-cells are suceptible, but only if infected by EBV. EBV-negative B-cell lines have not been found to support HHV-6 replication (109). Similar observations have been made regarding human immunodeficiency virus type 1 (HIV-1). HIV-1 favors T cells but can replicate in EBV-bearing B-cells. The replication of HIV-1 in such B-cells is markedly enhanced by coinfection with HHV-6. This finding, and others reviewed below, lead some to speculate that HHV-6 is a cofactor in the progression of AIDS (109).

### *Site of Infection*

Nearly all persons from whom HHV-6 has been recovered are adults with severe acquired immunodeficiency disorders, including AIDS and lymphomas (105,107,108, 110,113). Virus has never been isolated from healthy seropositive people. Peripheral blood mononuclear cells are the predominant material from which HHV-6 is recovered; isolation from saliva has also been achieved (119). Its distribution in tissues is not known, except in the setting of lymphoproliferative diseases. Viral DNA has been detected in the blood, lymph nodes, and salivary glands by Southern hybridization, by *in situ* hybridization, and by polymerase chain reaction (120–122).

### *Latency and Reactivation*

The site and nature of HHV-6 latency is not known. As regards virus reactivation, two general comments can be made on the basis of current knowledge. First, HHV-6 has been recovered repeatedly from blood and tissues of immunodeficient patients but not yet from normal seropositives, indicating that virus reactivation is strongly influenced by cellular immune mechanisms, much as it is with the other human herpesviruses. Second, the decline in titer of antibodies to HHV-6 with increased age suggests that virus reactivation may be uncommon in healthy people. This is similar to VZV and quite different from that which occurs with EBV.

### *Epidemiology*

Nothing is known of the incidence or prevalence of HHV-6 infection. That HHV-6 is associated with a common exanthematous infection of childhood (roseola infatum; see below) suggests that direct contact or exchange of body fluids must be capable of spreading the virus (123). Recovery of HHV-6 from saliva is compatible with this assertion (119). The incubation period of HHV-6 infections, as estimated from older studies of roseola, is 5–15 days (124,125).

Using relatively insensitive assays, the seroprevalence of HHV-6 was noted initially to be higher in immunocompromised patients (70–80%) than in normal age-matched adults (15–40%) (126; and H. Z. Streicher, unpublished observations, 1988). More sensitive assays revealed the higher seroprevalence in certain patient groups to reflect only a relatively higher antibody titer; nearly all adults are seropositive. Studies of sera from many different age groups suggest passive maternal transfer of antibody (127). The proportion of persons infected rises rapidly after 6 months of life and is nearly universal by mid-childhood (127,128). That HHV-6 antibodies wane after many years implies that virus reactivation is not sufficiently common in healthy people to boost the titers.

The prevalence of roseola infantum in early childhood and the low secondary attack rate among house contacts older than 3 years of age are compatible with these emerging seroepidemiologic data.

## Diagnosis

HHV-6 infection cannot be routinely diagnosed. The pace of research in the field and the desire to exploit this virus commercially, however, will likely encourage the development and widespread use of serologic assays and nucleic acid-based hybridization tests within 2–4 years. Virus isolation will remain cumbersome and the province of specialized laboratories. At present, acute infections can only be diagnosed definitively in research laboratories equipped to detect virus and seroconversion.

The current serologic assays are of two general types. Most serologic work to date has relied on immunofluorescence (IF) microscopy with either anticomplement or indirect IF reactions (126,128). HHV-6-infected cells are affixed to slides and used as a substrate to bind antibodies that react with viral capsid antigens (VCA) (127). The second type of serologic assay is based upon an enzymed-linked immunosorbent assay (ELISA) using purified virions as antigens. Neither of these serologic assays have been standardized. Efforts to do so for the purposes of supporting a number of research groups are underway (P. Levine, unpublished observations).

### Clinical Manifestations

There remain no clinical diseases that are proved to be caused by HHV-6. There are four syndromes, however, that have been associated with HHV-6 infection.

#### *AIDS*

HHV-6 has been recovered most frequently from patients with AIDS (105,107, 108,110,111). As with the other five human herpesviruses, HHV-6 may be more likely to reactivate in this setting of severe immune impairment. Such reactivation events could be asymptomatic or may contribute to AIDS-associated disease manifestations.

The association of HHV-6 with AIDS may be more than a mere epiphenomenon of immune deficiency. First, as a lytic, lymphotropic herpesvirus, HHV-6 has the potential for inducing lymphoproliferation and for causing lymphopenia, both of which are seen in AIDS. Second, HHV-6 infection enhances the replication and cytopathogenicity of HIV-1 (109). Thus, reactivation of latent HHV-6 in the setting of AIDS could accelerate disease progression, both directly and indirectly.

#### *Lymphoproliferative Disorders*

As noted earlier, HHV-6 sequences were detected in B-cell lymphomas (120,121). Interestingly, some of the HHV-6-containing lymphomas were also positive for EBV. This observation and the fact that HHV-6 does not transform B lymphocytes imply that HHV-6 has no direct role in lymphomagenesis.

The association of HHV-6 with lymphomas, therefore, may merely reflect an enhanced likelihood of virus reactivation in the setting of immune deficiency. An alternative possibility is that malignant transformation could favor HHV-6 replication, much as EBV transformation has been shown to do in B cells. Finally, HHV-6 could promote lymphomagenesis without directly causing it, by influencing the regulation and expression of endogenous and exogenous oncogenes.

HHV-6 may contribute more directly to the development of polyclonal lymphoproliferative disorders (121). In this regard, several cases of heterophile-negative mononucleosis associated with HHV-6 seroconversion have been observed (G. Pearson, unpublished observations). If HHV-6 were proven to cause a mononucleosis syndrome, one would have to presume that its pathogenesis is immunologically mediated, much as is EBV-induced infectious mononucleosis.

#### *Roseola Infantum*

Roseola infantum (*Exanthem subitum*) is a mild, acute febrile illness of infants and young children (124,125). The illness is heralded by 3–5 days of fever to 104°C, but with strikingly few other physical or constitutional complaints. There may be minimal coryza, pharyngitis, and adenopathy. The diagnosis is suggested when a maculopapular rash appears as the child defervesces. The rash is often evanescent, but it can persist or relapse repeatedly over the period of several days. Complications are rare.

Yamanishi et al. (123) recently reported that roseola is associated with primary HHV-6 infection. Careful study of four cases exhibiting classical features of roseola revealed that virus could be isolated from the blood during the acute illness. Moreover, recovery was associated with HHV-6 seroconversion. The combined data do not rule out other causes of roseola, but HHV-6 is one very likely cause.

### *Chronic Fatigue Syndrome*

As indicated in the section on EBV above, chronic fatigue syndrome is a heterogenous disorder that can be precipitated by acute infections (13). Several groups have suggested that there is a link between chronic fatigue syndrome and HHV-6 (109,126,129). The association is based predominantly on the observation that serologic titers to HHV-6 are higher in chronic fatigue syndrome patients than in controls. These observations might only reflect nonspecific immunological differences between normals and chronic fatigue syndrome patients, ones that lead to a greater propensity for asymptomatic virus reactivation and stimulation of antibody synthesis. Similar nonspecific elevations of antibody titers have been seen for both EBV and HHV-6 in sarcoidosis and a variety of lymphoproliferative malignancies (121,130,131).

### Treatment

There are no specific treatments for HHV-6-associated infections. Fortunately, most infections probably warrant nothing more than symptomatic care. Preliminary studies indicate HHV-6 to be resistant *in vitro* to clinically attainable concentrations of ACV and DHPG (132). Since both of these agents are activated by deoxypyrimidine (thymidine) kinases, their failure to inhibit HHV-6 replication suggests that this virus lacks the enzyme and fails to induce further expression of the cellular kinase. HHV-6 replication in cultured lymphocytes is impaired, however, by DNA polymerase inhibitors that do not require enzymatic activation. In preliminary studies, Streicher et al. (132) showed complete prevention of HHV-6 late protein synthesis in HSB-2 cells treated with 20 μg/ml of foscarnet.

## REFERENCES


1. Burkitt D. A sarcoma involving the jaws in African children. *Br J Surg* 1958;46:218–23.
2. Epstein MA, Achong BG, Barr YM. Virus particles in cultured lymphoblasts from Burkitt's lymphoma. *Lancet* 1964;1:702–3.
3. Henle G, Henle W. Immunofluorescence in cells derived from Burkitt's lymphoma. *J Bacteriol* 1966;91:1248–56.
4. Henle G, Henle W, Diehl V. Relation of Burkitt's tumor-associated herpes-type virus to infectious mononucleosis. *Proc Natl Acad Sci USA* 1968;59:94–101.
5. Evans AS, Niederman JC, McCollum, RC. Seroepidemiologic studies of infectious mononucleosis with EB virus. *N Engl Med* 1968;279:1121–7.
6. Sawyer RN, Evans AS, Niederman JC, McCollum RW. Prospective studies of a group of Yale University freshmen. I. Occurrence of infectious mononucleosis. *J Infect Dis* 1971;123:263–9.
7. Miller G, Niederman JC, Andrews LL. Prolonged oropharyngeal excretion of EB virus following infectious mononucleosis. *N Engl J Med* 1973;288:229–32.
8. Zur Hausen H, Schulte-Holthausen H, Klein G, et al. EBV DNA in biopsies of Burkitt's tumors and anaplastic carcinoma of the nasopharynx. *Nature* 1970;228:1056–8.
9. Purtilo DT, DeFlorio D, Hutt LM, et al. Variable phenotypic expression of an X-linked recessive lymphoproliferative syndrome. *N Engl J Med* 1977;297:1077–81.
10. Hanto DW, Frizzera G, Gajl-Peczalska KJ, Simmons RL. Epstein-Barr virus, immunodeficiency, and B cell lymphoproliferation. *Transplantation* 1985;39:461–72.
11. Andiman W, Gradoville L, Heston L, et al. Use of cloned probes to detect Epstein-Barr viral DNA in tissues of patients with neoplastic and lymphoproliferative diseases. *J Infect Dis* 1983;148:967–77.
12. Schooley RT, Carey RW, Miller G, et al. Chronic Epstein-Barr virus infection associated with fever and interstitial pneumonitis. Clinical and serological features and response to

antiviral chemotherapy. *Ann Intern Med* 1986; 104:636–43.
13. Straus SE. The chronic mononucleosis syndrome. *J Infect Dis* 1988;157:405–12.
14. Greenspan JS, Greenspan D, Lennette ET, et al. Replication of Epstein-Barr virus within the epithelial cells of oral "hairy" leukoplakia, an AIDS-associated lesion. *N Engl J Med* 1985;313:1564–71.
15. Swartz MN. The chronic fatigue syndrome—one entity or many? *N Engl J Med* 1988; 319:1726–8.
16. Roizman B. The family herpesviridae: general description, taxonomy, and classification. In: Roizman B, ed. *The herpesviruses, vol. 1*. New York: Plenum Press, 1982:1–23.
17. Miller G. Epstein-Barr virus. In: Fields BN, ed. *Virology*. New York: Raven Press, 1985: 563–89.
18. Epstein MA, Achong BG. *The Epstein-Barr virus: recent advances*. New York: John Wiley, 1986.
19. Baer R, Bankier AT, Biggin MD, et al. DNA sequence and expression of the B95-8 Epstein-Barr virus genome. *Nature* 1984;310:207–11.
20. Hummel M, Kieff E. Epstein-Barr virus RNA. VIII. Viral RNA in permissively infected B95-8 cells. *J Virol* 1982;43:262–72.
21. Adams A, Lindahl T. Epstein-Barr virus genomes with properties of circular molecules in carrier cells. *Proc Natl Acad Sci USA* 1975;72:1477–81.
22. Dillner J, Kallin B. The Epstein-Barr virus proteins. *Adv Cancer Res* 1988;50:95–158.
23. Littler E, Zeuthen J, McBride AA, et al. Identification of an Epstein-Barr virus-coded thymidine kinase. *EMBO J* 1986;5:1959–66.
24. Edson CM, Thorley-Lawson DA. Epstein-Barr virus membrane antigens: characterization, distribution, and strain differences. *J Virol* 1981;39:172–84.
25. Tanner J, Weiss J, Fearon D, Whang Y, Kieff E. Epstein-Barr virus gp350/220 binding to the B lymphocyte C3d receptor mediates adsorption, capping and endocytosis. *Cell* 1987; 50:203–13.
26. Lung ML, Chang RS, Jones JH. Genetic polymorphism of natural Epstein-Barr virus isolates from infectious mononuclear patients and healthy carriers. *J Virol* 1988;62:3862–6.
27. Alfieri C, Ghibu F, Joncas JH. Lytic, nontransforming Epstein-Barr virus (EBVO from a patient with chronic active EBV infection. *Can Med Assoc J* 1984;131:1249–52.
28. Dambaugh T, Hennessy K, Chamnankit L, et al. U2 region of Epstein-Barr virus DNA may encode Epstein-Barr nuclear antigen 2. *Proc Natl Acad Sci USA* 1984;81:7632–6.
29. Miller G, Enders JF, Lisco H, Kohn HL. Establishment of lines from normal human blood leukocytes by co-cultivation with a leukocyte line derived from a leukemic child. *Proc Soc Exp Biol Med* 1969;132:247–52.
30. Strauch B, Siegel N, Andrews L, Miller G. Oropharyngeal excretion of Epstein-Barr virus by renal transplant recipients and other patients treated with immunosuppressive drugs. *Lancet* 1974;1:234–7.
31. Young LS, Clark D, Sixbey JW, Rickinson AB. Epstein-Barr virus receptors on human pharyngeal epithelia. *Lancet* 1986;1:240–2.
32. Sixbey JW, Lemon SM, Pagano JS. A second site of Epstein-Barr virus shedding: the uterine cervix. *Lancet* 1986;2:1122–4.
33. Jones JF, Shurin S, Ambramowsky C, et al. T cell lymphomas containing Epstein-Barr virus DNA in patients with chronic Epstein-Barr virus infections. *N Engl J Med* 1988;318:733–41.
34. Stevenson M, Volsky B, Hedenskog M, et al. Immortalization of human T lymphocytes after transfection of Epstein-Barr virus DNA. *Science* 1986;233:980–3.
35. Dambaugh T, Hennessey H, Fennewald S, Kieff E. The virus genome and its expression in latent infection. In: Epstein MA, Achong BG, eds. *The Epstein-Barr virus: recent advances*. London: W Heinemann, 1986:13–45.
36. Yates JL, Warren N, Sugden B. Stable replication of plasmids derived from Epstein-Barr virus in various mammalian cells. *Nature* 1985;313:812–5.
37. Rickinson AB, Young LS, Reive M. Influence of the Epstein-Barr virus nuclear antigen EBNA 2 on the growth phenotype of virus-transformed B cells. *J Virol* 1987;61:1310–7.
38. Liebowitz D, Kopan R, Fuchs E, et al. An Epstein-Barr virus transforming protein associates with Vimentin in lymphocytes. *Mol Cell Biol* 1987;7:2299–308.
39. Lenoir G, Bornkamm G. Burkitt's lymphoma, a human cancer model for the study of the multistep development of cancer. *Virol Oncol* 1987;6:173–206.
40. Yao QY, Rickinson AB, Epstein MA. A reexamination of the Epstein-Barr virus carrier state in seropositive individuals. *Int J Cancer* 1985;35:35–42.
41. Countryman J, Miller G. Activation of expression of latent Epstein-Barr herpesvirus after gene transfer with a small cloned subfragment of heterogenous viral DNA. *Proc Natl Acad Sci USA* 1985;82:4085–9.
42. Sumaya CV, Boswell RN, Ench Y, et al. Enhanced serological and virological findings of Epstein-Barr virus in patients with AIDS and AIDS-related complex. *J Infect Dis* 1986; 154:864–70.
43. Haynes BF, Fauci AS. Immunoregulatory control of Epstein-Barr virus infections. In: Hook J, Jordan G, eds. *Viral infections in oral medicine*. Amsterdam: Elsevier North Holland, Inc., 1982:111–2.
44. Fleischer GR, Straus SE. Epidemiology and pathogenesis. In: Schlossberg D, ed. *Infectious mononucleosis*. New York: Praeger Scientific (in press).
45. Hoagland RJ. The transmission of infectious mononucleosis. *Am J Med Sci* 1955;229:262–72.
46. Evans AS. Infectious mononucleosis in Uni-

versity of Wisconsin students: report of a 5-year investigation. *Am J Hyg* 1960;72:342–62.
47. Nye FS, Lambert HP. Epstein-Barr virus antibody in cases and contacts of infectious mononucleosis: A family study. *J Hyg* 1973;71:151–9.
48. Storrie MC, Sphar R, Sawyer RN, et al. Seroepidemiological studies of Polaris submarine crews. II. Infectious mononucleosis. *Milit Med* 1976;141:30–4.
49. Chin TDY. Diagnostic criteria and differential diagnosis. In: Schlossberg D, ed. *Infectious mononucleosis*. New York: Praeger Scientific, 1983:181–95.
50. Okano M, Thiele GM, Davis JR, Grierson HL, Purtilo DT. Epstein-Barr virus and human diseases: recent advances in diagnosis. *Clin Microbiol Rev* 1988;1:300–12.
51. Paul JR, Bunnell WW. The presence of heterophile antibodies in infectious mononucleosis. *Am J Med Sci* 1932;183:90–104.
52. Evans AS. Infectious mononucleosis and related syndromes. *Am J Med Sci* 1978;276:325–39.
53. Henle W, Henle G, Horowitz CA. Epstein-Barr virus specific diagnostic tests in infectious mononucleosis. *Hum Pathol* 1974;5:551–65.
54. Henle W, Henle G. Epstein-Barr virus-specific serology in immunologically compromised individuals. *Cancer Res* 1981;41:4222–5.
55. Horwitz CA, Henle W, Henle G, et al. Long-term serological follow-up of patients for Epstein-Barr virus after recovery from infectious mononucleosis. *J Infect Dis* 1985;151:1150–3.
56. Reedman BM, Klein G. Cellular localization of an Epstein-Barr virus-associated complement-fixing antigen in producer and non-producer lymphoblastoid cell lines. *Int J Cancer* 1973; 11:499–520.
57. Miller G, Grogan E, Rowe E, et al. Selective lack of antibody to a component of EB nuclear antigen in patients with chronic active Epstein-Barr virus infection. *J Infect Dis* 1987;156:26–35.
58. Chang RS, Golden HD. Transformation of human leukocytes by throat washings from infectious mononucleosis patients. *Nature* 1971; 234:359–60.
59. Andersson J, Britton S, Ernberg I, et al. Effect of acyclovir in infectious mononucleosis: a double-blind, placebo-controlled study. *J Infect Dis* 1986;153:283–90.
60. Diaz-Mitoma F, Preiksaitis JK, Leung WC, et al. DNA-DNA dot hybridization to detect Epstein-Barr virus in throat washings. *J Infect Dis* 1987;155:297–303.
61. De-The G. Epidemiology of Epstein-Barr virus and associated diseases in man. In: Roizman B, ed. *The herpesvirus, vol. I*. New York: Plenum Publishing Company, 1982:25–103.
62. Schlossberg D, ed. *Infectious mononucleosis*. New York: Praeger Scientific, 1983.
63. Sumaya CV, Ench Y. Epstein-Barr virus infectious mononucleosis in children. II. Heterophil antibody and viral-specific responses. *Pediatrics* 1985;75:1011–9.
64. Horwitz CA, Henle W, Henle G, et al. Clinical and laboratory evaluation of infants and children with Epstein-Barr virus-induced infectious mononucleosis: report of 32 patients (aged 10–48 months). *Blood* 1981;57:933–9.
65. Horwitz CA, Henle W, Henle G, et al. Infectious Mononucleosis in patients aged 40 to 72 years: report of 27 cases, including 3 without heterophil-antibody responses. *Medicine* 1983; 62:256–62.
66. Sheldon P, Papamichael M, Hemsted E, Holborow E. Thymic origin of atypical lymphoid cells in infectious mononucleosis. *Lancet* 1973; 1:1153–5.
67. Straus SE. Relapsing, recurrent, and chronic infectious mononucleosis in the normal host. In: Levine PH, Ablashi DV, Pearson GR, Kottaridis SD, eds. *Epstein-Barr virus and associated diseases*. Brouten: Martines Nijhoff Publishing Co., 1985:18–33.
68. Ho M, Miller GT, Atchinson RW, et al. Epstein-Barr virus infections and DNA hybridization studies in posttransplantation lymphoma and lymphoproliferative lesions: the role of primary infection. *J Infect Dis* 1985;152:876–86.
69. Erikson J, Finan J, Nowell PC, Croce CM. Translocation of immunoglobulin $V_H$ genes in Burkitt's lymphoma. *Proc Natl Acad Sci USA* 1982;79:5611–5.
70. Henle W, Ho JHC, Henle G, et al. Antibodies to Epstein-Barr virus related antigens in nasopharyngeal carcinoma. Comparison to active cases and long term survivors. *JNCI* 1973; 51:361–9.
71. Leyvraz S, Henle W, Chahinian AP, et al. Association of Epstein-Barr virus with thymic carcinoma. *N Engl J Med* 1985;312:1296–9.
72. Purtilo DT, Sakamoto K, Barnabei V, et al. Epstein-Barr virus-induced diseases in boys with the X-linked lymphoproliferative syndrome (XLP). *Am J Med* 1982;73:49–56.
73. Sullivan JL, Byron K, Brewster F, et al. Deficient natural killer cell activity in the X-linked lymphoproliferative syndrome. *Science* 1980;210:543–5.
74. Purtilo DT. Malignant lymphoproliferative diseases induced by Epstein-Barr virus in immunodeficient patients, including X-linked, cytogenetic, and familial syndromes. *Cancer Genet Cytogenet* 1981;4:251–68.
75. Hanto DW, Frizzera G, Gail-Peczalska KJ, et al. Epstein-Barr virus-induced B cell lymphomas after renal transplantation. Acyclovir therapy and transition from polyclonal to monoclonal B cell proliferation. *N Engl J Med* 1982;306:913–8.
76. Resnick L, Herbst JS, Ablashi DV. Regression of oral "hairy" leukoplakia after orally administered acyclovir therapy. *JAMA* 1988;15:384–8.
77. DuBois RE, Seeley JK, Brus I, et al. Chronic mononucleosis syndrome. *South Med J* 1984; 77:1376–82.
78. Jones JF, Ray CG, Minnich LL, et al. Evidence for active Epstein-Barr virus infection in patients with persistent, unexplained illnesses: el-

evated anti-early antigen antibodies. *Ann Intern Med* 1985;102:1–7.
79. Straus SE, Tosato G, Armstrong G, et al. Persisting illness and fatigue in adults with evidence of Epstein-Barr virus infection. *Ann Intern Med* 1985;102:7–16.
80. Salit IE. Sporadic postinfectious neuromyasthenia. *Can Med Assoc J* 1985;133:659–63.
81. Caligiuri M, Murray C, Buchwald D, et al. Phenotypic and functional deficiency of natural killer cells in patients with chronic fatigue syndrome. *J Immunol* 1987;139:3306–13.
82. Straus SE. EB or not EB—that is the question. *JAMA* 1987;257:2335–6.
83. Kerns DL, Shira JE, Go S, et al. Ampicillin rash in children: relationship to penicillin allergy and infectious mononucleosis. *Am J Dis Child* 1973;125:187–90.
84. Neel EU. Infectious mononucleosis: death due to agranulocytosis and pneumonia. *JAMA* 1976; 236:1493–4.
85. Bender CE. The value of corticosteroids in the treatment of infectious mononucleosis. *JAMA* 1967;199:529–31.
86. Bolden KJ. Corticosteroids in the treatment of infectious mononucleosis. *J R Coll Gen Pract* 1972;22:87–95.
87. Andersson J, Ernberg I. Management of Epstein-Barr virus infections. *Am J Med* 1988; 85:107–15.
88. Colby BM, Shaw JE, Elion GB, Pagano JS. Effect of acyclovir [9-(2-hydroxyethoxymethyl) guanine] on Epstein-Barr virus DNA replication. *J Virol* 1980;34:560–8.
89. Lin JC, Smith MC, Pagano JS. Prolonged inhibitory effect of 9-(1,3-dihydroxy-2-propoxymethyl) guanine against replication of Epstein-Barr virus. *J Virol* 1984;50:50–5.
90. Lin JC, Smith MC, Pagano JS. Comparative efficacy and selectivity of some nucleoside analogs against Epstein-Barr virus. *Antimicrob Agents Chemother* 1985;27:971–3.
91. Kure S, Tada K, Wada J, Yoshie O. Inhibition of Epstein-Barr virus infection *in vitro* by recombinant human interferons α and γ. *Virus Res* 1986;5:377–90.
92. Andersson J, Skoldenberg B, Henle W, et al. Acyclovir treatment in infectious mononucleosis: a clinical and immunological study. *Infection* 1987;15(suppl 1):514–21.
93. Sullivan JC, Medveczky P, Forman SJ, Baker SM, Monroe JE, Mulder C. Epstein-Barr virus-induced lymphoproliferation. *N Engl J Med* 1984;311:1163–7.
94. Shofer H, Ochsendorf F, Helm F, Milbrandt R. Treatment of oral hairy leukoplakia in AIDS patients with vitamin A acid (topically) or acyclovir (systemically). *Dermatologica* 1987; 174:150–1.
95. Katz BZ, Niederman JC, Olson BA, et al. Fragment length polymorphisms among independent isolates of Epstein-Barr virus from immunocompromised and normal hosts. *J Infect Dis* 1988;157(2):299–308.
96. Kure S, Tada K, Wada J, et al. Inhibition of Epstein-Barr virus infection *in vitro* by recombinant human interferons α and γ. *Virus Res* 1986;5:377–90.
97. Aronson FR, Dempsey RA, Allegretta M, et al. Malignant granular lymphoproliferation after Epstein-Barr virus infection: partial immunologic reconstitution with Interlukin-2. *Am J Hematol* 1987;25:427–39.
98. Epstein MA, Morgan AJ. Clinical consequences of Epstein-Barr virus infection and possible control by an anti-viral vaccine. *Clin Exp Immunol* 1983;53:257–71.
99. Patrascu IV, Tache M. Epstein-Barr virus (EBV). IV. Studies on experimental inactivated vaccine against human EBV infection. *Virology* 1988;39:29–33.
100. Emini EA, Schleif WA, Armstrong ME, et al. Antigenic analysis of the Epstein-Barr virus major membrane antigen (gp350/220) expressed in yeast and mammalian cells: implications for the development of a subunit vaccine. *Virology* 1988;166:387–93.
101. Epstein MA, Morgan AJ, Finerty S, et al. Protection of cottontop tamarins against Epstein-Barr virus-induced malignant lymphoma by a prototype subunit vaccine. *Nature* 1985; 318:287–9.
102. Morgan AJ, Finerty S, Lovgren K, et al. Prevention of Epstein-Barr (EB) virus-induced lymphoma in cottontop tamarins by vaccination with the EB virus envelope glycoprotein gp340 incorporated into immune-stimulating complexes. *J Gen Virol* 1988;69:2093–6.
103. Lowe RS, Keller PM, Keech BJ, et al. Varicella-zoster virus as a live vector for the expression of foreign genes. *Proc Natl Acad Sci USA* 1987;84:3896–900.
104. Morgan AJ, Mackett M, Finerty S, et al. Recombinant vaccinia virus expressing Epstein-Barr virus glucoprotein gp340 protects cottontop tamarins against EB virus-induced malignant lymphomas. *J Med Virol* 1988;25:189–95.
105. Salahuddin SZ, Ablashi DV, Markham PD, et al. Isolation of a new virus, HBLV, in patients with lymphoproliferative disorders. *Science* 1986;234:596–601.
106. Josephs SF, Salahuddin ZS, Ablashi DV, Schachter F, Wong-Staal F, Gallo RC. Genomic analysis of the human B-lymphotrovic virus (HBLV). *Science* 1986;234:601–3.
107. Downing RG, Sewankambo N, Serwadda D, et al. Isolation of human lymphotropic herpesviruses from Uganda. *Lancet* 1987;2:390.
108. Tedder RS, Briggs M, Cameron CH, Honess R, Robertson D, Whittle H. A novel lymphotropic herpesvirus. *Lancet* 1987;2:390–2.
109. Ablashi DV, Josephs SF, Buchbinder A, et al. Human B-lymphotropic virus (human herpesvirus-6). *J Virol Methods* 1988;21:29–48.
110. Biberfeld P, Kramarsky B, Salahuddin SA, Gallo RC. Ultrastructural characterization of a new human B lymphotropic DNA virus (human herpesvirus 6) isolated from patients with lymphoproliferative disease. *JNCI* 1987;79: 933–41.
111. Lopez C, Pellett P, Stewart J, et al. Character-

istics of human herpesvirus-6. *J Infect Dis* 1988;157:1271–3.

112. Josephs SF, Ablashi DV, Salahuddin SZ, et al. Molecular studies of HHV-6. *J Virol Methods* 1988;21:179–90.
113. Efstathiou S, Gompels UA, Craxton MA, Honess RW, Ward K. DNA homology between a novel human herpesvirus (HHV-6) and human cytomegalovirus. *Lancet* 1988;1:63–4.
114. Kishi M, Harada H, Takahashi M, et al. A repeat sequence, GGGTTA, is shared by DNA of human B lymphotropic virus (HHV-6 or HBLV) and Marek's disease virus (MDV). *J Virol* 1988;62:4824–7.
115. Albashi DV, Salahuddin SZ, Josephs SF, Imam F, Lusso P, Gallo RC. Replication of HBLV (or HHV-6) in human cell lines. *Nature* 1987;329:207.
116. Lusso P, Salahuddin SZ, Ablashi DV, Gallo RC. Diverse tropism of human B lymphotropic virus (human herpesvirus 6). *Lancet* 1987; 2:743–4.
117. Lusso P, Markham PD, Tschachler E, et al. *In vitro* cellular tropism of human B lymphotropic virus (human herpesvirus-6). *J Exp Med* 1988; 167:1659–70.
118. Lopez C, Pellett P, Stewart J, et al. Characteristics of human herpesvirus-6. *J Infect Dis* 1988;157:1271–3.
119. Pietroboni GR, Harnett GB, Bucens MR, et al. Isolation of human herpesvirus-6 from saliva. *Lancet* 1988;1(8593):1059.
120. Josephs SF, Buchbinder A, Streicher HZ, et al. Detection of human B lymphotropic virus (human herpesvirus 6) sequences in B cell lymphoma tissues of three patients. *Leukemia* 1988;2:132–5.
121. Biberfeld P, Petren A-L, Eklund A, et al. Human herpesvirus-6 (HHV-6, HBLV) in sarcoidosis and lymphoproliferative disorders. *J Virol Methods* 1988;21:49–59.
122. Buchbinder A, Josephs SF, Ablashi D, et al. Polymerase chain reaction amplification and in situ hybridization for the detection of human B-lymphotropic virus. *J Virol Methods* 1988;21:191–7.
123. Yamanishi K, Okuno T, Shiraki K, Takahashi M, *et al.* Identification of human herpesvirus-6 as a causal agent for *Exanthem subitum*. *Lancet* 1988;1:1065–7.
124. Berenberg W, Wright S, Janeway CA. *Roseola infantum (Exanthem subitum). N Engl J Med* 1949;241:253–9.
125. Cherry JD. Roseola infantum (*Exanthem subitum*) In: Feigris RD, Cherry JD, eds. *Textbook of pediatric infectious diseases*. Philadelphia: W.B. Saunders, 1987:1842–5.
126. Krueger GRF, Kock B, Ramon A, et al. Antibody prevalence to HBLV (human herpesvirus-6, HHV-6) and suggestive pathogenicity in the general population and in patients with immune deficiency syndromes. *J Virol Methods* 1988; 21:125–31.
127. Saxinger C, Polesky H, Eby N, et al. Antibody reactivity with HBLV (HHV-6) in U.S. populations. *J Virol Methods* 1988;21:199–208.
128. Linde A, Dahl H, Wahren B, et al. IgG antibodies to human herpesvirus-6 in children and adults both in primary Epstein-Barr virus and cytomegalovirus infections. *J Virol Methods* 1988;21:117–23.
129. Komaroff AL. Chronic fatigue syndromes: relationship to chronic viral infections. *J Virol Methods* 1988;21:3–10.
130. Yirshaut Y, Glade P, Octavio L, et al. Sarcoidosis, another disease associated with serologic evidence for herpes-like virus infection. *N Engl J Med* 1970;283:502–6.
131. Johansson B, Klein G, Henle W, et al. Epstein-Barr virus (EBV)–associated antibody patterns in malignant lymphoma and leukemia. I. Hodgkin's disease. *Int J Cancer* 1970;6:450–62.
132. Streicher HZ, Hung CL, Ablashi DV, et al. *In vitro* inhibition of human herpesvirus-6 by phosphonoformate. *J Virol Methods* 1988; 21:301–4.
133. Schooley RT, Dolin R. Epstein-Barr virus (infectious mononucleosis). In: Mandell, Douglas, Bennett, eds. *Principles and practice of infectious diseases*. New York: John Wiley & Sons, 1979:1324–41.
134. Schofer H, Ochsendorf FR, Helm EB, et al. Treatment of oral "hairy" leukoplakia in AIDS patients with vitamin A acid (topically) or acyclovir (systemically). *Dermatologica* 1987; 174:150–1.
135. Friedman-Kien AE. Viral origin of hairy leukoplakia. *Lancet* 1986;2:694–5.

*Antiviral Agents and Viral Diseases of Man, 3rd Edition,* edited by G. J. Galasso, R. J. Whitley, and T. C. Merigan, Raven Press, Ltd., New York 1990.

# 17

# Cytomegalovirus and the Immunosuppressed Patient

Judith Falloon and Henry Masur

*Critical Care Medicine Department, Warren G. Magnuson Clinical Center, National Institutes of Health, Bethesda, Maryland 20892*



The human cytomegalovirus (CMV), a herpesvirus named for the effect it produces in cell culture, is a double-stranded DNA virus approximately 200 nm in diameter. An icosahedral capsid composed of 162 capsomeres surrounds the DNA-containing core and is itself surrounded by an envelope. The CMV genome is large, but the number of proteins produced is not known. Different CMV strains can be distinguished by restriction endonuclease analysis of viral DNA (1).

*In vivo* CMV infects a wide range of host tissues (2). After primary human infection, the CMV DNA becomes incorporated into host cells in latent form and persists lifelong (3). Although the sites of latency are uncertain, some evidence suggests that peripheral blood leukocytes are latently infected (4).

Latent CMV infection is assumed in the seropositive person. Other types of CMV infection are active infection, usually defined as the presence of culturable virus and/or of significant rises in the titer of antibody to CMV, and CMV disease, defined as the presence of signs or symptoms attributable to CMV infection. CMV infection can be primary, occurring in the previously uninfected, seronegative host, or recurrent, occurring in the previously infected, seropositive host. Recurrent infections can be caused either by the reactivation of latent virus or by reinfection from an exogenous source.

## EPIDEMIOLOGY

### Routes of Transmission

Humans are the only known reservoir for human CMV. Modes of transmission are not fully elucidated, but presumed routes include congenital, sexual, parenteral (through blood transfusion or organ transplantation), and close contact with a person who is excreting the virus (5–7). Transmission through saliva, either directly or possibly through contamination of environmental surfaces such as toys, is thought to occur (8). After CMV infection, the excretion of virus in urine, oral secretions, or genital fluids can be prolonged or recurrent, even in the absence of symptoms, accounting for the wide exposure of humans to CMV. This prolonged or recurrent excretion of CMV can occur in both immunocompetent and immunosuppressed individuals.

Congenital infection occurs as a consequence of either maternal primary infection or, more commonly, of maternal CMV reactivation (9). Perinatal CMV infection can also occur, either through contact of the baby during delivery with infected maternal genital secretions or through the ingestion of infected breast milk (9). Because of the frequency with which infected young children shed CMV in urine and saliva, CMV transmission is common in childhood, and the virus often spreads throughout such groups as children in daycare and families with young children (5,10,11).

Sexual transmission has been suggested by the presence of CMV in semen and in secretions of the uterine cervix, by the association of CMV infection with infection of the sexual partner (including evidence that the same strain infects partners), by the correlation of CMV seropositivity with sexual activity, and by the high incidence and prevalence of CMV infection in male homosexuals (12–14). Passive anal intercourse has been implicated as a risk factor for CMV seroconversion in homosexual men (14).

### Incidence and Prevalence

Serologic studies indicate that infection can be acquired throughout life. The percentage of a population that is seropositive depends on the socioeconomic setting, geographic location, and childrearing practices (breastfeeding, group care, etc.). By adulthood, more than 45–70% of the population of the United States has been infected with CMV (5). In contrast, 100% of adult women in the Ivory Coast are CMV-infected (9). In young adult populations in the United States and England, seroconversion rates of 0.6–5.5% per year have been reported (15,16).

## CLINICAL MANIFESTATIONS

### Immunocompetent Hosts

Immunocompetent hosts infected after birth typically are asymptomatic, but they can be symptomatic with such syndromes as CMV mononucleosis or postperfusion syndrome (17,18). Clinical manifestations of CMV mononucleosis include fever, myalgia, malaise, headache, sore throat, rash, splenomegaly, pharyngeal erythema, and adenopathy. The average duration of fever in one study was 19 days (17). Laboratory manifestations include lymphocytosis and the presence of atypical lymphocytes, elevations in serum transaminases, and the presence of antibodies such as rheumatoid factor, antinuclear antibodies, cryoglobulins, and cold agglutinins. Complications attributed to CMV disease in immunocompetent patients include pneumonia, myocarditis, pericarditis, central nervous system (CNS) abnormalities including meningoencephalitis and Guillain-Barré syndrome, granulomatous hepatitis, jaundice, and hematologic abnormalities including hemolysis; however, these complications are rare. The diagnosis is made by the use of CMV serology and culture, with CMV viremia, seroconversion, and/or the presence of immunoglobulin M (IgM) antibody to CMV most strongly suggesting the diagnosis. The absence of IgM antibody in this population argues against a diagnosis of CMV disease.

### Immunocompromised Hosts

Immunocompromised patients with defects in cell-mediated immunity can also have asymptomatic infection or mild disease, but they are at greater risk of developing devastating and life-threatening disease. Patients at greatest risk for severe disease are those with a history of organ or bone marrow transplantation and those with immunologic defects caused by infection with the human immunodeficiency virus (HIV). Active CMV infection in the immunocompromised patient can result from the reactivation of the patient's own latent infection, the acquisition of CMV from transfused blood products or from the donor organ or bone marrow, or, less likely, from contacts with other people. Although primary infection is more likely to be symptomatic, active infection caused by reactivation (or exogenous reinfection) is more common, both because of the high proportion of patients who are seropositive prior to transplant and because the risk of active infection is greater in the seropositive than in the seronegative patient (19–22).

In an immunocompromised host, illness caused by CMV can be manifested as dysfunction of one specific organ or as dysfunction of multiple organ systems. Although certain patterns of infection are more represented in some groups of patients, the types of infections caused are similar despite the specific etiology of the immunosuppression. The clinical course and prognosis, however, differ among the groups at risk.

### Pulmonary Disease

CMV pneumonitis is most commonly seen among bone marrow transplant patients, but it is also seen in other transplant recipients and in patients with HIV infection (22–24). The pneumonitis presents with fever, nonproductive cough, dyspnea, tachypnea, hypoxemia, and sometimes rales (23,25). Radiographs usually show an interstitial pneumonia, although occasional patients have localized alveolar infiltrates, nodules, or cavities on chest radiograph (25,26). Because CMV pneumonitis often occurs in conjunction with other infections, especially *Pneumocystis carinii* pneumonia (PCP), the contribution of CMV to these more unusual radiographic patterns is difficult to determine (23,25,27). The mortality of CMV pneumonitis in the bone marrow transplant patient is very high (more than 80%), although precise estimations of mortality in various populations are difficult to obtain because the definition of CMV pneumonia is based on different criteria in various published series. Although the mortality of CMV pneumonia is probably lower in patients with renal transplants, pneumonia is usually present in fatal CMV infection in these patients.

The clinical and radiographic manifestations of the pneumonitis are not specific for CMV, so that a firm diagnosis of CMV pneumonitis must be based on laboratory criteria. Because the shedding of CMV from the oropharynx is common in the immunocompromised patient, the isolation of CMV from sputum, bronchoalveolar lavage fluids, or biopsy specimens does not necessarily mean that CMV is the cause of the pneumonitis. There is no general agreement in the literature as to the precise definition of CMV pneumonia, i.e., as to what laboratory evidence suffices to prove that CMV is the cause of pulmonary dysfunction in a patient. A clear-cut, unequivocal diagnosis of CMV pneumonia depends on the recognition of extensive typical histologic findings of CMV in the lung tissue and the exclusion of other pathogens. Although an interstitial pneumonitis in the setting of CMV seroconversion or of the detection of virus, viral antigens, or viral nucleic acids in fluids or tissues can be suggestive, patients at risk for CMV pneumonitis are also at risk for other pneumonias, and the significance of these findings is less certain. It is possible that many undiagnosed cases of interstitial pneumonitis in the immunocompromised host in which the histologic findings of CMV are not seen are in fact caused by CMV, but it is currently impossible to prove or disprove such a possibility.

### Retinitis

Although CMV retinitis is now most commonly seen in the HIV-infected patient, it has occasionally been recognized in other immunosuppressed patients as well (24,28,29). It can occur late after renal transplantation (29). Symptoms of CMV retinitis are absent or nonspecific, with patients noting blurred vision, scotomata, or decreased visual acuity, but not ocular pain (28,30). The typical fundoscopic appearance is that of progressive, opaque, yellow-white lesions in the retina, generally in a vascular distribution, sometimes with vessel sheathing and hemorrhage (30) (Fig. 1). Progression is centrifugal with an active advancing edge and central atrophic scarring (30). If there is coexisting uveitis or vitritis, it is usually mild. Foci can be single or multiple within each eye, and the disease can be uniocular or bilateral (30). In transplant patients, spontaneous resolution has occurred (29), but in HIV-infected patients, untreated disease appears to be inexorably progressive with few exceptions. CMV retinitis may cause visual loss and blindness (24,28). Even with successful therapy, retinal detachment can result in new visual loss (24). Although CMV retinitis sometimes occurs in the presence of more widely disseminated CMV disease, it alone can be the major clinical manifestation of the patient's CMV infection so that the impetus for treatment is usually the sparing of vision rather than the saving of life.

CMV retinitis is diagnosed by clinical criteria, because biopsy of the retina risks retinal detachment and cultures of ocular specimens are often not helpful (24,28). The fundoscopic appearance is so typical that clinical diagnosis by an experienced ophthalmologist is generally accurate. Early lesions can be confused with cotton wool spots, but repeat examination usually demonstrates the difference because CMV retinitis tends to advance rapidly. Culturing CMV from other sites such as blood supports, but is not necessary for diagnosis, especially when therapy is being considered, because culture results can take an unacceptable amount of time to obtain.

### Gastrointestinal Disease

CMV infection of the gastrointestinal tract has been described in transplant patients, but most of the experience has been in the HIV-infected patient. CMV can cause disease in any part of the gastrointestinal tract; it can be manifested as esophagitis, gastritis, enteritis, or colitis (24,31). Gastrointestinal disease can be the only manifestation of CMV disease, or it may be a part of a multi-organ process. Patients with gastrointestinal CMV disease usually have fever and weight loss. Esophagitis or gastritis is manifested as dysphagia, odyn-

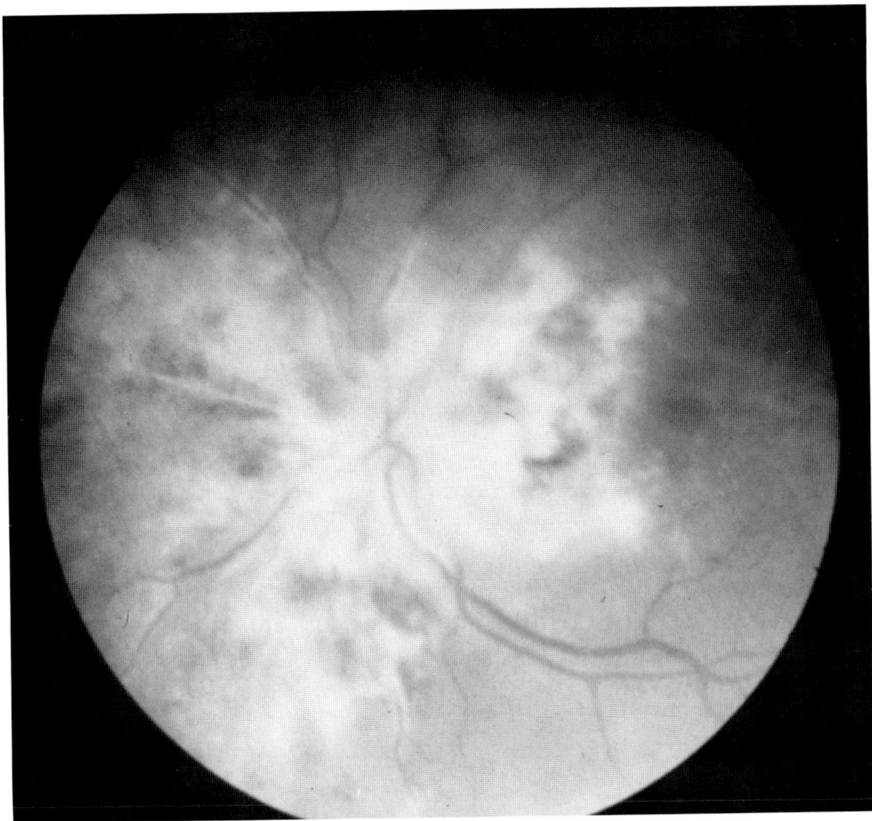

**FIG. 1.** CMV retinitis in a patient with HIV infection.

ophagia, and substernal or epigastric pain. The symptoms of colitis include abdominal pain and diarrhea, which can be copious or bloody (32,33). A wide spectrum of clinical manifestations can occur. Some patients with histologically proven disease can be asymptomatic, but the course is generally one of prolonged symptoms in the untreated patient (24). Serious hemorrhage and mucosal perforation occur but are not common (24,26). Endoscopy may reveal mucosal erythema, edema, hemorrhage, and erosions or ulcerations.

Although endoscopic findings can suggest the diagnosis, they are nonspecific, as are the abnormalities that can be demonstrated radiographically (Fig. 2). The diagnosis must be confirmed by biopsy. Because histologic findings may be patchy, multiple biopsies may be needed (32). Occasionally, histologic findings of CMV infection are found in biopsies from visually normal mucosa (32). Culturing CMV from rectal swabs, stool, or tissue is not sensitive or specific enough to provide a diagnosis, although culturing CMV from tissue can help confirm a histologic diagnosis (24,32). As in CMV pneumonitis, a precise and generally accepted set of criteria for the diagnosis of CMV esophagitis, gastritis, enteritis, or colitis have not been established. Other treatable pathogens need to be sought in cases of suspected CMV gastrointestinal disease. If symptoms or signs do not resolve when these other pathogens are treated, then therapy for CMV can be considered. Those patients with characteristic symptoms, inflamed or ulcerated mu-

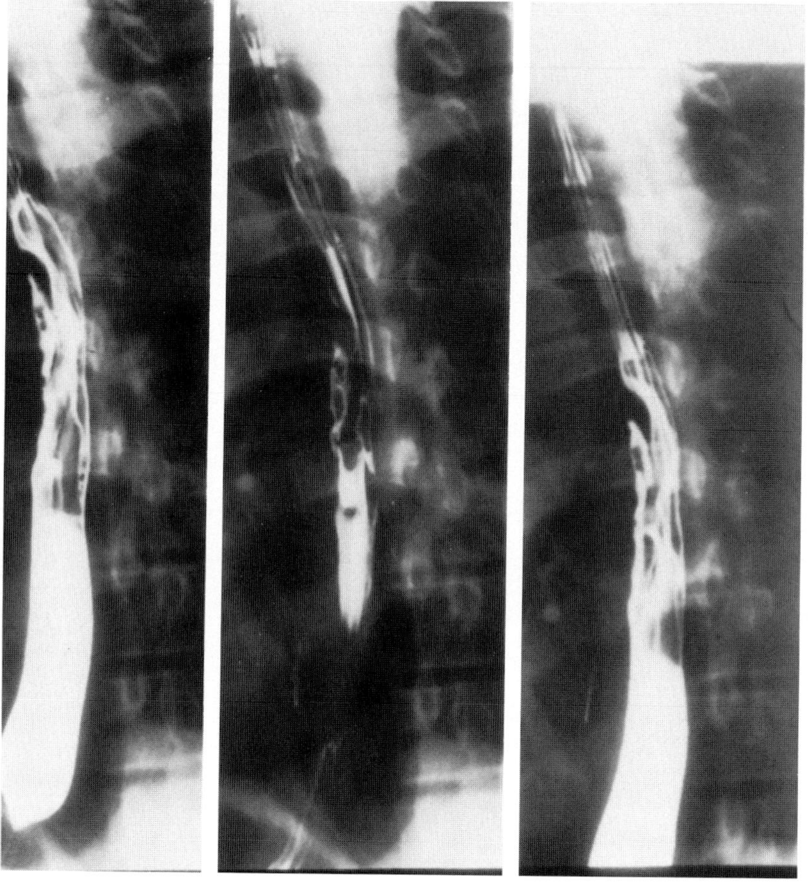

**FIG. 2.** Barium swallow demonstrating esophagitis in a patient with HIV infection. On endoscopic biopsy, CMV inclusion bodies were found.

cosa seen on endoscopy, and CMV inclusions on histology appear to be the most likely to respond to anti-CMV therapy.

### Other Manifestations of CMV Infection

Fever is characteristic of CMV disease in the immunocompromised host, and CMV disease in the transplant patient can be manifested exclusively as a self-limited febrile illness. Other findings in transplant patients are some combination of leukopenia, atypical lymphocytes and lymphocytosis, myalgia, arthralgia, increased hepatic transaminases, thrombocytopenia, abdominal pain, pneumonia, hepatosplenomegaly, gastrointestinal bleeding, or diarrhea (19,20,26,34–36). Although CMV is associated with the febrile wasting syndrome seen in some HIV-infected patients, its role in causing this syndrome is not yet clarified. The diagnosis of disseminated CMV disease remains a clinical one, supported by laboratory evidence of seroconversion, viral shredding or viremia, or CMV in tissues.

CMV is thought to cause a variety of other clinical entities. Hepatitis, seen predominantly in transplant patients, is manifested as hepatic dysfunction that can be chronic and even fatal (37,38). Hepatitis is diagnosed by the occurrence of hepatic dysfunction that is temporally linked to

CMV infection or, with greater certainty, by liver biopsy in which histologic evidence for CMV is found (26,31,37,38). CMV adrenalitis has been described in HIV-infected patients. It was initially an autopsy finding, but associated hypoadrenalism has been documented (24). Occasional cases of CMV encephalitis in adults have occurred, generally but not exclusively in HIV-infected patients. Because CMV encephalitis is a difficult diagnosis to make, its incidence is uncertain, although it appears to be rare (39,40). CMV encephalitis is manifested by abnormalities of mentation. Because symptoms, scans, and spinal fluid findings, including CMV cultures, are not specific, CMV encephalitis is diagnosed by biopsy or autopsy with the demonstration of histologic changes caused by CMV. The fact that some HIV-infected patients with encephalitis have responded to anti-CMV therapy suggest that CMV or other herpesvirus has played a role in the brain disease in these patients (24,41). CMV myelopathy has occurred in a few patients infected with HIV, and spinal fluid grew CMV in some of these cases (40). Also in HIV-infected patients, a syndrome of papillary stenosis and sclerosing cholangitis in which CMV may play some role has been described (42). Since there are no clear-cut criteria for the diagnosis of CMV hepatitis, adrenal disease, and CNS disease, the contribution of CMV infection to these entities can be difficult to determine. These are not commonly diagnosed clinical entities.

Active CMV infection may itself be immunosuppressive, and there is a correlation between active CMV infection and an increased risk of other serious infections in renal and heart transplant patients (43–45). CMV may also be a cofactor in the progression of HIV infection, and it has been proposed as a cofactor in the development of Kaposi's sarcoma in HIV-infected homosexual men (46). There is speculation that CMV may be oncogenic, but firm evidence supporting this hypothesis does not exist.

## CMV INFECTION IN SPECIFIC PATIENT POPULATIONS

### Renal Transplant Recipients

Active CMV infection is common among the recipients of transplanted kidneys (19, 20,22,26,27,34,47). Overall, 38–96% of renal transplant patients will develop active CMV infection as manifested by rises in complement fixation titers or by the recovery of virus from any site in the first 7 months after transplantation (5). The variability in infection rates is caused by differences in the study methods, the populations studied, and the immunosuppressive regimens used (22,26). From pooled data, Glenn (22) estimated that 53% of seronegative and 85% of seropositive patients will develop active infection after transplantation. Of seronegative recipients receiving a kidney from a seropositive donor, 77% will develop active infection (22). In contrast, only 8% of seronegative patients whose kidney donors were also seronegative developed active CMV infection, attesting to the importance of the donor kidney in the development of primary CMV infection after renal transplantation. The acquisition of infection from the donor kidney probably occurs in seropositive recipients of kidneys from seropositive donors as well, since exogenous reinfection has been demonstrated by restriction enzyme analysis of strains shed before and after transplantation (48); however, the contribution of exogenous reinfection versus reactivation of latent infection to active infection of CMV disease in seropositive transplant recipients is difficult to determine.

Although many actively infected renal transplant recipients are asymptomatic, 40–50% of those actively infected (38–96% of all recipients) will have associated clinical illness; thus, approximately 30% of all recipients will have symptomatic CMV disease (22,26). Fever is almost always present in symptomatic patients, and active CMV infection may be the most common cause of fever after kidney transplantation (26). Pneumonia occurs in 42% of patients with symptomatic infection (26). Active CMV infection in renal transplant recipients also causes a glomerulopathy that can result in allograft dysfunction (49) and is associated with decreased allograft survival, although its direct role in causing graft rejection is controversial (5,22,26,47). Risk factors for the development of CMV disease include the transplantation of a kidney from a seropositive donor into a seronegative recipient and the use of more immunosuppressive regimens, particularly those that employ antithymocyte globulin. CMV disease is becoming less common as cyclosporine replaces other immunosuppressive regimens.

CMV infection in renal transplant recipients has a mortality of approximately 2–20% and is an important contributor to mortality after renal transplantation (22,26,27,47). The inability to mount an antibody response or to develop CMV-specific cytotoxic lymphocyte responses appears to be a poor prognostic sign (21). The period of greatest risk for active CMV infection in the renal transplant patient is the first 3–4 months after transplantation (26,27), but delayed and recurrent CMV disease occur (22,26).

### Bone Marrow Transplant Recipients

CMV is the single most important infectious cause of death in bone marrow transplant recipients (23,50,51). Approximately 50% of bone marrow transplant recipients develop active CMV infection (51). Of these, 64% have recurrent infection. The most important form of CMV disease in this population is CMV pneumonitis, which occurs in approximately 16% of patients and has a mortality of 80–90% (50,51). Risk factors for the development of CMV disease in bone marrow transplant patients include older age, seropositive antibody status prior to transplantation, transplantation for hematologic malignancy rather than aplastic anemia, more immunosuppressive preparative regimen, and the development of graft-versus-host disease, especially if it is treated with antithymocyte globulin (23,27,50,51). The failure to develop CMV-specific cytotoxic responses is a poor prognostic finding in patients with CMV disease (52). The receipt of granulocyte transfusions or of bone marrow from a seropositive donor also increases the risk of the development of CMV infection in the seronegative patient (51); however, the role of the donor marrow is complicated by the possibility of the adoptive transfer of immunity. In one report, seropositive recipients who received marrow from seronegative donors were more likely to have severe CMV disease than were those who received marrow from a seropositive donor (53). CMV disease is most likely to occur within the first 3 to 4 months after marrow transplantation (23,51).

### Heart and Liver Transplant Recipients

Active CMV infection occurs in 73% or more of patients after heart transplantation and is also common after heart-lung transplantation (5,36). In this setting, CMV leads to morbidity, especially fever and pneumonia, in approximately 40% of patients. It is also associated with an increased risk of other types of infections (27,43,45). Although the donor organ is an important source of CMV infection, the multiple blood transfusions required in liver and heart transplantation could also be an important source of infection (27,45,54,55). Active CMV infection occurred in 59% of 121 liver transplant recipients (55). The majority of patients with primary infection (88%) were symptomatic. Although seropositive recipients were more likely to develop active CMV infection, fewer patients (32%) with reactivated disease were symptomatic.

### HIV-Infected Patient

CMV is a common infection in populations at risk for the development of HIV infection. Nearly all homosexual men have serologic evidence of recently acquired or reactivated CMV infection, and 30% shed CMV in the urine at least intermittently (14). Thus, in the HIV-infected homosexual man, the intermittent shedding of CMV in urine or saliva is common. In patients severely immunocompromised by HIV infection, i.e., those with the acquired immunodeficiency syndromes (AIDS), CMV viremia occurs in the majority of patients, and 69–90% have histologic evidence of CMV at autopsy (24,56–59). Although CMV is found in many organs at autopsy, its role in causing illness or death is often unclear (57,58). The diagnosis of CMV disease is made in life in less than 10% of AIDS patients. Retinitis is the first and gastroenteritis the second most commonly recognized manifestation (24). True CMV pneumonitis appears to be uncommon in AIDS patients, although culturing CMV from bronchoalveolar lavage fluid is not uncommon; CMV is often present when PCP is diagnosed. Encephalitis is a difficult diagnosis to make, but it, too, appears to be uncommon (40).

Serious CMV infection is seen after the immune system has been greatly compromised by HIV infection, so that it is usually accompanied by other opportunistic infections and occurs when the number of circulating helper T cells is quite low (less than 100/mm$^3$) (59). Thus, survival after the diagnosis of serious CMV disease in this population is typically measured in months. In one group of untreated patients with CMV retinitis, the median survival was 4 months (59). Since HIV-infected patients cannot reconstitute their immune systems, spontaneous cures of CMV disease in this setting probably do not occur, although the natural history of CMV disease in HIV-infected patients has not been conclusively documented. CMV disease in this population can respond to therapy; however, as in other infections in these patients, relapses occur after treatment is completed unless an adequate maintenance regimen can be devised.

### Other Immunosuppressed Patients

Other immunosuppressed patients have been less extensively studied but are thought to be at risk for active CMV infection and, less commonly, CMV disease (5,22). The incidence of active CMV infection and of CMV disease in patients with malignant neoplasms is not clearly established, although patients with cancer and CMV disease are seen (25). Pneumonia seems to be the primary clinical consequence of CMV disease in these patients, but it is not frequently documented by biopsy or autopsy (25). In patients with cancer, the role of their underlying malignancy in predisposing to active CMV infection and disease is difficult to distinguish from the role of the immunosuppressive therapies and blood transfusions they receive (2,5,60,61). Cytotoxic agents appear to play a role in the reactivation of CMV infection, however. In a group of patients in a rheumatology clinic, those receiving cytotoxic agents were more likely to be shedding CMV than those receiving glucocorticoid therapy, and there was a temporal relationship between the onset of virus shedding and beginning cytotoxic therapy (62). None of these patients had CMV disease.

## DIAGNOSIS

The presence of CMV can be documented directly by viral isolation, electron microscopy (EM), histologic or cytologic evaluation of specimens, or by the demonstration of CMV genome or antigen within specimens (63,64). CMV infection can also be diagnosed by demonstrating the production of antibody to CMV. Because of the ubiquity of this virus, it can be difficult to demonstrate a causal relationship between the detection of virus or serologic response and the development of clinical illness. In addition, diagnostic methods such as conventional cultures and paired serology result in a delay in diagnosis, providing an impetus for the development of more rapid, sensitive, and specific tests for the diagnosis of CMV infection and disease.

### Histopathology, Cytology, and Electron Microscopy

CMV is documented in tissues by the demonstration of characteristic enlarged (cytomegalic) cells with large nuclear inclusions separated from the nuclear membrane by a prominent clear halo ("owl's eye") and/or small cytoplasmic inclusions (2) (Fig. 3). The true sensitivity of histology in making the diagnosis of CMV disease cannot be determined. It has been shown that CMV can be cultured from tissues approximately four to six times more frequently than typical inclusions are seen (2,61). The demonstration of CMV inclusions, however, remains the most substantial evidence of the role of CMV in causing dysfunction of the biopsied organ. In some cases, CMV inclusions are sparse and difficult to find. The presence in a biopsy specimen of many cells with CMV inclusion bodies may indicate more clinically important CMV disease than the presence of only a single CMV inclusion-containing cell, but there is no consensus on this issue.

Urine specimens can be examined cyto-

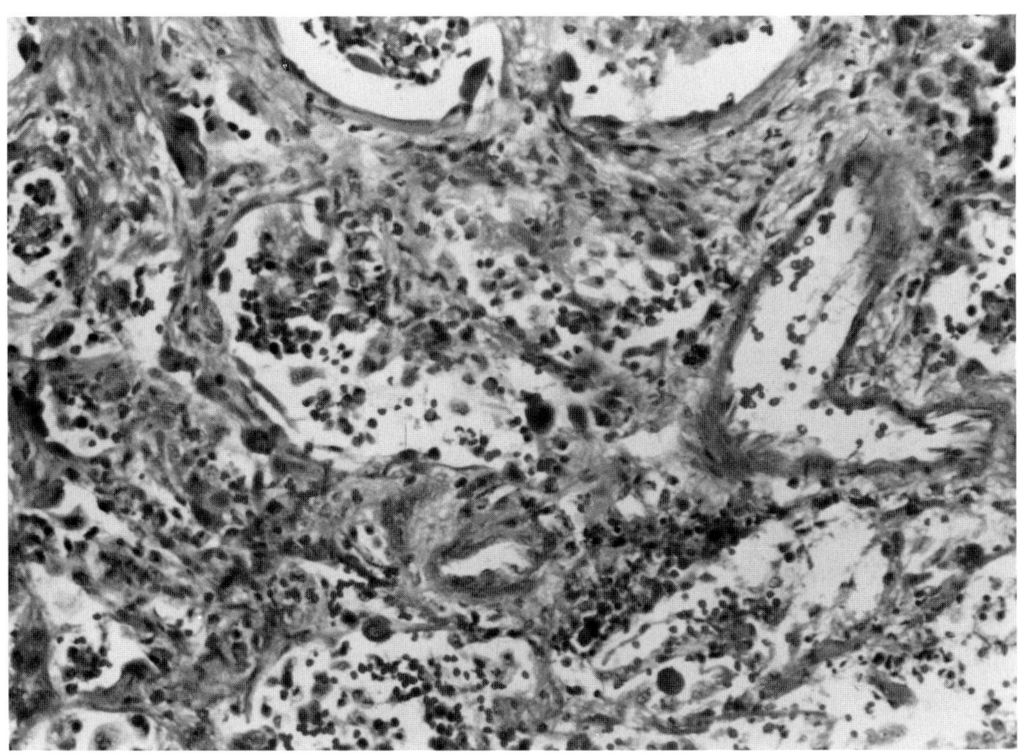

**FIG. 3.** Pulmonary tissue obtained from a patient with HIV infection and CMV pneumonitis demonstrating an inflammatory cell infiltrate and enlarged (cytomegalic) cells with inclusion bodies.

logically for CMV-infected cells, but this test is neither specific nor sensitive (63). Cytologic examination of specimens obtained by bronchoalveolar lavage can rapidly provide evidence of CMV infection. The cytologic demonstration of CMV is specific, although it is probably less sensitive than culture (65,66). The role of cytology in making the diagnosis of CMV pneumonitis remains to be clarified. Although EM has been used to demonstrate CMV in the urine of infected infants, this technique is less useful in the immunosuppressed patient because the titer of CMV is lower and because human herpesviruses cannot be distinguished from each other by EM (63,67,68). In addition, the demonstration by EM of a herpesvirus in the urine would have the same significance as a positive culture from that site; however, the results of EM are obtained more rapidly than are those of conventional cultures.

### Culture

CMV can be cultured only in human fibroblast cells, and growth in these cell cultures can be slow when the inoculated specimen has a low titer of virus. At least 4–6 weeks are required before determining that a culture is negative by the absence of cytopathic effect (CPE) (63,64). Culture is thus tedious, and its reliability depends on the correct acquisition and handling of specimens and on the experience of the laboratory. Techniques to detect CMV in culture more rapidly than the conventional demonstration of CPE are being developed. In one such test, conventional cultures are stained for the detection of early antigen fluorescent foci (DEAFF) that precede the development of CPE (67,69). Another method now being used in some laboratories is a centrifugation culture assay in which monoclonal antibodies and immunofluorescence (IF) techniques are used to detect CMV antigens in overnight shell vial cell cultures (66,70). This test is rapid and appears to be both sensitive and specific.

Specimens from which CMV can most often be cultured include urine, blood or buffy coat, saliva or throat washings, bronchoscopy or bronchoalveolar lavage specimens, tissue specimens, and cervical fluid or semen. The isolation of CMV from any site does not provide a diagnosis of CMV disease, since such isolates are frequently present in the absence of disease. The detection of CMV in blood may be a more significant finding, although again it can be found in asymptomatic patients (24,26,36,49,71).

### Antigen Detection

CMV can be demonstrated within infected cells in tissues or in body fluids by the use of antibodies to CMV and IF techniques (63–66). Because CMV infection induces the appearance of an Fc receptor with a high affinity for human IgG, mouse monoclonal antibodies are particularly useful for this testing (72). Mouse monoclonal antibodies have been demonstrated to be sensitive for the detection of CMV in respiratory tract specimens when IF is compared with culture, but the true sensitivity and specificity of this technique for identifying infection or disease are difficult to determine (65,66,70,73). For example, in some cases where IF is positive and culture is negative, the IF result appears likely to be valid. This technique can be performed on bronchoalveolar lavage specimens and may prove useful in the diagnosis of CMV pneumonitis, but the detection of CMV antigen may have the same significance as CMV detected by culture: it is generally present when CMV pneumonitis is present, but it can also be seen in the absence of pneumonitis caused by CMV.

Enzyme-linked immunosorbent assay (ELISA) systems to detect CMV antigen may become a useful diagnostic tool, but current ELISA methods are of limited sensitivity and specificity (64). In urine, poor sensitivity can be caused by the coating of CMV with $\beta_2$-microglobulin (74).

### Identification of Nucleic Acids

CMV nucleic acid probes have been developed for the detection of CMV in cell cultures and in clinical specimens such as urine, blood, and tissue (75–77). The role of polymerase chain reaction nucleic acid amplification, a new technology, in the diagnosis of CMV infection is being evaluated (78). These procedures are currently cumbersome, and they remain a research technique. Because some areas of the CMV genome are homologous with regions of human chromosomal DNA, probes must be carefully evaluated for specificity (79). If the probes used are strain specific, multiple probes may be required for adequate sensitivity. The significance of the identification of viral DNA in the absence of histological changes is not known. DNA hybridization may ultimately prove useful for the quantitation of virus within specimens, a procedure that currently cannot be done with accuracy (75). The role that nucleic acid identification may play in diagnosing CMV disease by improving the specificity of CMV culture and the sensitivity of identifying CMV inclusions in tissues is not yet known.

### Serologic Detection of Immune Response to CMV

Primary CMV infection in the immunocompetent host results in the development of both IgG and IgM antibodies. IgG antibodies persist lifelong, but IgM antibodies generally persist for 6–9 months in immunocompetent people (68). Thus, acute CMV infection can be serologically demonstrated by either a fourfold increase in IgG antibody or by the presence of IgM antibody to CMV. The presence of IgG antibody is used to estimate the numbers of previously infected persons in a population.

Many different techniques have been used to measure IgG antibodies against CMV. The complement fixation (CF) test is commonly used, but depending on the antigen employed can be less sensitive than tests such as neutralization, IFA, indirect hemagglutination (IHA), or immune adherence hemagglutination (IAHA) (63,80). Radioimmunoassay (RIA) and ELISA are particularly sensitive (21,80). Because CF antibody titers can diminish or fluctuate with time and because the CF test can miss low levels of antibody, CF seroconversion may represent only fluctuation in titer in a previously infected person. The use of a fourfold rise in CF titer to define CMV infection is also of low sensitivity; for example, of 81 patients with CMV mononucleosis, a fourfold rise in CF titer was observed in only 48% (18).

In the IF test, false-positive reactions and interpretation difficulties can be caused by the induction by CMV of a cytoplasmic Fc receptor for human immunoglobulin. The anticomplementary IF (ACIF) test, read as nuclear fluorescence, is more specific and thus preferable (68). IHA methods are rapid but have been inadequately tested (64). Neutralization antibody testing appears to be quite specific, but rises may be delayed when compared to other IgG methods (21). IgG antibodies to CMV early antigens can be detected, but they do not appear to be diagnostically useful because they can persist and can be found in the absence of clinical evidence of active infection (81).

IgM antibodies to CMV can be detected by RIA after the absorption of rheumatoid factor, by ELISA assays, or, less reliably, by IF (64,82). The presence of IgM antibodies to CMV in the immunocompetent host suggests recent acute CMV infection. IgM antibodies to CMV were detected in 81 of 82 nonimmunocompromised patients with CMV mononucleosis (18), but in some of these patients these antibodies persisted for over 1 year. IgM testing is less useful in homosexual men, since IgM is intermittently present in 95% of CMV seropositive homosexual men, probably reflecting frequent reactivation or reexposure (14). IgM testing is also less useful in immunosuppressed patients because they may fail to produce IgM antibodies to CMV, or they may have IgM responses to recurrent infection (21,32). For example, approximately one-third of renal transplant patients produce IgM antibodies to CMV during recurrent infections (21). In addition, IgM antibodies to CMV can persist for over 1 year in these patients (21).

Because it is often readily available, antibody testing is commonly used to define active CMV infection and to infer CMV disease, but this method of diagnosis lacks specificity and sensitivity, particularly in immunosuppressed patients. In the immunocompetent patient, the detection of IgM antibodies of CMV provides strong evidence for recent infection.

## THERAPY

The first line of treatment for CMV disease in patients receiving immunosuppressive therapies is the reversal of immunosuppression by discontinuing these therapies. For some patients, such as renal transplant recipients, this is feasible (26); in other patients, it is not.

A variety of agents, either singly or in combination, have been used to treat patients with serious CMV disease without any change in survival or consistent evidence of antiviral activity. These agents include transfer factor, vidarabine (adenine arabinoside), interferon-α, acyclovir (ACV), and CMV immune globulin (83–93). Recently, two promising investigational agents, ganciclovir (DHPG) and Foscarnet, have been used for the treatment of CMV disease.

### Ganciclovir

Ganciclovir [also known as dihydroxypropoxymethyl guanine (DHPG)] is an agent that appears to be an effective treatment for some forms of CMV disease (94–101), although studies have been uncontrolled. The drug has recently been approved for use by the Food and Drug Administration (FDA) of the United States. Virologic responses to ganciclovir occur in the majority (80–90%) of treated patients, but the impact on clinical illness varies according to the patient population treated and the site of infection. For example, although some renal transplant and HIV-infected patients with CMV pneumonitis have been reported to respond to ganciclovir therapy, the mortality of CMV pneumonitis in the bone marrow transplant population has not clearly been reduced by the use of ganciclovir (95,96,99,101,102). Differences in efficacy may relate to the degree of tissue damage present at the time that therapy is instituted or, in the case of pneumonia in the bone marrow transplant patient, to concomitant immunologically mediated lung damage (103).

One recent study has demonstrated the best ganciclovir response in the bone marrow transplant population, with 48% (10 of 21) of treated patients surviving the initial episode of CMV pneumonitis (three survivors and three nonsurvivors were treated concomitantly with CMV immune globulin) (104). The addition of corticosteroids to ganciclovir therapy in bone marrow transplant patients with pneumonitis did not improve efficacy (105). Several reports suggest that ganciclovir combined with immune globulin therapy improves survival in bone marrow transplant patients with CMV pneumonia. In one study, 52% of 25 patients treated with this combination of therapies survived (106) and, in another, 70% of 10 treated patients survived (107). Neither study included a control group; the diagnostic criteria for CMV pneumonia varied, patients who were ventilator-dependent were not studied, and the globulin preparations and dosing schedules differed between the two. Thus, the relative contributions of each therapy to improved outcome are uncertain, but these survival data appear impressive when compared to the mortality in historical controls. In a preliminary report, all of four ventilator-dependent patients with CMV pneumonia who were treated with ganciclovir and immune globulin died, suggesting that delayed therapy decreases survival (108).

The most promising data suggesting that ganciclovir is effective come from patients with CMV retinitis and HIV infection. Initial improvement or stabilization occurred in approximately 80% of treated patients (24,101). Subsequent relapse occurred after discontinuation of therapy, but relapsed patients often responded to a second course, again suggesting a role of ganciclovir therapy in controlling CMV infection. Intravenous maintenance therapy appeared to prolong the time to relapse in treated retinitis (24). Gastrointestinal disease in HIV-infected patients also responds to therapy (97). The role of treatment for other sites of disease such as adrenalitis and encephalitis is less clear (41).

Ganciclovir is a toxic drug, with granulocytopenia generally being the dose-limiting toxicity. Thrombocytopenia also occurs. Bone marrow suppression usually reverses after discontinuing therapy. Other toxicities include CNS abnormalities, especially confusion; gastrointestinal symptoms such as nausea, anorexia, or diarrhea; rash; fever; phlebitis; and, possibly, suppression of reproductive function (24,101). The use of ganciclovir can be difficult in patients with poor marrow reserves or in patients on other marrow suppressive agents such as zidovudine [azidothymidine (AZT)]. In order to decrease systemic toxicity, intravitreal use of ganciclovir in the treatment of retinitis has been attempted and may ultimately prove to be effective and safe. Because ganciclovir is given intravenously, maintenance therapy requires frequent intravenous infusions. The use of an oral preparation of the drug for maintenance therapy may be feasible, but such a preparation is not available (24).

Ganciclovir is now available only on a compassionate use basis from the manufacturer. Patients with normal renal function currently are treated with an initial therapeutic dose of 5 mg/kg body weight intravenously every 12 hr for 14 to 21 days. Patients at high risk of relapse receive a maintenance regimen of 5 mg/kg body weight once daily given indefinitely.

### Foscarnet

Foscarnet (trisodium phosphonoformate) is another investigational antiviral agent that has been used in open trials for the treatment of CMV disease in immunocompromised patients. Preliminary evidence suggests that it is likely to be useful (24,109,110). The toxicities of Foscarnet differ from those of ganciclovir, suggesting that each drug will be useful in a different subset of patients. Foscarnet is nephrotoxic, and can cause anemia, phlebitis, seizures and other nervous system side effects, and alterations in serum calcium levels. Foscarnet therapy does not, however, result in the leukopenia that is so commonly seen in ganciclovir therapy. Thus, it may be feasible to use Foscarnet simultaneously with AZT. Because of poor bioavailability, Foscarnet is used intravenously by continuous or bolus infusion, making its use as a maintenance regimen difficult.

## PROPHYLAXIS AND PREVENTION

### Interruption of Transmission

Prevention of infection is preferable to the treatment of established disease, especially when therapy requires the use of toxic agents such as ganciclovir or Foscarnet. An interruption of transmission is one conceptually simple way to prevent infection. For example, seronegative renal allograft recipients could receive kidneys only from seronegative donors, and seronegative immunocompromised patients could receive blood products only from seronegative donors (7,22). The use of leukocyte poor or frozen deglycerolized red blood cells may also decrease blood-borne transmission (7). Unfortunately, these plans are not always practical because of the high prevalence of CMV infection in donors and the difficulty and expense involved in matching donors and recipients. Handwashing is always in order to decrease any potential nosocomial spread (5). Sexual transmission might be decreased by the appropriate use of condoms and safer sex practices, where the unprotected exchange of body fluids is avoided (111).

### Prophylactic Use of Antiviral Agents

Once effective therapy is available for CMV, there will still be a need for antiviral prophylaxis. Prophylaxis may be more effective than therapy in patients whose period of risk is well known, such as in transplant patients. Prophylaxis using vidarabine, interferon-α, ACV, and immune globulins has been studied, but studies of the use of Foscarnet or ganciclovir have not yet been reported (71,112–115). In a placebo-controlled trial, human leukocyte interferon delayed the onset of CMV excretion and decreased the incidence of viremia after renal transplantation but did not affect the incidence of CMV disease (71). A second study using a longer course suggested that interferon decreased both CMV disease and superinfections with other agents. In this study, seven of 22 placebo recipients and one of 20 interferon recipients had CMV disease (113). A third study suggested that interferon prophylaxis provided no benefit after bone marrow transplantation, although interferon was not initiated until a median of 18 days after transplantation (114). A recent study suggested that ACV may play a role in prophylaxis even though it is not effective as therapy for CMV disease (115). ACV (500 mg/m$^2$ q 8 hr) was given after allogeneic marrow transplantation to patients who were seropositive for both herpes simplex virus (HSV) and CMV; CMV seropositive patients who were seronegative for HSV served as controls. Thus, the study of populations were not randomly selected. CMV infection as detected by the isolation of virus developed in 59% of 86 ACV recipients and in 75% of 65 control patients, and viral excretion was delayed in the treated patients. CMV disease developed in 22% of ACV recipients and 38% of controls; survival during the first 100 days was also better among treated patients. Further studies are required to confirm these results and to determine the optimal use of prophylactic ACV or interferon-α.

### Passive Immunization

The efficacy of the prophylactic use of various forms of CMV immune plasma or globulin is controversial, and their cost is high. The studies performed are difficult to compare and interpret because they differ in such points as the patient population studied (seronegative or seropositive, bone marrow or renal transplant patients); the techniques used for virologic surveillance; the definition of and diagnostic basis for CMV infection or disease; the use of placebo; and, most importantly, in the type, quantity and route of administration of the immunoglobulin preparation. Preparations used have included hyperimmune CMV globulin or plasma and standard intravenous immunoglobulin preparations. The most effective preparation to study and the correlation between various measurements of anti-CMV activity in the preparations and efficacy are not known. In bone marrow transplant recipients, beneficial effects have generally been seen only in patients not receiving prophylactic granulocyte transfusions. Moreover, the effects have been modest and not seen in all studies. The reported results of prophylactic immunoglobulin include decreases in symptomatic disease but not active infection, decreases in active infection but not symptomatic disease, and no effect (116–122). In one study in seronegative renal transplant patients who received transplants from seropositive donors, CMV immune globulin reduced serious CMV disease but not active infection (123). Thus, it is not yet possible to judge the utility of this therapy, although these studies leave the impression that high doses of an optimal antibody preparation would ameliorate CMV disease, although not completely or uniformly.

### Vaccines

Because primary CMV infection is more likely to be associated with CMV disease in the immunosuppressed patient or with the development of symptomatic congenital infection, the use of vaccines against CMV has been studied in both seronegative patients prior to renal transplantation and in seronegative fertile women. Although both subunit and live attenuated vaccines have been studied for the prevention of CMV infection or disease, only the live attenuated vaccine has been tested in humans. Obvious concerns related to the use of a live attenuated vaccine include oncogenic potential and the potential for causing disease either initially after vaccination or through the reactivation of latent vaccine virus. Two vaccine strains, AD 169 and the Towne strain, have been administered to a limited number of normal volunteers and renal transplant recipients (124–131). The vaccines are immunogenic and result in the production of antibody and lymphocyte blastogenic responses in normal hosts, although antibody responses wane with time (127,128). The immune response of renal transplant recipients to the Towne vaccine is diminished (126,127,129). Although vaccine recipients were not protected from active CMV infection after renal transplantation, vaccination may have decreased the severity of symptomatic illness (126,129). The toxicity from these vaccines appears limited to prolonged local reactions and rare fever in seronegative recipients; reactivation of vaccine virus has not been noted (130,131). The role of vaccination in preventing disease in both seronegative and seropositive patients remains to be determined.

## SUMMARY

Infection with CMV is common and results in latency. In immunocompromised patients, primary infection, exogenous reinfection, or reactivation of latent virus despite the presence of antibody can result in serious illness. Disease manifestations and the effects of prophylaxis and therapy differ among the various populations (HIV-infected and renal, bone marrow, or other transplant patients) at greatest risk for active infection. Available therapies include reduction of immunosuppression in patients receiving exogenous immunosuppressive agents, and the use of experimental agents that appear promising but whose efficacy and appropriate use remain uncertain. Such agents include DHPG and Foscarnet, both drugs with established toxicity. Because of the potential for therapy, sensitive diagnostic techniques that can differentiate between active CMV infection and CMV disease requiring therapy are needed. The prevention of CMV disease has been attempted in selected populations with the use of vaccines, passive immunization with immunoglobulin preparations, and prophylactic antiviral agents. There are no definitive studies, and where prophylaxis appears promising, its effect is only to partially protect patients at risk. Thus, CMV prophylaxis remains an experimental therapy. The development of effective prophylaxis and therapy strategies is anticipated.

## REFERENCES


1. Huang E-S, Alford CA, Reynolds DW, Stagno S, Pass RF. Molecular epidemiology of cytomegalovirus infections in women and their infants. *N Engl J Med* 1980;303:958–62.
2. Macasaet FF, Holley KE, Smith TF, Keys TF. Cytomegalovirus studies of autopsy tissue. II. Incidence of inclusion bodies and related pathologic data. *Am J Clin Pathol* 1975;63:859–65.
3. Jordan MC. Latent infection and the elusive cytomegalovirus. *Rev Infect Dis* 1983;5:205–15.
4. Schrier RD, Nelson JA, Oldstone MBA. Detection of human cytomegalovirus in peripheral blood lymphocytes in a natural infection. *Science* 1985;230:1048–51.
5. Onorato IM, Morens DM, Martone WJ, Stansfield SK. Epidemiology of cytomegaloviral infections: recommendations for prevention and control. *Rev Infect Dis* 1988;7:479–96.
6. Pass RF. Epidemiology and transmission of cytomegalovirus. *J Infect Dis* 1988;152:243–8.
7. Adler SP. Transfusion-associated cytomegalovirus infections. *Rev Infect Dis* 1983;5:977–93.
8. Hutto C, Little EA, Ricks R, Lee JD, Pass RF. Isolation of cytomegalovirus from toys and hands in a day care center. *J Infect Dis* 1986;154:527–30.
9. Stagno S, Pass RF, Dworsky ME, Alford CA Jr. Maternal cytomegalovirus infection and perinatal transmission. *Clin Obstet Gynecol* 1982;25:563–76.
10. Pass RF, Hutto C, Ricks R, Cloud GA. Increased rate of cytomegalovirus infection among parents of children attending day-care centers. *N Engl J Med* 1986;314:1414–8.
11. Pass RF, Hutto C. Group day care and cytomegaloviral infections of mothers and children. *Rev Infect Dis* 1986;8:599–605.
12. Chandler SH, Holmes KK, Wentworth BB, et al. The epidemiology of cytomegaloviral infection in women attending a sexually transmitted disease clinic. *J Infect Dis* 1985;152:597–605.
13. Handsfield HH, Chandler SH, Caine VA et al. Cytomegalovirus infection in sex partners: evidence for sexual transmission. *J Infect Dis* 1985;151:344–8.
14. Mintz L, Drew WL, Miner RC, Braff EH. Cytomegalovirus infections in homosexual men: an epidemiological study. *Ann Intern Med* 1983;99:326–9.
15. Dworsky ME, Welch K, Cassady G, Stagno S. Occupational risk for primary cytomegalovirus infection among pediatric health-care workers. *N Engl J Med* 1983;309:950–3.
16. Griffiths PD, Baboonian C. A prospective study of primary cytomegalovirus infection during pregnancy: final report. *B J Obstet Gynecol* 1984;91:307–15.
17. Cohen JI, Corey GR. Cytomegalovirus infection in the normal host. *Medicine* 1985;64:100–14.
18. Horwitz CA, Henle W, Henle G, et al. Clinical and laboratory evaluation of cytomegalovirus-induced mononucleosis in previously healthy individuals. *Medicine* 1986;65:124–34.
19. Betts RF, Freeman RB, Douglas RG Jr., Talley TE. Clinical manifestations of renal allograft derived primary cytomegalovirus infection. *Am J Dis Child* 1977;131:759–63.
20. Suwansirikul S, Rao N, Dowling JN, Ho M. Primary and secondary cytomegalovirus infection. Clinical manifestations after renal transplantation. *Arch Intern Med* 1977;137:1026–9.
21. Pass RF, Griffiths PD, August AM. Antibody response to cytomegalovirus after renal transplantation: comparison of patients with primary and recurrent infections. *J Infect Dis* 1983;147:40–6.
22. Glenn J. Cytomegalovirus infections following renal transplantation. *Rev Infect Dis* 1981;3:1151–78.
23. Meyers JD, Spencer HC Jr. Watts JC, et al. Cytomegalovirus pneumonia after human marrow transplantation. *Ann Intern Med* 1975;82;181–8.
24. Jacobson MA, Mills J. Serious cytomegalovirus disease in the acquired immunodeficiency syndrome (AIDS). Clinical findings, diagnosis, and treatment. *Ann Intern Med* 1988;108:585–94.
25. Abdallah PS, Mark JBD, Merigan TC. Diagnosis of cytomegalovirus pneumonia in compromised hosts. *Am J Med* 1976;61:326–32.
26. Peterson PK, Balfour HH Jr, Marker SC, Fryd DS, Howard RJ, Simmons RL. Cytomegalovirus disease in renal allograft recipients: a prospective study of the clinical features, risk factors, and impact on renal transplantation. *Medicine* 1980;59:283–300.
27. Rubin RH, Russell PS, Levin M, Cohen C. Summary of a workshop on cytomegalovirus infections during organ transplantation. *J Infect Dis* 1979;139:728–34.
28. Murray HW, Knox DL, Green WR, Susel RM. Cytomegalovirus retinitis in adults. A manifestation of disseminated viral infection. *Am J Med* 1977;63:574–84.
29. Pollard RB, Egbert PR, Gallagher JG, Merigan TC. Cytomegalovirus retinitis in immunosuppressed hosts. I. Natural history and effects of treatment with adenine arabinoside. *Ann Intern Med* 1980;93:655–64.
30. Egbert PR, Pollard RB, Gallagher JG, Merigan TC. Cytomegalovirus retinitis in immunosuppressed hosts. II. Ocular manifestations. *Ann Intern Med* 1980;93:664–70.
31. Aldrete JS, Sterling WA, Hathaway BM, Morgan JM, Diethelm AG. Gastrointestinal and hepatic complications affecting patients with renal allografts. *Am J Surg* 1975;129:115–24.
32. Culpepper-Morgan JA, Kotler DP, Scholes JV, Tierney AR. Evaluation of diagnostic criteria for mucosal cytomegalic inclusion disease in the acquired immune deficiency syndrome. *Am J Gastroenterol* 1987;82:1264–70.

33. Weber JN, Thom S, Barrison I et al. Cytomegalovirus colitis and esophageal ulceration in the context of AIDS: clinical manifestations and preliminary report of treatment with Foscarnet (phosphonoformate). *Gut* 1987;28:482–7.
34. Rubin RH, Cosimi AB, Tolkoff-Rubin NE, Russell PS, Hirsch MS. Infectious disease syndromes attributable to cytomegalovirus and their significance among renal transplant recipients. *Transplantation* 1977;24:458–64.
35. Luby JP, Ware AJ, Hull AR et al. Disease due to cytomegalovirus and its long-term consequences in renal transplant recipients. *Arch Intern Med* 1983;143:1126–9.
36. Dummer JS, White LT, Ho M, Griffith BP, Hardesty RL, Bahnson HT. Morbidity of cytomegalovirus infection in recipients of heart or heart-lung transplants who received cyclosporine. *J Infect Dis* 1985;152:1182–91.
37. Luby JP, Burnett W, Hull AR, Ware AJ, Shorey JW, Peters PC. Relationship between cytomegalovirus and hepatic function abnormalities in the period after renal transplant. *J Infect Dis* 1974;129:511–8.
38. Ware AJ, Luby JP, Hollinger B, et al. Etiology of liver disease in renal-transplant patients. *Ann Intern Med* 1979;91:364–71.
39. Dorfman LJ. Cytomegalovirus encephalitis in adults. *Neurology* 1973;23:136–44.
40. Morgello S, Cho E-S, Nielsen S, Devinsky O, Petito CK. Cytomegalovirus encephalitis in patients with acquired immunodeficiency syndrome: an autopsy study of 30 cases and a review of the literature. *Hum Pathol* 1987;18:289–97.
41. Fiala M, Cone LA, Cohen N, et al. Responses of neurologic complications of AIDS to 3′-azido-3′-deoxythymidine and 9-(1,3-dihydroxy-2-propoxymethyl) guanine. I. Clinical features. *Rev Infect Dis* 1988;10:250–6.
42. Jacobson MA, Cello JP, Sande MA. Cholestasis and disseminated cytomegalovirus disease in patients with the acquired immunodeficiency syndrome. *Am J Med* 1988;84:218–24.
43. Rand KH, Pollard RB, Merigan TC. Increased pulmonary superinfections in cardiac-transplant patients undergoing primary cytomegalovirus infection. *N Engl J Med* 1978;298:951–3.
44. Schooley RT, Hirsch MS, Colvin RB, et al. Association of herpesvirus infections with T-lymphocyte-subset alterations, glomerulopathy, and opportunistic infections after renal transplantation. *N Engl J Med* 1983;308:307–13.
45. Preiksaitis JK, Rosno S, Grumet C, Merigan TC. Infections due to herpesviruses in cardiac transplant recipients: role of the donor heart and immunosuppressive therapy. *J Infect Dis* 1983;147:974–81.
46. Drew WL, Conant MA, Miner RC, et al. Cytomegalovirus and Kaposi's sarcoma in young homosexual men. *Lancet* 1982;2:125–7.
47. Marker SC, Howard RJ, Simmons RL, et al. Cytomegalovirus infection: a quantitative prospective study of three hundred twenty consecutive renal transplants. *Surgery* 1981;89:660–71.
48. Chou S. Acquisition of donor strains of cytomegalovirus by renal-transplant recipients. *N Engl J Med* 1986;314:1418–23.
49. Richardson WP, Colvin RB, Cheeseman SH, et al. Glomerulopathy associated with cytomegalovirus viremia in renal allografts. *N Engl J Med* 1981;305:57–63.
50. Meyers JD, Flournoy N, Thomas ED. Nonbacterial pneumonia after allogenic marrow transplantation: a review of ten years' experience. *Rev Infect Dis* 1982;4:1119–32.
51. Meyers JD, Flournoy N, Thomas ED. Risk factors for cytomegalovirus infection after human marrow transplantation. *J Infect Dis* 1988;153:478–88.
52. Quinnan GV Jr, Kirmani N, Rook AH, et al. Cytotoxic T cells in cytomegalovirus infection. HLA-restricted T-lymphocyte and non-T-lymphocyte cytotoxic responses correlate with recovery from cytomegalovirus infection in bone-marrow-transplant recipients. *N Engl J Med* 1982;307:7–13.
53. Grob JP, Grundy JE, Prentice HG, et al. Immune donors can protect marrow-transplant recipients from severe cytomegalovirus infections. *Lancet* 1987;1:774–6.
54. Gorensek MJ, Stewart RW, Keys TF, McHenry MC, Goormastic M. A multivariate analysis of the risk of cytomegalovirus infection in heart transplant recipients. *J Infect Dis* 1988; 157:515–22.
55. Singh N, Dummer JS, Kusne S, et al. Infections with cytomegalovirus and other herpesviruses in 121 liver transplant recipients: transmission by donated organ and the effect of OKT3 antibodies. *J Infect Dis* 1988;158:124–31.
56. Quinnan GV, Masur H, Rook AH, et al. Herpesvirus infections in the acquired immune deficiency syndrome. *JAMA* 1984;252:72–7.
57. Macher AM, Reichert CM, Straus SE, et al. Death in the AIDS patient: role of cytomegalovirus. *N Engl J Med* 1983;309:1454.
58. Welch K, Finkbeiner W, Alpers CE, et al. Autopsy findings in the acquired immunodeficiency syndrome. *JAMA* 1984;252:1152–9.
59. Palestine AG, Rodrigues MM, Macher AM, et al. Ophthalmic involvement in acquired immunodeficiency syndrome. *Ophthalmology* 1984; 91:1092–9.
60. Duvall CP, Casazza AR, Grimley PM, Carbone PP, Rowe WP. Recovery of cytomegalovirus from adults with neoplastic disease. *Ann Intern Med* 1966;64:531–41.
61. Smith TF, Holley KE, Keys TF, Macasaet FF. Cytomegalovirus studies of autopsy tissue. I. Virus isolation. *Am J Clin Pathol* 1975;63:854–8.
62. Dowling JN, Saslow AR, Armstrong JA, Ho M. Cytomegalovirus infection in patients receiving immunosuppressive therapy for rheumatic diseases. *J Infect Dis* 1976;133:399–408.
63. Reynolds DW, Stagno S, Alford CA. Labora-

tory diagnosis of cytomegalovirus infections. In: Lennette EH, Schmidt NJ, eds. *Diagnostic procedures for viral, rickettsial, and chlamydial infections*. Washington D.C.: American Public Health Association, 1979:399–439.
64. Griffiths PD. Diagnostic techniques for cytomegalovirus infection. *Clinics in Haematology* 1984;13:631–44.
65. Cordonnier C, Escudier E, Nicolas J-C, et al. Evaluation of three assays on alveolar lavage fluid in the diagnosis of cytomegalovirus pneumonitis after bone marrow transplantation. *J Infect Dis* 1987;155:495–500.
66. Crawford SW, Bowden RA, Hackman RC, Gleaves CA, Meyers JD, Clark JG. Rapid detection of cytomegalovirus pulmonary infection by bronchoalveolar lavage and centrifugation culture. *Ann Intern Med* 1988;108: 180–5.
67. Lee FK, Nahmias AJ, Stagno S. Rapid diagnosis of cytomegalovirus infection in infants by electron microscopy. *N Engl J Med* 1978;299:1266–70.
68. Drew WL. Diagnosis of cytomegalovirus infection. *Rev Infect Dis* 1988;10:S468–75.
69. Stirk PR, Griffiths PD. Use of monoclonal antibodies for the diagnosis of cytomegalovirus infection by the detection of early antigen fluorescent foci (DEAFF) in cell culture. *J Med Virol* 1987;21:329–37.
70. Gleaves CA, Reed EC, Hackman RC, Meyers JD. Rapid diagnosis of invasive cytomegalovirus infection by examination of tissue specimens in centrifugation culture. *Am J Clin Pathol* 1987;88:354–8.
71. Cheeseman SH, Rubin RH, Stewart JA, et al. Controlled clinical trial of prophylactic human-leukocyte interferon in renal transplantation. *N Engl J Med* 1979;300:1345–9.
72. Keller R, Peitchel R, Goldman JN, Goldman M. An IgG-Fc receptor induced in cytomegalovirus-infected human fibroblasts. *J Immunol* 1976;116:772–77.
73. Hackman RC, Myerson D, Meyers JD, et al. Rapid diagnosis of cytomegaloviral pneumonia by tissue immunofluorescence with a murine monoclonal antibody. *J Infect Dis* 1985; 151:325–9.
74. McKeating JA, Grundy JE, Varghese Z, Griffiths PD. Detection of cytomegalovirus by ELISA in urine samples is inhibited by $beta_2$ microglobulin. *J Med Virol* 1986;18:341–8.
75. Chou S, Merigan TC. Rapid detection and quantitation of human cytomegalovirus in urine through DNA hybridization. *N Engl J Med* 1983;308:921–5.
76. Spector SA, Rua JA, Spector DH, McMillan R. Detection of human cytomegalovirus in clinical specimens by DNA-DNA hybridization. *J Infect Dis* 1984;150:121–6.
77. Myerson D, Hackman RC, Meyers JD. Diagnosis of cytomegaloviral pneumonia by *in situ* hybridization. *J Infect Dis* 1984;150:272–7.
78. Shibata D, Martin WJ, Appleman MD, Causey DM, Leedom JM, Arnheim N. Detection of cytomegalovirus DNA in peripheral blood of patients infected with human immunodeficiency virus. *J Infect Dis* 1988;158:1185–92.
79. Ruger R, Bornkamm GW, Fleckenstein B. Human cytomegalovirus DNA sequences with homologies to the cellular genome. *J Gen Virol* 1984;65:1351–64.
80. Booth JC, Hannington G, Bakir TMF, et al. Comparison of enzyme-linked immunosorbent assay, radioimmunoassay, complement fixation, anticomplement immunofluorescence and passive haemagglutination techniques for detecting cytomegalovirus IgG antibody. *J Clin Pathol* 1982;35:1345–8.
81. Friedman AD, Furukawa T, Plotkin SA. Detection of antibody to cytomegalovirus early antigen in vaccinated, normal volunteers and renal transplant candidates. *J Infect Dis* 1982; 146:255–60.
82. Demmler GJ, Six HR, Hurst SM, Yow MD. Enzyme-linked immunosorbent assay for the detection of IgM-class antibodies to cytomegalovirus. *J Infect Dis* 1986;153:1152–5.
83. Paganelli R, Soothill JF, Marshall WC, Hamblin AS. Transfer factor and cytomegalovirus viruria. *Lancet* 1981;1:273–4.
84. Ch'ien LT, Cannon NJ, Whitley RJ, et al. Effect of adenine arabinoside on cytomegalovirus infections. *J Infect Dis* 1974;130:32–9.
85. Rytel MW, Kauffman HM. Clinical efficacy of adenine arabinoside in therapy of cytomegalovirus infections in renal allograft recipients. *J Infect Dis* 1976;133:202–5.
86. Marker SC, Howard RJ, Groth KE, Mastri AR, Simmons RL, Balfour HH Jr. A trial of vidarabine for cytomegalovirus infection in renal transplant patients. *Arch Intern Med* 1980; 140:1441–4.
87. Meyers JD, McGuffin RW, Neiman PE, Singer JW, Thomas ED. Toxicity and efficacy of human leukocyte interferon for treatment of cytomegalovirus pneumonia after marrow transplantation. *J Infect Dis* 1980;141:555–62.
88. Balfour HH Jr, Bean B, Mitchell CD, Sachs GW, Boen JR, Edelman CK. Acyclovir in immunocompromised patients with cytomegalovirus disease: a controlled trial at one institution. *Am J Med* 1982;73:241–8.
89. Wade JC, Hintz M, McGuffin RW, Springmeyer SC, Connor JD, Meyers JD. Treatment of cytomegalovirus pneumonia with high-dose acyclovir. *Am J Med* 1982;73:249–56.
90. Reed EC, Bowden RA, Dandliker PS, Gleaves CA, Meyers JD. Efficacy of cytomegalovirus immunoglobulin in marrow transplant recipients with cytomegalovirus pneumonia. *J Infect Dis* 1987;156:641–5.
91. Meyers JD, McGuffin RW, Bryson YJ, Cantell K, Thomas ED. Treatment of cytomegalovirus pneumonia after marrow transplant with combined vidarabine and human leukocyte interferon. *J Infect Dis* 1982;146:80–4.
92. Wade JC, McGuffin RW, Springmeyer SC, Newton B, Singer JW, Meyers JD. Treatment of cytomegaloviral pneumonia with high-dose

acyclovir and human leukocyte interferon. *J Infect Dis* 1983;148:557–62.
93. Shepp DH, Newton BA, Meyers JD. Intravenous lymphoblastoid interferon and acyclovir for treatment of cytomegaloviral pneumonia. *J Infect Dis* 1984;150:776–7.
94. Masur H, Lane HC, Palestine A, et al. Effect of 9-(1,3-dihydroxy-2-propoxymethyl) guanine on serious cytomegalovirus disease in eight immunosuppressed homosexual men. *Ann Intern Med* 1986;104:41–4.
95. Collaborative DHPG Treatment Study Group. Treatment of serious cytomegalovirus infections with 9-(1,3-dihydroxy-2-propoxymethyl)guanine in patients with AIDS and other immunodeficiencies. *N Engl J Med* 1986; 314:801–5.
96. Erice A, Jordan MC, Chace BA, Fletcher C, Chinnock BJ, Balfour HH. Ganciclovir treatment of cytomegalovirus disease in transplant recipients and other immunocompromised hosts. *JAMA* 1987;257:3082–7.
97. Chachoua A, Dieterich D, Krasinski K, et al. 9-(1,3-Dihydroxy-2-propoxymethyl)guanine (ganciclovir) in the treatment of cytomegalovirus gastrointestinal disease with the acquired immunodeficiency syndrome. *Ann Intern Med* 1987;107:133–7.
98. Laskin OL, Cederberg DM, Mills J, Eron LJ, Mildvan D, Spector SA. Ganciclovir for the treatment and suppression of serious infections caused by cytomegalovirus. *Am J Med* 1987; 83:201–7.
99. Keay S, Bissett J, Merigan TC. Ganciclovir treatment of cytomegalovirus infections in iatrogenically immunocompromised patients. *J Infect Dis* 1987;156:1016–21.
100. Hecht DW, Snydman DR, Crumpacker CS, Werner BG, Heinze-Lacey B, The Boston Renal Transplant CMV Study Group. Ganciclovir for treatment of renal transplant-associated primary cytomegalovirus pneumonia. *J Infect Dis* 1988;157:187–90.
101. Buhles WC, Mastre BJ, Tinker AJ, Strand V, Koretz SH, The Syntex Collaborative Ganciclovir Treatment Study Group. Ganciclovir treatment of life- or sight-threatening cytomegalovirus infection: experience in 314 immunocompromised patients. *Rev Infect Dis* 1988; 10:3495–503.
102. Shepp DH, Dandliker PS, de Miranda P et al. Activity of 9-[2-hydroxy-1-(hydroxymethyl)-ethoxymethyl]guanine in the treatment of cytomegalovirus pneumonia. *Ann Intern Med* 1985;103:368–73.
103. Grundy JE, Shanley JD, Griffiths PD. Is cytomegalovirus interstitial pneumonitis in transplant recipients an immunopathological condition? *Lancet* 1987;2:996–9.
104. Crumpacker C, Marlowe S, Zhang JL, Abrams S, Watkins P, the Ganciclovir Bone Marrow Transplant Treatment Group. Treatment of cytomegalovirus pneumonia. *Rev Infect Dis* 1988;10:S538–46.
105. Reed EC, Dandliker PS, Meyers JD. Treatment of cytomegalovirus pneumonia with 9-[2-hydroxy - 1 - (hydroxymethyl)ethoxymethyl] guanine and high-dose corticosteroids. *Ann Intern Med* 1986;105:214–5.
106. Emanuel D, Cunningham I, Jules-Elysee K, et al. Cytomegalovirus pneumonia after bone marrow transplantation successfully treated with the combination of ganciclovir and high-dose intravenous immune globulin. *Ann Intern Med* 1988;109:777–82.
107. Reed EC, Bowden RA, Dandliker PS, Lilleby KE, Meyers JD. Treatment of cytomegalovirus pneumonia with ganciclovir and intravenous cytomegalovirus immunoglobulin in patients with bone marrow transplants. *Ann Intern Med* 1988;109:783–8.
108. Aulitzky WE, Tilg H, Niederwieser D, Hackl M, Meister B, Huber C. Ganciclovir and hyperimmunoglobulin for treating cytomegalovirus infection in bone marrow transplant recipients. *J Infect Dis* 1988;2:488–9.
109. Ringden O, Lonnqvist B, Paulin T, et al. Pharmacokinetics, safety and preliminary clinical experiences using foscarnet in the treatment of cytomegalovirus infections in bone marrow and renal transplant recipients. *J Antimicrob Chemother* 1986;17:373–87.
110. Walmsley SL, Chew E, Read SE, et al. Treatment of cytomegalovirus retinitis with trisodium phosphonoformate hexahydrate (Foscarnet). *J Infect Dis* 1988;157:569–72.
111. Katznelson S, Drew WL, Mintz L. Efficacy of the condom as a barrier to the transmission of cytomegalovirus. *J Infect Dis* 1984;150:155–7.
112. Kraemer KG, Neiman PE, Reeves WC, Thomas ED. Prophylactic adenine arabinoside following marrow transplantation. *Transplant Proc* 1978;10:237–40.
113. Hirsch MS, Schooley RT, Cosimi AB, et al. Effects of interferon-α on cytomegalovirus reactivation syndromes in renal-transplant recipients. *N Engl J Med* 1983;308:1489–93.
114. Meyers JD, Flournoy N, Sanders JE, et al. Prophylactic use of human leukocyte interferon after allogeneic marrow transplantation. *Ann Intern Med* 1987;107:809–16.
115. Meyers JD, Reed EC, Shepp DH, et al. Acyclovir for prevention of cytomegalovirus infection and disease after allogeneic marrow transplantation. *N Engl J Med* 1988;318:70–5.
116. Winston DJ, Pollard RB, Ho WG, et al. Cytomegalovirus immune plasma in bone marrow transplant recipients. *Ann Intern Med* 1982; 97:11–8.
117. O'Reilly RJ, Reich L, Gold J, et al. A randomized trial of intravenous hyperimmune globulin for the prevention of cytomegalovirus (CMV) infections following marrow transplantation: preliminary results. *Transplant Proc* 1983; 15:1405–11.
118. Meyers JD, Leszczynski J, Zaia JA, et al. Prevention of cytomegalovirus infection by cytomegalovirus immune globulin after marrow transplantation. *Ann Intern Med* 1983;98: 442–6.

119. Winston DJ, Ho WG, Lin C-H, Budinger MD, Champlin RE, Gale RP. Intravenous immunoglobulin for modification of cytomegalovirus infections associated with bone marrow transplantation. *Am J Med* 1984;76:128–33.
120. Condie RM, O'Reilly RJ. Prevention of cytomegalovirus infection by prophylaxis with an intravenous, hyperimmune, native, unmodified cytomegalovirus globulin. Randomized trial in bone marrow transplant recipients. *Am J Med* 1984;76:134–41.
121. Bowden RA, Sayers M, Flournoy N, et al. Cytomegalovirus immune globulin and seronegative blood products to prevent primary cytomegalovirus infection after marrow transplantation. *N Engl J Med* 1986;314:1006–10.
122. Winston DJ, Ho WG, Lin C-H, et al. Intravenous immune globulin for prevention of cytomegalovirus infection and interstitial pneumonia after bone marrow transplantation. *Ann Intern Med* 1987;106:12–8.
123. Snydman DR, Werner BG, Heinze-Lacey B, et al. Use of cytomegalovirus immune globulin to prevent cytomegalovirus disease in renal-transplant patients. *N Engl J Med* 1987;317:1049–54.
124. Elek SD, Stern H. Development of vaccine against mental retardation caused by cytomegalovirus infection *in utero*. *Lancet* 1974;1:1–5.
125. Plotkin SA, Farquhar J, Hornberger E. Clinical trials of immunization with the Towne 125 strain of human cytomegalovirus. *J Infect Dis* 1976;134:470–5.
126. Glazer JP, Friedman HM, Grossman RA, et al. Live cytomegalovirus vaccination of renal transplant candidates: a preliminary trial. *Ann Intern Med* 1979;91:676–83.
127. Starr SE, Glazer JP, Friedman HM, Farquhar JD, Plotkin SA. Specific cellular and humoral immunity after immunization with live Towne strain cytomegalovirus vaccine. *J Infect Dis* 1981;143:585–9.
128. Fleisher GR, Starr SE, Friedman HM, Plotkin SA. Vaccination of pediatric nurses with live attenuated cytomegalovirus. *Am J Dis Child* 1982;136:294–6.
129. Plotkin SA, Smiley ML, Friedman HM, et al. Towne-vaccine-induced prevention of cytomegalovirus disease after renal transplants. *Lancet* 1984;1:528–30.
130. Quinnan GV, Delery M, Rook AH, et al. Comparative virulence and immunogenicity of the Towne strain and a non-attenuated strain of cytomegalovirus. *Ann Intern Med* 1984;101:478–83.
131. Plotkin SA, Huang E-S. Cytomegalovirus vaccine virus (Towne strain) does not induce latency. *J Infect Dis* 1985;152:395–7.

*Antiviral Agents and Viral Diseases of Man, 3rd Edition,* edited by G. J. Galasso, R. J. Whitley, and T. C. Merigan, Raven Press, Ltd., New York 1990.

# 18

# RNA Viruses that Cause Hemorrhagic, Encephalitic, and Febrile Disease

John W. Huggins

*Virology Division, Department of Antiviral Studies, United States Army Medical Research Institute of Infectious Diseases, Fort Detrick, Maryland 21701-5011*



A group of small RNA viruses belonging to the families *Togaviridae, Bunyaviridae, Arenaviridae,* and *Filoviridae* cause hemorrhagic, encephalitic, or febrile disease throughout large areas of the world. All are associated with insect or rodent vectors whose interaction with humans defines the mode of disease transmission. Because these viruses occur primarily in Asia, Africa, and South America they are typically considered in the context of "tropical medicine" and are considered as "exotic viruses," both because of their unusual biology of transmission and the increased level of biohazard protection, biosafety level BL2 to BL4, required for their safe handling in the laboratory. Because they tend to occur either in underdeveloped countries, or with such low frequencies, the development of antiviral therapies has not been a commercial priority. Further, funding for studying many of these viruses is difficult to obtain from traditional sources. Research on them is focused in a few research institutes specializing in tropical medicine. Traditionally, the United States Army has been a major contributor to such research efforts, with laboratories both in the United States and overseas in several endemic areas, and through an extramural contract/grant system to support such work. The Centers for Disease Control (CDC) also conducts significant work in this field. Summarizing the field of clinically important viral diseases in tropical medicine is beyond the scope of this chapter, and the reader is referred to major reviews in the references for further information (1–3). Where several of these diseases represent either significant health

The views of the authors do not purport to reflect the position of the Department of Defense.

threats to large numbers of individuals or are useful prototype illnesses, significant work on antiviral chemotherapy has been done. The United States Army Medical Research Institute of Infectious Diseases (USAMRIID) has, for several years, had the only major drug discovery program directed specifically at many of these viruses, with a screening capacity of 1,500 compounds per year against 11 viruses, as well as animal models for studying many of the diseases.

The task of drug development is hampered by our limited understanding of many of the diseases and the viruses that cause them, due often to the remote location of outbreaks and the inherent problems in conducting sophisticated studies in such locations. Drug discovery is constrained by the requirement of utilizing biocontainment facilities, to include BL3 and BL4 or "spacesuit" laboratories, with their associated support facilities. This has significantly limited the number of laboratories able or willing to participate in development. In spite of these difficulties, significant progress has been made in developing therapy for the viral hemorrhagic fevers and several lead compounds are now being studied for febrile and encephalitic illnesses.

## VIRAL HEMORRHAGIC FEVERS

Viral hemorrhagic fevers cause severe clinical illness and represent a significant health threat in several areas of the world, as seen in overview in Table 1. They are caused by small enveloped RNA viruses transmitted by specific vectors or contact with rodent host. Their clinical presentation is similar although they are caused by members of the *Togaviridae, Bunyaviridae, Arenaviridae,* and *Filoviridae* families. Successful clinical trials of ribavirin have been completed against two of these diseases.

### Bunyaviruses

The *Bunyaviridae* family comprises more than 200 named viruses divided into five genera. Many of the *Bunyaviridae* members are firmly established as human pathogens. Three of these diverse array of viruses stand out as significant global problems: Rift Valley Fever, Crimean Congo hemorrhagic fever, and hemorrhagic fever with renal syndrome (4).

#### *Hemorrhagic Fever with Renal Syndrome*

##### *Etiologic Agent*

Following the propagation of hantaan virus in *Apodemus* (5) and its adaptation to cell culture (6), the agent was identified as a bunyavirus by immunoelectron microscopy (IEM) (7–9) and described as spherical, enveloped virions, with an average diameter of 95 nm. Biochemical characterization revealed that hantaan, like other members of the *Hantavirus* genus of the family bunyaviridae, possesses a single-stranded RNA genome of tripartite antisense message enclosed in a ribonuclease-sensitive nucleocapsid surrounded by a lipid envelope containing two virus-specified glycoproteins (10–13). No serological relationship can be demonstrated between hantaan virus and any other member of the *Bunyaviridae* (14).

##### *Epidemiology*

Hemorrhagic fever with renal syndrome (HFRS) is a group of closely related diseases known by several synonyms (epidemic hemorrhagic fever, Churilov disease, epidemic nephritis, epidemic nephroso-nephritis, hemorrhagic nephroso-nephritis, Songo fever, Korean hemorrhagic fever, Far Eastern hemorrhagic fever, nephropathia epidemica, endemic benign nephropathy, virus hemorrhagic fever, muroid virus nephropathy) (15). HFRS is caused by three of the four distinct viruses in the genus *Hantavirus* of the family *Bunyaviridae* (16,17) and is acquired by contact with chronically infected rodent hosts. Hantaan viruses, the cause of Korean hemorrhagic fever in Korea (18,19) and epidemic hemorrhagic fever (Songo fever) in China (20,21) and Japan (22), and hemorrhagic nephroso-nephritis in the Soviet Union (23–27) are associated with the rodent host *Apodemus agrarius* (striped field mouse) (5,28). Puumala virus, the cause of nephropathia epidemica in Scandinavia, is transmitted by *Clethrionomys glariolus* (bank vole) (29), and Seoul virus, the cause of a less severe form of HFRS in China and Korea, is associated with *Rattus rattus* and *Rattus norvegicus* (urban rats) (30). A severe form of HFRS is recognized across Asia including Korea (5), People's Republic of China (31,32), Japan (33), Hong Kong, Malaysia, Singapore (34), and the Eastern USSR (24–28). A milder form, nephropathia epidemica (35), occurs west of the Ural mountains in Scandinavian countries of Sweden (36), Finland (29), Norway (37), and Denmark (38), associated with puumula virus. Isolated cases of a mild form of HFRS have been reported in France (39), West Germany, Belgium (40), Scotland (41), and Italy, whereas a severe form occurs seasonally in Hungary (42), Czechoslovakia (43), Rumania (44), Bulgaria (45), Albania, Yugoslavia (46), and Greece (47,48).

Unlike other vectorborne *Bunyaviridae*, infection with hantaviruses is apparently associated with contacting chronic, asymptomatically infected rodent hosts. Transmission is believed to occur via aerosolized urine or feces of rodents (49,50); infection from contact with bodily fluids of infected individuals has not been documented. It is apparent that the epidemiology of hantaviruses is intimately associated with the complex ecology of their principal vertebrate hosts. Disease in China is variously estimated from 100,000 to more than 500,000 cases per year and occurs predominantly in rural areas among farmers, foresters, and soldiers stationed in the field. It is most prominent in males (60–80%). In Korea, 1,000 cases are seen each year. The disease has two seasonal peaks: one in late fall (October through January) and a smaller peak in early summer. In addition to infection from natural sources, more than 200 laboratory-acquired infections have been noted, both in laboratories working on HFRS and among animal handlers in laboratories (due to persistently infected rats). Several infections have been traced to infected animal colonies, although the scientific community has now taken steps to control infection through testing of breeding stocks.

### *Clinical Features of Severe Form*

The characteristic features of HFRS are a triad of fever, hemorrhagic phenomena, and renal insufficiency. Disease severity ranges from mild to grave based upon discriminators of severity, but no simple prognostic indicators of clinical severity are available on admission to predict outcome. In most patients, the clinical course can be divided into five often overlapping stages, but individual patients can be quite variable, skipping some stages entirely (16,44, 51–56). The specific diagnosis of classical HFRS depends on recognition of its characteristic multiphasic features together with an appropriate exposure history. Serologic confirmation of specific immunoglobulin M (IgM) can be made (within 8 hr) in most patients on admission [>95% in People's Republic of China (PRC) study (57)] either by indirect immunofluorescence (IF) on hantaan-infected Vero E6 cells or by an IgM enzyme immunosorbent assay (ELISA) (57,58).

*Febrile Phase*. A prodrome is rare. The incubation period of HFRS ranges from 1 to 4 weeks, with an average of 14 days, and extremes of 4 and 60 days. The febrile stage

**TABLE 1.** *Viral hemorrhagic fevers: etiologic and epidemiologic considerations*

| | Causative agent | Vector(s) | Vertebrate host(s) | Geographical distribution | Epidemiologic features of involvement of humans | Control | Remarks |
|---|---|---|---|---|---|---|---|
| YF (urban) | YF virus—a flavivirus | *Aedes aegypti* in cities | Humans | Human populations (usually urban) in tropics of South and Central America and Africa | Person-to-person passage by *Aedes aegypti* | *Aedes aegypti* control; vaccination | Sylvan YF can spread to cities |
| YF (sylvan) | YF virus—a flavivirus | *Haemagogus* mosquitoes in new world; *Aedes* species in Africa | Monkeys of several genera and species | Forests and jungles of South and Central America and West, Central, and East Africa | Humans infected by exposure in jungle (e.g., woodcutters, hunters) | Vaccination | Human cases sporadic and unpredictable; disease often a "silent" epizootic in forests |
| Dengue hemorrhagic fever | Dengue viruses of four types; flaviviruses | *Aedes aegypti* | Humans (involvement of other primates has been postulated) | Tropical and subtropical cities of Southeast Asia and Philippines | Small children usually involved in cities where *Aedes aegypti* densities are high | *Aedes aegypti* control; mosquito repellent, screens, etc. | Disease may represent an immunologic overresponse to a sequential infection with a different dengue strain |

| | | | | | | | |
|---|---|---|---|---|---|---|---|
| OHF | OHF virus—a flavivirus | Ticks of genus *Dermacentor* | Small rodents and muskrats | Omsk region of USSR; northern Rumania | People exposed in fields and wooded lands | Tick repellents and protective clothing | |
| KFD | KFD virus—a flavivirus | Ticks of several species in genus *Haemaphysalis* | Monkeys (rhesus and langur) and small rodents and birds | Mysore State, India | People exposed in fields and wooded lands | Tick control; tick repellents and protective clothing | Monkey mortality signals epidemic activity |
| AHF | Junin virus—an arenavirus | None recognized | Small rodents; *Akodon; Calomys laucha, musculinus* | Argentina: Northwest of Buenos Aires extending west to Province of Cordoba | Field workers at harvest time are particularly at risk | None practical | Infected rodents contaminate environment with urine |
| Bolivian hemorrhagic fever | Machupo virus—an arenavirus | None recognized | Small rodent, *Calomys callosus* | Beni Province of Bolivia | Residents of small, rodent-infested villages and homes; 1971 nosocomial outbreak in Cochabamba, Bolivia | Rodent control in villages | High mortality in humans |
| Lassa fever | Lassa virus—an arenavirus, LCM-related | None required | Small rodent, *Mastomys natalensis* | West Africa; Nigeria, Liberia, Sierra Leone | Residents of small rodent-infested villages; dramatic nosocomial outbreaks | None known; possibly rodent control | High mortality in humans |
| Crimean hemorrhagic fever | CCHF virus—a nairovirus | Ticks of several genera | Larger domestic animals implicated; also African hedgehog | Southern USSR, Bulgaria, East and West Africa | Cowhands and field workers in USSR; nosocomial outbreaks reported | Tick control relating to livestock; full isolation in patient care | Human disease important in USSR; importance to humans in Africa not known |

continued

**TABLE 1.** *Continued*

| | Causative agent | Vector(s) | Vertebrate host(s) | Geographical distribution | Epidemiologic features of involvement of humans | Control | Remarks |
|---|---|---|---|---|---|---|---|
| HFRS [Korean hemorrhagic fever hemorrhage nephrosonephritis] | Hantaan virus—a hantavirus | Not known | Small rodents: *Apodemus, Clethrionomys* | China, Korea; northern Eurasia to and including Scandinavia | Rural or sylvan exposure (military, forest occupations, farmers) | Rodent control in towns | Urban rats may be reservoirs |
| Ebola/Marburg | Ebola Marburg | Unknown | Unknown | Africa | Handling of infected primates; person to person during outbreak | Unknown | High mortality in humans |

OHF, Omsk hemorrhagic fever; KFD, Kyasamur Forest disease.
From ref. 130, with permission.

begins with abrupt onset of high fever (39°C to >40°C), chills, malaise, and myalgia, followed by headache, eye pain, dizziness, and anorexia. Within 1–3 days, large extravasation of plasma into the peritoneum and retroperitoneal space results in severe back and abdominal pain. Vascular dysregulation leads to characteristic flushing of the face, neck, and chest together with conjunctival hemorrhage. High white blood cell (WBC) counts are prognostic of severe disease. During the early febrile stage, the urine may contain small amounts of albumin, which increases abruptly in the late febrile phase. This stage lasts 3–7 days. Most patients seek medical care toward the end of this phase.

*Hypotensive Phase.* The hypotensive stage occurs coincident with defervescence; hypotension develops abruptly, lasting from several hours to 3 days. The classical picture of shock may occur, including tachycardia, narrowed pulse pressure, hypotension, cold and clammy skin, and dulled sensorium. Purpura and mucosal bleeding from respiratory, genitourinary, and gastrointestinal tracts may occur. Massive proteinuria is accompanied by a progressive fall in urinary specific gravity.

*Oliguric Phase.* The oliguric stage lasts 3–7 days. Blood pressure begins to normalize, but many patients become hypertensive due to relative hypervolemia. Prolonged periods of hypertension are predictive of poor prognosis. Bleeding tendencies increase in severity as manifested by extensive purpura, mucosal hemorrhage, and cerebral hemorrhage. Urine output, already compromised to a variable degree because of renal hypoperfusion, falls to oliguric or even anuric levels associated with increasing uremia. Serum creatinine levels may increase dramatically to greater than 10 mg/dl, with blood urea nitrogen (BUN) increasing to over 200 mg/dl. Central nervous system (CNS) symptoms and pulmonary edema may occur in severe cases. Nearly 50% of deaths occur in this stage, generally associated with renal failure, pulmonary edema, and electrolyte abnormalities.

*Diuretic Phase.* Clinical recovery begins with the onset of the diuretic stage, which may last for days to weeks. Diuresis may be delayed due to dehydration, electrolyte imbalance, and infection in some patients. Diuresis of 3–6 liters daily is the rule and can give rise to marked, life-threatening shifts in fluid and electrolyte balance. The convalescent stage lasts for several months and is characterized by progressive recovery of glomerular filtration rate, renal blood flow, and urine concentrating ability. In China, most patients return to light duty during this period, but anemia and hypothaenuria may persist for months to years.

### *Clinical Features of Mild Form (Nephropathica Epidemica)*

The characteristic features of nephropathica epidemica (NE) are biphasic, consisting of fever and renal insufficiency (29). Mortality in NE is low (<1%). The incubation period of NE averages 1 month (range 3 days to 6 weeks), and a prodrome is rare. The febrile stage begins with abrupt onset of high fever (39–40°C), chills, malaise, and headache, which last 2–9 days. Between the third and fourth days, somnolence, nausea, vomiting, back pain, and occasionally joint pain appear, heralding the onset of the renal phase. Restlessness and blurred vision are seen in one-fourth of patients, whereas characteristic severe abdominal pain, sometimes diffusely localized to the right lower quadrant, occurs in some patients. Renal involvement generally appears with lysis of fever. Clinical signs are accompanied by proteinuria (100%, peaking at 1 week), oliguria (>50%), and azotemia (>85%). Elevations of serum creatinine of 2–10 mg/dl and BUN of 50–200 mg/ml may be accompanied by mild electrolyte derangements. Mild hypotension is seen in 40% of patients during the first week, but hypertension is not seen. Oliguria is short lived and is followed by polyuria of 3–4 liters per day for 7–10 days. Hypothenuria is universal. Cylindruria, pyuria, and microscopic hematuria are seen in most patients, but gross hematuria is rare. Mild leukocytosis and thrombocytopenia occur during the renal phase of illness. With the onset of polyuria, clinical recovery begins. Patients are subjectively well within 14–17 days following onset of fever.

### *Prevention and Treatment of Severe Form*

No prevention is currently available, although efforts to develop both conventional and recombinant vaccines are underway. Treatment consists of supportive care, with careful attention to fluid balance. Mortality of untreated disease ranges from 15% to greater than 50%, and with best supportive care without renal dialysis varies from 5% to more than 30%. In facilities with intensive care, including aggressive use of renal dialysis, a mortality rate of 2–3% is associated primarily with hemorrhage.

### *Experimental Therapeutics*

*Preclinical Studies. In vitro* studies have shown that hantaan virus is among the most sensitive of RNA viruses to ribavirin. By way of comparison, plaque reduction 50% effective dose ($ED_{50}$) values for Rift Valley Fever (RVF) virus ($ED_{50}$ = 80 μg/ml) and sandfly fever [SF (Sicilian)] virus ($ED_{50}$ = 77 μg/ml) are substantially higher than for hantaan virus ($ED_{50}$ = 25 μg/ml).

Early studies showed that ribavirin could prevent the appearance of hantaan antigen in the lungs of experimentally infected rodents belonging to the species *Apodemus agrarius*, the natural viral host (59). Subsequently, ribavirin has been evaluated in suckling mice infected with hantaan virus at 24 hr of age (60). These mice develop viremia, detectable viral antigen in tissues, and a clinical syndrome marked by weight loss, depressed activity, hind limb paralysis, and ultimately death (61).

Ribavirin treatment of infected suckling mice was initiated at different stages postinoculation, with doses ranging from 0 to 100 mg/kg continued over 14 days. Treatment started at the onset of viremia on day 6 or at the appearance of viral antigen in tissues on day 10, resulted in a decrease in signs of illness, an increase in survival, and an increase in mean time to death (MTD) in mice that died. The effects of ribavirin were dose-dependent. To characterize the mechanism of protection produced by ribavirin in the suckling mouse model, a serial sacrifice study was performed employing the most promising treatment regimens: 25 mg/kg begun on day 6, and 50 mg/kg begun on day 10, with corresponding controls of placebo treatment and no treatment (60). This study established that protection was associated with decreased viremia and decreased tissue antigen in multiple organs, including liver, spleen, lung, kidney, and brain. The fluorescent antibody response, although delayed by 2 days in ribavirin-treated animals, followed a course similar to control animals. Neutralizing antibody appeared at the same time in both treated and control groups. The favorable effects of ribavirin on hantaan viral infection in suckling mice are especially impressive because drug toxicity peculiar to suckling mice limits drug doses to levels that are suboptimal for cures in other bunyavirus mouse models. Attempts to develop an adequate primate model for HFRS have not been successful.

*Clinical Trials.* The success of these preclinical studies prompted a clinical trial in the PRC from 1985 to 1987 (57,58,60). A prospective, randomized, double-blind, placebo-controlled clinical trial of intravenous ribavirin therapy of HFRS (33 mg/kg loading dose; 16 mg/kg every 6 hr for 4 days; 8 mg/kg every 8 hr for 3 days) was conducted in a nine-site study in Hubei Province, PRC (57). During two epidemic seasons, 244 patients met the study criteria for analysis (enrollment within 4 days of fever onset, extended to 6 days the second season, with clinical diagnosis serologically confirmed by IgM ELISA). Statistical analysis demonstrated random assignment of patients between treatment groups. Reduction in mortality was the most important (primary) determinant of the drug efficacy. Treatment significantly reduced mortality from 10 of 118 in the placebo group to 3 of 126 in the ribavirin-treated group ($p$ = 0.041 by a stratified Fisher's exact test). A stratified analysis of all valid patients entered in both years of the study showed mortality was significantly reduced among ribavirin-treated, compared to placebo-treated patients when comparisons were adjusted for baseline risk estimators of mortality [total serum protein and AST (SGOT) identified in the placebo group by logistic regression], utilizing a stepwise logistic procedure [$p = 0.02$ (two-tailed)]. This improvement in survival may be partially explained by the reduction in kidney damage seen in the drug-treated group. Ribavirin treatment decreased: maximum serum creatinine ($p = 0.05$), duration and magnitude of hypertension, fraction of patient entering oliguria ($p = 0.02$). Ribavirin therapy decreased the fraction of patients experiencing hemorrhagie ($p = 0.03$). Ribavirin shortened the duration of each postfebrile clinical phase. The only significant side effect was a reversible anemia.

Ribavirin is currently an investigational new drug for HFRS and has not been licensed. Intravenous ribavirin therapy at appropriate doses has provided the first effective therapy for early treatment of HFRS in this study. Treatment reduced mortality and improved several important aspects of the clinical course. An ongoing clinical trial for the treatment of all patients is continuing among United States troops who contract the disease in Korea and Okinawa.

A similar study was also conducted in Wuhan, PRC (62) to evaluate recombinant interferon-α therapy of HFRS. Although hantaan virus is sensitive to interferon-α *in vitro* (63), mortality was not reduced and no significant treatment effect was found at doses of $1 \times 10^7$ U per day for 5 days, although indications of reduction in bleeding tendencies were noted. Higher doses were not tested due to dose-limiting toxicity.

### *Prevention and Treatment of NE*

No prevention is currently available, and treatment consists of supportive care with renal dialysis when required. Ribavirin has not been evaluated in this form of the disease.

## *Rift Valley Fever*

### *Etiologic Agent*

RVF, an old-world phlebovirus, shares with other members of the *Bunyaviridae* family a lipid-enveloped spherical structure with a diameter of 90–120 nm, with 5–10 nm surface projections. They mature by budding into the cisternae of the Golgi region. The virion contains two surface glycoproteins, G1 and G2, which are the hemagglutinin (HA) and neutralization targets. It has a negative stranded segmented tripartite genome composed of three RNA species designated large (L), medium (M), which codes for G1 and G2, and small (S), which codes for the nucleocapsid protein and may be of "ambisense" polarity.

### *Epidemiology*

RVF, distributed throughout sub-Saharan Africa, causes serious and occasionally fatal infections in humans (64–68). Epizootics have been documented in Kenya, South Africa, Namibia, Mozambique, Tanzania, Uganda, Zimbabwe, Sudan, Central African Republic, Rhodesia, and Egypt as widely spaced outbreaks during the rainy season that infrequently extend to the next, then disappear for several years. RVF first appeared in Egypt in 1977 when an estimated 200,000 cases occurred with 598 reported deaths. Most cases had a typical febrile illness, but predominant complications included hemorrhagic fever, encephalitis, and exudative retinitis. RVF is also a significant pathogen of sheep and cattle. The virus has been isolated from several genera of mosquitoes. *Culex* and *Aedes* have been implicated during epizootics. Recent findings from Kenya that *Aedes* mosquitoes emerging from flooded depressions called "damboes" are already infected with virus provide strong evidence for transovarial transmission (3,69). RVF can also be transmitted by aerosol.

### *Clinical Features*

Human infection is usually (95%) a severe but self-limiting disease. In less than 5% of cases, disabling or life-threatening complications can occur. Following an incubation period of 2–6 days, back and muscle pain, anorexia, and incapacitating prostration occur. Physical findings are limited to conjunctival and pharyngeal injection. Epistaxis may occur, and a "saddle-back" fever is not uncommon. Initial leukocytosis is followed by leukopenia, composed mainly of lymphocytes. The illness usually lasts 2–5 days, and recovery is without complications (2,65,69,70).

A hemorrhagic form may develop in 1% of patients by the second to fourth day but cannot be predicted on admission. These patients develop petechiae, ecchymosis, hematemesis, melena, and bleeding of the gums. Liver function tests, including prothrombin, bilirubin, transaminase, and alkaline phosphatase, are elevated. Patients become jaundiced and die in shock. The prognosis is poor for patients with hemorrhagic disease and approaches 50% mortality. Recovery is slow but without sequelae (65,67).

Encephalitis can occur 5–10 days after the acute febrile episode, with a presentation of headache, meningismus, vertigo, confusion, hallucinations, and recrudescence of fever. The case fatality rate is unknown but has been estimated at 10% (3). Recovery is slow but without sequelae.

Ocular complications occur late in otherwise asymptomatic patients 1–3 weeks after acute illness, with brisk onset of impairment of visual acuity resulting from retinal hemorrhages, exudates, macular and paramacular edema, vasculitis, retinitis, and vascular occlusion. Lesions were bilateral in 50% of patients, and 40–50% suffer some permanent loss of visual acuity (69).

### *Prevention and Treatment*

No specific treatment exists, and uncomplicated disease is best managed by symptomatic treatment and observation. Hemorrhagic complications should be managed by standard techniques, but anticoagulation therapy of disseminated intravascular coagulation may be ill-advised due to virus-induced liver damage (69).

### *Experimental Therapeutics: Preclinical Studies*

Experimental infections of RVF in mice or hamsters result in death due to hepatitis on days 4–6 in virtually all animals (71,72). Ribavirin is very effective prophylactically and shows a bell-shaped dose response curve with 100% survival produced by 100 mg/kg/day (71). Punta Toro serves as a lower biohazard model for RVF in routine antiviral screening in the USAMRIID program. Ribavirin treatment of Punta-Toro-virus infected hamsters with 100 mg/kg/day on days 0–4 increased survival from 10% to 90% and MTD from 5 to over 45 days (72). Similar results are obtained in a murine model routinely used for testing antiviral drugs *in vivo* (73). Rhesus monkeys challenged with RVF virus intravenously (IV) and treated with ribavirin initially 2 hr after virus inoculation by the intramuscular (IM) route (50 mg/kg loading dose followed by 10 mg/kg tid) had significantly lower viremia ($p < 0.001$) compared to those of sham-treated control monkeys. All infected monkeys had serum neutralizing antibody titers of 1:80 or greater by day 7, even though two of four ribavirin-treated monkeys were not detectably viremic (74). Interferon in this same model is also protective (75). Poly(ICLC) is effective in the murine model, as are combinations of ribavirin and poly(ICLC).

### Crimean-Congo Hemorrhagic Fever

#### Etiologic Agent

Caused by a nairovirus genus of the family *Bunyaviridae,* the properties of Crimean-Congo hemorrhagic fever (CCHF) are similar to those of Rift Valley Fever.

#### Epidemiology

CCHF, transmitted by ticks, occurs over a wide area of the world, mainly in steppe, savannah, semi-desert, and foothill biotropes where the tick parasites are present on both domestic and wild animals in a large area of East and West Africa. Human disease has been documented as sporadic focal infection in the Union of Soviet Socialist Republics, Bulgaria, Pakistan, Dubai, Iraq, the Emirate of Sharjah, Zaire, Uganda, Mauritania, Burkina Faso, Upper Volta, Union of South Africa, Ethiopia, Nigeria, Senegal, Greece, Tanzania, Namibia, and the People's Republic of China (3). The distribution of virus is the second widest of all arboviruses and its distribution, based on virus isolation or serological studies, is from southern Europe to China. CCHF virus has been isolated from many species of ticks, and members of three genera have been shown to be capable of transmitting infection, but ticks of the genus *Hyalomma* have always been regarded as the main vectors (76). Disease is related to the interaction of ticks and their vertebrate hosts, which is complex. Secondary infections are common in a hospital setting. A nosocomial outbreak in Tygerberg Hospital illustrates the potential where an index case resulted in eight infections and two deaths. Typically, a severely ill patient presents to the hospital with severe hemorrhagic disease, but the diagnosis is not made on admission so proper isolation procedures are not initiated until after infection of medical personnel has occurred through contact with blood. The diagnosis is first suggested when 3–7 days later medical personnel involved in direct care, laboratory workers, patients in nearby beds, and/or close family members present with hemorrhagic disease and often a high mortality rate.

#### Clinical Features

The disease in the Soviet Union has been described in detail (24,77–79). The incubation period is estimated to be 3–12 days based on recall of tick exposure, and 3–6 days in nosocomially acquired cases. Onset is abrupt in virtually all cases, with severe headache, fever over 39°C, myalgia, weakness, anorexia, back and abdominal pain, and nausea, often accompanied by vomiting. There is hyperemia, most notable on the face, mucous membranes, and upper part of the body. The illness generally follows a biphasic course, early nonspecific symptoms being followed after the sixth day of illness by hemorrhage from the nose, mouth, and gastrointestinal tract. The appearance of large ecchymotic areas on the limbs is a particularly noticeable feature. Large purpuric areas sometimes occur. Most cases are apathetic or obtunded with halting speech; dizziness and mild meningeal signs are common. Severe cases will be delirious or comatose. Shock and death from circulatory collapse often occur. Laboratory findings include leukopenia and thrombocytopenia to 30,000/mm$^3$. Hematocrit is normal or elevated on presentation but falls with hemorrhage to less than half of normal values in severe cases. The case fatality rate has reached as high as 30–50% in nosocomial outbreaks (69,80–82) but typically is 9–40%. Differences in clinical course are described, with the Middle Eastern form yielding extensive nosocomial secondary and even tertiary spread, and there is a high prevalence of severe liver involvement with clotting abnormalities.

### *Prevention and Treatment*

There is no proven specific therapy. Convalescent immune plasma may be useful, but controlled studies have not been reported. Hospitalization, including careful attention to proper isolation procedures to avoid potentially devastating nosocomial spread, can be effectively implemented without the requirement for specialized treatment facilities. Laboratory and nursing staff must exercise care to avoid generation of aerosols. Recommendations for handling of cases have been published (83).

### *Experimental Therapeutics*

*Preclinical Studies.* Development of animal models has proven difficult. Available models utilize suckling mice infected on days 1–5, with the notable exception of one Russian report of a lethal adult mouse model, in which successful ribavirin therapy is reported. Ribavirin appears to be uniformly effective *in vitro* (84) and increases both the number of survivors and MTD in suckling mouse models (G. Tignor and B. Shope, unpublished observations).

*Clinical Studies.* During an outbreak of CCHF at the Tygerberg hospital (80,81), a large 2,000-bed teaching hospital near Cape Town South Africa, six of nine inoculation contacts were given ribavirin prophylactically (83). One patient had a mild clinical course, whereas the other five developed neither clinical CCHF nor antibodies to the virus. Although two of three needle contacts not treated with ribavirin developed a severe clinical course, one needle contact and 42 proven blood contacts who did not receive ribavirin also did not show any signs of clinical disease. Thus, no firm conclusions could be drawn about the prophylactic use of the drug. No obvious treatment failures were observed, but an opportunity to evaluate efficacy of the drug does not appear to have been present, because of the low attack rate among patients with blood contact. Due to the toxicity of interferon ($1.7 \times 10^7$ U), which was also tested, ribavirin remains the best available prospect for therapy.

## Arenaviruses

Arenaviruses include four human pathogens of which three produce hemorrhagic disease (4). The virulent new-world arenaviruses predominantly cause disease in men and are acquired in rural areas in the fall, when agricultural products are harvested. Transmission is thought to occur by contact with chronically infected rodent hosts (84). In West Africa, the arenavirus Lassa fever has also been found to be sensitive to ribavirin (85,86). Over the last several years, primate models have been developed to study the pathogenesis and treatment of each of these viruses. Studies in experimental animal models of guinea pigs and monkeys infected with either Machupo, Junin, or Lassa viruses have shown both prophylactic and therapeutic efficacy of ribavirin.

### ***Lassa Fever***

#### *Etiologic Agent*

Lassa virus is an enveloped, single-stranded, bisegmented RNA virus classified in the family *Arenaviridae*. Negative-staining electron microscopy (EM) shows the presence of pleomorphic particles ranging from 80 to 150 nm. The envelope is formed by budding from the plasma membrane of infected cells. The virus contains three major structural proteins: two glycoproteins and a nucleocapsid.

### Epidemiology

Lassa fever is a severe disease of West Africa, caused by Lassa virus, one of two pathogenic old-world arenaviruses. The natural host is the multimammate rat *Mastomys natalensis,* which is ubiquitous across sub-Saharan Africa and occupies ecological niches in both forest and savannah regions. Evidence suggests only one species is involved in infections (84). They are infected and shed high levels of virus throughout their life. The epidemiology of all arenaviruses is defined by the factors that determine maintenance and spread of the agents among rodents, which in turn spread virus into the environment. This African rodent, which lives in close association with humans, is found in and around most dwellings, the most important locations for transmission of the virus to humans. Under natural conditions, infection occurs via contact with *M. natalensis* or its excreta within the household (83). Naturally occurring infections, often associated with subsequent nosocomial outbreaks, have been recognized in Nigeria, Sierra Leone, and Liberia (1) and less frequently in Guinea, Senegal, Mali, and the Central African Republic (1,88). Several cases have been imported into the United States and Europe (89,90), but secondary transmissions have not been documented. Person-to-person spread required close personal contact or contact with blood or excreta. Proper barrier infection control procedures appear adequate to control nosocomial spread. Of infections, 70–90% result in mild or asymptomatic infections. Overall mortality of recognized infections is 1–2%, a major revision of initial impressions based on nosocomial outbreaks (91). The mortality of hospitalized patients is 15–20%. In West Africa, 50,000–150,000 infections occur each year and account for 5–15% of febrile illness.

### Clinical Features

The clinical spectrum of Lassa fever is quite variable, and the ratio of infection to illness is 9–26%. After an incubation period of 1–3 weeks, Lassa fever presents as an insidious onset of progressive fever, malaise, and myalgia, and a sore throat. At time of hospitalization, patients are toxic and mildly hypotensive. Pain is seen in the joints and lower back, along with headache, and a nonproductive cough. Retrosternal or epigastric pain, vomiting, diarrhea, and abdominal discomfort are also common. Frank bleeding tendencies may develop during the course of the illness, particularly in severely ill patients. Illness may last 3–4 weeks. Poor prognostic signs include sustained fever, bleeding diathesis, severe hypotension or shock, coma, and convulsions (89,92–100). Various degrees of permanent sensorineural deafness result in 25% of patients. Adverse prognostic factors are AST elevations above 150 IU/liter and high levels of viremia during hospitalization. The latter are not measurable in time to be clinically useful (83).

### Prevention and Treatment

Treatment is supportive and may require intensive care facilities. Attention must be paid to fluid and electrolyte balance, maintenance of blood pressure and circulatory volume, and control of seizures (83).

### Experimental Therapeutics

*Preclinical Studies.* Infection of rhesus monkeys with $10^6$ PFU of Lassa virus resulted in six of 10 deaths between 10 and 14 days after inoculation. The six lethally infected animals had viremia titers that significantly exceeded $10^4$ PFU/ml, whereas none of the surviving monkeys developed viremia in excess of this apparently critical titer. These results are quite similar to the human disease in which admission viremia is a predictor of survival (101). In four monkeys treated with ribavirin (50 mg/kg loading dose, followed by 10 mg/kg three times daily), from day 0 through day 18, the onset of detectable viremia was delayed until day 7, and peak viremia titers were significantly lower ($10^2$ PFU/ml) than those of surviving control monkeys. Clinical illness was mild and brief in monkeys that received ribavirin beginning on day 0. Some monkeys exhibited no clinical signs at all, whereas others became only slightly depressed and developed a minimal facial rash during the second week. All treated monkeys survived, even when ribavirin therapy was delayed until day 5. Four monkeys receiving ribavirin first on day 5 experienced a moderately severe disease course. However, all monkeys treated therapeutically with ribavirin by day 5 eventually recovered with no evident sequelae, and viremia titers never reached the critical level. Thus, therapeutic administration of ribavirin can reverse the hemorrhagic component of the disease (85). In cynomolgus monkeys, 13/14 untreated monkeys died, whereas ribavirin treatment begun at 0, 4, and 7 days resulted in 0/4, 0/4, and 4/8 deaths (102). Combination therapy with immune plasma possessing a log neutralizing index of greater than 2 was also evaluated with very promising results (102). These studies led to a clinical trial of ribavirin treatment of Lassa fever in Africa.

*Clinial Trials.* Ribavirin chemotherapeutic trials in Lassa fever patients were initiated in 1979 in Sierra Leone. An open, nonplacebo controlled trial of oral ribavirin was begun first, followed by a trial of higher dose intravenous ribavirin (2 g loading dose, then 1 g every 6 hr for 4 days, then 0.5 g every 8 hr for 6 days) in an attempt to improve survival over that observed with oral ribavirin. The mortality of patients hospitalized with acute Lassa fever in Sierra Leone is 16%, based on data from over 400 Lassa fever cases seen in two hospitals during the 3-year period preceding the drug study. Patients with Lassa fever may be subdivided by two indicators of mortality risk: admission levels of AST (SGOT) and viremia. An admission serum and AST over 150 carries a risk of mortality of 50%, whereas an admission viremia over $10^{3.6}$ $TCID_{50}$/ml carries a mortality rate of 76%. This high-risk group allowed for demonstration of drug efficacy, based solely on survival. Patients treated with IV ribavirin who had an admission viremia over $10^{3.6}$ $TCID_{50}$/ml had a mortality of 32% compared with 76% in patients who were untreated. The time of initiation of treatment, in relationship to the clinical course of the disease, was also determined retrospectively. Patients who began treatment early, before day 7 of clinical signs, had a significantly improved chance of survival, compared to late initiation of treatment. This observation of the need for early initiation of treatment is shared with all antiviral drugs currently in use (101).

### *Argentine Hemorrhagic Fever and Bolivian Hemorrhagic Fever*

#### *Etiologic Agent*

Bolivian hemorrhagic fever is caused by Machupo virus. Argentine hemorrhagic fever (AHF) is caused by Junin virus. Both are members of *Arenaviridae*, with properties similar to Lassa virus.

#### *Epidemiology*

Bolivian hemorrhagic fever is localized to the sparsely populated tropical savannah in the northeast of Bolivia. As with all arenaviruses, the epidemiology is influenced by the rodent host *Calomys callousus,* which causes focal house-related outbreaks. Rodent control programs have resulted in no outbreaks since 1974 although isolated cases are still seen (J. Miaztegui, unpublished observations). AHF occurs in the farmland of the humid pampa, predominantly in Buenos Aires and Cordoba Provinces. AHF is an occupational disease predominantly affecting men harvesting grain crops, principally maize. The primary rodent vector is *Calomys muscullinus*. Its density fluctuates widely over a 3–5-year period and correlates with human disease rates.

### *Clinical Features*

Insidious onset of fever, headache, asthenia, and myalgia after an incubation period averaging 7–14 days characterizes this syndrome. Mild or subclinical infection is unusual in contrast to Lassa and lymphocytic choriomeningitis (LCM) virus infection. Back pain, epigastric discomfort, retroorbital pain, photophobia, constipation, and occasionally mild diarrhea appear during the following 2–5 days. During this interval, patients are progressively toxic and lethargic with flushed face and trunk, conjunctival inflammation, and by the fourth to the sixth day of illness, fine petechiae in the axillary region. There may be lymphadenopathy and a palatine or faucial exanthem comprised of petechiae or fine vesicles. Pharyngitis is uncommon. Dysesthesia of the skin may be severe. Panleukopenia (to 1,000/mm$^3$) and thrombocytopenia (to 25,000/mm$^3$) are always present. Protein may appear in the urine along with cylindrical casts and erythrocytes.

At the end of approximately 1 week of fever and just prior to its resolution by lysis, patients begin to improve clinically (approximately 60%) or enter into a clinical crisis consisting of either a bleeding-shock phase lasting no more than 3 days or a neurological syndrome that may last up to 1 week. Mixed forms are commonly noted in AHF. The bleeding disease is heralded by petechiae, a rising hematocrit, and increasing proteinuria. If not treated promptly and, in some instances, irrespective of intervention, hypotension and disturbances in consciousness ensue. When clinical shock appears, the prognosis is grave. Pulmonary edema is a common complication, and bleeding from the gastrointestinal tract and mucous membranes is always evident.

In both Argentina and Bolivia, case fatality rates are approximately 15%, with neurologic disease more common in the former country and hemorrhagic disease predominant in the latter. Patients surviving this disease require several weeks for convalescence, and paroxysmal and orthostatic hypotension, asthenia, and mild anorexia are common (84,103).

### *Prevention and Treatment*

Administration of specific antibody (2 U of immune plasma) has been proven effective (mortality reduced from 16% to 1%) if given within 8 days in a double-blind trial of normal and convalescent plasma (104).

### *Experimental Therapeutics*

*Preclinical Studies with Machupo*. Junin, the causative agent of Argentine hemorrhagic fever, is sensitive to ribavirin *in vitro* (71,105), as is closely related to Machupo, which causes Bolivian hemorrhagic fever (72,86). The therapeutic potential of ribavirin was first evaluated in the treatment of Machupo-infected guinea pigs. Only 1/15 untreated animals survived, whereas 12/15 ribavirin-treated animals survived. Treatment was significant at the $p < 0.001$ level (72). Ribavirin was next evaluated using a rhesus monkey model (106–108). Sham-treated virus control monkeys reached peak viremia by days 12–14 and began to die. Treatment of individual monkeys was initiated at the time of onset of fever with 25 mg/kg and continued every 8 hr for 10 days. Quite remarkably, viremia responses of treated monkeys were lower by day 7 compared to sham-treated control monkeys and virtually undetectable by day 10. Regardless of the time of initial treatment or regimen of therapy, ribavirin prevented death during the acute phase of illness. The late neurological syndrome, seen in 20% of infected, untreated control monkeys, however, was not prevented in 4/5 treated animals. It is presumed that the late neurological phase of the disease results from the inability of ribavirin to reach the CNS in sufficient concentration (72).

*Preclinical Studies with Junin.* Prophylactic as well as therapeutic studies of ribavirin in Junin virus infection of rhesus macaques also have been performed (109). Sham-treated control animals infected with $10^{4.8}$ plaque-forming units (PFU) of the highly lethal Espindola strain of Junin virus showed 100% mortality with a classical hemorrhagic diathesis during the third and fourth weeks. Monkeys administered ribavirin on a prophylactic schedule (60 mg/kg/day for 4 days, 30 mg/kg/day for 3.5 days, then 15 mg/kg/day for 11 days) seroconverted, but failed to develop viremia or clinical signs of illness. In animals receiving ribavirin therapeutically beginning on day 6 postinfection (60 mg/kg/day for 1.5 days, then 15 mg/kg/day for 14 days), viremia was detected until the time of drug administration, then disappeared for the duration of observation. These animals had early signs of bleeding abnormalities (redness around eyes, circular ocular redness, dried blood in nose) and decreased platelet counts prior to onset of therapy. Treatment resulted in reversal of clinical disease including resolution of hemorrhage, petechiae, and restoration of platelet counts. As occurred in Machupo-treated animals, however, a late-onset neurological syndrome appeared in all animals, and was fatal in two of three. Similar studies in *Callithrix jacchus* (cotton-eared marmoset) revealed similar results (110).

*Clinical Trials.* A clinical trial of ribavirin is currently underway at the Instituto Nacional de Estudios sobre Virosis Hemorragicas, Pergamino, Argentina. A specific treatment is available for AHF, which consists of the administration of immune plasma with defined neutralizing antibody titers. However, this treatment is only effective when given within the first 8 days after onset of symptoms. Immune plasma therapy is not effective after 8 days of illness (104,111,112). An open study was therefore undertaken in this group of late patients to determine tolerance and antiviral activity. Six patients were treated during the epidemic season. Ribavirin treatment resulted in significant reduction in viremia and a drop in endogenous interferon (high interferon levels are indicators of poor prognosis) and an increase in average time to death (113). This prompted a placebo controlled study that has enrolled 18 patients to date.

## *Filoviridae*

The *Filoviridae* family of viruses was first identified in 1967 when an outbreak associated with laboratory workers harvesting tissues from wild caught African green monkeys developed Marburg disease. The two members of this family, Ebola and Marburg, cause the most severe of the viral hemorrhagic fevers (VHF), but outbreaks have been rare and research must be conducted in BL 4 containment laboratories.

### *Ebola/Marburg*

#### *Etiologic Agent*

The morphology of Ebola and Marburg is unique. Particles range from 130 to 14,000 nm in length but are more uniform in diameter (80 nm). The nucleocapsid is surrounded with a lipid envelope and contains a single-stranded RNA. Five polypeptides are associated with the virion (54).

*Epidemiology*

Marburg and Ebola represent two recently recognized viral hemorrhagic fevers of Africa. Marburg was first recognized in 1967 when seven deaths, which occurred among 31 cases in Germany and Yugoslavia, were traced to direct contact with blood, organs, or tissue culture cells from a group of African green monkeys caught in Uganda. In 1976, outbreaks of Ebola occurred in Sudan and Zaire with over 500 cases and 400 deaths, respectively. The disease occurs in all age groups, but with a predominance in adults. Transmission from person to person requires close contact, particularly with blood or body fluids. The method of maintenance in nature is not known.

*Clinical Features*

The clinical picture of Marburg and Ebola is indistinguishable. Following an incubation period of 4–16 days (average of 7 days), clinical illness begins suddenly with fever, malaise, headache, and myalgia followed by nausea, vomiting, and watery diarrhea. A maculopapular rash appears between days 5 and 7 and is most marked on the buttocks, trunk, and outer aspects of the upper arms, and conjunctivitis is common. Liver function is impaired by the second week of illness, but jaundice is not observed. Renal damage has been observed. Disseminated intravascular coagulopathy is a major feature of the disease, and bleeding occurs in the majority of cases, mainly from the gastrointestinal tract. Case fatality rates from 29% to 89% in outbreaks have been reported (114–116).

*Experimental Therapeutics: Preclinical Studies*

Ebola is not significantly inhibited *in vitro* by ribavirin in Vero, MRC-5, or FRhL cells. Ribavirin prophylaxis (20 mg/kg/day) of Ebola utilizing the guinea pig model with either the Zaire or Sudan strain resulted in no change in survivors but a significant prolongation of MTD with the Sudan strain. A study utilizing 100 PFU of Zaire strain of Ebola in cynomolgus monkeys was conducted. Animals were treated with ribavirin at 50 mg/kg loading dose, 4 hr prior to infection, followed by 20 mg/kg tid until time of death. No significant effect of the drug was seen (H. Lupton and J. Moe, unpublished observations).

**Flaviridae**

Two flaviviruses cause viral hemorrhagic fevers (VHFs) and are widely distributed in nature. Yellow fever (YF) often presents as a VHF, whereas Dengue fever is primarily a febrile illness with outbreaks or isolated cases of VHF.

***Yellow Fever***

*Etiologic Agent*

As all flaviviruses, YF virus is a positive, single-stranded RNA virus with a spherical, host-cell-derived lipid envelope. The structural proteins consist of a major glycosylated envelope protein (E) exposed on the virion surface that contains most immunologic determinates. A small nonglycosylated envelope protein (M) is not exposed on the surface, and a nonglycosylated nucleocapsid protein (C) is found in association with the viral RNA. The morphology of all flaviviruses is quite similar, being spherical with a mean diameter of 43 nm (37–50 nm), a unit membrane envelope with surface projections, and a 30-nm diameter core. The entire genomic RNA has been sequenced for the 17D and Asibi (vaccine parent) strain.

### *Epidemiology*

YF occurs throughout much of tropical South America and sub-Saharan Africa. The epidemiology of YF is explained by different transmission cycles of the virus among humans, mosquitoes, and monkeys. The vector mosquito, which belongs to one of several species, becomes infected by feeding on a viremic host (human or monkey) and then transmits the virus to another susceptible host. YF occurs in two major forms, urban and jungle (or sylvatic) with very different results. Sylvatic (jungle) YF circulates in a cycle involving nonhuman primates and forest or canopy mosquitoes. In Africa, the infection is not usually fatal to nonhuman primates, whereas in South America it is frequently fatal, a useful clue in identifying areas of viral transmission. In this area, YF is endemic with a year-round transmission cycle between monkeys and mosquitoes. Humans are infected when exposed to the enzootic cycle, and sporadic cases occur on a continuous basis. In the savanna surrounding the forest zone, YF is endemic. Human infections may occur at varying frequencies as vector populations expand during the rainy season. In this emergence zone, epidemics may occur, involving both monkey-to-human and interhuman transmission by sylvatic vectors. These epidemics are often characterized by focal outbreaks separated by areas without human cases. Urban YF, the oldest described viral hemorrhagic fever, is capable of explosive epidemics and still constitutes an important cause of viral hemorrhagic fevers. Urban YF is transmitted in a human-mosquito-human cycle involving domestic *Aedes aegypti*. The potential geographic distribution of urban YF is the range of *Aedes aegypti,* which includes Africa, South America, Central America, the Caribbean, and the Gulf coast of the United States. Disease incidence is modified by the presence of existing antibody, either through natural infection or by vaccination. The last major urban outbreak in a major city in the Americas occurred in Rio de Janeiro in 1928 and 1929. The outbreak in Ethiopia in 1960–62 involved over 100,000 cases and 30,000 deaths. An outbreak in Nigeria in 1987, although not fully described, involved over 30,000 cases.

### *Clinical Features*

YF is an acute infectious disease. The incubation period is usually 3–6 days following the bite of an infected mosquito. The clinical spectrum varies from very mild, nonspecific febrile illness to a fulminating, often fatal disease with pathognomonic features. The mild form is characterized by sudden onset of fever and headache without other symptoms, lasting 48 hr or less. The clinical diagnosis is almost impossible in most settings and must rely on serological diagnosis. In other patients, fever is higher, the headache severe, and there is myalgia, slight albuminuria, and bradycardia in relation to the height of fever (Faget's sign). The illness lasts several days with uneventful recovery (1). The so-called classical YF is characterized by a biphasic disease course. The febrile phase is characterized by abrupt onset of fever (39–40°C), chills, severe headache, lumbosacral pain, and general myalgia. The patient appears distressed and anxious, the conjunctiva is congested, and the face and neck are flushed. The tongue is reddened at the tip and edges, and the breath is foul-smelling. Anorexia, nausea, vomiting, and minor gingival hemorrhage or epistaxis may occur. Despite a persistent or rising temperature, the pulse may fall (Faget's sign). Proteinuria is minor initially but can become marked on day 3–4. This syndrome, lasting 3–4 days, corresponds to the period of viremia. This is followed by a remission with defervescence and improvement in the general condition of the patient, which lasts only a few to 24 hr. This is followed by a period of intoxication, the hepatorenal phase, characterized by rising temperature, reappearance of symptoms with more frequent vomiting, epigastric pain, prostration, and the appearance of jaundice. Prolongation of the clotting, prothrombin, and partial prothrombin times is marked in patients with jaundice. Total and conjugated serum bilirubin levels can be very high. Serum AST and ALT levels are markedly elevated in all icteric patients, and hypoglycemia has been noted with severe liver damage. Bleeding diathesis is manifested by coffee-grounds hematemesis, melena, metroohagia, petechiae, ecchymosis, and diffuse oozing from the mucus membrane. Dehydration results from vomiting and insensible losses. Renal dysfunction is marked by a sudden increase in albuminuria and decreased urinary output. Death usually occurs on day 7–10 and is preceded by deepening jaundice, hemorrhages, rising pulse, hypotension, oliguria, and azotemia. Hypothermia, agitated delirium, intractable hiccups, stupor, and coma are terminal events. Death is largely attributable either to an early fulminating hemorrhagic fever syndrome with hepatitis and clinical jaundice or to a later renal tubular lesion with renal insufficiency reminiscent of that seen in HFRS. Convalescence is often prolonged, but complete recovery of the liver function usually occurs. An atypical, fulminant form occurs with death on the second or third day without hepatic or renal signs (reviewed in detail in refs. 1 and 117–119).

### *Prevention and Treatment*

YF 17D is a safe and efficacious live attenuated viral vaccine prepared from infected chicken embryos under standards developed by the World Health Organization. Travel to endemic areas requires vaccination, which is valid for 10 years although immunity is probably life-long. Serious adverse reactions are extremely uncommon. Fewer than 10% of vaccinees experience headache and malaise. An immune response can be demonstrated in 95% of recipients within 7–10 days. Vector control in urban areas directed against *Aeges aegypti* should include elimination of breeding places, which is difficult in many locations due to local practices, and the use of insecticides and larvacides. Such measures are only effective in coordination with vector surveillance programs. Despite the effectiveness of mosquito eradication programs and the availability of a safe and effective vaccine, sporadic epidemics of YF still occur in South America and Africa.

### *Experimental Therapeutics: Preclinical Studies*

YF is sensitive to ribavirin *in vitro,* but, comparing YF sensitivity to other viruses that can be successfully treated with ribavirin in primates or humans, three strains of YF are 10- to 20-fold less sensitive in two lines of Vero cells than Lassa, HFRS, RVF, and sandfly fever (SF) (J. W. Huggins, unpublished observations). Because of differences in drug uptake and metabolism between cell lines, sensitivity comparisons must utilize the same cell for valid comparisons. This may explain why a series of primate experiments has yielded equivocal results. No acceptable rodent model is available. YF in rhesus monkeys produces a fulminate disease with a condensed disease course. This prompted a study with the well-characterized lethal model of Dakar 1279 strain of YF in rhesus monkeys (120) to evaluate ribavirin, utilizing the optimum primate dosing schedule (85). Two groups of eight rhesus monkeys were infected with $1 \times 10^3$ PFU of Dakar 1279 strain of YF and treated simultaneously with ribavirin (30 mg/kg loading 10 mg/kg t.i.d. for 7 days). No effect on either survival, MTD, or viremia titers was seen between the two groups. It is postulated that the relative insensitivity of YF to ribavirin may result from tissue levels of drug below those required to inhibit viral replication. Ribavirin hematopoietic toxicity in monkeys precluded testing significantly higher doses (J.W. Huggins, P.B. Jahrling, C.J. Peters, and T.M. Cosgriff, unpublished observations).

### Dengue Fever

#### Etiologic Agent

Four serologically distinct types of Dengue fever can be recognized (DEN 1–4). See section YF for a description of physical properties. Differences exist in the molecular weight of the structural proteins. DEN 1 and 3 form a subcomplex defined by monoclonial antibodies.

#### Epidemiology

Dengue fever, which had been advancing for several years toward the United States from Mexico and the Caribbean, crossed the border into Texas in 1980, making dengue outbreaks possible in areas of the United States where suitable vectors exist. Since 1977, hundreds of cases have been imported into the United States by travelers from the Caribbean (117). Dengue exists as four distinct serotypes (DEN 1–4) transmitted by *Aeges* mosquitoes, principally in tropical areas of Asia, Oceania, Africa, Australia, and the Americas. Dengue is a prevalent health problem in Southeast Asia, the Caribbean, Central America, northern South America, and Africa (1). Hundreds of thousands of cases occur each year in epidemic or endemic form around the world. Outbreaks have involved over 1 million individuals, with attack rates during epidemics in focal areas of high transmission reaching 50–90% (1). During the 1978 DEN 1 epidemic in Puerto Rico, 13% of the island population was infected (121). Dengue exists in a human-mosquito-human cycle, with *Aeges aegypti* being the most important vector. All four types can coexist in the same area. Protection against homotypic reinfection is complete and probably lifelong, but cross-protection between dengue types lasts less than 12 weeks. In Southeast Asia, children are infected by all four serotypes in childhood. The background of immunity of human populations determines the incidence and age distribution of infections.

#### Clinical Features

Dengue virus can produce two types of disease: classical dengue and dengue hemorrhagic fever (DHF). The clinical features of classical or uncomplicated dengue fever frequently depend on the age and gender of the patient, and whether it is an initial or secondary (other serotype) dengue infection. Infants and young children may have an undifferentiated febrile disease with maculopapular rash, an acute respiratory illness, or a gastrointestinal illness. Older children and adults infected with dengue for the first time will display more classical signs. In a typical case, after an incubation of 2–7 days, the disease begins abruptly with high fever, frontal headache or retroorbital pain, retrobulbar pain, and lumbosacral aching pain. Fever may be sustained for 6–7 days or be biphasic (saddle-back). Initial symptoms are followed by generalized myalgia or bone pain that increases in severity, anorexia, nausea, vomiting, weakness, and prostration. The pulse rate may be slow in relation to the fever. A rash may appear or reappear after defervescence (day 3–5) and be maculopapular or morbilliform in nature. Generalized lymphadenopathy may occur. The peripheral WBC count is depressed, and the platelet count may fall to less than 100,000/mm$^3$. Hemorrhagic phenomena are noted in a few cases and include petechiae, epistaxis, intestinal bleeding, menorrhagia, and a positive tourniquet test (reviewed in refs. 1 and 117). Myocarditis and various neurologic disorders have been associated with dengue fever. Central neurologic disorders appear to be more common in DHF than in classic dengue. Convalescence may be prolonged, with generalized weakness, depression, bradycardia, and ventricular extrasystoles (1).

A more severe form of dengue recognized during outbreaks is DHF. It is generally agreed that DHF is an immunologically mediated disease, as first proposed by Halstead (122). It is proposed that nonneutralizing antibodies, naturally acquired by previous dengue infection or passively acquired as maternal antibody, enhance *in vivo* replication in mononuclear phagocytes and lymphatic tissues. Increased replication of the virus in these cells may be associated with a secondary reaction in the host's attempt to eliminate dengue-infected cells, resulting in immune-mediated disease and shock. This concept is supported by the observation that DHF rarely occurs in primary dengue infection. Typical cases are characterized by four major clinical manifestations: high fever, hemorrhagic phenomena, hepatomegaly, and often circulatory failure. Moderate to marked thrombocytopenia with concurrent hemoconcentration is a finding that differentiates DHF from dengue. Two gradations are recognized, dengue hemorrhagic fever without shock (DHF) and dengue shock syndrome (DSS) that adds shock to DHF. The World Health Organization (WHO) has established guidelines to differentiate DHF/DSS from dengue. Typical cases are characterized by four major manifestations: high fever, hemorrhagic phenomena, hepatomegaly, and often circulatory failure. Moderate to marked thrombocytopenia with concurrent hemoconcentration is a distinct clinical laboratory finding that differentiates DHF from dengue, including dengue with hemorrhagic manifestations. A grading system has been established by the WHO and grading has been found clinically useful in DHF epidemics in children in Southeast Asia and the Western Pacific region, but its usefulness in adults is not fully established. The disease is initially similar to classical dengue, with a high continuous fever lasting 2–7 days. Hemorrhagic manifestations include, as a minimum, a positive tourniquet test and any of the following: petechiae, purpura, ecchymosis, epistaxis, gum bleeding, hematemesis, and/or melena. The liver is usually palpable early in the febrile phase. Patients usually recover spontaneously or after fluid and electrolyte therapy. If signs of shock are present, the disease is classified as DSS. Severe cases, after 2–5 days, rapidly progress with prostration and signs of shock (restlessness, irritability, cold clammy extremities, peripheral cyanosis, and narrowed pulse pressure). Patients in shock are in danger of dying if appropriate therapy is not given promptly. The duration of shock is short, and patients may die within 12–24 hr or recover rapidly following appropriate antishock therapy (1,117,123).

### *Prevention and Treatment*

The major pathophysiological abnormality seen in DHF/DSS is an acute increase in vascular permeability that leads to leakage of plasma. Hypovolemic shock, as a consequence of a critical level of plasma loss, leads to tissue anoxia, metabolic acidosis, and death, if uncorrected. In most cases, early and effective replacement of lost plasma results in a favorable outcome. The consistent finding that a drop in platelet count usually signals the onset of plasma leakage is of great diagnostic and prognostic value. There is no specific antiviral therapy, but symptomatic and supportive measures are effective (see ref. 124 for complete recommendations).

### *Experimental Therapeutics: Preclinical Studies*

DEN 1–4 are sensitive to ribavirin *in vitro*. Using a lethal murine intracranial (IC) model of DEN 2, Halstead et al. (125) were able to demonstrate activity of a lipophilic derivative of ribavirin thought to have improved capability to cross the blood-brain barrier, both on survival and MTD. Ribavirin was not effective, but it has been established that ribavirin does not cross the blood-brain barrier in significant quantities. Useful primate models that mimic the human disease do not exist at present; however, viremia in primates can be reproducibly measured utilizing mosquito cells (peak average viremia of $10^5$ PFU/ml), prompting a ribavirin trial for suppression of viremia (126). Treatment with an optimum ribavirin schedule in a blinded, placebo-controlled primate study resulted in no suppression of viremia compared to controls.

## ENCEPHALITIS

Encephalitis is the serious outcome of a number of viral illnesses that usually cause inapparent or febrile illness but with a varying frequency of patients who develop encephalitis, ranging from mild, with no sequelae, to fatal. All are associated with insect vectors (Table 2). It is especially difficult to develop antiviral drugs against the encephalitic forms because of problems with drug penetration through the blood-brain barrier to the site of viral replication. Prospects for antiviral chemotherapy are uncertain, and no successful trials have been conducted.

### *Flaviridae*

### *California Serogroup Viruses*

#### *Etiologic Agent*

LaCross, snowshoe hare, Jamestown Canyon, and California encephalitis virus are members of the California serogroup of the genus *Bunyavirus*, family *Bunyaviridae*. Properties are similar to Rift Valley Fever.

#### *Epidemiology*

LaCross is the most frequently reported arboviral encephalitis in North America. All of the viruses are focal and are associated with culicine mosquitoes, usually *Aedes* species.

#### *Clinical Features*

LaCross infection may be inapparent or a mild febrile illness following a 1-week incubation period. LaCross encephalitis is a disease of children. Onset is sudden, with fever and headache, followed within 12–14 hr by seizures. Convulsions are present in 50% of cases. The acute illness lasts typically 7 days with gradual recovery. The case fatality rate is 0.5%. Seizure disorders are the main sequelae of LaCross.

Jamestown Canyon encephalitis, in contrast, is usually a disease of adults. Prodromal fever and respiratory illness are followed by signs of meningitis or encephalitis (2).

#### *Prevention and Treatment*

No specific antiviral therapy is available.

### *Japanese Encephalitis*

#### *Etiologic Agent*

Japanese encephalitis (JE), a flavivirus, is a member of the West Nile antigenic group that includes Saint Louis encephalitis, Murry Valley encephalitis, West Nile, Ricio, and Ilheus. Properties of JE are similar to those of other flaviviruses.

#### *Epidemiology*

JE is a public health problem of major concern in Asia, Southeast Asia, and the Indian subcontinent. JE is endemic in Japan, the eastern Union of Soviet Socialist Republics, Korea, China, Indo-China, Indonesia, and India. In terms of morbidity and mortality, JE is by far the most important of the arboviral encephalitides. The incidence has decreased in recent years in Japan, Korea, and Taiwan through vaccination and vector control, but thousands of cases are seen annually in Thailand. The principal amplification cycle for JE involves pigs in a transmission cycle involving *Culex* and *Aedes spp.* mosquitoes and domestic animals, birds, bats, and reptiles. Two patterns of disease occurrence are observed based on the biology of the insect vector. In temperate zones, explosive outbreaks are associated with seasonal increases in vector populations. In subtropical and tropical regions, cases occur throughout the year. JE produces a high inapparent-to-apparent infection ratio of 25–500 infections to each case of encephalitis. The mortality among cases with encephalitis is 20–50%, with permanent sequelae in many survivors (2).

#### *Clinical Features*

Clinical manifestations of JE vary from asymptomatic infection to a fulminant course leading to death. Following an incubation of 5–15 days, illness is manifested by a febrile headache syndrome, aseptic meningitis, or encephalitis. Severe encephalitis begins with a 2–4-day long phase of headache, fever, chills, anorexia, nausea and vomiting, dizziness, and drowsiness of rapid onset. In children, abdominal pain and diarrhea are common. This is followed by nuchal rigidity, photophobia, altered states of consciousness, hyperexcitability, and varying objective neurological signs (1). Death occurs on the fifth to ninth day or during a more prolonged course with pulmonary complications (1). A poor prognosis is associated with respiratory dysfunction, positive Babinski signs, frequent or prolonged seizures, prolonged fever, and albuminuria.

#### *Prevention and Treatment*

The current vaccines were produced in Japan from the Nakayama-NIH strain, and because of antigenic variation there are questions about its effectiveness against current wild strains of JE, although a recent study demonstrates efficacy in Thailand (127). A live attenuated strain is currently undergoing evaluation in the People's Republic of China (Y. Yu, unpublished observations), and the WHO has called for new efforts to select relevant strains for development of new vaccines. No specific therapy is available.

#### *Experimental Therapeutics: Preclinical Studies*

Most antiviral drugs that inhibit JE *in vitro* do not cross the blood-brain barrier. Several natural products, however, appear to be protective in a prophylactic murine model and will be evaluated further (J.W. Huggins, M. Ussery, B.J. Gabrielsen, M. Hollingshead, and B. Shannon, screening data from USAMRIID antiviral drug development program).

### **Saint Louis Encephalitis**

#### *Etiologic Agent*

Saint Louis encephalitis (SLE) is a member of the West Nile antigenic subgroup. Properties of SLE are similar to those of other flaviviruses.

#### *Epidemiology*

SLE occurs in endemic and epidemic form through the Americas and is the most important arboviral disease in North Amer-

**TABLE 2.** *CNS Arthropod-borne viruses that cause acute infection and encephalitis*

| Virus | Taxonomic group | Mode of transmission | Geographic distribution | Disease in domestic livestock |
|---|---|---|---|---|
| Viruses principally associated with the encephalitis syndrome; epidemic and endemic | | | | |
| EEE | *Togaviridae, alphavirus* | Mosquito | Eastern North America, Caribbean, South America | Equines, penned pheasants |
| WEE | *Togaviridae, alphavirus* | Mosquito | Western North America, South America | Equines |
| VEE | *Togaviridae, alphavirus* | Mosquito, possibly other modes (see text) | Florida, Central and South America | Equines |
| St. Louis encephalitis | *Togaviridae, flavivirus* | Mosquito | North America, Caribbean, Central and South America | None |
| JE | *Togaviridae, flavivirus* | Mosquito | East, Southeast Asia; India | Equines, swine |
| Rocio encephalitis | *Togaviridae, flavivirus* | Mosquito | Brazil | None |
| Murray Valley encephalitis | *Togaviridae, flavivirus* | Mosquito | Australia | (Equines)[a] |
| California encephalitis and La Crosse | *Bunyaviridae,* California serogroup | Mosquito | North America | None |
| TBE: Russian spring-summer and Central European encephalitis | *Togaviridae, flavivirus* | Tick, ingestion of milk | Europe, USSR | None |
| Louping ill | *Togaviridae, flavivirus* | Tick | British Isles | Sheep, equines, cows |
| Powassan | *Togaviridae, flavivirus* | Tick | Eastern North America | None |

| | | | | |
|---|---|---|---|---|
| **Viruses principally associated with other syndromes, but occasionally causing encephalitis; epidemic and endemic** | | | | |
| Sindbis (febrile illness with rash) | *Togaviridae, alphavirus* | Mosquito | Africa, Europe | None |
| West Nile (febrile illness with rash) | *Togaviridae, flavivirus* | Mosquito | Africa, Middle East | (Equines)[a] |
| YF (hemorrhagic fever) | *Togaviridae, flavivirus* | Mosquito | Africa, tropical America | None |
| Rift Valley fever (febrile illness, hemorrhagic fever) | *Bunyaviridae,* phlebotomus fever group | Mosquito, direct contact | Africa | Sheep, cows, goats |
| Colorado tick fever (febrile illness) | *Reoviridae, orbivirus* | Tick | Western North America | None |
| Tick-borne hemorrhagic fevers | | | | |
| KFD | *Togaviridae, flavivirus* | Tick | India | None |
| OHF | *Togaviridae, flavivirus* | Tick | Central Asia | None |
| CCHF | *Bunyaviridae, nairovirus* | Tick | Eastern Europe, USSR, Africa | None |
| **Rare and sporadic infections associated with encephalitis** | | | | |
| Semliki Forest[b] | *Togaviridae, alphavirus* | Mosquito | Africa, Southeast Asia | (Equines)[a] |
| Ilheus | *Togaviridae, flavivirus* | Mosquito | South America | None |
| Negishi | *Togaviridae, flavivirus* | Tick | Japan | None |
| Langa[b] | *Togaviridae, flavivirus* | Tick | Asia | None |
| Thogoto | *Bunyaviridae* | Tick | Africa | None |

[a]Disease suspected but not well documented.
[b]Encephalitis recorded in laboratory infections or experimental infections of cancer patients only; significance in naturally acquired infections unknown.
From ref. 130, with permission.

ica. SLE is closely related antigenically to JE in Asia and Murry Valley encephalitis in Australia. Since first recognized in 1933, there have been numerous outbreaks in the western United States (Pacific coast states, primarily California), Texas, the Ohio-Mississippi Valley, Kansas, Colorado, and Florida. Two vectors have been implicated: In the western United States, *Culex tarsalis*, and in the eastern United States *Culex pipiens*. The largest outbreak occurred in 1975, with over 2,000 recognized cases. SLE occurs in epidemic form at approximately 10-year intervals, and attack rates from 1 to 800 per 100,000 population. The disease appears in July with peak incidence in August and September (1,117).

*Clinical Features*

The clinical picture of SLE ranges from inapparent infection to fulminant encephalitis and death. Three clinical syndromes are described: encephalitis, aseptic meningitis, and febrile headache. The severity of illness increases with increasing age, and persons over 60 are at increased risk (1). The incubation period is 4–32 days. The syndrome of febrile headache presents as an acute febrile illness with headache, frequently accompanied by nausea and vomiting. Onset is characterized by general malaise, chilliness, anorexia, nausea, myalgia, and sore throat or cough. No signs of meningeal irritation or localized neurologic abnormalities are found. The aseptic meningitis presentation is one of an acute febrile illness associated with acute or subacute meningeal signs (a stiff neck). The syndrome of encephalitis includes presentations of meningoencephalitis and encephalomyelitis. It is characterized by altered levels of consciousness, abnormal reflexes, tremor, and signs of thalamic, brain stem, and cerebellar dysfunction (1,117). A prolonged period of convalescence from a disorder called "convalescent fatigue syndrome" occurs in 30–50% of cases, lasting up to 3 years. In 20% of patients, symptoms of altered gait and speech disturbances, sensor motor impairment, psychoneurotic complaints, and tremors persist for extended periods.

*Prevention and Treatment*

Treatment is supportive, and no effective antiviral therapy exists.

***Tick-Borne Encephalitis***

*Etiologic Agent*

The tick-borne encephalitis (TBE) is a flavivirus belonging to the TBE virus complex, which consists of six members that cause human disease: TBE, Omnsk hemorrhagic fever, Kyasanur Forest disease, Negishi, Powassan, and louping-ill. There are two subtypes of TBE: Russian spring-summer encephalitis and Central European encephalitis, which differ in their tick vector and clinical expression. TBE shares the properties of other flaviviruses except for its resistance to acidic pH, a feature that makes the virus resistant to gastric acid and allows infection from ingesting contaminated milk.

*Epidemiology*

TBE occurs in western and eastern Europe (Austria, Denmark, Finland, East and West Germany, Hungary, Poland, Sweden, Yugoslavia, Czechoslovakia), the Soviet Union, and China in a pattern corresponding to the Ixodid tick vector. The virus is maintained in nature by a cycle involving ticks and several wild rodent vectors. *Ixodes ricinus* is responsible for transmission of the Central European encephalitis in Europe, whereas *Ixodes persulcatus* is responsible for Russian spring-summer encephalitis. Other tick species are also implicated in areas that do not support *Ixodes* ticks. Infection of goats, cattle, and sheep results of shedding of virus into the milk, and inactivation by pasteurization requires the relatively high temperature of 65°C for 30 min. The epidemiology of TBE is greatly influenced by whether the disease is tick-borne or milk-borne. Cases that are tick-borne tend to be sporadic and are influenced by occupations that increase exposure to ticks. The incidence is highest spring through early fall, corresponding to periods of tick activity. Milk-borne outbreaks tend to involve whole families and are determined by milk consumption patterns (1,117).

#### *Clinical Features*

The incubation period for TBE is 7–14 days, but the clinical course differs between the two strains. The Far East form (Russian spring-summer encephalitis) is more severe, with a case fatality rate of 20%. Onset is more often gradual than acute, with a prodromal phase including fever, headache, anorexia, vomiting, and photophobia. This is followed by a stiff neck, sensorial changes, visual disturbances, and variable neurological dysfunction. In fatal cases, death occurs within 7 days. Disease is more severe in children than adults. Neurologic sequelae occur in 30–60% of survivors, especially residual flaccid paralyses of the shoulder girdle and arms. The central European form is milder, with a case fatality rate of 1–5%. The typical disease is biphasic. The first phase is nonspecific and grippe-like, lasting approximately 1 week followed by a 1–3-day remission. The second phase begins abruptly and may take the form of benign meningitis or, in more severe cases, encephalitis. Approximately 20% of survivors have sequelae, which tend to be minor (1,117).

#### *Prevention and Treatment*

A formalin-inactivated vaccine is used in the Soviet Union, and a joint Austrian-British developed vaccine is available in Europe, but is only covered by an investigational new drug (IND) in the United States. Vaccination is recommended for high-risk occupations, as is avoidance of ticks by the use of tick repellants. Unpasteurized milk should be avoided. Treatment is supportive, and no specific antiviral therapy exists.

## Alphaviruses

### *Eastern Equine Encephalitis/ Western Equine Encephalitis/ Venezuelan Equine Encephalitis*

#### *Etiologic Agent*

Alphaviruses have a similar uniform and spherical appearance (50–65 nm), with a somewhat fuzzy outer surface that is icosahedral, with surface spikes composed of glycoproteins. The viral particle contains a nucleocapsid that ranges from 28 to 49 nm with a single-stranded infectious RNA of $4.1 \times 10^6$ daltons (2).

#### *Epidemiology*

Eastern equine encephalitis (EEE) is maintained in a natural transmission cycle between *Culiseta melanura* mosquitoes and birds in swampy and forested areas of New Jersey and Massachusetts. For transmission to humans, it is necessary for the virus to become established in *Aedes spp.* mosquitoes before human and equine cases occur. Western equine encephalitis (WEE) is maintained in nature by *Culex tarsalis* and *Culiseta melanura* and wild passerine birds in the western United States. Venezuelan equine encephalitis (VEE) is maintained in nature by a cycle involving *Culex ssp.* and

*Aedes aegypti* in a mosquito-rodent-mosquito cycle. Seasonal periods of peak transmission of VEE coincide with peak rainfall (2).

### *Clinical Features*

EEE is clinically the most severe encephalitis in North America. Onset of illness is usually rapid with high fever, vomiting, stiff neck, and drowsiness. Coma can occur by the second day. Children commonly manifest edema, either generalized, facial, or periorbital. Paralyses are common during the acute phase, and EEE seems to produce a greater disturbance in autonomic functions than other togaviral encephalitides. Case fatality rates vary from 50% to 75% of symptomatic patients. Up to 30% of patients surviving the acute infection will have neurologic sequelae, often of a severe nature, requiring permanent institutional care. Inapparent infections and milder clinical forms have been described.

The incubation period for WEE is 5–10 days, and the clinical symptoms observed depend on the age of the patient. A large number of asymptomatic infections or undifferentiated febrile illnesses occur. Illness usually begins with headache, followed rapidly by fever, which can be so high as to be life-threatening. Various manifestations of altered sensorium can progress to coma. Most infants will suffer convulsions. Most adults, even with a severe clinical course, will recover completely if death does not occur. Children under 1 year of age frequently suffer permanent sequelae ranging from minimal brain dysfunction to epilepsy or severe psychomotor disorders.

Very few people infected with VEE virus will have inapparent infection, but only a small percentage develop neurologic involvement. Many patients will have an undifferentiated febrile illness but, more typically, exhibit an influenza-like illness. Symptoms are sudden onset with fevers, chills, myalgia, generalized malaise, headache, nausea, and vomiting. Lumbosacral pain is a frequent complaint, and occasionally patients will also complain of sore throat and diarrhea. Some patients with mild CNS involvement will show lethargy, somnolence, or even mild confusion but do not develop seizures or other localizing signs. VEE infection rarely progresses to encephalitis in adults and is most common in children under 15 years of age. Case fatality rates are highest in children 5 years of age and under (35%) and decrease to less than 10% for older children and young adults. Patients who survive VEE may have permanent neurologic sequelae, but this outcome is less likely with VEE than encephalitis associated with other togaviruses (e.g., EEE) (1,117).

### *Prevention and Treatment*

Treatment is supportive. No effective antiviral therapy is known. VEE is part of the USAMRIID drug discovery program and Poly(ICLC) is effective early in the infection in the murine and primate model. Ribavirin and its triacetate are not effective, however (J.W. Huggins and USAMRIID Antiviral Drug Screening Program).

## PRIMARY FEBRILE ILLNESS

Undifferentiated febrile illness is characteristic of the majority of infections caused by arboviruses (Table 3). Dengue causes a significant number of febrile cases each year and is reviewed in the section of VHFs because of its significant complication. Sandfly fever, although not a serious clinical disease, is included because a ribavirin prophylactic study has been conducted.

### ***Bunyaviridae***

#### ***Rift Valley Fever***

Rift Valley Fever causes a febrile disease in 95% of all cases but is reviewed in the

**TABLE 3.** *Etiologic and epidemiologic features of undifferentiated* arbovirus *fevers*

| Fever | Virus type | Principal vector(s) | Vertebrate host(s) | Geographic distribution | Human epidemiologic features |
|---|---|---|---|---|---|
| Dengue | *Flavivirus* (Group B) | *Aedes aegypti, Ae. albopictus* | Humans | Tropics and subtropics; old and new world | Varies from continuous endemic to sporadic epidemic pattern based on human-*Aedes* population cycles |
| West Nile | *Flavivirus* (Group B) | *Culex* mosquitoes | Birds | Africa, Mediterranean basin, central Asia | Continuously endemic (tropics) to annual epidemic in Mediterranean climates |
| Phlebotomus | *Phlebovirus* | *Phlebotomus, Lutzomyia* sandflies | Wild rodents? | Southern Europe, Africa, central Asia, tropical America | Annual seasonal transmission to children; epidemic whenever large numbers of susceptible adults introduced; forest-associated infections in American tropics |
| Rift Valley | *Phlebovirus* | *Aedes, Culex* mosquitoes | Large wild and domestic animals | Egypt, sub-Saharan Africa | Sporadic transmission to humans; many contact infections during livestock epizootics |
| Chikungunya | *Alphavirus* (Group A) | *Aedes aegypti, Ae. africanus, Ae. furcifer* | Humans, monkeys? | Africa, southern Asia, Philippines | Basically similar to dengue |
| O'nyong-nyong | *Alphavirus* (Group A) | *Anopheles funestus, An. gambiae* | Humans | East Africa | Singular massive epidemic; malaria control may affect pattern |
| Mayaro | *Alphavirus* (Group A) | *Haemagogus* mosquitoes | Monkeys and/ or rodents? | Tropical South America | Endemic, forest-associated infection; localized outbreaks during forest destruction |
| Ross River | *Alphavirus* (Group A) | *Aedes vigilax, Ae. polynesiensis, Culex annulirostris* | Wild mammals, humans? | Australia, New Guinea, Oceania | Endemic to epidemic, depending on mosquito abundance and immunity level in human population |
| Colorado tick | *Orbivirus* | *Dermacentor andersoni* ticks | Ground squirrels, chipmunks | Rocky Mountains of North America | Sporadic and focal summer infections during recreational and occupational activity |

From ref. 130, with permission.

section on viral hemorrhagic fevers because of its sequelae.

### Naples and Sicilian Sandfly Fever

#### Etiologic Agent

Sandfly fever (SF) is an old-world *Phlebovirus;* its properties are similar to RVF.

#### Epidemiology

Naples and Sicilian SF occurs in Africa, Europe, and Asia. The epidemiology is closely associated with the habitats of the vector *P. papatasi,* which is found throughout the Mediterranean, extending as far east as India and Transcaucasia.

#### Clinical Features

SF is an acute, self-limiting febrile illness normally transmitted by the bite of the sandfly. The disease was recognized in 1887, and in 1908 an Austrian military commission reproduced the disease in humans by inoculation of healthy individuals with blood obtained from patients in the first day of fever. The clinical manifestations of sandfly fever were studied beginning in 1944 by Dr. Albert Sabin in more than 100 cases of experimentally induced disease (127). Following intravenous inoculation, the incubation period is 1.5–3.5 days. SF is sudden in onset with fever, lasting 2–4 days, and characterized by frontal and retroorbital pain, headache, photophobia, generalized malaise, arthralgia and low back pain. Anorexia, nausea, and, not infrequently, vomiting are associated with ill-defined abdominal distress. Approximately 65% of patients have fever over 102°F but not above 104.5°F. Fever above 100°F is seen in all patients who complain of a flu-like illness. The disease is self-limiting with complete recovery; no deaths have occurred among thousands of clinically diagnosed cases.

#### Experimental Therapeutics: Clinical Trials

It has not been possible to conduct a clinical trial against Rift Valley fever; however, a controlled trial was conducted at USAMRIID against SF (Sicilian), which is useful in evaluating potential clinical efficacy of the drug against RVF. This model has been used at USAMRIID since 1964 to study the effects of viral infection in humans. Ribavirin was evaluated in a double-blind, placebo-controlled study of prophylactic efficacy in prevention of sandfly fever (Sicilian) virus infection in human volunteers (C. Macdonald, K. Mckee, J. Huggins, and P. Canonico, unpublished observations). Twelve adult human volunteers were inoculated IV on day 0 with diluted human plasma containing sandfly fever (Sicilian) virus. Six subjects received oral ribavirin, 400 mg each 8 hr for a total of 1,200 mg/day beginning 1 day before infection and continuing for 8 days. Six subjects received placebo in an identical manner. Four of six placebo controls became ill with fever, chills, myalgia, prostration, and headache lasting 3 days. Serum chemistries were unaffected, but leukopenia (mean WBC = 2,870) and decreased platelet (mean = 140,000) were seen. All four had fever of greater than 100°F for 3 days, at the same time as clinical illness. During this time, sandfly antigen was detected by ELISA. Serum interferon levels were elevated in clinically ill patients. These four placebo-treated patients showed positive serological evidence of infection as demonstrated by specific IgM and IgG. All ribavirin treated subjects remained healthy without clinical signs during the course of the study, and five of six seroconverted. The failure to infect some subjects, as judged by seroconversion, is believed to be caused by the long storage of the inoculum virus, which had lost infectivity. To provide meaningful comparisons, analysis concentrated on these patients with positive serological evidence in infection. All four seropositive placebo patients became ill, with fever, clinical signs and symptoms, and circulating viral antigen. All five seropositive ribavirin-treated patients remained asymptomatic during the entire study, providing evidence that ribavirin can prevent the infection by a bunyavirus in humans (128).

## Flaviviruses

Many flavivirus infections produce an uncomplicated febrile disease in a significant percentage of patients; those that are capable of causing significant sequelae are covered in the section associated with those sequelae.

### *Dengue*

Dengue causes a febrile illness in the vast majority of cases, but is capable of causing severe hemorrhagic disease under certain conditions. Dengue is reviewed in the section on hemorrhagic fevers.

## Alphaviruses

### *Chikungunya Virus*

#### *Etiologic Agent*

Chikungunya virus is an alphavirus, with properties similar to other members of the family. It is serologically related to o'Nyong-Nyong.

#### *Epidemiology*

Chikungunya virus is transmitted among monkeys and baboons by forest *Aedes* mosquitoes. Large epidemics of chikungunya occur in urban and semiurban settings where the virus is transmitted by *Aedes aegypti*. Such epidemics can be explosive, involving, almost simultaneously, large populations. The geographic distribution is sub-Saharan Africa, India, and southeast Asia. Infections in southeast Asia have coincided with outbreaks of dengue from the same vector (1).

#### *Clinical Features*

Chikungunya is characterized by fever, rash, and arthritis. Following an incubation of 3–12 days, the disease presentation is strikingly abrupt, with intense pain in one or more joints, followed by high fever and myalgia. Rash develops on day 2–5 after onset and is maculopapular. The acute disease lasts 3–10 days, but convalescence may include prolonged joint swelling and pain lasting weeks to months (1).

#### *Prevention and Treatment*

No specific therapy is available.

## DISCUSSION

Significant progress has been made in the development of antiviral chemotherapy for hemorrhagic fevers. Much of this success must be attributed to the good fortune of the discovery of ribavirin, because studies of over 100 close analogs have revealed few with similar or significantly increased antiviral activity in animal models (J.W. Huggins and USAMRIID Antiviral Drug Screening Program) and none is at a state of development to allow for clinical trials.

Intravenous ribavirin is currently an investigational new drug for hemorrhagic fever with renal syndrome and is not approved for general human use by the United States Food and Drug Administration (FDA). In clinical trials, ribavirin has demonstrated therapeutic benefit against two hemorrhagic fevers, Lassa fever and HFRS. Animal models have demonstrated increased rates of survival and inhibition of viral replication for several hemorrhagic fever viruses belonging to the bunyavirus and arenavirus families. The weight of the evidence supports the merit of further studies of ribavirin in patients with Crimean-Congo hemorrhagic fever. It argues against a beneficial effect of the drug in dengue and yellow fever. The toxicity of ribavirin appears to be manageable and is fully reversible. It has not prevented treatment of hemorrhagic fever patients with effective levels of drug. Several new drugs, natural products and analogs of ribavirin, with improved therapeutic ratios are under evaluation, as are possible combinations of ribavirin or an analog with an interferon inducer to improve the overall efficacy. Such combinations may ultimately yield improved therapy, but are not yet ready for clinical trials.

The clinical trials necessary to establish new therapies for these viral diseases are particularly difficult for many reasons, including their predominant occurrence in the Third World where the medical infrastructure is much less developed and funding for health care is limited. Some of these diseases occur in an unpredictable fashion, making planning particularly difficult. Rapid and accurate diagnosis is also a requirement of any useful clinical trial. Despite these difficulties, given the impact of these diseases on the world community, additional clinical trials are clearly needed to achieve effective treatment of life-threatening diseases. Whenever possible, these trials should be prospective, blinded, and placebo-controlled to maximize the value of the results.

## REFERENCES


1. Monath TP. Flaviviruses. In: Fields BN, Knipe DM, Chanock RM, Melnick JL, Roizman B, Shope RE, eds. *Virology*. New York: Raven Press, 1985:955–1004.
2. Shope RE. Bunyaviruses. In: Fields BN, Knipe DM, Chanock RM, Melnick JL, Roizman B, Shope RE, eds. *Virology*. New York: Raven Press, 1985:1055–82.
3. Shope RE. Alphaviruses. In: Fields BN, Knipe DM, Chanock RM, Melnick JL, Roizman B, Shope RE, eds. *Virology*. New York: Raven Press, 1985:931–53.
4. Peters CJ, Johnson KM. Hemorrhagic fever viruses. In: Notkins AL, Oldstone MBA, eds. *Concepts in viral pathogenesis*. Berlin, Heidelberg, New York: Springer, 1985:325–37.
5. Lee HW, Lee PW, Johnson KM. Isolation of the etiologic agent of Korean hemorrhagic fever. *J Infect Dis* 1978:137:298–308.
6. French GR, Foulke RS, Brand OA, et al. Korean hemorrhagic fever: propagation of the etiologic agent of in a cell culture line of human origen. *Science* 1981;21:1046–8.
7. White JD, Shirley FC, French GR, Huggins JW. Hantaan virus, an etiologic agent of Korean Hemorrhagic fever, has a bunyaviridae-like morphology. *Lancet* 1982;1:768–71.
8. McCormick JB, Sasso DR, Palmer EL. Morphological identification of the agent of Korean hemorrhagic fever (Hantaan virus) as a member of *Bunyaviridae*. *Lancet* 1982;1:765–8.
9. Hung T, Xia SE, Song G, et al. Viruses of classical and mild forms of haemorrhagic fever with renal syndrome isolated in China have similar bunyavirus-like morphology. *Lancet* 1983; 1:589–91.
10. Schmaljohn CS, Hasty SE, Harrison SE, Dalrymple JM. Characterization of Hantan virions, the prototype virus of Hemorrhagic fever with renal syndrome. *J Infect Dis* 1983; 148:1005–12.
11. Schmaljohn CS, Dalrymple JM. Analysis of Hantaan virus RNA: evidence for a new genus of bunyaviridae. *Virology* 1983;131:482–91.
12. Schmaljohn CS, Dalrymple JM. In: Compans RW, Bishop DHL, eds. *Segmented negative stranded viruses*. Orlando, Florida: Academic Press, Inc., 1984:117–24.
13. Eliot LH, Kiley MP, McCormick JB. Hantaan virus: identification of virion proteins. *J Gen Virol* 1984;65:1284–93.
14. Tsai TF, Bauer SP, Sasso DR, et al. Serological and virological evidence of a Hantaan virus-related enzootic in the United States. *J Infect Dis* 1985;152:126–36.
15. Gajdusek DC, Goldgaber D, Millard E. *Bibliography of hemorrhagic fever with renal syndrome (muroid virus nephropathy)*. NIH publication no. 83-2603. Bethesda, Maryland, 1983.
16. World Health Organization. Hemorrhagic fever with renal syndrome: memorandum from a WHO meeting. *Bull WHO* 1983;61:269–75.
17. Schmaljohn CS, Hasty SE, Dalrymple JM, et al. Antigenic and genetic properties of viruses linked to hemorrhagic fever with renal syndrome into a newly defined genus of *Bunyaviridae*. *Science* 1985;277:1041–4.
18. Earle DP, ed. Symposium on epidemic hemorrhagic fever. *Am J Med* 1954;16:617–709.

19. Smadel JE. Epidemic hemorrhagic fever. *Am J Public Health* 1953;43:1327–30.
20. Ishii S, Ando K, Watanabe N, Murakami R, Nagayama T, Ishikawa T. Studies on Songo fever. *Jpn Army Med J* 1942;355:1755–1758.
21. Kashahara S, Kitano M, Kikuchi H, et al. Studies on epidemic hemorrhagic fever. *J Jpn Pathol* 1944;34:3–5.
22. Tamura M. Occurrence of epidemic hemorrhagic fever in Osaka City: first case found in Japan with characteristic features of marked proteinuria. *Biken J* 1964;7:79–94.
23. Smorodintsev AA, Dunaevski MI, Kazbintsev LI, Kakhreidze KA, Neutroev VD, Churilov AU. Ethiology and clinics of Hemorrhagic nephroso-nephritis. *Moscow Medgiz* 1944;26–47.
24. Smorodintsev AA, Kazbintsev LI, Chumakov VG. Virus hemorrhagic fevers. In: *Gimiz Gosndrastvennse Isdatel'stro Mdicitsinskoi Literaury*. Leningrad, 1963 [Israel program for scientific translation, Jerusalem, 1964]. Springfield, Virginia: Clearing House, 1964:19–25.
25. Casals J, Hoogstraal H, Johnson KM, Shelokov A, Wiebenga NH, Work TA. A current appraisal of hemorrhagic fevers in the U.S.S.R. *Am J Top Med Hyg* 1966;15:751–64.
26. Casals J, Henderson BE, Hoogstraal H, Johnson KM, Shelokov A. A review of Soviet viral hemorrhagic fevers. *J Infect Dis* 1969;122:437–53.
27. Chumakov M, Gavrilovskaja IN, Bopiko V, et al. Detection of hemorrhagic fever with renal syndrome (HFRS) virus in the lungs of bank voles *Clethrionomys glareous* redbacked voles Clethrionomys rutilus trapped in HFRS foci in the European part of U.S.S.R., and serodiagnosis of this infection in man. *Arch Virol* 1980;9:295–300.
28. Lee HW, Lee PW. Korean hemorrhagic fever. I. Demonstration of causitive antigen and antibodies. *Korean J Intern Med* 1976;19:371–83.
29. Lahdevirta J. Nephropathia epidemica in Finland. A clinical, histological, and epidemiological study. *Ann Clin Res* 1971;3(suppl 8):1–154.
30. Lee HW, Baek LJ, Johnson KM. Isolation of Hantaan virus, the etiologic agent of Korean hemorrhagic fever, from wild urban rats. *J Infect Dis* 1982;146:638–44.
31. Lee PW, Gajdusek DC, Gibbs CJ, et al. An ethiological relationship between Korean haemorrhagic fever and haemorrhagic fever with renal syndrome in People's Republic of China. *Lancet* 1980;1:1025–6.
32. Jiang YT. A preliminary report on hemorrhagic fever with renal syndrome in China. *Chin Med J* [Engl] 1983;96:265–8.
33. Lee HW, Lee PW, Tamura M, Tamura T, Okuno Y. Ethiologic relation between Korean hemorrhagic fever and epidemic hemorrhagic fever in Japan. *Biken J* 1979;22:41–5.
34. Wong TW, Cheong CY, Lee HW. Haemorrhagic fever with renal syndrome in Singapore: a case report. *Southeast Asian J Trop Med Public Health* 1985;16:525–7.
35. Lee HW, Lee PW, Lahdevirta J, et al. Etiological relation between Korean haemorrhagic fever and nephropathica. *Lancet* 1979;22:41–5.
36. Nystrom K. Incidence and prevalence of endemic benign (epidemic) nephropathy in AC County, Sweden in relation to population density and prevalence of small rodents. In: *Umea University medical dissertations, new series, no 30*. Umea: Umea University, 1977.
37. Lahdevita J, Enger E, Hunderi OH, et al. Hantaan virus is related to haemorrhagic fever with renal syndrome in Norway. *Lancet* 1982;1:794–5.
38. Traavik T, Mehl R, Berdal BP, Lund S, Dalrymple J. Nephropathia epidemia in Norway: description of serological response in human disease and implication of rodent reservoirs. *Scand J Infect Dis* 1983;15:11–6.
39. Dournon E, Morinere B, Matheron S, et al. HFRS after a wild rodent bite in the Haute-Savoir and risk of exposure to Hantaan-like viruses in a Paris laboratory. *Lancet* 1982;1:676–7.
40. Van Ypersele de Strihou C, Vandenbroucke JM, Doyen C, Cosyns JP, Van der Groen G, Desmyter J. Diagnosis of epidemic and sporastic interstitial nefritis due to Hantaan-like virus in Belgium. *Lancet* 1983;2:1493.
41. Walker E, Pinkerton IW, Lloyd G. Scottish case of hemorrhagic fever with renal syndrome. *Lancet* 1984;2:982.
42. Trenscenti T, Keleti B. Clinical aspects and epidemiology of hemorrhagic fever with renal syndrome. In: *Akademiai kiado*. Budapest, Hungary, 1971:103–28.
43. Lee HW. Korean hemorrhagic fever. *Prog Med Virol* 1982;28:96–113.
44. Gadjusek DC. Virus hemorrhagic fevers. Special reference to hemorrhagic fever with renal syndrome (epidemic hemorrhagic fever). *J Pediatr* 1962;60:841–57.
45. Gavrilovskaja I, Vasilenkaja S, Gumakov M, Sindarov K, Kacarov G. Hemorrhagic fever with renal syndrome in Bulgaria: spreading and serologic proof. *Epidemiolog Mikrobiolog I Infeck Bol* 1984;21:17–22.
46. Gaon J, Karlovac M, Gresikova M, et al. Epidemiological features of Haemorrhagic fever. *Folia Med Facult Med Univ Saraviensis* 1968;3:23–41.
47. Antoniadis A, Pyrpasopoulos M, Sion M, Daniels S, Peters CJ. Two cases of hemorrhagic fever with renal syndrome in northern Greece. *J Infect Dis* 1984;149:1011–3.
48. Antoniadis A, Le Duc JW, Daniel-Alexiou S. Clinical and epidemiological aspects of hemorrhagic fever with renal syndrome (HFRS) in Greece. *Eur J Epidemiol* 1987;3:295–301.
49. Lee HW, Lee PW, Baek LJ, Song CK, Seong IW. Intraspecific transmission of Hantaan virus, etiologic agent of Korean hemorrhagic fever, in the rodent *Apodemus agarius*. *Am J Trop Med Hyg* 1981;30:1106–12.
50. Yanagihra R, Amyx HL, Gajdusek DC. Experimental infection with Puumala virus, the etiologic agent of nephropathica epidemica, in

bank voles (*Clethrionomys galareolus*). *J Virol* 1985;55:34–8.
51. Katz S, Leedham CL, Kessler WH. Medical management of hemorrhagic fever. *JAMA* 1952; 150:1363–6.
52. Epidemic hemorrhagic fever. In: *Department of the army technical bulletin*. TB MED 240. 1953:5.
53. Sheedy JA, Froeb HF, Batson HA, et al. The clinical course of epidemic hemorrhagic fever. *Am J Med* 1954;16:619–28.
54. McKee KT, Peters CJ, Craven RB, Francy DB. Other viral hemorrhagic fevers and Colorado tick fever. In: Belshe RB, ed. *Textbook of human virology*. Littleton, Massachusetts: PSG Publishing Co., 1984:649–77.
55. McKee KT, MacDonald C, LeDuc JW, Peters CJ. Hemorrhagic fever with renal syndrome—a clinical perspective. *Milit Med* 1985;150:640–7.
56. Cosgriff TM, Huggins JW, Hsiang CM, et al. Prospective clinical evaluation of hemorrhagic fever with renal syndrome (HFRS). *Trans R Soc Trop Med Hyg* (in press).
57. Huggins JW, Hsiang CM, Cosgriff TM, et al. Intravenous ribavirin therapy of hemorrhagic fever with renal syndrome (HFRS) [Abstract]. *Antiviral Res* 1988;9:131.
58. Huggins JW, Hsiang CM, Cosgriff TM, et al. Clinical therapeutic efficacy of intravenous ribavirin treatment of hemorrhagic fever with renal syndrome (HFRS): randomized, double-blind, placebo controlled trial in the People's Republic of China [Abstract]. Presented at the VII International Congress of Virology, Edmonton, Canada. August 1987.
59. Lee HW, Seong IW, Baek LF, Lee JI. The effects of Virazole on Hantaan virus infection in *Apodemus agarius*. *Korean J Virol* 1981;11:13–9.
60. Huggins JW, Kim GR, Brand OM, McKee KT. Ribavirin therapy for Hantaan virus infection in suckling mice. *J Infect Dis* 1986;153:489–97.
61. Kim GR, McKee KT. Pathogenesis of Hantaan virus infection in suckling mice: clinical, virologic and serologic observations. *Am J Trop Med Hyg* 1985;34:388–95.
62. Huggins JW, Hsiang CM, Cosgriff TM, et al. Double-blind, placebo controlled clinical trial of ribavirin in the treatment of epidemic hemorrhagic fever: open phase for dose setting. Presented at the IX International Congress of Infectious and Parasitic Diseases, Munich. July 1986.
63. Gui XE, Ho M, Cohen MS, Wang QL, Huang HP, Xie QX. Hemorrhagic fever with renal syndrome: treatment with recombinant alpha interferon. *J Infect Dis* 1987;155:1047–51.
64. Canonico PG, Kende M, Luscri BJ, Huggins JW. *In vitro* activity of antivirals against exotic RNA viral infections. *J Antimicrob Chemother* 1984;14(suppl a):27–41.
65. McIntosh BM, Russell D, Dos Santos I, et al. Rift Valley fever in humans in South Africa. *S Afr Med J* 1980;58:803–6.
66. Van Velden DJJ, Meyer JD, Olivier J, Greer JHS, McIntosh B. Rift Valley fever affecting humans in South Africa: a clinicopathological study. *S Afr Med J* 1977;29:867–87.
67. Swanepoel R, Manning B, Watt JA. Fatal Rift Valley fever on man in Rhodesia. *Cent Afr J Med* 1979;25:1–8.
68. Laughlin LW, Meegan JM, Strausbaugh LJ, Morens DM, Watten RH. Epidemic Rift Valley fever in Egypt: observations of the spectrum of human illness. *Trans R Soc Trop Med Hyg* 1979;73:630–3.
69. Abdel-Wahab KSEI-D, El Baz LM, Tayeb EM, Omar H, Ossman MAM, Yasin W. Rift Valley fever virus infections in Egypt: pathological and virological findings in man. *Trans R Soc Trop Med Hyg* 1978;72:392–6.
70. Peters CJ, LeDuc JW. Bunyaviruses, phleboviruses and related viruses. In: Belshe RB, ed. *Textbook of human virology*. Littleton, Massachusetts: PSG Publishing Co., 1984:547–98.
71. Meegan JM, Watten RH, Laughlin LW. Clinical experience with Rift Valley fever in humans during the 1977 Egyptian epizootic. In: Swartz TA, Klingberg MA, Goldblum AM, eds. *Contributions to epidemiology and biostatistics. vol 3*. Basel: S Karger, 1981:114–23.
72. Stephen EL, Jones DE, Peters CJ, Eddy GA, Loizeaux PS, Jahrling PB. Ribavirin treatment of toga-, arena-, and bunyavirus infections in subhuman primates and other animal species. In: Smith RA, Kirkpatrick W, eds. *Ribavirin: a broad spectrum antiviral agent*. New York: Academic Press, 1980:169–83.
73. Huggins JW, Jahrling PB, Kende M, Canonico PG. Efficacy of ribavirin against virulent RNA virus infections. In: Smith RA, Knight V, Smith JAD, eds. *Clinical applications of ribavirin*. New York: Academic Press, Inc., 1984:49–63.
74. Sidwell RW, Huffman JH, Barnett B, Pifat DY. In vitro and in vivo phlebovirus inhibition by ribavirin. *Antimicrob Agents Chemother* 1988;32:331–6.
75. Peters CJ, Reynolds JA, Slone TW, Jones DE, Stephen EL. Prophylaxis of Rift Valley fever with antiviral drugs, immune serum, an interferon inducer, and a macrophage activator. *Antiviral Res* 1986;6:285–97.
76. Morrill JC, Jennings GB, Cosgriff T, Gibbs P, Peters CJ. Interferon alpha prevents Rift Valley fever in rhesus monkeys. *Rev Infect Dis* 11:(Supp 4)S815 25.
77. Swanepoel R, Shepherd AJ, Leman PA, et al. Epidemiology and clinical features of Crimean-Congo Hemorrhagic fever in Southern Africa. *Am J Trop Med Hyg* 1987;36:120–32.
78. Leshchinskaya BV. Differential diagnosis of hemorrhagic fever of the Crimean type. Mater II. Nauchn. Sess. Inst. Polio Virus Entsefalitov. Acad. Med. Nauk. SSSR. 1964:268–70.
79. Leshchinskaya BV, Chumakov MP. Comprehensive study of Crimean hemorrhagic fever in different endemic foci of similar diseases in central Asia. Sborn. Trudy Inst. Polio Virus

Entsefalitov. Acad. Med. Nauk. SSSR, 1965; 7:315–25.
80. Lazarev VN, Reunova NM, Manukyan NS, et al. Certain clinical laboratory features of Crimean hemorrhagic fever in Rostov Oblast. In: Eldridge BF, ed. *Miscellaneous publications of the Entomological Society of America*. Baltimore, Maryland: Geo W King Printing Company, 1974:170–2.
81. Van Eeden PJ, Joubert JR, Van de Wal BW, King JB, de Kock A. A nosocomial outbreak of Crimean-Congo hemorrhagic fever at Tygerberg hospital. Part I. Clinical features. *S Afr Med J* 1985;68:711–7.
82. Van Eeden PJ, Van Eeden SF, Joubert JR, King JB, Van de Wal BW, Michell WL. A nosocomial outbreak of Crimean-Congo hemorrhagic fever at Tygerberg hospital. Part II. Management of patients. *S Afr Med J* 1985;68:718–28.
83. Centers for Disease Control. Management of patients with suspected viral hemorrhagic fever. *MMWR* 1988;37(suppl 3):2–3.
84. Watts DM, Ussery MA, Nash D, Peters CJ. Inhibition of Crimean-Congo hemorrhagic fever viral infectivity yields in vitro by the antiviral drug ribavirin. (submitted).
85. Van de Wal BW, Joubert JR, Van Eeden PJ, King JB. A nosocomial outbreak of Crimean-Congo hemorrhagic fever at Tygerberg hospital. Part III. Preventive and prophylactic measures. *S Afr Med J* 1985;68:718–28.
86. Johnson KM. Arenaviruses. In: Fields BN, Knipe DM, Chanock RM, Melnick JL, Roizman B, Shope RE, eds. *Virology*. New York: Raven Press, 1985:103–5.
87. Jahrling PB, Hesse RA, Edy GA, Johnson KM, Calis RT, Stephens EL. Lassa virus infection of rhesus monkeys: pathogenesis and treatment with ribavirin. *J Infect Dis* 1980;141:580–9.
88. Peters CJ, Jahrling PB, Liu CT, Kenyon RH, McKee RK, Barrera Oro JG. Experimental studies of arenaviral hemorrhagic fevers. *Curr Top Microbiol Immunol* 1987;143:5–68.
89. Monath TP. Lassa fever: review of epidemiology and epizootiology. *Bull WHO* 1975;52:577–92.
90. Frame JD. Surveillance of Lassa fever in missionaries stationed in West Africa. *Bull WHO* 1975:52:593–8.
91. Frame JD, Baldwin JM Jr, Gocke DJ, Troup JM. Lassa fever, a new virus disease of man from West Africa: clinical description and pathological findings. *Am J Trop Med Hyg* 1970;19:670–6.
92. McCormick JB, Webb PA, Krebs JW, Johnson KM, Smith ES. A prospective study of epidemiology and ecology of Lassa fever. *J Infect Dis* 1987;155:437–44.
93. Leifer E, Goeke DJ, Bourne H. Lassa fever, a new disease of man from west Africa. II. Report of a laboratory-acquired infection treated with plasma from a person recently recovered from the disease. *Am J Trop Med Hyg* 1970; 19:677–9.
94. Keane E, Gilles HM. Lassa fever in Panguma hospital, Sierra Leone, 1973–1976. *Br Med J* 1977;16(73):1399–402.
95. Knobloch J, McCormick JB, Webb PA, Dietrich M, Schumacher HH, Dennis E. Clinical observations in 42 patients with Lassa fever. *Trop Med Parasitol* 1980;31(4):389–98.
96. White HA. Lassa fever. A study of 23 hospital cases. *Trans R Soc Trop Med Hyg* 1972;66:390–8.
97. Monath TP, Maher M, Casals J, et al. Lassa fever in the eastern province of Sierra Leone, 1970–1972. II. Clinical observations and virological studies on selected hospital cases. *Am J Trop Med Hyg* 1974;23:1140–9.
98. Mertens PE, Patton R, Baum JJ, Monath TP. Clinical presentation of Lassa fever cases during the hospital epidemic at Zorzor, Liberia, March–April 1972. *Am J Trop Med Hyg* 1973; 22:780–4.
99. Bowen GS, Tomori O, Wulff H, Casals J, Nooran A, Downs WG. Lassa fever in Onitsha, East Central State, Nigeria, in 1974. *Bull WHO* 1975;52:599–604.
100. McCormick JB, King IJ, Webb PA, et al. A case-control study of the clinical diagnosis and course of Lassa fever. *J Infect Dis* 1987;155:445–55.
101. Johnson KM, McCormick JB, Webb PA, Smith ES, Elliot LH, King IJ. Clinical virology of Lassa fever in hospitalized patients. *J Infect Dis* 1987;155:456–64.
102. McCormick JB, King IJ, Webb PA, et al. Lassa fever. Effective therapy with ribavirin. *N Engl J Med* 1986;314:20–6.
103. Jahrling PB, Peters CJ, Stephen EL. Enhanced treatment of Lassa fever by immune plasma combined with ribavirin in cynomolgus monkeys. *J Infect Dis* 1984;149:420–7.
104. Peters CJ. Arenaviruses. In: Belshe RB, ed. *Textbook of human virology*. Littleton, Massachusetts: PSG Pub., Co, 1984:513–45.
105. Miaztegui JI, Fernandez NJ, de Damilano AJ. Efficacy of immune plasma in treatment of Argentine hemorrhagic fever and association between treatment and a late neurological syndrome. *Lancet* 1979;2:1216–7.
106. Kenyon RH, Canonico PG, Green DE, Peters CJ. Effects of ribavirin and tributylribavirin on Argentine hemorrhagic fever (Junin virus) in guinea pigs. *Antimicrob Agents Chemother* 1986;29:521–3.
107. Kastello MD, Eddy GA, Kuehne RW. A rhesus monkey model for the study of Bolivian hemorrhagic fever. *J Infect Dis* 1976;133:57–62.
108. Eddy GA, Scott SK, Wagner FS, Brand OM. Pathogenesis of Machupo virus infection in primates. *Bull WHO* 1975;52:517–21.
109. Eddy GA, Wagner FS, Scott SK, Mahlandt BG. Protection of monkeys against Machupo virus by the passive administration of Bolivian hemorrhagic fever immunoglobulin (human origin). *Bull WHO* 1975;52:723–7.
110. McKee KT, Huggins JW. Ribavirin prophylaxis and therapy for experimental Argentine hemorrhagic fever. *Antimicrob Agents Chemother* 1988;32:1304–9.

111. Weissenbacker MC, Calello MA, McCormick JB, Rodrigues M. Therapeutic effects of the antiviral agent ribavirin in Junin virus infection of primates. *J Med Virol* 1986;20:261–7.
112. Rugiero HA, Magnoni C, Cintora FA, et al. Tratamiento de la fiebre hemorragia argentina con plasma de convaleciente. *La Prensa Medica Argentina* 1972;59:1569–78.
113. Montardit AI, Fernandez NJ, De Sensi MRF, et al. Neutrilizaacion de la viremia en enfermos de fiebre hemorragica argentina tratados con plasma immune. *Medicina (Buenos Aires)* 1979; 39:799.
114. Enria DA, Briggiler AM, Levis S, Vallejos E, Maiztegui JI, Canonico PG. Tolerance and antiviral effect of ribavirin in patients with Argentine hemorrhagic fever. *Antiviral Res* 1988;32:353–9.
115. Howard CR. Viral haemorrhagic fevers: properties and prospects for treatment and prevention. *Antiviral Res* 1984;4:169–85.
116. Martini GA, Siegert R. In: Martini GA, Siegert R, eds. *Marburg virus disease*. New York Springer-Verlag, 1971.
117. Pattyn SR. *Ebola virus hemorrhagic fever.* Amsterdam: Elsevier/North-Holland Biomedical Press, 1978.
118. Craven RB. Togaviruses. In: Belshe RB, ed. *Textbook of human virology.* Littleton, Massachusetts: SPG Publishing Company, 1984:599–648.
119. Pan American Health Organization, World Health Organization. *Report: seminar on treatment and laboratory diagnosis of yellow fever.* Brasilia, Brazil. April 1984.
120. World Health Organization. *Prevention and treatment of yellow fever in Africa. Technical report series*. Geneva: WHO.
121. Monath TP, Brinker KR, Chandler FW, Kemp GE, Cropp CB. Pathologic correlations in a rhesus monkey model of yellow fever. With special observations on the acute necrosis of B cell areas of lymphoid tissues. *Am J Trop Med Hyg* 1981;30:431–43.
122. *1978 annual report, San Juan Laboratories.* San Juan, Puerto Rico: Centers for Disease Control, 1978.
123. Halstead SB. Dengue hemorrhagic fever—a public problem and a field of research. *Bull WHO* 1980;58:1–21.
124. World Health Organization. *Guide for diagnosis, treatment and control of dengue haemorrhagic fever.* 2nd ed. Geneva: WHO.
125. Koff WC, Prat JL, Elm JL, Venkateshan, Halstead SB. Treatment of intracranial dengue virus infection in mice with a lipophilic derivative of ribavirin. *Antimicrobial Agents Chemother* 1983;24:134–6.
126. Malinoski FJ, Hasty S, Dalrymple J, Canonico PG. Prophylactic ribavirin treatment of dengue type 1 infection in rhesus monkeys [Abstract]. *Antiviral Res* 1988;9:131.
127. Hoke CH, Nisalak A, Sangwhipa N, et al. Protection against Japanese Encephalitis by Inactivated Vaccines. *N Engl J Med* 1988;319:608–61.
128. Sabin A. In: Rivers TM, ed. *Viral and rickettsial infections of man*. Philadelphia, Pennsylvania: Lippincott, 1948.
129. MacDonald C, McKee K, Huggins JW, et al. Ribavirin prophylaxis of Sandfly fever Sicilian infection in human volunteers (in preparation).
130. Wyngaarden JB, Smith LH Jr. *Cecil: Textbook of Medicine*, 16th ed. Philadelphia: W.B. Saunders Company, 1982.

*Antiviral Agents and Viral Diseases of Man, 3rd Edition,*
edited by G. J. Galasso, R. J. Whitley, and
T. C. Merigan, Raven Press, Ltd., New York 1990.

# 19

# Immunization Against Viral Diseases

Gerald V. Quinnan, Jr.

*Center for Biologics Evaluation and Research, Food and Drug Administration, United States Public Health Service, Bethesda, Maryland 20892*



The public health importance of vaccines against viral diseases is immense. To most of the world, the need for vaccines is apparent from the commonplace occurrence of death from measles or diarrhea, polio, rabies, congenital disease, and numerous other problems. Even in developed countries where widespread vaccination is the rule and many of these maladies have been nearly eliminated, viral diseases in need of prevention remain prevalent and visible problems. Technologies that can be applied to vaccine production have evolved rapidly such that it is generally possible to produce candidate vaccines by a variety of techniques, and the principal hurdles in vaccine development relate to basic research needs for defining principles by which to select one approach or another. Developments in immunology and viral structure/function relationships allow for more rigorous evaluation of various approaches than has been possible in the past. The scientific excitement of the times is a reflection of the immense public health accomplishments and initiatives to extend these benefits of developed countries to the rest of the world. The collective scientific disciplines that contribute to understanding immunological approaches to prevention of infections are sometimes referred to as "vaccinology" and span all the biological sciences. Principles of immunotherapy and prophylaxis of viral diseases will be reviewed in this chapter.

## TYPES OF IMMUNOGENS AGAINST VIRAL DISEASES

Products currently in use for active immunization against viral infections are live attenuated virus, killed virus, or virus subunit vaccines. Those viral vaccines currently available in the United States are listed in Table 1. A variety of novel approaches to vaccine development are under investigation, as summarized in Table 2, such as the use of live, recombinant viruses, antiidiotype monoclonal antibodies, and synthetic peptides. Passive immunization can employ standard immune globulin (IG) for intramuscular (IM) or intravenous (IV) use, as well as a variety of specific IGs.

### Live Viral Vaccines

#### *Advantages and Disadvantages*

A number of advantages and disadvantages can be ascribed to live-virus vaccines. In general, the intent of vaccination is to expose the immune system to the same stimuli that induce critical immune responses in the course of natural infection. Since live-virus vaccines cause infection, they expose the immune system to stimuli more nearly resembling those accompanying natural challenge than do other types of viral vaccines. Concerns regarding whether antigens are presented in the "correct" or natural way are obviated, and there is less chance that viral antigens necessary for protection will be missing from the product. Experience with live-virus vaccines is that protective immunity tends to be life-long. As a rule, this durability is greater than that seen with noninfectious vaccines. Live virus-vaccines also tend to be less expensive to produce. A few thousand infectious vi-

**TABLE 1.** *Licensed viral vaccines currently in distribution in the United States*

| Vaccine | Manufacturer |
|---|---|
| Smallpox | Wyeth Laboratories, Inc. |
| Rabies | Institut Merieux |
| Influenza, split virus | Connaught Laboratories, Inc. |
| | Parke Davis, Division of Warner Lambert Company |
| | Wyeth Laboratories, Inc. |
| Influenza, whole virus | Connaught Laboratories, Inc. |
| Influenza, subunit | Evans, Ltd./Lederle Laboratories |
| Poliovirus vaccine, live, oral | Lederle Laboratories |
| Poliovirus vaccine, inactivated | Connaught Laboratories, Ltd. |
| Yellow Fever vaccine | Connaught Laboratories, Inc. |
| Measles vaccine | Merck, Sharp & Dohme, Inc. |
| Mumps vaccine | Merck, Sharp & Dohme, Inc. |
| Rubella vaccine | Merck, Sharp & Dohme, Inc. |
| Measles and rubella vaccine | Merck, Sharp & Dohme, Inc. |
| Measles, mumps, and rubella vaccine | Merck, Sharp & Dohme, Inc. |
| Adenovirus vaccine, type 4 | Wyeth Laboratories, Inc. |
| Adenovirus vaccine, type 7 | Wyeth Laboratories, Inc. |
| Hepatitis B vaccine, plasma derived | Merck, Sharp & Dohme, Inc. |
| Hepatitis B vaccine, recombinant | Merck, Sharp & Dohme, Inc. |

**TABLE 2.** *Types of viral vaccines*

| Vaccine type | Examples |
|---|---|
| Living | |
| Jennerian | Smallpox |
| Selected mutant | Live oral poliovirus |
| Host range adaptation mutant | Measles |
| Reassortant | Experimental rotavirus |
| Chemically or physically mutagenized | Experimental dengue virus |
| Recombinant DNA-produced | Experimental recombinant vaccinia |
| Noninfectious | |
| Whole virus, inactivated | Rabies, influenza |
| Inactivated, disrupted | Influenza |
| Viral subunit | Influenza, hepatitis B |
| Recombinant-DNA-derived protein | Hepatitis B |
| Synthetic peptide | Experimental vaccines |
| Antiidiotype monoclonal antibody | Experimental vaccines |

ruses may be a sufficient dosage for a live vaccine, whereas millions of inactivated viruses may be needed in a killed virus vaccine. Thus, production costs of live vaccines may be very low. Concerns about quality, quantity, and durability of immune response and cost are reasons for continued interest in the development of live-virus vaccines.

Disadvantages associated with the use of live-virus vaccines include the risk of complications from infection in vaccinees or their contacts, and possibilities of vaccine failure due to interference from prior immunity or concurrent infection with other viruses. Complications from virus infection may be the result of residual virulence of the vaccine virus, reversion of the virus back to the virulent state, or unique susceptibility of the vaccinated host. Smallpox vaccine can cause complications attributable to replication of this virus, as exemplified by the sometimes severe local reaction typical of a primary "take" in vaccinees or in contacts of vaccinees (1). Special examples of host susceptibility being a contributing factor are provided by experience with smallpox vaccine, as well. Specifically, eczema vaccinatum occurs in children with underlying eczema and progressive vaccinia, a fatal disease, can occur in people who are immunosuppressed (2).

Reversion of vaccine virus to a more virulent state is rare, since genetic stability is one of the factors considered in assessment of clinical data to determine which vaccines should be placed in general use. Changes in neurovirulence of Sabin strain polioviruses occur during replication in the human intestine, and this partial reversion may contribute to the occurrence of vaccine-associated poliomyelitis in contacts of vaccinees (2).

Failure of live-virus vaccines to induce immunity is sometimes related to loss of potency, but also may result from preexisting immunity or from interfering virus infections (3,4). Appropriate stabilization and storage of vaccines and targeting usage to local circumstances can usually overcome problems of reduced efficacy.

### *Bases for Attenuation*

The safety and effectiveness of live viral vaccines is based on the balance obtained between the organism's ability to stimulate protective immunity and its virulence. The objective of efforts to produce virus strains suitable for use in live-virus vaccines is to develop virus strains that infect recipients with high efficiency, inducing potent and durable immune responses, without causing disease. A variety of approaches have been used to develop attenuated viruses. The Jennerian approach, exemplified by smallpox vaccine, uses an animal virus to protect humans from a human virus (5). Smallpox vaccine is the only virus vaccine that has been in general use that was based on this method of attenuation, but other efforts at vaccine development have been based on similar principles.

Adaptation of viruses to alternate host systems has been used successfully for virus attenuation. Repeated passage of viruses in cell culture, embryonated eggs, or animals can result in such adaptation. Positive selection of viruses with avirulent characteristics after serial passage in cell culture was used by Sabin for the development of attenuated polioviruses (6). Virus clones were identified that did not cause poliomyelitis when inoculated into the central nervous system (CNS) of monkeys. Intentional mutation of viruses may also be of value. Methods that result in useful mutations may involve selection of temperature sensitive or cold-adapted viruses, or use of chemical mutagens (7–9).

Reassortment is a technique also used for production of vaccine viruses. If two viruses of the same type with segmented genomes infect the same cell, the progeny viruses produced will contain mixtures of the RNA segments normally present in each parent virus. The technique is used to produce viruses with surface antigens of one virus and nonsurface antigens of the other. Selection of progeny with surface antigens of one type is accomplished using antibodies against the unwanted antigens, whereas selection of viruses containing the internal genes of the other is accomplished using selective growth conditions. For example, the internal genes of rhesus rotavirus serotype 3 have been used for *in vitro* growth advantage of the rhesus virus to make rhesus-human rotavirus reassortants containing the surface genes of human types 1, 2, and 4 rotaviruses (10).

Molecular biological techniques have been applied in a variety of ways for producing nonvirulent viruses. For example, they have been used to interrupt expression of specific genes in vaccinia and herpes simplex viruses (HSVs) that code for virulence factors (11,12). In the case of vaccinia virus, interruption of the expression of the thymidine kinase (TK) gene is associated with this effect, whereas in HSV the gene is one of unknown function. In addition to modification of virulence, recombinant DNA techniques can be used to delete or add genes to these viruses. Moss et al. (11) used the TK promoter sequence in vaccinia virus to control expression of hepatitis B surface antigen and other antigens. Roizman et al. (13) modified HSV type 1 (HSV-1) in similar ways. Adenoviruses have also been constructed that express foreign genes (14,15). Site-directed mutagenesis can be used to modify virus virulence. Gene sequence analyses of polioviruses have demonstrated that the more stable attenuation of the type 1 Sabin strain compared to the type 3 Sabin strain may be because it has many more mutations throughout the viral genome (16,17). An effort is underway to produce a stable attenuated type 1 Sabin virus that induces immunity to type 3 virus as a result of many site-directed mutations. The opportunities to develop new candidate vaccines using recombinant DNA techniques will continue to be explored.

### *Reversion and Virulence*

It is an inherent characteristic of live-virus vaccines that they replicate in the recipient and have the potential, therefore, however remote, to produce disease. For vaccines in general use, safety in large numbers of people has been established in clinical trials, such that serious disease in recipients and person-to-person transmission with serious disease in contacts should occur rarely. The likelihood that serious adverse events may occur in vaccine recipients depends on a number of factors, including (a) inherent genetic stability of the virus, (b) relative attenuation or nonvirulence of the virus; (c) amount and duration of virus replication that normally occurs; (d) host susceptibility including immunity and immune deficiency, and other host factors, such as age and gender; and, (e) opportunity for transmission based on site of replication (i.e., whether or not virus's shed in secretions). Genetic stability of the virus is a critical issue. If attenuation is based on a single or limited number of point mutations, back mutation or suppressor mutations elsewhere in the genome may readily render the virus virulent. Thus, the basis for attenuation of viruses in general use as vaccines is likely to be highly complex at the molecular level. When vaccine virus replicates extensively and for a long duration, there may be sufficient opportunity for reversion of even highly attenuated, very stable viruses. Immune deficiency may enhance the opportunity for reversion by allowing for extensive replication to occur and may provide the setting in which disease may be produced by a minimally virulent virus. It is unrealistic to expect absolute safety from live viral vaccines.

## Noninfectious Viral Vaccines

### *Advantages and Disadvantages*

Noninfectious vaccines have the obvious advantage that they do not contain virus capable of replicating to produce disease. Moreover, it is potentially possible to establish precisely the amount of each antigen or even epitope contained in the vaccine. It is normally possible to establish immunization regimens with noninfectious vaccines such that very high levels of immunity are obtained, even if the regimen is begun while maternal antibodies are still present in the circulation.

The disadvantages or difficulties associated with noninfectious vaccines are several. In comparison to live vaccines, large amounts of virus are needed and production costs may be high. Multiple doses of noninfectious vaccines are usually needed in people who have not been previously primed with the virus, and the durability of immunity is often less than after live vaccines. Noninfectious vaccines are normally given by injection and do not usually induce secretory immunity. Such vaccines are generally considered less effective at inducing cell-mediated immunity than live vaccines, perhaps because the injected antigen is processed by antigen presenting cells less efficiently than antigens of replicating viruses. Until the effectiveness of a new inactivated vaccine is shown, there is always theoretical concern that noninfectious vaccines may not fully mimic the antigenic exposures occurring during natural infection and may induce ineffective immune responses or even immunopathology. Allergy is more likely to be a problem with these than with live-virus vaccines because of the role of chemicals involved in inactivation and because of the relatively large amounts of foreign protein in the inoculum.

### *Types of Noninfectious Vaccines*

The most common type of noninfectious viral vaccines are killed, or inactivated, vaccines. The first vaccines of this type were the formalinized animal brain-derived rabies vaccines developed in the late 19th century. In more recent times, influenza and poliovirus vaccines were early examples of inactivated viral vaccines. All inactivated viral vaccines in general use depend on inactivation with formaldehyde or β-propiolactone. These agents inactivate viruses by chemical reactions that result in covalent linkage of the inactivating moiety to the viral proteins, a process known as "derivatization." The reactions are performed with excess derivatizing agent so that complete irreversible inactivation occurs. Residual live virus can only be present if some particles escape exposure to the inactivating agent. One such example was the incomplete inactivation of poliovirus in inactivated vaccine resulting in the transmission of poliomyelitis via vaccination, an event commonly referred to as the "Cutter incident" (18). It was learned soon thereafter that viral aggregation was the reason for failure of formaldehyde to gain access to some viral particles. No other basis for failure of action of formaldehyde or β-propiolactone on cell-free viruses has ever been noted. Complete inactivation with these agents can thus be assured by proper attention to inactivating conditions. Derivatization of vaccine proteins may result in formation of new haptens, although this has been a problem infrequently (19,20). The selection of either formaldehyde or β-propiolactone for use in inactivation of a specific virus is largely empiric, based on which chemical results in the best preservation of viral antigenicity.

Solubilizing agents, particularly detergents, are often of interest in vaccine preparation (21). In no case to date has a solubilizing agent been used alone successfully as the only method of inactivation. Other physical-chemical methods such as heat and radiation have been applied in some cases (22).

Subunit vaccines are comprised of disrupted, killed viruses or of one or a few proteins, usually derived by purification from virus particles. The subunit vaccines currently in use include influenza and hepatitis B vaccines. Subunit influenza vaccines were developed because of the pyrogenicity and other adverse effects that were attributed to whole-virus inactivated influenza vaccines. It is now known that adverse reactions attributable to the whole inactivated virus can be eliminated by virus solubilization or by appropriate standardization of vaccine potency. However, the safety and effectiveness of influenza vaccines consisting mostly of the surface glycoproteins, hemagglutinin (HA) and neurominidase (NA), has been established (23). The first HBV surface antigen vaccine was a subunit vaccine derived from human plasma because attempts to propagate the virus *in vitro* had not been successful (24,25).

Recombinant DNA techniques are applicable to the production of viral vaccines consisting of purified proteins. The first such vaccine to become generally available was hepatitis B surface antigen vaccine produced *in vitro* in *Saccharomyces cerevisiae* (26,27). Bacteria, yeast, and eukaryotic cells, including invertebrate cells, can all be used for this purpose, potentially. Viruses are essential in this technology as expression vectors or components of expression vectors. A baculovirus expression vector has been used to infect cells derived from the Fall Army worm (*Spodoptera frugiperda*) to produce an experimental acquired immunodeficiency syndrome (AIDS) vaccine (28).

The potential for using other recently developed technologies to produce noninfectious vaccines has evoked interest. Peptides of approximately 20 amino acids or fewer in length can be synthesized using solid-phase techniques quickly and inexpensively in large amounts. In theory, this approach can allow for the selection of specific epitopes as vaccines. Limitations inherent to the approach are that it can be used only for conformationally independent linear epitopes, there are always impurities in the products of the synthetic reactions, and there is usually a need for presentation by carrier proteins or in complex adjuvants (30,31). Antiidiotype monoclonal antibodies are also of interest, although they have not been used as candidate viral vaccines subject to extensive experimentation (32).

### Immune Globulin and Virus-Specific Immune Globulins

The introduction of antibacterial antibiotics led to the nearly complete disappearance of serotherapy, treatment by passive immunization, as a form of treatment of infectious diseases. However, IG is used rather extensively for prophylaxis of viral diseases and to a limited extent for treatment. Hyperimmune animal sera were once the mainstay of passive immunization against viruses. Although often effective, these products are highly allergenic on repeated exposure (33). Human IG has, therefore, been applied progressively more broadly.

Standard IG is produced from pools of plasma derived from thousands of donors and contains antibodies typical of the population from which the donors were derived. Thus, IG produced from donors in the United States would contain antibodies to common viruses, low levels of antibodies to less common viruses, such as HBV, and no antibodies to exotic viruses, such as Lassa fever virus. It is required that IG produced by United States' licensed manufacturers be tested and shown to contain antibodies to polio and measles viruses (34). Specific IGs are produced from plasma from selected donors to obtain higher titers of specific antibodies than is the norm for the population. In some cases, the donors are selected after specific immunization, such as for vaccinia, rabies, or hepatitis B immune globulin (VIG, HRIG, or HBIG, respectively) (1,35).

Another way to produce globulins with high titers of antibodies to a specific infectious agent is to select plasma by screening large numbers of normal donors to find those in the higher part of the normal range of distribution of titers against the specific virus. Examples of such products are cytomegalovirus and varicella-zoster virus IG (CMVIG and VZIG) (36,37). Lastly, donors may be selected from populations where exotic diseases are endemic, such as for Lassa IG.

The types of IG available in the United States are listed in Table 3 along with a description of their indications for use. With the exception of VIG, they are used for prophylaxis, either preexposure, as in the case of IG and CMVIG, or postexposure (HRIG, HBIG, VZIG).

**TABLE 3.** *Immune globulins approved for prevention or treatment of viral diseases in the United States*[a]

| Product | Indication |
|---|---|
| IG | Congenital or acquired hypogammaglobulinemia<br>Preexposure prophylaxis for hepatitis A |
| VIG | Therapy of progressive vaccinia, eczema vaccinatum and vaccinia opthalmicus |
| HRIG | Postexposure prophylaxis (administered with vaccine) |
| HBIG | Postexposure prophylaxis for parenteral exposures to blood<br>Neonatal active/passive immunization with vaccine in high-risk infants |
| VZIG | Postexposure prophylaxis of high-risk individuals |
| CMVIG | Passive immunization of renal transplant recipients |

[a]Products not currently in distribution have been omitted.

## PRODUCTION AND TESTING OF VACCINES

In general, the quality of a vaccine is highly dependent on manufacturing techniques. The risks associated with vaccination are related to manufacturing methods, and product consistency is directly related to process controls. Two central features of viral vaccine production are the virus strain used and the substrate in which the vaccine is produced (38). The principles involved in managing these aspects of production are generally relevant even to products produced by recombinant DNA techniques, where the expression vector would be analogous to the virus strain, and the cell used for expression, be it bacterial, fungal, or eukaryotic, would be the substrate (39). A common scheme for vaccine production is shown in Fig. 1. The scheme is based on a cell banking system and a seed virus system (40). A virus strain selected for specific characteristics that make it desirable as a vaccine strain is used to prepare a master seed virus. The master seed is stored in ali-

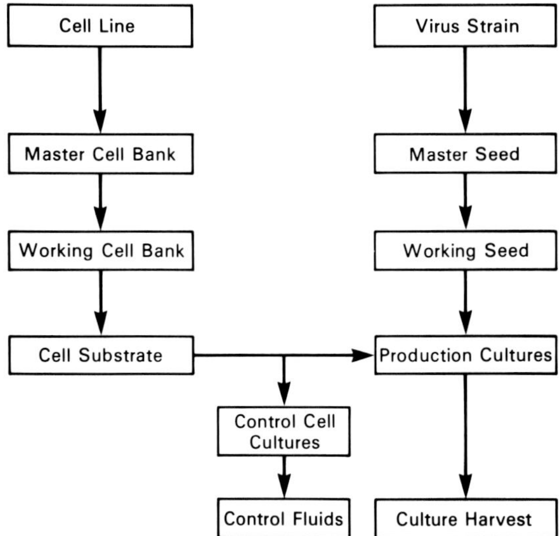


**FIG. 1.** Schematic description of the master and working virus seed and cell bank systems for process control in viral vaccine production.

quots that are used for characterization of the master seed and for preparation of working seed virus. The working seed is stored similarly in aliquots that are used for testing and for preparation of batches of vaccine. This approach, thus, involves the use of a highly pedigreed and characterized virus strain to produce qualified master and working seeds. In parallel, for vaccines produced in cell lines, a cell banking system is used. A suitable cell line is used to produce a master and working cell bank, the latter being used to produce batches of cell substrate for vaccine production. Cell banks at each level and cell substrates are qualified by specific tests to assure safety and quality. This approach allows for rigorous control of vaccine consistency.

## IMMUNE RESPONSES TO VIRAL VACCINES

Immune responses to viral vaccines may vary as a result of many factors that differ according to whether the vaccine is living or nonliving. Inoculation of a healthy nonimmune person with a single dose of a live viral vaccine will result in an adequate immune response if infection of sufficient magnitude and duration is established. It is critical that the mechanism used to attenuate the virus not reduce infectivity excessively.

### Interference

A number of interfering factors can interfere with establishment of infection by a suitably attenuated virus, including passively acquired antibodies, cross-reactive immunity acquired by infection with another related virus, and concurrent infection with another virus. Passively acquired antibodies are most often of maternal origin but may be acquired from Ig administration. Antibodies of maternal origin acquired transplacentally can interfere with responses to measles, mumps, and rubella vaccine (41–43). For example, currently available measles vaccine will induce protective immune responses in more than 95% of recipients in the United States if administered at or after 15 months of age (43). When administered at younger ages, lower response rates are observed. Antibodies acquired from IG are particularly relevant to travelers who may need to receive IG and live-virus vaccines in relation to the same trip.

Interference between viruses is a significant issue with regard to other live vaccines, including oral poliovirus vaccines (44). Enteric viral infections are relatively common in developing countries, and infection with other enteric viruses can prevent establishment of infection with polio vaccine virus. The dosage regimen currently used for the live vaccine was selected in part because interference occurred even between the different vaccine virus types, such that it was unlikely that all three poliovirus types would establish infection after a single dose. After two doses, more than 90% of vaccines will have had takes with each type (45).

## Immunization Regimens and Booster Effects

Responses to nonliving viral vaccines vary according to the dose, numbers, and timing of vaccinations. Dose-response relationships for inactivated polio and influenza vaccines were studied by Salk (46). The response to a single dose varied such that a 10-fold increase in amount of vaccine given resulted in approximately a twofold increase in mean antibody titers induced. At doses less than those that induce optimum responses after a single inoculation, multiple inoculations may induce adequate responses if a certain minimal potency is retained (47). The potency of the inactivated polio vaccines in use in the United States until 1988 were such that three doses 2 months apart were recommended for the primary immunization series (48). The new vaccine introduced in 1988 is more potent and induces adequate responses after a two-dose primary series (49).

Recommended regimens for immunizing with nonliving vaccines routinely include booster doses. After completion of a successful priming immunization regimen, if a sufficient amount of time is allowed to pass before giving a booster dose, the effect is a much greater response than would be obtained by giving an additional dose in the priming series. With inactivated polio vaccine, an optimum booster effect is obtained if at least 6 months is allowed to elapse between the completion of the primary series and the booster dose, as shown in Fig. 2 (46). Similar results have been obtained with hepatitis B surface antigen vaccine and rabies vaccine (50–52).

Persistence of immunity after vaccination varies according to the type of vaccine used, living or nonliving, and the response to the priming and booster regimen. A single infection with a live vaccine virus may induce immunity which lasts many years and which parallels that occurring after natural infection. After a killed vaccine, such as influenza, the effect of a single vaccine dose may last less than 1 year (53). When dosage regimens are used that involve an adequate priming series and induction of a good booster effect, high levels of antibodies can be induced, which typically show an initial period of relatively rapid decline, followed by stabilization at a relatively high level and persistence for many years.

## Route of Administration

The nature of the immune response obtained varies according to the route of inoculation. In general, parenteral administration of a vaccine induces relatively little secretory antibody, whereas intranasal or oral administration will result in such a response (54). Because of the mobile nature of gut-associated lymphoid tissue, enteric immunization may result in secretory immunity in the respiratory system (55). The intradermal (ID) route of administration is of interest, since amounts of antigen can be used that do not induce adequate responses when given subcutaneously (SC) or IM

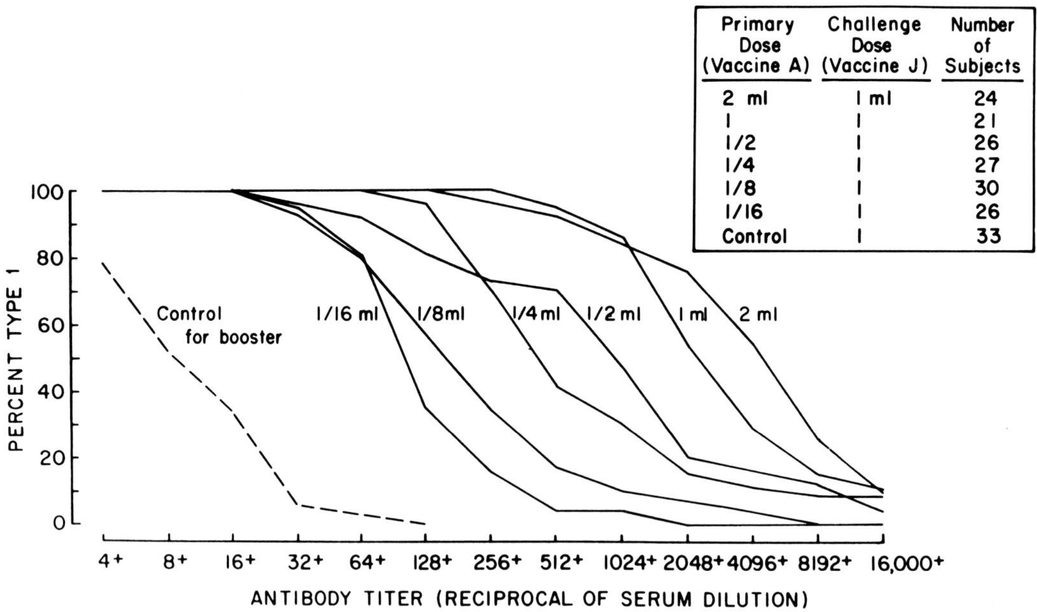


**FIG. 2.** Degree of immunological memory induced by vaccination. Data are expressed in terms of percentage of individuals with titers of type 1 antibody at or above the indicated levels 2 weeks after a uniform challenge dose of vaccine J given 1 year after a two-dose primary series (2 week interval). Groups were given different quantities of reference vaccine A for primary immunization. (From J. Salk et al., ref. 174, with permission.)

(56,57). The reason for this increased immunogenicity is unclear. It could reflect greater persistence of antigen because of lesser proteolysis or otherwise more efficient utilization by the immune system. Finally, it has become practice to administer nonliving vaccines in anatomic sites where delivery of vaccine IM is accomplished easily, such as into the deltoid muscle instead of the buttock. Poor responses to hepatitis and rabies vaccines have been observed when given in the buttock, presumably because of deposition into fat (58,59).

### Cell-Mediated Immunity

The traditional and most direct approach to monitoring immune responses to vaccines is by serology. Induction of cell-mediated responses by vaccination is undoubtedly important but generally more difficult to measure than antibody responses. Since B-cell responses reflected by antibody production depend on immunoregulatory T-cell responses, the tests for antibodies indicate the integrity of certain helper and suppressor cell responses (60). Experimentation in animals has demonstrated that cytotoxic T-cell responses occur more readily after live-virus infection than after administration of killed virus, leading to the general belief that nonliving vaccines are poor inducers of cell-mediated immunity. In fact, relatively few studies of vaccine-induced cytotoxic T-cell responses of humans have been performed. Those that have indicated that adequate doses of either live or nonliving vaccines can induce changes in lymphocyte proliferation responses and cytotoxic T-cell responses (61–64). The other major effector T-cell arm, delayed type hypersensitivity, can also be induced by both live and nonliving antigens (65,66). Cytotoxic T-cell responses are short-lived after infection or vaccination,

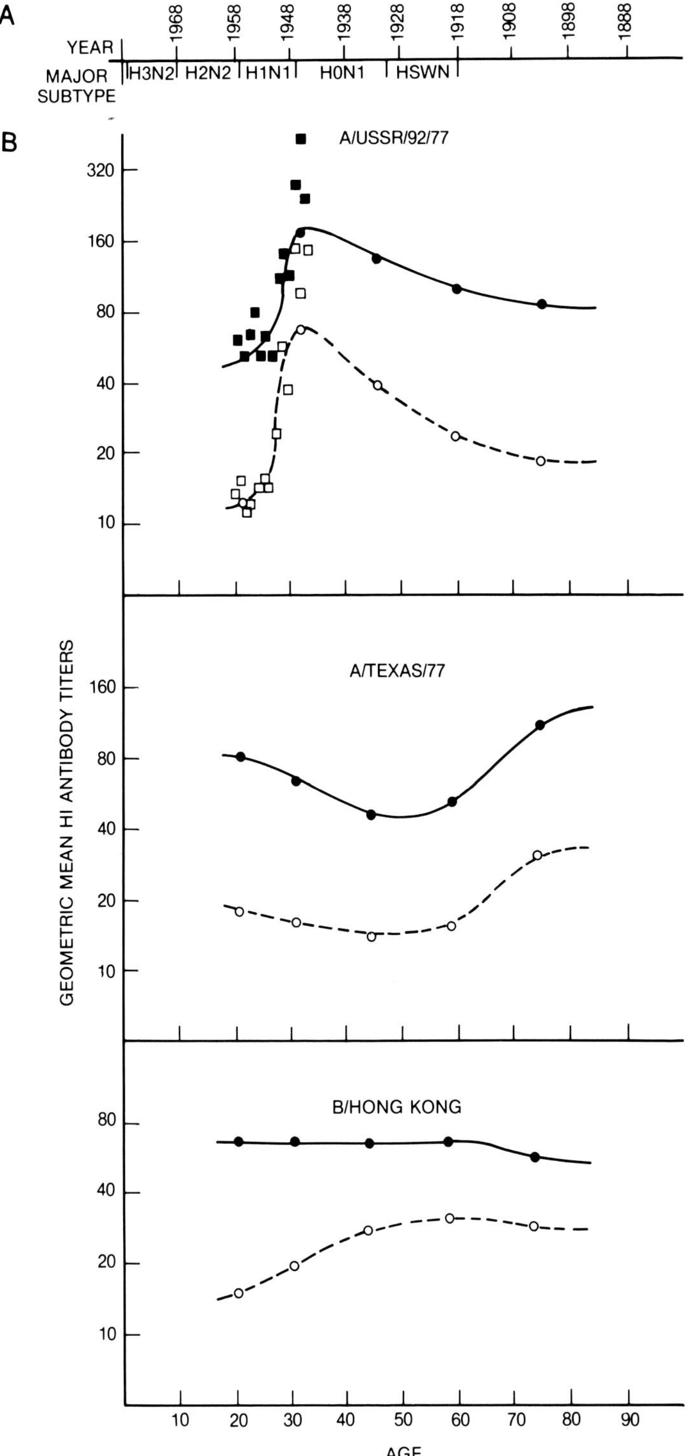


**FIG. 3. A**: Years of known or inferred major antigenic shifts of the HA of influenza A viruses. **B**: Geometric mean titers of HI antibody to the three influenza antigens in serum obtained from recipients of medium- and low-dose vaccine combined, by age groups before and after initial vaccination and by year of age before and after initial vaccination. Titers are expressed as reciprocals of the highest serum dilution producing HI. For calculating geometric mean titers, serum producing no reaction at a dilution of 1:10 was assigned a titer of 1:5. (From ref. 69, with permission.)

but priming for accelerated secondary cytotoxic T-cell responses persists as does delayed type hypersensitivity (62,65). In general, antibodies tend to be critical for prevention of establishment of infection, whereas the integrity of cellular immunity may be critical for recovery from infection to occur. The induction of both by vaccination is probably important, but the failure of a vaccine to induce protective immunity because it failed to induce cellular immunity has never been demonstrated.

### "Original Antigenic Sin"

An extraordinary example of the intricate nature of immune regulation is seen in the concept of "original antigenic sin," advanced by Davenport et al. (67). They noted that individuals would consistently develop and maintain throughout life high levels of antibodies against viruses of the influenza A subtype to which they were exposed first. Davenport et al. (68) applied this principle to interpret that high levels of preexisting antibodies to viruses of the H3N2 subtype in elderly individuals in 1968 were indicative of a probable H3N2 influenza epidemic around the end of the last century. This phenomenon influences the effects of vaccine. For example, elderly people were extensively exposed to both H1N1 and H3N2 strains of influenza prior to 1977, as shown in Fig. 3 (69). At that time, they tended to have high prevaccination titers against H3N2 strains and responded minimally to H3N2 vaccine antigens, but tended to have low prevaccination titers to H1N1 strains with good responses to vaccine as a result of prior priming (70,71). In contrast, individuals in the 25–35-year-old age range in 1977 had high prevaccination titers against H1N1 and low titers against H3N2 strains, but showed little increase in H1N1 antibodies with large increases in H3N2 antibodies. Original exposure results in persistently high levels of antibodies, whereas subsequent exposure primes for a good secondary response.

## ADVERSE EFFECTS OF VACCINES

The majority of adverse effects of vaccines are directly related to the nature of the product. For example, a complication of live oral poliovirus vaccine is vaccine-associated poliomyelitis (72). In general, live-virus vaccines cause adverse effects that are similar to those occurring during natural infection, but at lower frequencies and of lesser severity. These adverse effects are more likely to occur in recipients who are immunodeficient. Nonliving vaccines may be associated with other characteristic effects, such as fever attributable to high doses of whole-virus inactivated influenza vaccines (73). Other types of adverse effects include allergy, idiosyncratic (unexplained) reactions, and induction of immune status associated with pathology on subsequent natural infection (74–76).

### Allergy

The components of vaccines associated with allergy include animal proteins, antibiotics, and human proteins. Animal serum proteins are highly allergenic if administered in adequate amounts. Allergic reactions to animal serum proteins, such as fetal bovine serum, are rare if the concentration in the vaccine is limited to less than one part per million (77). Nonhydrolyzed gelatin of bovine origin has been used as a vaccine stabilizer and may be allergenic. Egg proteins are present in vaccines produced in hens' eggs, such as influenza and yellow fever vaccines. Despite the presence of significant levels of egg proteins in these vaccines, serious allergic reactions are extremely rare (78,79). People with histories of minor forms of intolerance to eggs tolerate these vaccines well, and only a history of anaphylactic hypersensitivity is considered a contraindication to use.

The antibiotics normally used in vaccine production are rarely associated with serious allergic reactions. Penicillins are not used in any stage of vaccine production, because proteins may be derivatized by penicillin byproducts and may remain allergenic even if all free penicillin is removed (80). Neomycin is commonly used in vaccine production. Minor skin test reactions to neomycin are quite common, but these reactions are not predictive of anaphylactic hypersensitivity (79). Serious reactions to neomycin are rare.

Allergic reactions to unmodified human or nonhuman primate proteins in vaccines have not been observed. Primary monkey kidney cells and human diploid cells have been used extensively without problems. Recent experiences with rabies vaccines have indicated that proteins derivatized with β-propiolactone, including human serum albumin, can be implicated in induction of a serum sickness-like reaction (20,81). The specific immunization regimen used for rabies prophylaxis, an intensive primary immunization regimen followed by an extended interval prior to booster immunization, may be critical to induction of this response.

### Demyelinating Diseases

Adverse neurological events following vaccination receive a great deal of attention. Among viral vaccines currently in use in the United States, the only neurological complication proven to be caused by the vaccine is vaccine-associated poliomyelitis attributable to live oral poliovirus vaccine (72). Otherwise there was one episode when a defective lot of a vaccine caused problems. Soon after introduction of the inactivated polio vaccine, the children receiving one lot of inactivated polio vaccine developed poliomyelitis, because the lot was incompletely inactivated (19). The reason for the problem was corrected, and no similar events have occurred since.

It is clear that some rabies vaccines not in use in the United States can cause neurologic complications including Guillain-Barré syndrome and transverse myelitis (82–86). These complications are summarized in Table 4. Vaccines prepared from sheep or mouse brain and containing large amounts of brain protein cause these complications with a high frequency (83,84). The vaccine produced in duck embryo tissues caused transverse myelitis and Guillain-Barré syndrome, but with a much lower frequency (85). Since the amount of rabies antigen in the duck embryo product was probably equivalent to or greater than that in the brain-derived products, it is likely that nonviral proteins or other antigens, particularly of neural origin, are the components that cause these reactions. It is not clear whether or not human diploid cell-derived rabies vaccine (HDCV) causes these problems, but if so it does so very rarely (86). It is of interest that Japanese encephalitis (JE) vaccine produced in mouse brain is rarely associated with neurological adverse events (87). This vaccine contains highly purified viral antigens and very little, if any, mouse brain protein.

There is specific interest in the potential of vaccines to cause Guillain-Barré syndrome because of its established relationship to rabies vaccine and because the syndrome normally occurs as a postinfectious event, possibly as an immunopathologic complication (88). In 1976, the incidence

**TABLE 4.** *Adverse neurological effects of various rabies vaccines*

| Vaccine type | Incidence of Guillian-Barré syndrome or transverse myelitis in recipients |
|---|---|
| Semple | 1/611–1/9,073 |
| Suckling mouse brain | 1/4,615–1/8,628 |
| Duck embryo derived | 1/32,615 |
| Diploid cell-derived (human and other) | <1/200,000 |

of Guillain-Barré syndrome was slightly greater in recipients of the swine influenza vaccine than in the general population (89). No cause-effect relationship was established, but the strength of the association of Guillain-Barré syndrome with vaccine receipt was sufficiently strong that it was considered likely that such a relationship did exist (90). No association with receipt of other influenza vaccines has been observed (91,92). Neural antigens from brain or embryos, and possibly viral antigens in some cases (e.g., swine influenza vaccine-associated Guillain-Barré syndrome occurred through an unknown mechanism), can induce Guillain-Barré syndrome and transverse myelitis (83–86).

### Encephalitis and Encephalopathy

Encephalitis and encephalopathy are potential vaccine complications of great concern, but are rarely if ever actually observed as an effect of viral vaccines currently in use in the United States. Encephalitis and encephalopathy have both been considered complications of smallpox vaccine, and numerous studies have measured incidence rates (93,94). These rates are, however, similar to those in the general population, and vaccinia virus has never been demonstrated in the CNS of such patients. Other live viral vaccines have the theoretical potential to infect the nervous system. However, neuropathogenicity is evaluated prior to the introduction of vaccine virus strains, so this potential is low from the outset. Passive surveillance systems have not documented that live viral vaccines in general use cause encephalitis. The Centers for Disease Control (CDC) in the United States have identified very few cases of encephalitis following measles vaccination, and none has been clearly attributed to vaccine virus (95). Furthermore, a national registry of cases of subacute sclerosing panencephalitis has documented that mass vaccination with measles vaccine has nearly eliminated this disease (96). Similarly, encephalitis due to rubella vaccine has not been documented, even in babies born to women vaccinated in relation to the first trimester of pregnancy (97,98). Aseptic meningitis is occasionally recognized in recipients of mumps vaccine, but it is impossible to distinguish these infections from wild-type virus or other virus infections (99). There have been no reports of encephalitis following adenovirus vaccine. Yellow fever virus vaccines have rarely been associated with encephalitis (100).

### Immunopathology

A potential adverse effect of vaccination is induction of an immune state that disposes the recipient to development of atypical and/or more severe disease on subsequent exposure to wild-type virus. Such an effect has been observed with regards to two vaccines, formaldehyde inactivated measles virus vaccine and formaldehyde inactivated respiratory syncytial virus (RSV) vaccine (101,102). The inactivated measles virus vaccine was in general use in the United States between 1963 and 1967 (103). When more attenuated live measles vaccine was introduced, its use was largely discontinued (104). Beginning approximately 10 years after the introduction of killed measles vaccine, the occurrence of "atypical measles" was recognized, consisting of an atypical rash and a relatively more severe illness, including pneumonia, compared to natural measles (105). The RSV vaccine was used experimentally in an efficacy trial in infants when it was observed that severe pneumonia was more common in the vaccines than placebo recipients (106). The pathogenesis of these types of immunopathology is not certain, but the most favored hypothesis in each case is that of a disseminated *Arthus* reaction (107,108). Theoretically, formaldehyde treatment destroyed antigenicity of critical virus antigens, and an imbalanced, nonprotective

to protect themselves from influenza (154). A single dose is usually given each year, unless an individual has not been vaccinated since 1977 and has probably not been previously infected with virus related to the vaccine components, in which case two doses are given. Annual vaccination is important.

A great deal of effort has been expended toward development of live influenza vaccines. Attempts at development of temperature-sensitive mutants did not result in stable attenuated strain production (157). Cold adaptation has been used successfully to produce stable attenuation, and a parent donor virus can be used to produce cold-adapted reassortant viruses that have the stable phenotype and express antigens of interest for inclusion in current experimental vaccines (157). Field trials of cold-adapted reassortants have shown efficacy in some situations, and additional circumstances and target groups are under study.

### Poliomyelitis

The development of polio vaccine followed closely on the discovery by Enders et al. (158) that polio virus could be propagated *in vitro* in tissue culture. It was, thus, one of the first major successes of modern virology and has become one of the most significant public health accomplishments of this century. Current poliomyelitis prevention programs incorporate the use of inactivated poliovirus vaccine (IPV) and live oral poliovirus vaccine (OPV). The widespread use of these vaccines has resulted in the virtual elimination of poliomyelitis in many countries and the potential for global control of the disease.

Industrialization in the Northern hemisphere led to dramatic changes in the epidemiology of polio viruses during the late nineteenth and early twentieth centuries (159). In countries where sanitation is poor and polio is endemic, infections are transmitted to most children during the first year of life while they are still protected by maternal antibodies and infection is unlikely to lead to paralysis. The incidence of endemic poliomyelitis is reflected in lameness surveys, but epidemics are not recognized. With the advent of better sanitation, the number of susceptible older children and adults increased and polio epidemics occurred of progressively increasing severity. By the time IPV became available, there were approximately 20,000 cases per year of paralytic poliomyelitis in the United States (160).

The potential for successful immunization against polio was suggested by the impact of maternal antibodies on the likelihood of disease occurring. In addition, a field trial of IG prophylaxis demonstrated protection by antibodies and studies in monkeys demonstrated that immunity induced by immunization could be protective (161,162). In 1953, Salk et al. (163) prepared IPV by formalin inactivation of virus grown in monkey kidney cell cultures and performed human immunogenicity studies. In 1954 and 1955, a large nation-wide vaccine trial in more than 1,800,000 people was conducted by Francis et al. (164). The study demonstrated protection against polio, which was more likely to occur if lots were relatively more immunogenic. This study formed the basis for introduction of IPV in 1955.

Efforts to attenuate polio viruses by passage in cell cultures were carried out successfully by Sabin (165). After a series of laboratory manipulations, clonal isolates were prepared by terminal dilutions and plaque purifications. Viruses for further development were selected by neurovirulence testing. These strains proved to be less neurovirulent than strains being developed in parallel at the time by Koprowski and Cox, and the Sabin strains were identified for use in vaccine production (166,167). The safety and immunogenicity of the Sabin strains were demonstrated in clinical trials involving more than 100,000,000 volunteers, mostly in Russia and eastern Europe (168).

No cases of vaccine-associated polio due to Sabin strains were recognized during that time. OPV was first approved in the United States in 1961 and came into general use by 1963.

The so-called Salk-Sabin debate over the relative merits of public health programs incorporating one or the other vaccine is one of the most celebrated controversies in public health. The relative success of different approaches is revealing. In the United States, vaccination programs have relied primarily on OPV. Certain characteristics of OPV have been recognized as a result. Immunization with OPV induces secretory immunity in the gastrointestinal tract. In addition, vaccine virus can be transmitted from person to person, so that nonimmune people continue to be exposed and infected, but with attenuated virus. As a result, nearly 100% of the population is immune to all three types of poliovirus, sustained transmission of wild polioviruses does not occur, and the only cases of poliomyelitis that have been observed for several years have been vaccine-associated or imported (169). The changes in incidence of poliomyelitis in relation to vaccine use are shown in Fig. 5.

In countries such as Finland and Holland, public health programs have relied on IPV. Vaccine-associated polio has not occurred. In Finland, polioviruses were not present in the environment for several years until 1987 when an outbreak occurred (170). It was not clear why polioviruses had been excluded from the environment. The last polio outbreak in Holland was in 1977 when type 1 virus spread through a religious community that had objections to vaccination (171). In both countries, OPV was used to interrupt the epidemics. In Finland, the epidemic probably resulted from use of subpotent vaccine, whereas in Holland it was the result of failure to use vaccine.

A significant advantage of IPV over OPV is the absence of vaccine-associated polio. In the United States, there are approximately eight cases per year of vaccine-associated polio, or approximately one case per 4,000,000 doses distributed. The rate associated with administration of first dose of vaccine is approximately 1 in 400,000 (171). Current policy in the United States is based on estimates that the total number of cases of polio would increase if IPV was used primarily. It has been estimated that the number of susceptible people would increase because secondary spread of vac-

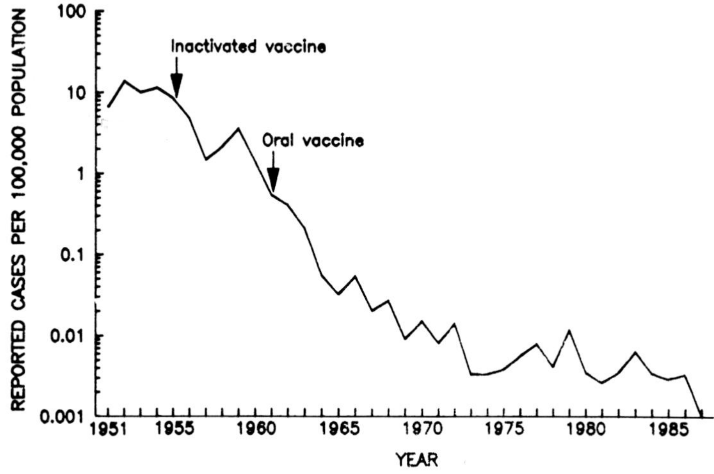


**FIG. 5.** Reported paralytic poliomyelitis attack rates, by year, United States, 1951–1976. (From ref. 310.)

cine virus infections would not occur. Until recently, there was also concern that more doses were needed of IPV than OPV to induce high response rates. Since wild polio viruses are continuously carried into the country, the potential for spread with lower rates of immunity leaves concern that the number of cases of polio might increase. This policy was recently reviewed by a group convened by the Institute of Medicine that recommended consideration of a program incorporating use of IPV and OPV be explored, especially as polio incidence in the Americas is reduced and if combined IPV-diphtheria, tetanus toxoids, and pertussis vaccine becomes available (172).

The number of cases of paralytic polio reported in the United States annually has decreased from approximately 20,000 in 1954, prior to the introduction of IPV, to 1,000 in 1962 prior to the introduction of OPV, to approximately eight at present, as shown in Fig. 5 (169). The presence of serum-neutralizing antibodies corresponds with protection against viremia involved in spread to the CNS.

The OPV currently used in the United States is manufactured from the Sabin strains. However, the seed virus used for type 3 vaccine production is a derivative of the Sabin strain developed by Pfizer, Ltd., in efforts to develop a more stable attenuated seed virus free of SV-40 virus. It was selected as an RNA clone of a fifth passage of the Sabin strain. Each lot of vaccine is tested for neurovirulence by inoculation of it into the CNS of macaque monkeys. Routine recommendations for vaccine administration are for doses to be given at 2, 4, and 15–18 months of age. Using this regimen, approximately 95–100% of children develop antibodies that neutralize all three types of poliovirus (173).

Significant developments in the manufacture of IPV occurred over the past 15 years. Van Wezel and colleagues developed a successful breeding program for African green monkey (*Cercopithecus*) species in which animals were screened for the presence of antibodies to foamy virus, and kidney cells from these monkeys were then suitable for serial propagation. They were thus able to use tertiary monkey kidney cells, which they produced by a large-scale fermentation technique, growing cells in suspension of microcarriers (174,175). The concentrations of poliovirus obtained by infecting such cultures are much greater than in conventional monolayer cultures. These modifications were supplemented by virus purification and improved standardization of vaccine potency (176). Vaccine manufactured by these improved techniques was introduced in the United States in 1987. This so-called enhanced potency vaccine is administered at 2, 4, and 15–18 months of age and induces antibody responses to all three types of polio virus in nearly 100% of recipients (177).

The potential for eradication of poliomyelitis worldwide is very real. There have been no endemic cases of wild polio virus disease in the United States for several years, and polio has come under control in a progressively increasing number of countries. Universal immunization against polio is a major objective of the Expanded Program on Immunization of the WHO, and the Pan American Health Organization has set 1991 as the target date for eradication of polio from the Americas.

Current research on polio vaccines is heavily focused on finding ways of further improving the safety of OPV. Type 3 poliovirus is the least stable of the three vaccine strains with respect to potential for reversion to neurovirulence and likelihood of causing vaccine-associated poliomyelitis. Gene sequence analysis of Sabin strains, wild type strains, and virus isolates from vaccinees indicates that the type 3 Sabin strain is more like the parent virus than the type 1 or 2 strains are like their parents (178). In addition, point mutations can result in partial reversion to neurovirulence (179). Other recent research findings of great interest have resulted in the mapping of epitopes of the polio virus capsid proteins to three distinct regions on the surface of the virus so that the involvement of individual amino acids in the antigenic site can be predicted (180). This information and data regarding the genetic basis of neurovirulence are being used together to guide experimental construction of viruses of potentially lower virulence. For example, amino acids of type 3 virus are being substituted to form type 3 epitopes on the surface of type 1 virus (181). Conversely, noncoding regions of type 1 can be used to replace noncoding regions of type 3 virus. Regardless of whether new vaccine strains result, studies on genetics and structure/function relationships of polio viruses are dramatic examples of the power of recently developed technologies to reveal important aspects of the biology of these viruses.

### Yellow Fever

The impact of epidemics of yellow fever (YF) on public health and on world history is as dramatic as that of any infectious disease. Rapidly mounting, devastating epidemics were typical in the early years of this country, as exemplified by the death of 10% of the population of Philadelphia in 4 months in 1793 (182). Epidemics have influenced the course of wars, one killing 40,000 French troops in 1802, and the impact of YF on French colonialism is thought to have influenced the decision of Bonaparte to sell Louisiana to the United States (183,184). The histories of the definition of the etiology of the disease and vaccine development are equally dramatic. In 1901, Walter Reed and his colleagues reported on the etiology of YF, describing studies performed in Havana that demonstrated the disease was caused by a heat-sensitive, filterable agent that was present in blood of acutely infected patients and was transmitted by the *Aedes aegypti* mosquito, and not by fomites as had been thought to be important (185,313). The virus is now recognized as a flavivirus. These studies opened opportunities for preventing epidemics by mosquito control and for attempting to develop vaccines.

Efforts to develop YF vaccine began with attempts to "fix" (develop into a stable, nonpathogenic strain) yellow fever virus by repeated passages of the virus in monkeys, mice, and chick embryo (186). The 17D strain of virus was derived from a virus isolated from a patient in Senegal in 1927. The virus was passaged in animals a total of 232–236 times between 1927 and 1939 when vaccines based on the 17D strain were introduced into general use in several countries. In 1951, the 17D strain was recommended as the only strain for general use by the WHO. YF vaccine was initially made in many countries using virus at different passage levels. Characteristics of the vaccine virus varied as increasing number of passages occurred. This behavior was the basis for the first recommendation by the WHO that vaccine viruses should be handled in seed lot systems.

Original seeds of the 17D virus contained avian leukosis virus because the virus had been passaged in hens' eggs containing this virus (187). After the discovery of the avian virus, contaminant was found to be present in the vaccine and an extensive case-control study was performed comparing 2,659 vaccine recipients who died of cancer to 2,659 controls (188). There was no evidence that receipt of vaccine was a risk factor for development of any particular cancer. Seeds of 17D virus have been produced subsequently that are avian leukosis virus-free.

Clinical trials of vaccine produced from the 17D strain were performed by Smith et al. (189) involving 59,000 vaccinees. Optimum doses of vaccine induce responses in more than 95% of vaccinees. Dose-response studies demonstrated that the magnitude and frequency of antibody responses were greater as the dose administered was increased over a wide range. However, when doses several-fold greater than the minimum amount that induced an optimum response were administered, the magnitude of the antibody response was less, indicating that interference occurred (190). The potency of yellow fever vaccines is established by testing in mice by IC inoculation (191). The minimum potency required by the WHO is 1,000 $LD_{50}$. The potency of some vaccines can be determined in plaque-forming units.

Viremia occurs typically approximately 3–5 days after immunization, but is not associated with illness (192). Significant adverse effects of YF vaccine are very unusual. Two cases of encephalitis have been reported in recipients of the 17D strain in the United States (193,194); in only one of these was YF virus recovered from the CNS.

YF vaccine is indicated for travelers to and residents of areas where the disease is prevalent (195). Most cases of YF occur in tropical areas and the southern hemisphere, but the potential for transmission exists wherever the *Aedes aegypti* mosquito breeds. The WHO publishes a description of the geographic distribution of YF virus periodically (196). Immunity induced by YF vaccine persists for at least 10 years (197).

## Measles

Measles virus is a paramyxovirus (198). It spreads rapidly among susceptible people, even with extremely casual contact. In populations where vaccine is not used widely, most children will be infected in the first few years of life (199). Changes in incidence of measles in the United States are shown in Fig. 6. In times prior to vaccine availability in developed countries where infant nutrition and medical care were good, measles was typically a moderately severe illness resulting in several days of fever, rash, prostration, and other symptoms (200). Prior to the introduction of vaccine, almost all children became infected; few cases occurred during the late teens (201). More severe complications occurred occasionally, including pneumonia and encephalitis. Approximately one per 1,000 infected children developed encephalitis (202). The mortality rate from measles in the United States in 1960–1965 was less than 1% (203). Presently, there are only a few thousand cases per year of measles in the United States (204). In developing countries, particularly where nutrition and medical care are poor, measles is a devastating illness.

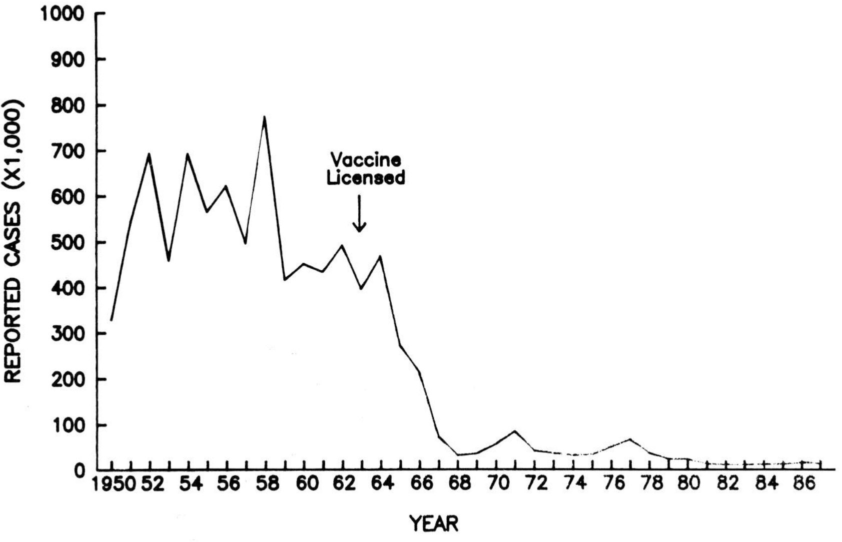


**FIG. 6.** Reported measles cases, United States, 1950–1987. (From ref. 311.)

Mortality rates can be as high as 5–15%, with nearly all children becoming infected in the first years of life (205).

Inactivated measles vaccine was first introduced in the United States in 1963. The vaccine did not induce durable immunity and was associated with the development of atypical measles upon later exposure to wild virus (206,207). Live measles virus vaccine development was begun by Enders (208), who first propagated the virus in cell culture in 1954. Extensive tissue culture passage was used to produce an attenuated virus, designated the Edmonston B strain (209,210). This virus induced fever and systemic symptoms in the majority of vaccinees, and was usually given in combination with IG or as part of a regimen involving killed measles vaccine (211,212). This original live measles vaccine was first approved in the United States in 1963 (213). More attenuated measles viruses were developed from the Edmonston B strain over the next few years (214,215). The two such viruses used in the United States were designated the Schwartz and Moraten strains. The Edmonston-Zagreb strain, developed in Yugoslavia, is of current interest as well, because of potentially greater immunogenicity in children under 1 year of age (216).

The only vaccine currently available in the United States is based on the Moraten strain and is produced in chick embryo cell culture (213). Its potency is established by *in vitro* infectivity titration. The vaccine is recommended for routine administration at 15 months of age (213). Immunization before 12 months of age is associated with reduced response rates because of interfering effects of maternal antibodies. In a setting where measles exposure is infrequent, withholding vaccination until 15 months of age is not problematic. In developing countries, maternal antibody titers wane more quickly, exposure is more common, and a high proportion of cases occur in the first year of life (217). Thus, vaccination at 6–9 months of age is often critical.

The vaccine currently available in the United States is produced from the Moraten strain in chick embryo cell culture. Its potency is determined by *in vitro* infectivity titration. It induces protective antibody responses in more than 95 percent of recipients (218). Fever occurs in approximately 10% of recipients (219). Minor rash is less common, and vaccine virus is not transmissible. Efforts at measles elimination in the United States have not been successful yet, in part because of the extreme transmissibility of wild virus.

### Mumps

Mumps virus is a paramyxovirus that causes, as its principal manifestations, parotitis, fever, and associated systemic symptoms (220,221). Complications of mumps virus infection include orchitis, pancreatitis, meningitis, and encephalitis (222). In adult males, orchitis may lead occasionally to sterility (223). Encephalitis is rarely associated with mortality. Prior to the introduction of vaccine, most children experienced mumps virus infection and there were approximately 1,000 cases of encephalitis reported annually in the United States (224). Since the introduction of widespread use of live mumps virus vaccine in 1967, the number of cases of mumps occurring annually in the United States has been reduced to several thousand, and serious complications of mumps have been nearly eliminated, as shown in Fig. 7 (224).

The first mumps vaccine was developed by Enders (225) and consisted of formalin-inactivated virus grown in chick embryos. It was introduced commercially in 1950, but was not widely used because efficacy was relatively poor and of short duration. He went on to demonstrate attenuation of mumps virus by *in vitro* passage (225). This finding was the basis for the work of Hilleman et al. (226), who developed the Jeryl Lynn strain, which is used for mumps vac-

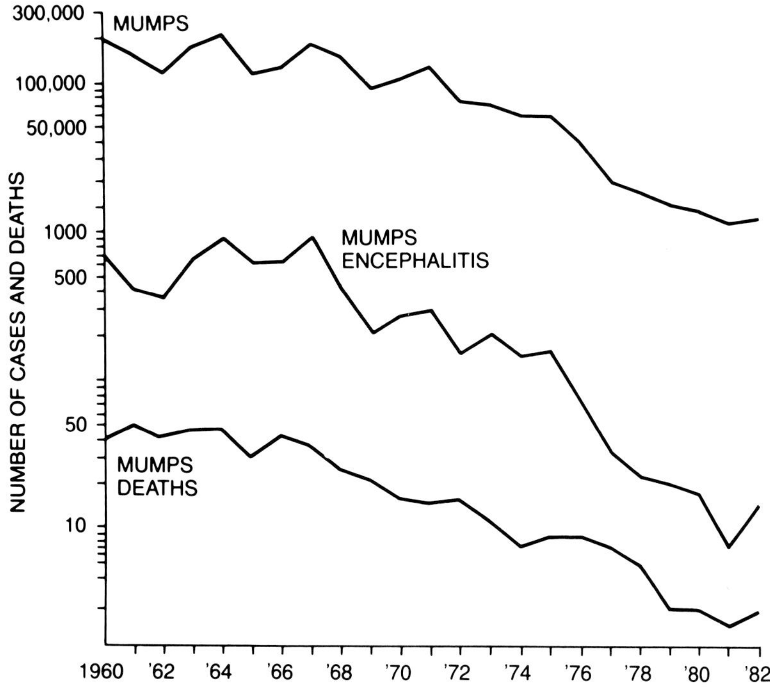


**FIG. 7.** Mumps incidence rates—United States, 1922–1985 (provisional data). (From ref. 312.)

cine currently in use in the United States. This vaccine is produced in chick embryo cell culture. Its potency is based on *in vitro* infectivity testing, and it induces neutralizing antibodies in approximately 98% of vaccinees (227). Adverse effects of mumps vaccine are rare. It is recommended for routine immunization of susceptible adults and children over 12 months of age (228). Immunity persists in most children vaccinated in the second year of life, at least into early adulthood. The vaccine virus is not communicable.

### Rubella

Rubella virus is a togavirus transmitted directly from person to person with no arthropod vector and no animal reservoirs (229). Prior to the introduction of vaccine for widespread use, rubella occurred as an endemic and epidemic disease (230). The majority of infections occurred in children under 10 years of age, but nearly 25% occurred after 15 years of age (231). The typical illness caused by rubella virus is a mild illness with rash and fever lasting approximately 3 days (232). Arthritis and arthralgia may occur and are more common in adults and females. Encephalitis is rare. The most significant effects of rubella are associated with infection occurring during the first trimester of pregnancy (233). *In utero* infection results in a variety of fetal abnormalities referred to as congenital rubella syndrome (CRS). The most common manifestations of CRS are cataracts, heart defects, and deafness, the so-called triad of CRS. A wide range of other neurological, cardiac, ophthalmic, and auditory problems may also occur. During the epidemic that occurred in the United States in 1963–1964, it is estimated that there were more than 30,000 infants born with CRS (231). Since the introduction of vaccine in 1969, CRS has been nearly eliminated in this country, as shown in Fig. 8 (234).

The first isolation of rubella virus was reported simultaneously by Parkman et al. (235) and Weller and Neva (236) in 1962. Its growth in monkey kidney cell cultures was detected by its interference with enterovirus replication (235). Antibodies are measured by neutralization, HI, and other techniques (237,238). Vaccine strains were attenuated by serial *in vitro* propagation. The first strain introduced in 1969 was the HPV-77 strain developed by Meyer et al. (239) in monkey kidney cell culture. This vaccine was produced subsequently for commercial distribution in dog kidney cell or duck embryo cell cultures (239,240). The Cendehill strain introduced in 1970 was produced in rabbit kidney cell cultures (241). The RA 27/3 strain was developed by Plotkin et al. (242) and was introduced in the United States in 1979. It is produced in human diploid fibroblast cell cultures. The RA 27/3 strain was considered slightly superior to the HPV-77 strain with respect to adverse reactions and immunogenicity. Neither strain appears to have the capacity to produce CRS even when administered intentionally during the first trimester of pregnancy (243). The RA 27/3 strain is the only one currently in use in the United States.

Various strategies have been employed for prevention of rubella and CRS. In some countries, vaccination efforts have been directed toward adolescent girls. This approach has had limited success, because adolescents do not consistently visit physicians for vaccination. In the United States, routine childhood immunization over a number of years has resulted in a highly immune population of adolescents and young adults, and the virtual elimination of CRS (244). Routine childhood immunization against rubella is becoming a more widespread practice in other countries.

Rubella vaccine induces neutralizing and HI antibodies in nearly 100% of vaccinees (245). It may induce mild symptoms similar to those caused by natural infection in a low percentage of recipients. The frequency of symptoms is age-related (246). Approximately 50% of adult women may be symptomatic, 25% may develop arthralgia or arthritis, and an occasional person may develop peripheral neuritis (247). These reactions are usually self-limited; rarely, there is persistence of arthritic or neuralgic symptoms. Other adverse events possibly due to vaccine virus have been reported rarely. Rubella vaccine is recommended for children 15 months of age, susceptible pre- or postadolescent females, and susceptible postpartum women (248). Children vacci-

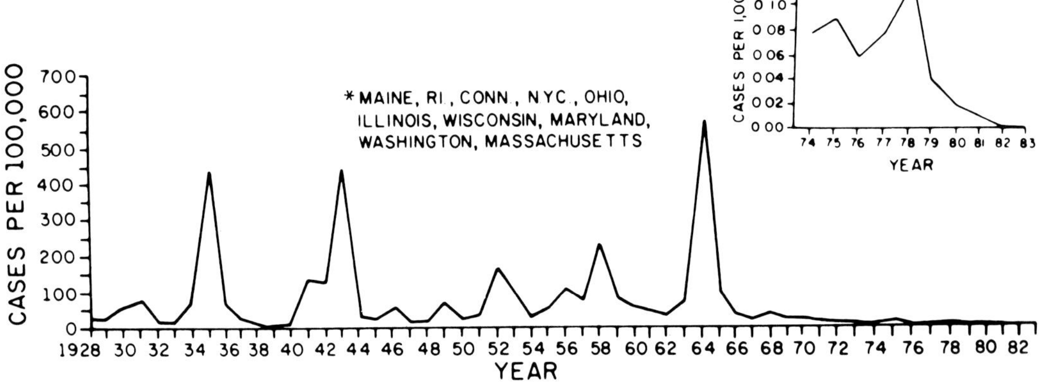


**FIG. 8.** Rubella incidence in 10 selected areas of the United States, 1928–1983. (From Williams and Preblud, ref. 244, with permission.)

nated in the second year of life remain immune into adulthood.

### Combinations of Measles, Mumps, and Rubella Vaccines

Routine immunization against these diseases is recommended using combined vaccine in the United States. The use of the combined vaccine allows for prevention of all three diseases with a single injection, an example of the importance of simplicity of vaccine regimen in the success of vaccination programs. Bivalent vaccines including measles and mumps, and measles and rubella are also produced.

### Adenovirus Acute Respiratory Disease

Adenoviruses are a group of 41 related virus serotypes, the first of which was isolated in 1933 (249). These viruses are generally divided into five groups. Group A includes three viruses, types 12, 18, and 31, which are highly oncogenic in hamsters and rarely associated with human disease (250). They are of interest with respect to study of viral oncogenesis. The nuclear "t antigen" of these viruses was used as a transformation marker and has been studied for its possible role in the transformation process (251). Group B includes types 3, 7, 11, 14, 16, 21, and 35. These viruses and types 4 (Group E) and 19 (Group D) are important causes of acute respiratory disease (ARD) in young adults. Types 11, 14, 16, and 21 are sporadic causes of disease, whereas types 3, 4, 7, 19, and 35 are often associated with epidemics. Group C includes types 1, 2, 5, and 6, which are important causes of ARD and gastrointestinal illness in children. Group D consists of 14 types (including type 19), which are associated with epidemic keratoconjunctivitis in addition to ARD. Type 4 is the only member of Group E. Types 38, 40, and 41 are ungrouped.

In children, adenoviruses account for approximately 5% of ARD, including the common cold, pharyngitis, and tonsillitis (252). The infections are often associated with fever and systemic symptoms. Gastroenteritis is a common manifestation. Intestinal intussusception due to mesenteric lymphadenopathy is often caused by adenovirus (253). Pneumonitis and hospitalization are not uncommon.

In young adults, particularly military recruits, epidemics have been common, often affecting approximately 80% of a group, with approximately 20% requiring hospitalization for care of febrile illnesses (254). The viruses most commonly associated with these epidemics are types 3, 4, and 7 (255). Vaccination using live adenovirus vaccines has effectively controlled epidemics of type 4 and 7 disease in the United States military.

A formalin-inactivated trivalent (types 3, 4, and 7) adenovirus vaccine was commercially available beginning in 1957 and was used primarily in the United States military (256). The vaccine was moderately effective. In 1963, it was learned that the vaccine was contaminated with SV-40 virus, a simian virus oncogenic in hamsters; the vaccine was withdrawn (257).

Chanock et al. (258) demonstrated the potential for adenovirus immunization by the establishment of gastrointestinal infection and investigated a type 4 adenovirus strain for this purpose. They showed that human diploid cells could be used for production of virus, a finding that allowed for preparation of SV-40 virus free adenoviruses. These efforts involved the following: (a) development of numerous human diploid cell adapted adenovirus strains (259); (b) identification of nontransforming variants and establishment of criteria for suitable evidence of lack of oncogenicity (259); (c) substantial contributions to the development of generally accepted criteria for use of human diploid cells as vaccine substrate (260); (d) extensive characterization of neurotropic properties of adenoviruses (261); (e) performance of clinical trials involving more than 5,000,000 vaccinees over a period of 15 years (262) and (f) development of a novel approach for manufacture of an enteric-coated tablet necessary for oral use (259). One of the studies involved vaccination of 5,000 military recruits whose names were entered into a computerized data base available for follow-up indefinitely (259). No unusual events have been observed in that study group that raised concern about vaccine safety. During this time, Green et al. (263) carried out extensive studies showing the absence of adenovirus DNA in a wide range of human tumors. These efforts led to the approval of adenovirus vaccines for limited use in this country in 1980.

When adenovirus vaccine is administered orally, it does not spread to infect the respiratory tract to produce ARD, but does induce systemic immunity. The vaccine viruses do not spread from person to person, a finding considered evidence of attenuation (259). It is likely a combination of bypassing the susceptible respiratory tract and attenuation with respect to gastrointestinal disease and person-to-person transmission both underlie the success of these vaccines.

The type 4 and type 7 adenovirus vaccines currently available are produced from the strains developed by Rubin et al. in the human diploid fibroblast cell line, WI 38 cells (259). Potency is established by *in vitro* determination of tissue culture infectivity. The vaccine is formulated as an enteric-coated tablet that is comprised of lyophilized virus surrounded by starch and binders and covered with a triple layer of enteric coating. Each type has similar characteristics with regard to safety and efficacy. No adverse effects are known. They are each at least 95% effective in preventing ARD caused by the homologous virus. The formulations are only suitable for administration to adults and are only used in military personnel in the United States. Prevention of ARD epidemics due to these adenoviruses is of substantial value both from a cost-benefit point of view and with regard to disease burden removed.

Adenoviruses are of future interest as potential live recombinant virus vaccines. Initial work focused on inserting foreign genes under the control of early gene promoters (14). Since these recombinant viruses are defective, coinfection with replication-competent helper viruses is needed. Recently, there has been success in using a late gene promoter to express the hepatitis B surface antigen gene and, in another construct, the envelope antigen of HIV (15). These recombinant viruses are replication competent and are of great interest because they may be capable of inducing potent systemic and secretory immunity.

### Hepatitis B

Transmission of hepatitis B virus (HBV) can occur as a result of parenteral exposure to contaminated blood, through sexual activity, and between mother and child at or soon after birth (264–266). Parenteral exposure was once the leading cause of transfusion-associated hepatitis; the implementation of routine blood screening has substantially eliminated this problem (266). People presently at high risk of HBV infection include intravenous drug abusers, homosexual men, medical care workers, hemodialysis patients, and children born to carrier mothers (266). The frequency of transmission from mother to newborn is approximately 95% if the mother's blood contains HBV surface antigen ($HB_sAg$) and e antigen, and is lower but still significant if the blood is only $HB_sAg$ positive. Approximately 5% of infected adults develop chronic active hepatitis and are at risk for development of cirrhosis, hepatic failure, and primary hepatocellular carcinoma. The frequency of chronic infection developing in newborns who acquire hepatitis B neonatally is approximately 95%. In many countries in the Far East, the maternal chronic carrier rate is very high, their infants become chronic carriers, and the prevalence of chronic HBV infection remains high.

Both active and passive immunization are important for prevention of HBV infection. The potential for vaccine development was demonstrated by Krugman (267,268), who found that heat-treated, plasma-derived $HB_sAg$ could be used to induce protective immunity in chimpanzees and antibodies to $HB_sAg$ in people. Since plasma of chronic carriers may contain high concentrations of $HB_sAg$, human plasma was a practical source of antigen for vaccine manufacture, a fortunate situation since the virus has not yet been propagated *in vitro*. Plasma-derived hepatitis B vaccines were introduced commercially in many countries in 1982 (266). The $HB_sAg$ gene has been cloned into cell lines by recombinant DNA techniques and antigen produced in cell cultures expressing the gene. *Saccharomyces cerevisiae,* brewers yeast, is used to produce the recombinant DNA-derived $HB_sAg$ vaccines that were introduced in the United States and Europe in 1987 (269,270). Both vaccines are available as alum-adsorbed purified protein preparations and are given by IM injection.

Hepatitis B immune globulin (HBIG) is produced from pooled human plasma collected from donors known to have antibodies to $HB_sAg$. Presently, the plasma donors are people who were immunized with hepatitis B vaccine.

Recommendations for immunoprophylaxis against hepatitis B vary with the target group. The target groups in the United States include medical care personnel, patients with need for frequent receipt of blood or blood products, hemodialysis patients, homosexual men, infants born to high-risk mothers, and residents and personnel at institutions for the mentally handicapped. In the United States, the plasma and yeast-derived vaccines are administered in three dose regimens. The second and third doses are given 1 and 6 months after the first. For healthy adults, the recommended dose is 20 mcg of the plasma-derived or 10 mcg of the yeast-derived vaccine. Pediatric doses are one-half the adult doses. Hemodialysis patients are given 40 mcg per dose. Newborn infants with high-risk mothers should receive HBIG at birth as well as a full vaccination series. HBIG is also used for postexposure prophylaxis of medical care personnel. Efficacy rates of these regimens vary. Efficacy in newborn infants is greater than 95%, in homosexual men is 90–95%, and in hemodialysis patients is approximately 80% (266,271,272). Levels of anti-$HB_sAg$ greater than or equal to 10 mIU are generally associated with protective immunity (273). Immunity persists in most vaccines for at least 5 years.

### Japanese Encephalitis

The Japanese encephalitis (JE) virus is a flavivirus that is endemic in many parts of the Far East and southern Asia (274,275). Infections are most common in childhood and are usually asymptomatic. Encephalitis occurs in approximately 1% of infections. Severe epidemics were noted in military personnel during the Vietnam War, suggesting that adults may be at greater risk than children. Cases in travelers to the Far East are extremely rare, but do occur. A common reservoir for the virus is swine, and the vector is the mosquito.

Control of JE has been accomplished in Japan through a program of routine vaccination and monitoring of the swine population for the presence of antibody to eliminate this reservoir of infection (277). Reduction of disease burden in a population after introduction of widespread vaccination is usually considered an important manifestation of vaccine efficacy. A similar vaccine has been used in China (278). Evidence of efficacy of the Chinese vaccine consists of observation of disease incidence in vaccinated and unvaccinated provinces. Until recently, no randomized, controlled studies of efficacy had been performed. Using a vaccine manufactured in Japan by the Biken Institute, Hoke et al. (279) performed a study in 300,000 children in Thailand that demonstrated a high level of effectiveness, efficacy of a vaccine strain from Japan against Southeast Asian strains, and a high level of safety.

The vaccine produced by the Biken Institute in Japan is derived by intracerebral inoculation of young mice (277). Brain tissue is harvested and virus purified so that no detectable brain antigen remains. The results of the study by Hoke et al. (279) clearly demonstrate that this purification process is effective in reducing the risk of neurological complications compared to risks of suckling mouse brain-derived rabies vaccine.

No JE vaccine is commercially available in the United States. The Biken Institute vaccine was used on a restricted basis for several years and is now available for military use only. Contingent upon availability, it has been considered appropriate to vaccinate travelers who will be in rural parts of endemic areas for more than 2 weeks during summer months. Regimens used for United States travelers have usually involved three doses.

### Varicella-Zoster and Chicken Pox

Varicella-zoster virus (VZV) is a herpes group virus that infects approximately 95% of people, usually in childhood (278). The manifestations of primary infection are generally self-limited consisting of the characteristic chicken pox rash and associated systemic symptoms (280). In certain immunodeficient people, and rarely otherwise, disseminated infections with pneumonitis or encephalitis may occur. Visceral involvement is particularly common in children with leukemia (281). Herpes zoster is a common self-limited disease that usually affects the elderly and is common in certain disease states, specifically Hodgkin's disease and HIV infection (282). In the presence of suppressed immunity, zoster may also progress to involve the viscera. At present, immunoprophylaxis has a role in prevention of primary disease but not reactivation of herpes zoster.

Tissue culture adaptation of VZV has been used to produce an attenuated vaccine. Takahashi et al. (283) isolated the OKA strain that was capable of infecting guinea pigs. After passage in embryonic guinea pig cell cultures and several tissue culture passages, the OKA strain was found to be immunogenic and attenuated, and well tolerated even by children with leukemia in remission (283). Extensive rash due to vaccine is an uncommon reaction in children with leukemia, and when it has occurred it has been responsive to antiviral therapy (284). Vaccines made from the OKA strain have been effective in preventing primary infection in healthy children as well. OKA strain vaccines are available in Japan and Europe and under study in the United States. It seems likely that their principal use will continue to be to prevent life-threatening infections in children with depressed immunity, but they may be used in healthy children to a limited extent.

Varicella-zoster immune globulin (VZIG) is prepared from pooled plasma collected from donors with high levels of antibody to VZV (286). The potency is established by testing for fluorescent antibody to membrane antigen (FAMA) (287). The presence of serum antibody detectable in this test corresponds with immunity to infection. The basis of VZIG development was work by Brunell (288), who showed that passive immunization with standard doses of Ig could prevent chicken pox when given postexposure to healthy children and that larger doses modified infection in children with leukemia. Efficacy of VZIG was demonstrated in children with leukemia, by Zaia et al. (286). VZIG is recommended for use as postexposure prophylaxis for people at increased risk of serious complications of primary varicella virus infection, including patients on immunosuppressive chemotherapy or with immunodeficiency disease, pregnant women, and infants born within 5 days of onset of varicella-form rash in the mother.

### Cytomegalovirus

Congenital mental retardation and opportunistic infection resulting in interstitial pneumonitis or other complications in patients undergoing organ transplantation are the most important manifestations of cytomegalovirus (CMV) infection (289). Efforts at live-virus vaccine development have been ongoing for a number of years, with the focus of efforts being renal transplant recipients and young women. The vaccine is produced from a tissue culture adapted virus named the Towne strain, developed by Plotkin et al. (290). The Towne strain is well tolerated and immunogenic (291). Reduced rates of complications of CMV infection were observed in renal transplant recipients vaccinated before transplantation, but the apparent protective effects were only partial (292,293). Studies of prevention of congenital diseases have not been done.

A CMV immune globulin (CMVIG) has been developed by Snydman et al. (37) using an approach similar to that used for VZIG. Studies in renal transplant recipients demonstrated protection against disease complications in susceptible recipients of grafts from immune or cadaveric donors.

### Hepatitis A

Efforts are in progress to develop live, killed, and subunit vaccines for prevention of hepatitis A virus (HAV) infection (294,295). Standard Ig is indicated for prophylaxis of HAV infection in travelers to developing countries (296).

## EXPERIMENTAL VACCINES

In addition to those vaccines under development described above, numerous candidate vaccines are at various stages of evaluation. Some infections for which vaccines may have important impact and for which experimental products are under active evaluation include RSV (297), HIV (298,299), rotaviruses (300,301), HSV (302), and Epstein-Barr virus (EBV) (303). Particularly with regard to AIDS vaccines, recently developed technologies are being applied extensively for viral vaccine development. Some approaches being evaluated include the production of purified proteins by recombinant DNA techniques in mammalian cells, insect cells, bacteria and yeast, the use of live viruses as *in vivo* expression vectors, synthetic peptides, and antiidiotype monoclonal antibodies. Perhaps more important than the application of new technologies to vaccine production is the potential to apply advanced technologies to understanding virus structure/function relationships, immune responses, and disease pathogenesis.

Among the aspects of virology that have been advanced markedly in recent years, viral immunology is outstanding. These developments reflect extraordinary advances in immunology in general. Studies of vaccine adjuvants are approaching biochemical definition of aspects of antigen presentation that may be critical to enhancement of immune responses to vaccines. Some specific adjuvants of current interest are muramyl dipeptide, micelles, and immune stimulating complexes (304–306). The functions of lymphokines in immune responses have also been extensively defined (307). The potential for modulating immune responses by combined use of antigens and lymphokines is an emerging possibility (308,309).

## CONCLUSION

The three decades that have elapsed since Enders and colleagues first propagated viruses in cell culture (208) and Salk pioneered the development of inactivated influenza vaccine (141) have been an extraordinary period in the history of virology. One viral disease has been eradicated, and the potential exists for global control and even elimination of many others. Highly effective vaccines have been developed and used for prevention of many diseases. Exciting opportunities ahead include clarification of the role of viruses and vaccines in the cause and prevention of cancer, the coordination of worldwide efforts to deliver existing vaccines to those in need, and development of effective vaccines against additional diseases that still devastate many populations. The AIDS epidemic has emerged as an immense challenge to vaccine developers at a time of great progress and accomplishment. It is likely that efforts at AIDS vaccine development will teach us a great deal about vaccine development generally. Future efforts at vaccine development should be much less empirical than in the past, giving cause to hope that progress will be even more rapid in the future than it has been recently.

## REFERENCES


1. Arita I, Fenner F. Complications of smallpox vaccination. In: Quinnan GV, ed. *Vaccinia viruses as vectors for vaccine antigens.* New York: Elsevier, 1985:49–60.
2. World Health Organization Consultative Group. The relationship between acute persisting spinal paralysis and poliomyelitis vaccine (oral): results of a WHO enquiry. *Bull WHO* 1986; 53:319.
3. Cherry JD, Feigen RD, Lobes JA Jr, et al. Urban measles in the vaccine era: a clinical, epidemiologic, and serologic study. *J Pediatr* 1972;31:217–30.
4. Ogra PL, Fishaut M, Gallagher MR. Viral vaccination via the mucosal routes. *Rev Infect Dis* 1980;2:353–69.
5. Jenner E. Reprinted in: Camac CNB, ed. *Classics of medicine and surgery. An inquiry into the causes and effects of the variolae vaccinae, a disease discovered in some of the western counties of England, particularly Gloucestershire and known by the name of the cow pox.* New York: Dover, 1959.
6. Melnick JL. Live attenuated poliovaccines. In: Plotkin SA, Mortimer EA Jr, eds. *Vaccines,* Philadelphia: WB Saunders, 1988:115–57.
7. Mills J, Chanock V, Chanock RM. Temperature-sensitive mutants of influenza virus. I. Behavior in tissue culture and in experimental animals. *J Infect Dis* 1971;123:145–57.
8. Murphy BR, Chanock RM. Genetic approaches to the prevention of influenza A virus infection. In: Nayak DP, ed. *Genetic variation among influenza virus.* New York: Academic Press, 1981.
9. Maassab HF, DeBorde DC. Development and characterization of cold-adapted viruses for use as live virus vaccines. *Vaccine* 1985;3:355–69.
10. Matsuno S, Hasegawa A, Mukoyama A, et al. A candidate for a new serotype of human rotavirus. *J Virol* 1985;54:623–4.
11. Buller RML, Moss B. Genetic basis for vaccinia virus virulence. In: Quinnan GV, ed. *Vaccinia viruses as vectors for vaccine antigens.* New York: Elsevier, 1985:37–46.
12. Roizman B, Arsenakis M. Genetic engineering of herpes simplex virus genomes for attenuated and expression of foreign genes. In: Quinnan GV, ed. *Vaccinia viruses as vectors for vaccine antigens.* New York: Elsevier, 1985:211–23.
13. Roizman B, Jenkins FJ. Genetic engineering of novel genomes of large DNA viruses. *Science* 1985;229:1208–14.
14. Davis AR, Kostek B, Mason BB, et al. Expression of hepatitis B surface antigen with a recombinant adenovirus. *Proc Natl Acad Sci USA* 1985;82:7560.
15. Morin JE, Lubeck MD, Barton JE, et al. Recombinant adenovirus induces antibody response to hepatitis B virus surface antigen in hamsters. *Proc Natl Acad Sci USA* 1987; 84:4626–30.
16. Kohara M, Abe S, Kuge S, et al. An infectious cDNA clone of the poliovirus Sabin strain could be used as a stable repository and inoculum for the oral polio live vaccine. *Virology* 1986;151:21–30.
17. Racaniello VR, Baltimore D. Cloned poliovirus complementary DNA is infectious in mammalian cells. *Science* 1981;214:915–9.
18. Nathanson N, Langmuir AD. The Cutter incident: poliomyelitis following formaldehyde-inactivated poliovirus vaccination in the United States during the spring of 1955. I. Background. *Am J Hyg* 1963;78:16–28.
19. Quinnan GV Jr. Protein contaminants in biologic products derived from cell substrates. In: Hopps HE, Petricciani JC, eds, *Abnormal cells, new products and risk.* Gaithersburg, Maryland: Tissue Culture Association, 1985: 41–7.
20. Anderson MC, Baer H, Frazier DJ, et al. The role of specific IgE and β-propiolactone in reactions resulting from booster doses of human diploid cell rabies vaccine. *J Allergy Clin Immunol* 1987;80:861–8.
21. Crawford CF, Faiza-Mukhlis FA, Jennings R,

et al. Use of zwitterionic detergent for the preparation of an influenza virus vaccine. 1. Preparation and characterization of disrupted virions. *Vaccine* 1984;2:193–8.

22. Krugman S, Giles JP, Hammond J. Hepatitis virus: effect of heat on the infectivity and antigenicity of the MS-1 and MS-2 strains. *J Infect Dis* 1970;122:432.
23. Wise TG, Dolin R, Mazur MH, et al. Serologic responses and systemic reactions in adults after vaccination with bivalent A/Victoria/75-A/New Jersey/76 and monovalent B/Hong Kong/72 influenza vaccines. *J Infect Dis* 1977; 136(S):S507–17.
24. McAleer WJ, Buynak EG, Maigetter RZ, et al. Human hepatitis B vaccine from recombinant yeast. *Nature* 1984;307:178–80.
25. Krugman S. Hepatitis B vaccine, In: Plotkin SA, Mortimer EA Jr, eds, *Vaccines*. Philadelphia: WB Saunders, 1988:458–73.
26. Davidson M, Krugman S. Recombinant yeast hepatitis B vaccine compared with plasma-derived vaccine: immunogenicity and effect of a booster dose. *J Infect* 1986;13(suppl A):31–8.
27. Emini EA, Ellis RW, Miller WJ, et al. Production and immunological analysis of recombinant hepatitis B vaccine. *J Infect* 1986;13(suppl A):3–9.
28. Katzenstein DA, Sawyer LA, Quinnan GV Jr. Human immunodeficiency virus. In: Plotkin SA, Mortimer EA Jr, eds. *Vaccines*. Philadelphia: WB Saunders, 1988:558–67.
29. Merrifield B. Solid phase synthesis. *Science* 1986;232:341–6.
30. Lerner RA, Green N, Alexander H, et al. Chemically synthesized peptides predicted from the nucleotide sequence of the hepatitis B virus genome elicit antibodies reactive with the native envelope protein of Dane particles. *Proc Natl Acad Sci USA* 1981;78:3403–7.
31. Emini EA, Jameson BA, Wimmer E. Priming for and induction of anti-poliovirus neutralizing antibodies by synthetic peptides. *Nature* 1983;304:699–703.
32. Dressman GR, Kennedy RC. Anti-iodiotypic antibodies—implications of internal images based on vaccines for infectious diseases. *Infect Dis* 1985;151:761–75.
33. Wiktor T, Plotkin SA, Koprowski H. Rabies vaccine. In: Plotkin SA, Mortimer EA Jr, eds. *Vaccines*. Philadelphia: WB Saunders, 1988: 474–91.
34. *Code of Federal Regulations*. Title 21, Part 640.104(a).
35. Gerety RJ, Smallwood LA, Tabor E. Hepatitis B immune globulin and immune serum globulin. *N Engl J Med* 1980;303:529.
36. Zaia JA, Levine MJ, Wright GG, et al. A practical method for preparation of varicella-zoster immunoglobulin. *J Infect Dis* 1978;137:601.
37. Snydman DR, Werner BG, Heinze-Lacey B, et al. Use of cytomegalovirus immune globulin to prevent cytomegalovirus disease in renal-transplant recipients. *JAMA* 1988;317:1049–54.
38. Hopps HE, Meyer BC, Parkman PD. Regulation and testing of vaccines. In: Plotkin SA, Mortimer EA Jr, eds. *Vaccines*. Philadelphia: WB Saunders, 1988.
39. Wittek AE, Quinnan GV Jr. Regulatory aspects of AIDS vaccine development. In: Bolognesi D, Putney S, eds. *AIDS Vaccines*. (in press).
40. Petricciani JC. Cell substrates for biologics production: factors affecting acceptability. In: Petricciani JC, Hopps HE, Chapple PJ, eds. *Cell substrates: their use in the production of vaccines and other biologicals, vol. 118*. New York: Plenum Press, 1978:9–21.
41. Hilleman MR, Buynak EG, Weibel RE, et al. Live attenuated mumps-virus vaccine. *N Engl J Med* 1968;278:227–32.
42. Vaananen P, Makela P, Vaheri A. Effect of low level immunity on response to live rubella virus vaccine. *Vaccine* 1986;4:5–8.
43. Sato H, Albrecht A, Reynolds DW. Transfer of measles, mumps, and rubella antibodies from mother to infant. *Am J Dis Child* 1979; 133:1240–3.
44. John TJ, Christopher S. Oral polio vaccination of children in the tropics. III. Intercurrent enterovirus infections, vaccine virus take and antibody response. *Am J Epidemiol* 1975;102: 422–8.
45. Pan American Sanitary Bureau. *Live poliovirus vaccines*. Special publication of the Pan American Sanitary Bureau, no. 44, 1959.
46. Salk J, Salk D. Control of influenza and poliomyelitis with killed virus vaccines. *Science* 1977;195:834–47.
47. Francis TM Jr, Korns RF, Voight RB, et al. An evaluation of the 1954 poliomyelitis vaccine trials (summary report). *Am J Public Health* 1955;45.
48. American Medical Association Reference Committee on Public Health and Occupational Health, American Medical Association. The present status of poliomyelitis vaccination in the United States—summary statement of the Council on Drugs (supplementary report P of Board of Trustees). *Am Med Assoc* 1961;June 20.
49. McBean AM, Thoms ML, Albrect P, et al. Serologic response to oral polio vaccine and enhanced-potency inactivated polio vaccines. *Am J Epidemiol* 1988;128:615–28.
50. Hadler SC, Francis DP, Maynard JE, et al. Long-term immunogenicity and efficacy of hepatitis B vaccine in homosexual men. *N Engl J Med* 1986;315:209–14.
51. Zajac BA, West DJ, McAleer WJ, et al. Overview of clinical studies with hepatitis B vaccine made by recombinant DNA. *J Infect* 1986; 13(suppl A):39–45.
52. Plotkin SA. Rabies vaccine prepared in human cell cultures: progress and perspective. *Rev Infect Dis* 1980;2:433–47.
53. Gross PA, Quinnan GV, Weksler ME, et al. Immunization of elderly people with high doses of influenza vaccine. *Am Ger Soc* 1988;36:209–12.
54. Ogra PL, Kerr-Grant D, Umana G, et al. Antibody response in serum and nasopharynx after

naturally acquired and vaccine-induced infection with rubella virus. *N Engl J Med* 1971;285:1333–9.

55. Chen KS, Burlington DB, Quinnan GV. Active synthesis of protective hemagglutinin-specific IgA by lung cells of mice that were immunized intragastrically with inactivated influenza virus vaccine. *J Virol* 1987;July;61:2150–4.
56. Nicholson KG, Prestage H, Cole PJ, et al. Multisite intradermal antirabies vaccination: immune responses in man and protection of rabbits against death from street virus by post-exposure administration of human diploid-cell strain rabies vaccine. *Lancet* 1981;2:915–8.
57. Burridge MJ, Baer GM, Sumner JW, et al. Intradermal immunization with human diploid cell rabies vaccine. *JAMA* 1982;248:1611–14.
58. ACIP. Update on hepatitis B prevention. *MMWR* 1987;36:353–66.
59. Fishbein DB, Sawyer LA, Reid-Sanden FL. Administration of human diploid-cell rabies vaccine in the gluteal area. *N Engl J Med* 1988;318:124–5.
60. Quinnan GV Jr. Immunology of viral infections. In: Belshe RB, ed. *Textbook of human virology.* Littleton, Massachusetts: PSG Publishing Company, Inc., 1984:103–38.
61. Quinnan GV, Ennis FA, Tuazon C, et al. Cytotoxic lymphocytes and antibody dependent complement-mediated cytotoxicity induced by administration of influenza vaccine. *Infect Immun* 1980;30:362–9.
62. Daisy JA, Tolpin MD, Quinnan GV, et al. Cytotoxic cellular immune responses during influenza A infection in human volunteers. In: Bishop DHL, Compans RW, eds. *The replication of negative strand viruses.* 1981:443–8.
63. Quinnan GV, Rook AH. The importance of cytotoxic cellular immunity in the protection from cytomegalovirus infection. In: Plotkin SA, ed. *Pathogenesis and prevention of cytomegalovirus infections.* New York: Alan R. Liss, 1984:245–62.
64. Ennis FA, Yi-Hua Q, Schild GC. Antibody and cytotoxic T lymphocyte responses of humans to live and inactivated influenza vaccines. *J Gen Virol* 1982;58:273–81.
65. Glazer JP, Friedman HM, Grossman RA, et al. Live cytomegalovirus vaccination of renal transplant candidates. *Ann Intern Med* 1979; 91:676–83.
66. Baba K, Yabuuchi H, Takahashi M, et al. Seroepidemiologic behavior of varicella zoster virus infection in a semiclosed community after introduction of VZV vaccine. *J Pediatr* 1984; 105:712–6.
67. Davenport FM, Hennessy AV. Determination by infection and by vaccination of antibody response to influenza virus vaccine. *J Exp Med* 1957;106:835.
68. Davenport FM, Hennessy AV, Francis T Jr. Epidemiologic and immunologic significance of age distribution of antibody to antigenic variants of influenza virus. *J Exp Med* 1953;98:641–56.
69. Wittek AE, Phelan MA, Wells MA, et al. Detection of human immunodeficiency virus core protein in plasma by enzyme immunoassay: association of antigenemia with symptomatic disease and T-helper cell depletion. *Ann of Int Med* 1987;107:286–92.
70. LaMontagne J, Noble G, Ennis F, et al. Serologic responses and systemic reactions in adults after vaccination with monovalent A/USSR/77 and trivalent A/USSR/77, A/Texas/77, B/Hong Kong/72 influenza vaccines. *Rev Infect Dis* 1983;5:748–57.
71. Quinnan GV, Schooley R, Dolin R, et al. Serologic responses and systemic reactions in adults after vaccination with monovalent A/USSR/77 and trivalent A/USSR/77, A/Texas/77, B/Hong Kong/72 influenza vaccines. *Rev Infect Dis* 1983;5:748–57.
72. WHO Consultative Group on Poliomyelitis Vaccines. *Report to World Health Organization.* 1985.
73. LaMontagne J, Noble G, Ennis F, et al. Summary of clinical trial of inactivated influenza vaccine-1978. *Rev Infect Dis* 1983;5:723–36.
74. Bierman CW, Shapiro GB, Pierson WE, et al. Safety of influenza vaccination in allergic children. *J Infect Dis* 1977;136:S652–5.
75. Sharp DS, MacDonald H. Use of medroxyprogesterone acetate as a contraceptive in conjunction with early postpartum rubella vaccination. *Br Med J* 1973;4:443–6.
76. Krause PJ, Cherry JD, Naiditch, et al. Revaccination of previous recipients of killed measles vaccine: clinical and immunologic studies. *J Pediatr* 1978;93:565–71.
77. *Code of Federal Regulations.* Title 21, Part 610.15(b).
78. Bierman CW, Shapiro GG, Pierson WE, et al. Safety of influenza vaccination in allergic children. *J Infect Dis* 1977;136:S652–5.
79. Yellow fever vaccine: recommendations of the Immunization Practices Advisory Committee. *Ann Intern Med* 1984;100:540–2.
80. *Code of Federal Regulations.* Title 21, Part 610.15(c).
81. Dreesen DW, Bernard KW, Parker RA, et al. Immune complex-like disease in 23 persons following a booster dose of rabies human diploid cell vaccine. *Vaccine* 1986;4:45–9.
82. Boe E, Nyland H. Guillain Barré syndrome after vaccination with human diploid cell rabies vaccine. *Scand J Infect Dis* 1980;12:231–2.
83. Assis JL. Neurological complication of antirabies vaccination in São Paulo, Brazil. *J Neurol Sci* 1975;26:593–8.
84. Held JR, Adaros HL. Neurological disease in man following administration of suckling mouse brain antirabies vaccine. *Bull WHO* 1972;46:321–7.
85. Briggs GW, Brown WM. Neurological complications of antirabies vaccine. *JAMA* 1960;173:802–4.
86. Bernard KW, Smith PW, Kader FJ, et al. Neuroparalytic illness and human diploid cell rabies vaccine. *JAMA* 1982;3136–8.

87. Monath TP. Japanese encephalitis—a plague of the orient. *N Engl J Med* 1988;319:641–3.
88. Miller HG, Stanton JB, Gibbons JL. Parainfectious encephalomyelitis and related syndromes. *Q J Med* 1956;25:427–505.
89. Langmuir AD, Bregman DJ, Kurland LT, et al. An epidemiologic and clinical evaluation of Guillain-Barré syndrome reported in association with the administration of swine influenza vaccines. *J Epidemiol* 1984;119:841–79.
90. Schonberger LD, Bregman DJ, Sullivan-Bolyai JZ, et al. Guillain-Barré syndrome following vaccination in the national influenza, immunization program US, 1976–1977. *Am J Epidemiol* 1979;110:105–23.
91. Hurwitz ES, Schonberger LB, Nelson DB, et al. Guillain-Barré syndrome and the 1978–1979 influenza vaccine. *N Engl J Med* 1981; 304:1557–61.
92. Langmuir AD, Bregman DJ, Kurland LT, et al. An epidemiologic and clinical evaluation of Guillain-Barré syndrome reported in association with the administration of swine influenza vaccines. *J Epidemiol* 1984;119:841–79.
93. Kempe CH. Studies on smallpox and complications of smallpox vaccine. *Pediatrics* 1960;26:176–89.
94. Stuart G. Memorandum on post-vaccinal encephalitis. *Bull WHO* 1947–1948;1:36–53.
95. Centers for Disease Control. *Adverse events following immunization surveillance, report no. 1, 1979–1983*. August 1984.
96. Centers for Disease Control. Subacute sclerosing panencephalitis surveillance—United States. *MMWR* 1982;31:585–8.
97. Sheppard S, Smithells RW, Dickson A, et al. Rubella vaccination and pregnancy: preliminary report of a national survey. *Br Med J* 1986;292:727.
98. Centers for Disease Control. Rubella vaccination during pregnancy—United States 1971–1986. *MMWR* 1987;36:457–61.
99. Centers for Disease Control. *Mumps surveillance, report no. 2*. September 1972.
100. Joint statement. Fatal viral encephalitis following 17D yellow fever vaccine inoculation. *JAMA* 1966;198:203–4.
101. Kapikian AZ, Mitchen RH, Chanock RM, et al. An epidemiologic study of altered clinical reactivity to respiratory syncytial virus (RSV) infection in children seriously vaccinated with an inactivated RSV vaccine. *Am J Epidemiol* 1969;89:405–21.
102. Nader PR, Horowitz MS, Rousseau J. Atypical exanthem following exposure to natural measles: eleven cases in children previously inoculated with killed vaccine. *J Pediatr* 1968; 72:22–8.
103. Nichols EM. Atypical measles syndrome: a continuing problem. *Am J Public Health* 1979; 69:160–2.
104. Modlin JF. Measles virus. In: Belshe RB, ed. *Textbook of human virology*. Littleton, Massachusetts: PSG Publishing Co., Inc., 1984;333–60.
105. Fulginiti VA, Arthur JM. Altered reactivity to measles virus: skin test reactivity and antibody response to measles virus antigens in recipients of killed measles virus vaccine. *J Pediatr* 1979;75:604–16.
106. Parrott RJ, Kim HW, Arrobio JO, et al. Respiratory syncytial and parainfluenza virus vaccines; experience with inactivated respiratory syncytial and parainfluenza virus vaccines in infants. *PAHO Sci Pub* 1967;147:35–41.
107. Belshe RB, Bernstein JM, Dansby. In: Belshe RB, ed. *Textbook of human virology*. Littleton, Massachusetts: PSG Publishing Co., Inc., 1984: 361–83.
108. Bellanti JA, Sanga RL, Klutinis B, et al. Antibody responses in serum and nasal secretions of children immunized with inactivated and attenuated measles-virus vaccines. *N Engl J Med* 1969;280:628–33.
109. Halstead SB, Nimmannitya S, Cohen SN. Observations related to the pathogenesis of dengue hemorrhagic fever. VI. Hypotheses and discussion. *Yale J Biol Med* 1970;42:311–28.
110. Halstead SB. Immunological parameters of togavirus disease syndromes. In: Schlesinger RW, ed. *The togaviruses*. 1st ed. New York: Academic Press, 1980:107–73.
111. Halstead SB, Udomsakdi S, Singharaj P, et al. Dengue and chikungunya infection in man in Thailand, 1962–1964. III. Clinical, epidemiologic and virologic observations on disease in non-indigenous white persons. *Am J Trop Med Hyg* 1969;18:984–96.
112. Plotkin SA. A short history of vaccination. In: Plotkin SA, Mortimer EA Jr, eds. *Vaccines*. Philadelphia: WB Saunders, 1988:1–7.
113. Baxby D. *Jenner's smallpox vaccine. The riddle of the origin of vaccinia virus*. London: Heinemann, 1981.
114. Metzgar DP. Smallpox vaccine *in vivo* production and testing. In: Quinnan GV, ed. *Vaccinia viruses as vectors for vaccine antigens*. New York: Elsevier, 1985:109–16.
115. Henderson DA. Smallpox and vaccinia. In: Plotkin SA, Mortimer EA Jr, eds. *Vaccines*. Philadelphia: WB Saunders, 1988:8–30.
116. Kempe CH, Fulginiti V, Minamitani M, et al. Smallpox vaccination of exzema patients with a strain of attenuated live vaccinia (CVI-78). *Pediatrics* 1968;42:980–9.
117. Benenson AS. Immediate (so-called immune) reaction to smallpox vaccination. *JAMA* 1950; 143:1238–49.
118. Fenner F. Global eradication of smallpox. *Rev Infect Dis* 1982;4:916–30.
119. Stuart-Harris C, Western KA, Chamberlayne EC, eds. Can infectious diseases be eradicated? A report on the International Conference on the Eradication of Infectious Diseases. *Rev Infect Dis* 1982;4:913–84.
120. Centers for Disease Control. Recommendations of the Immunization Practices Advisory Committee: smallpox vaccine. *MMWR* 1985; 35:341–2.
121. Moss B. Molecular biology of vaccinia virus:

Strategies for cloning and expression of foreign genes. In: Quinnan GV, ed. *Vaccinia viruses as vectors for vaccine antigens*. New York: Elsevier, 1985:27–36.

122. Paoletti E, Perkus ME, Piccini A, et al. Vaccinia vectored vaccines. In: Quinnan GV, ed. *Vaccinia viruses as vectors for vaccine antigens*. New York: Elsevier, 1985:137–51.
123. Koff WC, Hoth DF. Development and testing of AIDS vaccines. *Science* 1988;241:426–32.
124. Centers for Disease Control. Rabies prevention—United States. *MMWR* 1984;33:393–408.
125. Ajjan N, Strady A, Roumiantzeff M, et al. Effectiveness and tolerance of rabies post-exposure treatment with human diploid cell rabies vaccine in children. In: Kuwert EK, Merieux C, Koprowski H, et al, eds. *Rabies in the tropics*. Berlin: Springer-Verlag, 1985:85–90.
126. Fishbein DB, Bernard KW, Miller KD, et al. The early kinetics of the neutralizing antibody response after booster immunizations with human diploid cell rabies vaccine. *Am J Trop Med Hyg* 1986;35:663–70.
127. Fermi C. Uber die immunisierung gegen wutkrankheit. *Zietscher Hyg u Infectionskrankh* 1908;58:233–76.
128. Semple D. The preparation of a safe and efficient antirabic vaccine. *Sci Mem Med Sanit Dep India,* 1911, India, no. 44.
129. Fuenzalida E, Palacios R, Borgono JM. Antirabies antibody response in man to vaccine made from infected suckling-mouse brains. *Bull WHO* 1964;30:431–6.
130. Peck FB, Powell HM. Duck-embryo rabies vaccine: study of fixed virus vaccine grown in embryonated duck eggs and killed with β-propiolactone. *JAMA* 1956;162:1373–6.
131. Wiktor TJ, Sokol F, Kuwert E, et al. Immunogenicity of concentrated and purified rabies vaccine of tissue culture origin. *Proc Soc Exp Biol Med* 1969;131:799–805.
132. Berlin BS, Mitchell JR, Burgoyne GH, et al. Rhesus diploid rabies vaccine (adsorbed): a new rabies vaccine using FRhL-2 cells. *J Infect Dis* 1985;152:204–10.
133. Bijok U, Vodopija I, Smerdel S, et al. Purified chick embryo cell (PCEC) rabies vaccine for human use: clinical trials. *Behring Inst Mitt* 1984;76:155–64.
134. Winkler WG. Current status of use of human diploid cell strain rabies vaccine in the United States—May 1984. In: Vodopija I, Nicholson KG, Smerdel S, et al., eds. *Improvements in rabies post-exposure treatment*. Zagreb Institute of Public Health, 1985.
135. Plotkin SA, Wiktor TJ, Koprowski R, et al. Immunization schedules for the new human diploid cell vaccine against rabies. *Am J Epidemiol* 1976;103:75–80.
136. Nicholson KG, Prestage H, Cole PJ, et al. Multisite intradermal antirabies vaccination: immune responses in man and protection of rabbits against death from street virus by post-exposure administration of human diploid-cell strain rabies vaccine. *Lancet* 1981;2:915–8.
137. Mertz GJ, Nelson KE, Vithayasai V, et al. Antibody responses to human diploid cell vaccine for rabies with and without human rabies immune globulin. *J Infect Dis* 1982;145:720–7.
138. Bahmanyar M, Fayaz A, Nour-Salehi S, et al. Successful protection of humans exposed to rabies infection. Post exposure treatment with the new human diploid cell rabies vaccine and antirabies serum. *JAMA* 1976;236:2751–4.
139. Wattanastri S, Boonthai P, Thongcharoen P. Human rabies after late administration of human diploid cell vaccine without hyperimmune serum. *Lancet* 1982;2:870–96.
140. Smith W, Andrewes CH, Laidlaw PP. A virus obtained from influenza patients. *Lancet* 1933; 2:66–8.
141. Salk JE. Reactions to concentrated influenza vaccines. *J Immunol* 1948;58:369–95.
142. Horsfall FL Jr, Lennette EH, Rickard ER, et al. Studies on the efficacy of a complex vaccine against influenza A. *Public Health Rep* 1941;56:1863–75.
143. Van Voris LP, Young JF, Bernstein JM, et al. Influenza viruses. In: Belshe RB, ed. *Textbook of human virology*. Littleton, Massachusetts: PSG Publishing Co., Inc., 1984:267–97.
144. Laidlaw PP. Epidemic influenza: a virus disease. *Lancet* 1935;1:1118–24.
145. Burnet FM, White DO. Influenza. In: *Natural history of infectious disease*. 4th ed. London, New York: Cambridge University Press, 1972: 202–12.
146. Webster RG, Laver WG. Studies on the origin of pandemic influenza. *Virology* 1972;48:433–44.
147. Kilbourne ED. Influenza pandemics in perspective. *JAMA* 1977;237:1225–8.
148. Webster RG, Laver WG. Antigenic variation of influenza viruses. In: Kilbourne ED, ed. *The influenza viruses and influenza*. New York, San Francisco, London: Academic Press, 1975: 269–314.
149. Choi K, Thacker CB. Improved accuracy and specificity of forecasting deaths attributed to pneumonia and influenza. *J Infect Dis* 1981; 144:606–8.
150. Eickhoff TC. Immunization against influenza: rationale and recommendations. *J Infect Dis* 1971;123:446–54.
151. Hobson P, Curry RL, Beare AS, et al. The role of serum haemagglutination-inhibiting antibody in protection against challenge infection with influenza A2 and B viruses. *J Hyg (Camb)* 1972;70:767–77.
152. Gross PA, Rodstein M, LaMontagne J, et al. Epidemiology of acute respiratory illness during an influenza outbreak in a nursing home. A prospective study. *Arch Int Med* 1988;148: 559–61.
153. Ennis FA, Ruth WA, Wella MA. Host defense mechanisms against infection with influenza virus. I. Effect of sensitized spleen cells in infection *in vitro*. *J Infect Dis* 19XX;130:248–256.
154. Gross PA, Ennis FA, Gaerlan PF, et al. A controlled double-blind comparison of reactoge-

nicity, immunogenicity, and protective efficacy of whole virus and split-product influenza vaccines in children. *J Infect Dis* 1977;136:623–32.
155. Ennis FA, Mayner RE, Barry DW, et al. Correlation of laboratory studies with clinical responses to A/New Jersey influenza vaccines. *J Infect Dis* 1977;136:S397–406.
156. Centers for Disease Control. Recommendations of the Immunization Practices Advisory Committee: prevention and control of influenza. *MMWR* 1988;37:361–73.
157. Maassab HF, LaMontagne JR, DeBorde DC. Live influenza virus vaccine. In: Plotkin SA, Mortimer EA Jr, eds. *Vaccines*. Philadelphia: WB Saunders, 1988:435–57.
158. Enders JF, Weller TH, Robbins FC. Cultivation of the Lansing strain of poliomyelitis virus in cultures of various human embryonic tissues. *Science* 1949;109:85–7.
159. Melnick JL, Paul JR, Walton M. Serologic epidemiology of poliomyelitis. *Am J Pub Health* 1955;45:429–37.
160. Paul JR. *A history of poliomyelitis*. New Haven: Yale University Press, 1971.
161. Morgan IM. Immunization of monkeys with formalin-inactivated poliomyelitis viruses. *Am J Hyg* 1948;48:394–406.
162. Hammon WM, Coriell LL, Wehrle PF, et al. Evaluation of Red Cross gamma globulin as a prophylactic agent for poliomyelitis. Final report of results based on clinical diagnoses. *JAMA* 1953;151:1272–85.
163. Salk J, Bennett BL, Lewis LF, et al. Studies in human subjects on active immunization against poliomyelitis. 1. A preliminary report of experiments in progress. *JAMA* 1953;151:1081–98.
164. Francis TM Jr, Napier JA, Voight RB, et al. Evaluation of the 1954 field trial of poliomyelitis vaccine (Final report). Ann Arbor: University of Michigan, 1957.
165. Sabin AB, Hennessen WA, Winsser J. Studies on variants of poliomyelitis virus. I. Experimental segregation and properties of avirulent variants of three immunologic types. *J Exp Med* 1954;99:551–76.
166. Sabin AB. Present position of immunization against poliomyelitis with live virus vaccines. *Br Med J* 1959;i:663–80.
167. Koprowski H. Live poliomyelitis virus vaccines. Present status and problems for the future. *JAMA* 1961;178:1151–5.
168. Sabin AB. Oral poliovirus vaccine—recent results and recommendations for optimum use. *Roy Soc Health J* 1962;82:51–9.
169. Kim-Farley RJ, Schonberger LB, Nkowane BM, et al. Poliomyelitis in the USA: Virtual elimination of disease caused by wild virus. *Lancet* 1984;ii:1315–7.
170. Hammon W McD, Coriell LL, Wehrle PF. Evaluation of Red Cross gamma globulin as a prophylactic agent for poliomyelitis. IV. Final report of results based on clinical diagnosis. *JAMA* 1953;151:1272–85.
171. Centers for Disease Control. Poliomyelitis—Pennsylvania, Maryland. *MMWR* 1979;28:49–50.
172. Centers for Disease Control. Poliomyelitis prevention, supplemental statement. *MMWR* 1987;36:385–7.
173. World Health Organization Consultative Group. Evidence on the safety and efficacy of live poliomyelitis vaccines currently in use, with special reference to type 3 poliovirus. *Bull WHO* 1969;40:925–45.
174. Salk J, vanWezel AL, Stoeckel P, et al. Theoretical and practical considerations in the application of killed poliovirus vaccine for the control of paralytic poliomyelitis. *Dev Biol Stand* 1981;47:181–98.
175. Salk J, Drucker J. Noninfectious poliovirus vaccine. In: Plotkin SA, Mortimer EA Jr, eds. *Vaccines*. Philadelphia: WB Saunders, 1988:158–81.
176. Singer C, Knauert F, Bushar G, et al. Quantitation of poliovirus antigens in inactivated viral vaccines by enzyme-linked immunosorbent assay using animal sera and monoclonal antibodies. *J Biol Stand* 1989;17:37–150.
177. Centers for Disease Control Recommendations of the Immunization Practices Advisory Committee. Supplemental statement on poliomyelitis. *MMWR* 1987;36:373–80.
178. Benyesh-Melnick M, Melnick JL, Rawls WE, et al. Studies of the immunogenicity, communicability and genetic stability of oral poliovaccine administered during the winter. *Am J Epidemiol* 1967;86:112–36.
179. Minor PD, Schild GC, Cann AJ, et al. Studies on the molecular aspects of antigenic structure and virulence of poliovirus. *Ann Inst Pasteur Microbiol* 1986;137:107.
180. Wimmer E, Emini EA, Jameson BA. Peptide priming of poliovirus neutralizing antibody response. *Rev Infect Dis* 1984;6:S505–9.
181. Almond JW, Stanway G, Cann AJ, et al. New poliovirus vaccines: a molecular approach. *Vaccine* 1984;2:179–84.
182. Woodruff AW. Benjamin Rush, his work on yellow fever and his British connections. *Am J Trop Med Hyg* 1977;26:1055–9.
183. Geggus D. Yellow fever in the 1790's: the British army in occupied Saint Domingue. *Med Hist* 1979;23:38–58.
184. Woodward TE, Beisel WR, Faulkner RD. Marylanders defeat Philadelphia: yellow fever updated. *Trans Am Clin Climatol Assoc* 1976;87:69–101.
185. Downs WG. The known and the unknown in yellow fever ecology and epidemiology. *Ecol Dis* 1982;1:103–10.
186. Lloyd W, Theiler M, Ricci NI. Modification of the virulence of yellow fever virus by cultivation in tissues *in vitro*. *Trans R Soc Trop Med Hyg* 1936;29:481–529.
187. Harris RJC, Dougherty RM, Biggs PM, et al. Contaminant viruses in two live virus vaccines produced in chick cells. *J Hyg (Camb)* 1966;64:1–6.
188. Waters TD, Anderson PS, Beebe GW, et al.

Yellow fever vaccination, avian leukosis virus, and cancer risk in man. *Science* 1972;177:76–7.
189. Smith HH, Penna HA, Paoliello A. Yellow fever vaccination with cultured virus (17D) without immune serum. *Am J Trop Med* 1938;18:437–68.
190. Mason RA, Tauraso NM, Ginn RK, et al. Yellow fever vaccine V: antibody response in monkeys inoculated with graded doses of the 17D vaccine. *Appl Microbiol* 1972;23:908–13.
191. World Health Organization. *Requirements for biological substances (requirements for yellow fever vaccine). Technical report series, no. 179.* Geneva, 1959.
192. Wheelock EF, Sibley WA. Circulating virus, interferon and antibody after vaccination with the 17-D strain of yellow-fever virus. *N Engl J Med* 1965;273:194–8.
193. Feitel M, Watson EH, Cochran KW. Encephalitis after yellow fever vaccination. *Pediatrics* 1960;25:956–8.
194. Joint Statement. Fatal viral encephalitis following 17D yellow fever vaccine inoculation. *JAMA* 1966;198:203–4.
195. World Health Organization. Yellow fever vaccine. *Weekly Epidemiol Rec* 1984;59:94–96.
196. Freestone DS. Yellow fever vaccine. In: Plotkin SA, Mortimer EA Jr, eds. *Vaccines*. Philadelphia: WB Saunders, 1988:387–419.
197. Fox JP, DaCunha JF, Kossobudzki SL. Additional observations on the duration of humoral immunity following vaccination with the 17D strain of yellow fever virus. *Am J Hyg* 1948;47:64–70.
198. Beatty DW, Handzel ZT, Pecht M, et al. A controlled trial of treatment of acquired immunodeficiency in severe measles with thymic humoral factor. *Clin Exp Immunol* 1984; 56:479–85.
199. Morely D, Woodland M, Martin WJ. Measles in Nigerian children. A study of the disease in West Africa and its manifestations in England and other countries during difficult epochs. *J Hyg (Camb)* 1963;61:115–34.
200. Robbins FC. Measles: clinical features. Pathogenesis, pathology, and complications. *Am J Dis Child* 1962;103:266–73.
201. Langmuir AD. Medical importance of measles. *Am J Dis Child* 1962;103:224–6.
202. Black FL. Measles. In: Evans AS, ed. *Viral infections of humans. Epidemiology and control.* 2nd ed. New York: Plenum Medical Book Co., 1982.
203. Barkin RM. Measles mortality: a retrospective look at the vaccine era. *Am J Epidemiol* 1975;102:341–9.
204. Centers for Disease Control. Goal to eliminate measles from the United States. *MMWR* 1978;41:391.
205. International Conference on Measles Immunization. *Am J Dis Child* 1962;103:213–531.
206. Warren J, Gallian MJ. Concentrated inactivated measles-virus vaccine. *Am J Dis Child* 1966;103:418–23.
207. Fulginiti VA, Kempe CH. Measles exposure among vaccine recipients. *Am J Dis Child* 1963;106:450–61.
208. Enders JF, Peebles TC. Propagation in tissue cultures of cytopathogenic agents from patients with measles. *Proc Soc Exp Biol Med* 1954;86:277–86.
209. Katz SL, Enders JF, Holloway A. Studies on an attenuated measles-virus vaccine. II. Clinical, virologic and immunologic effects of vaccine in institutionalized children. *N Engl J Med* 1960;263:159–61.
210. Kempe CH, Ott EW, St Vincent L, et al. Studies on an attenuated measles-virus vaccine. III. Clinical and antigenic effects of vaccine in institutionalized children. *N Engl J Med* 1960;263:162–5.
211. McCrumb FR, Kress S, Saunders E, et al. Studies with live attenuated measles-virus vaccine. I. Clinical and immunologic responses in institutionalized children. *Am J Dis Child* 1961;101:689–700.
212. Kress S, Schluederberg AE, Hornick RB, et al. Studies with live attenuated measles-virus vaccine. II. Clinical and immunologic response of children in an open community. *Am J Dis Child* 1961;101:701–7.
213. Ad Hoc Advisory Committee on Measles Control. Statement on the status of measles vaccines. *JAMA* 1963;183:1112–3.
214. Schwarz AF, Boyer PA, Zirbel LW, et al. Experimental vaccination against measles. I. Tests of live measles and distemper vaccine in monkeys and two human volunteers under laboratory conditions. *JAMA* 1960;173:861–7.
215. Hilleman MR, Buynak EG, Weibel RE, et al. Development and evaluation of the Moraten measles virus vaccine. *JAMA* 1968;206:587–90.
216. Ikic D, Juzasic M, Beck M, et al. Attenuation and characterization of Edmonston-Zagreb measles virus. *Ann Immunol Hung* 1972;16: 175–81.
217. Collaborative Study by Ministry of Health in Kenya and World Health Organization. Measles immunity in the first year after birth and the optimum age for vaccination in Kenyan children. *Bull WHO* 1977;55:21–31.
218. Krugman S. Present status of measles and rubella immunization in the United States: a medical progress report. *J Pediatr* 1971;78:1–16.
219. Preblud SR, Katz SL. Measles vaccine. In: Plotkin SA, Mortimer EA Jr, eds. *Vaccines*. Philadelphia: WB Saunders, 1988:182–222.
220. Wolinsky JS, Server AC. Mumps virus. In: Fields BN, ed. *Virology*. New York: Raven Press, 1985:1255–84.
221. Philip RN, Reinhard KR, Lackman DB. Observations on the mumps epidemic in a "virgin" population. *Am J Hyg* 1959;69:91–111.
222. Finkelstein H. Meningoencephalitis in mumps. *JAMA* 1938;111:17–9.
223. Werner CA. Mumps orchitis and testicular atrophy. II. A factor in male sterility. *Ann Intern Med* 1950;32:1075–86.
224. *Mumps surveillance*. Centers for Disease Control, September 1984.

225. Enders JF. Techniques of laboratory diagnosis, tests for susceptibility, and experiments on specific prophylaxis. *J Pediatr* 1946;29:129–42.
226. Buynak EB, Hilleman MR. Live attenuated mumps virus vaccine. I. Vaccine development. *Proc Soc Exp Biol Med* 1966;123:768–75.
227. Weibel RE, Stockes J, Buynak EB, et al. Live attenuated mumps virus vaccine. *N Engl J Med* 1967;276:256–61.
228. Centers for Disease Control. Mumps vaccine. *MMWR* 1977;26:393–4.
229. Pattersson RF, Oker-Blom C, Kalkkinen N, et al. Molecular and antigenic characteristics and synthesis of rubella virus structural proteins. *Rev Infect Dis* 1985;7:S140–9.
230. Witte JJ, Karchmer AW, Case G, et al. Epidemiology of rubella. *Am J Dis Child* 1969;118:107–112.
231. *Rubella surveillance*. National Communicable Disease Center, United States Department of Health, Education and Welfare (no. 1). June 1969.
232. Cooper LZ, Ziring PR, Ockerse AB, et al. Rubella: clinical manifestations and management. *Am J Dis Child* 1969;118:18–29.
233. Plotkin SA, Oski FA, Hartnett EM, et al. Some recently recognized manifestations of the rubella syndrome. *J Pediatr* 1965;67:182–91.
234. Centers for Disease Control. *CDC surveillance summaries*. 33 (no 4SS). 1984.
235. Parkman PD, Beuscher EL, Artenstein MS. Recovery of rubella virus from army recruits. *Proc Soc Exp Biol Med* 1962;111:225–30.
236. Weller TH, Neva FA. Propagation in tissue culture of cytopathic agents from patients with rubella-like illness. *Proc Soc Exp Biol Med* 1962;111:215–25.
237. Parkman PD, Hopps HE, Meyer HM Jr. Rubella virus. Isolation, characterization and laboratory diagnosis. *Am J Dis Child* 1969;118:68–77.
238. Plotkin SA. Rubella virus. In: Lennette EH, Schmidt NJ, eds. *Diagnostic procedures for viral and rickettsial infections*. 4th ed. New York: American Public Health Association, 1969.
239. Meyer HM, Parkman PD, Hobbins TE, et al. Attenuated rubella viruses: laboratory and clinical characteristics. *Am J Dis Child* 1969; 118:155–65.
240. Hilleman MR, Buynak EV, Whitman JE, et al. Live attenuated rubella virus vaccines: experiences with duck embryo cell preparations. *Am J Dis Child* 1969;118:166–71.
241. Prinzie A, Huygelen C, Gold J, et al. Experimental live attenuated rubella virus vaccine: clinical evaluation of Cendehill strain. *Am J Dis Child* 1969;118:172–7.
242. Plotkin SA, Farquhar JD, Katz M, et al. Attenuation of RA27/3 rubella virus in WI-38 human diploid cells. *Am J Dis Child* 1969;118:178–85.
243. Anonymous. Rubella vaccination during pregnancy—United States, 1973–1983. *MMWR* 1984; 33:363–373.
244. Williams NM, Preblud SR. Rubella and congenital rubella surveillance. *MMWR* 1983;33: 1S–10S.
245. Weibel RE, Carlson AJ, Villarejos VM, et al. Clinical and laboratory studies of combined live measles, mumps, and rubella vaccines using the RA27/3 rubella virus. *Proc Soc Exp Biol Med* 1980;165:323–6.
246. Meyer HM, Parkman PD. Rubella vaccination: a review of practical experience. *JAMA* 1971;215:613–9.
247. Ogra PL, Jerd JK. Arthritis associated with induced rubella infection. *J Immunol* 1971;107:810–3.
248. Centers for Disease Control (Department of Health and Human Services). Rubella prevention: recommendation of the immunization practices advisory committee. *Ann Intern Med* 1984;101:505–13.
249. Ishibashi M, Yasue H. Adenoviruses of animals. In: Ginsberg HS, ed. *The adenoviruses*. New York: Plenum Press, 1984.
250. Fujinaga K, Sawada Y, Sekikawa K. Three different classes of human adenovirus transforming DNA sequences: highly oncogenic subgroup A-, weakly oncogenic subgroup B-, and subgroup C-specific transforming DNA sequences. *Virology* 1979;93:578–81.
251. Foy HM, Grayson JT. Adenoviruses. In: Evans AS, ed. *Viral infections of humans*. 2nd ed. New York: Plenum Press, 1982.
252. Horowitz S. Adenovirus diseases. In: Fields BN, Knipe DM, Chanock RM, Melnick JL, Roizman B, Shope RE, eds. *Virology*. New York: Raven Press, 1985:477–96.
253. Straus SE. Adenovirus infections in humans. In: Ginsburg HS, ed. *The adenoviruses*. New York: Plenum Press, 1984.
254. Bryant RE, Rhoades ER. Clinical features of adenoviral pneumonia in Air Force recruits. *Am Rev Respir Dis* 1967;96:717–29.
255. Van der Veen J, Oki KG, Abarbanel MFW. Patterns of infection with adenovirus types 4, 7, and 21 in military recruits during a 9-year survey. *J Hyg* 1969;67:255–68.
256. Buescher EL. Respiratory disease and the adenoviruses. *Med Clin North Am* 1967;51:769–79.
257. O'Connor GT, Rabson AS, Berezesky LK, et al. Mixed infection with simian virus 40 and adenovirus 12. *JNCI* 1963;31:903–12.
258. Chanock RM, Ludwig W, Huebner RJ, et al. Immunization by selective infection with type 4 adenovirus grown in human diploid tissue culture. *JAMA* 1966;196:445–52.
259. Rubin BA, Rorke LB. Adenovirus vaccines. In: Plotkin SA, Mortimer EA Jr, eds. *Vaccines*. Philadelphia: WB Saunders, 1988:492–512.
260. Rubin BA, Minecci LC, Tint H. The karyologic characteristics of the WI-38 diploid cell system. *National Cancer Institute Monograph No. 29*. 1968;97:105.
261. Rorke LB, Rubin BA, Myers J. Neurovirulence of adenoviruses. *Neuropathol Exp Neurol* 1973;32:161–2.
262. Top FH, Buescher EL, Bancroft WH, et al. Im-

munization with live types 7 and 4 adenovirus vaccines. II. Antibody response and protective effect against acute respiratory disease due to adenovirus type 7. *J Infect Dis* 1971;124:155–60.

263. Green M. Oncogenic viruses. *Ann Rev Biochem* 1970;39:701–56.
264. Beeson PB. Jaundice occurring one to four months after transfusion of blood or plasma. *JAMA* 1943;121:1332.
265. Stevens CE, Toy PT, Tong MJ, et al. Perinatal hepatitis B virus transmission in the United States: prevention by passive-active immunization. *JAMA* 1985;253:1740–5.
266. Krugman S. Hepatitis B vaccine. In: Plotkin SA, Mortimer EA Jr, eds. *Vaccines*. Philadelphia: WB Saunders, 1988:458–73.
267. Krugman S, Giles JP, Hammond J. Hepatitis virus: effect of heat on the infectivity and antigenicity of the MS-1 and MS-2 strains. *J Infect Dis* 1970;122:432.
268. Krugman S, Giles JP, Hammond J. Viral hepatitis, type B (MS-2 strain): studies on active immunization. *JAMA* 1971;217:41.
269. Zajac BA, West DJ, McAleer WJ, et al. Overview of clinical studies with hepatitis B vaccine made by recombinant DNA. *J Infect* 1986;13(suppl A):39–45.
270. Valenzuela P, Medina A, Rutter WJ, et al. Synthesis and assembly of hepatitis B virus surface antigen particles in yeast. *Nature* 1982;298:347–50.
271. Hadler SC, Francis DP, Maynard JE, et al. Long-term immunogenicity and efficacy of hepatitis B vaccine in homosexual men. *N Engl J Med* 1986;315:209–14.
272. Beasley RP, Hwang L-Y, Lee GYC, et al. Prevention of perinatally transmitted hepatitis B virus infections with hepatitis B immune globulin and hepatitis B vaccine. *Lancet* 1983;2:1099–102.
273. ACIP. Update on hepatitis B prevention. *MMWR* 1987;36:353–66.
274. Rosen L. The natural history of Japanese encephalitis virus. *Annu Rev Microbiol* 1986;40:395–414.
275. Umenai T, Krzysko R, Bektimirov TA, Assaad FA. Japanese encephalitis: current worldwide status. *Bull WHO* 1985;63:625–31.
276. Matsuda S. An epidemiologic study of Japanese B encephalitis with special reference to the effectiveness of the vaccination. *Bull Inst Public Health* 1962;11:173–90.
277. Hsu TC, Chow LP, Wei HY, et al. A completed field trial for an evaluation of the effectiveness of mouse-brain Japanese encephalitis vaccine. In: Hammon WM, Kitaoka M, Downs WG, eds. *Immunization for Japanese encephalitis*. Baltimore: Williams & Wilkins, 1971:258–65.
278. Huang CH. Studies of Japanese encephalitis in China. *Adv Virus Res* 1982;27:71–101.
279. Schauf V, Tolpin M. Varicella-zoster virus. In: Belshe RB, ed. *Textbook of human virology*. Littleton, Massachusetts: PSG Publishing Co., Inc., 1984:829–51.
280. Takahashi M. Varicella vaccine. In: Plotkin SA, Mortimer EA Jr, eds. *Vaccines*. Philadelphia: WB Saunders, 1988:526–48.
281. Feldman S, Hughes WT, Daniel CB. Varicella in children with cancer: Seventy-seven cases. *Pediatrics* 1975;56:388–97.
282. Schimpff S, Serpick A, Stoler B, et al. Varicella-zoster infection in patients with cancer. *Ann Intern Med* 1972;76:241–54.
283. Takahashi M, Otsuka T, Okuno Y, et al. Live vaccine used to prevent the spread of varicella in children in hospital. *Lancet* 1974;2:1288–90.
284. Gershon AA, Steinberg SP, Gelb L, et al. Live attenuated varicella vaccine: efficacy for children and leukemia in remission. *JAMA* 1984;252:355–62.
285. Weibel RE, Neff BJ, Kuter B, et al. Live attenuated varicella virus vaccine efficacy trial in healthy children. *N Engl J Med* 1984;310:1409–15.
286. Grady GF, Leszcynski J, Wright GG. Varicella-zoster immune globulin—United States. *MMWR* 1981;30:15–23.
287. Zaia JA, Levin MJ, Wright GG, et al. A practical method for preparation of varicella-zoster immune globulin. *J Infect Dis* 1981;137:601–4.
288. Brunell PA, Gershon AA, Uduman SA, et al. Varicella-zoster immunoglobulins during varicella, latency, and zoster. *J Infect Dis* 1975; 132:49–54.
289. Naraqi S. Cytomegaloviruses. In: Belshe RB, ed. *Textbook of human virology*. Littleton, Massachusetts: PSG Publishing Co., Inc., 1984: 887–927.
290. Plotkin SA. Vaccination against herpes group viruses, in particular, cytomegalovirus. *Monograph Paediatr* 1979;11:58–74.
291. Quinnan GV, Delery M, Rook AH, et al. Comparative virulence and immunogenicity of the Towne strain and a nonattenuated strain of cytomegalovirus. *Ann Intern Med* 1984;101:478–83.
292. Plotkin SA, Friedman HM, Fleisher GR, et al. Towne vaccine-induced prevention of cytomegalovirus disease after renal transplants. *Lancet* 1984;1:528–30.
293. Balfour HH, Sach GW, Gehrz RC, et al. Cytomegalovirus vaccine in renal transplant candidates. Progress report of randomized placebo-controlled double-blind trial. In: Plotkin SA, Michelson S, Pagano JS, eds. *Pathogenesis and prevention of human infection*. New York: Alan R. Liss, Inc., 1984.
294. Provost PJ, Banker FS, Giesa PA, et al. Progress toward a live, attenuated human hepatitis A vaccine. *Proc Soc Exp Biol Med* 1982;170:8–14.
295. Provost PJ, Hughes JV, Miller WJ, et al. An inactivated hepatitis A viral vaccine of cell culture origin. *J Med Virol* 1986;19:23–31.
296. Deinhardt F, Gust ID. Viral hepatitis. *Bull WHO* 1982;60:661–91.
297. Belshe RB, Bernstein JM, Dansby KN. In: Belshe RB, ed. *Textbook of human virology*. Littleton, Massachusetts: PSG Publishing Co., Inc., 1984:361–83.
298. Katzenstein DA, Sawyer LA, Quinnan GV. Ed-

itorial review: issues in the evaluation of AIDS vaccines. *AIDS* 1988;2:151–5.

299. Chakrabarti S, Robert-Guroff M, Wong-Staal F, et al. Expression of the HTLV-III envelop gene by a recombinant vaccinia virus. *Nature* 1986;320:535–7.
300. Clark HF, Rurukawa T, Bell LM, et al. Immune response of infants and children to low-passage bovine rotavirus (strain WC3). *Am J Dis Child* 1986;140:350–6.
301. Kapikian AZ, Midthun K, Hoshino Y, et al. Rhesus rotavirus: a candidate vaccine for prevention of human rotavirus disease. In: Lerner RA, Chanock RM, Brown F, eds. *Molecular and chemical basis of resistance to parasitic, bacterial, and viral diseases*. Cold Spring Harbor: Cold Spring Harbor Laboratory, 1985.
302. Corey L, Holmes KK. Genital herpes simplex virus infections: current concepts in diagnosis, therapy, and prevention. *Ann Intern Med* 1983;98:973–83.
303. Thorley-Lawson DA. A virus-free immunogen effective against Epstein-Barr virus. *Nature* 1979;281:486.
304. Allison A, Gregoriadis G. Liposomes as immunological adjuvants. *Nature* 1974;252:252.
305. Morein B, Sundquist S, Hoglund K, et al. Iscom, a novel structure for antigenic presentation of membrane proteins from enveloped viruses. *Nature* 1984;308:457–60.
306. Skelly J, Howard CR, Zuckerman AJ. Hepatitis B polypeptide vaccine preparation in micelle form. *Nature* 1981;290:51–4.
307. Wittek AE, Quinnan GV. Regulatory aspects of AIDS vaccine development. In: Belshe RB, ed. *Textbook of human virology*. 2nd ed. Littleton, Massachusetts: PSG Publishing Co., Inc., 1988.
308. Weinberg A, Konrand M, Merigan TC. Regulation by recombinant interleukin-2 of protective immunity against recurrent HSV-2 genital infection in guinea pigs. *J Virol* 1987;61: 2120–7.
309. Weinberg A, Merigan TC. Recombinant interleukin-2 as an adjuvant for vaccine induced protection: immunization of guinea pigs with subunit HSV vaccine. *J Immunol* 1987;140: 294–9.
310. *Morbidity and Mortality Weekly Report* 1988; 36:35.
311. *Morbidity and Mortality Weekly Report* 1988; 36:30.
312. *Morbidity and Mortality Weekly Report* 1986; 35:216.
313. Reed W, Carroll J, Agramonte A. The etiology of yellow fever. *JAMA* 1901;36:431–40. (Reprinted 1983;250:649–58.)

# Subject Index